H-2 Antigens

Genes, Molecules, Function

NATO ASI Series

Advanced Science Institutes Series

A series presenting the results of activities sponsored by the NATO Science Committee, which aims at the dissemination of advanced scientific and technological knowledge, with a view to strengthening links between scientific communities.

The series is published by an international board of publishers in conjunction with the NATO Scientific Affairs Division

A	**Life Sciences**	Plenum Publishing Corporation
B	**Physics**	New York and London
C	**Mathematical and Physical Sciences**	Kluwer Academic Publishers Dordrecht, Boston, and London
D	**Behavioral and Social Sciences**	
E	**Applied Sciences**	
F	**Computer and Systems Sciences**	Springer-Verlag
G	**Ecological Sciences**	Berlin, Heidelberg, New York, London,
H	**Cell Biology**	Paris, and Tokyo

Recent Volumes in this Series

Volume 138—Chaos in Biological Systems
edited by H. Degn, A. V. Holden, and L. F. Olsen

Volume 139—Lipid Mediators in the Immunology of Shock
edited by M. Paubert-Braquet

Volume 140—Plant Molecular Biology
edited by Diter von Wettstein and Nam-Hai Chua

Volume 141—Nervous Systems in Invertebrates
edited by M. A. Ali

Volume 142—A Multidisciplinary Approach to Myelin Diseases
edited by G. Serlupi Crescenzi

Volume 143—Antiviral Drug Development: A Multidisciplinary Approach
edited by Erik De Clercq and Richard T. Walker

Volume 144—H-2 Antigens: Genes, Molecules, Function
edited by Chella S. David

Volume 145—Pharmacokinetics: Mathematical and Statistical Approaches to Metabolism and Distribution of Chemicals and Drugs
edited by A. Pecile and A. Rescigno

Series A: Life Sciences

H-2 Antigens

Genes, Molecules, Function

Edited by

Chella S. David

Mayo Clinic
Rochester, Minnesota

Springer Science+Business Media, LLC

Proceedings of a NATO Advanced Research Workshop on
Major Histocompatibility Complex—Genes/Molecules/Function,
held June 5-9, 1987,
in Bar Harbor, Maine

Library of Congress Cataloging in Publication Data

NATO Advanced Research Workshop on Major Histocompatibility Complex—Genes/Molecules/Function (1987: Bar Harbor, Me.)
H-2 antigens: genes, molecules, function / edited by Chella S. David.
p. cm.—(NATO ASI series. Series A, Life sciences; v. 144)
"Proceedings of an NATO Advanced Research Workshop on Major Histocompatibility Complex—Genes/Molecules/Function, held June 5-9, 1987 in Bar Harbor, Maine"—T.p. verso.
"Published in cooperation with NATO Scientific Affairs Division."
Includes bibliographies and index.

1. Histocompatibility antigens—Congresses. I. David, Chella S. II. North Atlantic Treaty Organization. Scientific Affairs Division. III. Title. IV. Title: H-two antigens. V. Series. [DNLM: 1. H-2 Antigens—genetics—congresses. 2. H-2 antigens—immunology—congresses. WO 680 N279 1987]
QR184.3.N38 1987
599′.029—dc19 87-35977
CIP

ISBN 978-1-4757-0766-3 ISBN 978-1-4757-0764-9 (eBook)
DOI 10.1007/978-1-4757-0764-9

To

PETER GORER

on the 50th anniversary of his discovery
of H-2 antigens

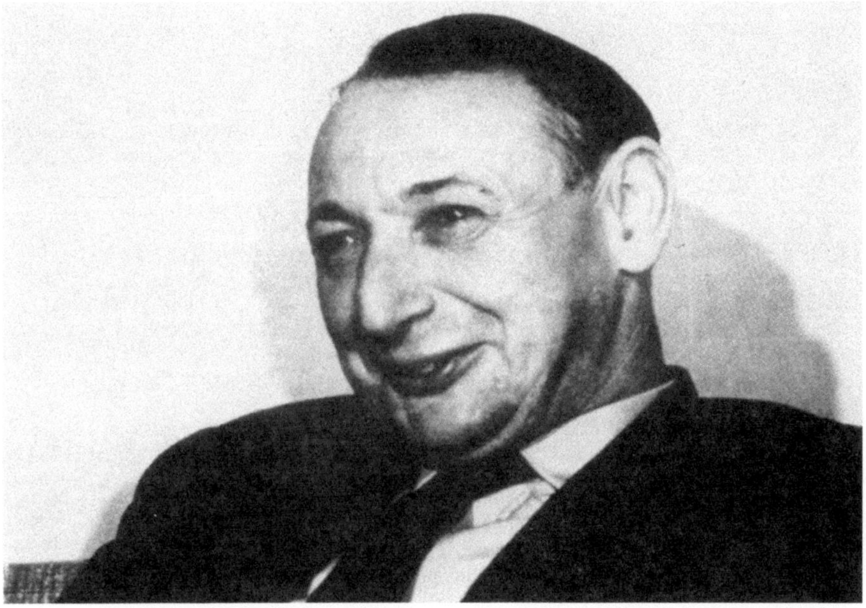

PREFACE

Approximately 50 years ago, a paper was published by Peter Gorer describing a blood group antigen system in the mouse. Little did anyone realize that this antigen system, later designated H-2 by George Snell, would play a central role in immune response and regulation. Today, the number of individuals pursuing studies on the H-2 system would run into the thousands. A meeting was organized in Bar Harbor, Maine, June 5-9, 1987, to commemorate the discovery of the H-2 antigens by Peter Gorer, to pay tribute to George Snell for his pioneering contributions in this antigen system and to bring together the young and the old scientists working in this field to look at current aspects of the H-2 gene complex.

The first session was devoted to the historical perspectives in the development of the H-2 system where Professor Jan Klein gave the opening address. The second session concentrated on the current organization and polymorphism of the genes in this chromosomal segment. The third session look at the structure of the genes and antigens controlled by this complex. The fourth session concentrated on the function of the H-2 in Immune Response and Regulation. The fifth session looked at the expression and the role of H-2 genes and their products on neoplastic cells. The sixth session brought in all aspects of the immune response which have bearing on the major histocompatibility genes. The final session looked at the role of H-2 genes in actual disease situations.

A good scientific conference is not comprised of only data presentation and discussion of scientific material in a formal setting. Poster sessions were presented by many young investigators. The participants were housed in the same hotel and all of them had their meals together such that there were many opportunities to renew old friendships, make new acquaintances, and to interact and exchange ideas. A scientific meeting also should not be all work and no fun. Many social functions were organized for the participants and their guests to enjoy the culinary specialities of the region and to enjoy the surroundings of Bar Harbor. A go-go mind functions much better in a go-go body than in a so-so body. Opportunities were available for both competition and friendly participation in athletic events such as tennis, running, and wind-surfing. A social room was available into the wee hours of the night stocked with libations and munchies, where conferees could gather and continue their discussions.

This volume presents the up-to-date studies on the H-2 Gene Complex and their role in immune function presented at this international congress. It is one of the few comprehensive proceedings which deals with all aspects of the H-2 gene complex, including the historical perspective in each aspect of the H-2 system. I thank the participants for promptly submitting the manuscripts for publication.

To organize this conference required a considerable amount of funds. The major sponsor of the conference was the NATO Scientific Affairs Council. The NATO grant enabled participation at this conference of many European scientists and scientists from other parts of the world to make it a truly international conference. It also enabled us to conduct this conference in a style that the participants will remember for a long time. A grant from the National Institutes of Health enabled us to provide complimentary hotel accomodations for all participants at this conference. Generous donations from non-profit organizations and private industry supported many of the other intangible expenses involved in organizing such a conference and the enjoyable social functions. The names of all of these organizations are listed separately. I thank all of these contributors for making it possible to hold this historic event.

Finally, I want to thank my co-chairperson, Dr. Barbara Sanford, and her staff at the Jackson Laboratories for being such wonderful hosts. I thank my secretary, Mrs. Mary Brandt, for efforts in putting together this conference and these proceedings. I thank the editorial staff at Plenum Press for their cooperation. These proceedings will be a reminder of a very important event in immunogenetics.

Chella S. David, Ph.D.
Editor

FINANCIAL SUPPORT

This conference would not have been possible without the generous contributions of the following organizations. We extend our sincerest gratitude.

NATO

National Institute of Allergy and Infectious Diseases
National Cancer Institute
National Institute of Child Health and Development

Sandoz
Hoffman LaRoche
Genentech, Inc.
National Multiple Sclerosis Society
The Upjoin Company

Quidel

Immunex Corporation
Lilly Research Laboratories
Monsanto Company
Ortho Pharmaceutical Corp.
Cetus Corporation
Biogen Research Corporation
DNAX Research Institute of Molecular and Cellular Biology, Inc.

Boehringer Ingelheim Pharmaceuticals, Inc.
Bristol-Myers Company
Schering Corporation

Miles Pharmaceuticals
Imperial Cancer Research Fund
Glaxco, Inc.
G.D. Searle R and D
Smith, Kline and French Laboratories
Ayerst Laboratories Research, Inc.
3M-Biosciences and Molecular Research
Ross Laboratories
Pfizer, Inc.
Technicon Instruments Corp.
Abbott Laboratories
LKB Instruments, Inc.
Mallinckrodt, Inc.
Pel-Freez

Burroughs-Wellcome

CONTENTS

SECTION I
HISTORIC PERSPECTIVES

SECTION II
POLYMORPHISM AND GENE ORGANIZATION

SECTION III
STRUCTURE OF H-2 GENES AND GENE PRODUCTS

SECTION IV
FUNCTION OF H-2 GENES AND GENE PRODUCTS

SECTION V
EXPRESSION OF H-2 GENES ON NEOPLASTIC CELLS

SECTION VI
ROLE OF H-2 GENES IN DISEASE

SECTION VII
IMMUNOGLOBULIN GENES AND NATURAL KILLER CELLS

SECTION I
HISTORIC PERSPECTIVES

RECOLLECTIONS

Gustavo Hoecker

Div. Ciencias Medicas; Norte Fac. Medicina, U. de Chile
Dept. Biol. Celular y Genetica; Santiago, Chile

I have been asked to recollect, that is, to evoke from the past those sections of space and time that our impressionistic brain mechanisms retain, but on coming back to find in this prestigious place so many of my friends from those days and so many others that I looked on with awe for their magnificent contributions, does not permit me to recollect but just to appraise my lucky destiny which made me a link between such monsters.

I started working on tumor immunity in 1944 in Chile and was therefore well aware of Snell through his beautiful, long and difficult theoretical paper of 1948 and of Peter Gorer's work on immunity against leukemic and tumor transplants.

My Professor, Gabriel Gasic, himself a student of Edwin Carleton McDowell at Cold Spring Harbor, met Peter Gorer in the 1952 World Cancer Congress in Paris, at which time we were presenting for the first time a demonstration of cell transmission of immunity against isogenic leukemic cells, i.e. adoptive immunity. He asked Gorer to take me as a postdoctoral student which he agreed.

I came to mighty London with its industrial melanism and cold, smoggy atmosphere about Christmas. The contrast with our mild, springy weather was shocking. But to compensate it, the Empire was still there after the war and I was supposed to come and work with the English master, i.e. the best place to learn in those days. Exciting indeed!

The old classical Victorian Guy's Hospital did not look impressive, but massive. I was taken there at 9 o'clock by a guide kindly produced by the British Council.

The first two persons I met were Barbara Mikulska, Gorer's Polish technician and his student, Bernard Amos, struggling then with the highly capricious reactions of mouse lymph node cells when tested with anti-E14, and other allotypic antibodies. They knew we Chileans were coming and immediately invited us to the inevitable English cup' o tea and a very enjoyable conversation.

Peter arrived as usual about 10:30. With his astute way of looking, half-smiling, he started probing our wits. Once satisfied, he took us around to meet the people and more cups of tea. He was developing his classical red cell agglutination technique which sometimes was as frustrating and unpredictable as Bernard's leukoagglutinations. After a year and lots of discussions I mastered it but could not publish with Peter. In spite of this he gave me a strong recommendation for the Guggenheim Foundation and to George Snell while he came to Europe. Thus, I came to Jackson Labs.

The clean atmosphere of Bar Harbor and those wonderful labs full of gleaming instruments was exciting. More so, was meeting that legend, Prexy Little, and his group from whom I had heard and studied so much.

George Snell impressed me as a lively, gentle and extremely generous man. He was then out on a sabbatical leave from the Jackson Labs. He accepted Gorer's judgement and also Medawar's because he left Av. Mitchison and myself his lab, his budget and his mice under the careful look of Priscilla Smith, his wonderful technician.

He showed me an enormous number of his splendid congenic mouse stocks which I already knew were a gold mine. We discussed the genetic requirements of our experiments and what we expected to find and he left Bar Harbor after a few days.

I started testing Snell's and the standard Jax inbred strains with antibodies I had from Gorer's lab and myself. but it was most useful in our purpose a small lot of alloantibodies prepared by Carl Cohen and some by Nat Kaliss.

The first surprising findings came out a couple of weeks after my arrival, when I found that DBA/1 and DBA/2 and C57BL/6 and C57BL/10 differed not in one, but at least in two antigens and that the A/Sn strain had a sum of the $H\text{-}2^d$ and $H\text{-}2^k$ antigens. And then, in a month and a half every day new H-2 antigens, public and private, came to exist like a real cornucopia. I wrote to George about this and he was so excited that he came to look at them.

At this time George had invited Sheila Counce, a brillant young Ph.D. from Waddington's lab at Edinborough to join his group, and he put her to work with us.

She was not an immunologist but caught very soon the intricacies of H-2 serology and with Priscilla Smith we made a good team. Sheila was trained in England as I was, but her main relationships were not with me but with Avrion Mitchison and the group of young cubs working under Tibby Russell.

After two months and a half, I gave my first seminar on the recently found complexity of H-2 antigens. It was well received.

From then on till today and in company with so many others from different countries I have worked in this tiny piece of a tiny chromosome of a tiny mammal finding all the time new aspects of H-2 a knowledge which has made the concept of MHC as one of a general commander of the immunological army comparable only to the genetic system responsible for immunoglobulin production.

For instance, in our laboratory Professor Alicia Ramos has found what looks like a new class of H-2 antigens whose function and biological meaning are still conjectural (Ramos et al., in press), and, not surprising, a control of the level of total immunoglobulin production and of some IgG subclasses are H-2 linked (Juri et al., submitted for publication).

Upon reflecting on these two extraordinary genetic systems, MHC and VDJ Ig, that make-up and take exquisite care of maintaining the individuality of vertebrates against foreign intrusions, I cannot but admire the perspicacity of these two main pillars of our discipline, Carl Landsteiner and George Snell.

They were able to see clearly through the mysteries inherent in that enormous heterogenities: the humoral response and the uniqueness of the self in tissue compatibility with their corresponding cellular immunity. They both reduced to the minimum these complexities with two simple and univocal approaches: the hapten for Landsteiner and the congenic lines for George Snell. However simple, these are very profound and general ideas that have opened the wide and deep vistas that biologists now have on the mechanistic basis of biological individuality.

Besides these main contributions, they and Peter Gorer provided us with the basic experimental tools of our trade, not only for immunology but for the understanding of the specificity of biological phenomena at large.

Albert Camus maintains that "no matter how we play with words, to understand is, first of all, to unify". But very few of us can unify problems of such mountainous proportions as Landsteiner and Snell have done.

This is the reason we pay now this homage.

PETER GORER COULD DISCOVER THE H-2 COMPLEX BY NATURALLY OCCURRING HUMAN ANTIBODIES

P. Ivanyi and T. Kloosterman

Central Laboratory of the Netherlands Red Cross Blood Transfusion Service, and Laboratory for Experimental and Clinical Immunology of the University of Amsterdam Amsterdam, The Netherlands

SUMMARY

Human sera, exceptionally, do contain lymphocytotoxic antibodies which detect polymorphic mouse lymphocyte membrane antigens whose expression is controled by the H-2 complex. In accordance with the original plans of Gorer, mouse transplantation antigens, namely the H-2 system, might have been discovered by naturally occurring human antibodies.

INTRODUCTION

After the discovery of human blood groups, various animal blood group antigens were also detected. Their function was unclear and it was suggested that they might have a role in tissue or tumor transplantation (for review see Klein 1986). Many studies on mammalian blood groups were performed with naturally occurring antibodies. Therefore Gorer (1936) examined human sera for natural antibodies which would detect mouse blood groups. The tests were done by haemagglutination (in saline) and three blood groups were detected on erythrocytes of inbred mouse strains. The nature of the observed polymorphism (negative, weak, strong haemagglutination) was not analysed in further details, as subsequently Gorer discovered the H-2 system by xeno- and allo-immune antibodies.

Here we describe the presence of naturally occurring lymphocytotoxic antibodies in normal human sera of healthy individuals who have never been allo-immunized and whose sera do not contain anti-HLA antibodies. Nevertheless these naturally occurring cytotoxic human antibodies detect murine lymphocyte membrane antigen polymorphism controled by the H-2 complex.

MATERIALS AND METHODS

C57Bl/10Sn (B10) H-2 congenic strains were maintained and bred at our Institue. Serology was described in a previous report (Ivanyi et al. 1983). In short, normal human sera (NHS) were tested in the routine microlymphocytotoxicity test on murine lymphnode cells. One complement batch was used in most of the tests. The human sera were tested in serial geometrical dilutions. The reaction in each well was recorded as 0, 1, 2, 3 or 4 corresponding to not more than 15, 30, 50, and 80% and more than 80% dead cells, respectively. The results are expressed either by titer (last dilution with positive reaction) or by the cytotoxicity scoring grade (CSG), which represents the sum of the pluses (0, 1, 2, 3, 4) obtained in a given titration.

RESULTS

We reported previously that among a total of 250 human sera 4 sera were found which showed a polymorphic reaction pattern on a panel of eight H-2 congenic strains on the B10 background (Table 1). These data show that the murine lymphocyte antigen(s) detected by natural cytotoxic antibodies in human sera are coded or controled by the H-2 complex. The specificity of these NHS antibodies was confirmed also on lymphocytes from B10 congenic strains with recombinant H-2 haplotypes and inbred strains on other backgrounds (BALB, C3H). Three of the sera were obtained from healthy human blood donors with no history of alloimmunization or anti-HLA antibodies in their serum. One serum was from a patient with multiple sclerosis also without anti-HLA antibodies (Ivanyi et al. 1983).

The antigens could be detected on mouse T cells. However, lysostrip experiments have shown, that the antibodies do not react with the classical H-2 Class i molecules (Ivanyi et al. 1983). We hypothesized, that the human naturally occurring cytotoxic antibodies are directed against lymphocyte membrane antigens controlled or modified by murine viruses (milk born or endogenous), whose expression is under the influence of the H-2 complex and that their production might have been stimulated by the products of human genes homologous to murine viruses.

Genetic studies have shown that the serum (IVA) detect an antigen (controled by $H-2^b$) for which a maternal effect influenced expression. Serum AGT detected an antigen (controled by $H-2^p$) which was inherited without maternal influence as was shown by progeny testing (Ivanyi et al 1983). However marked individual variations (among individual mice of identical H-2 genotype) were found for the expression of the murine lymphocyte antigen detected by serum AGT. While almost all B10 ($H-2^b$) mice were negative or reacted very weakly with serum AGT, most B10.Y ($H-2^p$) mice reacted strongly. This difference was inherited and segregated in (B10xB10.Y) F2 hybrids with the H-2 haplotypes. However in the F2 generation again a marked individual variation amongst individuals of the same genotype was observed. The original data were now extended to a large number of F2 individuals tested. It can be seen (Figure 1) that on a total of 133 $H-2^b/H-2^b$ F2 individuals the CSG is 4.8, but on a total of 136 $H-2^p/H-2^p$ F2 individuals the CSG (11.4) is almost three times higher and that the b/p heterozygots are intermediate (CSG 7.7). We made several efforts to breed (high x high) and low x low) individuals from these groups with the aim to obtain "substrains" with identical H-2 but high or low NHS antigen expression. While in the F3 generation indications were obtained that these individual differences are hereditary, and can be selected by serum AGT on the basis of phenotypic antigen expression, this could not be confirmed in further generations. Similar results were obtained with other sera. Serum NHS-MES "typed" for $H-2^k$ (similarly as MS11, see table 1). Progeny testing from breeding pairs selected in each generation for high and low expression of MES antigen on $H-2^k$ cells is shown in table 2. While a tendency in accordance with expectations was observed in the first and second generation, the differences were lost in F3 and F4 generations.

DISCUSSION

Further data confirm that human sera occasionally contain naturally occurring cytotoxic antibodies which are able to distinguish mice of various H-2 haplotypes amongst the series of B10 H-2 congenic strains. There are individual variations in the expression of the antigen detected by human sera. The reason of these variations is unclear. Further studies are needed to elucidate the precise nature of the antigen detected by the human antibodies the origin of the antibodies in the human sera.

These data illustrate that in accordance with the original plans of Gorer, naturally occurring antibodies in human sera might have discovered ultimately the H-2 system. However, the critical antibodies in the human sera are lymphocytotoxic and detect most probably an antigen not identical with the H-2 antigens but controled in expression by the H-2 complex. Moreover, the serological test suitable for this work was described by Gorer only much later.

Table 1. Polymorphic reaction pattern of cytotoxic antibodies in NHS sera (KLO, IVA, AGT) and one multiple sclerosis serum (MS11).

Inbred strain	H-2 haplotype	H-2 alleles K	1A	1E	S	D	Human sera KLO	IVA	AGT	MS11
B10	b	b	b	b	b	b	0	16	0	0
B10.D2/n	d	d	d	d	d	d	16	4	0	2
B10.M	f	f	f	f	f	f	0	2	16	0
B10.BR	k	k	k	k	k	k	2	4	2	16
B10.Y	p	p	p	p	p	p	0	2	32	0
B10.P	p	p	p	p	p	p	0	2	16	0
B10.Q	q	q	q	q	q	q	0	2	0	0
B10.RIII	r	r	r	r	r	r	0	2	0	0
B10.S	s	s	s	s	s	s	0	2	0	0
B10.A(4R)	b4	b	b	b	b	b			0	0

Table 2. Progeny testing of B10.BR mice selected for high and low expression of lymphocyte membrane antigen detected by human serum MES. For each generation breeding pairs of relatively high and low expression of MES antigen were selected.

Generation	Character of the breeding pairs LOW no. of progeny tested	LOW mean CSG	HIGH no. of progeny tested	HIGH mean CSG
F1	34	17.4	25	21.2
F2	17	16.2	29	21.3
F3	14	13.0	10	15.2
F4	15	21.2	16	21.3

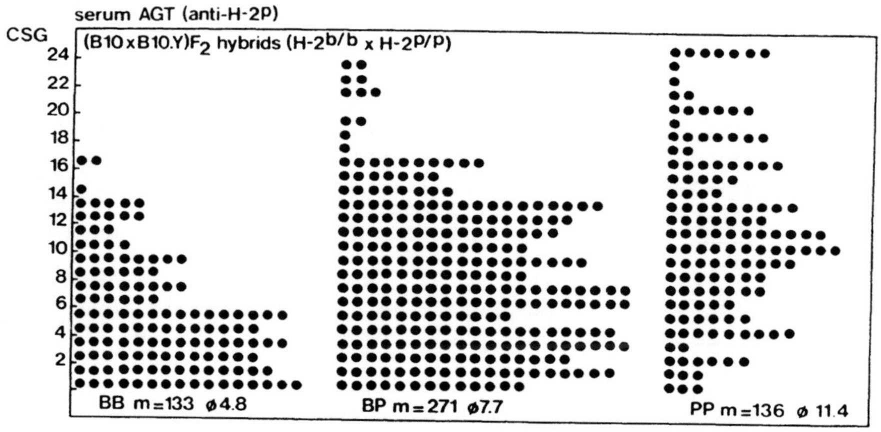

Figure 1. Reactivity of NHS-AGT on H-2 genotyped (B10xB10.Y)F2 hybrids.

References

Gorer, P.A.: The detection of a hereditary antigenic difference in the blood of mice by means of human group A serum. *J. Genetics*, 32: 17-31, 1936.

Ivanyi, P., Leupers, T., Mourik, P. van,: Naturally occurring cytotoxic human antibodies recognize H-2 controlled murine lymphocytotoxic antigens. *Proc.Nat.Acad.Sci.USA*, 80: 4479-4483, 1983.

Klein, J.: Natural History of the Major Histocompatibility Complex. *J. Wiley & Sons New York*, 198, 1968.

TRIBUTE TO GEORGE D. SNELL

Jack H. Stimpfling

The McLaughlin Research Institute

Great Falls, Montana

On this occasion when we have gathered to commemorate the fiftieth anniversary of a significant event and to honor the memory of the individual who is associated with that event, I wish to submit to this assembly the name of yet another investigator, Dr. George D. Snell who, likewise, has made very notable contributions to the study of immunogenetics.

The criteria by which we gauge the worthiness of our associates are, indeed, elusive and nearly impossible to define. Nonetheless, in some rare instances, individuals rise above uncertainty to stand as giants among their colleagues. The investigators that we honor at this conference, surely, are of such stature. If one were to measure Dr. Snell's accomplishments in terms of the number of graduate students or post-doctoral fellows he has supervised, the number of international conferences he has attended, the number of research grants that he has held or the number of publications he has authored, there are probably many investigators who surpass him. If his worthiness is regarded in terms of the influence he has had on the course of immunological research over the past 40 years, he has few peers.

I came to Bar Harbor 30 years ago as a post-doctoral fellow to work under the guidance of Dr. Snell and subsequently joined the staff of The Jackson Laboratory. I quickly grew to admire and respect Dr. Snell, a respect and admiration that has continued to grow over the intervening years. I know Dr. Snell as a quiet and unassuming man whose principal preoccupation was with science and research. He is a very modest man. Dr. Snell is easily embarrassed by honors and accolades. On the day that his Nobel award was announced, I called to congratulate him. He, instead, turned the conversation to a discussion of his flower garden in Bar Harbor. Dr. Snell was a patient and perservering investigator. In the pursuit of his research goals, patience was a virtue and an indispensable asset. In the course of his career, he experienced occasional setbacks which might easily have discouraged a less determined individual. Dr. Snell is also a very generous man. I rarely heard him raise his voice in anger or harshly criticize his colleagues. He was quick to respond to requests for advice or information. He frequently depleted his own animal colony in response to urgent requests for research animals from other investigators. Both Dr. Snell and Rhoda, his gracious wife and constant companion of many years, are caring individuals who often demonstrated a deep and sincere concern for the well-being of others.

Dr. Snell displayed remarkable foresight when he undertook the task of identifying individual histocompatibility genes and transferring them to uniform genetic backgrounds. It is worthwhile to note that this effort was initiated at a time when most immunologists regarded the laboratory mouse as the least desirable choice of creatures to use for the investigation of immunological mechanisms. However, the consequences of this undertaking shaped the character of immunological research for many years as it still does. For this we are deeply indebted to Dr. Snell. More recently, research involving the application of the methods of molecular biology to investigate the molecular genetics of the major histocompatibility complex and to explore the structure and function of its products has been very fruitful. Among other things, the results of these studies further establish the mouse as a creature of choice for the study of mammalian genetics. This also is a part of the legacy left to us by Dr. Snell.

Finally, I fondly recall the evenings when George and Rhoda would host receptions for visiting investigators in the warm and pleasant surroundings of their home. A camaraderie existed within the transplantation group at The Jackson Laboratory that is only rarely experienced.

I am honored to share with you this opportunity to acknowledge the singular accomplishments of Dr. Snell and the contribution he has made to the study of immunology.

BROTHER JUNIPER'S INCONCLUSIVE EXPERIMENT: A POETIC HISTORY OF THE *H-2* COMPLEX

Jan Klein

Max-Planck-Institut für Biologie, Abteilung Immungenetik, Correnstrasse 42, 7400 Tübingen Federal Republic of Germany

PRELUDE: THE BIOGRAPHER OF CHANCE

Brother Juniper, as every college graduate knows, is the hero of Thornton Wilder's novel *The Bridge of San Luis Rey*. As he witnessed the collapse of a centuries-old Inca bridge, which brought about the death of five travellers, he saw in this terrible accident a chance to prove that God has a reason for every disaster He sends. The poor fellow then spent the rest of his life collecting evidence to prove that the presence of the travellers on the bridge was not fortuitous. Alas, Brother Juniper failed in his experiment. He managed to convince himself, but his friends, not to mention his enemies and the Church authorities, remained unimpressed, and he was promptly burned at the stake for heresy.

Brother Juniper had been investigating chance events long before the fateful collapse of the bridge, and he had carried out these investigations scientifically, with proper controls and all. When pestilence raged in his village, he secretly drew up a chart in which he rated the qualities of fifteen victims and fifteen survivors, qualities such as goodness, piety, and usefulness. These he scored on a scale from zero to ten, then added up the totals and contrived an index of worthiness for each peasant. To his great dismay he discovered that the dead were five times more worth saving than the survivors. In the spirit of a true scientist, however, Brother Juniper was not at all discouraged by the outcome of his test, and he concluded that these data, far from disproving his hypothesis, confirmed it. Obviously, the wicked souls were called before their Creator for punishment and the good ones for a reward. This slight overinterpretation notwithstanding, Brother Juniper could be regarded as the first genuine investigator and biographer of Chance. He was obsessed with chance all his life and tried hard not only to explain it, but also to find evidence for his explanations.

What follows is a history of the *H-2* complex as Brother Juniper might have written it -- with an emphasis on chance, on fortuity, on the vicissitudes of fortune -- a history interpreted as a chain of circumstances. To Brother Juniper the events here narrated would amount to a demonstration of design; to me they are simply a cause for wonder and amazement. Just as Brother Juniper concentrated on five travellers in his magnum opus, in my story I will focus on five cities connected with breakthroughs in the history of the H-2 complex. It will be a drama in five acts.

ACT ONE: GRANDBY

If you take Highway 90 from Boston heading west and then, after Springfield, Route 202 heading south, you will hit upon a scattering of farmhouses, shops, and gas stations called Grandby, Massachussetts. By consulting your Encyclopedia Britannica, you will learn that the town is named after John Manners, the Marquis of Grandby, who on July 31, 1760 stormed the German city of Warburg at the head of the British cavalry, capturing fifteen hundred men and taking ten pieces of artillery. By consulting other sources[1] you may also learn that the town owes its existence to a quarrel, some 200 years back, over the location of a new church -- a meeting place, as it used to be called. After the court in Hadley had rejected several petitions from settlers east of the community to have the planned church built closer to their homes, the petitioners decided to erect their own meeting place. Around this church arose the town of Grandby.

As far as I could find out, no notables, whose reputation would extend beyond its borders, come from Grandby -- none that is, except one -- Abbie E.C. Lathrop, "the mouse woman of Grandby, Mass."[2]. Even Miss Lathrop, however, was actually born in Illinois, where her parents had moved earlier from Grandby. Both her mother and father were teachers, and for this reason there was no quirk of fate in her becoming a teacher too. The vicissitude of fortune, the first in a series in our story, happened only later, sometime around her thirtieth year, when she discovered that she was suffering from pernicious anemia. Forced to retire prematurely from her career, she tried her hand at poultry farming as a means of supporting herself, but without success. She then hit on the idea of raising and selling small animals as pets. It may have been her teaching experience that precipitated her decision, for she hoped that by selling pets to schools she could contribute to the children's knowledge of animal life. She started her business with a pair of waltzing mice and gradually expanded her collection by advertising to buy various coat color mutants. Some newspaper readers misunderstood her ads and thought that she was selling rather than buying mice. Thus, she began to receive her first mail orders. At some point, perhaps again through newspapers, several researchers learned about her collection, and they also began sending in orders. These were mainly for coat color variants, which they used in genetic studies. Soon Miss Lathrop was doing a brisk business with a number of laboratories all over the country, as well as with many private individuals. At the time of her death in 1918 at the age of 50, her animal colony consisted of some ten thousand mice, and a few rats, guinea pigs, and rabbits. All these animals were housed in a barn, part of which still stands by the side of the road near Five Corners in Grandby[3].

It is a pathetic sight, this small, white, decaying building -- the birthplace of so many inbred strains that are now in use. There is nothing to remind us of the old glory of this place: no plaque on the wall, no one around to tell tall tales, no oldtimers who proudly point out the site. But glory it once was -- at least in the eyes of someone tracing the roots of a discovery. As the setting autumn sun shimmers in the leaves of the magnificent elm tree towering over the house, and a thin haze rises from the meadow, it is easy to be tricked into hearing the rustle of thousands of mice rousing from their daytime lethargy for another night of feeding, fighting, and exploration. Wasn't that a carriage that just pulled up at the entrance of the barn to pick up the day's quota of boxes and deliver them to the local train station? Surely those are kids loitering around the building, hoping to earn a few pennies by helping out with washing the cages.

A slight tap on the shoulder interrupts the reverie: It is getting late, and we still want to find the tombstone. After some driving around, we finally locate the cemetery and then divide the territory amongst ourselves and begin a systematic search. Mladen is the first to find the stone, and we gather around it. The inscription reads simply:

Abbie E. C. Lathrop
1868 1918

The most famous, perhaps the <u>only</u> famous citizen of Grandby lies buried here without distinction. If Brother Juniper were standing here instead of us, he would undoubtedly be thinking of one particular day back in 1908, when another chance event brought together Abbie Lathrop and the second leading actor of our little drama.

On that day, the carriage delivered a box to the train station; it contained a single mouse and was addressed to Dr. Leo Loeb, Department of Pathology, University of Pennsylvania, Philadelphia. The mouse was sick, and Dr. Loeb was supposed to diagnose its illness. For some time, Miss Lathrop had noticed that her mice would occasionally come down with peculiar "skin lesions." These were almost invariably fatal, and she was therefore anxious to find the cause. After some inquiries, she was given Loeb's name, as an expert pathologist who might be able to help her. He graciously agreed to have a look at her sick mice.

Loeb was indeed qualified for the task. He had studied medicine at no less than eight European universities -- among them the Universities of Berlin, Basel, London, and Edinburgh[4]. He had also trained with some of the best pathologists of his time and, moreover, had carried out experiments on skin transplantation. He had been born in Germany, and the fact that he now held a position on the other side of the Atlantic was purely coincidental. Leo's brother Jacques also drifted from one university to another (some German students still do, so that by the time they have completed their studies, they are over thirty years old). While in Zurich, he met a young lady from Boston who was in Switzerland to study modern languages and literature. They eventually married and moved to the United States, where Jacques became a professor at the then newly-founded University of Chicago. Leo visited the newlyweds and was much impressed by the free spirit which dominated the United States at that time and was so different from the growing militarism and nationalism in his own country. Eventually he too decided to emigrate to the United States. He practiced medicine in Chicago for a while but was not quite content with this occupation and opted for an academic career. By this time, Jacques had become quite well-known for his studies on the physiology of instincts and involuntary action, and this was undoubtedly one of the factors that influenced Leo's decision.

Leo Loeb began his academic career at the University of Chicago. He then moved to Johns Hopkins University at Baltimore and from there to McGill University at Montreal. Finally, having found Montreal too cold for his liking, he went to the University of Pennsylvania, where he stayed from 1903 to 1910. When he received Abbie Lathrop's mouse in 1908, he immediately recognized that the "skin lesions" were in fact cancer, which he later identified histologically as mammary gland carcinoma. The letter in which he informed Abbie Lathrop of his diagnosis is lost, but one can imagine that it contained a number of questions: How frequently did these tumors occur in her mice? Were there differences in tumor incidence among the different mouse families? Did tumors appear at a particular age? These, at any rate, were some of the questions to which Abbie Lathrop later provided answers when the two of them embarked on a joint project investigating hereditary influences on the tumor incidence. The project resulted in ten research papers published by Lathrop and Loeb between 1914 and 1919, which (if nothing else) drew attention to the possible link between heredity and certain forms of cancer. The implications contained in those ten papers were not lost on researchers interested in the origin of cancer. The study also provided an impetus for the development of inbred strains, since several investigators realized that the reason why Lathrop and Loeb were able to demonstrate a genetic influence on cancer incidence was probably a result of the particular status of Lathrop's mice -- a status achieved by a high degree of inbreeding. Leo Loeb, however, is also linked to the discovery of the _H-2_ complex directly because of the work on tumor transplantation that he had done before he was contacted by Abbie Lathrop.

In 1903, Loeb came upon a Japanese waltzing mouse with a mammary adenocarcinoma. Where the mouse came from is not known, but it is unlikely that it was from Lathrop's farm, which was then only in its early stages. Nevertheless, the mice could well have come from the same stock that Lathrop carried in her colony, a stock that originated in China and reached the United States in the second half of the nineteenth century via Japan and England[5]. The waltzing trait of these mice, caused by a defect in the inner ear, is recessive, and the stock was therefore maintained by the mating of related animals. As a result, the stock was by that time almost inbred. Loeb transplanted the adenocarcinoma that had arisen spontaneously to other Japanese waltzing mice, as well as to mice of an unrelated stock and demonstrated that the tumor grew in the former animals but not in the latter[6]. This experiment was not the first demonstration of host factors influencing the growth of a transplanted tumor, but it was among the most convincing.

Loeb did not continue this line of investigation, but others, impressed by his results, did, and their work then led directly to the discovery of the _H-2_ complex. Each of the new actors in our drama were introduced into the play by accident. Ernest E. Tyzzer, who provided the first experimental proof that the outcome of tumor transplantation was determined by genetic factors from the host, was a country boy with natural curiosity, as he liked to describe himself[7]. While in his second year at Harvard Medical School, he noticed that some of the foxes he had trapped back on his father's farm were diseased. Curious about the illness, he brought them back to Harvard where the anatomist-pathologist William T. Councilman chanced upon them. The professor was impressed by young Tyzzer's "natural curiosity" and encouraged him to undertake experimental work on the potential relationship of parasitic protozoa to cancer. It was this chance encounter that launched Tyzzer on a distinguished career in pathology and led directly to the publication of his influential paper on the genetics of tumor transplantation in 1909 (ref 8).

It is not difficult to understand why Clarence C. Little, the next actor in our drama, became a biologist. As a boy in his father's house in Brookline, Massachusetts, he was continuously surrounded by dogs, cats, pigeons, and even mice[9]. Dogs, in particular, were part of the family, and his father is said to have introduced the longhaired dachshund to the United States. With this background, it is not surprising that Little became interested in genetics while at Harvard University, and that he subsequently went to work with William C. Castle at the Bussey Institute of Harvard University. It was, however, by pure chance that Little began working with mice. Castle apparently assigned each new student a different laboratory animal to study genetically, and Little's lottery ticket happened to have the name "house mouse" written on it. While working with Castle on the inheritance of coat colors in mice, Little heard of Tyzzer's experiments on tumor transplantation. His training in genetics, which Tyzzer lacked, helped him to come up with an interpretation of the puzzling observation that F_1 hybrids between susceptible and resistant mouse strains accepted the tumor transplants, whereas virtually all F_2 individuals rejected them. Little suggested that multiple genes determined susceptibility to tumor transplants and that among the F_2 individuals, only the very few that carried susceptibility alleles at <u>all</u> the loci accepted the graft[10]. Together with Tyzzer, he put this hypothesis to the test and demonstrated that a small proportion of the F_2 individuals did indeed fail to reject the tumor grafts. From the frequency of the survivors, they calculated that at least 15 segregating susceptibility genes determined the outcome of tumor transplantation[11].

This demonstration constituted a significant step toward the discovery of the <u>H-2</u> complex. Little, however, also influenced the plot of the play in another important way. At one stage in his career, he became the President of the University of Michigan at Ann Arbor and in this capacity came to know most of the automobile barons of nearby Detroit personally -- the captains of the industry, as they would be called today. When Little proved to be too liberal for such a conservative University, and the question arose of what he would do if he were to resign, a solution was found that seemed to suit everyone concerned. The barons owned great expanses of land in northern Maine, and obviously they were not short of money. They offered to donate some of the land and a certain amount of starting capital to set up a research laboratory near Bar Harbor on

Mount Desert Island. The laboratory was to be devoted to cancer and genetic research, and the mouse was chosen as the major experimental animal. Little was named as its first director. This decision was not only a deus ex machina for the thickening plot developing at the University of Michigan; it was also the beginning of a new act in the drama entitled "The discovery of H-2."

For the moment, however, we are still in Act One, and there are still more actors coming on stage, all pioneers in the development of inbred strains, which later proved to be so important in the study of the H-2 complex. They all entered the stage at the right moment, yet totally by chance, or at least so it seems. Leonell C. Strong got into cancer research and the project of developing inbred mouse strains via his family heritage. As a young man he was concerned that so many of his relatives died of cancer, and he resolved to study the genetic influences on the emergence of cancer in experimental animals[12].

John J. Bittner became involved in cancer research because he was in love with Strong's sister, whom he later married. Together with Strong, Bittner then became one of the founding members of the Jackson Laboratory at Bar Harbor.

Halsey J. Bagg, who provided the ancestors of the BALB/c strains, wanted to know whether there were smart and stupid mice and if so, whether the parents' stupidity was passed on to their children. He found that it was.

If I had the space, I could continue with this list and demonstrate how strange turns of fate brought all the other pioneers of mouse inbreeding, tumor transplantation, and cancer research into the play, and how chance molded their research careers and often played a decisive part in many of the crucial discoveries. I would then be digressing too much, however; instead, I shall move on to Act Two.

ACT TWO: LONDON

The scenery changes and the plot now moves from the United States to Great Britain. Strangely enough, had educators had their way, the main actor now on stage, Peter A. Gorer, would not have been in the play at all. He was branded as a slow learner who could not possibly make it through college, let alone become a scientist[13]. Having entered the university nonetheless, he might have become a practicing pathologist. Perhaps it was failing his exams in that subject which steered him toward a more research-oriented career. Having decided to become a scientist, however, he ought not to have gotten entangled with mice at all: One would have expected him to become an expert on hibernation -- the subject of his first paper[14] -- and work with bats, hedgehogs, bears and the like. Yet, Fortuna (God, in Brother Juniper's view) decided otherwise: Gorer's path accidentally crossed that of J.B.S. Haldane at a time when the latter was briefly flirting with the genetics of tumor transplantation.

That Haldane, who in the 1930s was already a well-known physiologist and public figure, would at some point undertake a trip to the United States was inevitable. What transpired on that trip, however, was not. Why, for example, should he have included Bar Harbor on his itinerary? True, the Jackson Laboratory was already emerging at that time as one of the foremost centers for genetic research in the country, but there were several others that were perhaps better known and that Haldane did not visit on this trip. Once in Bar Harbor, however, it was again inevitable that he would hear from Little about the work on tumor transplantation. Considering the broadness of Haldane's interests, it was then only to be expected that he would get hooked on this puzzle for at least a short while. He was certainly interested enough to carry breeding pairs of three of the inbred strains maintained at The Jackson Laboratory back to London. After giving the puzzle some thought, he came up with the idea that the tumor resistance factors might be either identical or similar to blood group antigens[15]. As Gorer happened to be in Haldane's laboratory at that time, he was chosen to test the idea. The coincidence in the Haldane-Gorer encounter is striking. Gorer was only in direct contact with Haldane for one year, and this year just so happened to coincide with his teacher's brief flirt with transplantation. Had he started in Haldane's laboratory any earlier than he actually did, he would have already been working on another project and thus probably not inclined to switch to something new. On the other hand, had Gorer joined Haldane later, the flirt would have been over and forgotten by then, or somebody else would have been working on the project. Brother Juniper, count the points for your tally!

The rest of the story is well known. I have narrated it on several occasions[16,17,18], and there is therefore no need to go into it again -- except, perhaps, for two points. One is that Gorer discovered, or at least thought to have discovered, mouse blood group antigen II (which eventually became H-2) with the help of natural antibodies present in human serum[19]. The serum he used was his own, and he happened to have blood group A[20]. For unexplained reasons, group A sera seemed to be the only ones with this peculiar activity. Luck, therefore, played straight into Gorer's hands. Even if the antibody in the serum had not been against antigen II, as defined later by rabbit antibodies against mouse erythrocytes and mouse antibodies against mouse cells[21,22,23,24], the positive reactions with the human sera were important for Gorer because they encouraged him to search further where others before him had failed[17]. The second point is that once Gorer discovered antigen II and proved that it was indeed one of the factors determining the outcome of tumor transplantation, he had the good fortune of being joined by several outstanding students, in particular D. Bernard Amos and Gustavo Hoecker. Here again, chance influenced the course of events. At that time, in the early post-war years, Gorer was not yet the international celebrity that he eventually would become. Students, therefore, did not come to him for a quick ride on the bandwagon; they came for other reasons. Bernard Amos joined Gorer because the latter was the only one who found his speculations so absurd as to be worth investigating. Amos began as a research technician and only later decided to study medicine. After the completion of his studies, he realized that he did not want to practice medicine but would rather carry out research, in particular, cancer research. From reading the literature he had an idea about the way in which immunity might work against tumors and wanted to test it. The pathology professor he approached told him "Why, this is a splendid hypothesis and worth testing, but since it concerns immunity, you should go to a microbiologist." The microbiology professor also found the hypothesis interesting but had no space in his laboratory. He recommended that Amos approach Peter Gorer, who was engaged in some kind of research on immunity in tumors. Gorer told Amos that his hypothesis was nonsense and accepted him on the spot.

Hoecker has a similar story to tell[25]. After taking a DVM degree at the University of Santiago, Chile, he was also dreaming of curing human leukemia by immunological means. Scanning the literature, he came across Gorer's papers and through his professor arranged to work with Gorer in London. The three of them -- Gorer, Amos, and Hoecker -- then laid the foundations for the immunogenetics of the H-2 complex and in more than one respect paved the way for the discovery of the human homologue of H-2, the HLA complex. Amos, of course, subsequently made many momentous contributions to the study of the HLA complex too.

ACT THREE: BAR HARBOR

The small crew that Little gathered together when he established The Roscoe B. Jackson Memorial Laboratory in the backwoods of Maine was quite homogeneous in its research orientation. Leonell Strong, John Bittner, Arthur Cloudman, Charles Green, Elizabeth Fakete, and Joseph and William Murray were all bound by a common interest in the study of cancer[26]. In 1935, however, the laboratory was joined by a young man who did not quite fit into the group. True, he had trained in mammalian genetics, but he had until then shown no particular curiosity as far as the investigation of cancer was concerned. Little, however, hoped that this slight handicap would be corrected with time. The young researcher was George D. Snell.

What brought Snell to Bar Harbor? The lack of better job offers, it seems. Snell owed his interest in mammalian genetics to his college professor at Dartmouth, who persuaded him to study with Castle at the Bussey Institute. Snell's lottery ticket at this institution, like that of Little before him, read "smelly mice" (the relatively non-smelly rabbits Castle apparently reserved for himself). His task was to investigate the linkage relationships between dilute, a coat color allele, and short ear (they proved to be very closely linked). By the time he took his Ph.D. degree, Snell had become interested in the effects of radiation on genetic material, because it was at this time that Muller discovered that X-irradiation can induce mutations in drosophila. Snell wanted to know what effect radiation would have on mammalian cells and went to Muller's laboratory at Austin, Texas to find an answer to this question. It turned out that Muller was hardly ever there (he was busy setting up a laboratory in the Soviet Union), but Snell found the answer anyway: Ionizing radiation induced chromosomal abberations -- primarily translocations -- in mouse germ cells. Snell thought this project worth pursuing and looked for a place where he could do so. At Austin they were willing to keep him but not his mice, and so he had to move on. After a few years of indecision, he wrote to Little, whom he knew from his Bussey Institute days, and was offered a position at Bar Harbor.

Little's gentle prodding, intended to involve Snell in the cancer project, did not seem to work. Snell continued working with his translocation stocks and at one point came up with the idea of editing a book that would summarize all the currently available knowledge about the biology of the laboratory mouse. Little was to contribute a chapter on tumor transplantation. It was while reading this chapter that Snell became interested in identifying the genes that determine the outcome of tumor transplantation and exploring the part immunity played in the rejection of the transplants by the host. This was back in 1939, a couple of years after Gorer had provided partial answers to some of these questions. Snell, however, was not aware of this, for Gorer was not mentioned in Little's review even though his papers were listed in the bibliography. Eventually, Snell hit on the idea of developing congenic lines that differed at a single tumor resistance locus and would thus serve as a means of identifying this locus. He formulated this idea in a theoretical paper that he submitted to the *Journal of Genetics*, edited by Haldane. The manuscript was accepted, but Haldane appended it with his own mathematical treatment of the problem[27]. However, he too failed to tell Snell about Gorer. It was only later, when Snell had developed the first set of congenic lines, that he learned about Gorer's work. Thus the time was right to merge the two streams that had trickled along independently until then. Gorer came personally to Bar Harbor in 1946 to attempt the merger. He brought with him antibodies specific for antigen II and the hope that the antibodies would react with the product of one of the tumor-resistance loci that Snell had separated with the help of his congenic lines and which he now called *histocompatibility* loci. Gorer left Bar Harbor with a new wife and the knowledge that antigen II was encoded in a histocompatibility gene linked to the *Fused* locus in linkage group IX[28] which was later found to be borne by chromosome 17. Antigen II thus became *histocompatibility-2* or *H-2*.

Snell was later joined at Bar Harbor by Jack Stimpfling, who initiated a systematic search for intra-*H-2* recombinants and with their help began constructing the genetic map of the *H-2* complex[29]. The first indication that *H-2* was not a single locus was provided by Snell in 1953 and was based on a chance observation. One of the inbred strains that Snell was working with happened to be A, whose *H-2*^{a} haplotype is a natural recombinant derived from haplotypes *H-2*^{d} and *H-2*^{k}. When Snell noticed that *H-2*^{a} tumors were accepted by *H-2*^{d}/*H-2*^{k} heterozygotes, he correctly concluded that the *H-2* "locus" consisted of at least two genetically separable elements[30]. Evidence for the additional genetic complexity of the *H-2* locus was obtained by Amos, Gorer, Hoecker, and now Stimpfling[29,31,32]. Before long the *H-2* became *too* complex and seemingly uninterpretable. For this part of the story, however, we have to change the scenery again and bring one more actor into the play.

ACT FOUR: ANN ARBOR

Donald C. Shreffler was born on a farm in Illinois. Since he did well in High School and then in college, his parents agreed that he should have a university education, tacitly or explicitly assuming that it should be an education in agriculture. He therefore began studying dairy cattle genetics but later decided that he needed a more general training in genetics, for which he went to the California Institute of Technology at Pasadena. Even when there, Shreffler tried to remain true to his background by choosing Ray D. Owen as his thesis advisor, an authority on blood groups in domestic animals and a prominent disciple of the famous Wisconsin immunogenetics school. Among the tasks of graduate students at Cal Tech was helping in practical courses taught to undergraduates. Shreffler's assignment was to demonstrate the immunodiffusion test in agar to the students. He duly immunized rabbits against mouse serum, obtained antibodies, and set up the assay. There was no shortage of precipitin bands on the agar slides, and the students were impressed by such a simple, yet dramatic demonstration of the power of immunological methods. Shreffler, however, noticed something that the students did not. When he tested sera from different mouse strains against the same rabbit antiserum, the *number* of bands was always the same, but the *position* of one band seemed to vary, suggesting a quantitative variation in the protein detected by the corresponding antibodies. At that time, in the early 1970s, there were still very few biochemical markers known in the mouse, and Shreffler, encouraged by his advisor, therefore decided to follow up this chance observation. This he did, even at the cost of being distracted from the subject of his Ph.D. work -- the genetics of transferrins in mouse serum. After testing sera of all the mouse strains available at Cal Tech, he noted a correlation between the quantitative variation of the serum substance or Ss and the *H-2* haplotype: All $H\text{-}2^k$ strains had a lower amount of Ss in comparison to the other strains[34]. This observation thus became Shreffler's entrance ticket to the exclusive *H-2* club. By attempting to map the *Ss* locus with respect to *H-2*, he was forced to learn how to *H-2* type mice, and having accomplished this, he realized that he had produced *H-2* recombinants in his crosses. From there it was only a small step to becoming a full time *H-2* immunogeneticist with a residence at the University of Michigan at Ann Arbor, where he was able to obtain a faculty position close enough to his native Illinois.

At Ann Arbor, Shreffler began to attract students, postdoctoral fellows, and research associates. Chella S. David and I were in this last category. It would be a long story to explain how I ended up in Ann Arbor. Suffice it to say that there have been many occasions in my life when the directions I have taken have depended solely on chance. Chella David was sent to the United States by his parents to learn agriculture so that he could then return to his native India as a master farmer. But Chella, being lazy by nature (as he describes himself), was not at all enthusiastic about working the whole day in the field at the agricultural station and therefore looked for an opportunity to work in the laboratory. He was eventually given the chance and became a Ph.D. student under the supervision of Arne W. Nordskog at Iowa State University, Ames, studying chicken allotypes. After taking his degree, he searched for a place to begin his postdoctoral work and had three offers -- from Owen, Steinberg, and Shreffler. He opted for Shreffler because he was the youngest of the three, and Chella thought he would be easiest to get along with. In Shreffler's laboratory, Chella David continued studying chicken allotypes for a while, but at the same time began work on H-2. Eventually he realized that chickens and mice do not mix and devoted himself entirely to H-2.

In the meantime, H-2 serology and genetics had grown so complex that there were only a few of us who could understand them. The rest of the world began to regard us as high priests of some secret doctrine that one spent years learning. Eventually, it became too complex even for us, especially when problems arose, such as the discovery that the same antigenic determinant mapped simultaneously into opposite ends of the H-2 complex. This fact disturbed us considerably, since we were not prepared to be like physicists, for whom the positioning of an electron simultaneously at two places is perfectly acceptable. We looked for a way out of this situation, especially since at that time there seemed to be only two segregant series in the HLA complex, while we, in the H-2 complex, had seven or eight regions.

In 1970, Don was asked by Göran Möller to contribute an article to Transplantation Reviews, and Don in turn asked me to coauthor it. At that time I was already more concerned about deadlines than Don, so when I saw Göran's letter at the bottom of the tall pile on his desk, I prepared a draft with a table in which the number of H-2 regions was reduced to two. We had discussed this possibility many times before, but knowing Don's conservative nature, I was afraid that he would not be willing to come into the open with such a radical "two-locus model of the H-2" as it later became known. Don, of course, spotted the table immediately. To my great surprise, however, his only comment was: "I see you got rid of A, E, V, and C," these being the regions that were causing us the greatest difficulties. As the paper came out[35], we learned that George Snell and Peter Démant had independently reached the same conclusion as we had[36]. Shortly afterwards, I separated from Don and established my own laboratory at the Dental Research Institute of the University of Michigan.

Time for the curtain to fall on Act Four.

ACT FIVE: PALO ALTO

This act actually begins in New York, at NYU. Enter Baruj Benacerraf. By his own account, Benacerraf became an immunologist because he suffered from asthma as a youngster, and he thought that by studying immunology he might come up with a cure. Instead, he ended up discovering Ir genes. The impulse that led to this discovery came from a disagreement with Elvin A. Kabat about the cause of delayed-type hypersensitivity. Kabat believed that DTH, like nearly everything else in immunology, was mediated by antibodies; Benacerraf, on the other hand, thought that cells were involved. To show that he was right, Benacerraf tried to prove that DTH and antibodies had different specificities. He therefore began to work with antigens of relatively defined structure, such as those containing haptens placed on synthetic polypeptides used as carriers. One of the simplest carriers then available was poly-L-lysine, PLL. When Benacerraf and his colleagues immunized guinea pigs against PLL, they discovered that some animals responded quite well to this antigen, while others did not respond at all[38]. By checking the literature, they realized that Paul Maurer and his coworkers had made a similar observation when he immunized rabbits against PLL[31]. Some of these animals were also responders to PLL, while others were nonresponders. The phenomenon, therefore, seemed to be worth following up.

The rest of the story is again well-known. Acting on this "tip," Benacerraf and his colleagues carried out genetic experiments and demonstrated that responsiveness to PLL is controlled by a single immune response or Ir gene. For the second part of the story, however, we now have to move to Stanford University at Palo Alto, California.

When Hugh O. McDevitt joined Stanford Universtiy in 1965, he also already knew that antibody response to certain antigens was genetically controlled. He came to this conclusion while studying with J.H. Humphrey at the National Institute for Medical Research, Mill Hill, London. The project that Humphrey assigned McDevitt was to test the template hypothesis of antibody production. He was to make the antigen so radioactive that it would kill the antibody-producing cell if it were indeed functioning as a template inside this cell. McDevitt heard that Michael Sela at the Weizman Institute at Rehovot, Israel, had succeeded in producing a synthetic poylpeptide, (T,G)-A--L, which could be made highly radioactive. He obtained some of this antigen, but when he immunized rabbits against it, he obtained no response. He complained to Sela, but the latter insisted that his rabbits did respond to (T,G)-A--L. At Humphrey's suggestion, McDevitt therefore immunized another breed of rabbits, and lo and behold, these rabbits readily produced antibodies. McDevitt realized that genes were probably involved in the control of the immune response but spent a year trying in vain to decipher this control in rabbits, in which the genetic status of the parents was largely unknown. He then decided to repeat these experiments in mice. The only two inbred mouse strains available at Mill Hill were CBA and C57. The former turned out to be nonresponders, but the C57 were responders to (T,G)-A--L (ref. 39). To appreciate McDevitt's incredible luck, we should realize that among virtually all the inbred strains, only $H\text{-}2^b$ mice like the C57 at Mill Hill are responders. Had McDevitt taken almost any other strain, the chances are that it too would have been a nonresponder, and he would have probably given up in frustration.

Mating studies with these two strains (carried out in part at Stanford University, to which McDevitt in the meantime had moved) again pointed to a rather simple genetic control of the immune response to (T,G)-A--L and related synthetic polypeptides. McDevitt and his colleagues then tried to find the reason for the nonresponsiveness of the CBA mice. Could it be that the antigen was, for some reason, degraded enzymatically in these but not in responder mice? To test this possibility, McDevitt and his associates attempted to transfer responsiveness with immune cells of the appropriate donor to an irradiated recipient. They encountered great difficulties, however, because of the graft-versus-host reaction. To reduce the GVHR, someone suggested the use of H-2 congenic lines to McDevitt. Presumably the response would be linked to the background, and matching the H-2 would lessen the incompatibility barrier between the donor and the recipient. To McDevitt's -- and everybody else's -- astonishment, the control of the response was not linked to the background but to the _H-2_ haplotype. A quick typing of a panel of _H-2_ congenic lines confirmed this observation: The immune response was controlled by the _H-2_ complex[40]. Mapping studies then revealed that the _Ir_ genes resided within the _H-2_ complex, between the _K_ and _D_ loci of the two-locus model[41].

The rest of the story is also well-known.

When the position of the _Ir_ genes became known, we all began to immunize all possible combinations of _H-2_ recombinant strains in the hope of producing antibodies against the hypothetical products of the _Ir_ genes. For a while, free communication among laboratories was suspended, and secrecy prevailed. Even between Shreffler's laboratory and my own, there was virtually no contact, although we were located only a few blocks apart. It was not until our papers were in press that we exchanged preprints.

Shreffler's group and mine were the first to identify the antibodies[42,43]. A few months later David Sachs came up with his antibody[44], followed by McDevitt and his colleagues with theirs[45]. The class II antigens and genes were thus identified. It then took several more years to establish that the antigens were the long sought-after products of the _Ir_ genes and that the _H-2_ and _Ir_ genes were the same. But that is another story, and so I end my account here.

To be honest, I would not enjoy relating part two of the story, because it is so different from part one. I like to think of the period before the discovery of the _Ir_ genes as the era of gentlemen. The group of _H-2_ researchers was then occasionally referred to as the "_H-2_ club," and in certain ways that's how it was: exclusive, small, intimate, and mutually compatible. Each member of the club knew the other members well, respected them, and considered them his friends. It was not that the members did not compete with one another; they did. It was never a fierce competition, however, and never transgressed the boundaries demarcated by respect for the others' work. Not that there was no disharmony occasionally in the realtionships among the members of the club. There was, but it never lasted very long. We found pleasure in our work and enjoyed the discoveries made by others almost as much as we did our own.

All this has changed in the post-_Ir_ period. The prospect of gold, Nobel gold, led to a real goldrush. People began streaming into the field in tremendous numbers and brought new rules and new ethics with them. The gentleman's era ended, and the era of power struggles, disrespect for others' work, commercialization, and salesmanship was ushered in. I presume that those who subscribe to this wild-west ethic enjoy the atmosphere. I do not, and that is why I end my story here.

I called this story "poetic" not for the style in which it was told (I lack the talent for that), but rather for its content. A true historian would have pursued the "logic of the scientific discovery" and sought the rational thread winding through the story. I have focused instead on the illogical, irrational, fortuitous, and adventitious. It was not the cause and consequence that interested me, but just the opposite, the chance and serendipity of the discovery. Irrationality, the absence of logic, and fortuity are all elements that interest poets, not historians. I confess that I find the web of chance from which the discovery of the H-2 complex stems tingling my spine in the same strange way that a good poem does.

BIBLIOGRAPHY

1. "Grandby Bicentennial 1768-1968," Town of Grandby, Mass., (1968).
2. E. C. Bowie, The mouse woman of Grandby, Mass., New England Homestead July:13,23 (1968).
3. H. C. Morse III, (ed.), "Origins of Inbred Mice," Academic Press, New York (1978).
4. L. Loeb, Autobiographical notes, Persp. Biol. Med. 2:1-23 (1958).
5. R. M. Yerkes, "The Dancing Mouse. A Study in Animal Behavior," McMillan, New York (1907).
6. L. Loeb, Über die Entstehung eines Sarkoms nach Transplantation eines Adenocarcinoms einer japanischen Maus, Zeitschr. Krebsforsch. 7:80-110 (1908).
7. E. E. Tyzzer, Harvard University Gazette April 30:204-205 (1966).
8. E. E. Tyzzer, A study of inheritance in mice with reference to their susceptibility to transplantable tumors, J. Med. Res. 21:519-573 (1909).
9. G. D. Snell, Clarence Cook Little, 1888-1971, Mem. Nat. Acad. Sci. USA 46:241-263 (1975).
10. C. C. Little, A possible Mendelian explanation for a type of inheritance apparently non-Mendelian nature, Science 40:904-906 (1914).
11. C. C. Little and E. E. Tyzzer, Further experimental studies on the inheritance of susceptibility to a transplantable tumor,carcinoma (J.W.A.) of the Japanese waltzing mouse, J. Med.Res. 33:393-453 (1916).
12. L. C. Strong, A Baconian in cancer research: Autobiographical essay, Cancer Research 36:3545-3553 (1976).
13. P. B. Medawar, Peter Alfred Gorer, Biograph. Rev. Fell. Roy. Soc. 7:95-109 (1961).
14. P. A. Gorer and M. S. Pembrey, Observations on the respiratory exchange in hibernation, J. Physiol. (Proc. Physiol. Soc.) 67:xxi-xxii (1929).
15. J. B. S. Haldane, The genetics of cancer, Nature 132: 265-267 (1933).
16. J. Klein, "The Biology of the Mouse Histocompatibility-2 Complex. Principles of Immunogenetics Applied to a Single System," Springer-Verlag, New York (1975).
17. J. Klein, Seeds of time: Fifty years ago Peter A. Gorer discovered the H-2 Complex, Immunogenetics 24:331-338 (1986).
18. J. Klein, "Natural History of the Major Histocompatibility Complex," Wiley, New York (1986).
19. P. A. Gorer, The detection of a hereditary antigenic difference in the blood of mice by means of human group A serum, J. Genet. 32:17-31 (1936).
20. B. D. Amos, The era of the immunogeneticist, J. Immunol. 127:1727-1734 (1981).
21. P. A. Gorer, The detection of antigenic differences in mouse erythrocytes by the employment of immune sera, Brit. J. Exp. Pathol. 17:42-50 (1936).

22. P. A. Gorer, The genetic and antigenic basis of tumor transplantation, J. Pathol. Bacteriol. 44:691-697 (1937).
23. P. A. Gorer, Further studies on antigenic differences in mouse erythrocytes, Brit. J. Exp. Pathol. 18:31-36 (1937).
24. P. A. Gorer, The antigenic basis of tumour transplantation. J. Pathol. Bacteriol. 47:231-252 (1938).
25. G. Hoecker, Recollections of a Chilean member of the very exclusive H-2 club, Immunogenetics 24:345-349 (1986).
26. J. Klein, A sentimental journey to Bar Harbor: Fifty years of the Jackson Laboratory, Immunogenetics 8:3-11 (1979).
27. G. D. Snell, Methods for the study of histocompatibility genes, J. Genetics 49:87-108 (1948).
28. P. A. Gorer, S. Lyman, and G. D. Snell, Studies on the genetic and antigenic basis of tumour transplantation; linkage between a histocompatibility gene and "fused" in mice, Proc. Roy. Soc.(Lond.) B 135:499-505 (1948).
29. J. H. Stimpfling and A. Richardson, Recombination within the histocompatibility-2 locus of the mouse. Genetics 51: 831-846 (1965).
30. G. D. Snell, The genetics of transplantation. J. Nat. Cancer Inst. 14:691-700 (1953).
31. D. B. Amos, P. A. Gorer, and Z. B. Mikulska, An analysis of an antigenic system in the mouse (the H-2 system), Proc. Roy.Soc. (Lond.) B 144:369-380 (1955).
32. P. A. Gorer and Z. B. Mikulska, Some further data on the H-2 system of antigens, Proc. Roy. Soc. (Lond.) B 151: 57-69 (1959).
33. G. Hoecker, S. Counce, and P. Smith, The antigens determined by the H-2 locus: A rhesus-like system in the mouse, Proc. Natl.Acad. Sci. USA 40:1040-1051 (1954).
34. D. C. Shreffler and R. D. Owen, A serologically detected variant in mouse serum: Inheritance and association with the histocompatiblity-2 locus, Genetics 48:9-25 (1963).
35. J. Klein and D. C. Shreffler, The H-2 model for major histocompatibility systems, Transplant. Rev. 6:3-29 (1971).
36. G. D. Snell, M. Cherry, and P. Démant, Evidence that H-2 private specificities can be arranged in two mutually exclusive systems possibly homologous with two subsystems of HL-A, Transplant.Proc. 3:183-186 (1971).
37. B. B. Levine, A. Ojeda, and B. Berracerraf, Studies on artificial antigens. III. The genetic control of the immune response to hapten poly-L-lysine conjugates in guinea pigs, J. Exp. Med. 118:953-975 (1963).
38. P. H. Maurer, B. F. Gerulat, and P. Pinchuk, Antigenicity of polypeptides. Studies in rabbits, J. Immunol. 90: 388-392 (1963).
39. H. O. McDevitt and M. Sela, Genetic control of the antibody response. I. Demonstration of determinant-specific differences in response to synthetic polypeptide antigens in two strains of inbred mice, J. Exp. Med. 122:517-531 (1965).
40. H. O. McDevitt and A. Chinitz, Genetic control of the antibody response: Relationship between immune response and histocompatibility (H-2) type, Science 163:1207-1208 (1969).
41. H. O. McDevitt, B. D. Deak, D. C. Shreffler, J. Klein, J. H. Stimpfling, and G. D. Snell, Genetic control of the immune response. Mapping of the Ir-1 locus, J. Exp. Med. 135:1259-1278 (1972).
42. C. S. David, D. C. Shreffler, and J. A. Frelinger, New lym-

phocyte antigen system (Lna) controlled by the *Ir* region of the mouse *H-2* complex, *Proc. Natl. Acad. Sci. USA* 70: 2509-2514 (1973).
43. V. Hauptfeld, D. Klein, and J. Klein, Serological identification of an Ir-region product, *Science* 181:167-170 (1973).
44. D. H. Sachs and J. L. Cone, A mouse B-cell alloantigen determined by gene(s) linked to the major histocompatibility complex, *J. Exp. Med.* 138:1289-1304 (1973).
45. G. J. Hämmerling, B. D. Deak, G. Mauve, U. Hämmerling, and H. O. McDevitt: B lymphocyte alloantigens controlled by the region of the major histocompatibility complex in mice, *Immunogentics* 1:68-81 (1974).

SECTION II
POLYMORPHISM AND GENE ORGANIZATION

THE MAJOR HISTOCOMPATIBILITY COMPLEX OF THE BALB/C MOUSE:
GENE ORGANIZATION AND RECOMBINATION

Michael Steinmetz[1] and Yasushi Uematsu[2]

[1] Central Research Units, F. Hoffmann-La Roche & Co.Ltd., CH-4002 Basel, Switzerland

[2] Basel Institute for Immunology CH-4058 Basel, Switzerland

INTRODUCTION

We have recently witnessed how efficiently a genetic region even as large as the major histocompatibility complex (MHC) of the mouse can be studied for structure and function using the powerful tools of molecular biology. The rapid progress was dependent, however, on the vast amount of genetic, serologic, biochemical and functional information that had been accumulated for the MHC genes over the past fifty years since their discovery by Peter Gorer (1936). In particular due to the availability of large numbers of inbred, congenic and recombinant congenic mouse strains (Snell, 1981) molecular genetic studies have advanced more rapidly for the mouse MHC as compared to man (for reviews see: Hood et al., 1983; Steinmetz and Hood, 1983; Möller, 1985a, b and c; Flavell et al., 1986; Klein, 1986).

The molecular dissection of the MHC began in 1980 with the isolation of cDNA clones, initially for human class I molecules in the laboratories of Strominger and Weissman (Ploegh et al., 1980; Sood et al., 1981) and subsequently for murine class I molecules in the laboratories of Hood, Dobberstein, Peterson and Kourilsky (Steinmetz et al., 1981a; Kvist et al., 1981). Soon thereafter cDNA clones for human class II (Kormann et al., 1982; Lee et al., 1982; Stetler et al., 1982; Wake et al., 1982; Wiman et al., 1982) and human and murine class III molecules (Woods et al., 1982; Carroll and Porter, 1983; Ogata et al., 1983) were isolated and together with the class I cDNA clones used to study the structure, complexity and organization of the corresponding murine genes (Steinmetz et al., 1981b, 1982a and b; Chaplin et al., 1983).

FIFTY GENES CLONED FROM THE MHC OF THE BALB/c MOUSE

The most efficient approach towards the analysis of the molecular organization of the mouse MHC has been the isolaton of MHC genes from cosmid libraries combined with chromosomal walking procedures (Steinmetz et al., 1982a and b; 1986; Chaplin et al., 1983; Weiss et al., 1984; Stephan et al., 1986). Gene cloning were combined with gene mapping studies in which polymorphic restriction sites were used as genetic markers to correlate genetic and physical maps in recombinant congenic mice (Winoto et al., 1983). More recently pulse field gradient gels have been used to extend the physical maps established by chromosomal walking and mapping techniques (Müller et al., 1987a). These efforts have provided us with a detailed picture of the molecular organization of the MHC of the BALB/c mouse as shown in Fig.1.

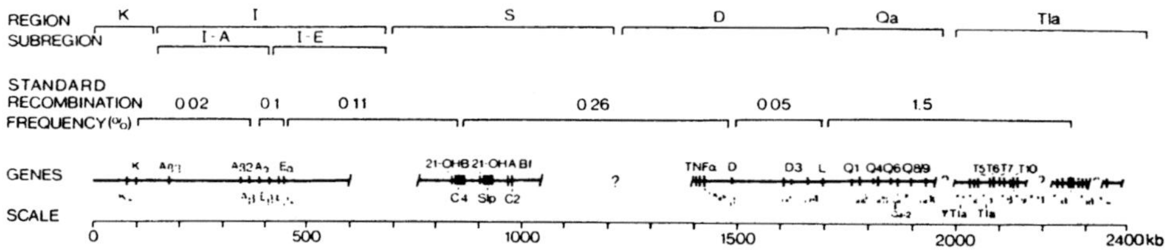

<u>Fig.1</u> Location of 50 genes in the MHC of the BALB/c mouse. Genes are indicated by vertical bars on six gene clusters that have been defined by overlapping cosmid clones. The order, orientation and spacing of the three gene clusters in the <u>Tla</u> region is not known. The complement gene cluster in the <u>S</u> region is separated from the <u>K-I</u> region gene cluster by about 170 kb while its distance to the <u>D-Qa</u> region gene cluster is at least 350 kb of DNA.

From the centromeric part of the MHC of the BALB/c mouse a 600 kb gene cluster has been cloned containing two class I (<u>K</u> and <u>K2</u>) and seven class II genes (<u>Aβ3</u> to <u>Eα</u>) (Steinmetz et al., 1986) (Fig.1). This cluster links the <u>K</u> to the <u>I</u> region at the molecular level. Following a gap of about 170 kb of so far uncloned DNA as second gene cluster of 330 kb in length has been cloned from the <u>S</u> region containing four genes (<u>C4</u>, <u>Slp</u>, <u>Bf</u>, <u>C2</u>) coding for complement or related components and two homologous genes (<u>21-OHA</u> and <u>21-OHB</u>), one of which codes for steroid 21-hydroxylase (Chaplin et al., 1983; Steinmetz et al., 1984; Müller et al., 1987a). The molecular map position and orientation of this gene cluster in the MHC has been determined by pulse field gradient gel electrophoresis (Müller et al., 1987a) and its orientation has been confirmed by genetic recombination analysis (Shiroishi et al., 1987). Following a gap of at least 350 kb (Müller et al., 1987a) a third gene cluster encompassing 500 kb of DNA has been isolated from the <u>D</u> and <u>Qa</u> regions and defines the location of 13 class I genes (<u>D</u> to <u>Q10</u>) (Stephan

	K	I	S	D	QA	TLA
NUMBER OF GENES	2	7	7-11	1-5	1-10	13-19
POLYMORPHISM	HIGH	HIGH	LOW	HIGH	LOW	LOW
EXPRESSION	ALL SOMATIC CELLS	B CELLS, MACROPHAGES, DENDRITIC CELLS	LIVER, MACROPHAGES	ALL SOMATIC CELLS	LIVER, HEMATO-POIETIC CELLS	THYMOCYTES, T LEUKEMIAS, AND OTHER CELLS
FUNCTION	ANTIGEN PRESENTATION TO $CD8^+$ T CELLS	ANTIGEN PRESENTATION TO $CD4^+$ T CELLS	COMPLEMENT, STEROID BIO-SYNTHESIS, CYTOTOXIN	ANTIGEN PRESENTATION TO $CD8^+$ T CELLS	?	?

Fig.2 The MHC of the mouse. Numbers of genes so far identified in six regions of the MHC in different mouse strains are given together with some of their characteristics. On this chart the border between the S and D regions is defined to be located between the TNF and D genes (see Fig.1).

et al., 1986), the TNF-α and -ß genes coding for two cytotoxins (Müller et al., 1987b) and a newly isolated gene of unknown function, which is located about 10 kb centromeric to TNF-α and is transcribed in B cells and macrophages but not in T cells, liver, brain and kidney (Tsuge et al., 1987). From the Tla region three gene clusters, 160, 90 and 40 kb in length, have been cloned with a total of 19 class I genes (Steinmetz et al., 1982a; Fisher et al., 1985; Transy et al., 1987). The order, orientation and spacing of the three class I gene clusters in the Tla region are not known.

In summary a total of 50 genes have so far been cloned and partially characterized from the MHC of the BALB/c mouse. Thirty-four of them are members of the class I gene family, seven are class II genes and nine prove to be structurally unrelated to class I and class II genes. All of these unrelated genes are clustered in the middle of the MHC but the significance of this location (if any) is not known. The MHC therefore covers at least 2.4 mega base pairs on chromosome 17. Future cloning efforts should fill in the remaining gaps and attempts should be made to identify additional genes presumably located in the MHC.

The MHC of the mouse is by no way a static structure. A lot of diversity signified by differences in gene numbers and allelic variation has been described and constitutes the molecular basis for the existence of a large number of different haplotypes (for a review see Geliebter and Nathenson, 1987). In addition to random point mutations, small insertions and deletions, two distinct recombinational mechanisms, namely gene conversion-like events and homologous but unequal crossovers, appear to be responsible for the generation of variability. Also homologous, equal recombination contributes to the generation of distinct haplotypes (see below). Fig.2 summarizes the extent of variation in gene numbers found in different regions of the MHC. With the exception of the K and I regions, evidence for gene expansion and contraction, presumably by unequal crossover, has been obtained for the S, D, Qa and Tla region genes. A function has been found so far for only three (K, D, L) of the 34 class I, four (Aα, Aß, Eα, Eß) of the seven class II and six (C2, Bf, C4, 21-OHB, TNF-α, TNF-ß) of the nine unrelated genes (Fig.2). Some of the unknowns are clearly non-functional genes. Also shown in Fig.2 is the degree of polymorphism observed at various gene loci. While the classical

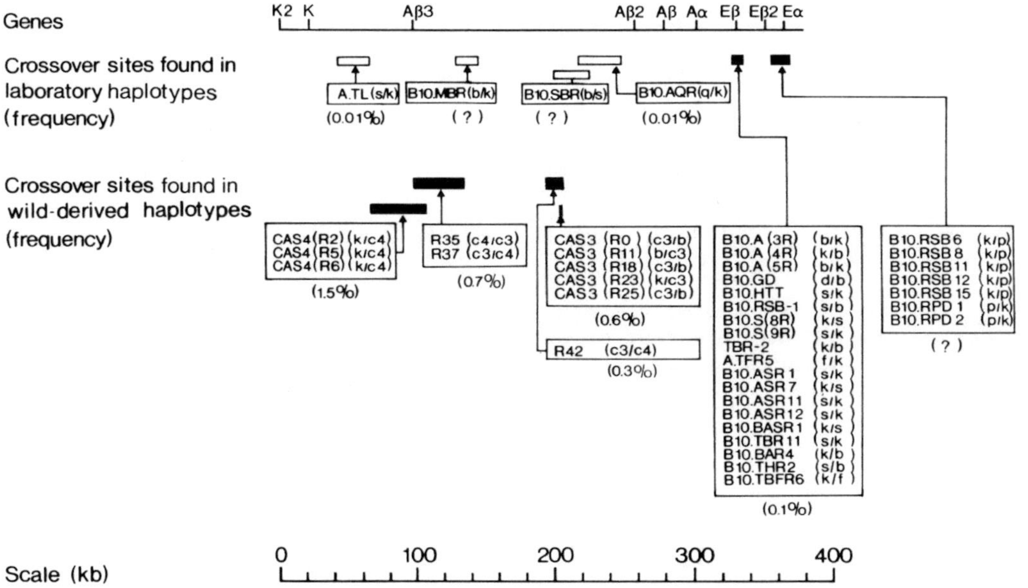

Fig.3 Location of recombinational breakpoints in the K-I interval. Crossovers located in recombinational hotspots have been confined to segments indicated by black boxes while those outside of hotspots have been mapped to the regions shown by open boxes. Only some of the recombinant mouse strains with known crossover breakpoints in the Eß or Eα hotspots are listed (Steinmetz et al., 1982b; Begovich and Jones, 1985; Lafuse and David, 1986; Lafuse et al., 1986; Saha and Cullen, 1986; Zimmerer et al., 1987).

class I genes (K, D, L) and three of the class II genes (Aα, Aß, Eß) are known to be highly polymorphic (presumably a result of mutation and positive selection mechanisms) all other genes do not appear to be unusually polymorphic.

FOUR RECOMBINATIONAL HOTSPOTS BETWEEN THE K AND Eα GENES

The cloning of extended segments of the MHC of the BALB/c mouse has made it possible to map meiotic recombinational breakpoints at the nucleotide level. Initially, nine intra-I region recombinant mouse strains were analyzed and surprisingly found to have undergone crossover within a segment of DNA at most 10 kb in length and covering part of the Eß gene (Steinmetz et al., 1982a) (Fig.3). This finding indicated that meiotic recombination events in the mouse MHC could be highly focal and that genetic and physical maps would not be congruent.

The discovery of a recombinational hotspot in the Eß gene raised interest to search for additional hotspots in the MHC. When molecular linkage of the K and I regions were obtained, a series of recombinant mouse strains with crossovers at unusually high frequencies in the K-A interval was analyzed. Such recombinant mouse strains had first been described by Shiroishi et al. (1982) and resulted from crossovers involving a Mus musculus (M.m.) molossinus haplotype. Subsequently Fischer Lindahl (1986) found high frequency crossover in the K-I interval when one of two different M.m. castaneus haplotypes were crossed with haplotypes from laboratory mouse strains. In contrast to the low frequency of recombination that is found for this segment of chromosome 17 when different laboratory strains are crossed, these crosses revealed a 50- to 100-fold higher recombination frequency (Shiroishi et al., 1982; Fischer Lindahl, 1986).

The molecular analysis of the castaneus recombinants identified the existence of two more recombinational hotspots, called K/Aß3 and Aß3/Aß2. While all three CAS4 recombinants have undergone crossover in the K/Aß3 hotspot, all five CAS3 recombinants mapped to the Aß3/Aß2 hotspot (Steinmetz et al., 1986; Uematsu et al., 1986) (Fig.3). In contrast four recombinational breakpoints in the K-A interval that were found at low frequency in crosses between distinct MHC haplotypes of laboratory mouse strains are not clustered (Steinmetz et al., 1986; Uematsu et al., 1986 and 1987) (Fig.3), indicating that laboratory haplotypes have lost these recombinational hotspots. A fourth recombinational hotspot was identified in the Eα gene (Lafuse and David, 1986; Lafuse et al., 1986).

The K/Aß3 and Aß3/Aß2 hotspots are not dependent on chiasma formation between haplotypes derived from the wild population and those from laboratory strains. Three recombinant mouse strains were recently found at a frequency of about 1%, in which crossovers had occurred between cas3 and cas4 haplotype DNA in the K-A interval (Uematsu et al., 1987). The molecular analysis of these recombinants showed that the three breakpoints again map to the K/Aß3 and the Aß3/Aß2 hotspots (Uematsu et al., 1987) (Fig.3). Thus the presence of recombinational hotspots in the K-A interval is an inherent feature of the cas3 and cas4 haplotypes. When recombinational hotspots are present they act in a dominant fashion.

The structural basis of recombinational hotspots is unknown. Repetitive sequences have been identified in the proximity of the Aß3/Aß2 and Eß hotspots and have been suggested to play a role based on their similarity to Chi, a recombinational hotspot in phage λ, and human hypervariable minisatellite sequences, constituting presumed hotspots in man (Steinmetz et al., 1987; Uematsu et al., 1986). Indeed Chi and MHC recombinational hotspots share a number of properties (Table 1) indicating that the mechanism of recombination might be similar in prokaryotes and eukaryotes. Sequence comparisons however can only suggest possibilities. Analysis of secondary recombinants and functional assays are needed to identify possible signal sequences involved (Steinmetz et al., 1987).

Table 1. Do MHC recombinational hotspots act like Chi?

Chi	MHC recombinational hotspots
GCTGGTGG	Tandem repeats related to Chi
Stimulates recombination near itself	Tandem repeats linked to clusters of crossover breakpoints
Stimulates recombination preferentially on one side	Tandem repeats might be located on one side of all crossover breakpoints
Acts in a dominant fashion	Act in a dominant fashion
Enhances only homologous recombination	Recombination is homologous and equal down to the nucleotide level
Recombination frequency drops if Chi is mutated	Show different recombination frequencies
Depends on a second site (Cos)	?

CONCLUSION

The molecular analysis of the mouse MHC over the past seven years has provided us with a detailed picture of its structural organization and variation during evolution. Fifty genes have so far been cloned from the MHC of the BALB/c mouse, fifty years after the discovery of the H-2 complex. Given the current interest in improving methodologies required for the studies of large gene complexes and eventually whole mammalian genomes it will not take another 50 years before the molecular organization of the MHC has been completely worked out.

ACKNOWLEDGEMENTS

We thank Ms. Anne Iff for typing the manuscript. The Basel Institute for Immunology was founded and is supported by F. Hoffmann-La Roche & Co. Ltd., Basel, Switzerland.

REFERENCES

Begovich, A. B., and Jones, P. P., 1985, Free Ia E_α chain expression in the $E_\alpha^+ : E_\beta^-$ recombinant strain A.TFR5, Immunogenetics, 22:523.

Carroll, M. C., and Porter, R. R., 1983, Cloning of a human complement component C4 gene, Proc. Natl. Acad. Sci. USA, 80:264.

Chaplin, D. D., Woods, D. E., Whitehead, A. S., Goldberger, G., Colten, H. R., and Seidman, J. G., 1983, Molecular map of the murine S region, Proc. Natl. Acad. Sci. USA, 80:6947.

Fischer Lindahl, K., 1986, Genetic variants of histocompatibility antigens from wild mice, Curr. Topics Microbiol. Immunol., 127:272.

Fisher, D. A., Hunt III, S. W., and Hood, L., 1985, Structure of a gene encoding a murine thymus leukemia antigen, and organization of Tla genes in the BALB/c mouse, J. Exp. Med., 162:528.

Flavell, R. A., Allen, H., Burkly, L. C., Sherman, D. H., Waneck, G. L., and Widera, G., 1986, Molecular biology of the H-2 histocompatibility complex, Science, 233:437.

Geliebter, J., and Nathenson, S. G., 1987, Recombination and the concerted evolution of the murine MHC, Trends in Genetics, 3:107.

Gorer, P. A., 1936, The detection of antigenic differences in mouse erythrocytes by the employment of immune sera, Br. J. Exp. Pathol., 17:42.

Hood, L., Steinmetz, M., and Malissen, B., 1983, Genes of the major histocompatibility complex of the mouse, Ann. Rev. Immunol., 1:529.

Klein, J., 1986, Natural History of the Major Histocompatibility Complex, John Wiley & Sons, New York.

Korman, A. J., Knudsen, P. J., Kaufman, J. F., and Strominger, J. L., 1982, cDNA clones for the heavy chain of HLA-DR antigens obtained after immunopurification of polysomes by monoclonal antibody, Proc. Natl. Acad. Sci. USA, 79:1844.

Kvist, S., Bregegere, F., Rask, L., Cami, B., Garoff, H., Daniel, F., Wiman, K., Larhammar, D., Abastado, J.P., Gachelin, G., Peterson, P. A., Dobberstein, B., and Kourilsky, P., 1981, cDNA clone coding for part of a mouse $H-2^d$ major histocompatibility antigen, Proc. Natl. Acad. Sci. USA, 78:2772.

Lafuse, W.P., and David, C.S., 1986, Recombination hot spots within the I region of the mouse H-2 complex map to the E_β and E_α genes, Immunogenetics, 24:352.

Lafuse, W. P., Berg, N., Savarirayan, S., and David, C. S., 1986, Mapping of a second recombination hot spot within the I-E region of the mouse H-2 gene complex, J. Exp. Med., 163:1518.

Lee, J. S., Trowsdale, J., and Bodmer, W. F., 1982, cDNA clones coding for the heavy chain of human HLA-DR antigen, Proc. Natl. Acad. Sci. USA, 79:545.

Möller, G., ed., 1985a, Molecular Genetics of Class I and Class II MHC Antigens 1, Immunol. Rev., 84.

Möller, G., ed., 1985b, Molecular Genetics of Class I and Class II MHC Antigens 2, Immunol. Rev., 85.

Möller, G., ed., 1985c, Molecular Genetics of Class III MHC Antigens, Immunol. Rev., 87.

Müller, U., Stephan, D., Philippsen, P., and Steinmetz, M., 1987a, Orientation and molecular map position of the complement genes in the mouse MHC, EMBO J., 6:369.

Müller, U., Jongeneel, C. V., Nedospasov, S. A., Fischer Lindahl, K., and Steinmetz, M., 1987b, Tumour necrosis factor and lymphotoxin genes map close to H-2D in the mouse major histocompatibility complex, Nature, 325:265.

Ogata, R. T., Shreffler, D. C., Sepich, D. S., and Lilly, S. P., 1983, cDNA clone spanning the α-γ subunit junction in the precursor of the murine fourth complement component (C4), Proc. Natl. Acad. Sci. USA, 80:5061.

Ploegh, H. L., Orr, H. T., and Strominger, J. L., 1980, Molecular cloning of a human histocompatibility antigen cDNA fragment, Proc. Natl. Acad. Sci. USA, 77:6081.

Saha, B. K., and Cullen, S. E., 1986, Molecular mapping of murine I region recombinants: Crossing over in the E_β gene, J. Immunol., 136:1112.

Shiroishi, T., Sagai, T., and Moriwaki, K., 1982, A new wild-derived H-2 haplotype enhancing K-IA recombination, Nature, 300:370.

Shiroishi, T., Sagai, T., Natsuume-Sakai, S., and Moriwaki, K., 1987, Lethal deletion of the complement component C4 and steroid 21-hydroxylase genes in the mouse H-2 class III region, caused by meiotic recombination, Proc. Natl. Acad. Sci. USA, 84:2819.

Snell, G. D., 1981, Studies in histocompatibility, Science, 213:172.

Sood, A. K., Pereira, D., and Weissman, S. M., 1981, Isolation and partial nucleotide sequence of a cDNA clone for human histocompatibility antigen HLA-B by use of an oligodeoxynucleotide primer, Proc. Natl. Acad. Sci. USA, 78:616.

Steinmetz, M., Frelinger, J. G., Fisher, D., Hunkapiller, T., Pereira, D. Weissman, S. M., Uehara, H., Nathenson, S., and Hood, L., 1981a, Three cDNA clones encoding mouse transplantation antigens: Homology to immunoglobulin genes, Cell, 24:125.

Steinmetz, M., Moore, K. W., Frelinger, J. G., Taylor Sher, B., Shen, F.-W., Boyse, E. A., and Hood, L., 1981b, A pseudogene homologous to mouse transplantation antigens: Transplantation antigens are encoded by eight exons that correlate with protein domains, Cell, 25:683.

Steinmetz, M., Winoto, A., Minard, K., and Hood, L., 1982a, Clusters of genes encoding mouse transplantation antigens, Cell, 28:489.

Steinmetz, M., Minard, K., Horvath, S., McNicholas, J., Frelinger, J., Wake, C., Long, E., Mach, B., and Hood, L., 1982b, A molecular map of the immune response region from the major histocompatibility complex of the mouse, Nature, 300:35.

Steinmetz, M., and Hood, L., 1983, Genes of the major histocompatibility complex in mouse and man, Science, 222:727.

Steinmetz, M., Malissen, M., Hood, L., Oern, A., Maki, R. A., Dastoornikoo, G. R., Stephan, D., Gibb, E., and Romaniuk R., 1984, Tracts of high or low sequence divergence in the mouse major histocompatibility complex, EMBO J., 3:2995.

Steinmetz, M., Stephan, D., and Fischer Lindahl, K., 1986, Gene organization and recombinational hotspots in the murine major histocompatibility complex, Cell, 44:895.

Steinmetz, M., Uematsu, Y., and Fischer Lindahl, K., 1987, Hotspots of homologous recombination in mammalian genomes, Trends in Genetics, 3:7.

Stephan, D., Sun, H., Fischer Lindahl, K., Meyer, E., Hämmerling, G., Hood, L., and Steinmetz, M., 1986, Organization and evolution of D region class I genes in the mouse major histocompatibility complex, J. Exp. Med., 163:1227.

Stetler, D., Das, H., Nunberg, J. H., Saiki, R., Sheng-Dong, R., Mullis, K. B., Weissman, S. M., and Erlich, H. A., 1982, Isolation of a cDNA clone for the human HLA-DR antigen α chain by using a synthetic oligonucleotide as a hybridization probe, Proc. Natl. Acad. Sci. USA, 79:5966.

Transy, C., Nash, R. S., David-Watine, B., Cochet, M., Hunt III, S. W., Hood, L. E., and Kourilsky, P., 1987, A low polymorhic mouse H-2 class I gene from the Tla complex is expressed in a broad variety of cell types, J. Exp. Med., in press.

Tsuge, I., Shen, F.-W., Steinmetz, M., and Boyse, E. A., 1987, A gene in the J-2S:H-2D interval of the major histocompatibility complex which is transcribed in B cells and macrophages, Immunogenetics, in press.

Uematsu, Y., Kiefer, H., Schulze, R., Fischer Lindahl, K., and Steinmetz, M., 1986, Molecular characterization of a meiotic recombinational hotspot enhancing homologous equal crossing-over, EMBO J., 5:2123.

Uematsu, Y., Fischer Lindahl, K., and Steinmetz, M., 1987, The same recombinational hotspots are active in wild/wild and wild/inbred chromosome crossovers, submitted.

Wake, C. T., Long, E. O., Strubin, M., Gross, N., Accolla, R., Carrel, S. and Mach, B., 1982, Isolation of cDNA clones encoding HLA-DR α chains, Proc. Natl. Acad. Sci. USA, 79:6979.

Weiss, E. H., Golden L., Fahrner, K., Mellor, A. L., Devlin, J. J., Bullman, H., Tiddens, H., Bud, H., and Flavell, R. A., 1984, Organization and evolution of the class I gene family in the major histocompatibility complex of the C57BL/10 mouse, Nature, 310:650.

Winoto, A., Steinmetz, M., and Hood, L., 1983, Genetic mapping in the major histocompatibility complex by restriction enzyme site polymorphisms: Most mouse class I genes map to the Tla complex, Proc. Natl. Acad. Sci. USA, 80:3425.

Wiman, K., Larhammar, D., Claesson, L., Gustafsson, K., Schenning, L., Bill, P., Böhme, J., Denaro, M., Dobberstein, B., Hammerling, U., Kvist, S., Servenius, B., Sundelin, J., Peterson, P. A., and Rask, L., 1982, Isolation and identification of a cDNA clone corresponding to an HLA-DR antigen ß chain, Proc. Natl. Acad. Sci. USA, 79:1703.

Woods, D. E., Markham, A. F., Ricker, A. T., Goldberger, G., and Colten, H. R., 1982, Isolation of cDNA clones for the human complement protein factor B, a class III major histocompatibility complex gene product, Proc. Natl. Acad. Sci. USA, 79:5661.

Zimmerer, E. J., Ogin, E., Shreffler, D. C., and Passmore, H.C., 1987, Molecular mapping of crossover sites within the I region of the mouse MHC, Immunogenetics, 25:274.

RECOMBINATION SITES WITHIN THE I REGION OF THE MOUSE H-2 COMPLEX

William P. Lafuse[1] and Chella S. David[2]

[1]Department of Medical Microbiology and Immunology, The Ohio State University, 333 W. 10th Avenue, Columbus, Ohio 43210
[2]Department of Immunology, Mayo Clinic and Medical School Rochester, Minnesota 55905

INTRODUCTION

Recombinant mouse strains have been important in the development of the genetic map of the H-2 complex and have been used to subdivide the H-2 complex into the K, D, Qa, Tla regions containing genes for class I MHC molecules; I region containing genes for class II MHC molecules; and S region containing genes for class III MHC molecules. A molecular map of the H-2 complex has also been developed with about 1,600 Kb of DNA having been cosmid cloned. The I region has been shown to consist of a 270 Kb segment of DNA that contains six class I genes: $A_{\beta 2}$, A_{β}, A_{α}, E_{β}, $E_{\beta 2}$ and E_{α} (Steinmetz et al. 1982). Over the last few years recombinant mouse strains with crossovers in the I region have been analyzed by DNA restriction fragment analysis and DNA sequencing (Steinmetz et al. 1982, 1986, Kobori et al. 1984, 1986, Lafuse et al. 1986, Lafuse and David, 1986, Begovich et al. 1985, Saha and Cullen 1986, Zimmerer et al. 1987). These studies have shown that recombination within the I region is not random but is limited to two specific locations. These sites which have been termed recombination hot spots are located within the E_{β} and E_{α} genes. In this report we will review these studies and discuss the implication that there are haplotype specific sequences that promote recombination at these two sites. We will also report studies on additional recombinants mapping within the I region.

RECOMBINANT MOUSE STRAINS WITH CROSSOVERS WITHIN THE E_{β} GENE

The first molecular studies of recombinant mouse strains were done by Steinmetz et al. 1982 and Kobori et al. 1984 using the technique of restriction fragment length polymorphism mapping. These studies showed that in six intra-I region recombinant mouse strains the crossovers occurred in the E_{β} gene. This first suggested that recombination within the H-2 complex is not random but localized to specific sites which have been termed recombination "hot spots". These studies mapped the recombination hot spot to a large intron between the second and third exons of the E_{β} gene. Kobori et al. 1986 sequenced the DNA from four of these recombinant mouse strains. Three of the four recombinants (B10.A(3R), B10.A(5R), B10.GD) recombined within a 1 Kb region of this intron. The fourth recombinant strain B10.A(4R) could not be precisely maped but occurred upstream of the crossovers in the other three recombinant strains.

Additional recombinant mouse strains have also been identified with crossovers within this recombination hot spot (Begovitch et al. 1985, Saha and Cullen 1986, Lafuse and David 1986, Zimmerer et al. 1987, Howard Passmore personal communication). The total number of recombinant mouse strains with crossovers in the E_β gene is 32. Table 1 lists the nine recombinant mouse strains which we mapped to the E_β recombination hot spot (Lafuse and David 1986). Eight of these recombinant mouse strains have the E_β negative f and q haplotypes as one of the parent haplotypes. When the functional haplotype (b or k) is 5' of the crossover, the E_β gene in the recombinant mouse strain is functional. When the nonfunctional haplotype (f or q) is 5' of the crossover, the E_β gene in the recombinant is not functional and the recombinant is I-E negative (Lafuse et al. 1987). This suggests the defect in f and q haplotypes is located 5' of the recombination hot spot.

Table 2 lists all the haplotype combinations in which E_β recombinant mouse strains have been found. Recombination at this site is reciprocal. For example, there are 2 recombinants with the k haplotype 5' of the crossover and the f haplotype 3' of the crossover and there are 3 recombinants with the f haplotype 5' of the crossover and the k haplotype 3' of the crossover. In all of the recombinant mouse strains one of the parental strains involved was from the b or k haplotype. This suggests the possibility that there is a DNA sequence present in these haplotypes that promotes recombination at this site. There are also haplotype combinations (k-p, k-d) in which no E_β recombinant mouse strains have been found. Recombinant mouse strains between the k and p haplotype crossover in the E_α gene. These recombinant mouse strains are reviewed later in this paper. There are two possible explanations for lack of E_β recombinants between the k and p haplotypes. A DNA sequence present in the E_α gene of the p haplotype might promote recombination in the E_α gene over recombination at the E_β gene. Alternately the sequence that promotes recombination at the E_β gene might be absent in the p haplotype. Restriction fragment analysis of the E_β gene has revealed that there is a deletion of about 1 Kb in the p haplotype (Lafuse and David, 1986). The exact nature and location of DNA sequences that might promote at the E_β gene is unknown. One possible sequence is a four-base repeat (AGGC)n located 50bp 5' of exon 3. This sequence is repeated 18 times in d haplotype and 10 times in the b and k haplotypes (Kobori et al. 1986). It has been suggested by Steinmetz et al. 1986 that this sequence could form Z-DNA. Z-DNA sequences has been suggested as a recombination signal in globin genes (Slightom et al. 1980, Kilpatrik et al. 1984). We are presently cloning the E_β gene from the p haplotype and will do sequence analysis to determine if this repeat sequence has been deleted.

RECOMBINANT MOUSE STRAINS WITH CROSSOVERS IN THE E_α GENE

There are seven recombinant mouse strains with crossovers in the E_α gene (Lafuse et al. 1986, Lafuse and David, 1986). These strains are listed in Table 3. These recombinant mouse strains were derived from crosses between strains with E_α genes from the p and k haplotypes. Like recombination at the E_β hot spot recombination in the E_α gene is reciprocal Five recombinant mouse strains crossed over k-p and two recombinant mouse strains crossed over p-k. The crossover points in these recombinants have been localized by restriction fragment mapping to a 5 Kb DNA segment within the E_α gene that extends from Dra I and Pst I sites in the intron between exons 4 and 5 to a Rsa I site that is 1 Kb 3' of the E_α gene. To further map this recombination hot spot we are currently cloning E_α genes from recombinant mouse strains and will sequence the DNA.

Table I

Recombinant Mouse Strains with E_β Crossovers

Strain	K	A_β	A_α	E_β	E_α	S	D
B10.RBF	b	b	b	b/f	f	f	f
B10.RKB	k	k	k	k/b	b	b	b
B10.RFB2	f	f	f	f/k	k	d	d
B10.RFB3	f	f	f	f/k	k	b	b
B10.RKF3	k	k	k	k/f	f	f	f
B10.RKD6	k	k	k	k/q	q	q	d
B10.RKD7	k	k	k	k/q	q	q	d
B10.RKQ2	k	k	k	k/q	q	q	q
B10.RQB3	q	q	q	q/k	k	d	b

Table 2

Recombinant Mouse Strains with E_β Crossovers

Haplotype Combination	No. of Recombinants
d/b	1
k/b	8
b/k	2
k/f	2
f/k	3
k/q	3
q/k	1
k/s	3
s/k	6
s/b	2
b/f	1
Total	32

Table 3

Recombinant Mouse Strains with E_α Crossovers

Strain	K	A_β	A_α	E_β	$E_{\beta 2}$	E_α Exons 5	4	3	2	1	S	D
B10.RSB6	s	s	s	s/k	k	k	———	———	———	p	b	b
B10.RSB8	s	s	s	s/k	k	k	———	———	———	p	b	b
B10.RSB11	s /	k	k	k	k	k	———	———	———	p	b	b
B10.RSB12	s	s	s	s/k	k	k	———	———	———	p	b	b
B10.RSB15	s /	k	k	k	k	k	———	———	———	p	b	b
B10.RPD1	p	p	p	p	p	p	———	———	———	k	d	d
B10.RPD2	p	p	p	p	p	p	———	———	———	k	d	d

Solid line represents DNA segment in which crossovers occurred.

We have also recently analyzed six secondary recombinant strains that were discovered during the initial breeding of E_α recombinant mouse strains B10.RPD1 and B10.RPD2. In the breeding program that yielded B10.RPD1 and B10.RPD2, F1 mice between B10.S(9R) $E_\alpha{}^k$ and B10.F(13R) $E_\alpha{}^p$ were crossed to B10.M (H-2^f). The resulting progeny were tested serologically for intra-H-2 recombinants. The two mice with recombination events were again crossed to B10.M. Chromosomes that have recently undergone a recombination event are unstable and with a high frequency undergo a second recombination in the next generation. Why this occurs is unknown. This was especially true with B10.RPD1 and B10.RPD2 as five secondary recombinants were found between B10.RPD1 and B10.M and one secondary recombinant was found between B10.RPD2 and B10.M. The serological typing of these secondary recombinant mouse strains is shown in Table 4. The E_α alleles of B10.RFD3, B10.RFD4, B10.RFD6, and B10.RFD7 were determined by F1 complementation (Lafuse et al. 1987). The serological typing showed that in four recombinants the crossover occurred in the interval between E_α and S region. In two recombinant mouse strains B10.RPF1 and B10.RFD7 the crossover occurred in the I region. We have mapped the recombination site in these two recombinant mouse strains by restriction fragment analysis. Restriction fragment analysis with E_β probes showed that the crossovers in these recombinant mouse strains did not map to the E_β gene (Lafuse and David, 1986). To determine if the crossovers map to the E_α recombination hot spot, DNA was digested with Rsa I and Dra I restriction endonucleases. Rsa I detects a f haplotype specific RFLP site between exons 1 and 2 of the E_α gene. B10.RPF1 types as f haplotype at this site and B10.RFD7 types as k haplotype. This maps the recombination site 5' of this RFLP site, consistent with crossovers being within the E_α gene. To confirm mapping within the E_α gene the restriction endonuclease Dra I was used. In the p haplotype there is a Dra I restriction site between exons 4 and 5, resulting in a E_α restriction fragment of 4.4 Kb. In all other haplotypes this site is absent, resulting in a 7.2 Kb E_α restriction

Table 4

Secondary Recombinants of B10.RPD1 and B10.RPD2

Strain	H-2 Complex					
	K	A_β	A_α	E_β	E_α	S	D
B10.RPF1	p	p	p	p /	f	f	f
B10.RPF2	p	p	p	p	p /	f	f
B10.RFD3	f	f	f	f	f /	d	d
B10.RFD4	f	f	f	f	f /	d	d
B10.RFD6	f	f	f	f	f /	d	d
B10.RFD7	f	f	f	f /	p	d	d

fragment. The Dra I restriction fragment is 7.2 Kb in the B10.RFD7 recombinant, indicating that this RFLP site is f haplotype in this recombinant. This places the recombination site in this strain within the E_α gene between the Dra I site located between exon 4 and 5 and the Rsa I site located between exon 1 and 2. Thus the crossover in B10.RFD7 maps within the E_α recombination hot spot.

The surprising result was obtained with the B10.RPF1 recombinant. The Dra I restriction fragment is about 500-600 kb smaller than the f haplotype fragment. There are two possible explanations for this finding. One is a unequal crossover in B10.RPF1 resulting in a deletion. If this occurred then the E_α restriction fragment pattern with other restriction endonucleases will also be different from parental haplotypes. DNA from B10.RPF1 was digested with Bam HI, Eco RI, Hind III and Tag I and probed with a E_α genomic DNA probe. The restriction pattern of B10.RPF1 was identical to parental haplotypes suggesting that B10.RPF1 does not have a deletion in the E_α gene. Another explanation is that there is a second p haplotype specific Dra I RFLP site 5' of the E_α gene. In the recombinant this site would be p haplotype origin and the Dra I RFLP site located between exon 4 and 5 would be absent, indicating f haplotype origin. This would place the recombination site in B10.RPF1 between these two Dra I restriction sites. To test this possibility we plan to clone this DNA segment from partial plasmid libraries of DNA from B10.RPF1 and parental strains B10.RPD1 and B10.M.

There is also haplotype specificity in this recombination hot spot. The recombinant mouse strains that we have mapped to the E_α gene were derived from crosses between strains with the p and k haplotypes at the E_α gene. Only these recombinants have been mapped to this site. This suggests that p haplotype has a sequence that promotes recombination at this site. The mapping of two secondary recombinant mouse strains to this recombination hot spot (B10.RFD7) or near this recombination hot spot (B10.RPF1) also suggests that the p haplotype sequence that promotes recombination is also present in the recombinants B10.RPD1 and B10.RPD2. This would place the promoting sequence 5' of the p/k crossover in B10.RPD1 and B10.RPD2.

SUMMARY

The location of crossovers in I region recombinant mouse strains has been determined for 42 recombinant mouse strains. There are also 3-5 other recombinants with possible I region crossovers which involve haplotype combinations for which we do not have RFLP sites for mapping. The recombination sites in these 42 recombinant mouse strains map to only two sites in the I region. These sites are the E_β gene and the E_α gene. There are indications that there is haplotype specificity in these recombination sites, suggesting that specific sequences promote recombination at these two sites. The location and nature of these sequences is still unknown. In order to define these sequences an in vitro recombination assay is needed.

Whether there is also other recombination hot spots elsewhere in the H-2 complex remains to be determined. There are fifteen recombinant mouse strains with crossovers in the E_α-S DNA segment and over 50 recombinant mouse strains with crossovers in the S-D DNA segment. We have recently started restriction fragment analysis to map crossovers in these two segments.

ACKNOWLEDGEMENTS

The authors thank Suresh Savariayan who produced and maintained the recombinant mouse strains. The authors also thank Dr. Lee Hood for providing the E_β and E_α DNA probes. This research was supported by grants AI-14764 from the National Institute of Allergy and Infectious Diseases and CA-24473 from the National Cancer Institute to CSD and grant IM-471 from the American Cancer Society to WPL.

REFERENCES

Begovich, A.B., and Jones, P.P.: Free Ia E_α chain expression in the E_α^+: E_β^- recombinant strain A.TFR5. Immunogenetics 22:523-532, 1985.

Kilpatrick, M.W., Klysik, J., Singleton, C.K., Zarling, D.A., Jovin, T.M., Harau, L.H., Erlanger, B.F., and Wells, R.D.: Intervening sequences of human fetal globin genes adopt left handed Z helices. J. Biol. Chem. 259:7269-7277, 1984.

Kobori, J.A., Winoto, A., McNicholas, J., and Hood, L.: Molecular characterization of the recombination region of six murine major histocompatibility complex (MHC) I-region recombinants. J. Mol. Cell. Immunol. 1:125-131, 1984.

Kobori, J.A., Strauss, E., Minard, K., and Hood, L.: Molecular analysis of the hot spot of recombination in the murine major histocompatibility complex. Science 234:173-179, 1986,

Lafuse, W.P., Berg, N., Savarirayan, S., and David, C.S.: Mapping of a second recombination hot spot within the I-E region of mouse H-2 gene complex. J. Exp. Med. 163:1518-1528, 1986.

Lafuse, W.P., Savarirayan, S., McCormick, J.F., and David, C.S.: Identification of I-E alpha genes in H-2 recombinant mouse strains by F1 complementation. Transplantation 43:297-302, 1987.

Lafuse, W.P., and David, C.S.: Recombination hot spots within the I region of the mouse H-2 complex map to the E_β and E_α genes. Immunogenetics 24:352-360, 1986.

Saha, B.K., and Cullen, S.E.: Molecular mapping of murine I region recombinants: Crossing over in the Eb gene. J. Immunol. 136:1112-1116, 1986.

Slightom, J.L. Bechl, A.E., and Smithies, O.: Human fetal Gy-Ay-globin genes: complete nucleotide sequences suggest that DNA can be exchanged between these duplicated genes. Cell 21:627-633, 1980.

Steinmetz, M., Minard, S., Horvath, S., McNicholas, J., Frelinger, J., Wake, C., Long, E., Mach, B., and Hood, L.: A molecular map of the immune response region from the major histocompatibility complex of the mouse. Nature 300:35-42, 1982.

Steinmetz, M., Stephan, D., and Lindahl, K.F.: Gene organization and recombination hot spots in the murine major histocompatibility complex. Cell 44: 895-904, 1986.

Zimmerer, E.J., Ogin, E., Shreffler, D.C., and H.C. Passmore: Molecular mapping of crossover sites within the I region of the mouse MHC. Analysis of ten recombinant chromosomes. Immunogenetics 25:274-276, 1987.

GENETIC ORGANIZATION OF THE *Qa* AND *Tla* REGIONS:

GENE MAPPING BASED ON THE ANALYSIS OF RECOMBINANT STRAINS

Howard C. Passmore and Joseph Romano

Department of Biological Sciences
Rutgers University
New Brunswick, N.J.

INTRODUCTION

Studies on the genetic organization of the mouse major histocompatibility complex (MHC) have been highly dependent on the development of intra-MHC recombinant inbred strains of mice (Klein 1979). For example, well over 200 recombinant strains have been developed for mapping the loci of the classically defined *H-2* complex (summarized in Klein *et al.*, 1983, and in *Mouse Newsletter* volumes 68, 70 and 74). Unfortunately however, only a handful of recombinant strains exist which carry crossover points associated with the *Qa* or *Tla* regions (Flaherty, 1981; O'Neill, 1986). In the past five years, the genetic analysis of the mouse MHC, has been highlighted by substantial advances in the molecular characterization and cloning of MHC genes including those of the *Qa* and *Tla* regions (Steinmetz *et al.*, 1982; Weiss *et al.*, 1985; Fisher *et al.*, 1985). This development, rather than detracting from the value of traditional analysis with intra-MHC recombinant strains, provides an opportunity to combine new and traditional approaches into a more powerful battery of tools for the examination of the organization, function and evolution of the class I genes of the *Qa* and *Tla* regions. Moreover, the advent of molecular genetics has even created new uses for intra-MHC recombinant strains including the study of the molecular character and distribution of meiotic recombination sites (Steinmetz *et al.*, 1986; Kobori *et al.*, 1986).

In the studies presented in this report, we have detailed a preliminary molecular characterization of 15 new recombinant strains which carry crossover points associated with the *Qa* and *Tla* regions. The data derived from these strains provide significant new information on the genetic organization of the mouse MHC distal to the *H-2D* locus, and provide a well-documented series of recombinant strains for future studies.

MATERIALS AND METHODS

Each of the recombinant inbred strains used in this study were developed at Rutgers University over the past six years. Strains on MA background were backcrossed five generations to MA/MyJ before intercrossing to establish a homozygous strain. These strains should be considered partially congenic. Strains B10.MR1, B10.MR2 and B10.MR3 were developed by nine generations of backcrossing to strain B10.K before intercrossing. The remainder of the strains were derived from hybrids in which both parental strains were congenic (B10.D2 x B10.K, or in one case B10.G x B10.K). These strains have been previously typed for serological and isozyme traits of the MHC (Shalders *et al*., 1983; Passmore and Shalders, unpublished).

Mouse DNA from recombinant and parental strains were prepared from liver according to Blin and Stafford with minor modifications. Agarose gel electrophoresis, transfer to nitrocellulose filters, nick translation, formamide hybridization and autoradiography were carried out essentially as described by Davis *et al*., (1980). All DNA probes used for the detection of restriction fragment length polymorphisms consisted of strain BALB/c genomic sequences originally derived from class I gene cosmids isolated and characterized by Steinmetz *et al*., 1982. These probes, many of which are described in more detail in Winoto *et al*., 1983 and Fisher *et al*., 1985, were as follows: Probe 50.21 - a 2.0-kb SmaI fragment from cosmid clone 50.2 subcloned into M13mp8 (this and other mp8 subclones were produced by A. Winoto), Probe 27.51 - a 375-bp EcoRI-BglII fragment subcloned into pBR322, Probe 46.21 - a 3.0-kb ClaI-SmaI fragment isolated directly from cosmid 46.2, Probe 36.21 - a 600-bp Sau3A fragment from cosmid 36.2 subcloned into mp8, Probe 47.11 - a 2.6-kb HpaI-XhoI fragment isolated directly from cosmid 47.1, Probe 22.11 - a 2.0-kb BamHI fragment from cosmid 22.1 subcloned into mp8, Probe 12.21 - a 2.0-kb EcoRI fragment from cosmid 12.2 subcloned into mp8, Probe 66.11 - a 2.0-kb KpnI-SmaI fragment isolated directly from cosmid 66.1, Probe pTLA.5 - a 641-bp PvuII-PstI genomic fragment containing the transmembrane and cytoplasmic exons of the *T13* gene from strain BALB/c subcloned into pBR322 (subcloned by D. Fisher), and Probe T9/T17 - a partial length cDNA derived from the *T9* gene (developed by S. Hunt).

RESULTS

This report presents the molecular characterization of fifteen new intra-MHC recombinant strains that carry crossover points between the *H-2D* locus and the locus controlling isozyme variants of kidney catalase (the *Ce-2* locus). Fourteen of these strains were derived from crossing over in (B10.D2 x MA/MyJ)F_1 or (B10.D2 x B10.K)F_1 hybrids. Since the MHC haplotype of MA/MyJ and B10.K appear to be identical for all serological, isozyme and molecular markers of the MHC, both crosses represent the same haplotype combination. These crosses are remarkable in that the two parental chromosomes carry different alleles at all of the known loci of the MHC with the exception of *Qa-1*, and importantly, differ at the isozyme loci located beyond the distal end of the MHC. Some of these differences are summarized in Table 1.

The principal approach used in the molecular characterization of these strains was to examine restriction fragment length polymorphism (RFLPs)

Table 1. Allelic differences for selected MHC traits. The alleles for strain MA/MyJ are identical to B10.K.

STRAIN	*H-2S*	*H-2D*	*Qa-2*	*Qa-3,4,5*	*Qa-6*	*Tla*	*Pgk-2*	*Ce-2*
B10.D2	*d*	*d*	*a*	*a*	*a*	*c*	*a*	*a*
B10.K	*k*	*k*	*b*	*b*	*b*	*b*	*b*	*b*

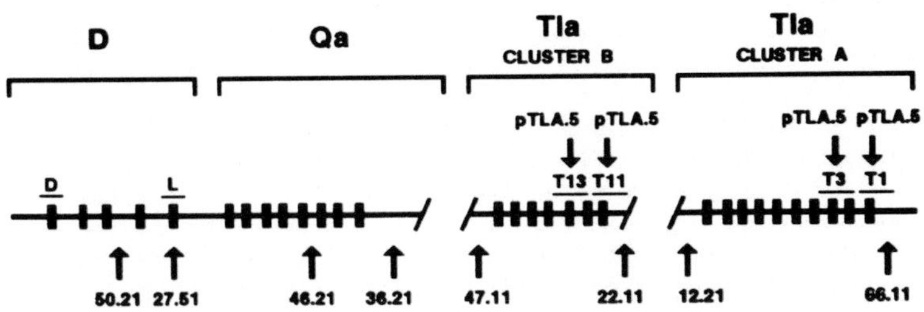

Figure 1. Class I genes of the *D*, *Qa* and *Tla* regions.

detected by DNA probes which hybridize with sequences located in the *D*, *Qa* and *Tla* regions. These low or single copies probes were selected to provide a general profile of the location of crossing over relative to the class I gene cosmid maps published for stain BALB/c (see Winoto *et al.*, 1983; Fisher *et al.*, 1985). In our hands the RFLP characteristics of the B10.D2 strain used in our recombinants were identical to BALB/c. Thus, since BALB/c and B10.D2 are serologically identical, these two strains are assumed to be identical in their MHC haplotype. The diagram in Figure 1 illustrates the positions of each of the nine DNA probes which were used to characterize these recombinants. Additional details of these probes can be found in METHODS. This diagram reflects our interpretation of the order of *Tla* gene clusters A and B based on the molecular analysis of recombinants strain B10.MR2. Probe pTLA.5 detects four *Tla* region genes, three of which (*T1*, *T11*, and *T13*) can be distinguished between parental haplotypes by RFLPs on Southern blots.

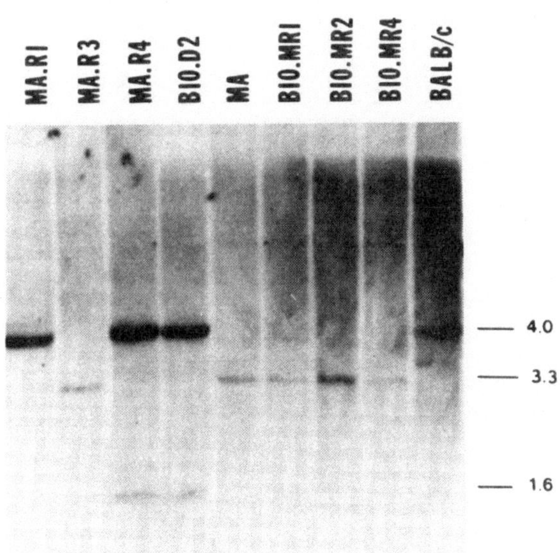

Figure 2. Southern blot analysis for Probe 46.21 using PstI.

Figure 2 illustrates a Southern blot using probe 46.21 which is derived from a sequence between the Q5 and Q6 genes of the BALB/c haplotype. This probe detects a 4.0-kb band in the lanes containing genomic DNA from BALB/c and B10.D2 digested with PstI. The 4.0-kb fragment was confirmed as the relevant target DNA by subjecting the BALB/c cosmid DNA from which the probe was derived (i.e. cosmid 46.2) to hybridization analysis after digestion with PstI. In contrast to the pattern seen in B10.D2, strains MA and B10.K lack this 4.0-kb band. It is unclear whether the homologous DNA sequence is missing in these strains or is represented by the lower molecular band apparent in the MA lane. The former interpretation is not unreasonable since a major portion of the Qa region has been shown to be deleted in $H\text{-}2^k$ strains (O'Neill, 1986). In any case, the characterization of recombinant strains with this probe was straight forward: 4.0-kb indicated a B10.D2 origin while lack of the 4.0-kb band demonstrated MA or B10.K origin. The RFLPs for four additional probes (50.21, 36.21, 22.11 and 12.21) are listed in Table 2. These probes have previously, been used to detect RFLPs among inbred strain of different MHC haplotypes (Winoto *et al.*, 1983).

Table 2. Restriction Fragment Length Polymorphisms (RFLPs) for Parental and Qa/Tla Recombinant Strains

	PROBE (ENZYME)			
STRAIN	50.21 (Kpn I) D Region	36.21 (Hind III) Qa Region	22.11 (Hind III) Tla Region	12.21 (Eco RI) Tla Region
PARENTAL:				
B10.D2	10.5 kb	8.8 kb	3.4 kb	2.1 kb
MA	5.2 kb	10.0 kb	-	MB
B10.K	5.2 kb	10.0 kb	-	MB
B10.G	10.5 kb	*	-	2.0 kb
RECOMBINANT:				
MA.R1	10.5 kb	8.8 kb	3.4 kb	2.1 kb
MA.R3	10.5 kb	10.0 kb	-	MB
MA.R4	10.5 kb	8.8 kb	-	MB
B10.MR1	5.2 kb	10.0 kb	3.4 kb	2.1 kb
B10.MR2	5.2 kb	10.0 kb	-	MB
B10.KR1	5.2 kb	10.0 kb	3.4 kb	2.1 kb
B10.KR3	5.2 kb	10.0 kb	3.4 kb	2.1 kb
B10.DR2	10.5 kb	8.8 kb	-	MB
B10.DR3	10.5 kb	8.8 kb	-	MB
B10.GR1	5.2 kb	10.0 kb	-	2.0 kb

* Not 8.8 or 10.0 kb MB = multiple bands
(-) = no band

Table 3 represents a summary of the 15 Qa/Tla region recombinant strains developed at Rutgers. The traits listed in this chart consist of serological markers (D, L, Qa-2 and Tla), RFLPs detected by DNA probes (50.21, 46.21, 36.21, pTLA.5, 22.11 and 12.21) as well as isozyme loci. These traits have been arranged left to right to reflect a consistent map order. To make this table easier to interpret, the chromosomal origin (MA, K, D2, G) of each marker has been indicated rather than the actual phenotype. Points of crossing over are indicated by the vertical lines. The last recombinant strain on this list, B10.GR1, carries a crossover from a different MHC haplotype combination (B10.K x B10.G) than was used for the fourteen previous strains. Many of the RFLPs that are characteristic of strains B10.G ($H-2^q$) are distinctly different from the other strains used in this study (see Table 2 and Figure 3).

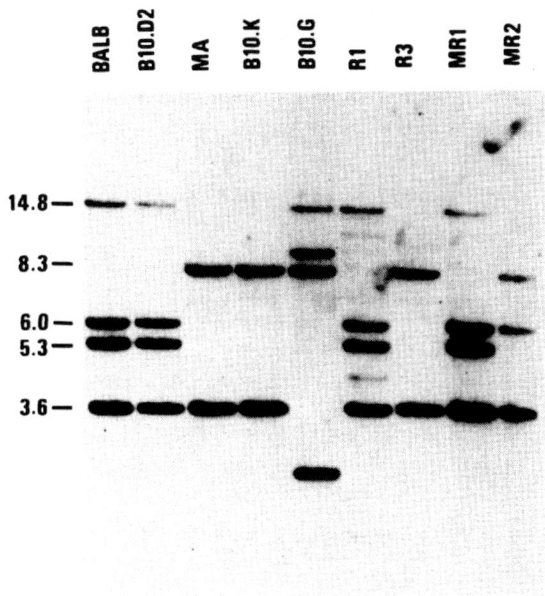

Figure 3. Southern blot analysis for probe pTLA.5 using EcoRI.

DNA probe pTLA.5 is particularly useful for characterizing the Tla region of our recombinant strains. This probe was produced by Douglass Fisher at the California Institute of Technology from the 3' end (including the transmembrane and cytoplasmic exons) of the Tla gene expressed in strain BALB/c. In Southern blots using genomic DNA, pTLA.5 hybridizes with four genes in strains BALB/c and with two genes in strain B6 (Fisher et al., 1985). The basis of this difference appears to be a large duplication present in BALB/c but absent in strain B6 (Fisher et al., 1985; Weiss et al., 1984). In our work, we have identified four distinct bands (14.8, 6.0, 5.3 and 3.6-kb) on Southern blots with B10.D2 and BALB/c DNA digested with EcoRI and two bands with strains MA and B10.K (8.3 and 3.6-kb). These patterns which clearly distinguish between the parental haplotypes are illustrated in Figure 3. Strain B10.G which is a parental haplotype for one of our recombinants has a four band pattern which is distinctly

Table 3. Summary of recombinant strains*

Strain	D			Qa			TL				Isozymes	
	H-2D	50.21	H-2L	46.21	Qa-2	36.21	Tla**	22.11	12.21	Tl**	Pgk-2	Ce-2
MA.R1	D2	D2	D2	D2	D2	D2	D2	D2	D2	D2	MA	MA
MA.R2	D2	(D2)	D2	(D2)	D2	D2	D2	D2	D2	D2	D2	MA
MA.R3	D2	D2	D2	MA	MA	MA	MA	MA	MA	MA	MA	MA
MA.R4	D2	D2	D2	D2	D2	D2	MA	MA	MA	MA	MA	MA
MA.R5	MA	(MA)	(MA)	MA	(MA)	MA	MA	MA	MA	MA	MA	D2
B10.MR1	MA	MA	MA	MA	MA	MA	D2	D2	D2	D2	D2	D2
B10.MR2	MA	MA	(MA)	MA	(MA)	MA	MA	MA	MA	D2	D2	D2
B10.MR3	MA	(MA)	(MA)	(MA)	(MA)	MA	(MA)	(MA)	(MA)	(MA)	MA	D2
B10.KR1	K	K	K	K	K	K	D2	D2	D2	D2	D2	D2
B10.DR1	D2	D2	(D2)	(D2)	(D2)	(D2)	D2	D2	D2	D2	D2	K
B10.KR2	K	(K)	(K)	(K)	(K)	K	K	K	K	K	K	D2
B10.KR3	K	K	(K)	K	(K)	K	D2	D2	D2	D2	D2	D2
B10.DR2	D2	D2	(D2)	D2	(D2)	D2	K	K	K	K	K	K
B10.DR3	D2	D2	(D2)	D2	(D2)	D2	K	K	K	K	K	K
B10.GR1	K	K	(K)	K	(K)	K	G	G	G	G	G	G

*Vertical line indicates crossover point. Chromosomal orgins: D2=B10.D2, MA=MA/MyJ, K=B10.K, G=B10.G
**Detected by pTLA.5. Some strains tested for the Tla serologically. ( ) = assumed not yet tested.

different from the four band pattern in B10.D2. Thus, the pTLA.5 probe can be used to type recombinant strains for Tla region genotype. Moreover, a change in the number of bands, the size of individual bands, or the combination of bands observed would be suggestive in intra-Tla region recombination. All but one of the recombinant strains (B10.MR2) have the expected four or two band pattern. The two and four band patterns seen in the parental strains in Figure 3 are very similar or identical to the patterns previously reported by Obata *et al.*, 1985.

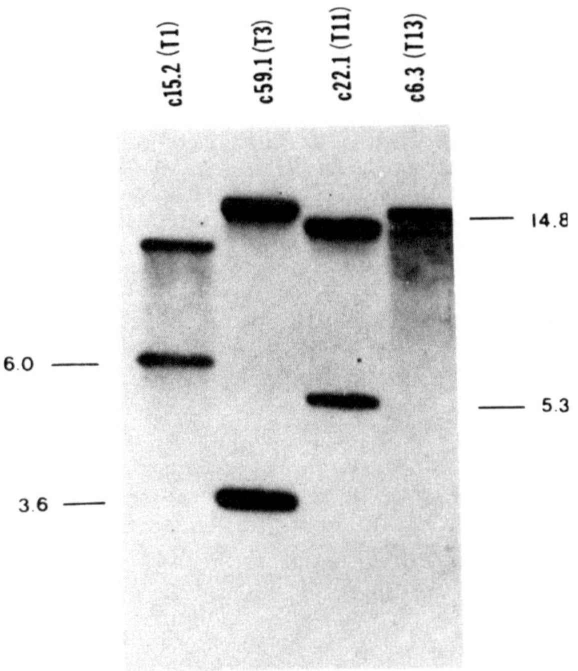

Figure 4. Clone blot of four class I BALB/c cosmids after digestion with EcoRI using probe pTLA.5.

In contrast to the patterns seen in most of the recombinant strains, B10.MR2 always gives a three-band pattern in Southern blots with pTLA.5 (see the last lane in Figure 3). Furthermore, the sizes of the EcoRI restriction fragments (8.3, 6.0 and 3.6-kb) indicate a contribution from both parental chromosomes (8.3-kb from MA, 6.0-kb from B10.D2, and 3.6-kb from both MA and B10.D2). Since this recombinant carries a new arrangement of Tla region genes, it was important to assign each of the bands seen on the Southern blot to a specific gene. Previous data indicated that pTLA.5 hybridizes with the T1, T3, T11, and T13 genes in BALB/c (Fisher *et al.*, 1985). Assignment of these genes to the bands seen in Figure 3 was accomplished by Southern blot analysis of the BALB/c cosmids that contain the appropriate target genes. These cosmids each contain one gene located within an EcoRI fragment that does not extend into the vector sequence. The autoradiograph from this hybridization analysis is illustrated in Figure 4. Since the B10.D2 chromosome appears to be identical to BALB/c, these gene assignments can be extended to the B10.D2 parental chromosome used in this study.

Table 4 summarizes the gene assignments for the two parental strains (B10.D2 and MA) and the B10.MR2 recombinant. The gene assignments for strain MA are based, in part, on the analysis of another *Tla*^{b} strain, C57BL/6 (Weiss *et al*., 1984; Pontarotti *et al*, 1986). An examination of Table 4 reveals that the recombinant B10.MR2 carries the *T1* genes from both MA (8.3-kb) and B10.D2 (6.0-kb). Further, a single band at 3.6-kb of greater intensity than the two larger bands suggests that the recombinant also carries the *T3* genes of both MA and B10.D2. Importantly, the two genes associated with cosmid cluster A (*T11* and *T13*) in the B10.D2 chromosome are missing in the recombinant. A similar analysis of B10.MR2 and the two parental strains with DNAs digested with BamHI and probed with pTLA.5 also revealed a unique Southern blot profile for the recombinant chromosome. This analysis with BamHI was fully consistent with the analysis done with EcoRI.

The most reasonable explanation for the unusual combination of genes in the B10.MR2 recombinant is unequal crossing over. Figure 5 represents a possible model for the unequal recombination event which is consistent with the data using pTLA.5 and other probes. Although this may not be the only model possible, it would seem that any other model would also need to invoke unequal crossing over. This model is based on the assumption that the *Tla* gene cluster of strain MA (carrying *T1* and *T3*) paired with *Tla* cluster B of the B10.D2 chromosome (carrying *T11* and *T13*) during meiosis rather than the more homologous cluster A. This "mispairing" is not unreasonable since *Tla* gene clusters A and B show considerable homology (Fisher *et al*., 1985; Pontarotti, *et al*., 1986).

Importantly, since the 14.8-kb band (which carries the expressed *Tla* gene - also designated *T13*) and the 5.3-kb band (designated as the *T11* gene) are absent in the recombinant, *Tla* cluster B must also be absent from B10.MR2. The only way both of these genes could have been excluded from the recombinant chromosome would be if *Tla* cluster B (carrying *T11* and *T13* is located to the left of (centromeric to) *Tla* cluster A (carrying *T1* through *T10*). Thus, B10.MR2 provides strong evidence for the order of the two *Tla* cosmid clusters identified bv Fisher *et al*., 1986.

Table 4. Assignment Of Genes To Fragments Seen On Southern Blots With Probe pTLA.5

STRAIN BALB/c	STRAIN MA	STRAIN B10.MR2
14.8 kb (*T13*)	-	-
-	8.3 kb (*T1*)	8.3 kb (*T1*)
6.0 kb (*T1*)	-	6.0 kb (*T1*)
5.3 kb (*T11*)	-	-
3.6 kb (*T3*)	3.6 kb (*T3*)	3.6 kb (*T3* + *T3*)

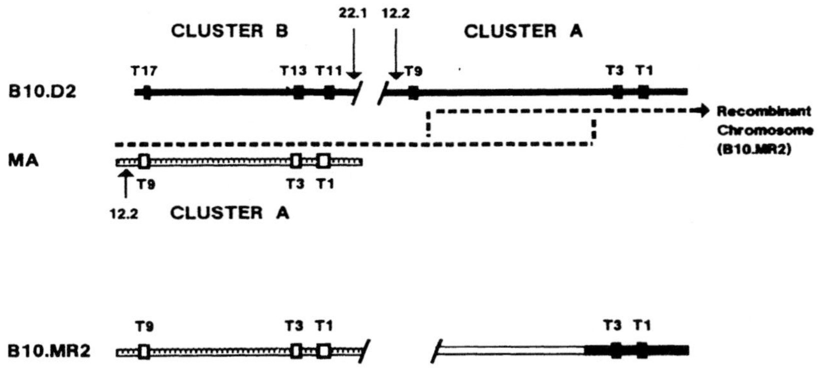

Figure 5. Model for the origin of the recombinant haplotype carried by strain B10.MR2.

DNA probes other than pTLA.5 gave data that were also consistent with the proposed model for B10.MR2 and provided additional valuable information. Two of these probes, 12.21 (a genomic sequence derived from an area flanking T10) and probe T9/T17 (a partial length cDNA derived from the T9 gene), detect RFLPs that distinguish between the haplotypes found in B10.D2 and MA. Southern blot analysis with these probes indicated that the B10.D2-specific sequences are missing in the B10.MR2 recombinant. This data indicate that only a portion of Tla gene cluster A from B10.D2 was retained in the recombinant, and that the crossover point occurred between T9 (deleted) and T3 (retained) relative to the B10.D2 chromosome. For this information to be consistent with the model, Tla gene cluster A of the B10.D2 haplotype must be oriented such that the end of the gene cluster carrying T9 and T10 are centromeric (left in the figure) relative to T1 through T3. No such constraints are necessary for the other clusters illustrated in the figure.

DISCUSSION

This study presents the molecular characterization of 15 new recombinant strains which carry crossovers associated with the Qa and Tla regions of the mouse major histocompatibility complex. Since these strains represent a variety of crossover points (with several in reciprocal directions), this series of recombinants should prove extremely valuable for genetic analysis and mapping of the distal end of the MHC. Six of the strains have recombination points which occur distal to the Tla cluster of genes and therefore can not be considered true intra-MHC recombinants. However, the utility of these recombinants has already been demonstrated in the mapping of the Mep-1 locus (controlling the activity of a kidney metalloendopeptidase) to a position between Pgk-2 and Ce-2 (Reckelhoff et al., submitted for publication). Furthermore, the recombinant carried by strain MA.R1 provides the first direct evidence for the complete separation of the Pgk-2 locus from the Tla region, and places the Pgk-2 locus distal to the Tla region.

Crossing over between the Qa and Tla regions appears to have occurred in seven of the recombinant strains. Although this is the most likely situation, it is still possible that the recombination sites in at least

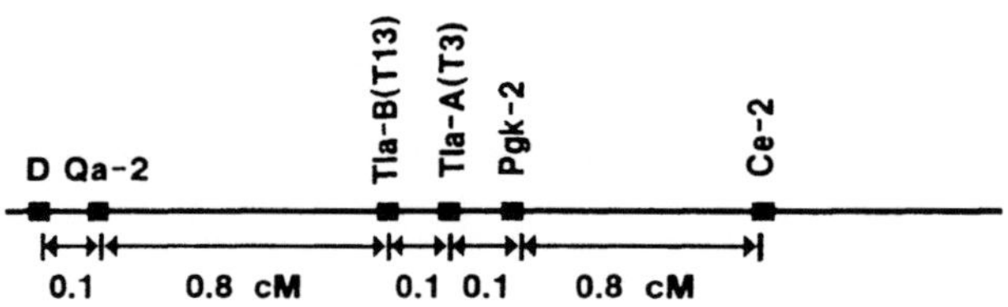

Figure 6. Recombination map of the mouse MHC distal to the *D* region.

some of these chromosomes lie within *Tla* cluster B. For example, if *Tla* clusters B and A are oriented in the manner depicted in Figure 1, it is possible that recombination may have occurred within Cluster B at a point to the left of the *T13* polymorphism detected by probe pTLA.5. Importantly, although probe 47.11 (see Figure 1) is a low copy probe, we have been unable to find a RFLP that distinguishes between the parental chromosomes at the sequence detected with this probe.

Only two of the recombinants in this series (MA.R3 and B10.MR2) can be mapped to a crossover point within the *Qa* or *Tla* clusters of genes. Thus, with the caution that our sample size may still be too small, no obvious hot spot of recombination can be demonstrated within these class I gene cluster. Although the seven recombinants that occurred between the *Qa* and *Tla* regions hold substantial future promise for the molecular characterization and mapping of crossover sites, the large gap of uncloned DNA between the *Qa* and *Tla* regions represents a formidable barrier to the present analysis of these crossover sites.

Since the 14 recombinants involving the B10.D2 chromosome were derived from carefully monitored backcrosses, it is possible to convert the information in Table 3 to a classical recombination map. This map, seen in Figure 6, represents the most precise and complete recombination map presently available for the area of the mouse MHC distal to the *D* locus. Importantly, all tentative recombinants identified in the original screening process were tested to confirm the recombinant event. This process contributed significantly to the accuracy of this map since it permitted the elimination of tentative recombinants that failed to breed true.

The most informative recombinant strain analyzed in this report is B10.MR2. This recombinant chromosome appears to have originated from unequal meiotic crossing over between the haplotypes carried by B10.D2 and MA. In this regard this recombinant is unique in that it represents a laboratory-derived case study of a mechanism that has been suggested as a major force in the evolution of the class I genes of the *Tla* and *Qa* regions, i.e., the expansion and contraction of the number of genes by duplication and deletion (Weiss *et al.*, 1984; Fisher *et al.*, 1985; Hammerling *et al.*, 1985; O'Neill, 1986; Stephan *et al.*, 1986). In addition, the analysis of this strain provides evidence that *Tla* gene cluster B (as defined by Fisher *et al.*, 1985) of the B10.D2 chromosome maps centromeric to *Tla* gene cluster A. This order of these *Tla* gene clusters is reflected on the MHC map in Figure 6.

ACKNOWLEDGEMENTS

This work was supported by grant AI14424 from the National Institutes of Health. J. Romano was supported by a predoctoral fellowship from the Charles and Johanna Busch Fund of the Bureau of Biological Research, and by a grant from the Anne and James Leathem Fund. We wish to thank S. Hunt, D. Fisher, A. Winoto, J. Kobori and L. Hood of the California Institute of Technology for providing DNA probes and BALB/c cosmids. We also wish to acknowledge M. Steinmetz for developing the BALB/c class I cosmids that made this analysis possible.

REFERENCES

Blin, N., and Stafford, D. W., 1976, A general method for isolation of high molecular weight DNA from eukaryotes, Nucleic Acids Res.; 3:2303.

Davis, R. W., Botstein, D., and Roth, J. R., 1980, "Advanced Bacterial Genetics," Cold Spring Harbor Laboratory, Cold Spring Harbor, New York.

Fisher, D. A., Hunt, S. W., and Hood, L., 1985, Structure of a gene encoding a murine thymus leukemia antigen and organization of Tla genes in the mouse, J. Exp. Med., 162:528.

Flaherty, L., 1981, Tla-region antigens, in: "The Role of the Major Histocompatibility Complex in Immunology," M. E. Dorf, ed., Garland Press, New York.

Hammerling, U., Ronne, H., Widmark, E., Servenius, B., Denaro, M., Rask, L., and Peterson, P. A., 1985, Gene duplications in the TL region of the mouse major histocompatibility complex, EMBO J., 4:1431.

Klein, J., 1979, The major histocompatibility complex of the mouse, Science, 203:516.

Klein, J., Figueroa, F., and David, C.S., 1983, H-2 haplotypes, genes and antigens: Second listing. II. The H-2 complex, Immunogenetics, 17:553.

Kobori, J. A., Strauss, E., Minard K., and Hood, L., 1986, Molecular characterization of the recombination region of six murine major histocompatibility complex (MHC) I region recombinants, Science, 234:173.

O'Neill, A. E., Reid, K., Garberi, J. C., Karl, M., and Flaherty, L., 1986, Extensive deletions in the Q region of the mouse major histocompatibility complex, Immunogenetics, 24:368.

Pontarotti, P. A., Mashimo, H., Zeff, R. A., Fisher, D. A., Hood, L., Mellor, A., Flavell, R.A., and Nathenson, S. G., 1986, Conservation and diversity in the class I genes of the major histocompatibility complex, Proc. Natl. Acad. Sci. USA, 83:1782.

Reckelhoff, J. F., Butler, P. E., Bond, J. S., Beynon, R. J., and Passmore, H. C., Mep-1 the gene regulations meprin activity, maps between Pgk-2 and Ce-2 on mouse chromosome 17, (submitted for publication).

Shalders, D. A., Flaherty, L., Hansen, T. H., and Passmore, H. C., 1983, Characterization of three new Tla region recombinant strains, Fed. Proc., 42:935.

Steinmetz, M., Winoto, A., Minard, K., and Hood, L., 1982, Clusters of genes encoding mouse transplantation antigens, Cell, 28:489.

Steinmetz, M., Stephan, D., and Fischer-Lindahl, K., 1986, Gene organization and recombinational hot spots in the murine major histocompatibility complex, Cell, 44:895.

Stephan, D., Sun, H., Fischer-Lindahl, K., Meyer, E., Hammerling, G., Hood, L., and Steinmetz, M., 1986, Organization and Evolution of D region class I genes in the mouse major histocompatibility complex, J. Exp. Med., 163:1227.

Weiss, E. H., Golden, L., Fahrner, K., Mellor, A. L., Devlin, J. J., Bullman, H., Tiddens, H., Bud, H., and Flavell, R. A., 1984, Organization and evolution of the class I gene family in the major histocompatibility complex of the C57BL/10 mouse, *Nature*, *310*:680.

Winoto, A., Steinmetz, M., and Hood, L., 1983, Genetic mapping in the major histocompatibility complex by restriction enzyme polymorphisms. Most mouse class I genes map to the *Tla* complex, *Proc. Natl. Acad. Sci. USA*, *80*:3425.

ORIGINS OF H-2 POLYMORPHISM

Felipe Figueroa[1] and Jan Klein[1,2]

[1] Max-Planck-Institut für Biologie, Abteilung Immungenetik, Correnssstr. 42, 7400 Tübingen, Federal Republic of Germany. [2] Department of Microbiology and Immunology, The University of Miami, School of Medicine, Miami, Florida 33101, USA

TWO FEATURES OF H-2 POLYMORPHISM

The two outstanding features of H-2 polymorphism are its extent and fragmentation. We still do not know how many alleles exist at appreciable frequencies in wild mouse populations, but we do know that the number is large as far as the functional loci [H-2K, H-2D(L), H-2A, and H-2E] are concerned (Klein and Figueroa 1981, 1986). We have thus far extracted 71 H-2K, 68 H-2D(L), 66 $H\text{-}2A_{\beta}$, and 53 $H\text{-}2E_{\beta}$ alleles from wild mouse populations (Klein and Figueroa 1986, Bukara et al. 1985, Nizetić et al. 1984). The polymorphism of the E_{α} locus is low, and we find no evidence for extensive polymorphism of the A_{α} locus, although the locus has been shown to vary among inbred strains (Benoist et al. 1983, Bukara et al. 1985). Among wild mice, however, many more alleles, exist. It is not at all difficult to extract new alleles simply through a random sampling of populations, but the probability of finding identical alleles in different populations is low, even when one uses reagents characterizing all of the already identified alleles. This situation is somewhat different from that encountered at the functional human HLA loci (Baur et al. 1984). Although many more HLA alleles than are presently known will undoubtedly be identified, most will probably turn out to be minor variants of the alleles already defined. The fact that identical or nearly identical HLA alleles are now being discovered even amongst different races indicates that the end of cataloging the major alleles is, if not near, at least within sight. The number of identified major Mhc alleles is already larger in the mouse than in man (Baur et al 1984, Klein 1986), and this difference is likely to grow even more with further typing. The difference can be explained by one or several of the following factors: the number of generations per unit of time, the age of the polymorphism, the rate of gene evolution, the social structure of the populations, the size of the original population from which each species arose, and the fluctuations in population size after the establishment of the two species. Whatever the reason, clearly the H-2 polymorphism is very high, even when measured by the Mhc standards, probably the highest of all the loci known, Mhc or others.

By fragmentation of the H-2 polymorphism we mean the fact that different populations occupying a single geographic area often differ dramatically in their H-2 alleles. An example of such a fragmentation is given in Figure 1, which shows the H-2 antigens found in two mouse populations from a single farm building in Giessen, West Germany. One population occupied the attic and the other the ground floor. We will refer to these two populations as "upstairs" and "downstairs," respectively. The upstairs population is characterized by the presence of antigens H-2K.m41, m90, 108, m154, and H-2D.m40, which the downstairs population lacks. The downstairs population, on the other hand, is characterized by the presence of antigens H-2K.m175, m155, H-2D.m84, m46, and m64, which the upstairs population lacks (F. Figueroa and J. Klein, unpublished data). Despite the sharing of a number of antigens, the differences between these two populations are so pronounced that by typing a mouse with three or four of the most informative reagents, it could be determined blindly and with 100% accuracy whether the mouse came from the upstairs or the downstairs population. In a building as small as this particular farmhouse, there must surely be contacts between the upstairs and the downstairs populations, yet clearly the two do not mix. The possibility of Georgina marrying Mr. Hudson is apparently also out of question in a stratified mouse population.

Although there are other mouse populations, which occupy a relatively large geographical area and are quite homogeneous (Neufeld et al. 1986, Figueroa et al. 1986), the above example is by no means unusual. We observed a similar fragmentation of the H-2 polymorphism among numerous local populations throughout most of Central Europe and the United States (Duncan et al. 1979, Figueroa et al. 1982, Götze et al. 1980, Klein 1970). The two main factors that undoubtedly contribute to this fragmentation are the rigid social structure within these population (the splintering of the population into small family units or demes) and the strongly developed territorial behaviour. The original cause of the fragmentation, however, may lie in the manner by which mice conquered the world -- on the heels of man. Travelling with man, they covered long distances in a short time and were transplanted into new territories. In those territories already occupied by mice

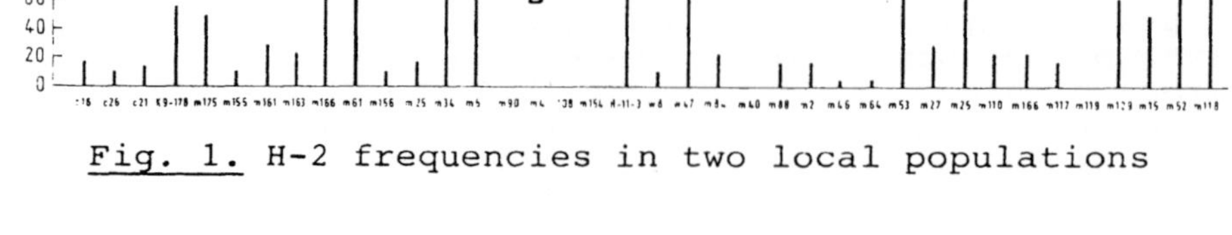

Fig. 1. H-2 frequencies in two local populations

introduced earlier, also by man, a mosaic pattern of populations developed in which unrelated populations coexist in a relatively small space without intermixing. This interpretation is supported by findings obtained in studies of other genetic systems, in particular the variation in chromosome numbers due to centromeric fusions (Adolph and Klein 1983, Tichy and Vucak 1987, Winking 1986). Both the extent of H-2 polymorphism and its fragmentation into local populations greatly complicate its analysis.

TWO VIEWS ON THE ORIGIN OF THE H-2 POLYMORPHISM

The study of H-2 polymorphism would be made easier if the multitude of alleles could be organized into a rational system reflecting the "affinities" of the individual genes, where "affinities" mean kinships based on the origin of the alleles. Ideally, all the alleles at a single locus would be organized into a genealogical tree showing their derivation from common ancestors. A slightly less ambitious grouping might organize the alleles into groups in which members of a given group are more related to one another than they are to the members of other groups. Is such a grouping of alleles at all possible?

The answer to this question depends on how one views the origin of Mhc polymorphism. The currently fashionable view is that Mhc polymorphism is generated by gene conversion, that is by a transfer of short segments of nucleotide sequences from one locus to another, often over a distance of at least 3000 kb (Weiss et al. 1983, Pease et al. 1983, Pease 1985). Gene conversion, according to this view, brings "foreign" sequences into an existing gene, thus diversifying it. If this were the explanation of Mhc polymorphism, it would be foolish to search for order among the alleles; for if the process of segmental transfer were random, it would be impossible to trace the origin of individual alleles. Each allele would be patched together from segments donated by different genes, so there would be no sense in trying to relate individual alleles to one another. If affinities were to be found, they would be the result of chance and not kinship.

We will put aside the question of whether gene conversion does or does not occur in Mhc (or other mammalian) genes; and if it does, to what degree it contributes to the generation of Mhc polymorphism. We have dealt with this question elsewhere (Klein and Figueroa 1986, Klein 1984). Suffice it to say that we find the so-called "evidence" for gene conversion unsatisfactory. The "evidence" is the observation that genes in multigene families share short segments of sequence similarity. This observation is just that -- an observation, and it needs to be to be explained. Gene conversion is one explanation, but there are other, equally, if not even more plausible explanations. To provide real evidence for gene conversion would mean setting up an experiment in which the intergenic sharing of segments, should it occur, could only be produced by the transfer of a segment from one locus to another and by no other means. To our knowledge, such an experiment has not been carried out. In its absence, the sharing of sequences should not be considered as evidence for gene conversion, and alternative explanations should be given an equal opportunity to explain the observation.

In the meantime, it is perfectly reasonable to assume that H-2 polymorphism has evolved in the same way as genes change from one species to another -- by the gradual accumulation of mutations. Assuming this, it should be possible to group the H-2 alleles according to their mutual affinities, which reflect their genealogical relationships. If such a grouping could be achieved, it could be used as an argument against gene conversion and for the mutational explanation of the generation of H-2 polymorphism. Here we shall provide the first evidence that a natural grouping of H-2 alleles is possible. However, before we do, we will consider the nature of the markers that could be used in the search for allele affinities.

MARKERS FOR ALLELIC GROUPS

The best potential markers for the genealogical classification of alleles are chromosomal mutations such as deletions and insertions. The frequency of such mutations is low, and the probability that precisely the same deletion or insertion will occur repeatedly is very low, especially when the mutation occurs in a coding sequence. In the noncoding segments of a chromosome, sequences that favor the recurrence of a particular chromosomal mutation are possible, but in a coding sequence selection against such mutations is strong, so that even if they were to occur repeatedly, chances are low that they would achieve appreciable frequencies. Hence, whenever two individuals are found in a population with identical deletions or insertions, one can be reasonably sure that their mutated alleles are related in origin. The same considerations apply to changes in the regulatory elements of a gene.

Otherwise, the grouping of alleles must rely on the structural similarity of genes or their products. At a time when both nucleotide and amino acid sequencing is still time consuming and expensive, the second best choice is serological analysis. The fact that serology can successfully predict affinities between allomorphs and alleles has been demonstrated most convincingly in the HLA system. Allomorphs found to be highly crossreactive by serologists turn out to be controlled by very similar alleles when they are sequenced (e.g., Cowan et al. 1987). However, one must, keep in mind that the sharing of antigenic determinants between allomorphs does not necessarily mean that these allomorphs are closely related. It all depends on what kind of determinants one is dealing with. The sharing of rare (private or semiprivate) determinants usually signifies an affinity between the corresponding alleles, whereas the sharing of common (public) determinants may not. In between these two categories, however, there is a continuous scale which is difficult to classify in terms of privacy versus nonprivacy. On the other hand, a combination of public determinants could be used to define affinities between alleles (Klein and Figueroa 1981).

Another marker for grouping alleles is linkage disequilibrium. If the same combination of alleles at closely linked loci occurs in two or more individuals, it is very likely that these individuals are related by descent from a common ancestor. Alleles in linkage disequilibrium that differ in minor ways from one another must clearly belong to the same genealogical group. Of course, repeated chance associations of alleles cannot be ruled out as an explanation of linkage disequilibrium.

The preamble now concluded, let us consider a few of the markers that could be used to group H-2 alleles. They are: the deletion of two codons in the A_{β} gene, the deletion of the promoter region in the E_{α} gene, unique restriction fragment length polymorphism (RFLP) in the vicinity of the C4 genes in the middle of the H-2 complex, and groups of class I and class II allomorphs defined by serological analysis.

DELETION IN THE A_{β} GENE

Sequencing of A_{β} genes derived from inbred and t strains has revealed that some of these genes have a deletion of two codons, while others do not (Estess et al. 1986, Larhammar et al 1983, Choi et al. 1983, Malissen et al 1983, Golubić et al. 1987). The deletions occur in exon 2 at positions 65 and 67, so that there is one nondeleted codon between the two deleted codons. The deletions shorten the A_{β} polypeptide by two amino acid residues without apparently affecting the functionality of the A molecules. There is no restriction endonuclease that could distinguish easily between the A_{β}^{Δ} and the A_{β}^{+} genes (we use these two designations for genes with and without the deletions, respectively), and which would therefore permit a large-scale typing of mice for the presence of the deletion. We have found, however, two A_{β}- specific monoclonal antibodies that correlate perfectly with the two types of A_{β} genes. The H-2A.m27 reacts with A_{β} chains that have the two deletions, and the H-2A.m25 antibody reacts with A_{β} chains that do not have the deletions. Although this correlation has thus far been demonstrated only for inbred and t-strain A_{β} molecules, it seems reasonable to assume that it also applies to wild mice. The generality of the correlation, however, will still have to be tested on a larger sample of A_{β} genes.

The testing of the 73 wild A_{β} allomorphs in our collection with the two antibodies has revealed a perfectly antithetical relationship between the determinants that these antibodies detect (Fig. 2). The allormorphs are either m25-positive and m27-negative or vice versa, but they are never positive or negative for both determinants at once (all strains tested were A_{β} homozygotes). This result gives further weight to the correlation of these determinants with the presence or absence of the deletions. Of the 191 wild mice that were typed with these two reagents, 44% were $m25^{+}m27^{-}$, 16% were $m25^{-}m27^{+}$, and 39% were $m25^{+}m27^{+}$; again, there were no $m25^{-}m27^{-}$ individuals in these populations. The presence or absence of these determinants behaved as an orthodox Mendelian trait present in the population in a Hardy-Weinberg equilibrium. There are thus two very large groups of A_{β} alleles, one (m27 positive) characterized by the presence and the other (m25 positive) by the absence of the deletions. All the alleles carrying the deletions can be assumed to have been derived from a common ancestral allele different from those ancestral alleles from which the A_{β} alleles not carrying the deletions were derived. (The A_{β} alleles not carrying the deletions could have been, and probably were, derived from several ancestral alleles.)

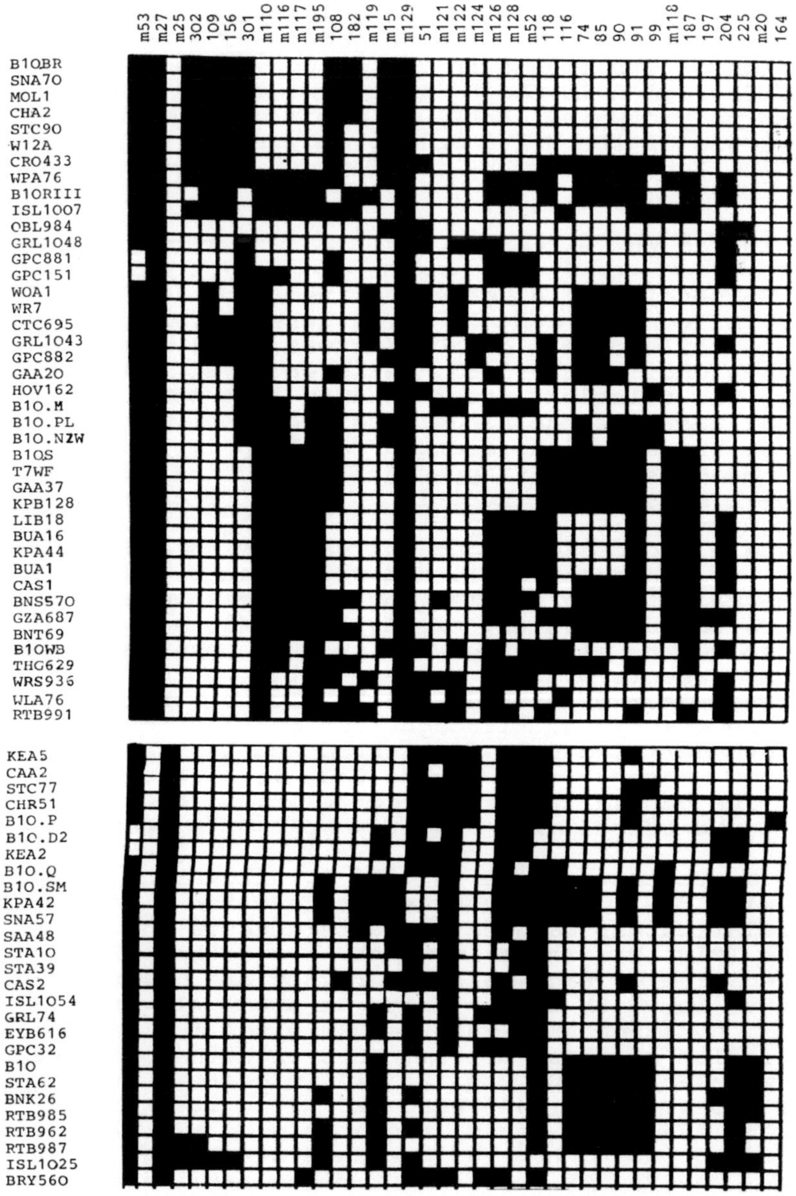

Fig. 2. Diagramatic representation of the reactivities of inbred and wild-derived strains with a panel of A_β-specific monoclonal antibodies. The antibodies are indicated at the top of the figure. Solid blocks indicate a positive reaction and blanks a negative reaction.

Table 1. Serological reactivities of monoclonal antibodies Ia.m27and Ia.m25 on species other than *Mus domesticus*

Species	Reactivity Ia.m27	Ia.m25
M. musculus	+/- *	+/- *
M. castaneus	+/-	+/-
M. spretus	+/-	+/-
M. molossinus	+	-
M. hortulanus	+	-
M. platythrix	+	-
M. cooki	+	-
Rattus norvegicus	+/-	+/-

* Some individuals are positive and others are negative.

Typing of other species and subspecies of the genus *Mus*, as well as of some other rodents (Table 1), suggests that the deletions might be present in *M. castaneus*, *M. molossinus*, *M. hortulanus*, *M. spretus*, *M. platythrix*, *M. cooki*, and the Norway rat; they are apparently absent in the mole-rat, *Spalax ehrenbergi*. In virtually all the typed species of *Mus*, the deletion is present as polymorphism, which means that some of the individuals of a given species have the A_β^Δ while others have the A_β^+ alleles. (The *M. molossinus* line carries the A_β^Δ allele, but we could not type other individuals of this species to check whether some of these carry the A_β^+ allele.)

These results are the first unequivocal demonstration of polymorphism older than the species. It appears that the A_β^Δ allele arose more than 10 million years ago before the separation of mice and rats from a common ancestor, somewhere in the Murinae branch of the evolutionary tree. It was then passed on, together with the A_β^+ allele, and hence as polymorphism, over a succession of species to the present-day respresentatives of the genus *Mus* (Fig. 3). There is no way that this polymorphism could have been generated by gene conversion, because there is no donor gene carrying the deletions, and it is extremely unlikely that the polymorphism arose independently more than once. We have argued elsewhere for the trans-species mode of generating Mhc polymorphism and have pointed out several examples that support it (Klein 1980,1982, Arden and Klein 1982, Arden et al. 1982). One could counterargue, however, that these examples represent cases either of convergent evolution or of introgression between interbreeding species such as *M. musculus* and *M. domesticus*. Since these arguments do not apply to the A_β^Δ-A_β^+ polymorphism (rats do not interbreed with mice), the conclusion must be that this polymorphism is more than 10 million years old, and that it arose long before the extant species of *Mus* had been established.

DELETION IN THE E_α GENE

Some E_α genes carry a deletion of 627 bp in the promoter region and the first exon, the consequence of which is nonexpression of these genes (Dembić et al. 1985). This deletion is

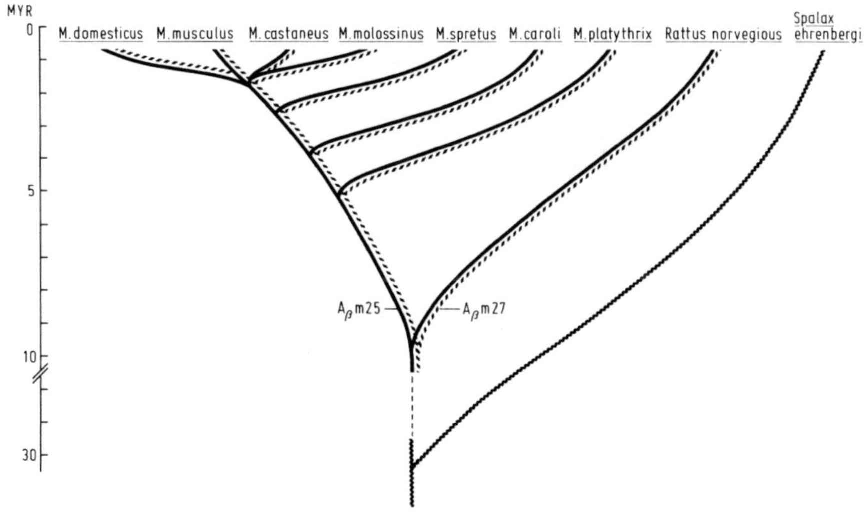

Fig. 3. Trans-species evolution of the A_β polymorphism as detected by the monoclonal antibodies Ia.m25 and Ia.m27. The defined polymorphism is estimated to be at least 10 million years old.

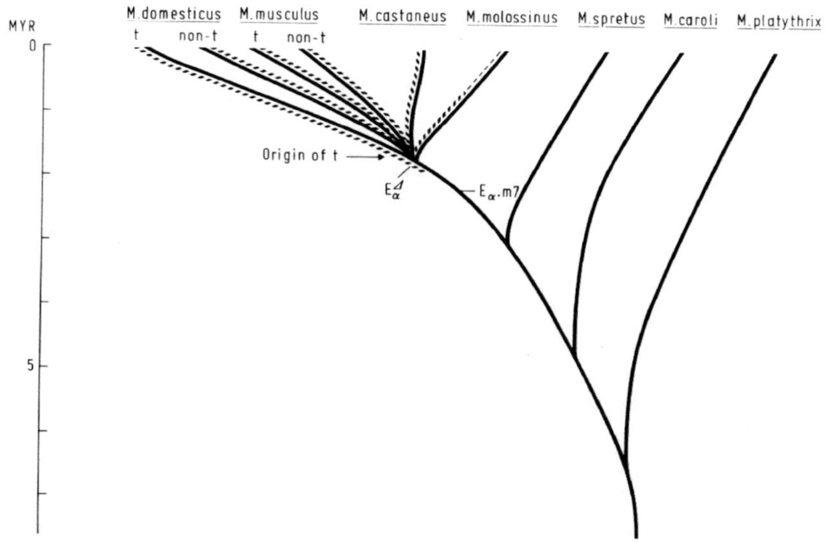

Fig. 4. Trans-species evolution of the Eα polymorphism. The 5' deletion in the Eα gene, indicated by the $E\alpha^\Delta$ symbol, is estimated to have occurred at least one million years ago. t stands for t-chromosomes.

present in 22 of the 85 E_α genes in our collection and is carried by about one half of the naturally occuring *t* haplotypes (Dembić et al. 1984). Its frequency in wild mice is estimated to be 5 - 20%. The E_α^Δ allele occurs in *M. domesticus*, *M. musculus*, and *M. castaneus* but is probably absent in all other species of the genus *Mus* (Dembić et al. 1984, F. Figueroa and J. Klein, unpublished data). Therefore, the deletion probably occured some one to two million years ago, shortly after the separation of *M. domesticus* and *M. musculus* from a common ancestor (Sage 1981). It may have occurred at the time when the *t* complex formed, or, alternatively, it may have arisen in an ancestral *t* haplotype and then been disseminated through mouse populations by the *t* complex (Fig. 4).

The E_α deletion, like the A_β deletions, divides the E_α genes into two groups, E_α^Δ and E_α^+, all the alleles in the E_α^Δ group being derived from a single ancestral gene. There is also a serological correlate to these two groups in that the determinant H-2E.m7 is present in all expressed E_α genes. The nonexpression of the E_α^Δ gene limits its value for grouping alleles, because serological typing cannot be used to determine affinities among the individual E_α^Δ alleles. Two E_α^Δ alleles, however, have been sequenced, and only very minor differences were found between them, all of which can be explained by the mutational differentiation of genes (Dembić et al. 1985, Kasahara et al. 1986). No evidence for the rapid evolution of alleles could be found in these genes, which are exempted from natural selection by virtue of their nonexpression.

RFLP IN THE VICINITY OF THE C4 GENES

The D17Tu2 probe was isolated from a cell line containing only two mouse chromosomes (17 and 18) and was mapped to the *S* region of the *H-2* complex (Kasahara et al. 1987, Figueroa et al. 1987). The probe contained the *C4* genes, in addition to unique, nonrepetative sequences recognized by restriction endonuclease Taq I. Depending on the origin of the DNA, Taq I digestion and hybridization with D17Tu2 resolves five patterns, designated *a* through *e* (Figueroa et al. 1987). The patterns found among the inbred strains correlate with the *H-2* haplotypes they carry (Table 2). All strains with *H-2* haplotypes *a*, *b*, *d*, *q*, *s*, and *u* have the D17Tu2-b pattern; strains with the *H-2*^{k} and *H-2*^{v} haplotypes have the D17Tu2-c pattern, which also occurs in *H-2* haplotypes *w1*, *w5*, *w7*, *w13*, *w16*, *w22*, and *w27* extracted from wild mice and related to *H-2*^{v}; strains with the *H-2*^{r}, *H-2*^{z} and *w8*, *w19* and *w24* haplotypes have the D17Tu2-d pattern. This clustering of *H-2* haplotypes reflects genealogical relationships among them. The haplotypes in the D17Tu2-b cluster are related in that the haplotypes *a*, *d*, and *u* carry the *H-2D*^{d} allele; the haplotypes *b*, *q*, and *s* all have the *E*-nonexpressor allele; and the class II loci of *H-2*^{b} and *H-2*^{d} are closely related in their nucleotide sequence. Among the *H-2* haplotypes in the D17Tu2-c cluster, haplotypes *v*, and *w1* are related serologically and by the fact that they both carry a rare allele at the *Neu-1* locus which maps in the middle of the *H-2* complex (Figueroa et al. 1982, Ayane et al. 1987). The *H-2* haplotypes *v*, *w1*, *w16*, *w22* and *w27* are related in that they code for antigens H-2.m153 and/ or H-2.m117, which are otherwise almost never found in other inbred or wild mice, with exception of those carrying certain *t* haplotypes (Klein

Table 2. Distribution of D17Tu2 pattern among laboratory mice: Correlation with *H-2* haplotypes.

Strain	D17Tu pattern	H-2 haplotype
A/J	b	*a*
C57L/J	b	*b*
LP/J	b	*b*
C57BL/10J	b	*b*
C57BL/6J	b	*b*
129/J	b	*b*
B6.K1	b	*b*
B6.K2	b	*b*
NZB/J	b	*d*
SEA/J	b	*d*
DBA/2J	b	*d*
BALB/cJ	b	*d*
THF	b	*d*
BUB/J	b	*q*
SWR/J	b	*q*
DBA/1J	b	*q*
SJL	b	*s*
PL/J	b	*u*
I/J	a	*j*
WB/J	a	*j*
WC/ReJ	a	*j*
BDP/J	a	*p*
P/J	a	*p*
B10.CAA2	a	*w11*
B10.GAA37	a	*w21*
B10.KPB128	a	*w19*
CE/J	c	*k*
MA/MyJ	c	*k*
RF/J	c	*k*
ST/bJ	c	*k*
AKR/J	c	*k*
C3H/HeJ	c	*k*
SM/J	c	*v*
B10.SM	c	*v*
B10.KPA42	c	*w1*
B10.BUA1	c	*w16*
B10.KEA5	c	*w5*
B10.WR7	c	*wr7*
B10.BUA16	c	*w22*
B10.STA62	c	*w27*
B10.STA10	c	*w13*
B10.STA12	c	*w13*
RIII/J	d	*r*
NZW/J	d	*z*
B10.LIB18	d	*w19*
B10.SNA70	d	*w8*
B10.KPA44	d	*w24*

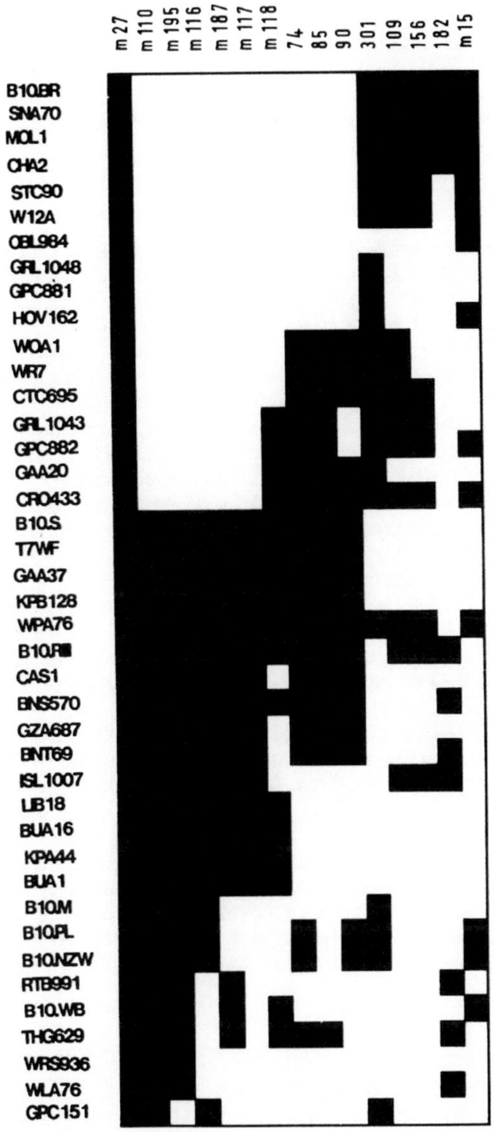

Fig. 5. Diagramatic representation of serological inclusions of the A_β.27 positive group. The antibodies are indicated at the top of the figure. Solid blocks indicate positive reactions and blanks negative reactions.

et al. 1983). The D17Tu2 polymorphism may thus help to detect linkage disequilibria between H-2 alleles in wild mice, which in turn could be used to establish genealogical relationships among these alleles. It should be possible to obtain many more such probes specific for the different regions of the H-2 complex, and with their help to trace the origins of at least some of the alleles.

SEROLOGICAL GROUPING

Figure 2 summarizes the results of serological typing in which a battery of A_β-specific monoclonal antibodies was tested against a panel of H-2 homozygous strains in our collection. Several affinities among the various A_β alleles are discernible from these data. The two largest groups are those defined by antibodies specific for determinants m25 and m27, which we have already discussed and which correlate with the presence or absence of the two small deletions within the A_β gene (note the antithetical relationship of the two determinants). As already mentioned, it is reasonable to assume that all the alleles in the m27-positive group derive from a common ancestor. This assumption is further supported by a series of inclusions observed within this group (Fig. 5). For example, all m110-positive allomorphs are within the group of m27-positive allomorphs, while virtually all m27-negative allomorphs are also m110-negative. Furthermore, all m116-positive allomorphs are within the group of m110-positive allomorphs, and so on. It is difficult to believe that these affinities are the result of chance. It seems to us far more likely that they reflect the fact that allomorphs have evolved in such a way that those showing higher mutual affinities are more closely related than the ones showing lower affinities. In Figure 6 we provide a speculative interpretation of the way in which the evolution might have occured for some of the determinants. Similar genealogical trees can be constructed for other determinants, and similar data are also available for the H-2E_β, H-2K, and H-2D(L) allomorphs. (The interpretation of the H-2K and H-2D typing data, however, is complicated by frequent crossreactivities between these two sets of allomorphs.)

GENERATION OF H-2 POLYMORPHISM

The data, only a small sample of which we could discuss here, lead us to two main conclusions concerning the origin of H-2 polymorphism. The first conclusion is that some of the polymorphism predated speciation so that not only loci, but also alleles at these loci evolve from species to species. Polymorphisms acquired by one species are often passed on to another, and then on to yet another, and so on, over periods of millions of years. This explanation removes the need for a special mechanism of rapid diversification of H-2 alleles. The assumption that H-2 alleles evolve over millions of years, allows enough time for all the multiple differences that distinguish extant alleles to accumulate. The evolution of the alleles need not be more rapid than that of the loci and may be achieved by the same mechanisms.

The second conclusion that follows from the data is that there is certain orderliness in the evolution of alleles, just as there is orderliness in the evolution of loci. Although it is still difficult -- because of the extent of H-2 polymorphism and because of our inadequate knowledge of it -- to arrange all the present-day alleles into evolutionary trees, groups of related alleles are beginning to emerge which we are confident will eventually grow into such trees. This orderli-

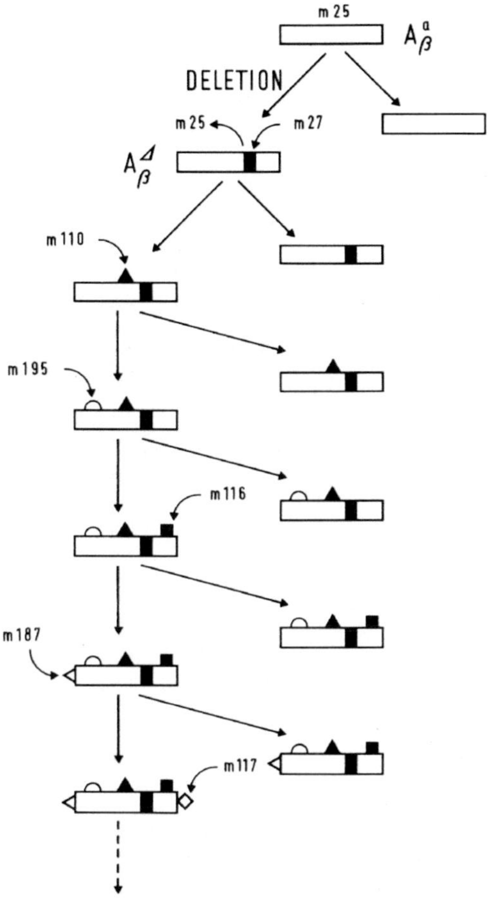

Fig. 6. Postulated mode of evolution of the A_β allomorphs (indicated by rectangles). A solid square within the rectangles indicates the deletions in the first domain of the allomorphs. Numbers refer to the different monoclonal antibodies, and small figures on the rectangles to the epitopes recognized by them.

ness, in turn, suggests to us that the main force behind the generation of H-2 polymorphism is a gradual accumulation of mutations rather than some hypothetical random scrambling process akin to gene conversion. Therefore, it does make sense to inquire into the evolution of Mhc polymorphism.

Acknowledgements: We thank Ms. Gudrun Labib and Ms. Beate Pömmerl for technical assistance in the generation of the data discussed in this communication. We also thank Ms. Jutta Gutknecht and Ms. Machell Buchmann for secretarial and editorial help. This work has been supported in part by grant No. AI 23667 from the National Institutes of Health, Bethesda, Maryland.

REFERENCES

Adolph, S. and Klein, J.: Genetic variation of wild mouse populations in southern Germany. I. Cytogenetic study. Genet. Res. Camb. 41: 117-134, 1983

Arden, B. and Klein, J.: Biochemical comparisons of major histocompatibility complex molecules from different subspecies of Mus musculus: Evidence for trans-specific evolution of alleles. Proc. Natl. Acad. Sci. USA 79: 2342-2346, 1982

Arden, B., Wakeland, E.K., and Klein, J. Minor structural variants of $H\text{-}2^k$-controlled molecules in wild mice. Immunogenetics: 16: 491-493, 1982

Ayane, M., Klein, D., Margetić, E., Figueroa, F., and Klein, J.: Neuraminidase-1 variation among mice carrying t chromosomes Immunogenetics, in press, 1987

Baur, M.P., Neugebauer, M., Deppe, H., Sigmund, M., Luton, T., Mayr, W.R., and Albert, E.D.: Population analysis on the basis of deduced haplotypes from random families. In E.D. Albert, M.P. Baur, and W.R. Mayr (eds.): Histocompatibility testing 1984, pp. 333-341, Springer-Verlag, Berlin, 1984

Benoist, C.O., Mathis, D.J., Kanter, M.R., Williams II, V.E., and McDevitt, H.O.: Regions of allelic hypervariability in the murine Aα immune response gene. Cell 34: 169-177, 1983

Bukara, M., Vincek, V., Figueroa, F., and Klein, J.: How polymorphic are class II loci of the mouse H-2 complex? Immunogenetics 21: 569-579, 1985

Choi, E., McIntyre, K., Germain, R.N., and Seidman, J.G.: Murine $I\text{-}A_\beta$ chain polymorphism: Nucleotide sequences of three allelic $I\text{-}A_\beta$ genes. Science 221: 283-286, 1983

Cowan, E.P., Jelachich, M.L., Biddison, W.E., and Coligan, J.E.: DNA Sequence of HLA-A11: Remarkable homology with HLA-A3 allows identification of residues involved in epitopes recognized by antibodies and T cells. Immunogenetics 25: 241-250, 1987

Dembić, Z., Ayane, M., Klein, J., Steinmetz, M., Benoist, C.O., and Mathis, D.: Inbred and wild mice carry identical deletions in their Mhc genes. EMBO J. 4: 127-131, 1985

Dembić, Z., Singer, P.A., and Klein, J.: E^0: a history of a mutation. EMBO J. 3: 1647-1654, 1984

Duncan, W.R., Wakeland, E.K., and Klein, J.: Histocompatibility-2 systems in wild mice. VIII. Frequencies of H-2 and Ia antigens in wild mice from Texas. Immunogenetics 9: 261-272, 1979

Estess, P., Begovich, A.B., Koo, M., Jones, P.P., and McDevitt, H.O.: Sequence analysis and structure-function correlations of murine q, k, u, s and f haplotype $I\text{-}A_\beta$ DNA clones. Proc. Natl. Acad. Sci. USA 83: 3594-3598, 1986

Figueroa, F., Kasahara, M., Tichy, H., Neufled, E., Ritte, U., and Klein, J.: Polymorphism of unique noncoding DNA sequences in wild and laboratory mice. Genetics, in press, 1987

Figueroa, F., Klein, D., Tewarson, S., and Klein, J.: Evidence for placing the Neu-1 locus within the mouse H-2 complex. J. Immunol. 129: 2089-2093, 1982

Figueroa, F., Tichy, H., Berry, R.J., and Klein, J.: Mhc polymorphism in island populations of mice. Curr. Top. in Microbiol. and Immunol. 127: 100-105, 1986

Golubić, M., Budimir, O., Schoepfer, R., Kasahara, M., Mayer, W.E., Figueroa, F., and Klein, J.: Nucleotide sequence analysis of class II genes borne by mouse _t_ chromosomes. _Genet. Res. Camb._, in press, 1987

Götze, D., Nadeau, J., Wakeland, E.K., Berry, R.J., Bonhomme, F., Egorov, I.K., Hjorth, J.P., Hoogstraal, H., Vives, J., Winking, H., and Klein J.: Histocompatibility-2 system in wild mice. X. Frequencies of _H-2_ and Ia antigens in wild mice from Europe and Africa. _J. Immunol._ _124_: 2675-2681, 1980

Kasahara, M., Figueroa, F., and Klein, J. Random cloning of genes from mouse chromosome 17. _Proc. Natl. Acad. Sci. USA_, in press, 1987

Kasahara, M., Stojlković, I., Mayer, W.E., Dembić, Z., Figueroa, F., and Klein, J.: The nucleotide sequence of the mouse _H-2_ E_{α}^{w28} gene. _Immunogenetics_ _24_: 324-327, 1986

Klein, J.: Histocompatibility-2 (_H-2_) polymorphism in wild mice. _Science_ _168_: 1362-1364, 1970

Klein, J.: Generation of diversity at MHC loci: Implications for T-cell receptor repertoires. _In_ M. Fougereau and J. Dausset (eds): _Immunology 80_, pp. 239-253, Acad. Press, London, 1980

Klein, J.: Evolution and function of the major histocompatibility complex. _In_ P. Parham and J. Strominger (eds.) _Histocompatibility Antigens: Structure and Function. Receptor and Recognition, Series B_ _14_: 223-239, Chapman and Hall Ltd, London, 1982

Klein, J.: Gene conversion in Mhc genes. _Transplant_ _38_: 327-329, 1984

Klein, J.: _Natural History of the Major Histocompatibility Complex_ Wiley, New York, 1986

Klein, J. and Figueroa, F.: Polymorphism of the mouse _H-2_ loci. _Immunol. Rev._ _60_: 23-57, 1981

Klein, J. and Figueroa, F.: Evolution of the major histocompatibility complex. _CRC Crit. Rev. Immunol._ _6_: 295-386, 1986

Klein, J., Figueroa, F., and David, C.S.: _H-2_ haplotypes, genes and antigens. Second listing. II. The _H-2_ complex. _Immunogenetics17_: 553-546, 1983

Klein, J., Tichy, H., and Figueroa, F.: On the origin of mice. _Ann. University of Chile_, in press, 1987

Larhammar, D., Hämmerling, U., Denaro, M., Lund, T., Flavell, R.A., Rask, L., and Peterson, P.A.: Structure of the murine immune response I-A_{β} locus: Sequence of the I-A_{β} gene and an adjacent β-chain second domain exon. _Cell_ _34_: 179-188, 1983

Neufeld, E., Ritte, U., Figueroa, F., and Klein, J.: Low H-2 polymorphism in some Israeli wild mouse populations. _Immunogenetics_ _24_: 374-380, 1986

Nizetić, D., Figueroa, F., and Klein, J.: Evolutionary relationships between the _t_ and _H-2_ haplotypes in the house mouse. _Immunogenetics_ _19_: 311-320, 1984

Pease, L.R., Schulze, D.H., Pfaffenbach, G.M., and Nathenson, S.G.: Spontaneous _H-2_ mutants provide evidence that a copy mechanism analogous to gene conversion generates polymorphism in the major histocompatibility complex. _Proc. Natl. Acad. Sci. USA_ _80_: 242-246, 1983

Pease, L.R.: Diversity in H-2 genes encoding antigen-presenting molecules is generated by interactions between members of the major histocompatibility complex gene family. _Transplant._ _39_: 227-231, 1985

Sage, R.D.: Wild mice. *In*: H.L. Foster, I.D. Small, and I.D. Fox (eds.): *The Mouse in Biomedical Research*, Vol. I, pp. 39-90, Academic Press, New York, 1981

Tichy, H. and Vucak, I.: Chromosomal polymorphism in the house mouse (*Mus domesticus*) of Greece and Yugoslavia. *Chromosoma* *95*: 31-36, 1987

Weiss, E.H., Mellor, A.L., Golden, L., Fahner, K., Simpson, E., Hurst, J., and Flavell, R.A.: The structure of a mutant H-2 gene suggest that the generation of polymorphism in H-2 genes may occur by gene conversion-like events. *Nature* (Lond.): *301*: 671-674, 1983

Winking, H.: Some aspects of Robertsonian karyotype variation in European wild mice. *Curr. Top. Microbiol. and Immunol.* *127*: 68-74, 1986

THE RELATIVE CONTRIBUTIONS OF GENE CONVERSION-LIKE SUBSTITUTIONS AND UNIQUE MUTATIONS TOWARD POLYMORPHISM AMONG MHC CLASS I GENES

L. R. Pease, D. E. Regnerus, B. K. Huntley and L. W. Duran

Department of Immunology, Mayo Medical School, Mayo Clinic
Rochester, MN 55905 USA

INTRODUCTION

One of the most intriguing characteristics of the murine major histocompatibility complex (MHC) is the high degree of polymorphism associated with the class I and class II loci mapping in the K, D, and I regions. This polymorphism has two components. The first is the large number of alleles identified in the wild (Klein and Figueroa, 1981). None of these alleles is present in the population at high frequencies and the total number of alleles is estimated at over 100 (Goetze et al., 1980). The second component of this extraordinary polymorphism is the extensive structural diversity distinguishing alleles. Whereas allelic variants at other loci typically differ by a single or a few amino acids (Gates et al., 1981; Perlmutter et al., 1984; Kimura and Nerbert, 1986), MHC alleles tend to differ by 5 to 10 percent of their amino acids. The amino terminal 273 amino acids, which compose the extracellular portion of four class I alleles of the H-2K locus, are shown in Figure 1. The sequences are divided into three 91 amino acid segments representing the exon structure of the K structural gene. Comparison of these sequences reveals the high degree of structural diversity which is most prominent in the first two segments encompassing amino acids 1 through 182, but also discernible in the more conserved regions of the glycoprotein represented here by amino acids 183 through 273. Diversity in the amino terminal 182 amino acids is known to influence function (see Duran and Pease, 1986 for review). Sequence variation within this segment of the H-2K glycoprotein may be influenced by natural selection. Conversely, no functional differences have been associated with diversity in the remainder of the glycoprotein. Many of these substitutions may be selectively neutral.

The structural characterization of a group of spontaneous variants derived from the H-2K^b allele defined one genetic process which may contribute to the generation of diversity in the MHC. All the characterized variants differed from the parental allele by a single cluster of amino acid substitutions (see Nathenson et al., 1986 for review). The nonrandom nature of the identified amino acid substitutions suggested a model based on a copy mechanism which substitutes sequences present in the parental H-2K gene with sequences present elsewhere in the genome (Pease et al., 1983). New variants arise at a low frequency (less than 1 per 1000 mice); each variant is presumed to represent a single genetic event. The copy-substitution model predicts a direct relationship between the structure

H-2K Consensus Sequence

```
                 10       20         30       40        50        60       70        80         90
CON     GPHSLRYF·TAVSRPGLG·PRFISVGYVDDT·FVRFDSDAENPRYEPRARWMEQ··PEYWERNTQIAKGNEQSFRVDLRT·LRYYNQSLGG
d               V         E    A       Q        D   F    P    EG     EQ  R  SD  W   S   AQ              (16)
k               H         K            Q                V     VE                I   N  A        A       (6)
t^w32           H         K       T    E                      VE            D    S     L                (7)
b               V         E  YME       E                      EG      E  K             L  G             (9)

               100        110      120       130       140       150       160       170       180
CON     SHT·QRM·GC·VGSD·RLLRGY·QYAYDGCDYIALNEDLKTWTAADMAALITKHKWEQAGDAER·RAYLEGTCVEWLRRYLKNGNATLLRT
d          F   F  D    W      Q F    R               T     RR         YY      E         EQ  E           (12.5)
k          F   Y  E    W      E                                        D                QL     P        (6.5)
t^w32      I   T  D    G      E V                                  A   R      A     S H                 (7.5)
b          I VIS  E    G      Q                                    E   L                                (5.5)

                190        200      210      220       230       240       250        260       270
CON     DSPKAHVTHHSRPEDKVTLRCWALGFTPADITLTWQLNGEELTQDMELVETRPAGDGTFQK·ASVVVPLGKEQYYTCHVYHQGLPQPLTLRW
d               Y P SQVD                       D                     Y A        N     H K               (11.5)
k               R                                                    W                                  (1.5)
t^w32                                                                W                        K         (1.5)
b                                                I                   Y                                  (1.5)
```

Fig. 1. Amino acid sequences of the amino terminal 273 residues of H-2K class I alleles. Amino acids are inferred from reported DNA sequences (Kvist et al., 1983; Arnold et al., 1984; Weiss et al., 1983a; Morita et al., 1985). Positions exhibiting no consensus are indicated •. Percent deviation from the consensus sequence is noted parenthetically.

of the variant K alleles and the hypothesized donor genes which are presumed to be located elsewhere in the genome. This model has been tested on two counts. First, the position and nature of amino acid and silent nucleotide substitutions were predicted on the basis of a representative set of donor gene sequences (Pease et al., 1983). Biochemical and molecular genetic analysis of previously uncharacterized variants supported the predictive model (Pease et al., 1983; Schulze et al., 1983a; Weiss et al., 1983b). Secondly, the prediction that sequences homologous to the variant substitutions are present elsewhere in the genome was substantiated by the identification of a Q10 sequence, identical to the substituted cluster in the bml variant, and a Q4 sequence, identical to the bm6 variant substitutions (Mellor et al., 1983 and Geliebter et al., 1986). Both Q10 and Q4 sequences were identified in the b-haplotype, the progenitor genotype of the spontaneous variants. Together these studies provided strong evidence that a genetic mechanism exists which can generate class I gene diversity.

As several investigators have proposed (Kvist et al., 1983; Weiss et al., 1983a; Lalanne et al., 1982), comparison of class I sequences such as those shown in Figure 1 suggests the possibility that the copy-substitution process represented by the spontanteous H-2K^b variants may be responsible in part for the extensive diversity distinguising alleles. This hypothesis has not been evaluated. Assessing the contribution of such events toward the observed diversity among mouse class I alleles is complicated by the unknown divergence time separating alleles and the presumption that multiple independent substitution events have accumulated in each allele since the time of their common ancestory. Nevertheless, we approached this question using a simple experimental strategy based on the following assumptions. We assumed that all variation in sequence among K-alleles arose either by unique mutation or by a nonrandom copy-substitution event. We assumed further that most donor sequences which may have given rise to the current K-alleles are still present within the MHC haplotypes common to standardly available inbred laboratory strains. By using allele specific oligonucleotides as probes, DNA sequences which distinguish alleles might be catagorized as unique or as common to potential donor genes. For the purpose of this analysis, only sequences mapping into the MHC were considered as potential donor sequences.

EXPERIMENTAL APPROACH

Definition of Allele Specific Sequences

Comparison of the DNA sequences of the H-2K b, d, and k alleles revealed extensive diversity among all three alleles (Schulze et al., 1983b; Weiss et al., 1983a; Kvist et al., 1983; Arnold et al., 1983). Three regions at which all three alleles differed from each other were selected for this study. These three segments encode amino acid positions 61 through 68, 79 through 86, and 152 through 158. Oligonucleotides 17 to 21 bases in length matching each of the allele specific sequences were synthesized to be used as probes. An oligonucleotide homologous to a highly conserved exon 4 sequence, spanning amino acids 201-207 and shared among all three H-2K alleles, was used as a positive control in the hybridization analysis.

Hybridization Studies

Oligonucleotides 17 to 21 bases in length can be used effectively as sequence specific probes (Conner et al., 1983; Schulze et al., 1983b; Wallace et al., 1979). In most cases, hybridization and washing conditions can be adjusted permitting reliable discrimination between targets exactly complementing the probe and targets differing by as few as one base from the exact sequence. The hybridization and washing procedures have been reported elsewhere (Schulze et al., 1983b). The hybridization temperature (Th) is determined by the imperical formula $Th = 2*(A+T) + 4*(C+G)$. The hybridization temperature can be systematically raised in a series of hybridization analyses to assess closeness of fit in ambiguous cases. The melting temperature of a probe is usually found within 2 to 4 degrees above the calculated Th. Tightly binding mismatched probes tend to have lower melting temperatures. However, in some circumstances we have failed to discriminate between two sequences known to differ by a single base, particularly when the mismatch is near the end of a probe.

In this analysis we have attempted to use stringent hybridization and washing conditions to maximize the homology required for hybridization. We strongly suspect that the sequences detected in these studies differ from the ideal target sequence by no more than one base and usually are exact matches. We are in the process of directly assessing this point by DNA sequence analysis of the detected targets. Sequence data for some of the target genes identified by the oligonucleotides are available and support this point of view (as described below). Furthermore, because the allelic sequences analyzed differ extensively from each other (greater than

Table 1. d Haplotype and b Haplotype Cosmids[a]

$H-2^d$ Cosmids	Genes	$H-2^b$ Cosmids	Genes
17.1	$K1K^d$	H24	K1
49.2	D^d	H21	K^b
4.1	$D_2{}^d$	B4.15	5′ flanking sequence of D^b
50.2	$D_2{}^dD_3{}^d$	B3.2	D^b
4.4	$D_4{}^d$	LSAW1	D^b
59.2	L^d	LSAW7(LSAW15)[c]	3′ flanking sequence of D^b
2.1	Q_1	B1.24	Q_1
6.3	$T_{14}T_{15}T_{16}T_{17}(T_{18})$[b]	H26	Q_2Q_3
8.1	A_f	B2.5	Q_4Q_5
19.1	$Q_{8/9}$	Bm1.2	Q_4Q_5
48.1	$T_7T_8T_9T_{10}$	B2.17	Q_6Q_7
12.2	$T_{10}T_{11}$	B4.8	Q_8Q_9
38.1	Q_6Q_7	B3.3	Q_7Q_8
59.1	T_2T_3	LSAW3	Q_{10}
15.3	T_{19}	H27	T_2T_3
65.1	Q_4Q_5	H11	$T_2T_3T_4T_5$
16.1	$D_4{}^d$	H10	$T_3T_4T_5T_6$
40.1	Q_4Q_5	LSK4	$T_6T_7T_8$
22.1	$T_{12}T_{13}T_{14}$	LSK14	$T_7T_8T_9T_{10}T_{11}$
66.1	T_1	LSK4.3	$T_{10}T_{11}T_{12}T_{13}$
64.1	Q_2	H6	$T_{12}T_{13}T_{14}$
15.1	Q_{10}		
52.3	$Q_7Q_{8/9}$		
9.1	$T_4T_6T_7$		
49.1	T_3T_4		

[a]The cosmids listed have been characterized previously (Steinmetz et al., 1982 and Weiss et al., 1984).

[b]We could not detect gene T18 on cosmid 6.3 by hybridization analysis.

[c]The map of cosmid LSAW7 (not published) is similar to the published map for cosmid LSAW15 (Steinmetz et al., 1982).

four base mismatches) the potential ambiguity resulting from the possibility that a single mismatch may not be detected would not alter our conclusions regarding the relative importance of unique and copy-substitution derived mutations.

Cosmid Class I Clone Banks

The recombinant cosmid clones used in these studies were gifts from Michael Steinmetz, Lee Hood, and Richard Flavell. The clones listed in Table 1 were described previously (Steinmetz et al., 1982; Stephan et al., 1985; and Weiss et al., 1984). Upon receipt of the cosmids, restriction maps were performed on DNA from each clone to confirm its identity using the published restriction maps. One microgram of each recombinant cosmid DNA, digested with the endonuclease Bam HI, was used to prepare Southern blots for hybridization analysis as described (Maniatis et al., 1982).

Genomic Southern Blots

The technique for using oligonucleotides in genomic Southern blot analysis was described previously (Geliebter et al., 1986).

Mice

All inbred strains tested were from the Immunogenetics colony at the Mayo Clinic and were generous gifts from Dr. Chella David. The strains tested were C57BL/10SnDV, B10.D2/SnDV, B10.S/SgDV, B10.P/SgDV, B10.WB/SnDV, B10.SM/SgDV, B10.M/SgDV, B10.BR/SnDV, B10.RVB/DV, B10.Q/SgDV, B10.RIII/SgDV.

RESULTS

Hybridization Analysis Using Recombinant Cosmid Clones

Cosmid clone banks containing 33 d-haplotype and 26 b-haplotype members of the class I multigene family were analyzed using the Southern blot technique. The H-2K alleles used as positive controls in each analysis were H-$2K^b$ from the plasmid R2.E1 (Schulze et al. 1983b), H-$2K^k$ from the plasmid 142 (unpublished) and H-$2K^d$ from the cosmid 17.1 (Steinmetz et al. 1982). Control hybridizations using probes to regions conserved (Steinmetz et al., 1982) among all characterized K-alleles as well as most murine class I genes identified each of the known class I genes in each haplotype (data not shown). Oligonucleotide probes representing allele specific coding sequences for the amino acid segments spanning amino acid positions 61 through 68 are shown in Figure 2. Typical hybridization results are shown in Figures 3 and 4. Several important points are illustrated. The sequence specific to the b-allele for this segment is shared with the several members of the class I gene family. Notably, the Q6 gene hybridizes in both the b and d haplotypes. A second gene hybridizes in each haplotype that is not present in the other, D2 in the d-haplotype and Q8 in the b-haplotype. The k-allele specific sequence is also present in a set of genes in the d-haplotype, D3, L, and Q2 (Figure 3). In contrast to the previous case, no b-haplotype gene in the cosmid bank hybridizes to the k-specific probe (Figure 4) even though a gene mapping to the Q2 position has been identified among the b-haplotype cosmids (Weiss et al., 1984). The absence of a detectable target sequence in the Q2 gene of the b-hapotype has been confirmed in separate analyses using varying temperatures of hybridization on blots containing both the d and b haplotype Q2 genes (data not shown). This finding is one of several observations made during this study (data not shown, see Table 2 for summary) suggesting considerable variation among Q region alleles. The final illustrated case is that of th d-specific

PROBES

	61							68
		**	* *	*		**		
K^b	GAG	CGG	GAG	ACA	CAG	AAA	GCC	AAG
	Glu	Arg	Glu	Thr	Gln	Lys	Ala	Lys
		**	* *	*		**		
K^d	GAG	GAG	CAG	ACA	CAG	AGA	GCC	AAG
	Glu	Glu	Gln	Thr	Gln	Arg	Ala	Lys
		**	* *	*		**		
K^k	GAG	CGG	AAC	ACG	CAG	ATC	GCC	AAG
	Glu	Arg	Asn	Thr	Gln	Ile	Ala	Lys

Fig. 2. Allele specific sequences corresponding to amino acid positions 61 through 68. The bases included in the oligonucleotide probes are underscored.

sequence. Only a single b-haplotype gene, T5, hybridized strongly (Figure 4). No T5 equivalent gene has been detected among the d-haplotype cosmids (Figure 3). All three allele specific sequences were identified in other members of the class I multigene family, and therefore, all three sequences are consistent with the copy-substitution model of class I gene diversification.

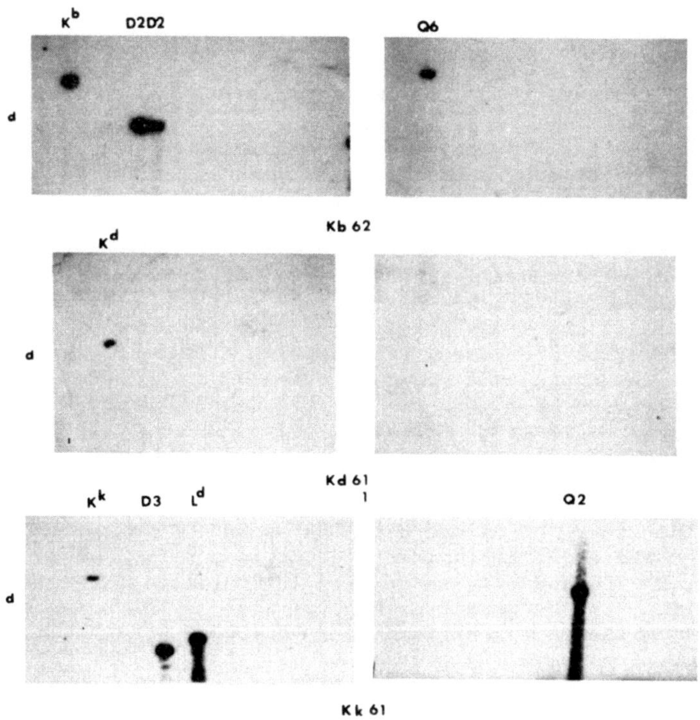

Fig. 3. Hybridization of d-haplotype class I genes with allele-specific oligonucleotides. The oligonucleotides shown in Fig. 2 were hybridized to 33 class I genes (see Table 1) under stringent hybridization and washing conditions. Only strongly hybridizing genes are identified.

Similar studies were conducted using allele specific probes derived from the gene segments encoding amino acid positions 79 through 86 and positions 152 through 158. As summarized in Table 2, in five of nine cases tested, matching sequences were detected. Four of the five matches occurred with Qa region gene even though a greater number of Tla region genes were analyzed. Note that in the case of the d-allelic sequence representative of amino acids 79-86 homologous Qa sequences are present in the b-haplotype but not in the d-haplotype. Although no exact matches were identified in either the d or b cosmid banks for four of the probes shown in Table 2, closely related genes were identified in three of these cases by lowering hybridization and washing stringency. In the case of the k-allelic sequence representing amino acids 79-86, the Kl genes in both the d and b cosmid banks hybridized upon lowering the hybridization temperature. The Kl^b gene

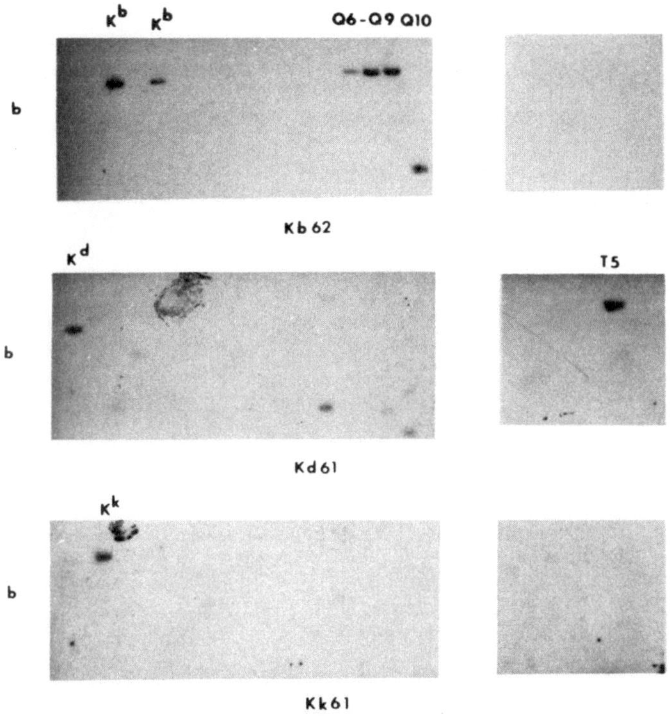

Fig. 4. Hybridization of b-haplotype class I genes with allele-specific oligonucleotides. Twenty-six b-haplotype genes were analyzed as in Fig. 3.

is known to differ from the target sequence by a single base (Weiss et al., 1983a). The d-haplotype specific sequence representing amino acid positions 152 through 158 hybridized to the L^d and Q10 genes and is only one base different from the L^d and $Q10^b$ gene sequences (Linsk et al., 1986; Mellor et al., 1984). Similarly, the Kk 152-158 sequence differs from the D^d sequence by a single base (Sher et al., 1985). Only the b allelic sequence representing amino acid positions 152 through 158 contains a sequence that is not closely matched (within one base) to sequences present in the d or b class I gene banks.

Genomic Southern Blot Analysis

Three possible explanations for the absence of a potential donor gene sequence in the cosmid clone banks for the b-allelic sequence were considered. The absence of hybridizing sequences could be attributed to incomplete gene banks used in the analysis, to the deletion of the donor sequence from the analyzed haplotypes by previous recombination events, or to the origin of the b-allelic sequence in question by unique mutation. To evaluate these possibilities the oligonucleotide probe was used to analyze a panel of standard laboratory haplotypes using a genomic Southern blot technique. The results are shown in Figure 5. The position of the 5.2 Kb gene fragment containing the relevant Kb gene sequence is indicated. Two other hybridizing sequences were also detected. A conserved band approximately 8 Kb in size is present in all haplotypes tested (and may not map to the MHC) and a single band 2.5 Kb in size was detected only in the v-haplotype. This band maps distal to the I region within the MHC because

Table 2. Summary of Hybridization Studies

Genes in Cosmid Banks Strongly Hybridizing with Probes:

Probe	d-haplotype	b-haplotype
Kb62-67	D2,Q6	Q6,Q8,Q10[a]
Kd61-67	none	T5
Kk61-67	D3,L,Q2	none
Kb79-84	T10	T10
Kd79-84	none	Q6,Q8
Kk79-84	none[b]	none
Kb152-157	none	none
Kd152-157	none[c]	none
Kk152-157	none[d]	none

[a]DNA sequence known to differ from probe by one base.

[b]Kk79-84 sequence differs from Kl^b by a single base.

[c]Kd152-157 sequence differs from L^d and Q10 by a single base.

[d]Kk152-157 sequences differ from D^d by a single base.

all the DNA preparations were prepared from congenic strains differing primarily at the MHC and the recombinant mouse line B10.RVB (K^v/D^b) does not contain the sequence in question (Data for B10.RVB not shown). The presence of these hybridizing sequences suggests that the b-allelic sequence representing amino acid positions 152 through 158 is related to a potential donor gene. Therefore, with the allowance of sporadic occasional point mutations, eight of the nine allelic sequences summarized in Table 1 are consistent with the copy-substitution hypothesis describing class I gene diversification. The ninth case involving the b-allelic sequences encoding amino acid positions 152 through 158 also appears to be closely related to a class I gene mapping in the D, Qa or Tla region of the $H\text{-}2^v$ haplotype.

DISCUSSION

The high degree of structural diversity identified among the polymorphic alleles of the H-2K gene must ultimately be explained in the context of the functional properties of the encoded H-2K glycoproteins. The allelic structures present in existing mouse populations presumably have been influenced by natural selection and represent a collection of changes that are selectively advantageous in some cases and neutral in others.

Extensive diversity among the alleles is not a compelling reason to postulate that a complex genetic mechanism must be generating diversity. Natural selection of rare variants alone can account for this observation. The hypothesis that a nonrandom copy-substitution mechanism generates MHC diversity is drawn from the unusual patterns of amino acid and silent base substitutions observed among the spontaneous variants of the $H\text{-}2K^b$ allele (Pease, 1985).

In this study we have attempted to determine whether sequence differences distinguishing polymorphic alleles, which are established in the populations, are consistent with the copy-substitution model. We reasoned

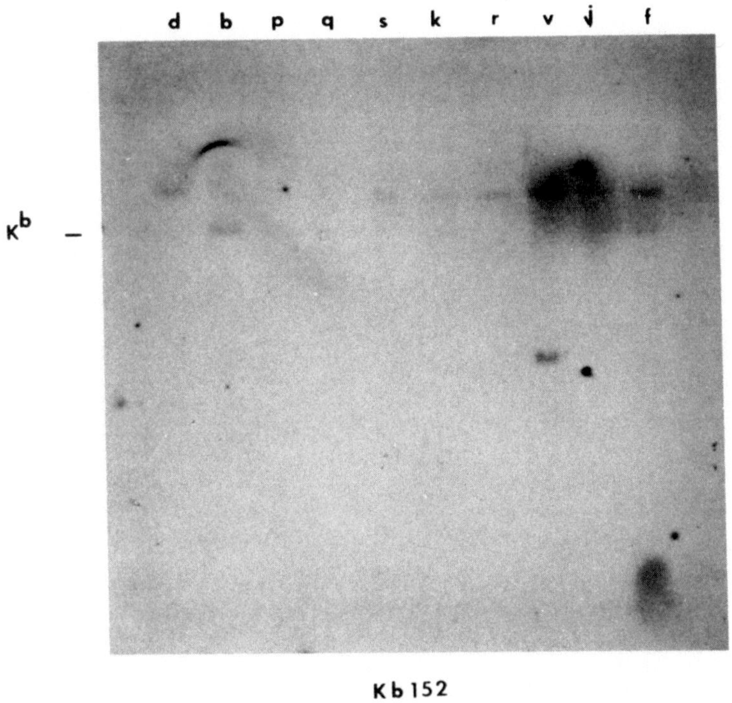

Fig. 5. Genomic Southern blot hybridized with K^b specific oligonucleotide derived from amino acid positions 152-158. All strains are B10 congenic lines differing at the MHC. Haplotypes tested are indicated. The position of the 5.2 Kb positive control band representing the K^b gene in the b-haplotype lane is labeled.

that random mutations would tend to generate unique sequences, even in the presence of natural selection. This result is the genetic consequence of the degenerate code which determines amino acid structure. By definition the copy-substitution model would tend to generate sequences shared among genes. Structural diversity is generated according to this model by the juxtaposition of novel arrangements of conserved structures within the interactive framework of the class I glycoprotein domains (see Duran and Pease, 1986 and Pease, 1987 for expanded discussion). Novel amino acid sequences apparently are not generated by the copy-substitution event because substituted regions tend to be flanked by highly conserved segments present in both the donor and acceptor genes (Mellor et al., 1983 and Geleibter et al., 1986). Therefore, the fossil record of the genetic events may be discernible in the structure of the polymorphic K-alleles. In this report, we have defined diversity segments which distinguish K-alleles and have divided them into two categories, common to other members of the class I gene family or unique. Sequences assigned to the former category would be most consistent with a nonrandom substitution mechanism. Sequences in the latter category would suggest a random mutation hypothesis. We argue that the copy-substitution model described for the spontaneous variants may be generalized and could be the major mechanism generating diversity at the H-2K locus. This conclusion is based on the observation that all nine allele-specific diversity sequences investigated appear to be closely related to other class I gene sequences mapping outside the K-locus. We do not argue that random point mutations do not generate diversity. However, random mutations do not appear to play a predominant role in determining the naturally occurring diversity which distinguishes H-2K alleles.

One consequence of our model is that the structure of non-K and presumably also non-L and -D gene sequences indirectly influences the nature of K, D, and L sequences. The sequences of the Q10 alleles tend to be closely related as reportedly are allelic sequences of gene Q7 (Mellor et al., 1984; Devlin et al., 1985). In the course of our analysis, we have uncovered several sequence differences among Qa alleles within the homologous segments representing amino acids 1 through 182. The pattern of differences suggests a history of genetic interactions resulting in the transfer of sequences among Qa genes. Diversity among Qa alleles may be more complex and extensive than suggested by the sequence analysis of the Q10 and Q7 alleles.

ACKNOLWEDGEMENTS

This works was supported in part by grants AI22420, AI00706, and CA09127-K from the National Institutes of Health. We would like to thank Ms. Theresa Lee for her contribution in preparing this manuscript.

REFERENCES

Arnold, B., Burget, H. G., Archibald, A. L., and Kvist, S., 1984, Complete nucleotide sequence of the murine H-K^k gene. Comparison of three alleles. Nucl. Acid. Res. 12:9473.

Conner, B. J., Reyes, A. A., Itakura, K., Teplitz, R. L., Morin, C., and Wallace, R. B., 1983, Detection of sickle cell β-globin allele by hybridization with synthetic oligonucleotides. Proc. Natl. Acad. Sci. (USA) 80:278.

Devlin, J., Weiss, E. H., Paulson, M. and Flavell, R. A., 1985, Duplicated gene pairs and alleles of class I genes in the Qa2 region of the murine major histocompatibility complex: a comparison. EMBO J. 4:3203.

Duran, L. W. and Pease, L. R., 1986, Relating the structure of major transplantation antigens to immune function. Transplantation 41:279.

Gates, F. T., III, Coligan, J. E. and Kindt, T. J., 1981, Complete amino acid sequence of murine β_2-microglobulin: Structural evidence for strain-related polymorphism. Proc. Natl. Acad. Sci. USA 78:554.

Geliebter, J., Zeff, R. A., Schulze, D. H., Pease, L. R., Weiss, E. H., Mellor, A. L., Flavell, R. A., and Nathenson, S. G., 1986, Interaction between K^b and Q4 gene sequences generates the K^{bm6} mutation. Molec. Cell. Biol. 6:645.

Gotze, D., Nadeau, J., Wakeland, E. K., Berry, R. J., Bonhomme, F., Egorov, I. K., Hjorth, J. P., Hoogstraal, H., Vives, J., Winking, H., and Klein, J., 1980, Histocompatibility-2 system in wild mice. X. Frequencies of H-2 and Ia antigens in wild mice from Europe and Africa. J. Immunol. 124:2675.

Kimura, S., and Nerbert, D. W., 1986, cDNA and complete amino acid sequence of mouse P2 (450): Allelic variant of mouse P3 (450) gene. Nucl. Acids Res. 14:6765.

Klein, J., and Figueroa, F., 1981, Polymorphism of the mouse H-2 loci. Immunologic Rev. 60:23.

Kvist, S., Roberts, L., and Dobberstein, B., 1983, Mouse histocompatibility genes: Structure and organization of a K^d gene. EMBO J. 2:245.

Lalanne, J. L., Bregegere, F., Delarbe, C., Abastado, J. P., Gachelin, G., and Kourilsky, P., 1982, Comparison of nucleotide sequences of mRNAs belonging to the mouse H-2 multigene family. Nucl. Acids Res. 10:1039.

Linsk, R., Vogel, J., Stauss, H., Forman, J., and Goodenow, R. S., 1986, Structure and function of three novel MHC class I antigens derived from a C3H ultraviolet-induced fibrosarcoma. J. Exp. Med. 164:794.

Maniatis, T., Fritsch, E. F., and Sambrook, J., 1982, Molecular cloning: A Laboratory Manual, Cold Spring Harbor Laboratory, Cold Spring Harbor, New York, 545 pp.

Mellor, A. L., Weiss, E. H., Ramachandvan, K., and Flavell, R. A., 1983, A potential donor gene for the bml gene conversion event in the C57BL mouse. Nature 301:792.

Mellor, A. L., Weiss, E. H., Kress, M., Jay, G., and Flavell, R. A., 1984, A nonpolymorphic gene in the murine major histocompatibility complex. Cell 36:139.

Morita, T., Delarbre, C., Kress M., Kourilsky, and Gachelin, G., 1985, An H-2K gene of the t^{w32} mutant at the T/t complex is a close parent of an $H-2K^q$ gene. Immunogenetics 21:367.

Nathenson, S. G., Geliebter, J., Pfaffenbach, G. M., and Zeff, R. A., 1986, Murine major histocompatibility complex class-I mutants: molecular analysis and structure-function implications. Ann. Rev. Immunol. 4:471.

Pease, L. R., 1985, Diversity in H-2 genes encoding antigen-presenting molecules is generated by interactions between members of the major histocompatibility complex gene family. Transplantation 39:227.

Pease, L. R., 1986, Relating diversity to function in the MHC. in: "Evolution and Vertebrate Immunity. The Antigen-Receptor and MHC Gene Families," G. Kelsoe and D. H. Schulze, eds., University of Texas Press, Austin, p. 329-347.

Pease, L. R., 1987, Relating diversity to function in the MHC. In Evolution and Vertebrate Immunity: The antigen-receptor and MHC gene families. G. Kelsoe and D. Schulze, eds. (The University of Texas Medical Branch at Galveston Press), pp. 329-347.

Pease, L. R., Schulze, D. H., Pfaffenbach, G. M., and Nathenson, S. G., 1983, Spontaneous H-2 mutants provide evidence that a copy mechanism analagous to gene conversion generates polymorphism in the major hitocompatibility complex. Proc. Natl. Acad. Sci. 80:242.

Perlmutter, R. M., Benson, B., Griffin, J. A., and Hood, L., 1985, Diversity in the germline antibody repertoire: molecular evolution of the T15 V_H gene family. J. Exp. Med. 162:1998.

Sher, B. T., Nairn, R., Coligan, J. E., and Hood, L. E., 1985, DNA sequence of the mouse $H-2D^d$ transplantation antigen gene. Proc. Natl. Acad. Sci. USA 82:1175.

Steinmetz, M., Winoto, A., Minard, K., and Hood, L., 1982, Clusters of genes encoding mouse transplantation antigens. Cell 28:489.

Stephan, D., Sun, H., Lindahl, K. F., Meyer, E., Hammerling, G., Hood, L., and Steinmetz, M., 1986, Organization and evolution of D region class I genes in the mouse major histocompatibility complex. J. Exp. Med. 163:1227.

Schulze, D. H., Pease, L. R., Geier, S. S., Reyes, A. A., Sarmiento, L. A., Wallace, R. B., and Nathenson, S. G., 1983a, Comparison of the cloned $H-2K^{bml}$ variant gene with the $H-2K^b$ gene showns a cluster of seven nucleotide differences. Proc. Natl. Acad. Sci. USA 80:2007.

Schulze, D. H., Pease, L. R., Obata, Y., Nathenson, S. G., Reyes, A. A., Ikuta, S., and Wallace, R. B., 1983b, Identification of the cloned gene for the murine transplantation antigen $H-2K^b$ by hybridization with synthetic oligonucleotides. Molec. Cell. Biol. 3:750.

Wallace, R. B., Shaffer, J., Murphy, R. F., Bonner, J., Hirose, T., and Itakura, K., 1979, Hybridization of synthetic oligodroxyribonucleotides to OX174 DNA: the effect of single base pair mismatch. Nuc. Acid Res. 6:3543.

Weiss, E., Golden, L., Zakat, R., Mellor, A., Fahrner, K., Kvist, S., and Flavell, R. A., 1983a, The DNA sequence of the H-2K^b gene: evidence for gene conversion as a mechanism for the generation of polymorphism in histocompatibility antigens. EMBO J. 2:453.

Weiss, E. R., Mellor, A., Golden, L., Fahrner, K., Simpson, E., Hurst, J., and Flavell, R. A., 1983b, The structure of a mutant H-2 gene suggests that the generation of polymorphism in H-2 genes may occur by gene conversion-like events. Nature 301:671.

Weiss, E. H., Golden, L., Fahner, K., Mellow, A. L., Devlin, J. J., Bullman, H., Tiddens, H., Bud, H., and Flavell, R. A., 1984, Organization and evolution of the class I gene family in the major histocompatibility complex of the C57BL/10 mouse. Nature 310:650.

CAN HETEROZYGOTE ADVANTAGE ACCOUNT FOR THE MAINTENANCE OF H-2 POLYMORPHISMS?

Wayne K. Potts°!, C. Jo Manning*, Ammon B. Peck°,
Marjorie Price-LaFace° and Edward K. Wakeland°

°Laboratory of Molecular Biology, Department of Pathology,
University of Florida, Gainesville, Florida 32610;
!Department of Zoology, *Department of Psychology,
University of Washington, Seattle, Washington 98195

ABSTRACT

Discovering the forces that maintain the extreme polymorphisms found at loci within the major histocompatibility complex (MHC) is critical to understanding the role of MHC gene products in nature. It is often assumed that MHC polymorphisms are maintained in natural populations by heterozygote advantage. The feasibility of this assumption is examined by applying population genetics models developed by Sewall Wright to relevant parameters for the MHC of Mus musculus (H-2). The parameters that affect the number of alleles that can be maintained (assuming random mating) are effective population size (N_e), mutation rate (μ), and the selection against homozygotes relative to heterozygotes (s). The number of alleles that can be maintained for various combinations of N_e, μ, and s are presented graphically. Even with extreme parameter values maximizing the number of alleles at equilibrium (N_e=100, $\mu=10^{-4}$, s=1) only about seven alleles can be maintained within local populations. More commonly accepted sets of parameters indicate that heterozygote advantage could only account for the maintenance of four to five alleles. An analysis of previously published data suggest that local populations carry approximately ten alleles at both the K and D loci. These results indicate that either our estimates of the relevant parameters and number of alleles actually maintained contain significant errors, or that factors other than heterozygote advantage contribute to the maintenance of H-2 polymorphisms. We briefly review a number of mechanisms other than heterozygote advantage that could play a role in the maintenance of MHC polymorphisms, including frequency dependent selection, variation in pathogen assemblages across space and time, mating preferences, and transmission distortion. We present data from a retrospective analysis of backcross and F_2 matings made during the early development of H-2 homozygous lines that show transmission distortion leading to a 52% deficiency of H-2 homozygotes (n=80, p<.002). This level of transmission distortion would contribute significantly to the maintenance of H-2 polymorphisms.

INTRODUCTION

The class I and II loci of the major histocompatibility complex (MHC) are among the most polymorphic loci in vertebrates. Some of these loci within the Mus MHC (H-2) are estimated to have over 100 alleles on a global scale (Duncan et al. 1979, Gotze et al. 1980, Klein and Figueroa 1981) and 5 to 15 alleles in local populations (Nadeau et al. 1981). Another remarkable feature of MHC polymorphisms is the degree of allelic divergence, with many alleles differing in nucleotide sequence by 5 to 10% (Benoist et al. 1983, Estess et al. 1986). Two basic questions arise concerning this unprecedented genetic diversity - what is the origin of the polymorphisms and what mechanisms maintain them in local populations. The question of origin is currently controversial. There is evidence that at least some class I and II genes experience segmental exchanges of blocks of nucleotides (Pease et al. 1983, Widera and Flavell 1984, Mengle-Gaw and McDevitt 1985). This discovery has led to the hypothesis that H-2 genes diversify rapidly via this gene conversion-like process. However, in this volume Figueroa and Klein, and Wakeland et. al. provide evidence that certain contemporary H-2 alleles diverged millions of years ago and have been maintained across subsequent speciation events. If existing polymorphisms tend to survive speciation events then rapid diversification processes are not required to explain the extensive diversification of MHC alleles. The importance of gene conversion-like events relative to normal mutational mechanisms will be elucidated as restriction fragment length polymorphisms (RFLP) and nucleotide sequences of more alleles and mutants are compared.

The question of what mechanisms maintain MHC diversity in local populations is potentially the more fundamental problem, because the answer will likely relate to the function of MHC gene products and their effect on individual fitness. It would be surprising if MHC allelic forms are found to be selectively neutral, i.e. have no effect on fitness, since these polymorphisms are known to affect immune responses. If MHC diversity is not neutral, then high mutation rates and/or some form of balancing selection must be responsible for the maintenance of MHC polymorphisms. Mean H-2 mutation rates of 4×10^{-5} (Klein 1978) are within the normal range and so are unlikely to be the major force. If balancing selection is the predominant mechanism responsible for the maintenance of MHC genetic diversity, then discovering the nature of this selection becomes a critical step in understanding the biological role of MHC genes in natural populations.

Heterozygote advantage has been the traditional answer to the question of what type of selection maintains MHC polymorphisms. This idea was proposed by Doherty and Zinkernagel (1975) after the discovery of MHC restriction. They proposed that MHC heterozygotes have effective immune responses against a wider range of pathogens and parasites than homozygotes because recognition of a specific antigen is more effective in association with some MHC allelic products than others. Thus, heterozygotes are able to recognize more antigens since they possess twice as many class I restriction elements and four times as many class II elements as homozygotes. This form of heterozygote advantage is commonly assumed to be the primary mechanism for maintaining MHC polymorphisms (Doherty and Zinkernagel 1975, Duncan et al. 1979, Treismann 1981, Zinkernagel 1979, Black and Salzano 1981, Klein 1986).

In this paper we briefly review the empirical evidence for and against heterozygote advantage at the MHC. Then we test the hypothesis that heterozygote advantage can account for the maintenance of H-2 polymorphisms, by applying population genetics models to relevant parameters for Mus. Finally, we overview some of the alternative forms of selection that may be involved in the maintenance of MHC polymorphisms and present preliminary data supporting one of these - transmission distortion leading to excess proportions of H-2 heterozygous progeny.

ARE MHC HETEROZYGOTES MORE FIT THAN HOMOZYGOTES?

The fundamental test of the heterozygote advantage hypothesis will be to compare fitnesses of MHC heterozygotes versus homozygotes in natural populations. Such evidence is currently unavailable. The following is a brief summary of indirect evidence, both for and against the hypothesis.

Restriction Element Diversity via Duplication

In as much as restriction element diversity due to duplication is analogous to that due to heterozygosity, the following line of evidence supports the heterozygote advantage hypothesis. DNA sequence homologies among class I and II genes indicate that they arose by duplication of a primordial gene (Larhammar et al. 1982, Malissen et al. 1983). Subsequent to duplication, MHC loci have diversified and specialized not only into the two classes, but within a class, specialization among loci occurs, such that recognition of a given antigen is often primarily in association with allelic products from one locus (Zinkernagel and Doherty 1974, Bubbers et al. 1977, Gomard et al. 1977, Baxevanis et al. 1980, Ishii et al. 1981). These duplication events suggest that restriction element diversity has been selectively advantageous over evolutionary time.

Similarly, the failure to express class II E restriction elements in mice has been associated with diminished immune responsiveness (Schwartz et al. 1976, Benacerraf and Dorf 1976, Solinger et al. 1979, Jones et al. 1981), another indication that restriction element diversity enhances immune responsiveness. However, the relatively high frequency (15%) of E non-expressing individuals in nature (Wakeland and Klein 1981) suggests there may be some advantage to non-expressors (see Kappler et al. 1987 for one possible advantage).

MHC Genotype and Immunological Responsiveness

Immune response genes generally map to Class II loci and non-responsiveness is recessive (Klein 1986 for review). There is also evidence of complementarity, i.e. two congenic strains that are both low responders to a specific antigen, may yield F_1 progeny that are high responders (Dorf and Benacerraf 1975, von Boehmer et al. 1977, Simpson and Gordon 1977, Matis et al. 1982), probably due to the new class II restriction elements generated by the additional combinations of alpha and beta chains present in F_1's. If non-responsiveness is both recessive and complementary, this would seem to be prima facie evidence for MHC heterozygote advantage. However, experiments demonstrating non-responsiveness generally require the use of antigens such as synthetic amino acid polymers that have extremely limited immunogenicity. It is unclear whether results from these experiments can be extrapolated to the effectiveness of the immune system in neutralizing immunogenically complex pathogens. The observation that susceptibility to specific pathogens is rarely related to specific MHC genotype (reviewed in Tiwari and Terasaki 1985, Klein 1986) suggests this extrapolation is inappropriate. If expressing additional restriction elements increases the number of pathogens to which an individual can effectively respond, then there should be a correlation between specific MHC alleles (in the homozygous condition) and susceptibility to infectious diseases. The failure to find such a correlation is perhaps the most damaging evidence to the heterozygote advantage hypothesis.

Even if MHC heterozygotes tend to have higher immune responsiveness, this may not always be beneficial due to the deleterious effects of autoimmunity and autoaggressive reactions. F_1 hybrids of inbred mice have a heightened immune response to the lymphocytic choriomeningitis virus.

Table 1. Data from one animal and two aboriginal human populations showing significant deficiencies of MHC (class I) homozygotes relative to Hardy-Weinberg expectations.

Population	MHC Homozygotes Expected	MHC Homozygotes Observed	p*	Study
Kel Kummer Taureg	10.0	1	<.005	Degos et al. 1974
South American Indians	73.4	46	<.001	Black and Salzano 1981
Rattus norvegicus	20.9	9	<.01	Shonnard et al. 1979

*Chi-square test

However, tissue damage from the heightened response results in greater mortality (Doherty and Zinkernagel 1975). Similarly, in humans, while class II DR3 and DR4 homozygotes suffer high susceptibility to insulin dependent diabetes mellitus (IDDM), DR3/DR4 heterozygotes have the highest level of susceptibility to this autoimmune disease (Henson et al. 1986).

MHC Genotype and Fitness

There have been some indirect measures of fitness in relation to MHC genotype. First, in mice, *H-2* heterozygotes have greater longevity than homozygotes (Williams et al. 1981, Yunis et al. 1984). Similar relationships have been observed in humans, although some studies have failed to show a relationship (reviewed in Tiwari and Terasaki 1986).

Second, during early attempts to inbreed rats there was failure to achieve histocompatibility after 67 generations of full sib matings. This occurred under the practice of removing the least vigorous individuals each generation (Loeb et al. 1943). These less vigorous individuals must have been MHC homozygotes because histocompatibility was achieved at normal rates (approximately 20 generations) when all individuals, independent of their vigor, were allowed to breed (Billingham and Silvers 1959). This potential case of MHC homozygotes suffering a significant reduction in vigor was never pursued.

Third, an extremely low level of MHC polymorphisms in cheetah (*Acinonyx jubatus*) populations, presumably due to recent population bottlenecks, has been associated with susceptibility to infectious disease (O'Brien et al. 1985). However, MHC monomorphic populations have been reported for house mice (Figueroa et al. 1986) suggesting MHC diversity and heterozygosity are not essential for survival in nature.

Fourth, heterozygote advantage could be responsible for the deficiency of MHC homozygotes (relative to Hardy-Weinberg expectations) in two human aboriginal populations (Degos et al. 1974, Black and Salzano 1981) and similar deficiencies revealed in an analysis of published data for wild populations of *Rattus norvegicus* (Shonnard et al. 1979) (Table 1). These deviations from Hardy-Weinberg expectations could be due to factors other than heterozygote advantage.

In summary, the evidence that MHC heterozygotes are more fit than homozygotes is on the whole positive, but the strength of the evidence is not yet compelling. The heterozygote hypothesis needs critical testing.

THE STRENGTH OF HETEROTIC SELECTION REQUIRED TO MAINTAIN *H-2* POLYMORPHISMS

The claim that MHC polymorphisms are maintained by heterozygote advantage (Bodmer 1972, Duncan et al. 1979, Treisman 1981, Klein 1986) is usually based on an uncritical extrapolation from infinite population models for two alleles, to the maintenance of multiple alleles in finite populations. This extrapolation is fraught with difficulties (Wright 1939, Kimura and Crow 1964, Lewontin et al. 1978). In this section we use finite population models to compare estimates of the actual number of alleles found in house mouse populations with estimates of the equilibrium number of alleles that theoretically could be maintained by heterozygote advantage.

Wright (1939, 1960; see also Kimura and Crow 1964, Watterson 1977) developed finite population models for the number of alleles (n) that can be maintained by heterozygote advantage. Three factors affect n - effective population size (N_e), mutation rate (μ), and the selective disadvantage of homozygotes relative to heterozygotes (s). Figure 1, derived from Wright's (1960) calculations, show the equilibrium number of alleles maintained for various combinations of these parameters. The model assumes that all heterozygotes have equal fitness as do all homozygotes. Relaxing these assumptions reduces the number of alleles maintained, causing the predicted n to be an overestimate (Wright 1969, Lewontin et al. 1978).

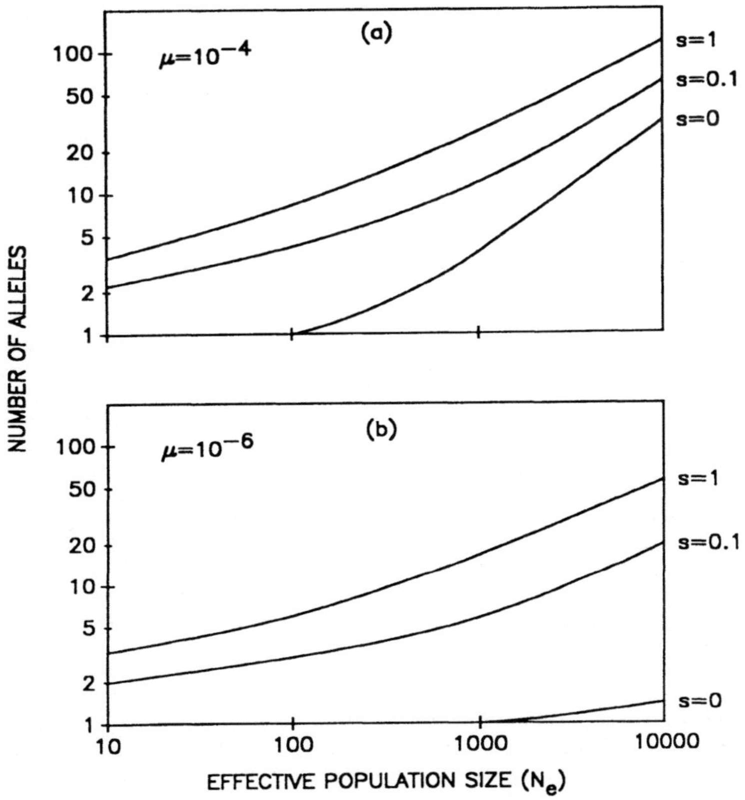

Figure 1. The equilibrium number of alleles at a heterotic locus for various values of selection (s), effective population sizes (N_e), and two mutation rates (μ) of (a) 10^{-4} and (b) 10^{-6}. These results should be treated as upper limits due to simplifying assumptions of the model that result in overestimates (see text and Table 3).

Table 2. The mean number of alleles at two H-2 loci in 13 populations of *Mus musculus* (from original data by Nadeau et al. 1981). The estimated mean number of alleles is derived by dividing the mean number of alleles identified, by their mean frequency (1 - mean frequency of blanks). This estimation assumes that the frequency distribution blanks is similar to that of the identified alleles.

Locus	Mean # of Alleles Identified	Mean Frequency of Blanks	Estimated Mean # of Alleles
K	6.5 ± 2.7	0.4 ± 0.2	10.2
D	6.2 ± 2.4	0.4 ± 0.2	9.9

Estimated ranges for these parameters in wild mice are as follows: 1) Most studies estimate the effective population size (deme size corrected for breeding sex ratios and gene flow between demes) of commensal wild house mice at less than 100 with "best" estimates centered around 10 (reviewed in Sage 1981, Berry 1981). 2) Mutation rates for H-2 loci have been determined by identification of mutants from skin graft rejections between individuals of an inbred strain and subsequent mapping of the mutants. The mean mutation rate is 4 x 10^{-5} per locus per generation (Klein 1978). 3) Unfortunately, there are not sufficient data to estimate the degree of selection against homozygotes, but it must be significantly less than 1, since approximately 10% of wild mice are homozygous at the three H-2 loci that have been studied (Duncan et al. 1979, Gotze et al. 1980).

Inspection of Figure 1a shows that even under the extreme values most favorable for the maintenance of genetic variation i.e. s=1 (homozygotes effectively lethal), N_e=100, and $\mu=10^{-4}$, only seven alleles can be maintained at equilibrium. Note that few alleles could be maintained if they were selectively neutral (s=0).

How does this compare to the number of alleles in wild mouse populations? It is difficult to get an accurate estimate of the number of alleles at H-2 loci for three reasons. 1) Sampling may occur across unknown population boundaries resulting in an overestimate of the number of alleles present. 2) Sampling will usually be incomplete. 3) Many of the alleles do not react with the available battery of antisera, producing "blanks". The total number of alleles may be estimated by assuming that identified and unidentified alleles ("blanks") have a similar frequency distribution. This assumption will usually cause an underestimate of the actual number of alleles because the battery of antisera is derived from animals sampled from wild populations, and therefore, likely to represent the more common alleles. Thus, the number of "blank" alleles will be underestimated because they are a subset of alleles with below average frequencies.

Nadaeu et al. (1981) sampled 13 house mouse populations by setting 30-50 traps in single farm buildings or fields for two consecutive nights. They demonstrated that with sample sizes of 10 to 12 mice, 90% of the existing identifiable alleles would be detected. Table 2 summarizes an analysis of these data, giving estimates of about ten for the mean number of alleles at both K and D loci. This estimated excess of two alleles above the seven expected at equilibrium (Figure 1a) is probably highly conservative because all of the assumptions used in this analysis, except one, cause either an underestimation of the number of alleles in natural populations or an overestimation of the number expected from a heterozygote advantage model (summarized in Table 3). If it is generally found that natural populations maintain more alleles than equilibrium expectations, as suggested by this analysis, then heterozygote advantage will be insufficient to account for the observed polymorphisms.

Table 3. Summary of assumptions and their effects on the comparison of the actual number of alleles in natural populations to the number expected from a heterozygote advantage model.

Model assumptions overestimating the expected number of alleles:
1. Fitness of all homozygotes is the same
2. Fitness of all heterozygotes is the same
3. Fitness of all heterozygotes > all homozygotes
4. Selection against homozygotes overestimated (s=1)
5. Effective population size overestimated (N_e=100)
6. Mutation rate overestimated ($\mu=10^{-4}$)

Factors underestimating the actual number of alleles:
1. Assumed similar frequency distributions for blanks and identified alleles
2. Sampling was incomplete

Factors overestimating the actual number of alleles:
1. Sampling may have occurred across population boundaries

Other Mechanisms that May Aid the Maintenance of H-2 Polymorphisms

Although there are numerous forces that could contribute to the maintenance of polymorphisms (Hartl 1980 for review) only a subset are likely to apply to the MHC. Six major mechanisms (other than heterozygote advantage) are likely candidates for the maintenance of polymorphism at the MHC - high mutation rates, neutrality, frequency dependent selection, variation in pathogen assemblages across space and time, mating preferences, and transmission distortion favoring MHC heterozygotes. The first two hypotheses are of doubtful significance. Mutation rates for MHC loci appear to be relatively normal (Klein 1978), HLA allelic frequencies are too uniform to conform to neutrality expectations (Hedrick and Thomson 1983, Klitz et al. 1984), and neutrality is too weak a force to explain the extent of H-2 polymorphisms in local populations of *Mus* (Figure 1).

Frequency dependent selection favoring rare alleles is a more potent force in maintaining polymorphisms than heterozygote advantage (Hedrick 1972). It is also theoretically attractive because rare and/or novel MHC alleles might enjoy an advantage in the molecular arms race against pathogens (Bodmer 1972). Most pathogen breakthroughs will be against the most common host genotypes, since these genotypes form the primary selective landscape. This will favor rare genotypes and help prevent their loss (Hamilton 1982). Documenting frequency dependent selection caused by pathogen evolution will be difficult because it will require long term studies to observe the cycles due to pathogen evolution.

If pathogen assemblages vary in space and time and specific MHC products are more effective against one subset of pathogens than others, then natural selection would favor different subsets of MHC alleles according to the current pathogen assemblage. This type of selection would contribute to the maintenance of MHC polymorphisms because different alleles would be favored in different populations (Wakeland and Nadeau 1980). The appropriate test for this hypothesis would be to characterize pathogen assemblages and see if similar assemblages are associated with similar MHC alleles. Unfortunately these data are unavailable due to our rudimentary knowledge of the pathogens for any species.

Disassortative mating according to MHC genotype would contribute to the maintenance of polymorphisms. In four of six strains tested, mice have been shown to prefer H-2 disparate mates (Yamazaki 1976, Boyce et al. 1983). The mechanism involves olfaction and the genes responsible map to the MHC.

Investigators have looked for human mating preferences based on MHC, but the evidence has generally been negative (Pollack et al. 1982, Rosenberg et al. 1983, Bischof et al. 1985).

The sixth possibility, proposed by Clarke and Kirby (1966), is transmission distortion (selective fertilization or abortion) that favors the production of MHC heterozygotes (reviewed below). It should be noted that mating preferences and transmission distortion superficially resemble heterozygote advantage in that they result in an excess proportion of heterozygotes. However, they are more effective at maintaining polymorphisms because rare alleles have an advantage in all genotypes, whereas under heterozygote advantage, rare alleles enjoy an advantage only in the heterozygous condition. In addition, heterozygote advantage carries a much higher genetic load than mating preferences or transmission distortion.

TRANSMISSION DISTORTION FAVORING MHC HETEROZYGOTES

In this final section we review the evidence for transmission distortion favoring MHC heterozygotes and present the first data from non-inbred animals in support of this hypothesis. The frequency of abortion in mammals is high, particularly in humans where it is estimated that 76% of all conceptions are spontaneously aborted (Drife 1983). In wild house mice, the mean loss of eggs and/or embryos between ovulation and live birth is 33.9% (Batten and Berry 1967). Some of this abortion is probably due to genetic abnormalities (Boue et al. 1975), but some may be due to selective abortion of particular genotypes. The following lines of evidence support the hypothesis that selective abortion of MHC homozygotes may be a general phenomenon in mammals.

Spontaneous Abortions in Humans

Recurrent abortion in humans is more frequent in couples who share MHC alleles (for reviews see Gill 1983, 1985, Beer et al. 1985, Thomas et al. 1985, Hunziker and Wegmann 1986). Similarly, Ober et al. (1983, 1984) showed in Hutterite communities that couples sharing two or more class I MHC alleles had greater median intervals between births than couples sharing one or no alleles. The most striking result came from couples who shared two or more class II alleles, who, when compared to couples sharing one or no alleles, had a smaller median completed family size (5 vs 8) and significantly higher early fetal loss (27% vs 10%).

Experimental Matings

Preferential production of MHC heterozygotes has been reported in mice (Hamilton and Hellstrom 1978) and in rats (Palm 1969, 1970, 1974, Hings and Billingham 1981, 1983; but see Hings and Billingham 1985). A particularly important aspect of these experiments is the reciprocal backcross design which provides a control for other sources of fetal wastage, especially recessive lethals. The experimental matings were between inbred A females and F_1(AxB) males. The control matings were the reciprocal - F_1(AxB) females and inbred A males. Mendelian genetics predicts equal proportions of MHC heterozygotes and homozygotes from both matings. Equal proportions were observed when the female was the F_1. But when the female was inbred, significantly more MHC heterozygotes were produced. This asymmetry in transmission distortion clearly demonstrates that recessive lethals alone are not responsible for the preferential loss of MHC homozygotes and suggests that the ability of the inbred female to respond to paternal antigens (unlike the F_1 female who recognizes all paternal antigens as self) is involved in the preferential production of heterozygotes.

These results indicate that selective abortion is not against MHC homozygotes per se, but rather, against embryos with relatively low immunogenicity. When the female is the F_1 and carries both haplotypes no distortion occurs, presumably because both heterozygous and homozygous embryos have similar histocompatibility to their mother. This immunogenic hypothesis is supported by the recent success in treating recurrent aborting couples by immunizing the female against paternal antigens, effectively making the fetus more immunogenic (Taylor and Faulk 1981, Beer et al. 1985, Mowbray et al. 1985, Takakuwa et al. 1986). If the most immunogenic fetuses are favored, then alleles that are relatively more immunogenic would be transmitted above Mendelian expectations. This may explain the preferential transmission in humans of DR3 and DR4 alleles (Vadheim et al. 1985) and A1-B8 and A2-B15-Cw3 haplotypes (Cudworth et al. 1979).

Inbreeding Depression in Litter Size

During full sib inbreeding in mice, decline in fecundity is gradual rather than abrupt and tends to decline more rapidly beginning around generation five (Bowman and Falconer 1960, Lynch 1977, Conner and Bellucci 1979, Wallace 1981). This eliminates recessive lethals as a major component of inbreeding depression in litter size, because half of the total lethality would be expressed in the first generation, causing a sharp decline in litter size. The cumulative expression of deleterious recessive alleles is the other conventional explanation of inbreeding depression, but selective abortion of MHC homozygotes could also explain the observed pattern. There are no data that distinguish between these two hypotheses.

Transmission Distortion Favoring *H-2* Heterozygotes in Wild Mice

The failure of some strain combinations to show transmission distortion favoring MHC heterozygotes (Palm 1974, Hings and Billingham 1985, Hamilton et al. 1986) may be due to the use of inbred strains. Green (1966) estimates that over 80% of all inbreeding attempts in *Mus* fail due to low litter size. Thus, lines having low levels of fetal loss are at a selective advantage during the inbreeding process. Furthermore, surviving lines show little if any decline in litter size during the entire inbreeding process (Bowman and Falconer 1960, Lynch 1977, Conner and Bellucci 1979) indicating they were initially a genetically unique subset, perhaps having abnormally low levels of selective abortion. It is unfortunate that all experiments on selective abortion have used inbred strains!

In an attempt to extend these experiments to non-inbred animals we performed a retrospective analysis of backcross and F_2 matings made during the early development of *H-2* homozygous lines from wild mice (Wakeland et al. 1987). Equal numbers of *H-2* heterozygotes and homozygotes are expected from all three types of matings. Table 4 shows that only in the first type of mating where *H-2* heterozygous and homozygous progeny differed in their relative histocompatibility to their mother, was there transmission distortion favoring *H-2* heterozygotes. In the second and third mating types all progeny are histocompatible (at *H-2*) to their mother. Progeny were *H-2* typed between 21 and 90 days of age, so differential post-natal mortality could not be eliminated as a factor. However, the significant deficiency of *H-2* homozygotes in the first mating type compared to the pooled results of the second and third mating types indicate that the observed differences were not simply due to high post-natal mortality of *H-2* homozygotes, since that would affect all mating types equally. These data are consistent with the hypothesis of transmission distortion favoring fetuses that are *H-2* disparate with their mother and they show about three times higher levels of distortion than reported in a previous study on inbred strains (Hamilton and Hellstrom 1978). We are currently repeating these matings and *H-2* typing the newborns to eliminate all effects of post-natal mortality.

Table 4. The numbers of H-2 heterozygous (Het's) and homozygous (Hom's) progeny from F_2 and backcross matings.

H-2 Genotypes of Mates ♂	♀	H-2 Genotypes of Offspring Het's	Hom's	Mendelian Expectations	Probability
a/b	a/a	54	26	1:1	.002
a/a	a/b	26	21	1:1	.46
a/b	a/b	75	69*	1:1	.62

*combined homozygote classes - a/a=38, b/b=31
Comparing the results from mating type 1 with the pooled results from mating types 2 and 3 gives $X^2=4.9$, $p<.05$.
Methods: Animals were H-2 typed using one way mixed lymphocyte responses between subjects and homozygous lines (details in Rodriguez et al. 1979).

CONCLUSIONS

The disparity between the number of alleles expected due to heterozygote advantage (Figure 1) and estimates of the number of H-2 alleles found in commensal *Mus* populations (Table 1) indicates that either there are significant errors in commonly accepted estimates of population size, H-2 mutation rates, and/or levels of H-2 polymorphisms in local populations, or, that forces other than heterozygote advantage must contribute to the maintenance of H-2 polymorphisms. A number of mechanisms other than heterozygote advantage could play a role in the maintenance of H-2 polymorphisms including frequency dependent selection, variation in pathogen assemblages across space and time, mating preferences, and transmission distortion. Data from Table 4 suggest that transmission distortion favoring fetuses histoincompatible with their mother may occur in *Mus* and could contribute to the maintenance of H-2 polymorphisms.

ACKNOWLEDGEMENTS

We thank J. Nadeau, S. Rohwer, M. Beecher, M. Hamilton, C. Muller, G. Orians, J. Felsenstein, S. Adolph, E. Thompson, R. Shaw for their contributions to this manuscript. This work was supported in part by NIH grant AI17966 to E.K.W. and partially conducted while W.K.P. was supported by NIH training grant T32CA09126.

BIBLIOGRAPHY

Batten, C.A. and R.J. Berry, 1967, Prenatal mortality in wild-caught house mice, *J. Anim. Ecol.*, 36:453-463.

Baxevanis, C.N., D. Wernet, Z.A. Nagy, P.H. Maurer, and J. Klein, 1980, Genetic control of T-cell proliferation responses to poly(glu40 ala60) and poly(glu51 lys34 tyr15): Subregion-specific inhibition of the responses with monoclonal Ia antibodies, *Immunogenet.*, 11:617-628.

Beer, A.E., A.E. Semprini, Z. Xiaoyu, and J.F. Quebbeman, 1985, Pregnancy outcome in human couples with recurrent spontaneous abortions: HLA antigen profiles; HLA antigen sharing; female serum MLR blocking factors; and paternal leukocyte immunizations, *Exp. Clin. Immunogenet.*, 2:137-153.

Benacerraf, B. and M.E. Dorf, 1976, Genetic control of specific immune responses and immune suppressions by I-region genes, *Cold Springs Harbor Symp. Quant. Biol.*, 41:465-475.

Benoist, C.O., D.J. Mathis, M.R. Kanter, V.E. Williams II, and H.O. McDevitt, 1983, Regions of allelic hypervariability in the murine A_α immune response gene, Cell, 34:169-177.
Berry, R.J., 1981, Population dynamics of the house mouse, pp. 395-425, in "Biology of the House Mouse", R.J. Berry, ed., Academic Press, N.Y.
Billingham, R.E. and W.K. Silvers, 1959, Inbred animals and tissue transplantation immunity, Transpl. Bull. (Plas. Recon. Surg.), 6:399-403.
Bischof, P., M. Jeannet, B. Bourrit, P. Vuagnat, W.L. Herrmann, and P.C. Sizonenko, 1985, Mating is random, Am. J. Reprod. Immunol. Microbiol., 7:124-126.
Black, F.L. and F.M. Salzano, 1981, Evidence for heterosis in the HLA system, Am. J. Hum. Genet., 33:894-899.
Bodmer, W.F., 1972, Evolutionary significance of the HL-A system, Nature 237:139-145.
von Boehmer, H., C.G. Fathman, and W. Haas, 1977, H-2 gene complementation in cytotoxic T-cell responses of female against male cells, Eur. J. Immunol., 7:443-447.
Boue, J., A. Boue, and P. Lazar, 1975, Retrospective and prospective epidemiological studies of 1500 karyotyped spontaneous human abortions, Teratol., 12:11-26.
Bowman, J.C. and D.S. Falconer, 1960, Inbreeding depression and heterosis of litter size in mice, Genet. Res. Camb., 1:262-274.
Boyce, E.A., G.K. Beauchamp, and K. Yamakazi, 1983, The sensory perception of genotypic polymorphism of the major histocompatibility complex and other genes: some physiological and phylogenetic implications, Hum. Immunogenet., 6:177-183.
Bubbers, J.E., K.J. Blank, H.A. Freedman, and F. Lilly, 1977, Mechanisms of the H-2 effect on viral leukemogenesis, Scand. J. Immunol., 6:533-539.
Clarke, B. and D.R.S. Kirby, 1966, Maintenance of histocompatibility polymorphisms, Nature, 211:999-1000.
Conner, J.L. and M.J. Bellucci, 1979, Natural selection resisting inbreeding depression in captive wild housemice (Mus musculus), Evol., 33:927-940.
Cudworth, A.G., E. Wolf, A.N. Gorsuch, H. Festenstein, 1979, A new look at HLA genetics with particular reference to Type-1 Diabetes, Lancet, ii:389-391.
Degos, L., J. Colombani, A. Chaventre, B. Bengston, and A. Jacquard, 1974, Selective pressure on HLA polymorphism, Nature, 249:62-63.
Doherty, P.C. and R.M. Zinkernagel, 1975, Enhanced immunological surveillance in mice heterozygous at the H-2 gene complex, Nature, 256:50-52.
Dorf, M.E. and B. Benacerraf, 1975, Complementation of H-2-linked Ir genes in the mouse, Proc. Natl. Acad. Sci., 72:3671-3675.
Drife, J.O., 1983, What proportion of pregnancies are spontaneously aborted? Brit. Med. Journal, 286:294.
Duncan, W.R., E.K. Wakeland, and J. Klein, 1979, Heterozygosity of H-2 loci in wild mice, Nature, 281:603-605.
Estess, P., A.B. Begovich, M. Koo, P.P. Jones, and H.O. McDevitt, 1986, Sequence analysis and structure-function correlation of murine q, k, u, s, and f haplotype I-A_b cDNA clones, Proc. Natl. Acad. Sci. USA, 83:3594-3598.
Figueroa, F., H. Tichy, R.J. Berry, and J. Klein, 1986, MHC polymorphism in island populations of mice, Curr. Top. Microbiol. Immunol., 127:100-105.
Gill, T.J., 1983, Immunogenetics of spontaneous abortions in humans, Transplan., 35:1-6.
Gill, T.J., 1985, Immunity and pregnancy, Crit. Rev. Immunol., 5:201-227.
Gomard, E., V. Duprez, T. Reme, M.J. Colombani, and T.P. Levy, 1977, Exclusive involvement of H-$2D^b$ or H-$2K^d$ product in the interaction between T-killer lymphocytes and syngeneic H-2^b or H-2^d viral lymphomas, J. Exp. Med., 146:909-922.
Gotze, D., J. Nadeau, E.K. Wakeland, R.J. Berry, F. Bonhomme, J.K. Egorov, J.P. Hjorth, H. Hoogstraal, J. Vives, H. Winking, and J. Klein, 1980,

Histocompatibility-2 system in wild mice. X. Frequencies of H-2 and Ia antigens in wild mice from Europe and Africa, J. Immunol., 124:2675-2681.
Green, E., 1966, Breeding systems, pp. 11-22, in "Biology of the Laboratory Mouse", 2nd ed., E.Green, ed., McGraw-Hill, N.Y.
Hamilton, B.L., A. Hamilton, and M.S. Hamilton, 1985, Maternal-fetal disparity at multiple minor histocompatibility loci affects the weight of the feto-placental unit in mice, J. Reprod. Immunol., 8:257-261.
Hamilton, M. and I. Hellstrom, 1978, Selection for histoincompatible progeny in mice, Biol. Reprod., 19:267-270.
Hamilton, W.D., 1982, Pathogens as causes of genetic diversity in their host populations, pp. 269-296, in "Population Biology of Infectious Diseases, Dahlem Konferenzen, R.M. Anderson and R.M. May, eds., Springer-Verlag, Heidelberg.
Hartl, D., 1980, "Principles of Population Genetics", Sinauer, Sunderland.
Hedrick, P.W., 1972, Maintenance of genetic variation with a frequency dependent selection model as compared to the overdominant model, Genetics, 72:771-775.
Hedrick, P.W. and G. Thomson, 1983, Evidence for balancing selection at HLA, Genet., 104:449-456.
Henson, V., N. Maclaren, W. Winter, W. Riley, J. Rotter, and E.K. Wakeland, 1986, Molecular genetics of insulin-dependent diabetes mellitus. Mol. Biol. Med., 3:129-136.
Hings, I.M. and R.E. Billingham, 1981, Splenectomy and sensitization of Fischer female rats favors histoincompatibility of R2 back-cross progeny, Transplan. Proc., 13:1253-1255.
Hings, I.M. and R.E. Billingham, 1983, Parity-induced changes in the frequency of RT1 heterozygotes in an R2 backcross, Transplan. Proc., 15:900-902.
Hings I. and R.E. Billingham, 1985, Maternal-fetal immune interactions and the maintenance of major histocompatibility complex polymorphism in the rat, J. Reprod. Immunol., 7:337-350.
Hunziker, R.D. and T.G. Wegmann, 1986, Placental immunoregulation, CRC Crit. Rev. Immunol., 6:245-285.
Ishii, N., C.N. Baxevanis, Z.A. Nagy, and J. Klein, 1981, Selection of H-2 molecules for the context of antigen recognition by T lymphocytes, Immunogenet., 14:283-292.
Jones, P., D. Murphy, and H. McDevitt, 1981, Variable synthesis and expression of E_α and $A_\varepsilon(E_\beta)$ Ia polypeptide chains in mice of different H-2 haplotypes, Immunogenet., 12:321-337.
Kappler, J.W., T. Wade, J. White, E. Kushnir, J. Bill, N. Roehm, and P. Marrack, 1987, A T cell receptor Vβ segment which imparts reactivity to a class II major histocompatibility complex product, Cell, 49:263-271.
Kimura, M. and J.F. Crow, 1964, The number of alleles that can be maintained in a finite population, Genetics, 49:725-738.
Klein, J.: H-2 mutations: Their genetics and effect on immune function. Adv. Immunol. 26:55-146, 1978
Klein, J., 1986, "Natural History of the Major Histocompatibility Complex", Wiley, N.Y.
Klein, J. and F. Figueroa, 1981, Polymorphism of the mouse H-2 loci, Immunol. Rev., 60:23-57.
Klitz, W., G. Thomson, and M.P. Baur, 1984, The nature of selection in the HLA region based on population data from the ninth workshop, pp. 330-332, in "Histocompatibility Testing 1984", E.D. Albert, M.P. Baur, and W.R. Mayr, eds., Springer-Verlag, Berlin.
Larhammar, D., L. Schenning, K. Gustaffson, K. Wiman, L. Claesson, L. Rask, and P.A. Peterson, 1982, Complete amino acid sequence of an HLA-DR antigen-like beta chain as predicted from the nucleotide sequence: similarities with immunoglobins and HLA-A, B, C antigens, Proc. Natl. Acad. Sci. USA, 79:3687-1500.
Lewontin, R.C., L. R. Ginzburg, and S.D. Tuljapurkar, 1978, Heterosis as an explanation for large amounts of genic polymorphism Genet., 88:149-170.

Loeb, L., H.D. King, and H.T. Blumenthal, 1943, Transplantation and individuality differences in inbred strains of rats, Biol. Bull., 84:1-12.
Lynch,C.B., 1977, Inbreeding effects upon animals derived from a wild population of *Mus musculus*, Evol., 31:526-537.
Malissen, M., T. Hunkapiller, L. Hood, 1983, Nucleotide sequence of a light chain gene of the mouse I-A subregion: A-beta, Science, 221:750-754.
Matis, L.S., P.P. Jones, D.B. Murphy, S.M. Hedrick, E.A. Lerner, C.A. Janeway, Jr., J.M. McNicholas, R.H. Schwartz, 1982, Immune response gene function correlates with the expression of an Ia antigen. II. A quantitative deficiency in $A_{\varepsilon}:E_{\alpha}$ complex expression causes a corresponding defect in antigen-presenting cell function, J. Exp. Med., 155:508-523.
Mengle-Gaw, L. and H.O. McDevitt, 1985, Genetics and expression of mouse Ia antigens, Ann. Rev. Immunol., 3:367-396.
Mowbray, J.F., H. Liddell, J.L. Underwood, C. Gibbings, P.W. Reginald, and R.W. Beard, 1985, Controlled trial of treatment of recurrent spontaneous abortion by immunisation with paternal cells, Lancet, i:941-943.
Nadeau, J.H., E.K. Wakeland, D. Gotze, and J. Klein, 1981, The population genetics of the H-2 polymorphism in European and North African populations of the house mouse (*Mus musculus*), Genet. Res. Camb., 37:17-31.
Ober, C., A. Martin, J. Simpson, W. Hauck, D. Amos, D. Kostyu, M. Fotino, and F. Allen, Jr., 1983, Shared HLA antigens and reproductive performance among Hutterites, Am. J. Hum. Genet., 35:994-1004.
Ober, C., W.W. Hauck, E. O'Brien, D.D. Kostyu, S. Elias, L. Cohen, R. Radvany, R. Anderson, J. Simpson, A.O. Martin, 1984, Decreased fertility among Hutterites sharing HLA-DR antigens, Amer. J. Hum. Genet., 36:130s.
O'Brien, S.J., M.E. Roelke, L. Marker, A. Newman, C.A. Winkler, D. Meltzer, L. Colly, J.F. Evermann, M. Bush, and D.E. Wildt, 1985, Genetic basis for species vulnerability in the cheetah, Science, 227:1428-1434.
Palm, J. 1969, Association of maternal genotype and excess heterozygosity for Ag-B histocompatibility antigens among male rats, Trans. Proc., 1:82-84.
Palm, J., 1970, Maternal-fetal interactions and histocompatibility antigen polymorphisms, Trans. Proc., 2:162-173.
Palm, J., 1974, Maternal-fetal histoincompatibility in rats: An escape from adversity, Can. Res., 34:2061-2065.
Pease, L.R., D.H. Schulze, G.M. Pfaffenbach, and S.G. Nathenson, 1983, Spontaneous *H-2* mutants provide evidence that a copy mechanism analogous to gene conversion generates polymorphism in the major histocompatibility complex, Proc. Natl. Acad. Sci. USA, 80:242-246.
Pollack, M.S., C.J. Wysocki, G.K. Beauchamp, D. Braun Jr., C. Callaway, and B. Dupont, 1982, Absence of *HLA* association or linkage for variations in sensitivity to odor of androstenone, Immunogenet., 15:579-589.
Rodriguez, G., G. Andersson, H. Wigzell, and A. Peck, 1979, Non-T cell nature of the naturally occurring, spleen associated suppressor cells present in the newborn mouse, Eur. J. Immunol., 9:737-746.
Rosenberg, L.T., D. Cooperman, and R. Payne, 1983, HLA and mate selection, Immunogenet., 17:89-93.
Sage, R.D., 1981, Wild mice, pp. 39-90, *in* "The Mouse in Biomedical Research", Vol.I, H.L. Foster, J.D. Small, J.G. Fox, eds., Academic, N.Y.
Schwartz, R.H., C.S. David, D.H. Sachs, and W.E. Paul, 1976, T lymphocyte-enriched murine peritoneal exudate cells III. Inhibition with anti-Ia antisera, J. Immunol., 117:531-540.
Shonnard, J.W., B.K. Davis, D.V. Cramer, S.F. Radka, and T.J. Gill III,1979, The association of immune responsiveness, mixed lymphocyte responses, and Ia antigens in natural populations of Norway rats, J. Immunol., 123:778-783.
Simpson, E. and R.D. Gordon, 1977, Responsiveness to H-Y antigen Ir gene complementation and target cells, Immunol. Rev., 35:59-75.

Solinger, A.M., M.E. Ultee, E. Margoliash, and R.H. Schwartz, 1979, T-lymphocyte response to cytochrome c. I. Demonstration of a T-cell heteroclitic proliferative response and identification of a topographic antigenic determinant on pigeon cytochrome c whose immune recognition requires two complementing major histocompatibility complex-linked immune response genes, J. Exp. Med., 150:830-848.
Takakuwa, K., K. Kanazawa, and S. Takeuchi, 1986, Production of blocking antibodies by vaccination with husband's lymphocytes in unexplained recurrent aborters: the role in successful pregnancy, Am. J. Reprod. Immunol. and Microbiol., 10:1-9.
Taylor, C. and W.P. Faulk, 1981, Prevention of recurrent abortion with leucocyte transfusions, Lancet, ii:68-70.
Thomas, M.L., J.H. Harger, D.K. Wagner, B.S. Rabin, and T.J. Gill, 1985, HLA sharing and spontaneous abortion in humans, Am. J. Obstet. Gynec., 151:1053.
Tiwari, J.L. and P.I. Terasaki, 1985, "HLA and Disease Associations", Springer-Verlag, N.Y.
Treisman, M., 1981, The significance of immunity restriction by the major histocompatibility complex, and of the occurrence of high polymorphism at MHC loci: Two hypotheses, J. Theor. Biol., 89:409-421.
Vadheim, C.M., J.I. Rotter, N.K. Maclaren, W.J. Riley, and C.E. Anderson: Selective transmission of insulin dependent diabetes genes? Pediat. Res., 19:A255.
Wakeland, E.K. and J. Klein, 1981, The polymorphism of I region encoded antigens among wild mice, Curr. Trends in Histocompatibility, 4:
Wakeland, E.K. and J.H. Nadeau, 1980, Immune responsiveness and polymorphism of the major histocompatibility complex: an interpretation, pp. 149-156, in "Strategies of Immune Regulation", E.I. Sercarz and A.J. Cunningham, eds., Academic Press, N.Y.
Wakeland, E.K., M. Price-LaFace, V. Henson, and A.B. Peck, 1987, Production of 35 H-2 homozygous strains from wild mice, Immunogenet. (in press).
Wallace, M.E., 1981, The breeding, inbreeding and management of wild mice, pp. 183-204, in "Biology of the House Mouse", R.J. Berry, ed., Academic Press, N.Y.
Watterson, G.A., 1977, Heterosis or neutrality? Genet., 85:789-814.
Widera, G. and R.A. Flavell, 1984, The nucleotide sequence of the murine I-Eβ^6 immune gene: evidence for gene conversion events in class II genes of the major histocompatibility complex, EMBO J., 3:1221-1225.
Williams, R.M., L.J. Kraus, P.T. Lavin, L.L. Steele, and E.J. Yunis, 1981, Genetics of survival in mice: localization of dominant effects to subregions of the major histocompatibility complex, pp. 247-266, in "Immunological Aspects of Ageing", E. Segre and L. Smith, eds., Marcel Dekker, N.Y.
Wright, S., 1939, The distribution of self-sterility alleles in populations, Genet., 24:538-552.
Wright, S., 1960, On the number of self-incompatibility alleles maintained in equilibrium by a given mutation rate in a population of a given size: A re-examination, Biometrics, 16:61-85.
Wright. S., 1969, "Evolution and the Genetics of Populations, Vol. 2, The Theory of Gene Frequencies", Univ. of Chicago Press, Chicago.
Yamakazi, K., E.A. Boyse, V. Mike, H.T. Thaler, B.J. Mathieson, J. Abbott, J. Boyse, Z.A. Zayas, and L. Thomas, 1976, Control of mating preferences in mice by genes in the major histocompatibility complex, J. Exp. Med., 144:1324-1335.
Yunis, E.J., A.L. Watson, R.S. Gelman, S.J. Sylvia, R. Bronson, M.E. Dorf, 1984, Traits that influence longevity in mice, Genet., 108:999-1011.
Zinkernagel, R.M., 1979, Associations between major histocompatibility antigens and susceptibility to disease, Ann. Rev. Microbiol., 33:201-213.
Zinkernagel R.M. and P.C. Doherty, 1974, Restriction of in vitro T-cell mediated cytotoxicity in lymphocytic choriomeningitis within a syngeneic or semiallogeneic system, Nature, 248:701-702.

HEMOPOIETIC HISTOCOMPATIBILITY (Hh-1) ANTIGENS: POLYMORPHISM AND MAPPING

Richard M. Rembecki[1], Michael Bennett[1], Vinay Kumar[1] and Chella S.David[2]

[1] Department of Pathology and Graduate Program in Immunology University of Texas Health Science Center at Dallas, Dallas TX, 75235

[2] Department of Immunology, Mayo Medical School, Rochester MN 55901

ABSTRACT

"Hybrid resistance" to grafts of parental strain bone marrow cells (BMC) by irradiated *H-2* heterozygous F1 hybrid mice suggested that Hh-1 antigens were inherited recessively. *H-2* homozygosity is required for optimal immunogenicity of BMC grafts. $H\text{-}2^b/H\text{-}2^d$ lymphoma cells are $Hh\text{-}1^{null}$, but variants which do not express $H\text{-}2D^d$ do express $Hh\text{-}1^b$. This suggests that *trans*-acting genes at or near *H-2D* down-regulate the expression of *Hh-1* antigens. NK cells mediate BMC graft rejection and immune response-like genes control the ability to reject BMC grafts in an Hh-1 determinant-specific manner. We have used a panel of recipient mice which reject certain strain BMC grafts in order to determine the Hh-1 phenotype of new strains of mice to be tested. When non-recombinant *H-2* types of independent origin were studied, six patterns of expression of four different Hh-1 determinants were detected. The extremely limited degree of polymorphism compared to *H-2* is interesting because NK cells do not rearrange immunoglobulin or T cell receptor genes and are expected to possess a paucity of receptor diversity. The great majority of more than 60 intra-*H-2* recombinant strain mice had *Hh-1* alleles predicted by *H-2D* or *L*. However, of the many *H-2S/D* recombinants, two strains expressed *Hh-1* alleles which did not correlate with *L*. A unique D^d/L^b recombinant, B10.RQDB, expresses the Hh-1 phenotype which is characteristic of the *d* haplotype, indicating that *Hh-1* maps to the left of *H-2L*. Since the L^b is the only *b* haplotype class I molecule at *H-2DL*, $Hh\text{-}1^b$ cannot be a class I gene. In another strain, *H-2S* is predictive of *Hh-1*. Even more interesting are several strains which express Hh-1 phenotypes different from both donor strains which generated the recombinant. We believe that these strains represent intra-*Hh-1* recombinants; furthermore, intra- *Hh-1* crossover events are not rare. Recombinants involving $H\text{-}2^f$ indicate that the structural genes for $Hh\text{-}1^f$ are linked to *H-2* and appear to map to the left of the regulatory genes (possibly centromeric of E_β). Other intra-*Hh-1* recombinants indicate that the structural genes of most haplotypes map just to the left of the regulatory genes in the *S/D* interval of *H-2*.

INTRODUCTION

Lethally irradiated mice are capable of rejecting bone marrow stem cell (BMC) grafts, and this rejection is mediated by natural killer (NK) cells which are capable of recognizing the Hemopoietic histocompatibility (Hh) antigens (Bennett, 1987). The expression of Hh antigens differs significantly from that of classical transplantation antigens. F1 hybrids between antigenically different strains codominantly express the Class I transplantation antigens of both parents, and F1s accept parental solid tissue grafts. However, F1 hybrids between strains of disparate Hh fail to express either parental Hh type. These F1 hybrids are capable of rejecting parental BMC grafts; conversely, grafts of F1 BMC are accepted by both parental strains. These observations gave rise to the term "hybrid resistance" to marrow grafts (Cudkowicz and Stimpfling, 1964).

Hh-1, the 'major' Hh antigen, is characterized as a non-codominantly inherited BMC antigen whose expression is regulated by genes which map to the *D* region of *H-2*. Early studies indicated that the serological *H-2D* type was predictive of the *Hh-1* type (Cudkowicz and Bennett, 1971a,b); the *Hh-1* genes have been mapped to the *H-2D* region for the *b* and *d* haplotypes. Recent experiments suggest that dominant, *trans*-acting down-regulatory genes map to this region (Rembecki et al. 1987) and the structural genes may be encoded elsewhere. Recent developments strongly suggest that Hh-1 antigens should not be conventional class I H-2 antigens. Firstly, murine NK cells do not functionally rearrange immunoglobulin or T cell receptor genes (Tutt et al. 1986,1987) and therefore should have a limited repertoire of receptors for antigens. Secondly, mice with severe combined immnunodeficiency (SCID) lack functional T or B cells and lack serum immunoglobulins, yet reject BMC grafts in an *H-2/Hh-1* specific manner (Murphy et al. 1987). The number of Hh-1 determinants so far detected is quite limited, consistent with the possibility that NK cells may express specific receptors for Hh-1 antigens.

To more precisely map *Hh-1* and to assess the polymprphism of this genetic system, we have analyzed the expression of Hh-1 antigens on BMC of numerous B10 and other congenic resistant inbred mouse strains. We present a model for *Hh-1* expression and regulation and show its evolution with recent findings. The model also has predictive value which will be valuable for the study of Hh-1 antigens in wild type strains as well as in recombinant strains. Studies of mice expressing intra-*H-2* recombinant haplotypes have allowed us to map *Hh-1* to the *S/D* interval of *H-2,* and to assign a possible gene order in the regulatory region. Furthermore, studies with recombinants have suggested that the *Hh-1* structural genes may also be linked to *H-2.*

MATERIALS AND METHODS

Bone Marrow Transplant Assay

The animals are exposed to to ^{137}Cs gamma irradiation . BALB/c congenic mice receive 700 cGy, B6 and B10 congenic inbred strains and recombinant mice, 780 cGy, and F1 hybrids 930 cGy. BMC suspensions are made by flushing out the marrow cavity of the tibias and femurs of donor mice with Hanks Balanced Salt Solution (HBSS). Inocula of 1.0 to 2.5×10^6 nucleated BMC are infused i.v. via the lateral tail vein in a volume of 0.5 ml. BMC growth is assessed five days later. The animals are injected with 0.2ml of $10^{-7}\underline{M}$ (25mg/100ml) 5-fluoro-2'-deoxyuridine i.p. to inhibit endogenous thymidylate synthetase. Thirty to sixty minutes later, the animals are injected with 0.5μCi ^{125}IUdR, a radioactive thymidine analog and DNA precurser. The spleens are removed 8-18 hours later and ^{125}I radioactivity is measured in a Packard crystal scintillation counter.The data is expressed as the geometric mean % IUdR uptake. Parametric and non-parametric analyses are performed on log transformed data to determine statistically significant differences between groups (Afifi et al. 1985). After determination of statistical significance, the data is normalized to yield 1.00% uptake as the value of the syngeneic control in order to faciltate camparison between experiments. Due to a shortage of certain mice, anti-asialo GM1 serum treated mice were utilized as positive controls in certain experiments.

Background For Analysis: Determination of the Hh-1 Phenotype

The criteria used to determine the Hh-1 phenotype of new mouse strains are presented in Table 1 and are based on the empirical and reproducible findings of hybrid and allogeneic resistance to BMC grafts. These rules are used to type the BMC Hh antigens of new strains . They are the basis of the assignment of *Hh-1* alleles to the various *H-2* haplotypes. The ability of mice to reject Hh-1 allogeneic BMC is under genetic control and is determinant-specific (Cudkowicz 1971). The determinants are assigned numbers (Bennett 1972) and the various *Hh-1* alleles have genes which result in the expression of zero, one, or combinations of determinants. We have utilized the strains of mice described in Table 2 to assemble a panel of recipients to analyze the determiants expressed by BMC of new mouse strains. We chose this panel of hosts because they allow the unequivocal assignment of the Hh-1 antigens expressed by a strain; each of the prototypic strains exhibits a unique pattern of acceptance and rejection in these hosts as shown in Table 3. $H\text{-}2^b$ grafts of B6 or B10 BMC proliferate well in syngeneic and C3H ($H\text{-}2^k$) hosts, but are rejected by B6xD2 and NZBxB6 hosts (hybrid resistance). This defines the Hh-1 phenotype *b* [determinant 1]. B10.D2, B10.BR, and B10.WB ($H\text{-}2^d$,$H\text{-}2^k$,$H\text{-}2^j$ respectively) also reject B6 BMC (allogeneic resistance, data not shown). *d* haplotype BMC grafts which are $Hh\text{-}1^d$ [determinant 2] are rejected by allogeneic B6 hosts and by NZBxB6 $H\text{-}2^{d/b}$ F1 hybrids. Note that B6xD2 mice, also *d* heterozygous, fail to reject parental $H\text{-}2^d$ grafts.

TABLE 1. DETERMINATION OF THE Hh-1 PHENOTYPE

1) Strains with identical Hh-1 antigens will not reject each other's BMC, but will reject BMC from donors which express non-identical Hh-1 antigens.

2) Strains with identical Hh-1 antigens will exhibit the same pattern of acceptance and rejection of BMC when transplanted into a panel of irradiated hosts.

3) F1 hybrids between strains with identical Hh-1 antigens retain the shared Hh-1 determinant and do not reject parental strain grafts.

4) F1 hybrids between strains with non-identical Hh-1 antigens will lose Hh-1 antigen expression and typically reject parental grafts.

TABLE 2. REJECTION CAPABILITIES OF IRRADIATED RECIPIENTS

STRAIN	*H-2*	EXPRESSES *Hh-1* DETERMINANT:	CAN REJECT BMC EXPRESSING DETERMINANTS:
B6,B10	*b*	1	2,3
B10.D2	*d*	2	1,3
B6xD2,B6xC	*b/d*	none	1,3 but not 2*
NZBXB6	*d/b*	none	1,2,3*
C3H	*k*	none	3, but not 1 or 2#
C3HxB6	*k/b*	none	1,2,3
B10.WB	*j*	2,3@	1

* (NZBxB6)F1 hybrids are capable of rejecting both *b* and *d* haplotype parental grafts (determinants 1 and 2); however, B6xD2 and B6xC F1's are only capable of rejecting $H\text{-}2^b$ [determinant 1] parental grafts.

\# C3H are only capable of rejecting grafts expressing determinant 3.

@ $H\text{-}2^j$ grafts share determinant 2 with the *d* haplotype and in addition express the unique determinant 3.

This differential ability of various $H\text{-}2^d$ heterozygous mice to reject parental *d* haplotype grafts is a consistent and interesting finding (probably due to a regulatory aspect of the effector system), but the genetic basis for the presence or absence of hybrid resistance has not been conclusively determined. $H\text{-}2^k$ BMC grafts were not rejected by any strains tested when we began these studies and were therefore thought to be $Hh\text{-}1^{null}$. B10.WB *(j)* BMC are rejected by allogeneic B6, B6xD2, C3H and NZBxB6 mice. The ability of C3H mice to reject *j* haplotype BMC defines the additional determinant 3 which *b* and *d* haplotype BMC lack. This operational definition of the Hh-1 phenotypes is crucial for the studies to be presented.

<u>A *Trans* Gene Regulatory Model To Explain Hemopoetic histocompatibility Antigen Expression</u>

A possible explanation for the non-codominant inheritance of Hh-1 antigens has been presented (Bennett 1987) and is based upon experiments utilizing *H-2* loss variants of ACCb, a pre-B cell lymphoma derived from BALB/cxBALB.B, $H\text{-}2^{d/b}$ (Rembecki et al. 1987). Briefly, the ACCb cells were used to inhibit hybrid resistance to $H\text{-}2^b$ BMC grafts by infusing large numbers of irradiated cells i.v. three hours before BMC transplantion. Control EL-4, $H\text{-}2^b$ homozygous cells, known to express $Hh\text{-}1^b$ (Clark and Harmon 1980), inhibited hybrid resitance to B6 BMC while ACCb cells failed to do so. The ACCb $H\text{-}2^{d-}$,$D^{d-}L^{d-}$, and D^{d-} loss variants were able to inhibit hybrid resistance, indicating that the cells expressed $Hh\text{-}1^b$ antigens (Rembecki et al. 1987). These results were the basis for a preliminary *trans*-gene model for regulation of Hh-1 antigen expression which is presented in Table 4.

TABLE 3. PATTERNS OF GROWTH AND REJECTION: OPERATIONAL DEFINITION OF Hh-1 PHENOTYPES

DONOR STRAIN		GROWTH IN IRRADIATED HOSTS*:					Hh-1
	H-2	SYNGENEIC	B6	B6xD2	C3H	NZBxB6	PHENOTYPE$
B6	*b*	++++	++++	-	++	-	*b*[1]
B10.D2	*d*	++++	-	++++	++++	-	*d*[2]
CBA	*k*	++++	++++	++++	++++	ND	*k*[null]
B10.WB	*j*	++++	-	-	-	ND	*j*[2,3]

* Growth in hosts is depicted as ++++ = >0.80 normalized %IUdR uptake ('growth'); ++ = >0.30,<0.70 normalized %IUdR uptake ('partial rejection'); - =<0.10 normalized %IUdR uptake ('rejection'). ND= not done.

$ $Hh\text{-}1^b$ [determinant 1] grafts are accepted by B6 and C3H, but are rejected by B6xD2 and NZBxB6 hosts.

$ $Hh\text{-}1^d$ [determinant 2] grafts are accepted by B6xD2 and C3H, but are rejected by B6 and NZBxB6 hosts.

$ $Hh\text{-}1^j$ [determinants 2+3] grafts are accepted only by syngeneic and anti-$ASGM_1$ treated animals, but are rejected by B6, B6D2F1, C3H, and NZBxB6 hosts.

$ $Hh\text{-}1^k$ [null] grafts are not rejected.

The model as presented in Table 4 consists of three regulatory genes (1',2',3',), which correspond to the structural determinants 1,2,3. each with two alleles (the regulatory gene is present or absent) and the Hh-1 phenotype is the composite of the regulatory genotype. The Hh phenotype of an F1 hybrid can be determined from Table 4 by seeing which regulatory genes would b present. The model also predicts the existence of other *Hh-1* alleles based on a random assortment of regulatory genes in the murine genome, and the discovery of any of these phenotypes would support the model.

POLYMORPHISM OF Hh-1 ANTIGENS

Discovery of New Hh-1 Phenotypes

Determinant 4. Our use of NZBxB6 F1 hybrid mice in the panel of recipients resulted in the detection of a new Hh-1 determinant expressed by $H\text{-}2^k$ BMC (Table 5). Our initial survey of standard *H-2* types had suggested that *k, q,* and *r* haplotype BMC grafts were *null,* but

TABLE 4. PRELIMINARY *TRANS* GENE REGULATORY MODEL OF *Hh-1* EXPRESSION

A: Assumptions used to construct the model:

1) The regulatory genes are dominant, *trans*-acting and map to the *Hh-1* locus near *H-2D*.

2) The *Hh-1* structural genes are present in all strains and may or may not be linked to *H-2;* the genes may be located on other chromosomes.

3) The Hh-1 phenotype (expression of determinants 1,2, or 3) is directly governed by the presence or absence of the corresponding *Hh-1* regulatory genes, 1',2', and 3'.

4) Bone marrow cells expressing determinants not present on host cells will be rejected provided that the host possesses the proper genetic background for a good rejection response.

5) The Hh-1 phenotype is determined as described in tables 1-3; the *Hh-1* regulatory genotype is inferred from it.

B: Hh-1 PHENOTYPES ALREADY OBSERVED

Hh-1	*H-2* Haplotypes	Regulatory Genes	Determinants Expressed
o null	*k,q,r*	1' 2' 3'	none
b	*b,*	2' 3'	1
d	*d,f,p*	1' 3'	2
j	*j*	1'	2 3

C: *Hh-1* PHENOTYPES PREDICTED BY THE REGULATORY MODEL

Hh-1	Regulatory Genes	Determinants Expressed
x1	1' 2'	3
x2	2'	1 3
x3	3'	1 2
x4	none	1 2 3

recently we observed that NZBxB6 hosts strongly rejected *H-2*^{k} BMC. We have also observed that NZB/BlNJ will reject *k* haplotype grafts(data not shown). By the criteria of rejection by NZB and its F1 hybrids but not any other strain we have defined a new determinant, 4. Since *q* and *r* BMC are not rejected by any host so far tested, they are at least tentatively considered *Hh-1*^{null}. C3H*(k)* mice were crossed with B6*(b)* or BALB/c*(d)*, and B6 mice crossed with C to obtain F1 hybrids. BMC from these heterozygous donors is tested for the expression of Hh-1 antigens by grafting cells into irradiated B6xD2 and NZBxB6 mice. We observe that C3H and C3HxB6 BMC are rejected by NZBxB6 hosts(Table 6). C3HxC and B6xC BMC are not rejected. We deduce from this that the *k* haplotype expresses determinant 4, and that the *b* and *k* haplotypes share that determinant. Additionally, *d* is able to down regulate determinant 4 expression in both the *b* and *k* haplotypes. In experiments not shown, we have demonstrated that the *k, q,* and *r* *Hh-1* types map to *H-2D* like the other alleles studied. Thus the regulatory model of expression would predict the presence of regulatory genes 2' and 3' in *H-2*^{b} strains which would allow the expression of determinants 1 and 4; *H-2*^{k} would possess genes 1',2' and 3' to allow the expression of determinant 4. These findings help to explain previous findings of Eastcott et al. 1981, which described an Hh-1 antigen on C3H lymph node cell grafts which resulted in rejection by NZBxB6 hosts; C3HxB6 lymph node cell grafts were also rejected, and this may also have been due to determinant 4 expression.

H-2^{s} exhibits a novel Hh-1 phenotype. A previous study of BMC grafts involving *s* haplotype grafts suggested that the Hh-1 phenotypes of *s* and *b* were similar (Cudkowicz 1978, Warner 1978). Our preliminary studies of *s* grafts demonstrated that B10.S *(H-2*^{s}*)* BMC were rejected by B6 and B6xD2 hosts but not by C3H (data not shown), suggesting that they expressed determinants 1 and 2 but not 3 (see Table 2). We crossed B10.S with B6*(b)*, DBA/2(D2,*d)*,or C3H*(k)* mice. The BMC of the F1 hybrid mice were infused into irradiated syngeneic, B6, B6xD2 or NZBxB6 hosts and the results are presented in Table 7. B10.SxB6 BMC grow in B6 and are rejected by B6xD2 hosts, indicating that such cells express determinant 1. B10.SxD2 BMC are rejected by B6 hosts and are accepted by B6xD2 hosts, suggesting that determinant 2 is expressed. Finally, B10.SxC3H BMC proliferate well in B6 and B6xD2 hosts but are strongly rejected by NZBxB6 recipients. Thus the BMC also express determinant 4. Since *Hh-1*^{s} maps to *H-2D* (data not shown), *H-2*^{s}*/Hh-1*^{s} represents a new *Hh-1* allele which differs from others by expressing determinants 1, 2 and 4. The discovery of a strain which co-expresses determinants 1 and 2 was predicted by the preliminary model in Table 4.

Modified Model for Trans Gene Regulation

The detection of determinant 4 has forced us to modify the model for regulation of expression of Hh-1 antigens(Table 8). We now have observed four Hh determinants and infer the existence of four corresponding regulatory genes which map to *Hh-1* near *H-2D*. All of the non-recombinant *H-2* types have been studied and thus far exhibit one of the six phenotypes presented in Table 8. The addition of determinant 4 and the corresponding regulatory gene 4' greatly expands the number of possible Hh-1 phenotypes now predicted by the model, and the analysis of wild type strains and recombinants in order to discover predicted phenotypes will be valuable in supporting the validity of this model.

TABLE 5. REJECTION OF *k* BUT NOT *q* or *r* HAPLOTYPE BMC BY NZBxB6: DEFINITION OF DETERMINANT 4

DONOR STRAIN	*H-2*	GROWTH IN IRRADIATED HOSTS*: SYNGENEIC	B6	B6xD2	NZBxB6	Hh-1 PHENOTYPE$
CBA/La	*k*	++++	++++	++++	-	*k*[4] ●
B10.Q	*q*	++++	++++	++++	++++	*q*[null] #
B10.RIII	*r*	++++	++++	++++	++++	*r*[null] #

* See Table 3.

$ The phenotype was determined as described in Tables 1-3.

● $H\text{-}2^k$ grafts proliferate well in syngeneic, B6, and B6xD2 hosts but are strongly rejected by NZBxB6 hosts.

$H\text{-}2^{q,r}$ grafts are null; they are not rejected by any of the hosts, even NZBxB6.

TABLE 6. EXPRESSION OF DETERMINANT 4 BY $H\text{-}2^b$ BUT NOT BY $H\text{-}2^d$ BMC GRAFTS

DONOR STRAIN	*H-2*	GROWTH IN IRRADIATED HOSTS*: SYNGENEIC	B6	B6D2F1	NZBxB6	Hh-1 PHENOTYPE$
C3H/HeJ	*k*	++++	++++	++++	-	*k*[4]
C3HxB6	*k/b*	++++	++++	++++	-	[4] #
C3HxC	*k/d*	++++	++++	++++	++++	*null* ●
B6xC	*b/d*	++++	++++	++++	++++	*null* ●

* See Table 3.

$ The phenotype was determined as described in Tables 1-3.

$H\text{-}2^b$ shares *Hh-1* determinant 4 with the *k* haplotype.

● $H\text{-}2^d$ does not express determinant 4, but is capable of down regulating its expression in the *b* or *k* haplotypes.

TABLE 7. ANALYSIS OF *H-2^s* GRAFTS: DESCRIPTION OF A NEW *Hh-1* PHENOTYPE

DONOR STRAIN	*H-2*	GROWTH IN IRRADIATED HOSTS*: SYNGENEIC	B6	B6D2F1	NZBxB6	Hh-1 PHENOTYPE$
B10.S	*s*	++++	-	-	ND	1+2#
B10.SxB6	*s/b*	++++	++++	-	ND	1#
B10.SxD2	*s/d*	++++	-	++++	ND	2#
B10.SxC3H	*s/k*	++++	++++	++++	-	4#

* See Table 3.

$ The phenotype was determined as described in Tables 1-3.

\# *H-2^s* grafts share determinants 1,2,4 with the *b, d, and k* haplotypes respectively.

MAPPING Hh-1

Association of *Hh-1* and *H-2D*

Approximately 60 strains from the Mayo Medical School mouse colony were analyzed for the Hh-1 phenotype by grafting BMC into the panel of hosts noted in Table 2. The BMC of the great majority of the strains tested expressed that Hh-1 phenotype predicted by *H-2D* (Table 9).

Evidence that Hh-1 maps to the left of H-2L

A new and unique recombination was detected between *H-2D* and *H-2L* in the strain B10.RQDB (Levy et al. 1985). The two parental strains were B10.A(2R) and B10.T(6R). B10.RQDB expresses both D^dD^b but does not express L^d. This indicates that D^b is allelic to L^d and the *b* haplotype has *L* as its only class I gene in the *H-2D* region. In Table 10, BMC from the parental strains and B10.RQDB were assessed for the Hh-1 phenotype as described in Tables 1-3. B10.A(2R) and B10.T(6R) are *b* and *d* respectively at *Hh-1*. RQDB BMC are accepted by B6xD2 hosts and are rejected by B6 hosts, indicating that the cells express the *d* allele, determinant 2, but not determinant 1. B6xRQDB BMC are not rejected by any type of host, indicating that the BMC had the null phenotype even though the donors are homozygous for L^b. RQDBxBALB/c(C) BMC are rejected by B6 hosts and are accepted by B6xD2 hosts, indicating that determinant 2 is expressed. Therefore B10.RQDB BMC express the *Hh-1^d* phenotype.

TABLE 8. MODIFIED *TRANS* GENE REGULATORY MODEL OF Hh EXPRESSION

A: Hh-1 PHENOTYPES ALREADY OBSERVED

Hh-1	*H-2* Haplotypes	Regulatory Genes	Determinants Expressed
o null	*q,r*	1' 2' 3' 4'	none
k	*k,z,w3*	1' 2' 3'	4
b	*b*	2' 3'	1,4
s	*s*	3'	1,2,4
d	*d,f,p*	1' 3' 4'	2
j	*j*	1'	2,3,4

B: Hh-1 PHENOTYPES PREDICTED BY THE REGULATORY MODEL*

Hh-1	Regulatory Genes	Determinants Expressed
x1	2' 3' 4'	1
x2	3' 4'	1 2
x3	1' 3'	2 4
x4	1'	2 3
x5	1' 2' 4'	3
x6	2' 4'	1 3
x7	4'	1 2 3
x8	1' 2'	3 4
x9	2'	1 3 4
x10	none	1 2 3 4

* The assumptions for determining the Hh-1 antigen phenotype and inferring the *Hh-1* genotype are as described in Table 4 with the addition of determinant 4 and the corresponding regulatory gene 4'.

These results indicate that the *b* allele of *Hh-1* must map to the left of *H-2L*, the only *b* haplotype class I gene in that region. Thus, we conclude that $Hh\text{-}1^b$, and presumably other Hh-1 types, are not class I genes. B10.RFDB is a recombinant near *H-2E* and is derived from B10.RQDB and B10.M ($H\text{-}2^f$). The BMC of RFDB also express the *d* phenotype (Table 10). Not shown in Table10 are results of BMC transplants using B10.RQDB, CxRQDB and B6xRQDB as recipients of RQDB, BALB/c and B6 BMC. B6 *(b)* BMC are rejected by RQDB, CxRQDB and B6xRQDB, even though B10.RQDB is homozygous for L^b. BALB/c and RQDB BMC are accepted by RQDB and CxRQDB hosts, as one would expect if both donors and hosts are $Hh\text{-}1^d$.

TABLE 9. A MAJORITY OF THE *H-2* RECOMBINANTS POSSESS THE *Hh-1* PREDICTED BY THE *H-2D* TYPE

STRAIN	*H-2* HAPLOTYPE	ORIGIN	*H-2* COMPOSITION									*Hh-1*
			K	A_β	A_α	E_β	$E_{\beta 2}$	E_α	*S*	*D*	*L*	
B10.D2-dm1	*dm1*	*d*	*d*	*d*	*d*	*d*	*d*	*d*	*d*		*d**	*d**
C-H-2 dm2	*dm2*	*d*	*d*	*d*	*d*	*d*	*d*	*d*	*d*	*d*	-	*d*
B10.A(5R)/SgDv	*i5*	*b/a*	*b*	*b*	*b*	*b*	/ *k*	*k*	:*d*	*d*	*d*	*d*
B10.S(9R)/Sg	*t4*	*s/a*	*s*	*s*	*s*	*s*	/ *k*	*k*	:*d*	*d*	*d*	*d*
B10.A,A/J	*a*	*k/d*	*k*	*k*	*k*	*k*	*k*	*k*	/*d*	*d*	*d*	*d*
B10.RFD3/DV	*ap12*	*f/td1*	*f*	*f*	*f*	*f*	*f*	*f*	/*d*	*d*	*d*	*d*
BSVS/WrDv	*t5*	*s/d*	*s*	*s*	*s*	*s*	*s*	*s*	/*d*	*d*	*d*	*d*
B10.RPD2/Dv	*td2*	*pb/t4*	*p*	*p*	*p*	*p*	*p*	*p*	/*k*	*d*	*d*	*d*
B10.RKD2/Dv	*a7*	*h2/y2*	*k*	*k*	*k*	*k*	*k*	*k*	/*q*	:*d*	*d*	*d*
A.AL/SfDv	*a1*	*k/d*	*k*	*k*	*k*	*k*	*k*	*k*	*k*	/*d*	*d*	*d*
B10.RKD1/Dv	*a3*	*h2/t3*	*k*	*k*	*k*	*k*	*k*	*k*	:*d*:	/*d*	*d*	*d*
B10.RKD3/Dv	*a8*	*h2/t3*	*k*	*k*	*k*	*k*	*k*	*k*	:*d*:	/*d*	*d*	*d*
B10.M(11R)/Dv	*ap1*	*f/a*	*f*	*f*	*f*	*f*	*f*	*f*	*f*	/*d*	*d*	*d*
B10.RFD1/Dv	*ap6*	*f/a8*	*f*	*f*	*f*	*f*	*f*	*f*	*f*/	*d*	*d*	*d*
B10.RFD2/Dv	*ap7*	*f/a8*	*f*	*f*	*f*	*f*	*f*	*f*	*f*/	*d*	*d*	*d*
B10.RSD1/Dv	*t11*	*s/ap9*	*s*	*s*	*s*	*s*	*s*	*s*	*s*	/*d*	*d*	*d*
B10.RSD2/Dv	*t12*	*s/ap9*	*s*	*s*	*s*	*s*	*s*	*s*	*s*	/*d*	*d*	*d*
B10.D2(R107)	*i7*	*b/d*	*b*	*b*	*b*	*b*	*b*	*b*	*b*	/*d*	*d*	*d*
B10.S(7R),A.TH	*t2*	*s/a*	*s*	*s*	*s*	*s*	*s*	*s*	*s*	/*d*	*d*	*d*
B10.PL/SgDv	*u*		*u*	*u*	*u*	*u*	*u*	*u*	*u*	/*d*	*d*	*d*
B10.T(6R)/SgDv	*y2*	*q/a*	*q*	*q*	*q*	*q*	*q*	*q*	*q*	/*d*	*d*	*d*
B10.F(14R)/SfDv	*b/p*	*b/p*	*b*	*b*	*b*	*b*	*b*	*b*	/*p*	*p*	*p*	*p*
B10.A(4R)/SgDv	*h4*	*a/b*	*k*	*k*	*k*	*k*	/ *b*	*b*	*b*		*b*	*b*
B10.RSB5/Dv	*at20*	*t4/pb*	*s*	*s*	*s*	*s*	*k*	*k*	/*b*		*b*	*b*
B10.RSB14/Dv	*at28*	*pb/t1*	*s*	*k*	*k*	*k*	*k*	*k*	/*b*		*b*	*b*
B10.F(13R)SgDv	*pb*	*p/b*	*p*	*p*	*p*	*p*	*p*	*p*	/*b*		*b*	*b*
B10.RVB/Dv	*vb1*	*v/h4*	*v*	*v*	*v*	*v*	*v*	*v*	/.		*b*	*b*
B10.RSB2/Dv	*at10*	*t4/h4*	*s*	*s*	*s*	*s*	*k*	*k*	*d*	/	*b*	*b*
B10.RSB3/Dv	*at11*	*t3/h2*	*s*	*s*	*s*	*s*	*k*	*k*	*k*	/	*b*	*b*
B10.RSB7/Dv	*at22*	*t3/h2*	*s*	*s*	*s*	*s*	*k*	*k*	*k*	/	*b*	*b*
B10.RSB10/Dv	*at24*	*t4/h4*	*s*	*s*	*s*	*s*	*k*	*k*	*d*	/	*b*	*b*
B10.RSB13/Dv	*at27*	*pb/t1*	*s*	*k*	*k*	*k*	*k*	*k*	*k*	/	*b*	*b*
B10.D2(R103)	*g3*	*d/b*	*d*	*d*	*d*	*d*	*d*	*d*	*d*	/	*b*	*b*
B10.BDR1/PsDv	*g4*	*d/b*	*d*	*d*	*d*	*d*	*d*	*d*	*d*	/	*b*	*b*
B10.A(2R)/SgDv	*h2*	*a/b*	*k*	*k*	*k*	*k*	*k*	*k*	*d*	/	*b*	*b*
B10.RKB3/Dv		*k/b*	*k*	*k*	*k*	*k*	*k*	*k*	*k*	/	*b*	*b*
B6.AKL/FlDv	*ak1*	*b/k*	*b*	*b*	*b*	*b*	*b*	*b*	*b*	/*k*	*k*	*k*
C3H.OH/SfDv	*o2*	*d/k*	*d*	*d*	*d*	*d*	*d*	*d*	*d*	/*k*	*k*	*k*
B6-H-2 oz1	*oz1*	*b/k*	*b*	*b*	*b*	*b*	*b*	*b*	*b*	/*k*	*k*	*k*
B10.ASR2/Dv	*as2*	*a/s*	*k*	*k*	*k*	*k*	*k*	*k*	:*d*	/*s*	*s*	*s*
B10.DA/SnDv	*qp1*	*q/s*	*q*	*q*	*q*	*q*	*q*	*q*	*q*	/*s*	*s*	*s*
B10.AKM/SgDv	*m*	*k/q*	*k*	*k*	*k*	*k*	*k*	*k*	*k*	/*q*	*q*	*q*
B10.RBQ1/Dv	*bq2*	*i2/q*	*b*	*b*	*b*	*b*	*b*	*b*	.	*q*	*q*	*q*

d* Represents the D-L fusion product of *dm1*.
: Indicates a previous recombination in one of the donor strains.
/ Indicates the most recent recombination.

TABLE 10. BMC TRANSPLANTS UTILIZING *H-2D/L* RECOMBINANTS: B10.RQDB AND B10.RFDB BMC DONORS EXPRESS DETERMINANT 2 ONLY

DONOR STRAIN	*H-2* COMPOSITION *K A E S D L*	GROWTH IN IRRADIATED HOSTS*: SYNGENEIC	B6	B6xD2	Hh-1 PHENOTYPE$
B10.A(2R)	*k k k :d / b*	++++	++++	-	*b*[1]
B10.T(6R)	*q q q q/d d*	++++	-	++++	*d*[2]
B10.RQDB	*q q q q:d/b*	++++	-	++++	*d*[2]
B10.RFDB	*f f f/q q:d:b*	++++	-	++++	*d*[2]
CxRQDB	*q q q q:d/b* *d d d d d d*	++++	-	++++	*d*[2]
B6xRQDB	*q q q q:d/b* *b b b b b*	++++	++++	++++	*null* #

* See Table 3.

$ The phenotype was determined as described in Tables 1-3. B10.T(6R), B10.RQDB, BALB/cxB10.RQDB, and B10.RFDB grow in syngeneic and B6xD2 but are rejected by B6, $C3B6F_1$, AND NZBxB6. This is an $Hh\text{-}1^d$ pattern of growth/rejection.

B6xB10.RQDB grafts are $Hh\text{-}1^{null}$ even though homozygous for $H\text{-}2L^b$.

B10.WB *(j)* mice were crossed with BALB/c *(d)* or with BALB.B *(b)* to produce F1 hybrids. $H\text{-}2^j$ BMC are rejected by B6, B6xD2 and C3H hosts (Table 11) confirming that determinants 2 and 3 are expressed. CxB10.WB BMC are rejected by B6 but not by B6xD2 hosts and therfore express determinant 2. BALB.BxB10.WB BMC grow well in B6 and B6xD2 hosts but are rejected by NZBxB6 hosts, detecting determinant 4. Thus the *b* and *j* haplotypes share determinant 4 but not 1. An examination of the *H-2* composition of B10.WB *(j)* in Table 11 reveals that this haplotype contains the L^b gene and may be an *H-2S/D* interval recombinant with the *Hh-1* allele donated by the *j* haplotype from the *S* side of the crossover site.

Possible Intra-*Hh-1* Recombination

The detection of Hh-1 phenotypes in intra-*H-2* recombinants which are different from both parents would constitute evidence that crossing over occurred within *Hh-1.* In fact, several such instances were detected when evaluating the *S/D* recombinants. B10.D2(R106) and B10.RSF5 represent two similar cases in which the resultant Hh-1 phenotype is distinct from the

TABLE 11. *j* HAPLOTYPE BMC TRANSPLANTS: *Hh-1* EXPRESSION PREDICTED BY *H-2S* NOT *H-2L*

DONOR STRAIN		GROWTH IN IRRADIATED HOSTS*:					Hh-1
	H-2	SYNGENEIC	B6	B6xD2	C3H	NZBxB6	PHENOTYPE$
B10.WB	*j*	++++	-	-	-	ND	3#
CxB10.WB	*d/j*	++++	-	++++	ND	ND	2**
BxB10.WB	*b/j*	++++	++++	++++	ND	-	4##

H-2 COMPOSITION									
K	A_β	A_α	E_β	$E_{\beta 2}$	E_α	*S*	*D*	*L*	*Hh-1*
j	*j*	*j*	*j*	*j*	*j*	*j*	/	*b*	*j*[2,3,4] @

* See Table 3.

$ The phenotype was determined as described in Tables 1-3.

\# B10.WB exhibits a unique *Hh-1* phenotype; *H-2* ^{j}(determinant 2,3,4) grafts are rejected by B6, B6xD2, and C3H.

** F1 hybrids with BALB/c *(H-2^d/Hh-1^d)* express determinant 2 but not 3.

\#\# F1 hybrids with BALB.B *(H-2/Hh-1^b)* are accepted by B6 and B6xD2 but are rejected by NZBxB6 indicating expression of determinant 4.

@ *Hh-1* maps left of *H-2L* in this strain.

alleles of the donor strains. The results of BMC transplants from B10.D2(R106) and B10.RSF5 donors are presented in Table 12A. In addition we show the *H-2/Hh-1* composition of the donor strains and the resultant recombinants. The parents of R106 were B6 *(Hh-1^b)* and B10.D2-*H-2dm1* *(Hh-1^d)* yet R106 BMC express the *null* phenotype. The parents of RSF5 are B10.RSB12 *(Hh-1^b)* and B10.M*(f)* but the BMC of RSF5 are also *null* for Hh-1. The model as presented in Table 8 consists of four regulatory genes (1',2',3',4'), each with two alleles (the regulatory gene is present or absent) and the Hh-1 phenotype is the composite of the regulatory genotype. Of 24 possible gene orders which represent all permutaions of the regulatory gene order within *Hh-1,* nine are compatible with a single crossover event within *Hh-1* to give rise to the phenotype expressed by both of these recombinants. In Table 12B, one possible gene order is presented as an example which is consistent with the data. The recombination could have produced a haplotype with all four regulatory genes and the resultant *null* phenotype.. A prediction that follows is that F1 hybrids between R106 or

TABLE 12. B10.D2(R106) AND B10.RSF5 BMC TRANSPLANTS

A: EVIDENCE FOR INTRA-*Hh-1* RECOMBINATION

STRAIN	*H-2*	ORIGIN	*H-2* COMPOSITION *K*	A_β	A_α	E_β	$E_{\beta 2}$	E_α	*S*	*D L*	*Hh-1* #
B6	*b*		*b*	*b*	*b*	*b*	*b*	*b*	*b*	*b*	*b*[1,4]
B10.D2-dm1	*dm1*	*d*	*d*	*d*	*d*	*d*	*d*	*d*	*d*	*d**	*d**[2]
B10.D2(R106)	*ia1*	*b/dm1*	*b*	*b*	*b*	*b*	*b*	*b*	*b*	/ *d**	*null*
B10.F(13R)	*pb*	*p/b*	*p*	*p*	*p*	*p*	*p*	*p*	/*b*	*b*	*b*[1,4]
B10.RSB12	*at26*	*t4/pb*	*s*	*s*	*s*	*s*	*k* /	*p*	*b*	*b*	*b*[1,4]
B10.M	*f*		*f*	*f*	*f*	*f*	*f*	*f*	*f*	*f f*	*f*[2]
B10.RSF5/Dv	*an6*	*at26/f*	*s*	*s*	*s*	*s*	*k*	*p*	*b*	/*f f*	*null*

\# Phenotype determined by grafting BMC into syngeneic, B6, B6xD2, and NZBxB6 irradiated hosts.

d* Refers to the fused D/L gene of the *dm1* mutant.

B: A POSSIBLE REGULATORY GENE ORDER CONSISTENT WITH INTRA-*Hh-1* RECOMBINATION +

STRAIN	*H-2*	*K*	A_β	A_α	E_β	$E_{\beta 2}$	E_α	*S*	*Hh-1* @ (2' 1' 4' 3')	*D L*
B6	*b*	*b*	*b*	*b*	*b*	*b*	*b*	*b*	-(2' 3')^{b}	*b*
B10.D2-dm1	*dm1*	*d*	*d*	*d*	*d*	*d*	*d*	*d*	(1' 4' 3')^{d}-	*d**
B10.D2(R106)	*ia1*	*b*	*b*	*b*	*b*	*b*	*b*	*b*	(2' 1' 4' 3')^{o}	*d** ++

\+ There are twenty-four possible gene orders (four genes, 2 alleles); this is one of nine gene orders which can explain the results with a single crossover.

@ See Table 9 for phenotypes.

d* Refers to the fused D/L gene of the *dm1* mutant.

++ If recombination has occurred within *Hh-1* to create a regulatory region which possesses all four genes, then F1 hybrids can be used to confirm this prediction.

TABLE 13. B10.D2(R106) F1 HYBRID BMC TRANSPLANTS

DONOR STRAIN	*H-2* *K*	*S*	*D L*	GROWTH IN IRRADIATED HOSTS#: SYNGENEIC	B6	B6xD2	NZBxB6	Hh-1 PHENOTYPE$
B10.D2	*d*	*d*	*d d*	++++	-	++++	-	*d*[2]
B10.D2dm1	*d*	*d*	*d**	++++	-	-	-	*d**[2]
R106	*b*	*b*	/ *d**	++++	++++	++++	++++	*null*
R106xD2	*b* / *d*	*b* / *d*	/ *d** / *d d*	++++	++++	++++	++++	*null* ●
R106xB6	*b* / *b*	*b* / *b*	/ *d** / *b*	++++	++++	++++	++++	*null* ●

\# See Table 3.

d* Refers to the fused D/L gene of the *dm1* mutant.

$ The phenotype was determined as described in Tables 1-3.

● These results support the predictions made in Table 12.

RSF5 with any other mouse strain would have BMC of the *null* phenotype. Data consistent with this prediction, using R106, are presented in Table 13. Both B10.D2 and B10.D2-*H-2dm1* BMC were strongly rejected by B6 hosts, as expected for *Hh-1*^{d}. However, R106, R106xD2 and R106xB6 BMC grow well in every host tested, including NZBxB6 mice. Similar results were obtained for BMC transplants of B10.RSF5 and F1 hybrids with C and B6 (data not shown). The relatively poor resistance by H-2^d heterozygous NZBxB6 hosts to grafts of H-2dm1 BMC has been previously noted (Bennett et al. 1980).

STRUCTURAL AND REGULATORY GENES

Hh-1^f Appears to Map to the Left of H-2S

Results of studies of BMC transplants recombinants involving *H-2*^{f} were quite surprising. The data in Table 14 indicate that crossing over to the left of *D*^{f} results in the loss of determinant 2 expression and the BMC have the *null* phenotype. Our initial interpretation of studies with RQF1, RKF1 and RKF2 was that *Hh-1* mapped just to the left of *H-2D*. However, the crossover events of RPF2, RKF3 and RBF are to the left of *H-2S*. This is the only haplotype to yield such data.

TABLE 14. TRANSPLANTS OF *f* HAPLOTYPE BMC

DONOR STRAIN	*H-2* COMPOSITION *K A E S D L*	GROWTH IN IRRADIATED HOSTS#: SYNGENEIC	B6	B6xD2	Hh-1 PHENOTYPE$
B10.M	*f f f f f f*	++++	-	+++	*f*[2]
B10.RKF1	*k k k d/f f*	++++	+++	+++	*null**
B10.RQF1	*q q q q/f f*	++++	++++	+++	*null**
B10.RKF2	*k k kb b/f f*	++++	+++	+++	*null**
B10.RPF2	*p p p /f f f*	++++	+++	+++	*null* @
B10.RKF3	*k k k/f f f f*	++++	+++	+++	*null***
B10.RBF	*b b b/f f f f*	++++	+++	+++	*null***

\# See Table 3.

$ Phenotype is determined as described in Tables 1-3.

* Results appear to map $Hh\text{-}1^f$ centromeric of *H-2D*.

@ Results appear to map $Hh\text{-}1^f$ centromeric of *H-2S*.

** Results appear to map $Hh\text{-}1^f$ centromeric of *H-2E*.

Evidence that *f* Regulatory Genes Map in the *H-2S/D* Interval

We analyzed other *S/D* recombinants involving $H\text{-}2^f$ in greater detail. The results with B10.M(17R) are described in Table 15. The parents of B10.M(17R) are B10.A $(Hh\text{-}1^d)$ and B10.M $(H\text{-}2^f)$, both of which have BMC expressing determinant 2 and presumably possess indistinguishable regulatory genotypes. However, BMC of $H\text{-}2^{aq1}$ are of the *null* phenotype. One interpretation is that a crossover has occurred which has reconstituted a functional regulatory gene 2'. A second possibliity is that $Hh\text{-}1^f$ maps far to the left of *D* (Table 14) and the recombination has failed to include either the *d* or *f Hh-1* regulatory region. Another explanation would have the structural genes for $Hh\text{-}1^f$ to the left of *H-2S* but the regulatory genes may still be in the *S/D* interval, and M(17R) may have retained the regulatory region without the structural genes. Each of these possibilities yields different predictions for the Hh-1 phenotype of M(17R) F1 hybrids. To test these possibilities, F1 hybrids between B10.M(17R) and BALB/c *(d)* or BALB.B *(b)* were bred. BMC from these donors were assessed for Hh-1 phenotype. If the entire *Hh-1* region was lost in this recombination, crosses of that haplotype with any strain would result in F1 hybrids expressing the Hh-1

TABLE 15. BMC TRANSPLANTATION OF B10.M(17R) AND F1 HYBRIDS: EVIDENCE FOR Hh STRUCTURAL GENE LOSS AND COMPLEMENTATION

A: B10.M(17R) EXPRESS A *null* PHENOTYPE

STRAIN	*H-2*	ORIGIN	*H-2* COMPOSITION *K*	A_β	A_α	E_β	$E_{\beta 2}$	E_α	*S*	*D*	*L*	*Hh-1**
B10.A	*a*	*k/d*	*k*	*k*	*k*	*k*	*k*	*k*	*/d*	*d*	*d*	*d*[2]
B10.M	*f*		*f*	*f*	*f*	*f*	*f*	*f*	*f*	*f*	*f*	*f*[2]
B10.M(17)R/Dv	*aq1*	*a/f*	*k*	*k*	*k*	*k*	*k*	*k*	*:d*	*/f*	*f*	*null*
A.AL	*al*	*k/d*	*k*	*k*	*k*	*k*	*k*	*k*	*k/*	*d*	*d*	*d*[2]
A.TL	*tl*	*s/al*	*s/*	*k*	*k*	*k*	*k*	*k*	*k:*	*d*	*d*	*d*[2]
A.CA	*f*		*f*	*f*	*f*	*f*	*f*	*f*	*f*	*f*	*f*	*d*[2]
A.TFR1/SfDv	*an1*	*tl/f*	*s*	*:k*	*k*	*k*	*k*	*k*	*k*	*/f*	*f*	*null*

* Phenotype determined by grafting into syngeneic, B6, B6xD2, and NZBxB6 irradiated hosts.

B: EVIDENCE FOR Hh STRUCTURAL GENE COMPLEMENTATION

DONOR STRAIN	*H-2* *K*	*S*	*D*	*L*	GROWTH IN IRRADIATED HOSTS#: SYNGENEIC	B6	B6xD2	NZBxB6	*Hh-1* PHENOTYPE$
B10.M(17R)	*k*	*:d*	*/f*	*f*	++++	++++	++++	++++	*null*
CxM(17R)	*d* *k*	*d* *:d*	*d* */f*	*d* *f*	++++	-	++++	ND	*d,f*[2]**
BxM(17R)	*b* *k*	*b* *:d*	*b* */f*	*b* *f*	++++	++++	++++	ND	*null* @

\# See Table 3.

$ Determined as described in Tables 1-3.

** C (BALB/c, $H\text{-}2^d$)xB10.M(17R) BMC expresses determinant 2 suggesting that the lack of an Hh structural gene in $H\text{-}2^{aq1}$ can be overcome by gene complementation.

@ B (BALB.B, $H\text{-}2^b$)xB10.M(17R) BMC display the *null* phenotype, suggesting that $H\text{-}2^{aq1}$ has the *Hh-1* regulatory genes of either the *f* or *d* haplotype (1'3'4').

TABLE 16. FREQUENCY OF RECOMBINATION NEAR *Hh-1*

FRACTION OF ALL INTRA-*H-2* RECOMBINANTS*	RECOMBINATION INTERVAL
3.1%	K/A_β
16.2%	A_β/E_α
16.3%	E_α/S
63.6%	*S/D*
0.8%	*D/L*

ANALYSIS OF THE *H-2S/D* INTERVAL RECOMBINANTS**

68.3%	Exhibit an *Hh-1* which correlates with *H-2D*
7.3%	Exhibit an *Hh-1* which correlates with *H-2S* or maps centromeric of *H-2L*
24.4%	Represent possible intra-*Hh-1* recombination

* Based on Klein et al, 1983.

** Based on Tables 9-15 and unpublished observations.

phenotype of the strain used in the cross. In contrast, the actual data indicates that the *f* or *d* *Hh-1* regulatory genes are maintained in $H\text{-}2^{aq1}$ (Table 15B). BALB/c x B10.M(17R) BMC express determinant 2 since they were rejected by B6 hosts but BALB.B x B10.M(17R) BMC expressed the *null* phenotype. Thus, gene complementation for the *Hh-1* structural gene of determinant 2 occurred in the cross with BALB/c, and the regulatory gene effects of *f* or *d* are evident in the cross with BALB.B,(i.e., B10.M(17R) has at least the 1' regulatory gene). In addition, analysis of A.TFR1 and B10.RBF (see Table 14) and their F1 hybrids indicates that other *f* recombinants retain the *Hh-1* regulatory but not the *Hh-1* structural region (data not shown). Other *S/D* recombinations also result in phenotypes different from both parental strains. The results can best be explained if the structural genes are to the left of the regulatory genes but near the *S/D* interval for haplotypes other than $H\text{-}2^f$ (data not shown).

CONCLUSIONS

We have used a panel of recipient mice which reject certain strain BMC grafts in order to determine the Hh-1 phenotype of new strains of mice to be tested. When non-recombinant *H-2* types of independent origin were studied, six patterns of expression of four different Hh-1 determinants were observed. The great majority of more than 60 intra-*H-2* recombinant strain mice had *Hh-1* alleles predicted by *H-2D or L.* However, of the many *H-2S/D* recombinants, two strains expressed *Hh-1* alleles which did not correlate with *D* or *L.* In addition, several strains which express Hh-1 phenotypes different from both donor strains which generated the recombinant. We believe that these strains represent intra-*Hh-1* recombinants.

TABLE 17. MODIFIED ASSUMPTIONS FOR THE *TRANS* GENE REGULATORY MODEL OF *Hh-1* EXPRESSION: *

1) The regulatory genes are dominant, *trans*-acting and map to the *Hh-1* locus near *H-2D*.

2) The *Hh-1* structural genes are differentially distributed among strains with dissimilar haplotypes and may be linked to *H-2* and the *Hh-1* regulatory locus.

3) The Hh-1 phenotype (expression of determinants 1,2,3, and 4) is directly governed by the presence or absence of the corresponding *Hh-1* regulatory genes, 1',2',3' and 4' and the appropriate structural genes.

4) The Hh-1 phenotype is determined as described in Tables 1-3; the *Hh-1* regulatory genotype is inferred from it. It is of critical importance to analyze F1 hybrids in order to assess the presence or absence of regulatory and structural genes.

5) Bone marrow cells expressing determinants not present on host cells will be rejected provided that the host possesses the proper genetic background for a good rejection response.

* See Tables 4 and 8 for previous models. The modified assumptions are based on the studies of the Hh-1 structural genes (Tables 14,15).

According to a recent listing of intra-*H-2* recombinant mouse strains (Klein et al. 1983), a majority of the crossover events have occurred in the *S/D* interval (Table 16). This could be due to the length of DNA in that interval or, as suggested by Kirsten Lindahl (personal communication), one or more recombinational "hot spots" may exist in this region. Of the *S/D* recombinants, approximately one fourth appear to involve *Hh-1* (Table 16) which may be part of the "hot spot". Because most *Hh-1* types correlate with *H-2DL,* we conclude that *Hh-1* much closer to *D* than to *S*. We are presently analyzing restriction fragment polymorphisms of strains of mice used in this study for the TNF_α tumor necrosis factor/cachectin gene, since the two tumor necrosis factor genes map 70 kilobases 5' of *H-2D* (Muller et al. 1987). This will serve to map *Hh-1* relative to the TNF locus.

The peculiar finding that the stuctural and regulatory genes have separated in the *f* haplotype (Tables 14, 15) supports the idea that the two loci are independent. Studies of the genetic composition of the *f* haplotype may help characterize the *Hh-1* stuctural locus. A modified set of assumptions to explain the genetic control of Hh-1 antigen expression which incorporates the linkage of the *Hh-1* structural loci to *H-2* and to the regulatory genes between *S* and *D* is presented in Table 17. A complete description of the rejection capabilities of various inbred and F1 hybrid mouse strains based on these and other recent experiments is presented in Table 18 to assist in the interpretation of the data presented in this manuscript.

TABLE 18. REJECTION CAPABILITIES OF IRRADIATED RECIPIENTS

STRAIN	*H-2*	EXPRESSES Hh-1 DETERMINANT:	CAN REJECT BMC EXPRESSING DETERMINANTS:
B6,B10	*b*	1,4	2,3
B10.D2	*d*	2	1,3
NZB/BlNJ	*d*	2	1,3,4#
B10.S	*s*	1,2,4	3
B10.Q	*q*	none	1,2,3, but not 4
B10.RIII	*q*	none	1,2,3, but not 4
CxB10.RIII	*d/r*	none	1,2,3, but not 4*
B6xD2,B6xC	*b/d*	none	1,3 but not 2 or 4*
NZBxB6	*d/b*	none	1,2,3,4*#
C3H	*k*	4	3, but not 1,2**
C3HxB6	*k/b*	4	1,2,3
B10.WB	*j*	2,3,4●	1

* (NZBxB6)F1 hybrids are capable of rejecting both *b* and *d* haplotype parental grafts(determinants 1 and 2); however, B6xDBA/2, B6xBalb/c, and B10xB10.D2 F_1's are only capable of rejecting $H\text{-}2^b$ [determinant 1] parental grafts. We recently observed that (BALB/cxB10.RIII)F1 $H\text{-}2^d/H\text{-}2^r$ mice are capable of rejecting *d* haplotype parental grafts.

(NZBxB6)F1 hybrids and NZB/BlNJ detect determinant 4 on $H\text{-}2^k$ BMC grafts which are not immunogenic in other strains.

** C3H are only capable of rejecting grafts expressing determinant 3.

● $H\text{-}2^j$ grafts share determinant 2 with the *d* haplotype and in addition express the unique determinant 3.

REFERENCES

Afifi, M.S., Kumar, V., and Bennett,M.: Stimulation of genetic resistance to marrow grafts in mice by interferon-α/β. *J. Immunol. 134:* 3739, 1985

Bennett, M.: Rejection of marrow allografts. Importance of *H-2* homozygosity of donor cells. *Transplantation 14:* 289, 1972

Bennett, M., Melvold, R.W. and Kohn, H.I.: Bone marrow cell grafts involving the *H-2D* and *H-2L* mutant haplotypes. *Immunogenetics 10:* 273, 1980

Bennett, M.: Biology and Genetics of Hybrid Resistance. *Adv. Immunol. 41:* 433-545, 1987

Eastcott, J.W., Broitman, S.A., and Bennett,M.: Immunogenetic differences between lymph node cell and bone marrow cell grafts in irradiated mice. *Cell. Immunol. 59:* 378, 1981

Clark, E.A., and Harmon, R.C.: Genetic control of natural cytotoxicity and hybrid resistance. *Adv. Cancer Res. 31:* 227, 1980

Cudkowicz, G.: Genetic control of bone marrow graft rejection I. Determinant-specific difference of reactivity in two pairs of inbred mouse strains. *J. Exp. Med. 134:* 281, 1971

Cudkowicz, G.: Natural resistance to foreign hemopoietic and leukemia grafts. *In* G. Cudkowicz, M. Landy, and G. M. Shearer (eds.): *Natural resistance systems against foreign cells, tumors, and microbes,* p.1, Academic Press, New York, 1978

Cudkowicz, G., and Stimpfling, J.H.: Deficient growth of C57BL marrow cells transplanted in F1 hybrid mice. Association with the *Histocompatibility-2* locus. *Immunology 7:* 291, 1964

Cudkowicz, G., and Bennett, M.: Peculiar immunobiology of bone marrow allografts. I. Grafts rejection by irradiated responder mice. *J. Exp. Med. 134:* 83, 1971a

Cudkowicz, G., and Bennett, M.: Peculiar immunobiology of bone marrow allografts. II. Rejection of parental grafts by resistant F1 hybrid mice. *J. Exp. Med. 134:* 1513, 1971b

Klein, J., Figueroa, F., and David, C.S.: *H-2* haplotypes, genes and antigens: Second listing II. The *H-2* complex. *Immunogenetics 17:* 553, 1983

Levy, N.E., Lafuse, W.P., Savarirayan, S., Duran,L., Pease,L. and David,C.S.: Gene order of the *H-2D* region. *Fed. Proc. 44:* 553, 1985

Murphy, W.J., Kumar,V., and Bennett, M.: Rejection of bone marrow allografts by mice with severe combined immune deficiency (SCID): evidence that natural killer cells can mediate the specificity of marrow graft rejection. *J. Exp. Med. 165:* 1212-1217, 1987

Muller, V., Jongeneel, C.V., Nedospasov, S.A., Lindahl, K.F., and Steinmetz,M.: Tumour necrosis factor and lymphotoxin genes map close to *H-2D* in the mouse major histocompatibility complex. *Nature 325:* 265-267, 1987

Rembecki, R.M., Bennett, M., Kumar, V., and Potter, T.A.: Expression of Hemopoietic histocompatibility antigens on *H-2* loss variants of F1 hybrid lymphoma cells: evidence consistent with *trans* gene regulation. *J. Immunol. 138:* 2734-2738, 1987

Tutt, M.M., Kuziel, W.A., Hackett, J.Jr., Bennett, M., Tucker, P.W., and Kumar,V.: Murine natural killer cells do not express functional transcripts of α-,β, or Γ- chain genes of the T cell receptor. *J. Immunol. 137:* 2998-3001, 1986

Tutt, M.M, Schuler, W., Kuziel, W.A., Tucker, P.W., Bennett, M., Bosma, M.J., Kumar, V.: T cell receptor genes do not rearrange or express functional transcripts in natural killer cells of *scid* mice. *J. Immunol. 138:* 2338-2344, 1987

Warner, N.L.: Natural resistance to foreign hemopoietic and leukemia grafts. *In* G. Cudkowicz, M. Landy, and G. M. Shearer (eds.): *Natural resistance systems against foreign cells, tumors, and microbes,* p.12, Academic Press, New York, 1978

INVOLVEMENT OF THE H-2 COMPLEX IN STEROID HORMONE METABOLISM

Marika Pla*, Anna Rocca*, Daniel Gillet*, Jean-Marie Villette**, Jean Fiet** and Laurent Degos*

*U 93 INSERM and **Laboratoire de Pharmacie
Hôpital St. Louis; 2, place du Dr A. Fournier
75010 Paris, France

ABSTRACT. We investigated DNA from mice with different H-2 haplotypes (b, d, f, j, k, p, q, r, s, u, v,). DNA was digested with five restriction enzymes (Eco RI, Taq I, Pvu II, Hind III, and Bgl II) and probed with human 21-OHase cDNA clone. Combined restriction fragment length polymorphism identify six different patterns of endonuclease fragment polymorphism of the murine 21-OHase region. Furthermore, we have investigated the serum level of two steroid hormones (progesterone and corticosterone) in the metabolic pathway involving the 21-OHase. Serum progesterone and corticosterone concentrations exhibit variations according to the H-2 haplotypes of the mice, suggesting that genetic factor(s) identical to or closely linked to the H-2 complex is involved in the control of their metabolism.

INTRODUCTION

Originally, the major histocompatibility antigens were found to be involved in transplantation. The experiments of Zinkernagel and Doherty (1979) expanded our understanding of the actual function of the MHC molecules demonstrating that T lymphocytes can recognize foreign antigens in the context of the major histocompatibility complex (MHC) molecules, a phenomenon called MHC restriction. Nevertheless, there is evidence that the MHC chromosomal segment contains genes which code for products of no known immunological function (class IV - enzyme encoding genes).

In the present report we have been interested in the study of one of these enzymes, the 21-hydroxylase (21-OHase), a key enzyme in the synthesis of glucocorticosteroid and mineralocorticosteroid hormones. The 21-OHase, a cytochrome P-450 enzyme, mediates the 21-hydroxylation of progesterone to desoxycorticosterone or of 17-hydroxyprogesterone to 11-desoxycortisol (Cooper et al. 1965). Mouse and human 21-OHase genes have been cloned and sequenced (Chaplin et al. 1986, Higashi et al. 1986, White et al. 1986).

Since 21-OHase genes are located at the MHC, a highly polymorphic region, information about the extent of their polymorphism is of great interest. The DNA blotting technique provides a simple method for recognizing genomic differences in the form of restriction fragment length polymorphism (RFLP). Furthermore, we have investigated the blood level of two steroid hormones (progesterone and corticosterone) in the metabolic pathway of which the 21-OHase is involved.

MATERIAL AND METHODS

Mice. All mice were bred in our animal house (Mouse Immunogenetics, U93 INSERM) and used at 10 to 16 weeks of age.

Detection of restriction fragment length polymorphism (RFLP). DNA extracted from mouse liver was digested with different restriction enzymes (Eco RI, Taq I, Pvu II, Hind III, and Bgl II). Restriction fragments were subjected to electrophoresis in 0,7 % agarose gel. The DNA fragments were depurinated, denaturated and neutralized before transfer to a hybridization membrane, according to the method of Southern (1975). The human 21-OHase cDNA clone pC21/3c (White et al. 1986), kindly provided by Dr. Bo Dupont (Laboratory of Human Immunogenetics, Memorial Sloan-Kettering Cancer Center, New York) was used for hybridization. Hybridizing restriction fragments were visualized by autoradiography.

Determination of progesterone and corticosterone levels in the mouse serum. Adult male mice were individually bled and equal volume of sera from 2 or 3 mice were pooled and stored at -20 °C. Determination of progesterone and corticosterone in sera were performed using direct radioimmunoassay. Labelled I^{125}-progesterone and progesterone antiserum were provided by Compagnie ORIS Industrie (Saint-Quentin-Yvelines, France). Iodination of corticosterone and production of corticosterone antiserum was performed in the Laboratoire de Pharmacie (Hôpital Saint-Louis, Paris). Corticosterone antiserum was obtained by immunization of rabbit with the hapten-conjugated mouse corticosterone.

Statistical analysis. The one-factor variance and the Student's t test analysis were used to determine the significance level of interstrain differences.

RESULTS AND DISCUSSION

Extensive genomic polymorphism at mouse 21-OHase region. Among the 11 haplotypes tested [$H\text{-}2^b$ (C3H.B10), $H\text{-}2^d$ (B10.D2), $H\text{-}2^f$ (B10.M), $H\text{-}2^j$ (B10.WB), $H\text{-}2^k$ (C3H), $H\text{-}2^p$ (B10.P), $H\text{-}2^q$ (B10.G), $H\text{-}2^r$ (B10.RIII), $H\text{-}2^s$ (B10.S), $H\text{-}2^u$ (B10.PL), $H\text{-}2^v$(B10.SM)] , no 21-OHase RFLP was observed with restriction endonucleases Hind III and Bgl II (data not shown). However, polymorphism of the 21-OHase probe hybridizing sequences was revealed using restriction enzymes Eco RI, Taq I, and Pvu II (Fig. 1, Table 1). Four Eco RI patterns are observed : (a) 3.5 kb, 3.8 kb and 30 kb bands in b and q haplotypes, (b) 3.5 kb, 3.8 kb and ~180 kb bands in d,s and u haplotypes, (c) 3.5 kb, 4 kb and ~180 kb bands in f, j, k, p and r haplotypes and (d) 3.5 kb, 4 kb and 30 kb bands in v haplotype. With Taq I, five patterns are observed : (a) 3.1 kb and 3.4 kb bands in b, d, q and u haplotypes, (b) 3.4 kb and 3.9 kb bands in f, j, k and p haplotypes, (c) 3.2 kb and 3.4 kb bands in r haplotype, (d) 3.4 kb and 3.6 kb bands in s haplotype and (e) 3.1 kb, 3.4 kb and 3.9 kb bands in v haplotype. Using Pvu II, two patterns are evident : (a) unique 2.2 kb band (b, d, f, j, k, p, q, s, u and v) and (b) 2.2 kb and 2.4 kb bands (r). Table 1 summarizes the findings of the genomic analysis. Combined RFLP identify six different patterns of endonuclease fragment length polymorphism at 21-OHase region : (I) in H-2^{b} and H-2^{q} haplotypes, (II) in H-2^{d} and H-2^{u} haplotypes, (III) in H-2^{f}, H-2^{j}, H-2^{k} and H-2^{p} haplotypes, (IV) in H-2^{r} haplotype, (V) in H-2^{s} haplotype and (VI) in H-2^{v} haplotype.

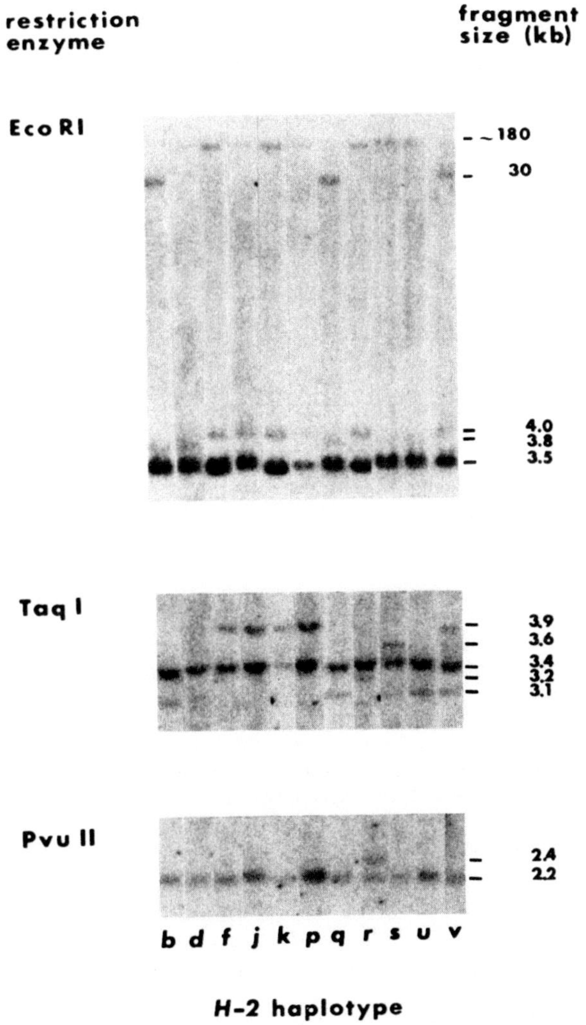

Fig. 1. Southern blot analysis of mouse genomic DNA digested with different restriction endonucleases (Eco RI, Taq I, and Pvu II) using a human 21-OHase probe. The H-2 haplotypes of mice from which DNA was extracted are indicated under the lanes

Table 1. Summary of RFLP patterns of <u>21-OHase</u> regions

Restriction enzyme	Fragment size (kb)	Allele of *S* region										
		b	*d*	*f*	*j*	*k*	*p*	*q*	*r*	*s*	*u*	*v*
Eco RI	~180	−	+	+	+	+	+	−	+	+	+	−
	30	+	−	−	−	−	−	+	−	−	−	+
	4	−	−	+	+	+	+	−	+	−	−	+
	3.8	+	+	−	−	−	−	+	−	+	+	−
	3.5	+	+	+	+	+	+	+	+	+	+	+
	Type	a	b	c	c	c	c	a	c	b	b	d
Taq I	3.9	−	−	+	+	+	+	−	−	−	−	+
	3.6	−	−	−	−	−	−	−	−	+	−	−
	3.4	+	+	+	+	+	+	+	+	+	+	+
	3.2	−	−	−	−	−	−	−	+	−	−	−
	3.1	+	+	−	−	−	−	+	−	−	+	+
	Type	a	a	b	b	b	b	a	c	d	a	e
Pvu II	2.4	−	−	−	−	−	−	−	+	−	−	−
	2.2	+	+	+	+	+	+	+	+	+	+	+
	Type	a	a	a	a	a	a	a	b	a	a	a
	Pattern	I	II	III	III	III	III	I	IV	V	II	VI

Since pC21/3c probe used in our study is a cDNA clone of about 2 kb, lacking only 15 bp of coding sequences on the 5' end (White et al. 1986), it can be argued that the genomic differences described here are those of the <u>C4</u> genes. We examined this possibility, by comparing the RFLP patterns of C4-hybridizing sequences previously described (Sackstein et al. 1984) with those of 21-OHase hybridizing sequences obtained with the same restriction endonucleases (Eco RI, Pvu II and Hind III). Eco RI shows extensive genomic variations with both C4 and 21-OHase probes, although, without any significant correlation. DNA digested with Pvu II shows RFLP when hybridized with 21-OHase probe and not with C4 probe. When DNA is digested with Hind III, the RFLP is obtained only when C4 probe is used for hybridization. Thus, the most straightforward interpretation is that the genomic differences observed may be assigned to variations of the <u>21-OHase</u> gene(s) and/or of flanking region(s).

<u>H-2</u>-associated differences of the steroid hormone levels in the mouse serum. In an attempt to assess the possible influence of the genomic differences at <u>21-OHase</u> region on the metabolism of steroid hormones, we have determined the level of progesterone, a substrate of 21-OHase, in the sera of male mice from various <u>H-2</u> congeneic strains with B10 genetic background (Table 2). Serum progesterone concentrations exhibit variations according to the <u>H-2</u> haplotypes of the mice ($P < 0.05$), suggesting that genetic factor(s) identical to or closely linked to the <u>H-2</u> complex is involved in the control of progesterone metabolism.

Table 2. Progesterone concentrations (ng/ml) in sera of *H-2* congeneic mice on the B10 genetic background

H-2 haplotype	Number of determinations	Serum progesterone concentration (ng/ml) mean	s.d.
b	5	0.531	0.34
d	5	0.773	0.27
f	5	1.148	0.58
j	5	1.891	1.16
k	5	1.488	0.55
p	17	2.670	0.66
q	15	1.602	0.63
r	5	1.585	1.06
s	5	1.288	0.82
u	5	1.224	0.74
v	5	1.725	0.74

Two *H-2* haplotypes (*p* and *q*) having a statistically significant difference in serum progesterone concentrations were chosen for the further investigation. Concentrations of corticosterone, a major 21-OHase dependent corticosteroid in mice, were determined in the sera of mice of these two haplotypes. The $H\text{-}2^p$ mice have significantly ($P < 0.05$) higher serum corticosterone concentrations (42.1 ± 7.4 ng /ml) in comparison with the $H\text{-}2^q$ mice (31.3 ± 3.0 ng/ml). In Figure 2, progesterone values are plotted against corticosterone values (serum samples in which both values were examined). In both haplotypes, higher progesterone values tend to be associated with higher corticosterone values.

The nature of the *H-2* associations with 21-OHase dependent steroid hormone concentrations has not yet been tested in *H-2* recombinant strains which would allow a more precise location within the *H-2* complex. *H-2*-associated variations in progesterone concentrations do not show any correlation with the polymorphic endonuclease fragment length patterns of 21-OHase region. Regardless of whether the *H-2* locus itself or some closely linked gene(s) are involved, these findings point to the frequently discussed nature of association of histocompatibility complex with a number of physiological and pathological traits. Corticosteroids are well-known lympholytic agents. There is increasing evidence that different populations of lymphoid cells vary markedly in their sensitivity to corticosteroids (Ahmed et al. 1985). Thus the genetic factor involved in the regulation of corticosteroid concentration might influence the heterogeneity of the lymphoid cell population and may thus participate in the complex phenomenon of *H-2* influenced immune responses.

A quantitative trait of non-immunological character influenced by the *H-2* complex was described by the pioneer work of Ivanyi and Mickova (1971), who showed that H-2 haplotypes influence vesicular gland weight, with the subsequent extension of this finding to testes, thymus, and lymph node weight (Ivanyi et al. 1972a).The vesicular gland is known to be a target organ for testosterone and indicator of sensitivity to its action. The H-2 associated gene was designated Hom-1 (Hormone metabolism-1) and located in the H-2K-end (Ivanyi et al. 1973, Gregorova and Ivanyi 1973). A more direct involvement of the H-2 complex in regulation of steroid hormone metabolism was indicated by the H-2 influence on blood testosterone and testosterone binding globulin level (Ivanyi et al. 1972, 1976). The H-2 complex has also

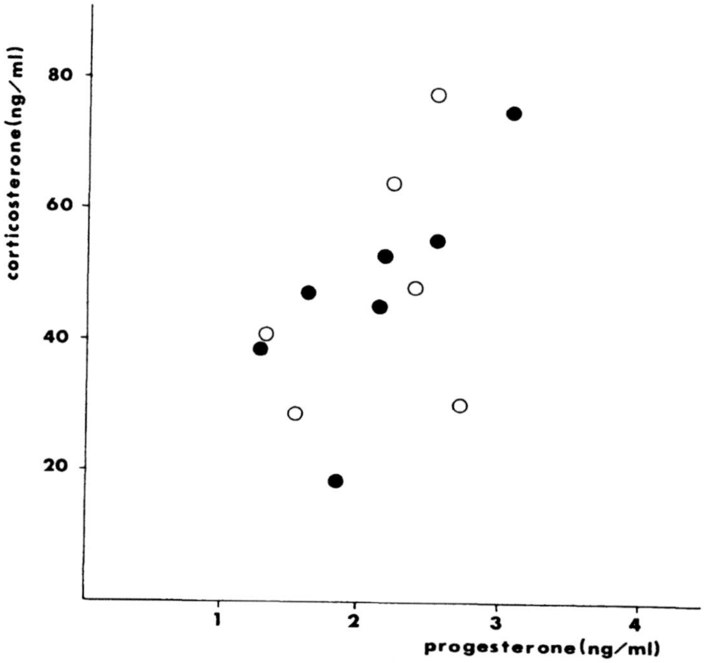

Fig. 2. Serum corticosterone concentration plotted against the serum progesterone concentration in H-2^p (●) and H-2^q (○) mice. Each determination represents pooled serum sample from 2 mice

been shown to influence target sensitivity to cortisone action (Pla et al. 1976), cytosol cortisol-binding protein levels (Goldman et al. 1977), cortisone induced cleft palate (Bonner and Slavkin 1975, Bonner and Tyan 1984) and glucocorticoid receptor levels (Gupta and Goldman 1982). The H-2-influenced traits involved in steroid hormone metabolism represent some acts in the endless list of H-2-phenotypic manifestation called very adequately by Klein (1978) "Théâtre de l'absurde". Quantitative variations in physiological and pathological traits influenced by the H-2 complex were exhaustively reviewed and their consequences thoroughly discussed by Ivanyi

(1978). The many traits found to be influenced by H-2 haplotypes are interrelated. However, some appear to be rather independent and it is quite difficult to find a common denominator. The consequences of these findings are far reaching. Undoubtedly, the genetic differences in such basic phenomena as for instance immune response and steroid hormone level influence also the susceptibility to disease. Described findings on non-immunological functions may be indicative of an area worthy of further study in terms of physiological and pathological functions of the MHC. The future will tell if the MHC belongs only to immunologists, or if it could be explored by many other biologists as well.

Acknowledgments. We thank Dr. Pavol Ivanyi for providing a starting point for this project and for his continued support and interest. We aknowledge Dr. B. Dupont for the kind gift of the probe. We are grateful to Dr. C. Sportes for helping in the manuscript preparation.

REFERENCES

Ahmed, S. A., Penhale, W. J., and Talal, N. : Sex hormones, immune responses, and autoimmune diseases. *Amer. J. Pathol. 121* : 531-551, 1985

Bonner, J. J., and Slavkin H. C. : Cleft palate susceptibility linked to histocompatibility-2 (H-2) in the mouse. *Immunogenetics 2* : 213-218,1975

Bonner, J. J., and Tyan, M. L. : Glucocorticoid-induced cleft palate genes in chromosome 17 : Genetic linkage and mapping analysis. *Immunogenetics 20* :169-183, 1984

Chaplin, D. D., Gailbraith, L. J., Seidman, J. G., White, P. C., and Parher, K. L. : Nucleotide sequence analysis of murine 21-hydroxylase genes : Mutations affecting gene expression. *Proc. Natl. Acad. Sci. U.S.A. 83* 9601-9605, 1986

Cooper, D. Y., Levin, S., Narasimhulu, S., Rosenthal, O., and Estabrook, R.W. : Photochemical action spectrum of the terminal oxydase of mixed function oxydase systems. *Science 147* : 400-402,1965

Goldman, A. S., Katsumata, M., Yaffe, S. J., and Gasser, D. L. : Palatal cytosol cortisol binding protein associated with cleft palate susceptibility and H-2 genotype. *Nature 265* : 643-645, 1977

Gregorova, S., and Ivanyi, P. : H-2 associated genetic differences in androgen-dependent traits. The effects of testosterone injections. *Folia Biol. (Praha) 19* : 337-345, 1973

Gupta, C., and Goldman, A. : H-2 histocompatibility region : Influence on the murine glucocorticoid receptor and its response. *Science 216* : 994-996, 1982

Higashi, Y., Yoshika, H., Yamane, M., Gotoh, O., and Fujii-Kuriyama, Y. : Complete nucleotide sequence of two steroid 21-hydroxylase genes tandemly arranged in human chromosome : A pseudogene and a genuine gene. *Proc. Natl. Acad. Sci. U.S.A. 83* : 2841-2845, 1986

Ivanyi, P. : Some aspects of the H-2 system, the major histocompatibility system in the mouse. *Proc. Roy. Soc. 202* : 117-158, 1978

Ivanyi, P., and Mickova, M. : Further studies on genetic factors in the ninth linkage group influencing reproductive performance in male mice. *In* A. Lengerova and M. Vojtiskova (eds.): *Immunogenetics of the H-2 system,* pp. 104-119, Basel, 1971

Ivanyi, P., Gregorova, S., and Mickova, M. : Genetic differences in thymus, lymph node, testes and vesicular gland weights among inbred mouse strains. Association with the major histocompatibility (H-2) system. *Folia Biol. (Praha) 18* : 81-97, 1972a

Ivanyi, P., Hampl, R., Starka, L., and Mickova, M. : Genetic association between H-2 gene and testosterone metabolism in mice. *Nature 238* : 280-281, 1972b

Ivanyi, P., Gregorova, S., Mickova, M., Hampl, R., and Starka, L. : Genetic association between histocompatibility gene (H-2) and androgen metabolism in mice. *Transplant. Proc. V (1)* : 189-191, 1973

Ivanyi, P., Hampl, P., Mickova, M., ans Starka, L. : The influence of the H-2 system on blood serum testosterone level. *Folia Biol. (Praha) 22* : 42-43, 1976

Klein, J. : H-2 mutations : Their genetics and effect on immune functions. *Adv. Immunol. 26* : 55-146, 1978

Pla, M;, Zakany, J; and Fachet, J. : H-2 influence on corticosteroid effects on thymus cells. *Folia Biol. (Praha) 22* : 49-50, 1976

Sackstein, R., Roos, M. H., Démant, P., and Colten, H. R. : Subdivision of the S region of the mouse major histocompatibility complex by identification of genomic polymorphism of the class III genes.*Immunogenetics 20* :321-330 1984

Southern, E. M. : Detection of specific sequences among DNA fragments separated by gel electrophoresis; *J. Mol. Biol. 98* : 503-517, 1975

White, P. C., New, M. I., and Dupont, B. : Structure of human steroid 21-hydroxylase genes. *Proc. Natl. Acad. Sci. U.S.A. 83* : 5111-5115, 1986

Zinkernagel, R. M., and Doherty, P. C. : MHC-restricted cytotoxic T cells : Studies on the biological role of polymorphic major transplantation antigens determining T cell restriction-specificity. *Adv. Immunol.27* : 51-77, 1979

SOME RECENT DATA ON THE Q-SUBREGION GENES AND THEIR PRODUCTS

Lorraine Flaherty

Wadsworth Center for Laboratories and Research
New York State Department of Health
Albany, New York 12201

INTRODUCTION

For the last ten years we have concentrated our studies on the Q genes of the murine major histocompatibility complex (MHC). These genes determine a series of class I molecules which are 80-90% homologous to the more classical H-2K and H-2D genes. Because of this homology, we have frequently hypothesized that these genes have an important function in the immune system. However, recent data showing large deletions in the Q subregion, without any overt effects on survival, have cast some doubt on this hypothesis.

In this report, I would like to survey some of the more recent data on the Q-subregion genes and their products. These data indicate that the Q region may have several unique characteristics.

MOLECULAR GENETICS

Genetic Loci

Both Weiss et al. (1984) and Steinmetz et al. (1982) have provided us with information on the genetic organization of the Q subregion. The Q subregion is defined by the recombinational events which have occurred in the B6.K1 and B6.K2 congenic strains (Flaherty et al., 1985b). Ten class I genes have been identified in the Q subregion of the B10 haplotype. These are numbered from Q1 to Q10. Most of these genes appear functional and are transcribed and translated into protein (Mellor et al., 1985). However, so far only two of these protein products (Q6/Q8 and Q7) have been found on the cell surface after gene transfection (Flaherty et al., 1985a; Waneck et al., 1987). Both of these cell surface products were identified with anti-Qa-2 reagents. Recent evidence from Widacki and Cook (1987) suggests that a product of the Q7 locus is the predominant molecule which appears on the normal lymphocyte cell surface. Table 1 gives a summary of our knowledge of these genes and their products.

Alleles and Polymorphism

Because of the high degree of homology among the Q subregion genes, it has been difficult to define allelism. This situation is especially

Table 1. Genes of the Q subregion of the murine MHC

Gene	Evidence for Transcription?	Protein Product?	Cell surface Expression?	Reference[a]
Q1	no	--	--	1
Q2	no	--	--	1
Q3	no	--	--	1,2
Q4	yes	yes	?	1,3
Q5	no	--	--	1
Q6[b]	yes	yes	yes	1,4
Q7	yes	yes	yes	1,5
Q8[b]	yes	yes	yes	1,4
Q9	yes	yes	?	1,6
Q10	yes	yes	no?	7

[a]References are as follows: (1) Mellor et al., 1984; (2) Weiss et al., 1984; (3) Robinson, 1985; Robinson and Mellor, 1986; Palmer and Frelinger, 1987; (4), Flaherty et al., 1985a; (5) Waneck et al., 1987; (6) Fahrner et al., 1987; (7) Cosman et al., 1982; Mellor et al., 1984; Kress et al., 1983.
[b]The *Q6* and *Q8* genes and their products appear identical.

evident when the *Q6/Q8* and *Q7/Q9* pairs are involved; *Q6* is indistinguishable from *Q8* by restriction-fragment-length-polymorphisms (RFLPs) or by preliminary sequence analysis and there is only one known base pair difference between *Q7* and *Q9* (Weiss et al., 1985, Devlin et al., 1985, Eastman O'Neill et al., 1986). (Because *Q6* cannot be distinguished from *Q8*, we often consider these two genes jointly.) Thus without knowledge of the order of these genes in a particular genotype, it is impossible to ascribe an allele to one member of a particular pair. Nevertheless certain principles can be noted. In RFLP analyses of Q-subregion families, certain Q genes appear to have allelic variants while others do not (Weiss et al., 1984, Siwarski et al.,1985; Palmer and Frelinger, 1987; Eastman O'Neill et al., 1986). Notably, the Q6 through Q10 region has the least variation. These data agree with the serological and biochemical data which show a low degree of polymorphism for this region.

Large deletions can also occur in this subregion and span several Q genes. For example, in the *H-2*^{f} haplotype, the area between *Q1* and *Q9* (and perhaps *Q10*) is deleted while in the *H-2*^{k} and *H-2*^{d} haplotypes shorter stretches are missing. These conclusions were based on Southern blot analyses with low-copy number probes which hybridize to specific families of Q-subregion genes (Eastman O'Neill et al., 1986).

Unfortunately it is difficult to correlate these individual genes and their alleles with previous data from serological studies. Qa-2 was the first serologically defined cell surface antigen known to be determined by this region. Subsequently several other Q-subregion serological specificities were defined and distinguished from Qa-2 by their different tissue and strain distributions. However, the co-immunoprecipitation experiments of Widacki et al (1985) have shown that most if not all of these specificities appear on the same molecule(s). Thus it is unclear whether separate genes determine these specificities or whether there are linked modifying genes. Conceivably, alternate splicing of the Q genes could also lead to the appearance of new specificities. Transfection experiments have still not clarified these relationships. Presumably some of the difficulties in these studies stem from our inability to distinguish between the highly homologous Q-subregion gene products.

RNA transcription studies

The transcription of several genes in the Q region have been extensively studied--Q10 (Cosman et al., 1982; Mellor et al., 1984; Lalanne et al., 1985), Q7/Q9 (Waneck et al., 1987; Fahrner et al., 1987), Q4 (Palmer and Frelinger, 1987) and Q6/Q8 (Elliott et al., 1987). Several of these genes appear to be transcribed in a manner different from H-2K and H-2D.

Q10. The Q10 gene was originally identified by its liver-specific mRNA transcript (Cosman et al., 1982). This transcript could be distinguished from other class I mRNAs by its somewhat smaller size (1.7kb instead of 1.8kb) and its tissue-specific expression. Further work has shown that there are at least two additional minor Q10 transcripts of sizes 1.6 kb and 1.4 kb. One of these shortened forms has been found in a cDNA library and is due to an alternate splice site which joins exon 2 to exon 4 (Lalanne et al., 1985). So far only the protein product of the predominant Q10 species has been found.

Q7/Q9. Similar to Q10, there are at least three different Q7 transcripts (Waneck et al., 1987; Fahrner et al., 1987). These are sized at 1.2 kb, 1.5 kb, and 1.8 kb; the predominant transcript is 1.2 kb in size and codes for an mRNA which is missing exons 4, 5, 7, and part of 8. However transfection experiments have shown that the larger 1.5 kb mRNA codes for the cell surface Qa-2 molecule detectable with monoclonal antibodies. It is not known whether the 1.2 kb RNA codes for a functional protein. Fahrner et al (1987) have also examined Q9 gene transcripts; these appear similar to the Q7 varieties.

Q4. The Q4 transcript has been examined in the $H\text{-}2^p$ haplotype (Palmer and Frelinger, 1987). This gene is transcribed in most tissues of the body but in varying amounts. Only one form of size 1.7 kb has so far been noted.

Q6/Q8. By use of a congenic strains and a Q4/Q6/Q8-specific probe, Elliott et al (1987) have identified a unique Q6/Q8 transcript. This transcript is 2.2 kb in size and is larger than any known class I mRNA. Probes to DNA segments located 3' to the normal polyadenylation signal have revealed that this larger size is due to an extension of the 3' end. Although transfection studies have shown that the Q6/Q8 gene can code for a cell surface Qa-2-like protein, no functional studies have yet been performed to determine if this longer transcript actually codes for this protein.

BIOCHEMISTRY

Six of the Q-subregion genes are known to determine protein products (Table 1). With the possible exception of Q10, all of these products are detectable with anti-Qa-2 antisera or monoclonal reagents. Early immunoprecipitation and serological studies suggested that the cell surface molecule (or molecules) detectable with these anti-Qa-2 reagents was distinct from other class I molecules (Michaelson et al., 1981). Qa-2 was significantly smaller in size than H-2K and H-2D (by approximately 5000 daltons). Moreover, it could be easily modulated off the cell surface by specific antibody (Flaherty et al., 1985b; Widacki et al., 1985). More recent work on the genetic structure of the Q-subregion genes have defined these distinctions more clearly. First, all of the known and functional Q-subregion genes have a stop codon in exon 5 (Steinmetz et al., 1981; Devlin et al., 1985; Mellor et al., 1984). This truncated state results in a somewhat smaller molecule with a shortened transmembrane domain and no cytoplasmic one.

Second, at least some of these molecules are secreted. Q10 appears in mouse serum while at least one of the Qa-2 antigen-bearing molecules is secreted after Concanavalin A stimulation (Maloy et al., 1984; Soloski et al., 1986; Robinson, 1987a and b). In the case of Qa-2 there is still some controversy on the origin of these secreted molecules, i.e. whether the cell surface and secreted molecules are derived from a single precursor or from two different ones. Alternate splicing of the Q gene mRNAs may also be involved.

Third, and perhaps more importantly, Stiernberg et al (1987) have recently found that the Qa-2 molecule(s) is anchored to the cell surface via phosphatidylinositol. This observation is in sharp contrast to that seen for other class I molecules which seem to span the cell membrane and possess no such anchorage. The significance of this cell surface attachment is not understood; however, this phenomenon may help to explain the unusual modulating capability of this molecule as well as its appearance in supernatants from mitogen-activated cell cultures.

Moreover, it is very tempting to speculate that this attachment to phosphatidylinositol has some functional significance. There are only a few molecules that are known to anchored in this manner. These include alkaline phosphatase, 5'nucleotidase, acetylcholinesterase, variant surface glycoprotein antigen of trypanosomes, Thy-1, decay-accelerating factor, RT-6 antigen, Ly-6, and ThB (Low et al., 1986). Phosphatidylinositol metabolism is intimately connected to growth regulation and lymphocyte activation. The cleavage of phosphatidylinositol-linked membrane proteins will lead to the liberation of 1,2-diacylglycerol which has been implicated as a second messenger for various cell surface receptors (Berridge, 1984). In light of this anchorage, it is certainly conceivable that activation signals may be mediated through Thy-1 or Qa types of molecules. This hypothesis is strengthen by the recent observation of Warner et al (1987a and b) that genes in the Q region seem to control the speed of early development in the pre-implantation mouse embryo. However, the identity of these Q-subregion genes is unknown.

ACKNOWLEDGMENTS

Some of the work reported from the author's laboratory was supported by NIH grant GM 37947 awarded by the National Institute of General Medical Sciences.

REFERENCES

Berridge, M. J., 1984, Inositol trisphosphate and diacylglycerol as second messengers, Biochem. J. 220:345.

Cosman, D., Kress, M., Khoury, G., and Jay, G., 1982, Tissue-specific expression of an unusual H-2 (class I)-related gene, Proc. Natl. Acad. Sci. USA, 79:4947.

Devlin, J. J., Weiss, E. H., Paulson, M., and Flavell, R. A., 1985, Duplicated pairs and alleles of class I genes in the Qa2 region of the murine major histocompatibility complex: a comparison, EMBO J, 4:3203.

Eastman O'Neill, A., Reid, K., Garberi, J. C., Karl, M., and Flaherty, L., 1986, Extensive deletions in the Q subregion of the murine major histocompatibility complex, Immunogenetics, 24:368.

Elliott, E., Karl, M., and Flaherty, L., 1987, Novel mRNA species from a Q-subregion class I gene of the murine major histocompatibility complex, Gene, in press.

Fahrner, K., Hogan, B. L. M., and Flavell, R. A., 1987, Transcription of H-2 and Qa genes in embryonic and adult mice. EMBO J., 6:1265.
Flaherty, L., DiBiase, K., Lynes, M. A., Seidman, J. G., Weinberger, O., and Rinchik, E. M., 1985a, Characterization of a subregion gene in the murine major histocompatibility complex. Proc. Natl. Acad. Sci USA, 82:1503.
Flaherty, L., Karl, M., and DiBiase, K., 1985b, The Qa series of antigens. in "Cell Biology of the Major Histocompatibility Complex," B. Pernis and H. J. Vogel, eds., Academic Press, New York.
Kress, M., Cosman, D., Khoury, G., and Jay, G, 1983, Secretion of a transplantation-related antigen, Cell 34:189.
Lew, A. M., McCluskey, J., Maloy, W. L., Margulies, D. H., and Coligan, J. E.,1987, Multiple class I molecules generated from single genes by alternative splicing of pre-mRNAs, Immunol. Res., 6:117.
Low, M. G., Ferguson, M. A. J., Futerman, A. H., and Silman, I., 1986, Covalently attached phosphatidylinositol as a hydrophobic anchor for membrane proteins, Trends Biochem. Sci., 11:212.
Mellor, A. L., Weiss, E. H., Kress, M., Jay, G., and Flavell, R. A., 1984, A nonpolymorphic class I gene in the murine major histocompatibility complex, Cell, 36:139.
Maloy, W. L., Coligan, J. E., Barra, J., and Jay, G., 1984, Detection of a secreted form of the murine H-2 class I antigen with an antibody against its predicted carboxyl terminus, Proc. Natl. Acad. Sci. USA, 82:5920.
Mellor, A. L., Antoniou, J., and Robinson, P. J., 1985, Structure and expression of genes encoding murine Qa-2 class I antigens, Proc. Natl. Acad. Sci. USA, 82:5920.
Michaelson, J., Flaherty, L., Bushkin, Y., and Yudkowitz, H., 1981, Further biochemical data on Qa-2. Immunogenetics, 14:129.
Palmer, M. J. and Frelinger, J. A., 1987, Widespread transcription of a Qa region gene in adult mice, J. Exp. Med., 166:95.
Robinson, P. J., 1985, Qb-1, a new class I polypeptide encoded by the Qa region of the mouse H-2 complex, Immunogenetics 22:285.
Robinson, P. J. and Mellor, A., 1986, Identification of a class I polypeptide encoded by the murine Q4 gene, Sixth Internatl. Congr. of Immunol., p.151.
Robinson, P. J., 1987a, Structure and expression of polypeptides encoded in the mouse Qa region, Immunol. Res., 6:46.
Robinson, P. J., 1987b, Two different biosynthetic pathways for the secretion of Qa region-associated class I antigens by mouse lymphocytes, Proc. Natl. Acad. Sci. USA, 84:527.
Siwarski, D. F., Barra, Y., Jay, G., Rogers, M. J., 1985, Occurrence of a unique MHC class I gene in distantly related members of the genus Mus, Immunogenetics, 21:267.
Soloski, M. J., Vernachio, J., Einhorn, G., and Lattimore, A., 1986, Qa gene expression: Biosynthesis and secretion of Qa-2 molecules in activated T cells, Proc. Natl. Acad. Sci. USA, 83:2949.
Steinmetz, M., Moore, K. w., Frelinger, J. G., Sher, B. T. Shen, F-W., Boyse E. A., and Hood, L., 1981, A pseudogene homologous to mouse transplantation antigens: transplantation antigens are encoded by eight exons that correlate with protein domains, Cell 25:683.
Steinmetz, M., Winoto, A., Minard, K., and Hood, L., 1982, Clusters of genes encoding mouse transplantation antigens, Cell, 28:489.
Stiernberg, J., Low, M. G., Flaherty, L., and Kincade, P. W., 1987, Removal of lymphocyte surface molecules with phosphatidylinositol-specific phospholipase C: Effects on mitogen responses and evidence that ThB and certain Qa antigens are membrane-anchored via phosphatidylinositol, J. of Immunol., 38:3877.

Waneck, G. L., Sherman, D. H., Calvin, S., Allen, H, and Flavell, R. A., 1987, Tissue-specific expression of cell-surface Qa-2 antigen from a transfected $Q7^b$ gene of C57BL/10 mice, J. Exp. Med., 165:1358.

Warner, C. M., Gollnick, S. O., and Goldbard, S. B., 1987, Lineage of pre-implantation-embryo-development (Ped) gene in the mouse major histocompatibility complex (MHC), Biol. of Reprod. 36:606.

Warner, C. M., Gollnick, S. O., Flaherty, L., and Goldbard, S. B., 1987, Analysis of Qa-2 antigen expression by preimplantation mouse embryos. Possible relationship to the Ped gene product, Biol. of Reprod. 36:611.

Weiss, E. H., Golden, L., Fahrner, K., Mellor, A. L., Devlin, J. J., Bullman, H., Tiddens, H., Bud, H., and Flavell, R. A., 1984, Organization and evolution of the class I gene family in the major histocompatibility complex of the C57BL/10 mouse, Nature 310:650.

Widacki, S. M., Flaherty, L., and Cook, R., 1985, Biochemical characterization of the molecules reactive with Qa-6 antiserum and monoclonal antibody 20-8-4. Evidence for structural similarity with the Qa-2 molecule. J. Immunol. 135:3333.

Widacki, S. M. and Cook, R. G., 1987, Evidence for multiple distinct Qa-2 antiserum reactive polypeptides, Federation Proceedings, 46:943.

THE EVOLUTION OF MHC CLASS II GENES WITHIN THE GENUS *MUS*

Edward K. Wakeland, Roy W. Tarnuzzer, Cheng-Chan Lu, Wayne Potts, Richard A. McIndoe, William S. Talbot, and Thomas J. McConnell

Laboratory of Molecular Biology
Department of Pathology
University of Florida
Gainesville, FL 32610

INTRODUCTION

The class II genes of the *I* region in the murine major histocompatibility complex (*H-2*) are a tightly-linked cluster of highly polymorphic genes which control immune responsiveness (reviewed by Klein 1986). A physical map of the *I* region has been produced, and the expressed class II genes (*A*α, *A*β, *E*α, and *E*β) are present on a segment of about 100 kilobases (kb) of DNA (Steinmetz *et al.* 1982). The *A*α, *A*β, and *E*β genes are remarkably polymorphic. About 30 alleles of each gene are estimated to be prevalent in natural mouse populations (Duncan *et al.* 1979, Wakeland and Klein 1981), with major alleles differing in 5 to 10% of their nucleotide sequence (Benoist *et al.* 1983, Estess *et al.* 1986). Serologic studies have demonstrated that many of these alleles are globally-distributed with frequencies ranging from 1% to 10% in wild mouse populations (Gotze *et al.* 1980, Nadeau *et al.* 1981). *H-2* polymorphism is thought to be advantageous in natural mouse populations due to the adaptive value of diversifying the capacities of individuals to respond to endemic microbial pathogen. However, the precise evolutionary mechanisms responsible for the production and maintenance of this polymorphism are unknown.

We have been studying the polymorphisms of class II genes in natural mouse populations with the hope of gaining some insights into the evolutionary mechanisms responsible for their generation and maintenance. In this review, we discuss three aspects of our findings. First, we describe our results on the evolutionary origins of contemporary *I* region alleles and present data supporting the notion that class II genes diversify via a transspecies mode of evolution. Second, we describe the distribution of class II alleles among local mouse populations and demonstrate that even small, local mouse populations are highly diversified for *H-2*. Finally, we discuss the role of recombination in the diversification of *I* region haplotypes and present data supporting the presence of a recombinational hot spot between the *A*α*A*β gene duplex and *E*β.

EVOLUTIONARY ORIGINS OF Aβ ALLELES

Two competing hypotheses currently dominate speculations about H-2 diversity. The first suggests that new alleles are generated by specialized hypermutational mechanisms (i.e. "gene conversion or segmental exchange") which operate on specific sites within H-2 genes (Pease 1985, Mengle-Gaw and McDevitt 1985). This mechanism rapidly diversifies those regions of H-2 genes which modify immune responsiveness and advantageous variants increase in frequency in natural mouse populations due to selective pressures mediated by endemic pathogens. The result is a dynamic state of diversification which can potentially adapt rapidly to changes in the antigenicity of endemic pathogens. The second hypothesis, commonly termed "transspecies evolution", proposes that several MHC alleles are commonly incorporated into the gene pools of new species (Klein 1980, Klein and Figueroa 1987). Consequently, the point of divergence between contemporary MHC alleles is not limited by the age of the species in which they are found, and the diversification of MHC allomorphs can occur by mutational and selective mechanisms operating for extremely long periods. This hypothesis emphasizes the importance of mechanisms operating to maintain MHC diversity in natural populations in the evolution of contemporary alleles and argues that no unique hypermutational mechanisms are required to explain MHC polymorphism. The two hypotheses generate different predictions concerning the age of H-2 alleles. The segmental exchange hypothesis predicts that most of the polymorphism will be generated within the lifetime of the species, whereas the transspecies hypothesis predicts that diversity is generated over much longer evolutionary periods, with polymorphisms persisting through speciation events.

The genus *Mus* is an excellent model system in which to assess the age of contemporary MHC alleles. Speciation within *Mus* has been extensively studied and a variety of closely-related species and subspecies have been characterized (Sage 1981, Ferris *et al.* 1983, Marshall 1986). Several subspecies of the commensal house mouse, *Mus musculus*, have been defined which include: *Mus m. musculus* in eastern Europe; *Mus m. domesticus* which originated in western Europe and subsequently spread to the Americas and many islands in association with the global movements of Europeans; and *Mus m. castaneus* in Asia. Biochemical and molecular genetic studies indicate that these subspecies diverged approximately 1-2 million years ago. Two "aboriginal" mouse species which are related to the *Mus musculus* complex have also been carefully studied: *Mus hortulanus* which are mound-building mice found in grain fields in the steppe of eastern Europe; and *Mus spretus* which are found in fields along the western rim of the Mediterranean Sea. Biochemical, molecular genetic, and fossil evidence indicate that these species diverged from the *Mus musculus* complex 3-4 million years ago.

We recently completed a molecular genetic analysis of the I region diversity in a collection of 49 H-2 haplotypes derived from these 5 *Mus* species (McConnell *et al.* 1987). The panel of H-2 haplotypes included 13 haplotypes of standard laboratory mice and 36 haplotypes extracted from wild mouse populations (Zaleska-Rutzynska and Klein 1979, Duncan and Klein 1980, Wakeland *et al.* 1987). Genomic DNA from each mouse strain or cell line was digested with each of 7 restriction endonucleases and analyzed by Southern blot hybridization. A total of 31 Aβ alleles were distinguished among the 49 independently-derived H-2 haplotypes by this restriction fragment length polymorphism (RFLP) analysis. The nucleotide sequence homologies among the 31 Aβ alleles were estimated by calculating the fraction of restriction fragments (F) shared by pairs of alleles according to the method described by Nei and Li (1979). The purpose of this analysis was to compare the sequence divergence of Aβ alleles between *Mus* species. As illustrated in Table 1, this analysis ordered the 31 Aβ alleles into 3 distinct groups. Alleles within a group shared on average 66% of their restriction fragments (mean $F=0.66 \pm 0.14$) while alleles in separate groups shared on average 15.4% (mean $F=0.154 \pm 0.06$, $p < 0.0001$). These results indicate that 3 structurally-distinct genomic forms of Aβ are prevalent among the alleles tested.

The Mus species from which these Aβ alleles were derived are presented in Table 1. The majority of the Aβ alleles (28/31) were in either Evolutionary group 1 or 2, and each group contained alleles derived from 4 separate Mus species. These findings are consistent with the transspecies evolution of Aβ and contrast with data obtained when other nuclear genes or mitochondrial DNA polymorphisms were analyzed in these populations (Sage 1981, Ferris et al. 1983). For example, an RFLP analysis of the class III

Table 1. Definition of 3 Evolutionary Groups of Aβ Allele by Quantitative RFLP Analysis

Evolutionary Group	No. of Aβ Alleles	F Values[a] Within Group	F Values[a] Between Groups	Mus species[b]
1	14	0.65 ± 0.14	0.15 ± 0.06	m. domesticus m. musculus m. castaneus hortulanus
2	14	0.66 ± 0.14	0.15 ± 0.06	m. domesticus m. musculus hortulanus spretus
3	3	0.66 ± 0.05	0.13 ± 0.07	m. domesticus

[a]F values were calculated as described previously (McConnell et al. 1986). The results are based on RFLP analysis with restriction endonucleases Bam HI, Eco RI, Hind III, Pst I, Pvu II, Bgl II, and Sac I. The mean ± S.D. values obtained when comparing all Aβ alleles within the same group, or when comparing all Aβ alleles in one group with all Aβ alleles in other groups are presented.
[b]The Mus species origins of these mouse strains are described in detail elsewhere (Sage 1981, Wakeland et al. 1987).

MHC genes in these same strains demonstrated that their diversity correlated closely with the species-origin of the genome (Falus et al. 1987). These results indicate that even closely-linked genes within the H-2 complex can evolve by distinct mechanisms.

The structural basis for the extensive sequence variation between Aβ alleles in Evolutionary groups 1 and 2 was determined by comparing the published genomic sequences of $A\beta^d$ (Evolutionary group 1, Malissen et al. 1983) and $A\beta^b$ (Evolutionary group 2, Larhammer et al. 1983). As shown in Figure 1, the majority of the genomic polymorphisms distinguishing these two alleles occur in the intron separating the Aβ1 and Aβ2 exons. The sequence homology in this intron is less than 90%, and $A\beta^b$ contains 861 bps of sequence which are absent in $A\beta^d$. Analysis of the inserted sequence demonstrated that it consists entirely of a combination of short interspersed repetitive elements (SINEs), flanked by 13 bp direct repeats of host-derived sequence. SINE elements are highly repetitive DNA sequences which are found randomly inserted at locations throughout the genome (Houck et al. 1979). SINE elements are commonly termed retrotransposons because

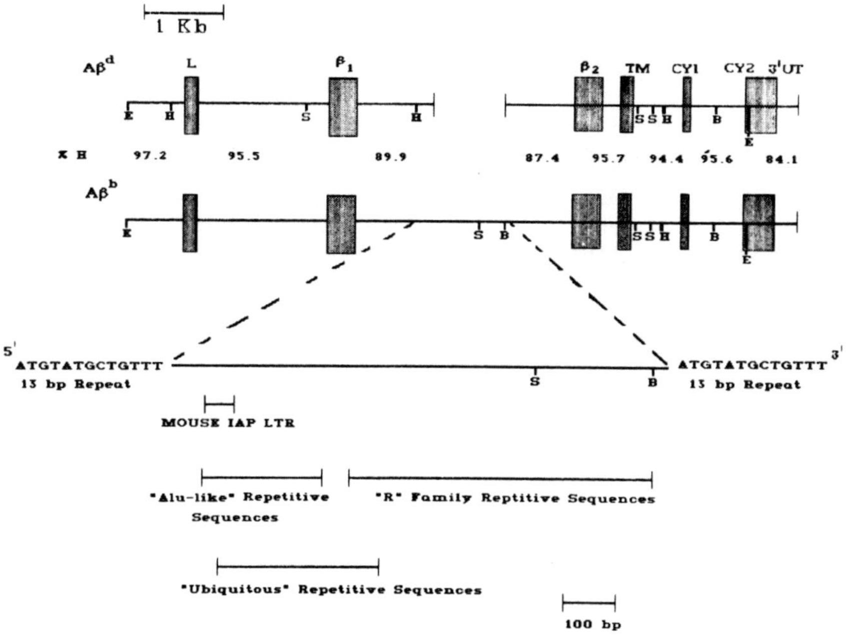

Fig. 1. An analysis of the sequence homology of $\underline{A}\beta^d$ (group 1) and $\underline{A}\beta^b$ (group 2) from sequences available in the Genetic Sequences Data Bank (Genbank). The sequence homologies (%H) of the introns and flanking regions are shown and the exons of each allele are identified by closed boxes. The area in $\underline{A}\beta^b$ between the dashed lines represents the 861 bp insertion sequence and an expanded version of this sequence is presented below $\underline{A}\beta^b$. The 13 bp host-derived direct repeats which flank the inserted sequence are presented on either side of the insert and the regions which are homologous to various SINEs are labelled.

they are thought to mobilize via RNA intermediates (Jagadeeswaran, 1981). The flanking direct repeats of host-derived sequences on either side of the retrotransposon in $\underline{A}\beta^b$ indicate that this SINE element inserted into this position as a random event during the evolutionary divergence of $\underline{A}\beta$.

Inspection of the restriction maps of $\underline{A}\beta^b$ and $\underline{A}\beta^d$ (Figure 1) suggests that this retrotransposon polymorphism is the major distinguishing characteristic of the genomic structures of $\underline{A}\beta$ alleles in Evolutionary groups 1 and 2. This possibility might be tested by probing the $\underline{A}\beta$ alleles in our panel with the inserted sequence, however, this experiment could not be performed because the insert consists entirely of repetitive sequences. Therefore, we searched for the presence of the retrotransposon by genomic restriction mapping of all the $\underline{A}\beta$ alleles in Evolutionary groups 1 and 2. Representative genomic restriction maps of alleles derived from separate Mus species are presented in Figure 2. The results indicate that the retrotransposon is characteristic of $\underline{A}\beta$ alleles in Evolutionary group 2, indicating that the Evolutionary groups defined by RFLP analysis represent alleles with different retrotransposon polymorphisms. This suggestion is consistent with the results of Choi et al. (1983), who demonstrated that the intron separating the $\underline{A}\beta1$ and $\underline{A}\beta2$ exons had different lengths in $\underline{A}\beta^d$ (group 1), $\underline{A}\beta^b$ (group 2), and $\underline{A}\beta^k$ (group 3).

In summary, our findings establish an evolutionary framework with which to interpret the polymorphism of Aβ. The presence of indistinguishable retrotransposon polymorphisms in multiple modern Mus species strongly supports a transspecies mode of evolution for Aβ. The divergence of the 3 Evolutionary groups defined by the retrotransposon polymorphisms is depicted in Figure 3. Our data indicate that Evolutionary group 2 was formed by a retrotransposon insertion into a group 1 Aβ allele. We propose that this

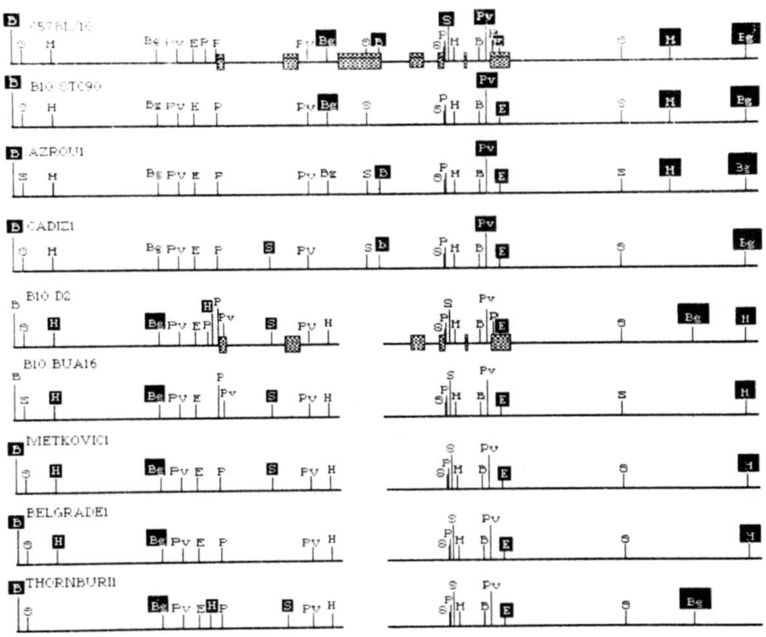

Fig. 2. Representative restriction maps of Aβ alleles in Evolutionary groups 1 and 2. The top 4 alleles are in group 1 and the bottom 5 are in group 2. The strain of origin of each allele is listed above each map on the left. The restriction maps of alleles in group 1 and 2 were aligned by inserting a gap in the group 1 alleles at the site of the insert in group 2 so that the overall homology outside of this region is more apparent. Restriction sites assayed: B, Bam HI; S, Sac I; H, Hind III; Bg, Bgl II; Pv, Pvu II; E, Eco RI; P, Pst I.

event occurred in an ancestral Mus species at least 3-4 million years ago. Subsequently, alleles with and without the retrotransposon persisted as Aβ polymorphisms through several speciations and now both forms are present in multiple modern Mus species. Evolutionary group 3, which we only found in laboratory H-2 haplotypes and Mus m. domesticus, appears to have been derived from an Evolutionary group 2 allele by an additional insertion and/or duplication event effecting the same intron (C.C. Lu, C. Zack, and E.K. Wakeland, unpublished results). These results suggest that

Evolutionary group 3 may have arisen in Mus m. domesticus, however, a larger sampling of H-2 haplotypes from other species would be required to rule out a more ancient origin.

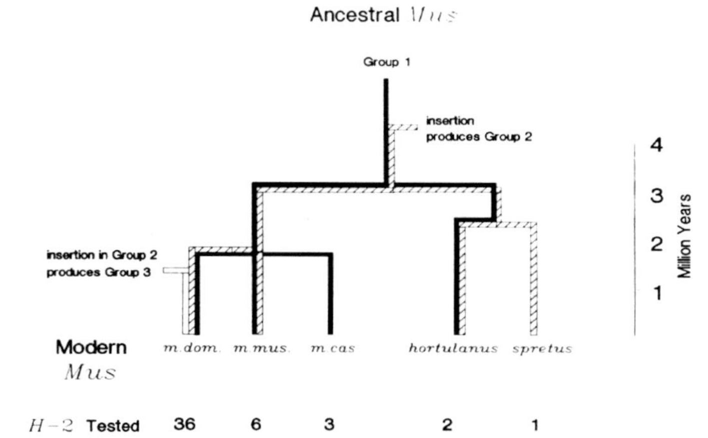

Fig. 3. Illustration of the evolutionary origins of 3 Evolutionary groups of Aβ alleles. The solid line represents group 1, the hatched line group 2, and the open line group 3 alleles.

THE DISTRIBUTION OF Aβ EVOLUTIONARY GROUPS IN WILD MOUSE POPULATIONS

Several features of Aβ diversity in wild mice can be assessed by analyzing the distribution of alleles among natural mouse populations. The retrotransposon polymorphism that distinguishes Evolutionary groups 1 and 2 is a convenient evolutionary tag with which to trace the distribution of these two large groups of Aβ alleles in natural mouse populations. We have categorized a large collection of Aβ alleles into Evolutionary groups 1 and 2. These alleles were derived from wild mouse populations trapped in a variety of geographical areas and from several specific local populations in Florida. In this section, we will discuss the distribution of these two forms of Aβ in wild mouse populations and discuss the data in the context of transspecies evolution, the maintenance of Aβ polymorphism, and the possible functional significance of the two evolutionary groups.

The persistence of genetic polymorphisms during speciation (i.e. transspecies evolution) simply requires that the polymorphisms be present in the founding gene pool and not lost via genetic drift during any population "bottlenecks" which accompany speciation. The critical factors that influence the loss of alleles during speciation are the size of the founding population and the distribution of alleles. If a species is founded by a single pair (the Adam and Eve mode of speciation), then a maximum of 4 alleles would be present at any locus and the probability of decreased polymorphism due to genetic drift would be high. However, if the founding population contained enough individuals so that most allelic forms were carried by a large number of individuals, then the persistance of allelic polymorphisms at highly polymorphic loci such as H-2 during speciation is quite probable (see Hartl 1980 for rates of loss of neutral alleles in relation to population size and allelic frequencies). For example, geological events such as glaciation would subdivide and isolate large populations of the parental species and consequently promote allopatric speciation events that could preserve much of the original genetic polymorphisms. Thus, as has been previously suggested (Klein and Figueroa 1987), a transspecies mode of evolution may be common.

Transspecies evolution predicts that Aβ alleles from both Evolutionary groups should be broadly distributed in the global population, since both forms would have been present prior to the global radiation of *Mus*. We assessed the distribution of Aβ alleles from these two groups in 80 independently-derived H-2 haplotypes from wild mice trapped at 22 separate geographic locations. Representative results are summarized in Table 2.

Table 2. Geographic distribution of wild mouse populations containing Aβ alleles derived from Evolutionary groups 1, 2, and 3

Geographic location of wild mouse populations	No. of Aβ alleles tested[a]	Aβ Evolutionary group found[b]
Rottenburg, W. Germany[c]	4	2
Viborg, Denmark	3	1
Metkovic, Yugoslavia	3	1, 2
Brno, Yugoslavia	2	1, 2
Pancevo, Yugoslavia	2	1, 2
Azrou, Morocco	2	2
Greece[c]	2	1
Faiyum, Egypt	2	2
Haifa, Israel[c]	3	1, 2
Jerusalem, Israel	3	2
Thonburi, Thailand	3	1
Santiago, Chili[c]	4	1, 2
Michigan, U.S.A.[c]	21	1, 2, 3

[a]This represents the number of independently-derived Aβ alleles tested.
[b]This column lists the Evolutionary groups represented in each sample.
[c]These data were obtained by interpreting RFLP data published by Bukara *et al.* (1985).

Evolutionary groups 1 and 2 were both detected in wild mice trapped in Europe, North Africa, the Mid East, South America, and North America. These findings indicate that these polymorphic forms of Aβ were present prior to the global radiation of *Mus* from the Mid East, and that alleles from both groups subsequently persisted as polymorphisms in natural mouse populations all over the world. The global distribution of these Evolutionary groups is consistent with a transspecies mode of evolution for Aβ alleles.

The distribution of Aβ alleles within local mouse populations provides information useful in resolving whether H-2 polymorphisms are maintained by selective forces or neutrality. In the absence of selection (i.e. neutrality among all alleles at H-2), the 2 evolutionary groups of Aβ

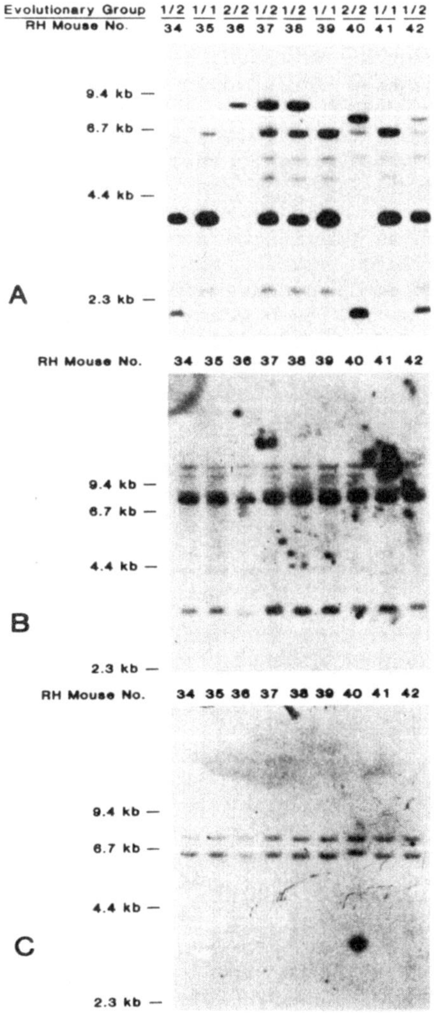

Fig. 4. RFLP analysis of 9 wild mice trapped at the RH dairy. The Evolutionary group assignments of the 2 alleles present and the mouse number are labelled at the top. The results are from sequential hybridizations of the same membrane and represent genomic DNAs digested with Bam HI. Panel A: Aβ; Panel B: Tcγ; and Panel c: Tcβ.

alleles would be expected to exhibit a "patchy" distribution among local mouse populations, particularly in light of the small deme size and the apparently limited gene flow between demes (reviewed by Sage 1981). Some local mouse populations would be expected to have Aβ alleles derived from both groups, some would have only group 1 alleles, and some only group 2 alleles. This type of distribution results when neutral polymorphisms undergo random genetic drift in a sub-divided population. In contrast, balancing selection would promote the maintenance of alleles from both Evolutionary groups in a high proportion of local populations. Thus, by sampling several local mouse populations, it is possible to determine whether the distribution of Aβ Evolutionary groups is consistent with the expectations of neutrality or balancing selection (see Hedrick and Thomson 1983 and Klitz et al. 1984 for similar analyses applied to the human MHC).

We have trapped wild mice at 6 separate locations near Gainesville and studied the polymorphisms for the Aβ, and T cell receptor constant chain genes Tcα, Tcβ, and Tcγ by RFLP analysis. Representative Southern blots are presented in Figure 4. The polymorphism of Aβ (top panel) is compared with that of the genes encoding the Tc subunits (middle panel) and the Tcβ subunits (bottom panel) in 9 wild mice trapped in a single barn at an isolated dairy near Gainesville, Florida. The results demonstrate that Aβ is very diversified in this population and that alleles from both Evolutionary group 1 and 2 are present. In contrast, both Tcγ (chromosome 13) and Tcβ (chromosome 6) were invariant among these mice, although both of these genes are polymorphic in wild mice (Huppi *et al*. 1986). The distribution of alleles for the Tcα, Tcβ, and Tcγ genes in the Gainesville populations is of the classical form where one allele is common with a few other alleles present at low frequencies (data not shown).

Table 3 summarizes the distribution and frequencies of Aβ Evolutionary groups 1 and 2 among 6 separate local mouse populations. The data indicate that Aβ alleles derived from both Evolutionary groups were present in all 6 populations at appreciable frequencies. Although a larger sampling will be necessary to rigorously demonstrate that this distribution deviates significantly from that predicted by neutrality, the data suggest that some type of balancing selection may be responsible for the maintenance of alleles from both Evolutionary groups in local demes. This is not totally unexpected in that the Aβ molecules encoded by alleles in group 1 are quite different from those in group 2 (McConnell *et al.* 1987), indicating that these groupings may have relevance to the functional properties of the expressed A molecules. We are in the process of expanding the data base to test for evidence of selection in the distribution of the Evolutionary groups in local mouse populations.

Table 3. Analysis of the frequencies Aβ alleles from Evolutionary groups 1 and 2 among local wild mouse populations near Gainesville, Florida.

Location	No. of Mice Tested	Frequency of alleles by Group[a] 1	2
HS	26	0.56	0.27
RH	23	0.54	0.33
SU	12	0.33	0.21
DR	8	0.56	0.38
BF	6	0.50	0.50
AH	5	0.70	0.30

[a] Aβ alleles were grouped into Evolutionary groups on the basis of results with Bam HI and Eco RI. It was not always possible to unambiguously assign one of the alleles in a heterozygote to either group based on only these enzymes. Consequently, the sums of the frequencies of alleles in both groups do not equal 1.0 for every population.

In summary, the global distribution of Aβ Evolutionary groups (Table 2) indicates that these groups existed prior to the global radiation of *Mus* and is consistent with a transspecies mode of evolution. The relatively uniform distribution of these groups among local demes (Table 3), particularly in relation to other polymorphic genes (Fig. 4), suggests that class II gene diversity among these two groups of alleles is maintained by balancing selection rather than neutrality. The selective mechanisms involved are unknown, however, several possibilities have been proposed including heterozygote advantage (Zinkernagel 1979), H-2-linked mating preferences (Yamazaki et al. 1976), and transmission distortion favoring H-2 heterozygous progeny (Clark and Kirby 1976) (see Potts et al. this volume for review). Further work on the nature of the selective mechanisms which operate on H-2 polymorphisms in natural mouse populations will be needed to unravel the forces responsible for the maintenance of H-2 polymorphisms in wild mice.

RECOMBINATION AND THE EVOLUTION OF I REGION HAPLOTYPES

Recombination within the I region has been extensively studied in intra-H-2 recombinant strains by RFLP analysis (Steinmetz et al. 1982, Kobori et al. 1984, Lafuse et al. 1985, Saha and Cullen 1986, Zimmerer et al. 1987). These studies demonstrated that meiotic recombination occurs at two specific recombinational hot spots (RHS) in the I region. One of these RHS, located in the central intron of Eβ, contains repetitive sequences which have limited homology with the "chi" sequences which regulate recombination in bacteriophage lambda (Steinmetz et al. 1986) A similar repetitive sequence was found in a highly active RHS located between H-2K and Aβ2 in an H-2 haplotype derived from *Mus m. castaneus* (Steinmetz et al. 1986). These observations suggest that meiotic recombination may be regulated by the positions of specific, cis-active DNA sequences which promote recombination.

Studies by Lafuse and co-workers suggest that the positions of RHS within the I region may be polymorphic (Lafuse et al. 1985). These investigators analyzed 7 recombinant I region haplotypes produced between I^p and I^k and found that the recombinational breakpoints occurred at a unique RHS proximal to Eα. These observations indicate that the RHS in the central intron of Eβ is not the only site at which recombination can occur in the I region, suggesting that different pairs of I region haplotypes may utilize distinct RHS during meiotic recombination.

The restriction of meiotic recombination to specific sites which exhibit positional polymorphisms within the I region could profoundly influence the evolution of class II gene haplotypes in wild mouse populations. Class II genes which are not separated by RHS would be predicted to accumulate mutations in a coordinate manner since they will remain linked throughout their evolutionary divergence. In contrast, class II genes which are separated by RHS would be expected to follow independent evolutionary paths and to occur in numerous cis-configurations.

The impact of RHS on the evolution of I region haplotypes can be tested by measuring the stability of linkage associations among alleles at specific sites in the I region. As shown in Figure 5, we have derived 9 separate probes from a collection of cosmids which contain the relevant portion of the I region (kindly supplied by M. Steinmetz) and have used these probes for RFLP analysis of 36 I regions from our collection of wild-mouse-derived H-2 haplotypes (Tarnuzzer et al. manuscript in preparation). The number of alleles and the average sequence divergence (F value from Nei and Li 1979) at each site assayed is presented below the position of the fragment in the I region.

These results reveal some interesting features of the diversity of this segment of the I region. Previous studies have suggested that the H-2 complex can be divided into tracts which exhibit either high or low degrees of sequence diversity (Steinmetz et al. 1984). The Aβ, Aα, and 5'Eβ genes are proposed to occupy a high divergence tract which terminates in or near the RHS in the central intron of Eβ, while the 3'Eβ, Eβ2, and Eα genes occupy a low divergence tract which extends telomeric from the Eβ RHS. Our analysis of 36 I region haplotypes essentially confirms these results. The diversity of sites within the high divergence tract was very high, with the number of alleles detected at each site ranging from 15 to 21 and average F values ranging from 0.29 to 0.52. The sites assayed included both expressed genes and regions of intervening DNA between these genes. The low diversity exhibited by a site about 10 kb centromeric to Aβ suggests that the high diversity tract may terminate close to the 5' end of Aβ, although further analysis with additional centromeric probes would be required to confirm this possibility. Sites telomeric to Eβ exhibit less diversity, with the number of alleles detected at each site ranging from 8 to 11 and average F values ranging from 0.48 to 0.68. These results support the presence of higher and lower diversity tracts on either side of the RHS in Eβ, although the difference in the diversity of these two segments of the I region is not great.

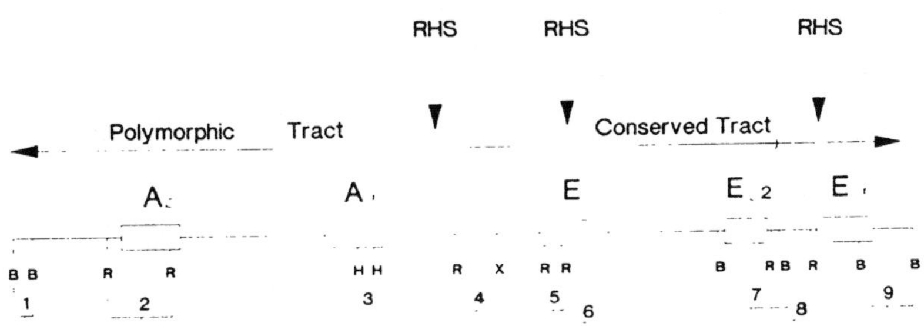

	1	2	3	4	5	6	7	8	9
# Alleles	16	21	16	15	15	21	9	11	8
Clusters	4	17	17	11	10	12	4	3	5
F Value	0.70	0.29	0.47	0.52	0.29	0.58	0.65	0.68	0.48

Fig. 5. A map of the I region illustrating the positions of the relevant class II genes and the DNA probes used for the analysis of I region haplotypes. The specific fragments used are numbered sequentially from the proximal side of the I region and the probes used are defined by brackets. A total of 36 independently-derived I regions were analyzed by RFLP with 5 restriction enzymes. The number of alleles detected with each probe, the number of clusters formed by these alleles, and the average F value are presented below each probe.

The role of recombination in the diversification of I region haplotypes was assessed by comparing the stability of linkage associations formed between alleles at each of the sites assayed. If recombination can only occur at the 2 RHS defined by analysis of laboratory recombinants, probes 1 through 5 should detect specific sets of alleles among our collection of I region haplotypes. In contrast, recombination within this segment of the I region would cause the reassortment of these alleles into multiple I region haplotypes. By comparing the allelic combinations found among the I region haplotypes in our panel, the positions of these recombinational events can be tentatively identified. However, the analysis of allelic combinations is complicated by the presence of minor variants among the alleles detected at each site. Therefore, we defined the term "allelic clusters" and organized all the alleles at each site into groups based on relatedness. Alleles were placed in the same cluster if they differed by only a single restriction enzyme site polymorphism from the prototypic allele of that cluster. The prototypic alleles differed by at least 25% of the fragment analyzed. The number of allelic clusters defined at each site are listed in Figure 5.

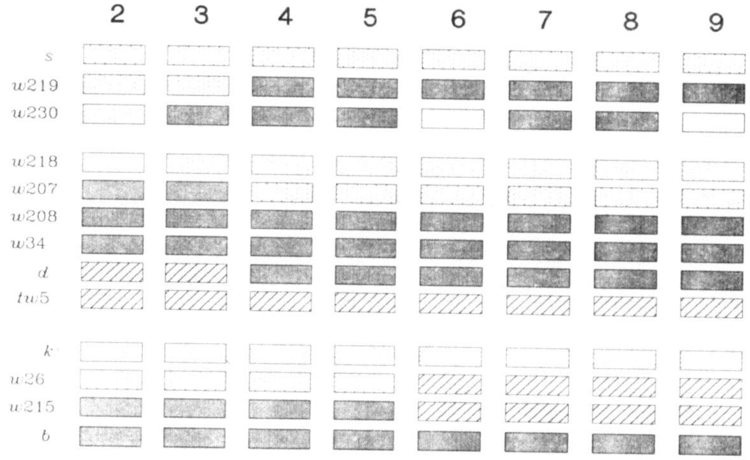

Fig. 6 A diagram illustrating potential intra-I region recombinants. The numbers at the top of each column refer to the probes defined in Figure 4. The specific I region haplotypes presented are listed on the left. The patterned boxes define the cluster-origins of the alleles at each site assayed. The top 3 I region haplotypes illustrate a putative recombinant between Aβ (probe 2) and Aα (probe 3). The middle 6 I region haplotypes illustrate putative recombinants between Aα (probe 3) and IVS1 (probe 4). The bottom 4 I region haplotypes illustrate recombination at the RHS between 5'Eβ (probe 5) and 3'Eβ (probe 6).

Since all the alleles within a cluster probably represent recent mutational variants of a single ancestral allele, scoring recombination based on such polymorphisms could be unreliable. Consequently, all alleles in a cluster were considered indistinguishable when searching for evidence of recombination. This type of analysis will underestimate the frequency of recombination since I region haplotypes will be scored as intra-I region recombinants only when the alleles bordering the putative recombination site came from separate allelic clusters of that I region segment.

The results indicate that intra-I region meiotic recombination has been restricted to a limited number of specific sites during the evolutionary divergence of the I region. Some of the results are diagrammed in Figure 6. The RHS in Eβ and the RHS between Eβ2 and Eα were the most active recombinational sites detected in our analysis. A minimum of 10 recombinational events were observed at each of these sites among the 36 independently-derived I region haplotypes assayed. The bottom 4 I region haplotypes in Figure 6 illustrate putative I region recombinants in the RHS in Eβ. I^{w26} and I^{w215} both have haplotypes which appear to be partially derived from I^b or I^k, with the switch occurring between probes 5 (5'Eβ) and 6 (3'Eβ). These findings are consistent with previous analyses of recombination among laboratory-derived H-2 haplotypes, and confirm that these RHS strongly influence linkage associations during the evolutionary divergence of this portion of the I region.

A new RHS between Aα (probe 3) and a probe derived from intervening DNA between Aα and Eβ (probe 4) was defined by 9 independently-derived intra-I region recombinants. The middle 6 I region haplotypes in Figure 6 illustrate these recombinants. The presence of "natural" recombinants between AαAβ and Eβ was first described on the basis of tryptic peptide fingerprinting (Singh et al. 1981, Wakeland and Darby 1983) Our analysis establishes that all the recombinants between AαAβ and Eβ in our panel occurred within a region of about 10-15 kb which is located close to the 5' end of Aα. These results suggest that another RHS must be present in this position in the I region haplotypes of some wild mice. The location and boundaries of this new RHS are defined in Figure 5.

Recombinational events at other sites in the I region were very rare in this analysis, with only 3 or 4 putative recombinants detected at any sites other than those listed as RHS in Figure 5. An example of one of these novel recombinants is illustrated by the top 3 I region haplotypes in Figure 6. When compared with 2 I region haplotypes derived from *Mus m. domesticus*, the *Mus spretus*-derived I^{w230} appears to have undergone recombination between Aβ and Aα. I^{w230} has an Aβ allele in the same cluster as those of I^s and I^{w219}, however, it is found in combination with an Aα allele which is unrelated to the Aα allele found in I^s or I^{w219}. These results suggest that recombination can occur between Aα and Aβ, although a more detailed analysis of the AαAβ duplexes in I^{w230} and I^{w219} would strengthen the argument for recombination.

In summary, our analysis of the stability of linkage associations among alleles at various sites in the I region establish that RHS play an important role in the formation of I region haplotypes. The two RHS which were defined through the analysis of laboratory intra-I region recombinants were found to be quite active in the formation of new I region haplotypes within our panel. In addition, we have identified a new RHS which mediates recombination between the AαAβ gene duplex and Eβ. The activity of this RHS was readily apparent within our panel of independently-derived I region haplotypes, although no laboratory recombinants have been detected at this position. We are in the process of refining the boundaries of this RHS with the hope of identifying sequence homologies between this region and other RHS in the I region.

ACKNOWLEDGEMENTS

We thank Marjorie Price-Laface for the maintenance of the mouse strains used in this study and Jan Klein for providing breeding pairs for some of the mouse strains analyzed. This work was supported in part by NIH grant AI-17966. T.J.M., R.W.T., and W.P. were supported by CA-09126.

REFERENCES

Benoist, C.O., D.J. Mathis, M.R. Kanter, V.E. Williams II and H.O. McDevitt, 1983, Regions of allelic hypervariability in the murine A_α immune response gene. Cell, 34:169-177.

Bukara, M., V. Vincek, F. Figueroa, and J. Klein, 1985, How polymorphic are class II loci of the mouse H-2 complex? Immunogenetics, 21:569-74.

Choi, E., K. McIntyre, R.N. Germain and S.G. Seidman. 1983, Murine-I-A chain polymorphism: nucleotide sequences of three allelic I-A genes. Science 221:283-85.

Clarke, B. and D.R.S. Kirby, 1966, Maintenance of histocompatibility polymorphims, Nature, 211:999-1000.

Duncan, W.R. and J. Klein, 1980, Histocompatibility-2 system in wild mice. IX. Serological analysis of 13 new B10.W congenic lines, Immunogenetics, 10:45-57.

Duncan, W.R., E.K. Wakeland, and J. Klein, 1979, Histocompatibility-2 System in Wild Mice. VIII. Frequencies of H-2 and Ia Antigens in Wild Mice from Texas. Immunogenetics 9:261-68.

Estess, P., A.B.Begovich, M. Koo, P.P. Johes, and H.O. McDevitt, 1986, Sequence analysis and structure-function correlation of murine q, k, u, s, and f, haplotype I-A^{b} cDNA clones, Proc. Natl. Acad. Sci. USA, 83:3594-3598.

Falus, A., E.K. Wakeland, T.J. McConnell, J. Gitlin, A.S. Whitehead, and H.R. Colten, 1987, DNA polymorphism of MHC III genes in inbred and wild mouse strains, Immunogenetics, 25:290-299.

Ferris, S.D., R.D. Sage, E.<. Prager, U.Ritte, and A.C. Wilson, 1983, Mitochondrial DNA evolution in mice. Genetics 105:681-721.

Gotze, D., J. Nadeau, E.K. Wakeland, R.J. Berry, F. Bonhomme, J.K. Egorov, J.P. Hjrth, H. Hoogstraal, J. Vives, H. Winking, and J. Klein, 1980, Histocompatibility-2 system in wild mice. X. Frequencies of H-2 and Ia antigens in wild mice from Europe and Africa. J. Immunology 124:2675-2680.

Hartl, D., 1980, "Principles of Population Genetics", Sinauer, Sunderland.

Hedrick, P.W. and G. Thomson, 1983, Evidence for balancing selection at HLA, Genetics 104:449-456.

Houck, C.M., F.P. Rinehart, and C.W. Schmid, 1979, A ubiquitous family of repeated DNA sequences in the human genome, J. Mol.Biol. 132:289-306.

Huppi, K., L. D'Hoostelaere, M. Kiefer, M. Steinmetz, E. Jouxin-Marche, 1986, The context of T-cell receptor gamma chain genes among wild mouse species, Immunogenetics 24:304-309.

Jaggedeewaren, P., B.G. Forget, and S.M. Weissman, 1981, Short interspersed repetitive DNA elements in eukaryotes: Transposable DNA elements generated by reverse transcription of RNA pol III transcripts, Cell 26:141-142.

Klein, J., Generation of diversity at MHC loci: implications for T-cell receptor repertoires, in:"Immunology 80," M. Fougereau and J. Dausset, eds., Academic Press, London (1980).

Klein, J., 1986, "Natural History of the Major Histocompatibility Complex", Wiley, N.Y.

Klein, J. and F. Figueroa, 1986, Evolution of the major histocompatibility complex, CRC Critical Review in Immunology, 6:295.

Klitz, W., G. Thomson, and M.P. Baur, 1984, The nature of selection in the HLA region based on population data from the ninth workshop, pp. 330-332, in "Histocompatibility Testing 1984", E.D. Albert, M.P. Baur, and W.R. Mayr, eds., Springer-Verlag, Berlin.

Kobori, J.A., E. Strauss, K. Minard, and L. Hood, 1986, Molecular analysis of the hotspot of recoombination in the murine major histocompatibility complex, Science, 234:173-76.

Lafuse, W.P., N. Berg, S. Savarirayan, and C.S. David, 1986, Mapping of a second recombination hot spot within the I-E region of the mouse H-2 gene complex, J. Exp. Med., 163:1518-29.

Larhammar, D., L. Schenning, K. Gustaffson, K. Wiman, L. Claesson, L. Rask, and P.A. Peterson, 1982, Complete amino acid sequence of an HLA-DR antigen-like beta chain as predicted from the nucleotide sequence: similarities with immunoglobins and HLA-A, B, C antigens, Proc. Natl. Acad. Sci. USA, 79:3687-1500.

Malissen, M., T. Hunkapiller, L. Hood, 1983, Nucleotide sequence of a light chain gene of the mouse I-A subregion: A-beta, Science, 221:750-754.

Marshall, J. T., 1986, Systematics of the Genus Mus, in,"Current Topics in Microbiology and Immunology, Vol. 127: The Wild Mouse in Immunology, M. Potter, J.H. Nadeau, and M.P. Cancro, eds., Springer-Verlag, New York.

McConnell, T.J., Darby, B. and Wakeland, E.K, 1986, Restriction fragment length polymorphisms of class II gene sequences in mice expressing minor variants of I-A^k or I-A^p, J. Immunol. 136:3076-3082.

McConnell, T.J., .S. Talbot, R.A. McIndoe, and E.K. Wakeland, 1987, The origin of MHC class II gene polymoorphism within the genus Mus, submitted for publication.

Nadeau, J.H., E.K. Wakeland, D. Gotze, and J. Klein, 1981, The population genetics of the H-2 polymorphism in European and North African populations of the house mouse (Mus musculus), Genet. Res. Camb., 37:17-31.

Nei, M. and W.H. Li, 1979, Mathematical model for studying genetic variation in terms of restriction endonucleases. Proc. Natl. Acad. Sci. USA 76:5269-5273.

Potts, W.K., C.J. Manning, A.B. Peck, M. Price-Laface, and E.K. Wakeland, 1987, Can heterozygote advantage account for the maintenance of H-2 Polymorphism?, this volume.

Sage, R.D., 1981, Wild mice, pp. 39-90, in "The Mouse in Biomedical Research", Vol.I, H.L. Foster, J.D. Small, J.G. Fox, eds., Academic, N.Y.

Saha, B.K. and .E. Cullen, 1986, Molecular mapping of murine I region recombinants: Crossing over in the Eβ gene, J. Immunol. 136:1112-16.

Singh, S.K., E.K. Wakeland, I. Vacek, Z.A. Nagy, and J. Klein, 1981, An H-2 haplotype possibly derived by crossing-over between the $(A_\alpha A_\beta)$ Duplex and the E_β locus, Immunogenetics 14:273-78.

Steinmetz, M., K. Minard, S. Horvath, et al., 1982, A molecular map of the immune response region from the major histocompatibility complex of the mouse, Nature 300:35.

Steinmetz, M., M. Mallissen, L. Hood, A. Orn, R.A. Maki, G.R. Dastoonikoo, D. Stephan, E. Gibb, and R. Romaniuk, 1984, Tracts of high or low sequence divergence in the mouse major histocompatibility complex. EMBO Journal. 3:2995-3001.

Steinmetz, M., D. Stephan, and K. Fisher Lindahl, 1986, Gene organization and recombinational hotspots in the murine major histocompatibility complex, Cell 44:895-902.

Tarnuzzer, R., McIndoe, R.A., McConnell, T.M., and E.K. Wakeland, 1987, Recombinational hot spots and the evolution of MHC class II gene haplotypes in the mouse, manuscript in preparation.

Wakeland, E.K. and B.R. Darby, 1983, Recombination and mutation of class II histocompatibility genes in wild mice, J. Immunol. 131:3052.

Wakeland, E.K. and J. Klein, 1981, The polymorphism of I region encoded antigens among wild mice, Curr. Trends in Histocompatibility, 4:289-305.

Wakeland, E.K., M. Price-LaFace, V. Henson, and A.B. Peck, 1987, Production of 35 H-2 homozygous strains from wild mice, Immunogenetics, in press.

Yamakazi, K., E.A. Boyse, V. Mike, H.T. Thaler, B.J. Mathieson, J. Abbott, J. Boyse, Z.A. Zayas, and L. Thomas, 1976, Control of mating preferences in mice by genes in the major histocompatibility complex, J. Exp. Med., 144:1324-1335.

Zimmerer, E.J., E. Ogin, D.C. Shreffler, and H.C. Passmore, 1987, Molecular mapping of crossover sites within the I region of the mouse MHC. Analysis of ten recombinant chromosomes, Immunogenetics, 25:274-276.

Zinkernagel, R.M., 1979, Associations between major histocompatibility antigens and susceptibility to disease, Ann. Rev. Microbiol., 33:201-213.

SECTION III
STRUCTURE OF H-2 GENES AND GENE PRODUCTS

TOWARD AN UNDERSTANDING OF THE BIOCHEMICAL NATURE OF H-2 MOLECULES: A HISTORICAL PERSPECTIVE

Stanley G. Nathenson

Department of Microbiology and Immunology
and Department of Cell Biology
Albert Einstein College of Medicine, Bronx, NY 10461

As part of an historical perspective of the development of our knowledge of the H-2 genes and products, this paper presents a brief, selected, personal account of those studies from my laboratory which were carried out with the objective to understand the biochemical nature of H-2 molecules. This work was performed with the goal of relating the structural features of what are now called class I MHC molecules to their biological function, in addition to expanding our understanding of the genetic organization and diversity of the H-2 region genes.

Our understanding of the biochemical nature of the H-2 region products began first with the localization of H-2 antigenic activity to membrane fractions. These studies in the late 1950s and early 1960s and were carried out in a number of laboratories (for discussion see ref. 1). Thus, the work of D.A. L. Davies, L. Herzenberg, A. Kandutsch and J. Stimpfling, J. Palm and L. Manson, R.E. Billingham, L. Brent, P.B. Medawar and M. Ruscewitz, and G. Haughton established that H-2 antigenic activity resided in a membrane bound form whether measured by accelerated graft rejection, tumor rejection, hemagglutination or cytotoxicity assays. It was clear that the next step in defining the biochemical nature of these antigens was to solubilize them and purify them to homogeneity.

I had obtained a fellowship from the Helen Hay Whitney Foundation, and had decided to study the problem of specific cell-cell recognition in mammal systems. Allen Davies had just moved to a transplantation unit at the Blonde Laboratory, East Grinstead, Sussex. Since he and his colleagues were leaders in the techniques for analysis and preparation of H-2 active membrane fractions, it seemed an ideal place to begin to pursue the study of the H-2 antigen system. Further, Hans Wigzell and Arnold Sanderson (2,3) had developed an accurate and rapid antibody mediated ^{51}Cr release cytotoxic assay which was available to me when I arrived in 1964, thus providing the crucial key for biochemical purification. The stage was set, therefore, for applying the tools of biochemistry to define the nature of transplantation antigens.

To provide clues as to the carbohydrate or protein nature of the antigenic activity, we first intended to use enzymes which would cleave either between carbohydrate residues, or at peptide bonds, to explore whether such treatment would destroy activity. Because we knew that blood group antigens were carbohydrate (H-2 antigens were originally reported as blood group substances) we expected the carbohydrases to destroy activity. However, we found that the proteolytic enzyme ficin destroyed antigenic activity while none of the carbohydrases we tried had any effect. In our obvious excitement, we proceeded to test the supernatant of the enzyme treated antigenic membrane suspension, and found to our delight that antigenic materials were now present in a soluble form. We had made the crucial breakthrough! An example of the proteolytic enzyme solubilization process is demonstrated in Fig. 1 which demonstrates that generation of H-2 antigenic activity in a soluble form was dependent upon amount of enzyme, length of incubation and did not occur in the absence of activation of the enzyme.

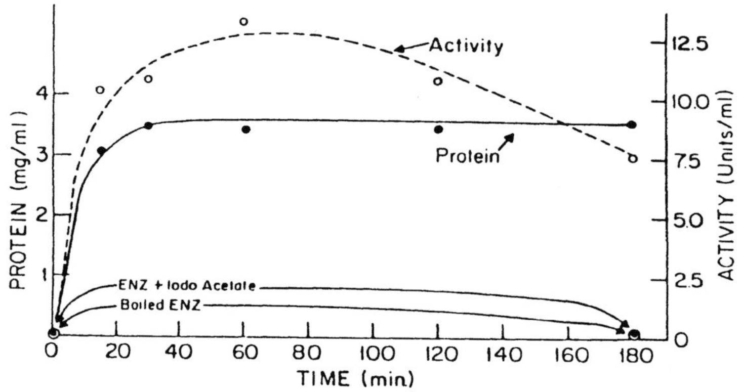

Fig. 1. A time course of release of H-2 soluble antigen and protein by ficin from a lipoprotein fraction.

The next step was to develop a purification scheme. The H-2 assay of inhibition of antibody mediated cytotoxicity was both straightforward and quantitative, and proved to be ideal to follow standard biochemical fractionation procedures. We were able to devise a purification scheme in our laboratory permitting us to purify the H-2 fragments by 700- or 800-fold, using a protocol including ammonium sulfate precipitation, Sephadex G-150, CM-Sephadex and DEAE Sephadex chromatography and PAGE (4). The purified enzyme generated molecules from H-2^b mice were found to exist in two sizes. The molecular weight of the molecule carrying specificity 5 and 33 was approximately 57,000 daltons (e.g. K^b plus β_2m), whereas that fragment expressing specificity 2 had a molecular weight of 34,000 daltons (4). Analysis of these preparations allowed us to definitively identify that transplantation antigens were glycoproteins containing nearly 90% protein and approximately 10% carbohydrate (4% neutral carbohydrate, 3% glucosamine, and 1% sialic acid).

From these studies also came the first evidence from Sephadex gel chromatography (Fig, 2) that some H-2 specificities resided in fragments separable from other fragments bearing different specificities. For example, Sephadex chromatography clearly separated the papain derived molecule carrying H-2.2 (now known to exist on D^b) from that expressing H-2.5 (now known to be expressed on K^d).

T. Muramatsu (5) was able to characterize the carbohydrate moieties in purified preparations and established that the glycopeptides were of the N-glucosamine linked type with a M.W. of about 3300 daltons. We postulated that two carbohydrate moeities were attached per polypeptide chain. Thus our first goal was attained, and we were able to define the transplantation antigens of the H-2 "locus" as glycoproteins. Our preliminary conclusion was that the antigenic activity resided in the protein portion of the antigen, and this has turned out to be the case for most antibodies directed to these products. While some antigenic sites may be carbohdyrate determined, it is clear from contemporary evidence that most monoclonal antibodies detect protein determined sites in H-2 molecules.

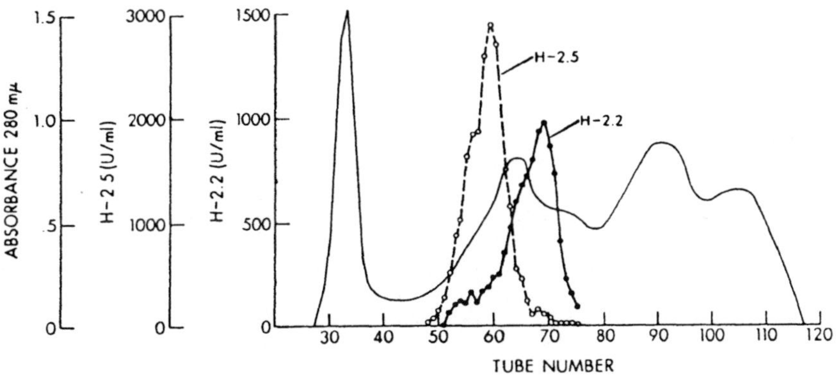

Fig. 2. Sephadex G150 column chromatography of ammonium sulfate fraction of papain solubilized H-2^b antigens showing separation of fragments bearing different specificities.

It is relevant to note that K. Yamane and A. Shimada in their studies with me in 1967 to 1969 (ref. 4 and unpublished observations) had noted a small molecular weight protein which co-purified with the antigenic glycoprotein fragment prepared from mouse spleens. This protein also seemed to co-precipitate in immune precipitates prepared with monospecific alloantisera. This was a variable finding because we did not find this small polypeptide in all preparations. We unfortunately did not pursue this problem actively. However a short time later several investigators reported (6,7) that a protein previously discovered in urine was in fact associated with the antigenic glycoprotein. This protein, called $\beta_2$microglobulin was therefore shown to be a subunit of the H-2 antigen. It is of interest that the interaction of $\beta_2$microglobulin with different class I heavy chains is quite variable; and had we studied only the K^b molecule which tightly binds $\beta_2$microglobulin we might have been able to unequivocally establish the subunit nature of the K^b antigen.

Once it was clear that the H-2 glycoprotein fragments carried antigenic activity we could attempt to answer our next question. What is the structural basis of the serologically defined polymorphism and diversity of the H-2 antigens? Since, until this time, we had only analyzed proteolytically derived H-2 fragments, we felt that before we could approach these questions we must clarify the size and nature of the intact gene product. We turned to the use of non-ionic detergents such as NP-40 to release intact class I molecules from their membrane location. B. Schwartz (8) spearheaded these studies by utilizing metabolically radiochemically labeled H-2 antigens isolated by immuno affinity techniques. In these studies we analyzed the antigens in denaturing solvents, which separated them from the non-covalently bound β_2m subunit. The intact H-2 molecule solubilized by NP-40 which we recovered was 44,000 daltons, only slightly larger (approximately 7,000 M.W.) than the papain solubilized molecule. Our conclusion of these studies was that the papain generated fragment was, in fact, the major stretch of polypeptide of the H-2 heavy chain. We speculated that the enzyme had cleaved at an amino acid residue in a stretch containing the membrane binding region of the H-2 molecule, in order to release the soluble, carbohydrate-bearing extracellular form (37,000 M.W.) which carried the antigenic determinants (8).

The NP-40 solubilized antigens became the source of material to approach the question of whether the H-2 complex determined multiple products. This question was particularly relevant at this time because concurrent genetic analysis of the H-2 region suggested that at least two loci, K and D, existed in what was thought previously to be a single, complex locus (9). If so, multiple separate products should be expressed on the cell surface. To resolve this question, S. Cullen B. Schwartz, M. Cherry and I utilized a pre-clearing approach to demonstrate the existence of separate K and D products. For example, after first pre-clearing a detergent cell lysate of the K^b product by a monospecific antiserum, we found that the D^b product still remained and could be precipited by an anti-D^b antiserum. Using all possible combinations of preclearing, we concluded that in homozygous animals at least one K and one D product was expressed. In heterozygous animals there were 4 products, 2 for the K end and 2 for the D end (Fig. 3).

As genetic and biological studies revealed an increasingly complex organization of the H-2 region, C. David, D. Shreffler, S. Cullen and I were able to biochemically define a second set of "H-2" gene products, those determined by genes of the I region (11). Alloantisera prepared between recombinant mouse strains which shared the K and D regions but differed at the I region, detected at least two sizes of radiolabeled materials. Thus, we in this field became aware of the possibility of many linked genes in the H-2 region which determined cell surface located glycoproteins important in the immune response.

Studies on the I region products expanded when new workers entered the H-2 field, and students from my laboratory, including S. Cullen, B. Schwartz and J. Freed, began analysis of these molecules. The historical development of the understanding of these glycoproteins is covered in a paper by P. Jones later on in this volume.

A Genetic level

Homozygous : $H\text{-}2^a/H\text{-}2^a$

	H-2K	H-2D
$H\text{-}2^a$	11	4
$H\text{-}2^a$	11	4

Heterozygous : $H\text{-}2^a/H\text{-}2^b$

	H-2K	H-2D
$H\text{-}2^a$	11	4
$H\text{-}2^b$	33	2

Homozygous : $H\text{-}2^b/H\text{-}2^b$

	H-2K	H-2D
$H\text{-}2^b$	33	2
$H\text{-}2^b$	33	2

B. Cellular level (membrane)

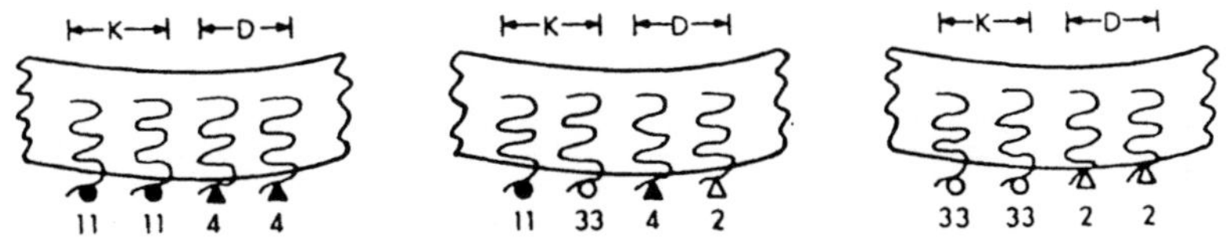

Fig.3. Summary of the molecular-genetic relationships for the H-2 system.

Monospecific antisera against K or D gene products were used in preclearing experiments as described in text and ref. 10. Under A. Genetic level, are listed the haplotypes of the two homozygous strains, and their heterozygous strain. Under the particular postulated H-2K gene and H-2D gene for each haplotype are listed the major or "private" specificities determined by that particular gene. For example, in the homozygote, $H\text{-}2^a/H\text{-}2^a$, the specificity of the $H\text{-}2K^a$ gene is 11 and the specificity of the $H\text{-}2D^a$ gene is 4. Under the heading, B. Cellular level, a schematic representation of the cellular membrane is shown. The H-2 polypeptide is depicted by the curving line that carries the antigenic site of the major specificity. For the homozygous cell, at least two types of alloantigens can be isolated. For example, in the $H\text{-}2^a/H\text{-}2^a$ cell, glycoproteins reactive for specificities 11 and 4 can be detected. In the $H\text{-}2^a/H\text{-}2^b$ heterozygote cell, on the other hand, there are at least four antigen molecules, each carrying exclusively the antigenic sites for one of the H-2 specificities, i.e., 11, 33, 4, or 2.

The next question which became a primary goal was to determine the basis of the observed serological complexity and the polymorphism of the H-2 genes at the level of the primary protein structure. The study on the diversity of the protein structure among alleles was approached through the development of an ion exchange peptide mapping technique for metabolically radiolabeled antigens. We perfected this radiochemical approach because only small amounts of the H-2 glycoproteins were available in cell extracts and in cell membranes. The use of tracer labeling paired with immunoaffinity isolation by monospecific allo-antibodies directed against either K or D gene products of a specific allele, proved not only to be a powerful approach for peptide comparisons, but also later, crucial for the determination of the primary sequence.

L. Brown in my laboratory established the methodology for comparing tryptic peptides using ion exchange chromatography. To our surprise a comparison of labeled peptides from allelic products such as K^b and K^d (labeled in either Arg or Lys) showed extraordinary diversity (12). This remarkable diversity is exemplified in Figure 4, which shows that a large number of the peptide peaks (approximately 60-70%) did not coincide.

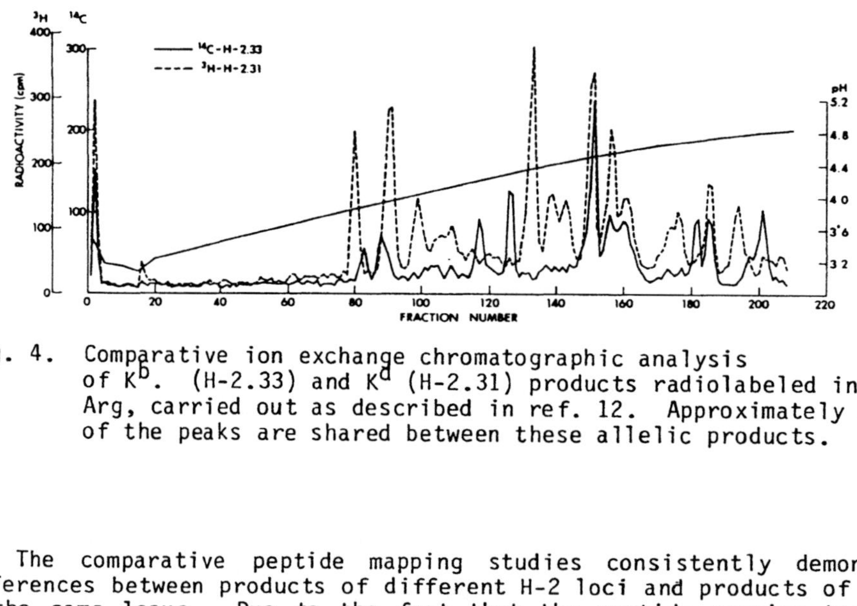

Fig. 4. Comparative ion exchange chromatographic analysis of K^b. (H-2.33) and K^d (H-2.31) products radiolabeled in Arg, carried out as described in ref. 12. Approximately 35% of the peaks are shared between these allelic products.

The comparative peptide mapping studies consistently demonstrated differences between products of different H-2 loci and products of alleles of the same locus. Due to the fact that the peptide mapping techniques tended to overestimate the number of actual sequence differences between the compared proteins, (since only a single amino acid difference in a peptide containing many unaltered amino acid residues can alter its chromatographic behavior), we predicted that about 30% of the primary structure of allelic proteins would be different. This turned out to be close to the results of nucleic acid and amino acid sequence data completed 8 to 10 years later which show divergencies of about 20-25% in the first and second domains. Thus the extraordinary number of serologically defined H-2 "specificities" expressed by H-2 products of different mouse haplotypes were found to be directly due to an unusually high degree of sequence diversity among alleles at the K or D loci.

It was clear that amino acid sequence analysis was now required to proceed to refine our understanding of the nature and location of the diversity and the intramolecular organization of the H-2 class I molecules. However, the major problem for approaching the sequencing of a protein estimated to be approximately 350 amino acids in length was how to obtain sufficient material in purified form for the complex fragmentation and sequence analysis techniques available at this time.

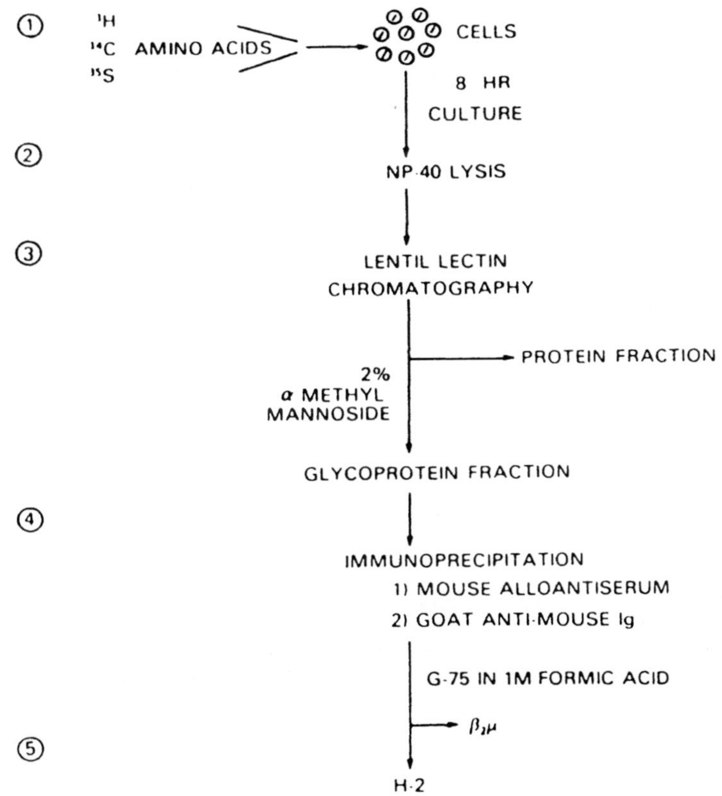

Fig. 5. General methodology for isolation of labeled H-2 alloantigens.

I approached this problem during a sabbatical in England in 1975 with L. Mole and R.R. Porter at which time we developed a sequencing strategy utilizing the radiochemical approach crucial for our previous studies. The general strategy for preparing radiolabeled K^b molecules is outlined in Fig. 5.

T. Kindt and J. Coligan, two excellent protein biochemists, joined in a collaboration with my group including B. Ewenstein, J. Martinko, R. Nairn and H. Uehara (13,14). To sequence the radiolabeled H-2K^{b} molecules isolated by immune affinity procedures, we adapted the classical techniques of fragmentation, separation and analysis of peptides. A major problem was the variable incorporation of different amino acids, but these and other problems were resolved and led us to the sequence of the first H-2 class I molecule (Fig. 6).

1 GPHSLRYFVTAVSRPGLGEPRYMEVGYVDDTEFVRFDSDAENPRY 45

46 EPRARWMEQEGPEYWERETQKAKGNEQSFRVDLRTLLGYYNQSKG 90

CHO

91 GSHTIQVISGCEVGSDGRLLRGYQQYAYDGCDYIALNEDLKTWTA 135

S—S

136 ADMAALITKHKWEQAGEAERLRAYLEGTCVEWLRRYLKNGNATLL 180

CHO

181 RTDSPKAHVTHHSRPDDKVTLRCWALGFYPADITLTWQLNGEELI 225

S—S

226 QDMELVETRPAGDGTFQKWASVVVPLGKEQYYTCHVYQQGLPQPL 270

Papain

271 TLRWDEPPSTVSNMATVAVLVVLGAAIVTGAVVAFVMKMRRRATG 315

Transmembrane

316 GKGGDYALAPGSQISDLSLPDCKVMVHPPHS 346

Fig. 6. Complete amino acid sequence of the H-2K^{b} molecule. Amino acid residues are indicated in the single letter amino acid code. (IUPAC-IUB Commission on Biochemical Nomenclature 1968). CHO, carbohydrate moeity; S-S, cysteine disulfide bridge. The prominent letters on the right side indicate: N,N-terminal 90 amino acid residues; C1, first disulfide loop region; C2, second disulfide loop region; TM, hydrophobic region and COOH-terminal hydrophilic region. (See ref. 14.)

Concurrent studies were completed by the group of J. Strominger on HLA class I molecules using non-radiolabeled techniques (15). Thus the features of both murine and human transplantation antigens could be compared. The information provided us the ingredients for understanding not only the relevant features of the protein structure, a significant advance in itself, but also provided the basis for determining and identifying cDNA and genomic clones (16), and hence the key to open the door for the application of the powerful tools of molecular genetics for the analysis of MHC genes.

The sequence information combined with the exact positioning of the disulfide bonding and positioning of the carbohydrate chain (14) allowed us to propose a model that the heavy chain was divided into 3 domains in the region external to the cell membrane which we called N, C-1 and C-2 (subsequently redesignated α1, α2 and α3 to conform to the HLA designations). These amino terminal outer domains were then followed by a postulated membrane binding region of approximately 23 hydrophobic amino acids and then by a cytophilic intracytoplasmic tail. Evidence on the quaternary relationships were provided by studies done by K. Yokoyama (17), in which $\beta_2$microglobulin in the K^b molecule could be shown to associate with a proteolytic fragment containing only the α3 region. This suggested that α3 and $\beta_2$microglobulin were in close, noncovalent apposition, as indicated in the orientation shown in Figure 7.

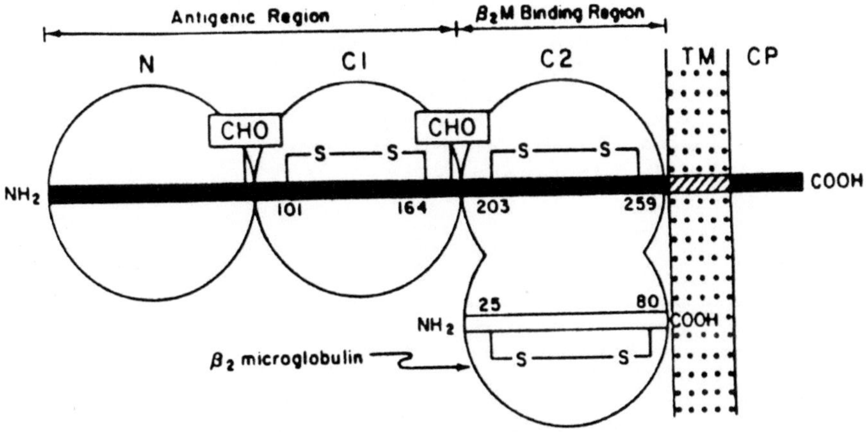

Fig. 7. Schematic representation of the H-2K^b molecule. The postulated three subregions, N, C-1, and C-2, comprise the extracellular portion of the H-2K^b, and each domain consists of about 90 amino acid residues. The alloantigenic determinants of H-2K^b are present on the first and second domains, and the β_2m is bound to the third domain. The transmembrane region (TM) is postulated to span the lipid bilayer of the cellular membrane, and intracellular cytoplasmic carboxy terminal tail (CP) is postulated to be present in the cytoplasma.

Another phase in our quest for understanding the structure/function relationships of the class I MHC molecules began in parallel with the amino acid sequence analysis (and in fact determined the choice of the K^b molecule to sequence), and focused on a unique resource -- the mutant mouse strains which apparently had mutations in their MHC class I K or D genes. The diversity which was noted among allelic products, (e.g. K^b and K^d differ by approximately 50 amino acids out of 350) made it impossible to attempt to define sites of allorecognition between such products. However the discovery in 1960s by I. Egorov (18) and H. Kohn and D. Bailey (19) that spontaneous mutations in the K or D genes occuring naturally in mice could be detected by transplantation techniques allowed us to approach such questions of structure/function in a highly refined manner. We reasoned that the H-2 products of the mutants should bear only a few differences from the parental gene products and chose for our studies a series of K^b mutants to analyze. The first strains discovered were the bm1 mutant isolated by Kohn and Bailey (19) and the bm3 line by Egorov (18). Subsequently a number of additional mutants were detected and isolated by Melvold and Kohn, and eventually there were about 15 mutant strains of the K^b gene and 3 mutant strains of the D^b gene available (20).

The radiolabeled tryptic peptide mapping technique allowed us to detect small differences between mutant and parent K^b molecules (21). For example, we could detect several changes in peptide peaks between the mutant K molecule of M505 (bm3) and wild type K^b while most of the peptides were identical in behavior. Once such differences were obtained we approached the localization of differences along the protein chain by tryptic peptide mapping separate longer cyanogen bromide fragments. Thus by these means we were able to localize the changes to certain specific CNBr fragments. Radiochemical sequencing, either of CNBr fragment itself or of derived tryptic peptides further localized the changes and allowed us to construct the map shown in Figure 8 representing our predictions for the amino acid changes in approximately 10 mutants.

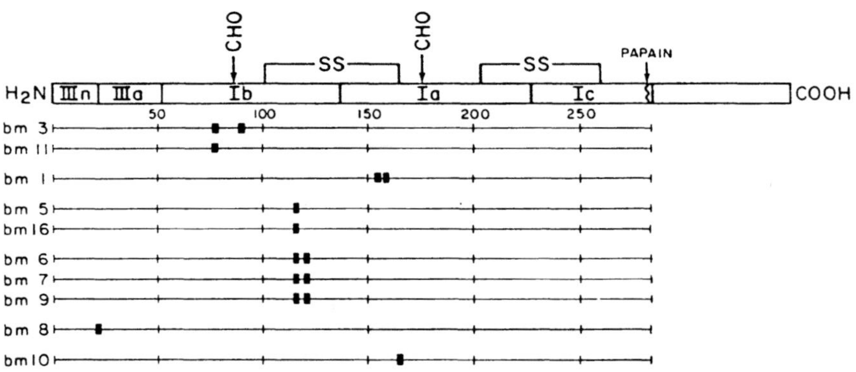

Fig. 8. Schematic outline of the overall structure of the H-$2K^b$ molecule with the positions of the known amino acid alterations in the H-2K molecules of the H-$2K^b$ mutants determined from protein analysis only (20). The positions of the disulfide bridges (SS) and the carbohydrate side chains (CHO) in H-$2K^b$ are shown along with the designations for the CNBr fragments. Numbering of the residues in the molecules is indicated. The location of the known amino acids altered from the H-2K molecule of the parent in the H-2K molecules of the mutants if given by a solid bar.

It was immediately obvious from such an analysis that the changes between parent and mutant K molecules were discretely localized to the first 180 amino acids, i.e. within the α1 and α2 domains. Such results suggested for the first time that the two amino terminal domains were of extreme importance in allorecognition, and appeared to form the sites which interacted with the T cell. Intriguingly, multiple amino acid changes were found in some of the mutants, and in addition some of the changes were complex, in that they could not be generated by a single nucleotide mutation. It was also found that some independently arising mutants carried the identical change (20) such as the Tyr to Phe alteration at position 116 of K^b from mutants bm5,16, and 6,7, and 9.

At this time additional class I sequences became available from protein sequencing as well as from cDNA clones. We noted that in many cases the mutant changes were in fact identical to stretches of amino acid residues in homologous positions in other class I genes. Thus we concluded that a mechanism involving recombination ("gene conversion") as a method of exchange of genetic information among class I genes could be potentially operating to generate the mutations (22).

The next step in the analysis of these mutants was then carried out at the molecular genetic level and these studies are reported in the companion paper by Geliebter et al.

In summary therefore, I've described a personal view of my part in the development of our understanding of the biochemistry, structure/function relationships and mechanisms for generating diversity of the H-2 genes and molecules. It has been an exciting period of research for me encompassing roughly 23 years, from 1964 when I began my studies, to 1987 the time of this conference celebrating the 50th anniversary of the discovery of the H-2 system.

Acknowledgement

I especially thank my secretary, C. Whelan, for her help in preparing this manuscript, and to all my colleagues and students who played key roles in the studies I have described. The research has been supported by NIH grants and ACS grants. I am a member of the Irvington House Institute for Medical Research.

References

1. Nathenson, S.G. Biochemical properties of histocompatibility antigens, Ann. Rev. Genetics 4:69 (1970).
2. Sanderson, A.R., Cytotoxic reactions of mouse isoantisera; scope of an assay using radiolabeled target cells, Transplantation 3:557 (1965).
3. Wigzell, R. Quantitative titration of mouse H-2 antibodies using Cr^{51} labeled target cells, Transplantation 3:423 (1965).
4. Shimda, A. and Nathenson, S.G., Murine histocompatibility-2 (H-2) alloantigens: Purification and some chemical properties of soluble products from $H-2^b$ and $H-2^d$ genotypes released by papain digestion of membrane fractions, Biochemistry 8:4048 (1969).
5. Muramatsu, T. and Nathenson, S. G., Studies on the carbohydrate portion of membrane-located mouse H-2 alloantigens, Biochemistry 9:4875 (1970).
6. Rask, L., Lindblom J.B. and Peterson, P.A., Subunit structure of H-2 alloantigens, Nature 249:833 (1974).
7. Silver, J. and Hood, L., Detergent-solubilized H-2 alloantigen is associated with a small molecular weight polypeptide, Nature 249:764 (1974).

8. Schwartz, B.D. and Nathenson, S.G., Isolation of H-2 alloantigens solubilized by the detergent NP-40, J. Immunol. 107:1363 (1971.
9. Snell, G.D., Cherry, M. and Demant, P., Evidence that H-2 private specificities can be arranged in two mutually exclusive systems possibly homologous with two subsystems of HL-A, Transpl. Proc. 3:183 (1971).
10. Cullen, S., Schwartz, B.D., Nathenson, S.G. and Cherry, M., The molecular basis of codominant expression of the histocompatibility-2 genetic region, Proc. Natl. Acad. Sci. USA 69:1394 (1972).
11. Cullen, S.E., David, C.S., Shreffler, D.C. and Nathenson, S.G., Membrane molecules determined by the H-2 associated immune response region: Isolation and some properties, Proc. Natl. Acad. Sci. USA 71:648 (1974).
12. Brown, L., Kato, K., Silver, J. and Nathenson, S.G. Notable diversity in peptide composition of murine H-2K and H-2D alloantigens, Biochemistry 13:3174 (1974).
13. Ewenstein, B.M., Freed, J.H., Mole, L.E. and Nathenson, S.G., Localization of the papain cleavage site of H-2 glycoproteins, Proc. Natl. Acad. Sci. USA 73:915 (1976).
14. Nathenson, S.G., Uehara, H., Ewenstein, B.M., Kindt, T.J. and Coligan, J.E., Primary structural analysis of the transplantation antigens of the murine H-2 major histocompatibility complex, Ann. Rev. Biochem. 50:1025 (1981).
15. Strominger J.L. Engelhard, V.H., Fuks, A., Guild, B.C., Hyafil, F., Kaufman, J.F., Korman, A.J., Kostyk, T.G., Krangel, M.S.., Lancet, D., Lopez de Castro, J.A., Mann, D.L., Orr, H.T., Parham, P., Parker, K.C., Ploegh, H.L., Pober, J.S., Robb, R.J., and Shackelford, D.A., Biochemical analysis of products of the MHC. in "The Role of the Major Histocompatibility Complex in Immunobiology," M.E. Dorf, ed., Garland, New York (1981).
16. Steinmetz, M., Frelinger, J.G., Fisher, D., Hunkapiller, T., Periera, D., Weissman, S.M., Uehara, H., Nathenson, S.G. and Hood, L., Three cDNA clones encoding mouse transplantation antigens: Homology to immunoglobulin genes, Cell 24:134 (1981).
17. Yokoyama, K. and Nathenson, S.G., Intramolecular organization of class I H-2 antigens: Localization of the alloantigenic determinants and the β_2 binding site to different regions of the H-2 K^b glycoprotein, J. Immunol. 130:1419 (1983).
18. Egorov, I., Genetic control of H-2 alloantigens as inferred from analysis of mutations, Immunogenetics 1:97 (1974).
19. Bailey, D.W. and Kohn, H., Inherited histocompatibility changes in progeny of irradiated and unirradiated inbred mice, Genet. Res. 6:330 (1965).
20. Nairn, R., Yamaga, K. and Nathenson, S.G., Biochemistry of the gene products from murine MHC mutants, Ann. Rev. Genetics 14:241 (1980).
21. Nathenson, S.G., Brown, J.L., Ewenstein, B.M., Nisizawa, T., Sears, D.W., and Freed, J.H. Structural differences between parent and variant H-2K glycoproteins from mouse strains carrying H-2 gene mutations, in Cold Spring Harbor Symposia on Quantitative Biology, Cold Spring Harbor Laboratory, New York, Vol. XLI, 1977, p. 343.
22. Pease, L.R., Schulze, D.H., Pfaffenbach, G.M. and Nathenson, S.G., Spontaneous H-2 mutants provide evidence that a copy mechanism analogous to gene conversion generates polymorphism in the major histocompatibility complex, Proc. Natl. Acad. Sci. 80:242 (1983).

THE ANALYSIS OF H-2 MUTANTS:

MOLECULAR GENETICS AND STRUCTURE/FUNCTION RELATIONSHIPS

Jan Geliebter, Richard A. Zeff, Rita Spathis, Gertrude Pfaffenbach*, Mayumi Nakagawa, Brigid McCue, Hiroshi Mashimo, Krishna Kesari, Silvio Hemmi, Kim Hasenkrug, Francescopaolo Borriello, P. Ajit Kumar and Stanley G. Nathenson

Departments of Cell Biology and Microbiology and Immunology
Albert Einstein College of Medicine, Bronx, NY 10461
*Present Address: Deptartment of Zoology
University of Texas at Austin, Austin, TX 78712

The class I genes of the murine major histocompatibility complex are located in four regions (K, D, Qa, Tla) along chromosome 17. The K and D regions contain the genes encoding the classical H-2 transplantation antigens (K, D, L). Alleles of each of the K, D and L loci exhibit substantial sequence diversity (1-3). Further, H-2 loci are highly polymorphic, with over 100 alleles identified per locus (3). The high sequence diversity and polymorphism of H-2 genes are thought to play a role in the function of their products as antigen presenting molecules, thus enabling a population to respond to many different pathogens. In contrast, Qa and Tla region loci are much less polymorphic and alleles of each locus appear to be much more conserved (4,5). Qa and Tla gene products have a limited tissue distribution and their function is unknown.

The study of structure/function relationships of H-2 molecules has been hampered by the extraordinary diversity among alleles. For example, functionally crucial amino acid differences between alleles are not conspicuous against a "background" of high amino acid sequence diversity. As described in the previous chapter, the biochemical analysis of mutant K^b molecules provided the first insights into the fine structure/function relationships of histocompatibility molecules (6). The limited amino acid alterations between the mutant and parental K^b molecules allows for the correlation of discrete structural differences with the observed functional differences of the mutant molecules such as the elicitation of graft rejection and altered H-2 restriction (see below). However, due to the nature of the amino acid sequencing techniques and the prevalent thought that the substitutions in the mutant K^b molecules were the result of spontaneous point mutations, the full extent of the alterations in the mutant glycoproteins escaped detection.

With the advent of DNA and RNA sequencing techniques all of the nucleotide and deduced amino acid alterations of several of the K^b mutants were determined (7-10). An amino acid substitution profile for the K^b mutants analyzed thus far is diagrammed in Figure 1a. The K^{bm10} molecule which was previously thought to contain a single amino acid alteration was found to have 4 substitutions (10). The K^{bm6} and K^{bm9} molecules contain the identical substitutions at positions 116 and 121 (9). Amino acid sequencing data indicate that K^{bm8} has at least 3 altered residues (11, and G. Pfaffenbach and S.G. Nathenson, unpublished data). K^{bm3} and K^{bm11} have the identical Asp to Ser alteration at position 77 but each contains one additional amino acid substitution at position 89 and 80, respectively (10).

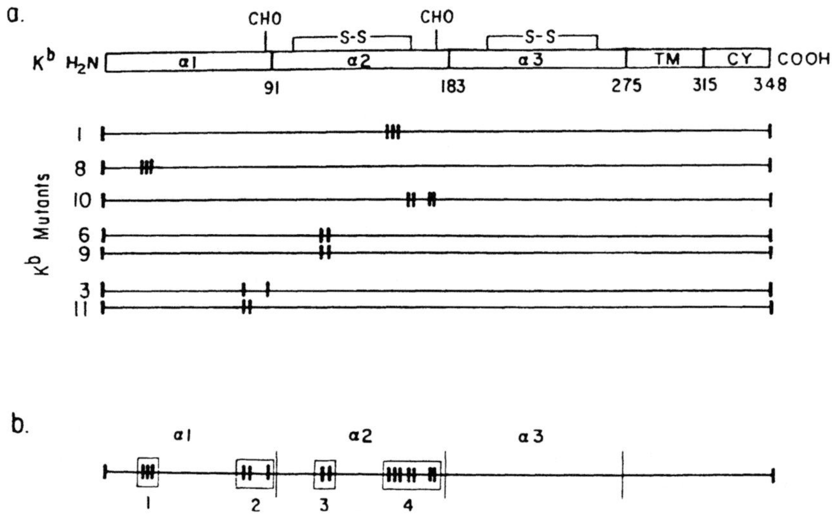

Fig. 1. a) Amino acid substitution profile of the K^b mutants. The K^b molecule is represented as an empty rectangle; K^b mutants are depicted as solid lines. Domain structure of K^b is according to exon-intron organization as described by Weiss et al. (27). The three extracellular domains are α1, α2 and α3; the transmembrane domain is abbreviated, TM; three cytoplasmic exons are presented in a single domain, CY. Amino acid residues are numbered according to Weiss et al. (27). Disulfide bridges are represented as S-S and carbohydrate moieties are represented by CHO. Vertical dashes represent known amino acid alterations. K^{bm1} from Weiss et al. (7) and Schulze et al. (8); K^{bm6} and K^{bm9} from Geliebter et al. (9); K^{bm3}, K^{bm11} and K^{bm10} from Geliebter and Nathenson (10); K^{bm8} alterations are from amino acid sequencing (11, and G. Pfaffenbach and S.G. Nathenson, unpublished data).
(b) Antigenically important regions of K^b. The positions of altered amino acids of all the K^b mutants are presented on a single molecule to localize immunologically important regions of K^b (open rectangles).

The sequence analyses of mutant K^b molecules has enabled us to identify 4 antigenically important regions within the α1 and α2 domains of the K^b molecule (Fig. 1b). Alterations in any of these regions results in the formation of new alloreactive epitopes (relative to K^b) which are detectable by graft rejection in vivo and by CTL in vitro (12,13). Further, at least some of these regions also appear to be involved in the presentation of viral products to the T cell receptor. For example, CTL directed against vesicular stomatitis virus antigens in association with K^b will not recognize VSV antigens in association with K^{bm3}, K^{bm11} or K^{bm1} (mutations in regions 2 and 4) (14). Lymphocytic choriomeningitis virus (LCMV) antigens in association with K^{bm8} (mutations in region 1) are poorly recognized by K^b restricted CTL against LCMV antigens (15). Thus, these portions of the K^b molecule probably play a major role in interactions with the T cell receptor and/or antigen presentation.

In addition to expanding our understanding of the structure-function relationships of H-2 molecules, the nature of the alterations in the K^b molecules and genes suggested that they were generated by a recombination mechanism (often referred to as gene conversion in the literature) rather than by random point mutations (11). The interesting characteristics of the K^b mutants that led to this suggestion include (Fig. 1):

1) All of the mutant molecules sequenced to date contain multiple amino acid substitutions. For example, K^{bm10} contains 4 amino acid replacements, at positions 163, 165, 173 and 174 (10). The K^{bm1} molecule is altered at 3 positions, 152, 155 and 156 (7,8).

2) The substituted amino acids of each mutant are grouped into small clusters, implying non-randomness. For example, the 3 amino acid substitutions in K^{bm1} are clustered within 5 residues (7,8).

3) Many of the altered amino acids contain multiple nucleotide substitutions per codon, again implying non-randomness and complexity in the mutation process. A dramatic example is codon 155 of K^{bm1} where the entire triplet is changed from AGA to TAT (7,8).

4) The identical alterations reoccur in mutant mice of independent origins. At least 5 independent mutant molecules (K^{bm5}, K^{bm6}, K^{bm7}, K^{bm9}, K^{bm16}) contain the identical Tyr to Phe substitutions at position 116 (16,17). K^{bm6} and K^{bm9} have been sequenced at the nucleotide level and contain the identical A to T substitution at position 116, as well as the same T to C alteration at position 121 (9).

5) As more sequence data became available for class I molecules and genes it was observed that the amino acids substituted into the mutant K^b molecules were also found in other class I molecules of various haplotypes (11,18). For example, the 3 amino acids substituted into K^{bm1} at positions 152, 155 and 156 (Ala, Tyr, Tyr) are identical to those already found at positions 152, 155 and 156 of the L^d molecule (11,18).

Taken collectively, these characteristics hinted that a recombination mechanism between K^b and other class I genes may be responsible for the generation of the K^b mutants. This idea was supported by the observation that both Southern blot hybridization analysis (19,20) and cosmid cloning (21,22) data indicated that the class I genes comprise a multigene family of approximately 30 homologous genes. The vast majority of these genes are non-H-2, mapping to the Qa and Tla regions. It was thought that the non-H-2 genes could serve as a reservoir of genetic information that could be recombined into and "mutate" H-2 genes.

The confirmation of the recombination theory required that "donor" DNA sequences, identical to those substituted into the mutant K^b genes be present elsewhere in the parental C57BL/6 genome. The use of mutant-specific oligonucleotide probes was instrumental in the identification of donor genes. Synthetic oligonucleotides, complementary to the altered nucelotides of the mutant K^b genes, were radiolabeled and hybridized to cloned class I genes (9,10,23). The identification of a potential donor gene was followed by the sequencing of the gene to ensure that it contained the identical sequence as substituted into the particular mutant K^b gene.

Genes from all 4 regions of the MHC (K, D, Qa, Tla) have been identified as donor genes for the various K^b mutants (Fig. 2). For example, the Qa region genes Q4 and Q10 have been demonstrated to be the donor genes for the $K^{bm6,9}$ and K^{bm1} mutants, respectively (9,23). The D^b gene contains the same sequence as substituted into the K^{bm11} gene (5). The K1 gene which is located approximately 15 kilobases centromeric to K^b is the donor gene for the K^{bm10} mutations (10). Thus, the flow of genetic information to K^b proceeds centromerically and telomerically along chromosome 17, across distances of hundreds of kilobases (21).

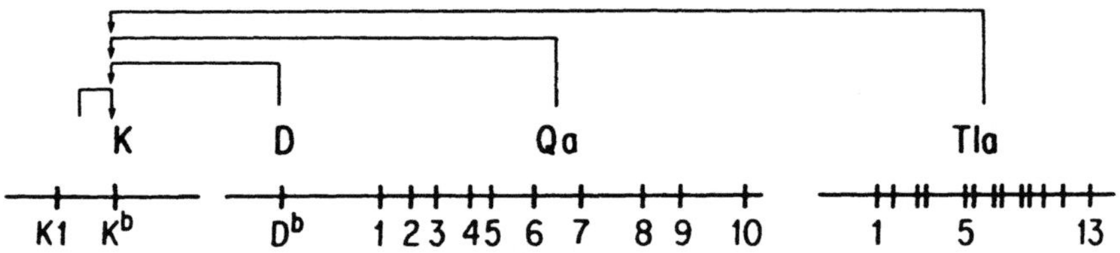

Fig.2. Generation of K^b mutants by micro-recombinations with other class I genes. Uppermost capital letters represent the K, D, Qa and Tla regions of the H-2^b MHC. K1 and K^b are indicated; Qa region genes are numbered 1-10; Tla region genes are numbered 1-13 according to Weiss et al. (27). Arrows indicate the transfer of genetic information from class I genes to K^b via micro-recombinations (Reprinted from Trends in Genetics 3, p. 110, 1987).

The segments of genetic information transferred from the various donor genes to K^b are less than 100 nucleotides (9,10,23). Thus, K^b-donor gene interactions can be considered "micro-recombinations", reflecting the transfer of tens of nucleotides between 2 class I genes. Interestingly, the MHC class II I-A_β^{bm12} mutant was also generated by a micro-recombination event in which less than 44 nucleotides were transferred between 2 class II genes (24,25). Mechanistically, micro-recombination products may result from double crossovers or gene conversion-like events, both of which are consistent with a small "foreign" segment of DNA being substituted into an otherwise wild type gene. The mutant K^b genes clearly do not result from single, reciprocal crossovers between the K^b and donor genes as this would result in K^b/donor hybrid genes, which are not observed. Such a single crossover and the resultant hybrid gene product has been demonstrated for the D^{dm1} mutant of the B10.D2 mouse (26).

Alleles of H-2 loci exhibit extreme sequence diversity from one another (1,2). For example, K^b and K^d differ from each other by 35 of the amino terminal 180 amino acids (27,28). Micro-recombinations may be the mechanism by which H-2 alleles achieve their diversity. The occurrence of many micro-recombination events accumulating within the K genes of a mouse population could, over time, produce the allelic sequence diversity observed among K alleles. As depicted in Fig. 3, repeated micro-recombinations would result in a hypothetical chimeric allele, K^x, which contains sequences from K, D, Qa and Tla region genes. Natural K alleles do indeed resemble K^x in that they appear to be mosaics of class I gene sequences from all 4 regions of the MHC. For example, compared to K^b, the K^d allele (from DBA/2 mouse) contains some of the same Q10, Q4 and K1 gene sequences as substituted into the K^{bm1}, $K^{bm6,9}$, and K^{bm10} genes (9,10,23). Thus, it appears that the K^d allele may have attained its present mosaic structure by several micro-recombinations with various class I genes.

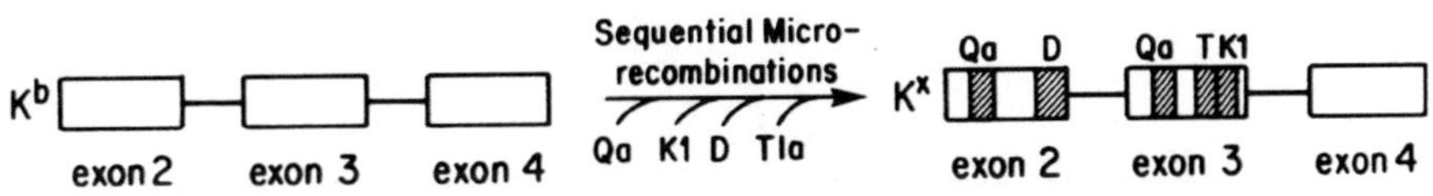

Fig.3. Micro-recombinations generate diversity in the K^b gene. The accumulation of several micro-recombinations within the same K^b gene generates a new K allele, K^x, which contains K, D, Qa and Tla region sequences. Open rectangle represents exons 2, 3 and 4 (domains α1, α2 and α3). Solid lines between exons represent introns. Hatched areas in K^x indicate non-K^b class I DNA and are in the regions of mutant K^b micro-recombination events. No micro-recombinations have been detected in exon 4 (Reprinted from Trends in Genetics 3, p. 110, 1987).

The maintenance and fixation of mutant alleles in the population is probably determined at the level of the gene product where the ability of the new allele to function as an antigen presenting molecule for contemporary pathogens is tested. The inability of a mutant allele to present the antigens of a pathogen would result in its elimination from the population. On the other hand, the substitution of new amino acid sequences into either of the 4 antigenically important regions of the K^b molecule (Fig. 1b) may result in a new allele that can more effectively present antigens than the parental K^b molecule. In this case, selection against the K^b allele would, de facto, favor the fixation of the new mutant allele. Thus, while micro-recombination events provide the raw materials for the sequence diversification of H-2 genes, natural selection at the product level probably provides the driving force for the maintenance of diverse and polymorphic H-2 genes and products in the population.

The possible role of selection as the driving force in the maintanance of diverse and polymorphic H-2 alleles may also explain the conservation of alleles of Qa and Tla region loci. Alleles of Qa and Tla region loci often exhibit greater than 99% sequence homology (4,5,29). While it is not known whether Qa and Tla region genes are the recipients of H-2 gene sequences, such recombination products, if they exist, may not be under the driving force of selection for diversity as postulated for H-2 genes. If so, such recombinant Qa and Tla genes might not become fixed in the population and be lost. In support of this idea is the finding that the number of Qa region genes varies dramatically among inbred mouse strains and thus may be dispensable (30), and therefore not be subject to strong selective pressures.

In summary, the concerted evolution of the MHC class I multigene family has been shown to include micro-recombination events between K^b and class I donor genes from all regions of the MHC. The diverse and polymorphic nature of H-2 genes can then be explained by the micro-recombination process coupled with selection for a large repertoire of diverse antigen presenting molecules. Further, the analysis of micro-recombinations at the product level has enabled us to localize those regions of the K^b molecule that are strategically involved in the presentation of foreign antigens to or interactions with the T cell receptor.

Acknowledgements

The authors would like to thank Ms. Catherine Whelan for secretarial assistance. The authors are supported by grants to S.G.N.: AI-10702, AI-07289 and NCI P30-13330 from NIH, ACS grant IM-236, and by the Irvington House Institute for Medical Research. J.G. is supported by NIH training grant CA-09173.

References

1. Steinmetz, M., and Hood, L., Genes of the major histocompatibility complex in mouse and man, Science 222:727 (1983).
2. Kimball, E. S., and Coligan, J. E., Structure of class I major histocompatibility antigens, Contemp. Topics Molec. Immunol. 9:1 (1983).
3. Klein, J., and Figueroa, F., Evolution of the major histocompatibility complex, Critical Reviews in Immunology 6:295 (1986).
4. Flavell, R. A., Allen, H., Burkly, L. C., Sherman, D. H., Waneck, G. L., and Widera, G., Molecular biology of the H-2 histocompatibility complex, Science 233:437 (1986).
5. Pontarotti, P., Mashimo, H., Zeff, R. A., Fisher, D., Hood, L., Mellor, A., Flavell, R. A., and Nathenson, S. G., Conservation vs. diversity in the class I genes of the major histocompatibility complex: Sequence analysis of the Tla^a gene and comparison with a Tla^c gene, Proc. Natl. Acad. Sci. USA 83:1782 (1985).
6. Nairn, R., Yamaga, K., and Nathenson, S.G., Biochemistry of the gene products from murine MHC mutants, Ann. Rev. Genet. 14:241 (1980).
7. Weiss, E. H., Mellor, A., Golden, L., Fahner, K., Simpson, E., Hurst, J., and Flavell, R. A., The structure of a mutant H-2 gene suggests that the generation of polymorphism in H-2 genes may occur by gene conversion-like events, Nature 301:671 (1983)
8. Schulze, D. H., Pease, L. R., Geier, S. S., Reyes, A. A., Sarmiento, L. A., Wallace, R. B., and Nathenson, S. G., Comparison of the cloned $H\text{-}2K^{bm1}$ variant gene with the $H\text{-}2K^b$ gene shows a cluster of seven

nucleotide differences, Proc. Natl. Acad. Sci. USA 80:2007 (1983).
9. Geliebter, J., Zeff, R. A., Melvold, R. W., and Nathenson, S. G., Mitotic recombination in germ cells generated two MHC mutants determined to be identical by RNA sequence analysis: K^{bm9} and K^{bm6}. Proc. Natl. Acad. Sci USA 83:3371 (1986).
10. Geliebter, J., and Nathenson, S. G., Micro-recombinations generate sequence diversity in the murine major histocompatibility complex: Analyses of the K^{bm3}, K^{bm4}, K^{bm10}, and K^{bm11} mutants, submitted.
11. Pease, L. R., Schulze, D. H., Pfaffenbach, G. M., and Nathenson, S. G., Spontaneous H-2 mutants provide evidence that a copy mechanism analogous to gene conversion generates polymorphism in the major histocompatibility complex, Proc. Natl. Acad. Sci. USA 80:242 (1983).
12. Melief, C. J. M., de Waal, L. P., van der Meulen, M. Y., Melvold, R. W., and Kohn, H. I., Fine specificity of alloimmune cytotoxic T lymphocytes directed against H-2K. A study of K^b mutants, J. Exp. Med. 151:993 (1980).
13. Sherman, L. A., Recognition of conformational determinants on H-2 by cytolytic T lymphocytes, Nature 997:511 (1982).
14. Clark, S. S., Geier, S., Nathenson, S. G., and Forman, J., Analysis of associative recognition determinants on class I $H\text{-}2K^b$ mutant molecules, Immunogenetics 22:391 (1985).
15. Blanden, R. V., Dunlop, M. B. C., Doherty, P. C., Kohn, H. I. and McKenzie, I. F. C., Effects of four H-2K mutations on virus-induced antigens recognized by cytotoxic T cells, Immunogenetics 3:541 (1976).
16. Yamaga, K. M., Pfaffenbach, G. M., Pease, L. R., McGovern, D., Nisizawa, T., Melvold, R. W., Kohn, H. I., and Nathenson, S. G., Biochemical studies of H-2K antigens from a group of related mutants. I. Identification of a shared mutation in $B6\text{-}H\text{-}2^{bm5}$ and $B6\text{-}H\text{-}2^{bm16}$, Immunogenetics 17:19 (1983).
17. Yamaga, K. M., Pfaffenbach, G. M., Pease, L. R., McGovern, D., Nisizawa, T., Melvold, R. W., Kohn, H. I., and Nathenson, S. G., Biochemical studies of H-2K antigens from a group of related mutants. II. Identification of a shared mutation in $B6\text{-}H\text{-}2^{bm6}$, $B6.C\text{-}H\text{-}2^{bm7}$, $B6.C\text{-}H\text{-}2^{bm9}$ (1983).
18. Evans, G. A., Margulies, D. H., Camerini-Otero, R. D., Ozato, K., and Seidman, J. G., Structure and expression of a mouse major histocompatibility antigen gene, $H\text{-}2L^d$, Proc. Natl. Acad. Sci. USA 79:1994 (1982).
19. Steinmetz, M., Frelinger, J. G., Fisher, D., Hunkapiller, T., Pereira, D., Weissman, S. M., Uehara, H., Nathenson, S. G., and Hood, L., Three cDNA clones encoding mouse transplantation antigens: Homology to immunoglobulin genes, Cell 24:125 (1981).
20. Pease, L. R., Nathenson, S. G., and Leinwand, L. A., Mapping class I gene sequences in the major histocompatibility complex, Nature 298:382 (1982).
21. Weiss, E. H., Golden, L., Fahrner, K., Mellor, A. L., Devlin, J. J., Bullman, H., Tiddens, H., Bud, H., and Flavell, R. A., Organization and evolution of the class I gene family in the major histocompatibility complex of the C57BL/10 mouse, Nature 310:650 (1984).
22. Steinmetz, M., Winoto, A., Minard, K., and Hood, L., Clusters of genes encoding mouse transplantation antigens, Cell 28:489 (1982).
23. Mellor, A. L., Weiss, E. H., Ramachandran, K., and Flavell, R. A., A potential donor gene for the bml gene conversion event in the C57BL mouse, Nature 306:792 (1983).
24. McIntyre, K. R., and Seidman, J. G., Nucleotide sequence of mutant $I\text{-}A\beta^{bm12}$ gene is evidence for genetic exchange between mouse immune response genes, Nature 308:551 (1984).

25. Widera, G., and Flavell, R. A., The nucleotide sequence of the murine I-Eβ^b immune response gene: Evidence for gene conversion events in class II genes of the major histocompatibility complex, EMBO J. 3:1221 (1984).
26. Sun, Y. H., Goodenow, R. S., and Hood, L., Molecular basis of the dml mutation in the major histocompatibility complex of the mouse: A D/L hybrid gene, J. Exp. Med. 162:1588, 1985.
27. Weiss, E. H., Golden, L., Zakut, R., Mellor, A., Fahrner, K., Kvist, S., and Flavell, R. A., The DNA sequence of the H-2K^b gene: Evidence for gene conversion as a mechanism for the generation of polymorphism in histocompatibility antigens, EMBO J. 2:453 (1983).
28. Kvist, S., Roberts, L., and Dobberstein, B., Mouse histocompatibility genes: Structure and organization of a K^d gene, EMBO J. 2:245 (1983).
29. Fisher, D. A., Hunt III, S. W., and Hood, L., The structure of a gene encoding a Murine Thymus Leukemia antigen and the organization of Tla genes in the BALB/c mouse, J. Exp. Med. 162:528 (1985).
30. O'Neill, A. E., Reid, K., Garberi, J. C., Karl, M., and Flaherty, L., Extensive deletions in the Q region of the mouse major histocompatibility complex, Immunogenetics 24:368 (1986).

SITE DIRECTED MUTAGENESIS IDENTIFIES ALLO-ANTIGENIC EPITOPES OF AN H-2 ANTIGEN RECOGNIZED BY ANTIBODIES AND BY CYTOTOXIC T-LYMPHOCYTES

Keiko Ozato,[1] David Koeller,[1] Ronald Lieberman,[1,3] Jun-ichi Miyazaki,[1] Ettore Appella,[2] Donald W Mann,[4] and James Forman[4]

[1]Laboratory of Developmental and Molecular Immunity, National Institute of Child Health and Human Development, [2]Laboratory of Cell Biology, National Cancer Institute, National Institutes of Health Bethesda, Maryland, 20892, [3]Division of Cardio-Reno Drug and Drug Products, Food and Drug Administration, Rockville, Maryland, and the [4]Department of Microbiology, University of Texas, Health Science Center at Dallas, Dallas, Texas, 25235.

ABSTRACT

To test our previous hypothesis that the segment between amino acid position 63 to 73 of the H-2D^d antigen forms a major allo-antigenic site, mutations were introduced into the H-2L^d gene in a sequential fashion, which replaced the codons for amino acid position 63, 65, 66, 70 and 73 of the H-2L^d antigen with those of the H-2D^d antigen. Gain and loss of serological and CTL epitopes specific for the H-2D^d and H-2L^d antigens were examined. The amino acid substitutions at position 63, 65, and 66 led to the acquisition of multiple serological H-2D^d specificities which were expressed in the mutant H-2L^d antigen. A further amino acid substitution at position 70 resulted in the gain of additional H-2D^d specificities, allowing to localize more than half of all the relevant H-2D^d serological epitopes to position 63 to 70. An allo CTL epitope of the H-2D^d antigen was also localized to this stretch of amino acid sequence, as one of several H-2D^d specific CTL clones reacted with the mutant molecule in which amino acids were replaced at position 63 to 70. Further, some H-2L^d specific allo CTL clones lost reactivity to the mutant molecules, demonstrating the presence of CTL epitopes in this region of the H-2L^d antigen. From these results we conclude that the amino acid sequence encompassing from position 63 to 70 of the H-2D^d and H-2L^d molecules forms major allo- antigenic epitopes recognized by multiple antibodies and CTLs.

INTRODUCTION

The polymorphic MHC class I antigens evoke unusually vigorous allo-immune responses among MHC disparate mice. There are an unexpectedly large number of precursor T-cells capable of recognizing allo-epitopes of H-2 antigens (Fisher-Lindahl and Wilson, 1977), which are greater in number than precursors for MHC antigens of other species. Allo-immunizations also lead to production of antibodies that are diverse in specificities and idiotypes. Analyses of the humoral and cell-mediated allo-responses pioneered by Gorer and Snell (Gorer 1937; Snell 1948), provided the foundation of genetics of murine major histocompatibility complex. However, T- and B-cell repertoire which constitutes allo-immune responses has not been fully elucidated, partly because the epitope organization of H-2 antigens have been difficult to dissect.

Recent studies on exon shuffled and mutant H-2 genes revealed that the majority of serological and CTL epitopes are localized in the first (α-1) and second (α-2) external domains of H-2 antigens, which show greater polymorphism than the third (α-3) external domain at the level of nucleotide and amino acid sequences (Nathenson et al., 1986; Koeller and Ozato, 1987; Forman, 1987). A number of conformational epitopes generated by the interaction of the α-1 and α-2 domains have been found, which comprise most of epitopes recognized by CTLs. Wheras a large proportion of antibodies have been found to react with determinants localized soley to the α-1 or the α-2 domain. These results illustrate the dichotomy of epitopes detected by antibodies and by CTLs.

We previously postulated that the amino acid sequence encompassing position 63 to 73 of the α-1 domain of the H-2D^d antigen constitutes a major serological allo-antigenic site (Ozato et al., 1985). This region is one of the most polymorphic region of all MHC class I antigens. Furthermore, this region shows the highest predicted local hydrophilicity in the H-2D^d antigen.

Mutagenesis

To address the role of amino acid sequence from position 63 to 73 of the H-2D^d and H-2L^d antigens for the formation of allo-epitopes, specific mutations were introduced into the H-2L^d gene (Koeller et al., 1987) by site directed mutagenesis. The mutations were designed to replace amino acid codons of position 63, 65, 66, 70 and 73 of the H-2L^d antigen with those of the H-2D^d type. The site directed mutagenesis procedure described by Smith and Zoller (1984) was employed with small modifications. A XbaI fragment containing the 5'coding region of a genomic H-2L^d gene cloned in a single stranded DNA vector, M13 was used as the original template (Shiroishi et al., 1985). Mutations were sequentially introduced by using 4 synthetic oligonucleotides containing several mismatches (Table 1). The first mutant M66 has substitutions at position 63, 65, and 66. The second mutant M70 has an additional substitution at position 70. The final mutant M73 has a further substitution at position 73, making this mutant identical to the H-2D^d antigen in amino acid sequence from position 53 to 76. Fig. 1 depicts DNA sequence of the final mutant M73. Due to the degeneracy of the amino acid codes the mutant sequence differs from that of the native H-2D^d gene, even though the two genes encode the same amino acids in this region. The mutant clones were ligated to the 3' coding region of the H-2L^d gene, and introduced into mouse L-cells by DNA mediated gene transfer. Clones expressing the H-2L^d antigens were detected by binding of a monoclonal antibody (mAb) specific for the α-3 domain of the H-2L^d antigen.

TABLE 1

[A] AMINO ACID SEOUENCES OF CLASS I MOLECULES

Molecule	61	62	63	64	65	66	67	68	69	70	71	72	73	74	75
H-2L^d	GLU	ARG	ILE	THR	GLN	ILE	ALA	GLY	LYS	GLY	GLN	GLU	TRP	PHE	ARG
H-2D^d	·	·	GLU	·	ARG	ARG	·	·	·	ASN	·	·	SER	·	·
M66	·	·	GLU	·	ARG	ARG	·	·	·	·	·	·	·	·	·
M70	·	·	GLU	·	ARG	ARG	·	·	·	ASN	·	·	·	·	·
M73	·	·	GLU	·	ARG	ARG	·	·	·	ASN	·	·	SER	·	·

[B] OLIGONUCLEOTIDES USED FOR MUTAGENESIS

					***					
LE2-1	ATA	ACC	CTC	GCC	CTC	TGC	GTC	TAG	CGG	
	59	60	61	62	63	64	65	66	67	

					*	**			
LE2-3	CTC	GCC	CTC	TGC	GCC	TCC	CGG	TTC	CCG
	61	62	63	64	65	66	67	68	69

			* *					
LE2-4	TTC	CCG	TTA	CTC	GTC	ACC	AAG	GCT
	68	69	70	71	72	73	74	75

					*			
LE2-7	CCG	TTA	CTC	GTC	AGC	AAG	GCT	CAC
	69	70	71	72	73	74	75	76

[A] Comparison of the amino acid sequences of the α-1 domains of the L^d, D^d and three mutant L^d antigens generated in this study. Mutations were introduced into the L^d gene at the underlined residues with the D^d amino acids.

[B] Sequences of the four oligomers used for site directed mutagenesis with the corresponding amino acid positions indicated. The positions of mismatched nucleotides are indicated by asterisks.

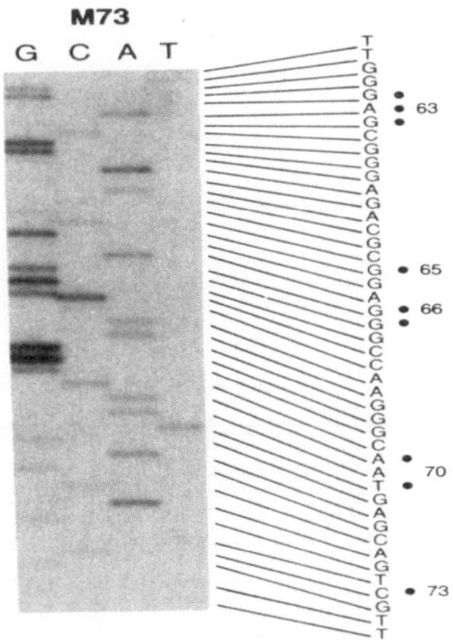

Figure l: Nucleotide sequence of the final mutant M73. DNA sequence of each mutant was determined by the method of Sanger et al. (1980). The relevant portion of DNA sequence is shown. Circles denote the position of the corresponding nucleotide substitution. Numbers indicate the corresponding amino acid position.

Multiple serological epitopes expressed in the mutant H-2L^d antigens.

Evaluation of serological specificities of each mutant molecule was carried out by cytofluorography analysis with a series of mAb reactive with the H-2D^d or H-2L^d antigen (Ozato et al., 1980; Ozato et al., 1985; Chătterjee-Das et al., 1987). Strain distribution and domain specificities of these antibodies have been previously characterized in detail. Table 2 shows 28 mAb representing unique specificities of the H-2D^d antigen. Epitopes of these mAb have been localized within the α-1 domain or to conformational determinants influenced by both the α-

1 and α-2 domains. The substitutions at position 63, 65, and 66 resulted in the gain of 9 H-2D^d serological specificities, indicating the involvement of these amino acids for formation of epitopes. The additional substitution at position 70 resulted in the further gain of additional 6 unique specificities, illustrating that a single amino acid can participate in the formation of multiple serological specificites. Thus, more than half of all epitopes in the α-1 domain or α 1-α/2-domain of the H-2D^d antigen are at least in part localized to amino acid sequence from 63 to 70: Epitopes of these mAb may be directly mapped into this region or they may be composed of discontinuous sets of amino acid sequences, one of which is governed by amino acids 63 to 70. Examples of mAb binding to the mutant antigens M66 and M70 expressed in L-cells are shown in Fig.2. The binding of anti-D^d mAb to the mutant molecules was, for most cases, comparable to that to the native H-2D^d antigen. The final mutation at position 73 (M73) did not lead to the gain of new specificities, indicating that this amino acid is not essential for the formation of H-2D^d seological specificities. Although most H-2D^d specificites expressed in M66 and M70 were retained in M73, a few mAb lost reactivity to this mutation (see Table 2). The basis of the loss of these specificites is not clear: It appears that the alteration at position 73 imparied the conformational structure expressed in M66 and M70, which was influenced by the α-2 domain of the H-2L^d molecule. Eight mAb previously assigned to the α-2 and α-3 domain of the H-2D^d antigen were all negative with the mutants, as expected. Six mAb specific for the H-2L^d antigen were tested, only one of which has been assigned to react with the α-1 domain. All 3 mutant molecules retained full reactivity to these anti-H-2L^d mAb.

TABLE 2

More Than Half of the H-2D^d Specificities Present in the

α-1 or α-1/α-2 Domain are Localized to Residue 63-70

	REACTIVITY TO				
Anti-D^d mAb	L^d	M66	M70	M73	D^d
T.O. 107	-	-	-	-	+
T.O. 111	-	-	-	-	+
T.O. 119	-	-	-	-	+
T.O. 120	-	-	-	-	+
T.O. 129	-	-	-	-	+
T.O. 131	-	-	-	-	+
T.O. 137	-	-	+	+	+
T.O. 124	-	+	+	+	+
34.4.21	-	+	+	+	+
34.1.2	-	+	+	+	+
T.O. 104	-	-	-	-	+
T.O. 115	-	-	-	-	+
T.O. 116	-	-	-	-	+
T.O. 125	-	-	-	-	+
T.O. 130	-	-	-	-	+
T.O. 138	-	-	-	-	+
T.O. 141	-	-	-	-	+
T.O. 108	-	-	+	+	+
T.O. 118	-	-	+	+	+
T.O. 126	-	-	+	+	+
23.5.21	-	-	+	-	+
T.O. 122	-	-	+	-	+

T.O. 145	-	-	+	-	+
T.O. 110	-	+	+	+	+
T.O. 127	-	+	+	+	+
T.O. 128	-	+	+	+	+
T.O. 132	-	+	+	+	+
T.O. 134	-	+	+	+	+

Anti-D^d mAb 108

Anti-D^d mAb 34-4-21

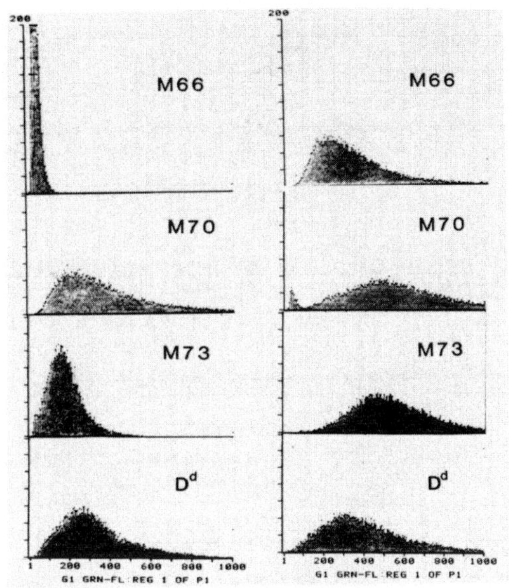

Figure 2: Cytofluorographic analysis of binding of anti-H-$2D^d$ mAb to the H-$2L^d$ mutant. Cells transformed with the mutant L^d genes were stained with mAb as described. Background staining with antibodies of unrelated specificities was indistinguishable from that shown in the top left panel.

Reactivity of anti-H-$2D^d$ and anti-H-$2L^d$ CTL clones with the mutant H-$2L^d$ molecules.

CTL clones specific for the H-$2D^d$ antigens were generated by the limiting dilution method (Forman et al., 1984) from a CTL culture of B10.D2 (R103) anti-BALB/cH-2^{dm2} or CBA anti-BALB/c H-2^{dm2}. Anti-H-$2L^d$ CTL clones were produced by stimulation of C3HxBALB/c.H-2^{dm2} with BALB/c or CBA with A.AL cells. Reactivity of mutant molecules to these CTL clones was tested in a 4 hr 51[Cr]-release assay at 25 to 1 or 5 to 1 effector to target cell ratio. As seen in Fig. 3 an anti-H-2D clone designated D.88.42 specifically lysed L cells expressing M66 and M70 mutant gene, demonstrating that a CTL epitope is localized in the amino acid sequence between 63 to 70 of the H-$2D^d$ molecule. Similar to the loss of serological epitopes seen in M73, this CTL clone did not react with M73. This again suggests conformational influence by the α-2 domain of the H-$2L^d$ antigen. As seen in Fig. 4, an anti-H-$2L^d$ CTL clone failed to react with all 3 mutant, M66, M70 and M73, even though this clone elicits a high level of cytolysis against the native H-$2L^d$ molecule, demonstrating that this region is essential for the formation of epitopes recognized by this clone. The presence of additional CTL epitopes in this region of the H-$2L^d$ molecule is indicated by clone L13D.8A-which was reactive with the native H-$2L^d$, M66, but not with M70. Clearly, amino acid position 70 is critically involved in generating H-$2L^d$ epitopes. These data show that some of H-$2L^d$ CTL epitopes are also mapped into this region of the molecule.

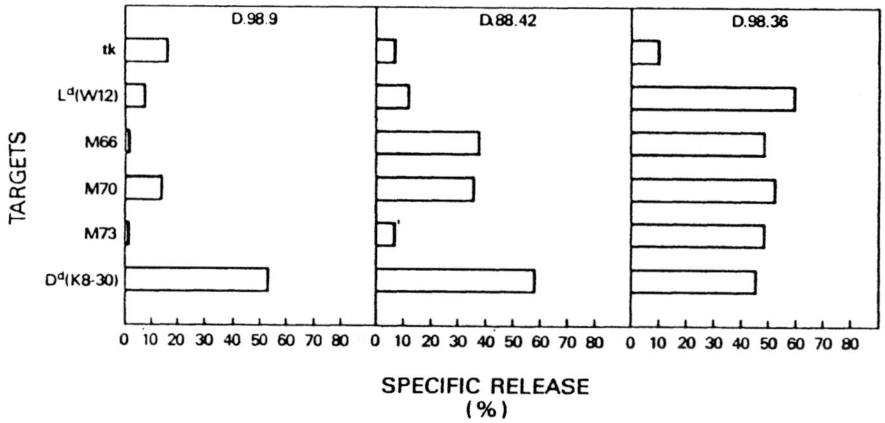

Figure 3: Reactivity of anti-H-$2D^d$ CTL clones to mutant H-$2L^d$ molecules. Clone D8.3 is from B10.D2 (R103) anti-BALB/c-H-2^{dm2} and the other three clones are from CBA anti-BALB/c-H-2^{dm2} cultures. Data shown for E/T=25.

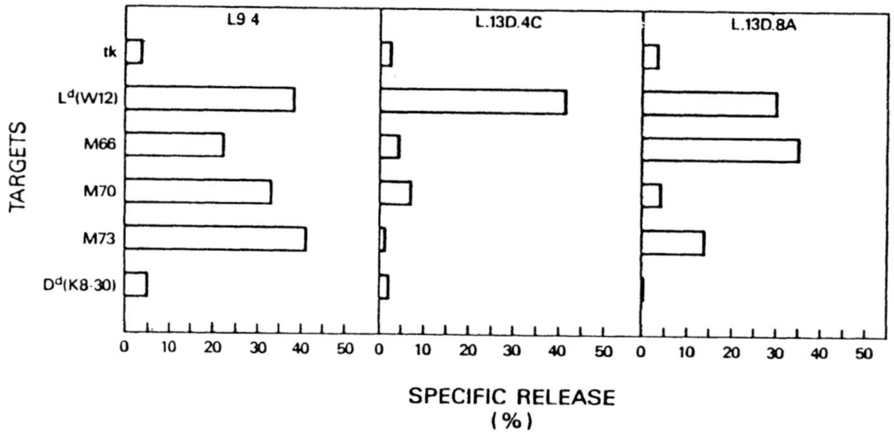

Figure 4: Reactivity of anti-$2L^d$ CTL clones to mutant H-$2L^d$ molecules. Clone L9.4 is from (C3H x BALB/c-H-2^{dm2})F_1 anti-BALB/c and clones L.13D.4C and L.13D.8A are from CBA anti-A.AL cultures. Data shown for E/T=25.

DISCUSSION

We have localized multiple allo-antigenic determinants of the H-$2D^d$ antigen defined both by antibodies and by CTLs to the amino acid sequence from position 63 to 70. The extensive serological epitopes clustered in this region of the H-$2D^d$ antigen indicates that it is an immunodominant area of the molecule. For serological epitopes of the H-$2L^d$ antigen, very few determinants have been localized to the α-1 domain of the molecule. The retension of all H-$2L^d$ specificities in the mutants and the paucity of serological epitopes in the α-1 domain suggest that neither the region from 63 to 70 nor the entire α-1 domain forms a major epitope structure. Analyses of anti-H-$2L^d$ CTL clones, however, show that this region of the molecule contains multiple allo-CTL specificities. Thus, there appears to be a certain level of dichotomy in the location of epitopes detected by mAb and by CTLs for the H-$2L^d$ molecule.

Exactly how the amino acid sequence of this region forms multiple serological and CTL -epitopes is not clear. Hopp and Woods (1981) have proposed that elevated local hydrophilicity within a protein molecule contributes to the formation of antigenic sites detected by antibodies. It is notable that amino acid position 63 to 66 of the H-2D^d antigen exhibits the highest predicted local hydrophilicity within the α-1 domain, while this region of the H-2L^d antigen is not particularly hydrophilic. Other factors such as those that influence local mobility of a protein may be a critical element for the formation of serological epitopes, as reported by Geysen (1987).

DeLisi and Bersofsky (1985) have proposed a model for epitopes uniquely recognized by T-cells, in which an amphipathic structure plays a determining role. Further understanding of the secondary and tertially structure of this region of various H-2 molecules should help reveal a structural basis of allo-immune responses.

REFERENCES

Chatterjee-Das, S., E.P. Lillihoj, D.M. Hernandez, J.E. Coligan and D.H. Sachs. 1987. Analysis of the D-region products of H-2^q using monoclonal antibodies reveals the expression of new class I like molecules. J. Immunogenet. (in press).

DeLisi, C. and J.A. Berzofsky. 1985. T-cell antigenic sites tend to be amphipathic structures. Proc. Natl. Acad. Sci. USA 82:7048.

Fisher-Landahl, K. and D.B. Wilson. 1977. Histocompatibility antigen-activated cytotoxic T-lymphocytes. II. Estimates of the frequency and specificity of precursors. J. Exp. Med. 145:508.

Forman, J. 1987. Determinants on major histocompatibility complex class I molecules recognized by cytotoxic T-lymphocytes. Adv. Immunol. (in press).

Forman, J., R. Riblet, K. Brooks, E.S. Vitteta and L.A. Henderson. 1984. H-40, an antigen controlled by an Igh-linked gene and recognized by cytotoxic T-lymphocytes. I. Genetic analysis of H-40 and distribution of its product on B-cell tumors. J. Exp. Med. 159:1724.

Geysen, H.M., J.A. Talner, S.J. Rodda, T.J. Mason, H. Alexander, E.D. Getzoff and R.A. Lerner. 1987. Chemistry of antibody binding to a protein. Science 235:1184.

Gorer, P.A. 1937. Further studies on antigenic differences in mouse erythrocytes. Brit. J. Exp. Pathol. 18:31-36.

Hopp, T.P. and K.R. Woods. 1981. Prediction of protein antigenic determinants from amino acid sequences. Proc. Natl. Acad. Sci. USA 78:3824.

Koeller, D. and K. Ozato. 1986. Evaluation of the structure function relationships of MHC class I antigens by molecular genetic techniques. Year Immunol. 2:195.

Koeller, D., R. Lieberman, J. Miyazaki, E. Appella, K. Ozato, D.W. Mann and J. Forman. 1987. Introduction of H-2D^d determinants into the H-2L^d antigen by site directed mutagenesis. J. Exp. Med. (in press).

Nathenson, S.G., J. Geliebter, G.M. Pfaffenbach and R.A. Zeff. 1986. Murine major histocompatibility complex class I mutants: Molecular analysis and structure function implications. Ann. Rev. Immunol. 4:471.

Ozato, K., T.H. Hansen and D.H. Sachs. 1980. Monoclonal antibodies to mouse MHC antigens. II. Antibodies to the H-2L^d antigen, the products of a third polymorphic locus of the mouse major histocompatibility complex. J. Immunol. 125:2473.

Ozato, K., H. Takahashi, E. Appella, D. Sears, C. Murre, J. Seidman, S. Kimura and N. Tada. 1985. Polymorphism of murine major histocompatibility class I antigens: Assignment of putative allodeterminants to distinct positions of the amino acid sequence within the first external domain of the antigen. J. Immunol. 134:1749.

Sanger, F., A.R. Coulson, B.G. Barrell, A.J.H. Smith and D.A. Roe. 1980. Cloning in single stranded bacteriophages in an aid to rapid DNA sequencing. J. Mol. Biol. 143:161.

Shiroishi, T., G. Evans, E. Appella and K. Ozato. 1985. In vitro mutagenesis of a mouse MHC class I gene for the evaluation of structure-function relationships. J. Immunol. 134:623.

Snell, G.D. 1948. Methods for the study of histocompatibility genes. J. Genet. 49:87-108.

Zoller, M. and M. Smith. 1984. Oligonucleotide directed mutagenesis: A simple method using two primers and a single-stranded DNA template. DNA 3:479.

TRANSACTING NUCLEAR PROTEINS THAT BIND TO THE UPSTREAM REGULATORY REGION OF A MHC CLASS I GENE

Keiko Ozato, Yasuaki Shirayoshi, Peter Burke, Ettore Appella * and Jun-ichi Miyazaki

Laboratory of Developmental and Molecular Immunity, National Institute of Child Health and Human Development, and the *Laboratory of Cell Biology, National Cancer Institute, National Institutes of Health, Bethesda, Maryland, 20892

ABSTRACT

Expression of MHC class I gene is regulated via the highly conserved 5' class I regulatory element (CRE) and interferon consensus sequence (ICS). The CRE exerts both negative and positive regulation that is responsible for developmental control of the MHC class I gene expression. The ICS is involved in elevating transcription of MHC class I gene in response to interferon treatment. We examined the presence of transacting nuclear factors which interact with these regulatory sequences in a variety of cells. In gel mobility shift analyses we show that in cells expressing MHC class I genes possess at least three distinct nuclear factors capable of binding to the CRE. These three nuclear factors bind DNA sequences comprizing precise direct- and inverted repeats within the CRE. F9 embryonal carcinoma cells lack one of the three factors, which may be relevant to the absence of MHC gene expression in these cells. We also show that the ICS binds a unique nuclear factor, independent of the above factors. Tests with a number of mutant duplex oligonucleotides allowed us to localize the binding site of the factor to the core region of the ICS.

INTRODUCTION

Developmental Regulation of MHC Class I Gene Expression

We previously studied expression of MHC class I genes during murine embryonic development, and found that MHC class I messages and the surface H-2 antigens begin to be detected after midsomite stage of embryonic development (Ozato, et al., 1985). The levels of MHC class I mRNA and the surface antigens remain very low during the entire period of gestation. The surface MHC class I antigens expressed after mid-somite stage are predominantly classic H-2 antigens: Extensive search for Qa antigen expression in embryos at various stages after blastocyst stage with monoclonal antibodies of different reactivities has not yielded the positive evidence for Qa surface expression (unpublished data). We found that a sharp increase in the levels of MHC class I gene expression occurs during the first week of postnatal development (Kasik, et al., 1987). Embryonal carcinoma cells, such as F9 cells, which have many traits characteristic of early embryos, do not express MHC class I genes in the undifferentiated state. The antigen expression can be induced in these cells by retinoic acid treatment, serving as a model to study MHC gene regulation. Recently, we have established a number cells derived from mid to late somite stage of mouse embryos after infection and transformation of the embryonic cells with murine retroviruses. These cells, distinct from embryonal cacinoma cells in morphology and other traits, express either no or very low levels of MHC class I mRNA. They are also very low in surface MHC class I antigens. These results are consistent with the very low expression of the MHC class I genes observed with in vivo embryos at these stages (Silverman, et al., 1987; submitted).

We tested regulation of transcription of a MHC class I gene in F9 cells by CAT assay (Gorman, et al., 1982), and identified a ~35 bp negative regulatory element in the 5' upstream region of a MHC class I gene (Miyazaki, et al.). This regulatory element, highly conserved among classical MHC class I genes (Kimura, et al., 1986) has been found to have a dual function. It exerts both positive and negative regulation in MHC Class I gene transcription depending on the state of development and expression of MHC class I genes. Figure 1 depicts CAT constructs tested for evaluating transcription of MHC class I gene in F9 and L cells. In F9 cells constructs containing the CRE consistently gave lower CAT

CAT CONSTRUCTS

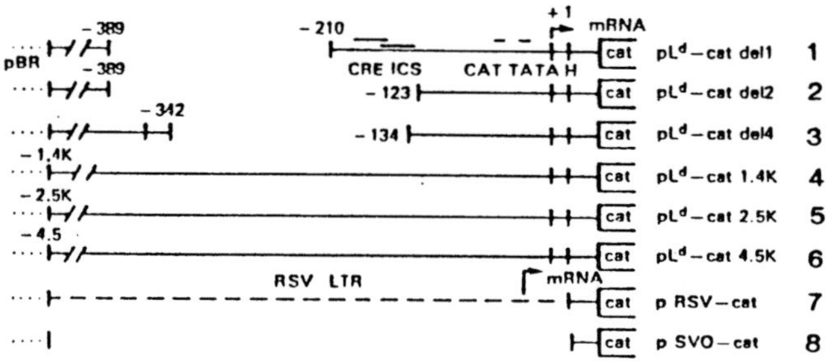

Figure 1. CAT constructs used for this study. H-2L^d CAT constructs in which chloramphenicol acetyl transferase reporter gene is under the control of the 5' flanking region of the H-2L^d gene were reported by Miyazaki, et al., 1986. The position of the CRE and ICS is indicated by a bar. CAT and TATA stand for CAT and TATA boxes present in the promoter region of the H-2L^d gene.

activity than those devoid of the CRE. The situation is reversed in L-cells which express MHC class I genes at a high level; the constructs with the CRE elicited higher CAT activity than those lacking it. These and the additional finding that the negative regulation is relieved upon retinoic acid induced differentiation of F9 cells, led us to postulate that developmental regulation of MHC class I gene expression is mediated via the CRE. In this hypothesis, a switching event would be anticipated during development, which shifts transcription from negative to positive regulation. Cells derived from mid-late somite stage embryos were also tested for CAT activity. Interestingly in those cells expressing negligible levels of MHC class I mRNA, the CRE showed neither negative nor positive regulation. These results suggest that there is an intermediate stage in the development during which the negative regulation ceases before attaining fully efficient positive regulation.

TABLE 1

Promoter Activity of H-2L^d 5' Upstream Region

CAT Construct	F9 EC	L-Cells
1	1.1	NT
2	10.9	0.2
3	8.1	0.3
4	1.0*	1.0*
5	0.6	1.3
6	1.1	1.4
7	13.9	3.8
8	0.3	0.1

CAT constructs shown in Figure 1 were introduced into undifferentiated F9 EC cells or L-cells, and transient CAT activity was measured 48 hrs later (Gorman, et al., 1982; Miyazaki, et al., 1986).

*Promoter activity of each construct is normalized by taking CAT values obtained by Construct 4 (containing the CRE) as 1.

NT: Not tested.

Regulation of MHC Class I Gene Expression by Interferons

It has been well established that interferons (both -γ and -α/β type) increase expression of MHC class I genes (Rosa, et al., 1987). Interferons are capable of inducing expression of MHC class I genes even in embryonic cells and neuronal cells that do not express the genes in normal conditions (Ozato, et al., 1985; Wong, et al., 1984). We and others (Israel, et al., 1986; Sugita, et al., 1987) noted that the conserved interferon consensus sequence (ICS) (Friedman and Stark, 1985) is responsible for elevating transcription of MHC classI genes in interferon treated cells. The ICS overlaps and juxtaposes with the CRE. Thus, the CRE and ICS are both involved in the regulation of transcription of MHC class I genes. These obvervations led us to examine transacting nuclear factors that interact with these regulatory sequences of MHC class I genes.

Specific Binding of Nuclear Factors to the CRE

Nuclear extracts were prepared according to the method of Dignam, et al. (1983) from L-fibroblasts, and T-cell line LH8, both of which express high levels of MHC class I genes, as well as from undifferentiated F9 EC cells which do not express to gene. Gel mobility shift analyses (Fried and Crothers, 1981; Garner and Rezvin, 1981) were carried out in the following fashion. A 32[P]-labeled H-2L^d fragment containing the CRE and ICS was incubated with nuclear extracts in the presence of poly (dI-dC), and electrophoresed in 3.5% polyacrylamide gel elecrophoresis. Retarded bands distinct from free fragment in the bottom of the gel represent DNA-factor complexes (Fig. 2). Nuclear extracts from LH8 T-cells and L-cells exhibited at least three major bands (arrowheads) in gel mobility shift experiments, all of which were eliminated by excess unlabeled fragment or duplex oligonucleotides corresponding to the CRE. Unrelated DNA fragments such as salomon sperm DNA or PBR sequence did not eliminate the retarded bands. The ICS also failed to eleminate any of the bands seen in Figure 2. Proteinase K treatment of nuclear extracts completely abolished the formation of the retarded bands, indicating that these factors are proteins. It is of note that nuclear extracts from F9 EC cells did not elicit the uppermost band which is a major in other cells (Fig. 2). Preliminary results indicate that embryonic cells established from mid-late somite stage embryos also lack the uppermost band. These results suggest that the factor that forms the uppermost band in the gel mobility shift experiments is important for the positive regulation of MHC class I genes.

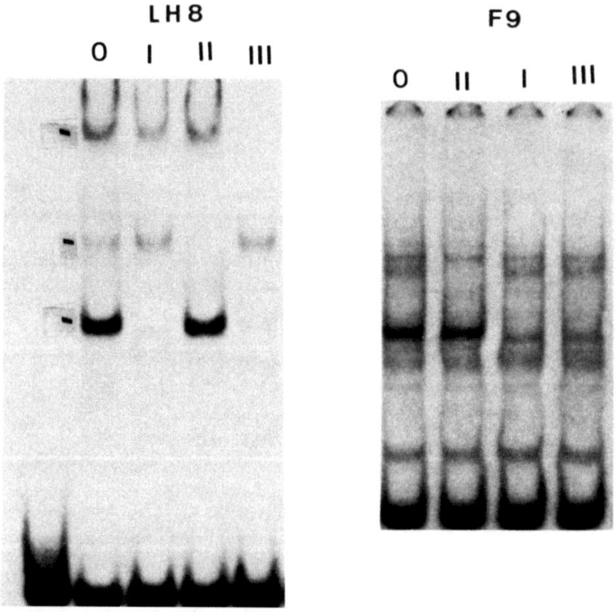

Figure 2. Detection of nuclear proteins that bind to the CRE region by gel mobility shift experiments. Nuclear extracts prepared from LH8 and F9 EC cells were mixed with a 32[P] labeled probe encompassing nucleotide sequence from -210 to -131. Binding of factors to the CRE in LH8 cells was tested with competitor duplex oligonucleotides corresponding to different portions of the CRE. Retarded bands were detected by electrophoresis of the reaction mixtures through 3.5% polyacrylamide gel. Note that the uppermost band is missing in the nuclear extract from F9 EC cells (arrow).

To further localize the binding site of each DNA-factor complex, competition experiments were performed with duplex oligonucleotides corresponding to three different parts of the CRE. Competitor oligonucleotides were added to the reaction mixture at 10 to 50 molar excess. Results obtained with LH8 T-cell extracts are shown in Figure 2. Three independent oligonucleotides depicted in Figure 4 competed for each of the three bands independently. Essentially the same results were obtained with L-cell and F9 extracts. In F9 cells the competitor corresponding to the sequence I and sequence II, but not sequence III, competed for the retarded bands. These results establish that there are at least three independent factors binding to distinct regions of the CRE in cells expressing MHC class I gene. As summarized in Figure 3, these three sequences precisely correspond to the direct repeat and inverted repeats present within the CRE. Our results extends the observations made by Baldwin and Sharp (1987) and Israel, et al. (1987) who reported the binding of a factor to sequence I shown in

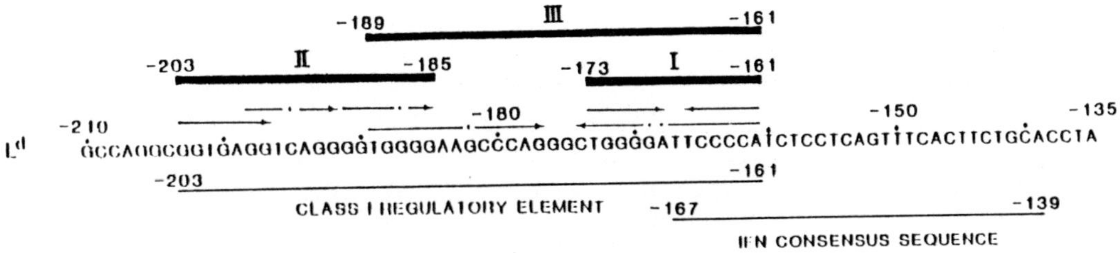

Figure 3. Three factor binding sites present within the CRE. Competition analyses revealed that there are at least three independent factors capable of binding to three distinct regions of the CRE as outlined.

Binding of a Nuclear Factor to the ICS.

In our hands DNA probes that contain both the ICS and CRE have not revealed any specific factor-binding to the ICS. We found, however, that a probe from which the 5' CRE sequence has been removed allows the detection of the binding of a factor(s) to the ICS. As seen in Figure 4 with the probe containing the ICS sequence. Also, one detects a retarded band which is competable by the homologous ICS, but not by the CRE (Fig 4). The basis of the failure to detect factor binding to the ICS with probes containing both the ICS and CRE is not clear. It is possible that binding of factors to the CRE inhibits the formation of an ICS- protein complex, perhaps due to competition for the sequence overlapping between the ICS and CRE (Fig. 4). As indicated in Figure 4 changes in peripheral nucleotides of the ICS did not impair the ability to bind the factor. However, nucleotide changes in the central portion of the ICS completely abolished the factor binding, suggesting that this core sequence is essential for the factor binding.

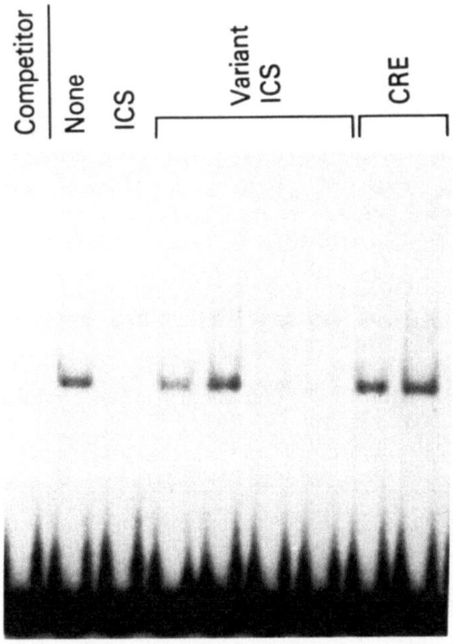

Figure 4. Binding of a nuclear factor to the ICS. Nuclear factor prepared from BW5147 T-cells were mixed with a 32[P]-labeled ICS probe, and gel mobility shift experiments were carried out as in Figure 2.

REFERENCES

Baldwin, A.S., Jr., and P.A. Sharp. 1987. Binding of a nuclear factor to a regulatory sequence in the promoter of the mouse H-2K^b class I major histocompatibility gene. Mol. Cell. Biol 7:305-313.

Dignam, J.D., R.M. Lobowitz, and R.G. Roeder. 1983. Accurate transcription initiation by RNA polymerase II is a soluble extract from isolated mammalian nuclei. Nucl. Acids Res. 11:1475-1489.

Fried, M., and D.M. Crothers. 1981. Equilibria and kinetics of lac repressor-operator interactions by polyacrylamide gel electrophoresis. Nucl. Acids Res. 9:6505-6525.

Friedman, R.L., and G.R. Stark. 1985. α-interferon-induced transcription of HLA and metallothionein genes containing homologous upstream sequences. Nature 314:637-639.

Garner, M.M., and A. Rezvin. 1981. A gel electrophoresis method for quantifying the binding of proteins to specific DNA regions. Applications to components of the E. coli lactose operon regulatory system. Nucl. Acids Res. 9:3047-3170.

Gorman, C.M., G.T. Merlino, M.C. Willingham, I. Pastan, and B.H. Howard. 1982. The Rous sarcoma virus long terminal repeat is a strong promoter when introduced into a variety of eukaryotic cells by DNA-mediated transfection. Proc. Natl. Acad. Sci. USA 79:6777-6781.

Israel, A., A. Kimura, M. Kieran, O. Yano, J. Kanellopoulos, O. LeBail, and P. Kourilsky. 1987. A common positive trans-acting factor binds to enhancer sequences in the promoters of mouse H-2 and β2-microglobulin genes. Proc. Natl. Acad. Sci. USA 84:2653-2657.

Israel, A., A. Kimura, A. Fournier, M. Fellous, and P. Kourilsky. 1986. Interferon response sequence potentiates activity of an enhancer in the promoter region of a mouse H-2 gene. Nature 322:743-746.

Kasik, J.W., Y-J.Y. Wan, and Ozato, K. 1987. A burst of c-fos gene expression in the mouse occurs at birth. Mol. Cell. Biol. (in press).

Kimura, A., A. Israel, B. LeBail, and P. Kourilsky. 1986. Detailed analysis of the mouse H-2K^b promoter: Enhancer-like sequences and their role in the regulation of class I expression. Cell 44:261-271.

Miyazaki, J., E. Appella, and K. Ozato. 1986. Negative regulation of the major histocompatibility class I gene in undifferentiated embryonal carcinoma cells. Proc. Natl. Acad. Sci. USA 83:9537-9541.

Ozato, K., Y.-J. Wan, and B.M. Orrison. 1985. Mouse major histocompatibility class I gene expression begins at midsomite stage and is inducible in earlier-stage embryos by interferon. Proc. Natl. Acad. Sci. USA 82:2427-2431.

Rosa, F.M., M.M. Cochet, and M. Fellous. 1986. Interferon and major histocompatibility complex genes: A model to analyze eukaryotic gene regulation? IN Interferon 7, Gresser, I. (ed.), Academic Press (London), pp. 48-84.

Sugita, K., J. Miyazaki, E. Appella, and K. Ozato. 1987. Interferons increase transcription of a major histocompatibility class I gene via 5' interferon consensus sequence. Mol. Cell. Biol. (in press).

Wong, G.H.W., P.F. Bartlett, I. Clark-Lewis, F. Battye, and J.W. Schrader. 1984. Inducible expression of H-2 and Ia antigens on brain cells. Nature 310:688-691.

THE PREVIOUSLY DEFINED R^d CLASS I MOLECULE IS A NON-β_2M ASSOCIATED CONFORMATIONAL VARIANT OF L^d

Ted H. Hansen, Nancy B. Myers, Jill B. Keeney and David R. Lee

Department of Genetics, Washington University School of Medicine, St. Louis, Missouri 63110

Abstract

Post-translational differences between murine class I molecules were compared. As determined in a pulse-chase experiment, the rate of N-linked oligosaccharide processing of L^d molecules was found to be 4-5 times slower than that of D^d, K^d or D^{dml} molecules. Furthermore, the relative molar ratio of β_2m to class I was found to be significantly lower with L^d than with D^d, K^d or D^{dml} molecules. Thus, both the slower processing and weaker β_2m association correlate with the previously reported lower cell surface expression of L^d compared to D^d, K^d or D^{dml} molecules. Since D^{dml} is a chimeric D^d/L^d molecule these results demonstrate that the amino terminus of the class I molecule influences processing, β_2m-association and cell surface expression.

The R^d molecule was initially defined by sequential immunoprecipitation using anti-L^d reactive mAbs 30-5-7 (α2 specific) and 28-14-8 (α3 specific). In contrast to L^d, the R^d molecule is only positive with mAb 28-14-8. In this communication we demonstrate that both L^d and R^d are products of the <u>H-2L^d</u> gene using an <u>H-2L^d</u> gene transfectant. Furthermore, the <u>30-5-7$^-$ L^d molecule (R^d) was</u> found not to be β_2m associated, in contrast to the 30-5-7$^+$ L^d molecule where β_2m was readily apparent. As much as 40% of the biosynthetically-labelled L^d molecules were found in this non-β_2m associated conformation. Thus, these studies suggest that L^d molecules have several unique properties that could all be related to an aberrant β_2m association. These properties include slower oligosaccharide processing, lower cell surface expression and detection of a non-β_2m associated conformational variant.

Introduction

Quantitative differences in the expression of class I major histocompatibility molecules are known to have profound effects on immune recognition of virus-infected or malignant cells. However, relatively little is known about the biosynthesis of class I molecules and the stages at which they are amenable to regulatory stimuli. Much of the published data on the biosynthesis of class I molecules has focused on the role of β_2m-microglobulin (β_2m), a relatively non-polymorphic light chain thought to be non-covalently associated with all class I molecules. Many of the initial findings regarding β_2m came from studies of Daudi cells. Daudi is a human Burkitt's lymphoma that does not synthesize β_2m protein (Goodfellow et al. 1975). As an apparent consequence of their β_2m^- phenotype, Daudi cells were found not to express class I antigens even though they were detected in the cytoplasm (Parnes and Seidman, 1982; Rose et al. 1983). Furthermore, pulse-chase experiments demonstrated that the class I molecules in Daudi have a significantly slower rate of carbohydrate processing compared with β_2m^+ cell lines, suggesting an impaired transport from the endoplasmic reticulum to the Golgi (Krangel et al. 1979). Thus, these studies employing Daudi cells provided evidence that β_2m plays a key role in the maturation and membrane expression of class I molecules. This supposition however has come under scrutiny because of recent reports using murine systems. A variant of the EL4 tumor (EL4/mar) has been described that expresses only D^b and not K^b antigens (Potter et al. 1984). Unexpectedly, no β_2m was detected on the surface of EL4/mar cells even though it was present in the cytoplasm. Similarly, a tumor line expressing only L^d antigens has been characterized that also lacks β_2m on the surface (Martinko et al. 1986). Perhaps the most surprising result was that of Allen et al. (1986) who transfected the D^b gene into a β_2m^- cell line and found D^b on the cell surface. However, the D^b expressed by these β_2m^- cells was in a conformation that could be recognized neither by allogeneic cytotoxic T lymphocytes nor by most monoclonal antibodies (mAbs) to D^b antigens. It is also noteworthy that the endogenous antigens K^k and D^k were not detected on this β_2m^- tumor variant. Thus, the absolute requirement of β_2m for processing and surface expression of at least certain class I molecules has come into question. Our laboratory is undertaking an extensive investigation of the biosynthesis of several D region encoded molecules, since these are the ones that appear to have unique properties. We report here the detection in normal splenic lymphocytes of a non-β_2m associated conformational variant of the L^d molecule that corresponds to the previously defined R^d molecule. This observation is presented in the context of our recent findings that L^d molecules have a slower processing, weaker β_2m association, and lower surface expression than D^d, D^b or K^d molecules (Beck et al. 1986).

Results and Discussion

Oligosaccharide processing of class I molecules and the role of β_2m. The synthesis and expression of different class I molecules were compared to define their post-translational regulatory differences. One of the criteria used for these comparisons was the rate of N-linked oligosaccharide processing. Glycosylation of class I molecules occurs in the presence of microsomal membranes. As commonly occurs with several glycoproteins, newly synthesized class I molecules on the rough endoplasmic reticulum have N-linked high mannose oligosaccharides (Krangel et al. 1979). After transport to the Golgi, high mannose residues are converted to complex type oligosaccharides, and only this mature form is thought to make it to the cell surface. These two different glycosylated forms of class I molecules were resolved by SDS-PAGE, using 10-15% linear polyacrylamide gradient slab gels (Beck et al. 1986). To compare the relative carbohydrate maturation times for different class I molecules, pulse-chase experiments were performed using ^{35}S-methionine labelled spleen cell antigen preparations. Specific monoclonal antibodies were used to precipitate each class I molecule, and densitometric tracings were used for quantitative comparisons. Experimental details of these procedures were described earlier (Beck et al. 1986), and the results are summarized in tabular format in Fig. 1.

Multiple independent calculations of processing time were made for L^d, D^d and D^{dml} molecules using two different mAbs for each of these products. One monoclonal antibody was specific for the $\alpha 2$ protein domain, whereas the other was specific for the $\alpha 3$ domain. The time required to convert one-half ($C_{1/2}$) of the L^d molecules to species bearing complex oligosaccharides was 282-300 minutes. This time was approximately 5 times longer than the $C_{1/2}$ for D^d molecules that ranged between 45 to 48 minutes. The chimeric molecule D^{dml} isolated from the B10.D2-H-2^{dml} mutant was found to have an oligosaccharide processing time similar to D^d molecules. This result indicated that the slower processing time of L^d molecules is determined by protein sequence in the amino terminus (see Fig. 1). Preliminary results also showed that K^d molecules have

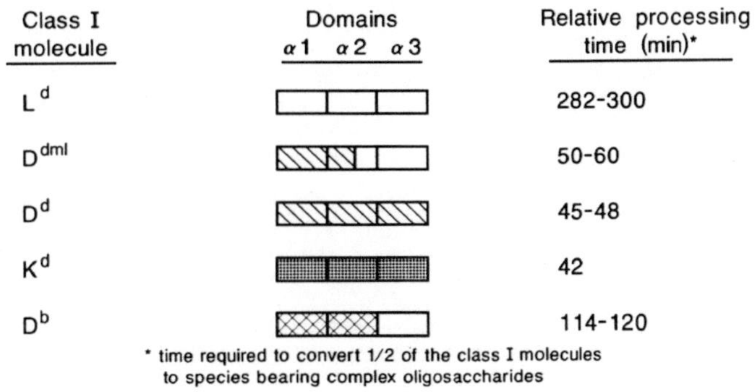

Fig. 1. Comparisons of the rates of oligosaccharide processing of different class I molecules

an equivalent processing time with D^d and that D^b molecules are processed at a rate intermediate between L^d and D^d molecules. Therefore in mice of the H-2^d haplotype the K^d and D^d molecules are processed relatively quickly, whereas the L^d molecule is processed significantly more slowly. It is noteworthy that K^d and D^d antigens are expressed on the cell surface at equivalent levels, whereas L^d antigens have been found to have a 4-fold lower surface expression (Potter et al. 1981). This correlation also applies to the H-2^{dml} haplotype where the K^d and D^{dml} molecules have both a comparable processing rate and cell surface expression (Beck et al. 1986). Thus, in the haplotypes studied thus far there is a striking correlation between rate of N-linked oligosaccharide processing and cell surface expression.

One hypothesis consistent with the aforementioned correlation is that class I molecules compete for a limiting cytoplasmic factor that is necessary for maturation and cell surface expression. A good candidate for such a limiting factor is β_2m that has been proposed to influence the transport of class I molecules from the endoplasmic reticulum to the Golgi (Krangel et al. 1979). To compare the amount of β_2m associated with L^d and D^d molecules, BALB/c or B10.D2 splenic lymphocytes were labelled continuously with ^{35}S methionine for 4 to 8 hrs. As indicated in Table 1, two different mAbs to L^d or D^d were independently used to precipitate each of these molecules. Fluorographs were traced by densitometry to compare relative molar ratios of β_2m associated with L^d or D^d molecules. The amount of β_2m associated with L^d was found to be significantly less than that associated with D^d molecules. Furthermore, this was true regardless of which mAb was used for the precipitation.

Strain	Molecule	mAb Used (domain recognized)	Relative β_2M Association[a]
BALB/c	L^d	28-14-8 (α3)	0.10
	L^d	30-5-7 (α2)	0.20
	D^d	34-2-12 (α3)	0.31
	D^d	34-5-8 (α2)	0.42
BIO.D2	L^d	28-14-8 (α3)	0.08
	L^d	30-5-7 (α2)	0.12
	D^d	34-2-12 (α3)	0.47
	D^d	34-5-8 (α2)	0.52

a. based on densitometer tracings of fluorographs and corrected for number of methionine residues in each molecule.

Table 1. β_2M association of L^d vs D^d molecules

In data not shown the D^{dml} molecule was found to have an even higher β_2m association than the D^d molecule (Beck et al. 1986). The simplest explanation of the data summarized thus far is that 1) the weak association of β_2m with L^d is responsible for the slower carbohydrate processing and ultimately the lower cell surface expression, and 2) all of these phenomona are determined by the amino terminus. This latter conclusion is supported by recent studies using constructs of exon shuffled genes that were expressed in L cells (Weiss and Murre, 1985). The differences in the synthesis and expression of D region encoded antigens underscore the importance of post-translational regulation of class I molecules. This contention is supported by recent studies of cells infected by adenovirus type 2 that has been found to affect intracellular transport and cell surface expression in a manner analogous to the locus specific differences defined above (Anderson et al. 1985).

Conformational maturation of class I molecules and the role of β_2m. In addition to the putative importance of β_2m for intracellular transport and surface expression, other findings suggest that β_2m plays an important role in the conformation attained by class I molecules. In support of this contention HLA class I molecules that are, or are not, β_2m associated were distinguished serologically or by susceptibility to proteolysis (Krangel et al. 1979; Ploegh et al. 1979). It was therefore surprising when studies in the murine system showed that the D^b and L^d class I molecules can be found on the surface of tumor cells in the absence of β_2m, even though β_2m is present in the cell (Potter et al. 1984; Martinko et al. 1986). Further, these β_2m^- class I molecules were recognized serologically and functionally in the expected manner. This finding implied that, at least for D^b and L^d, the continuous presence of β_2m was not necessary to maintain conformation. Extending this observation, Allen et al. (1986) transfected D^b into the β_2m^- cell line R1E and observed cell surface expression. It is noteworthy that neither R1E cells nor the R1E-D^b transfectant were found to express their endogenous K^k D^k antigens on the surface although this could be a false negative resulting from not having appropriate mAbs for their detection. In any case, these findings were interpreted as evidence that β_2m is not an absolute requirement for cell surface expression. However, the D^b antigens expressed by R1E were found to have a very different conformaton than the D^b antigens expressed by β_2m^+ cells. Indeed alloreactive and virus-specific cytotoxic T lymphocytes generated against bonafide D^b failed to lyse R1E-D^b targets; and all but one monoclonal antibody to D^b failed to bind R1E-D^b cells. The exceptional antibody, 28-14-8, was the only one tested that recognizes a determinant associated with the $\alpha 3$ molecular domain. These results thus provide unequivocal evidence that β_2m imparts conformation on class I molecules or at least the D^b antigens. When taken together, published reports of β_2m suggest that it instills a conformational alteration early in the synthesis of class I molecules and that once this conformation is attained, β_2m may dissociate or be exchanged. Reciprocally, if class I molecules fail to associate with β_2m during this critical time, then subsequent association with β_2m does not instill conformation and furthermore probably does not occur. This conclusion of non-reversibility is based on studies where β_2m is combined with class I molecules that maturated in the absence of β_2m *in vivo* (Krangel et al. 1979) or that grew in a cell free translaton system without β_2m (Ploegh et al. 1979).

These studies of β_2m raise interesting questions of the occurrence and expression of non-β_2m associated class I molecules in normal cells. Even though the finding of Allen and associates (1986) demonstrated that D^b molecules can be expressed after transfection into a β_2m^- cell line, this result does not necessarily imply that this occurs in normal cells. It is possible that the copy number or chromosomal location of a transfected gene could overload the *in vivo* translation system in such a manner that a molecule not normally expressed could be expressed.

The experiment shown in Fig. 2 is relevant to the question of whether class I molecules without a β_2m-associated conformational change can be detected in normal splenic lymphocytes. The data of Allen et al. (1986) suggest a strategy whereby non-β_2m conformed D^b molecules can be differentiated from those that were β_2m conformed. Specifically, their results imply that the β_2m-conformed D^b molecules should react with both mAbs B22/249 and 28-14-8, whereas the non-conformed D^b molecules should react only with 28-14-8. Thus, sequential immunoprecipitation techniques can be used to compare the relative amounts of these two conformational forms of D^b molecules.

Spleen cells from B6 (<u>H-2</u>^{b}) mice were cultured for 4 hrs <u>in vitro</u> in the presence of continuous ^{3}H-leucine. After solubilization in NP40, a glycoprotein pool was obtained by affinity chromatography using a lentil-lectin column. Antigens prepared by this protocol can contain radiolabelled class I molecules from inside and outside of the cell. As indicated in Fig. 2, this B6 antigen preparation was first treated with excess amounts of mAb B22/249 followed by protein A bearing SaCI. This precipitate is shown in the left hand panel of Fig. 2. To demonstrate complete clearance, a 2nd precipitation with B22/249 was performed and is shown in the middle panel. Finally, this preparation was treated with 28-14-8 to test for D^b molecules that were not conformed by β_2m. As shown in the right hand panel relatively few residual 28-14-8$^+$ molecules were detected. Thus in these continuously labelled splenic lymphocytes, less than 15% of the D^b molecule appeared not to have a β_2m induced conformation. This small percentage probably reflects how quickly or efficiently D^b molecules bind β_2m and furthermore may contain only cytoplasmic and not cell surface forms of D^b.

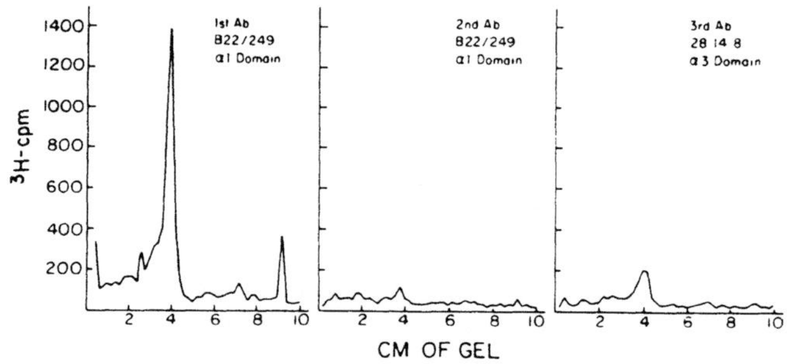

Fig. 2. Sequential precipitation of biosynthetically-labeled D^b antigens.

An analogous sequential immunoprecipitation experiment was performed using anti-L^d reactive mAbs and a BALB/c (<u>H-2</u>^{d}) antigen preparation. The antigen preparation was initially treated with an excess amount of mAb 30-5-7 that detects an epitope associated with the α2 domain. The result of this precipitation is shown in the left hand panel of Fig. 3. A second treatment of the antigen preparation with 30-5-7 was performed to demonstrate complete clearance (middle panel). The third treatment was with mAb 28-14-8 that is specific for an epitope in the α3 domain. As shown in the right hand panel, a significant peak of residual 28-14-8$^+$ class I molecules was detected. A sequential precipitation in the opposite direction showed that an initial treatment with mAb 28-14-8 cleared 30-5-7 reactive molecules (Hansen et al. 1981). Based on these results, we previously suggested that they define two separate molecules, one designated L^d that is $30\text{-}5\text{-}7^+$, $28\text{-}14\text{-}8^+$ and the other designated R^d is $30\text{-}5\text{-}7^-$, $28\text{-}14\text{-}8^+$ (Hansen et al. 1981). Further comparisons determined that L^d and R^d have minor differences that were resolved by 2D electrophoresis (Koch et al. 1983; Nichols et al. 1983), even though their peptide maps were found to be indistinguishable (Lillihoj et al. 1985). In addition, cocapping studies suggested that L^d and not R^d antigens are on the cell surface (Ivanyi and Demant 1983). Recently we have generated data which demonstrate that the R^d and L^d molecules are both products of the <u>H-2L^d</u> gene. This conclusion was indicated by studies using the <u>H-2L^d</u> gene transfectant T1.1.1 kindly provided by Dr. D. Margulies (NIH). An antigen preparation was made from T1.1.1 and a sequential immunoprecipitation experiment was performed that was analogous to the one shown in Fig. 3. Two antigenic forms of L^d were again detected, both of which were reactive with mAbs 28-14-8, but only one reacted with mAb 30-5-7. Thus, both L^d and R^d are encoded by the H-2L^d gene.

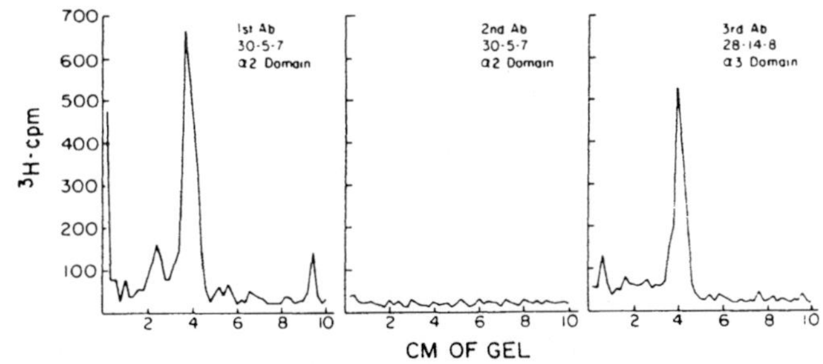

Fig. 3. Sequential precipitation of biosynthetically-labeled L^d antigens.

The L^d and D^b molecules are structurally very homologous including sharing an identical sequence in their α3 domains and a corresponding $28\text{-}14\text{-}8^+$ phenotype. Therefore, it seemed possible that L^d is like D^b and requires β_2m to attain a serologically recognizable conformation in the α1 - α2, but not its α3 domain. If this were the case, then the previously defined $30\text{-}5\text{-}7^-$, $28\text{-}14\text{-}8^+$ L^d molecules (R^d) would not be expected to be β_2m associated. Indeed, the $30\text{-}5\text{-}7^-$ L^d molecules were found to have no detectable β_2m associated with them in contrast to the $30\text{-}5\text{-}7^+$ L^d molecules where β_2m was readily observed. This finding is apparent in the analysis shown in Fig. 3 that used a tube gel containing 10% acylamide such that β_2m migrates between 8 to 9 cm into the gel.

However the differential β_2m association is more striking in Fig. 4 where the precipitates were analyzed in a 10-15% linear gradient acrylamide slab gel. A possible caveat to this conclusion is that mAb 28-14-8 dissociates β_2m from L^d. This possibility was ruled out since mAb 28-14-8 was shown to be capable of precipitating β_2m associated L^d. Evidence for this is shown both in Table 1 and in lane 2 of Fig. 4. It should be noted however that 30-5-7 precipitates contain approximately twice as much β_2m compared to the 28-14-8 precipitates (Table 1 and Fig. 4). This can now

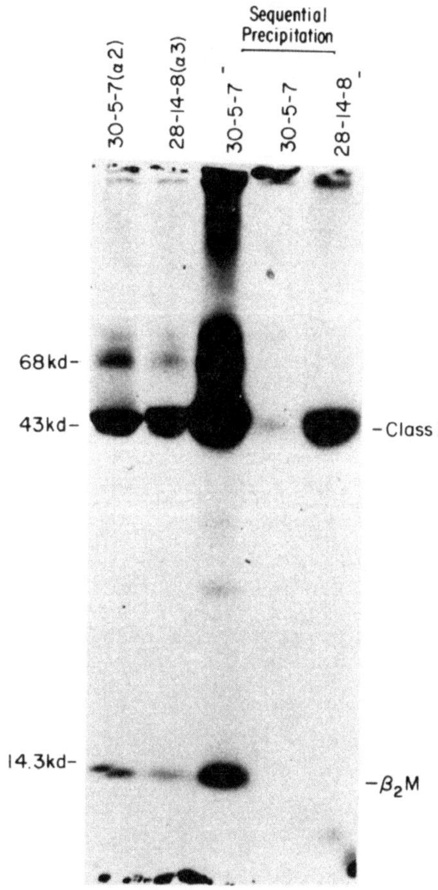

Fig. 4. ^{35}S-methionine labelled BALB/c antigen was purified by lentil-lectin affinity chromatography and precipitated with the indicated mAb. The first two lanes represent precipitates from test aliquots, whereas the next three lanes are sequential precipitations of a single antigen pool. These precipitates were analysed on a 10-15% linear gradient acylamide slab gel as described earlier (Beck et al. 1986).

be explained since as much as 40% of the 28-14-8 precipitate (or total biosynthetic L^d pool) is in a conformation that does not associate with β_2m. Alternatively, the differential association with these two forms of L^d could be explained by hypothesizing that 30-5-7 recognizes a combinatorial determinant on L^d:β_2m dimers, whereas 28-14-8 recognizes either free or associated L^d molecules. This however was ruled out since 30-5-7 can precipitate free L^d molecules (manuscript in preparation). Thus these results indicate that the previously defined R^d molecule is a variant of the L^d molecule that has a different conformation resulting from a failure to interact with β_2m.

Taken together with other recent reports, our results demonstrate that β_2m induces a conformation change early in the synthesis of at least L^d and D^b and perhaps other class I molecules. Furthermore this β_2m-induced alteration affects only the α1 and α2 domains of these class I molecules and not their α3 domain. It is not yet clear, whether this conformation change in the class I molecule is what facilitates intracellular transport or alternatively whether this is a second discrete function of β_2m. Unexpectedly, the critical regions on the class I molecules for both the conformation and transport appear to be the N terminal α1 and α2 domain, even though the α3 domain was previously proposed to contain the sites for β_2m association (Yokoyama and Nathenson 1983). Another question raised by these studies is whether non-β_2m associated forms of class I molecules normally make it to the cell surface, and if they do, whether this is a feature of all class I molecules or only ones with aberrant β_2m associations. Even if non-β_2m associated class I molecules do not make it to the cell surface in normal cells, it is possible that they could be expressed in malignant or transfected cells or cells from mice with a transgenic class I gene. In any case, further studies using this system should help define the precise role of β_2m for the intracellular transport, conformation and cell surface expression of class I molecules.

Acknowledgments

We thank Dr. David Margulies for the kind gift of the L^d-transfectant Tl.l.l, Dr. Susan Cullen for her advice in the analysis of the oligosaccharide processing assays, and Mrs. Karen Perks for expert secretarial help. This work was supported by NIH grants AI 19687 (THH) GM 07067 (JBK) and AI 23410 (DRL).

References

Allen, H., Fraser, J., Flyer, D., Calvin, S., and Flavell, R.: β_2-Microglobulin is not required for cell surface expression of the murine class I histocompatibility antigen H-$2D^b$ or of a truncated H-$2D^b$. Proc. Natl. Acad. Sci. USA 83: 7447-7451, 1986.

Anderson, M., Paabo, S., Nilsson, T., and Peterson, P.A.: Impaired intracellular transport of class I MHC antigens as a possible means for adenoviruses to evade immune surveillance. Cell 43: 215-222, 1985.

Beck, J.C., Hansen, T.H., Cullen, S.E., and Lee, D.R.: Slower processing, weaker β_2m association and lower surface expression of H-$2L^d$ are influenced by its amino terminus. J. Immunol. 137: 916-922, 1986.

Goodfellow, P.N., Jones, E.A., van Heyningen, V., Solomon, E., Bobrow, M., Miggiano, V., and Bodmer, W.F.: The β_2-microglobulin genes is on chromosome 15 and not in the HL-A region. Nature 254: 267-269, 1975.

Hansen, T.H., Ozato, K., Melino, M.R., Coligan, J.E., Kindt, T.J., Jandinski, J.J., and Sachs, D.H.: Immunochemical evidence in two haplotypes for at least three D region encoded molecules, D, L, and R. J. Immunol. 126: 1713-1716.

Ivanyi, D., and Demant, P.: Capping experiments fail to reveal H-$2R^d$ molecules in D^d region. Transplant. Proc. 15: 2039-2041, 1983.

Koch, S., Robinson, P.J., Koch, N., and Hammerling, G.J.: Separation of H-$2D^d$, H-$2L^d$ and H-$2R^d$ by two-dimensional gel electrophoresis. Immunogenetics 17: 215-218, 1983.

Krangel, M.S., Orr, H.T., and Strominger, J.L.: Assembly and maturation of HLA-A and HLA-B antigens in vivo. Cell 18: 979-991, 1979.

Lillehoj, E.P., Hansen, T.H., Sachs, D.H., and Coligan, J.E.: Primary structural evidence that the H-$2D^q$ encodes at least three distinct gene products: D^q, L^q and R^q. Proc. Natl. Acad. Sci. USA 81: 2499-2503, 1984.

Martinko, J.M., Anderson, S.J., and Potter, T.: A murine cell line defective in expression of several class I molecules. Immunogenetics 23: 64-66, 1986.

Nichols, E.A., Krakauer, T., and Hansen, T.H.: Two-dimensional gel comparisons of murine H-2D region-associated antigens of different H-2 haplotypes. J. Immunol. 131: 2440-2444, 1983.

Parnes, J.R., and Seidman, J.G.: Structure of wild-type and mutant mouse β_2-microglobulin. Cell 29: 661-669, 1982.

Ploegh, H.L., Cannon, L.E., and Strominger, J.L.: Cell-free translation of the mRNAs for the heavy and light chains of HLA-A and HLA-B antigens. Proc. Natl. Acad. Sci. USA 76: 2273-2277, 1979.

Potter, T.A., Hansen, T.H., Habbersett, R., Ozato, K., and Ahmed, A.: Flow microfluorometric analysis of H-2L expression. J. Immunol. 127: 580-584, 1981.

Potter, T.A., Boyer, C., Schmitt-Verhulst, A.M., Golstein, P., and Rajan, T.V.: Expression of H-$2D^b$ on the cell surface in the absence of detectable β_2-microglobulin. J. Exp. Med. 160: 317-322, 1984.

Rosa, F., Berissi, H., Weissenbach, J., Maroteaux, L., Fellous, M., and Revel, M.: The β_2-microglobulin mRNA in human Daudi cells has a mutated initiation codon but is still inducible by interferon. EMBO J. 2: 239-243, 1983.

Weiss, J.H., and Murre, C.: Differential expression of H-$2D^d$ and H-$2L^d$ histocompatibility antigens. J. Exp. Med. 161: 356-365, 1985.

Yokoyama, K., and Nathenson, S.G.: Intramolecular organization of the alloantigenic determinants and the β_2-microglobulin binding site to different regions of the H-$2K^b$ glycoprotein. J. Immunol. 130: 1419-1425, 1983.

REGULATORY ELEMENTS IN THE PROMOTER OF THE H-2D^d CLASS I GENE

Bette Korber, Leroy Hood, and Iwona Stroynowski

Division of Biology
California Institute of Technology
Pasadena, CA 91125

INTRODUCTION

Murine class I antigen expression undergoes modulation during development and adult life. Early embryonic cells do not transcribe detectable amounts of class I and β_2 microglobulin mRNA and express little, if any, H-2 antigens (1,2). In contrast, adult cells express class I mRNA constitutively and ubiquitously but the relative basal level of class I antigen expression varies on different cells and tissues (reviewed in 3). The quantity of various class I antigens expressed undergoes additional changes upon exposure to agents such as type I and type II interferons and tumor necrosis factor (4-6). Since quantitative variation in class I protein expression can influence the acquisition of tolerance, MHC restriction, and the efficiency of cell-mediated immune responses we were interested in identifying and characterizing the DNA elements and trans-acting factors which are important for the regulation of class I gene expression. This information may be eventually applied for therapeutic purposes to modulate class I protein levels and to affect the immune response in vivo.

Several laboratories have described regulatory elements in the promoters of class I genes (7-11). According to the present view of gene regulation (12) these short DNA sequences bind nuclear transcription factors and control the resulting level of promoter activity. Figure 1 shows a comparison of the published 5' flanking sequences of H-2 class I genes. The locations of cis-acting elements believed to be important for transcriptional regulation are indicated in the figure. Two fragments with enhancer activities (elements which potentiate transcription and act independently of their orientation) were identified upstream of the structural H-2K^b gene (7). A region required for interferon inducibility of the H-2K^b, D^d, and L^d genes, designated the interferon response sequence, or IRS (10), is shown overlapping the class I response element (CRE), which functions as an H-2L^d negative sequence in the embryonal teratocarcinoma F9 cells and as an enhancer in NIH 3T3 cells (8).

Four sequences within these functionally defined regulatory regions were found to bind nuclear factors (13-15). They are located in the enhancer A fragment, in the enhancer B fragment, and in the IRS (Figure 1). Bind A and bind B (designated bind A and bind B because they are regions within enhancer A and B that bind nuclear factors) are protected in a footprinting assay using nuclear extracts made from mouse myeloma MPC 11 cells (15), and are also recognized by the highly purified transcriptional activating protein called AP-1 (15). AP-1 also

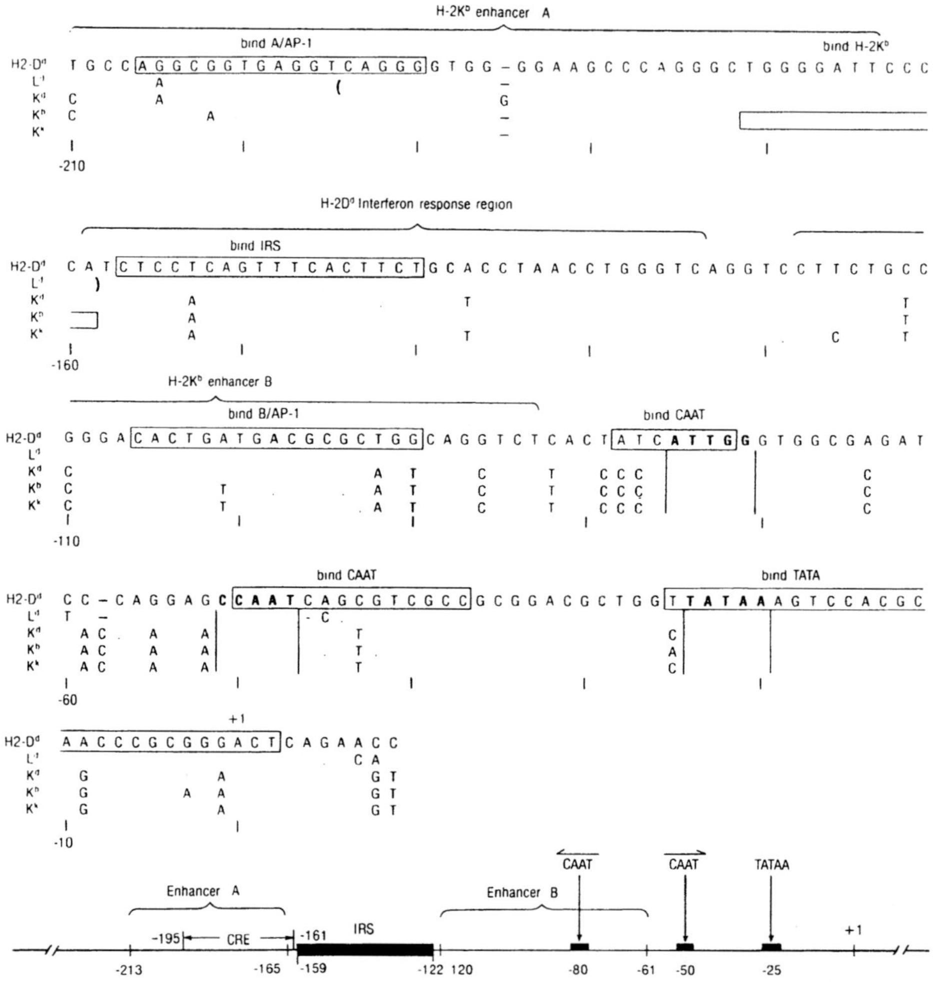

Fig. 1. Regulatory elements in the 5' flanking regions of H-2 class I genes. The sequences are aligned according to the transcription start site mapped for the H-2K^{d} gene (24). The cap sites for other H-2 genes were not determined experimentally. The locations of the sequences encoding the response to interferons (IRS) in the H-2D^{d} gene (10), and the enhancers A and B of the H-2K^{b} gene (7), are indicated. The class I regulatory element (CRE) (8) is enclosed in parentheses in the H-2L^{d} sequence. The DNA sequences, which bind nuclear factors are boxed. Bind A/AP-1, bind B/AP-1 and bind IRS were determined using the H-2D^{d} template (15), and bind H-2K^{b} using the H-2K^{b} template (13,14). The CCAAT and TATA boxes are indicated in bold letters. Vertical lines highlight the homology of the CCAAT and TATA elements in these H-2 genes. The DNA sequences are derived from references 7, 10, 25 and 26. A schematic representation of an H-2 5' flanking region and known regulatory elements is provided beneath the sequence.

interacts with the 12-0-tetradecanoyl-phorbol-13 acetate (TPA) inducible enhancers of the SV40 and metallothionein promoters (16). In these gene systems AP-1 acts as a positive transcription factor. An additional factor binds to a sequence which overlaps with enhancer A (13,14). The promoter of the H-2K^b gene was used to detect this binding activity, so we called the protected region bind H-2K^b (Figure 1). The factor that interacts with the IRS of the H-2 D^d gene may be involved in interferon regulation of class I genes (15). It has been suggested that these DNA binding factors may enhance transcription from H-2 promoters (13-15).

The class I promoter regions encode two CCAAT motifs as well as a TATA motif. These sequences are highly conserved elements found in the promoters of many eukaryotic genes. The TATA box element, in conjunction with the cap sequence, is believed to position the start site of the transcription (reviewed in 17); the CCAAT element is required for the maximum transcriptional activity of many promoters (18). Factors binding to these two elements have recently been partially characterized (19-20). In class I genes the canonical TATA element is located 24 nucleotides upstream of the putative transcription initiation site. Two CCAAT motifs are present 5' of the TATA box (Figure 1). They are arranged in a symmetrical palindrome with the two centers of the motifs spaced 20 nucleotides from each other. We report here that trans-acting factors can bind to both of the H-2D^d CCAAT motifs as well as to the region surrounding the H-2D^d TATA element.

METHODS

Nuclear extracts were prepared by adapting the procedure described in Parker and Topol (21) to MPC11 cells. Cells were seeded at a concentration of 5 x 10^4/ml and grown for three days in roller bottles in suspension. The nuclear extracts were prepared at 4°C by the following procedure. The cells were pelleted at 3,000 rpm for 6 min in a Beckman J6 centrifuge. The cellular pellet was washed in 10 times its volume buffer A: 15 mM KCl, 10 mM Hepes (pH = 7.6, Ultrol, Calbiochem), 2 mM $MgCl_2$, and .1 mM EDTA. The cells were repelleted at 6000 rpm for 6 min in a Sorvall RC-2B centrifuge in a SS34 rotor, and resuspended in 3 times the cellular volume of buffer A and fresh 1 mM DDT. The cells were lysed in a glass Dounce homogenizer. The salt concentration of the hypotonic buffer A was increased by adding 1/10 volume of buffer B: 1.5M KCl, 50 mM Hepes (pH 7.6), 30 mM $MgCl_2$, .1 mM EDTA and 1 mM DTT. The homogenate was centrifuged at 10,000 rpm for 10 min in the Sorvall SS34 rotor, and the crude nuclear pellet was resuspended in 3 times the cell volume of 9:1 buffer A:B. 1/10 of the total volume of 4 M ammonium sulfate (pH 7.9) was added to a final concentration of .36 M ammonium sulfate. The nuclei were lysed by gentle rocking for 30 min. The nuclear lysate was centrifuged at 35,000 rpm for 60 min in a Beckman SW41 rotor. The supernatant was retained, 0.25 g/ml ammonium sulfate was added, and the mixture was rocked for 30 min. The precipitated proteins were pelleted by centrifugation at 35,000 rpm for 15 min in a Beckman SW41 rotor. The supernatant was discarded and the protein pellet was resuspended in 1/2 the volume of the original cell pellet in buffer C: 10% glycerol (Mallinckrodt), 50 mM Hepes (pH 7.6), 20 mM KCl, .1 mM EDTA, and 1 mM DTT. The extract was dialyzed against 250x the extract volume buffer C for 3 hr, divided into aliquots and stored frozen at -80°C. The protein concentration of each extract was determined by BioRad protein assay.

The H-2D^d CAT deletion mutant Δ-262 (10) was used for the footprinting analysis. The DNA was labeled at the Eco RI site (located in pBR322 DNA adjacent to the deletion junction Δ-262) by end-filling with DNA polymerase I (Klenow fragment), or by T4 polynucleotide kinase phosphorylation. After labeling, the DNA was cut with the restriction enzyme Pvu II, at a site which lies in the chloramphenicol acetyl transferase (CAT) coding region, and the 3' or 5' end-labeled Eco RI-Pvu II fragment was gel purified.

The footprinting reactions were done in a 25 µl reaction volume. Twenty µl of nuclear extract or double distilled H_2O was incubated with 2-5 ng of end-labeled fragment, 100 µg/ml of poly(dI-dC) (Pharmacia), 5 mM $MgCl_2$, and 20 mM Hepes (pH 7.6) for 10 min at 4°C. Freshly diluted DNAase I (Worthington) was added to the final concentrations indicated in Figure 2 and allowed to react on ice for 30 sec. The appropriate amount of nuclear extract and DNAse I was determined by titration. The reactions were stopped by the addition of 50 µl of termination buffer (1% Sarkosyl, 100 mM NaCl, 100 mM Tris (pH 8), 10 mM EDTA, 100 µg/ml of proteinase K (Boehringer Mannheim), and 25 µg/ml calf thymus DNA). The tubes were then incubated at 37°C for 15 min, then at 90°C for 2 min. The final mixtures were extracted with 75 µl of phenol, then 75 µl of 50:50 phenol:chloroform. The DNA was precipitated, dried, resuspended in 10 µl of 90% formamide, TBE, and .1% dyes, denatured at 90°C for 5 min, and electrophoresed in a 5% polyacrylamide sequencing gel.

RESULTS

We have previously observed binding of nuclear factors to three DNA sequences in the 5' flanking region of the H-2D^d gene (15). Here we used the same approach of DNA footprinting (22) to identify additional sequences that may interact with nuclear transcription factors. The footprinting assay detects specific DNA/protein interactions by visualizing DNA regions that are protected from DNAase I degradation in the presence of nuclear extracts. The MPC 11 cell line was selected as a source of the nuclear extracts because it expresses high levels of the class I antigens (comparable to those on spleen cells of the parental BALB/c strain). Therefore, we reasoned, it may contain high levels of the class I gene specific transcription factors.

The results of the footprinting experiments on the H-2D^d template are shown in Figure 2. Three DNA regions, that have not been previously reported, are detectably "cleared". They are located at positions -71 to -78, -37 to -50 and -25 to +3 (on the coding strand). These footprinted sequences are also indicated schematically in Figure 1. Two of these regions coincide with the position of the CCAAT elements and the third one overlaps the canonical TATA box and extends into the sequences downstream from the putative transcription initiation site. These DNAse I protected regions are specific by the following criteria: first, they occur on both strands of the H-2D^d DNA template and second, the MPC 11 nuclear extracts used in all of the experiments do not footprint randomly selected fragments of the pBR322-CAT plasmid DNA.

DISCUSSION

We report here binding of nuclear proteins to two elements of the H-2D^d DNA promoter: the CCAAT and the TATA boxes. Based on the conserved nature of these two sequences in many RNA polymerase II promoters, we propose that the observed binding involves transcription factors that are similar to those whose interactions with other promoters have been previously characterized (19-21, 27-28). The following discussion will relate the footprinting patterns observed on the H-2D^d template to the properties of known CCAAT and TATA binding factors.

CTF can contribute to the transcriptional activation of eukaryotic promoters that contain the sequence CCAAT and, in addition, it can act as a cellular DNA binding protein required for the initiation of adenovirus DNA replication (19). CTF factor, purified by sequence-specific DNA affinity chromatography from HeLa cells, consists of a family of polypeptides with molecular weights between 52 and 66 kd. The nature of this heterogeneity in protein size is not presently understood. Purified CTF was shown to recognize CCAAT related sequences with

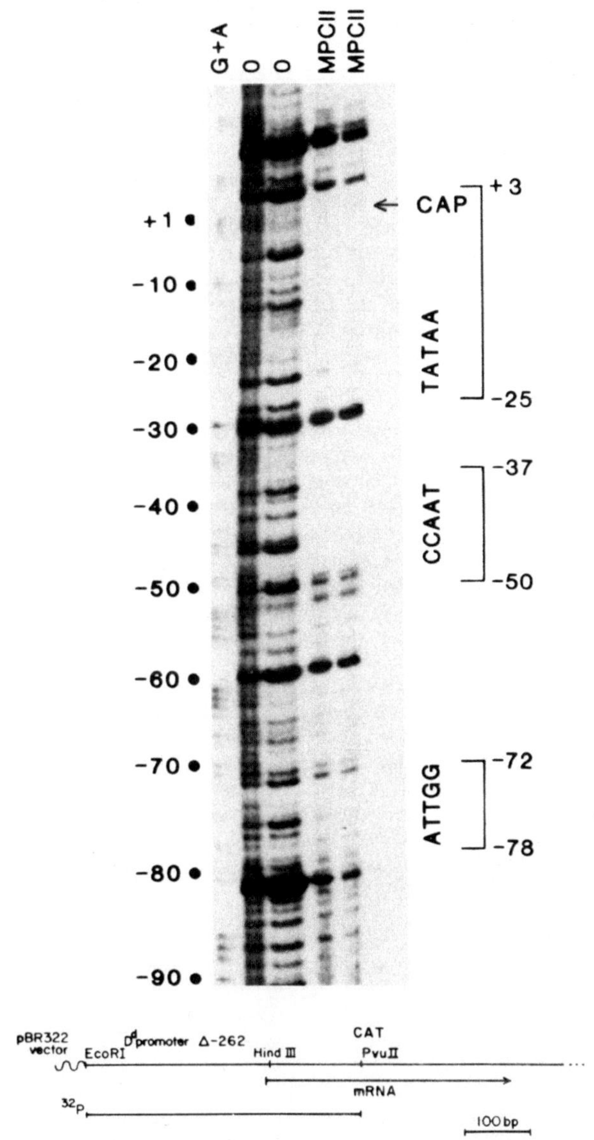

Fig. 2. Footprint analysis of the H-2D^d promoter region. The ^{32}P-kinased EcoRI-PVuII restriction fragment, which allows visualization of the coding strand, was either directly digested with DNAase I (the lanes labeled O, using 2.5 or 1 μg/ml of DNAse I) or first incubated with MPC 11 nuclear extract and then digested with DNAase I (the lanes labeled MPC 11, using 250 or 100 μg/ml of DNAase I). The G+A lane was generated by chemical cleavage reactions; the numbering is relative to the proposed cap site. The TATA and CAAT box sequences are indicated, and cleared regions are bracketed.

affinities that vary according to the extent to which the recognition sequence matches the consensus (AGCCAA) and whether or not the consensus is present in a 2-fold rotationally symmetric configuration. The symmetrical sequence TTGGCT (N_3) AGCCAA was proposed to be one of the highest affinity CTF sites (19). The H-2D^d gene encodes a related palindrome: TTGGGT (N_{14}) AGCCAA, which is strongly conserved in all the H-2 genes (Figure 1). Since these two recognition sequences vary only by a single nucleotide and a change in spacing between the putative target CTF sites (one helical turn in the consensus, two helical turns in the H-2 genes) it is possible that CTF can bind strongly to the H-2 promoter region. This is supported by observation that CTF can bind with high affinity even to a single AGCCAA sequence (19). Another important consideration is location of the CCAAT boxes in relation to other regulatory sites. In the H-2 promoters the CCAAT elements are located at positions centered around -50 and -80, upstream of the putative transcription initiation sites. In human β-globin promoter the functional CCAAT box is located at position -80, while the non-functional CTF binding sites are found further upstream (-125 to -300 region). Hence the location of the H-2 CCAAT boxes approximates sites predicted to be functionally active in promoting transcription.

A second CCAAT binding protein (CBP) has been partially purified from rat liver nuclear extracts (27). It interacts with a sequence closely related to the CTF target site in the HSV thymidine kinase promoter (27,28). CBP is thought to be distinct from CTF because the two proteins have different chromatographic and heat stability properties, and recognize related DNA sequences with different affinities. In particular, a C→G transversion in the first residue of the CCAAT pentanucleotide increases the binding affinity of CBP and substantially reduces the binding affinity at CTF. In addition, the two proteins have reproducibly different DNAase I protection patterns on the HSV-tk promoter (28).

The positions of the footprinted DNA regions in the H-2D^d template are different from the protection patterns predicted for either the CTF or the CBP factors. Whereas in other promoters the CCAAT motif is embedded within the CTF or the CBP binding sites, in the H-2D^d gene the CCAAT boxes are located assymmetrically at the edge of the MPC 11 cleared regions (Figs. 1 and 2). This difference may reflect species or tissue/cell-specific variability of closely related proteins having, otherwise, similar properties. Alternatively, the CTF, the CBP and the H-2D^d CCAAT binding factors may be unrelated to each other except for being able to recognize similar DNA sequences.

Several laboratories have identified factors which bind to the highly conserved TATA motif and are essential components in reconstituted in vitro transcription systems dependent on RNA polymerase II. One such protein, designated the B factor, was partially purified from Drosophila Kc cell nuclear extracts and was shown by DNAase I protection assays to bind to the Drosophila histone H3 and actin 5C promoters (21). Another TATA box binding protein, TFIID, was derived from HeLa cell nuclear extracts and was shown to interact with the adenovirus major late promoter (20). Both the B factor and TFIID protect large regions of their respective promoters' sequences in DNAase I footprinting experiments. The footprinted regions encompass ~30 base pairs upstream of the cap site, including the TATA box, as well as DNA sequences located downstream from the transcription initiation site. The more discriminative method of footprint analysis using methidiumpropyl-EDTA-Fe(II) as a DNA cleavage agent revealed a 10 bp long primary TFIID binding site centered on the TATA motif (23). The MPC 11 extracts also protect large regions of the H-2D^d promoter from DNAse I degradation. The protected regions include the TATAAA consensus as well as sequences downstream from the transcription initiation site. The results of these experiments suggest that the DNAase I protection we have observed using MPC11 extracts may be due to the murine equivalent of the human TFIID or the Drosophila B factor.

Our studies indicate that class I genes may be controlled in part by general transcription factors similar to CTF/CBP and TFIID/B. It should be emphasized, however, that proof of this assertion will require further studies involving DNA mutagenesis of the H-2 TATA and CCAAT sequences and functional analysis of the mutants, as well as assays with purified factors in an in vitro reconstituted transcription system.

Present-day knowledge of the H-2 5' flanking elements suggests a complex view of class I gene transcriptional regulation - the promoter region contains many potential target sequences which may interact with different regulatory proteins. It is possible that regulation during ontogeny, tissue specificity in the relative levels of expression, and adjustment of class I antigen expression during an immune response, bring about the observed complexity in the molecular structure of the H-2 promoters. Future years will likely lead to a better understanding of the mechanisms by which the cooperative protein-protein and protein-DNA interactions cause concerted and controlled expression of these genes.

REFERENCES

1. D. Morello, P. Duprey, A. Israel, and C. Babinet, Asynchronous regulation of mouse H-2D and beta-2-microglobulin RNA transcripts, Immunogenetics 22:441-452 (1985).
2. K. Ozato, Y.-J. Wan, and B. M. Orrison, Mouse major histocompatibility class I gene expression begins at midsomite stage and is inducible in earlier-stage embryos by interferon, Proc. Natl. Acad. Sci. USA 82:2427-2431 (1985).
3. H. W. Harris, and T. J. Gill III, Expression of class I transplantation antigens, Transplantation 42:109-116 (1986).
4. F. Rosa, and M. Fellous, The effect of gamma-interferon on MHC antigens, Immunology Today 5:261-262 (1984).
5. O. Yoshie, H. Schmidt, E. Shyam, P. Reddy, S. Weissman, and P. Lengyel, Mouse interferons enhance the accumulation of human HLA RNA and protein in transfected mouse and hamster cells. J. Biol. Chem/ 257:13169-13172 (1982).
6. T. Collins, L. A. Lapierre, W. Fiers, J. L. Strominger, and J. S. Pober, Recombinant human necrosis factor increases mRNA levels and surface expression of HLA-A,B antigens in vascular endothelial cells and dermal fibroblasts in vitro, Proc. Natl. Acad. Sci. USA 83:446-450 (1986).
7. A. Kimura, A. Israel, O. Le Bail, and P. Kourilsky, Detailed analysis of the mouse H-2K^b promoter: enhancer-like sequences and their role in the regulation of class I gene expression, Cell 44:261-272 (1986).
8. J. Miyazaki, E. Appella, and K. Ozato, Negative regulation of the major histocompatibility class I gene in undifferentiated embryonal carcinoma cells, Proc. Natl. Acad. Sci. USA 83:9537-9541 (1986).
9. A. Israel, A. Kimura, A. Fournier, M. Fellous, and P. Kourilsky, Interferon response sequence potentiates activity of an enhancer in the promoter region of a mouse H-2 gene, Nature (London) 322:743-746 (1986).
10. B. Korber, L. Hood, and I. Stroynowski, Regulation of murine class I genes by interferons is controlled by regions located both 5' and 3' to the transcription initiation site, Proc. Natl. Acad. Sci. USA 84:3380-3384 (1987).
11. J. Vogel, M. Kress, G. Khoury, and G. Jay, A transcriptional enhancer and and interferon-responsive sequence in major histocompatibility complex class I genes, Mol. Cell. Biol. 6:3550-3554 (1986).
12. T. Maniatis, S. Goodbourn, and J. A. Fischer, Regulation of inducible and tissue-specific gene expression, Science 236:1237-1244 (1987).
13. A. S. Baldwin, Jr. and P. A. Sharp, Binding of a nuclear factor to a regulatory sequence in the promoter of the mouse H-2K^b class I major histocompatibility gene, Mol. Cell. Biol. 7:305-313 (1987).

14. A. Israel, A. Kimura, M. Kieran, O. Yano, J. Kanellopoulos, O. Le Bail, and P. Kourilsky, A common positive trans-acting factor binds to enhancer sequences in the promoters of mouse H-2 and beta-2-microglobulin genes, Proc. Natl. Acad. Sci. USA 84:2653-2657 (1987).
15. B. Korber, L. Hood, and I. Stroynowski, Regulation of gene expression by interferons: cell-type and multi-site control of H-2 promoter responses (submitted) (1987).
16. W. Lee, P. Mitchell, and R. Tjian, Purified transcription factor AP-1 binds to TPA-inducible enhancer elements, Cell 49:741-752 (1987).
17. R. Breathnach, and P. Chambon, Organization and expression of eukaryotic split genes, Ann. Rev. Biochem. 50:349-383 (1981).
18. P. Mellon, V. Parker, Y. Gluzman, and T. Maniatis, Identification of DNA sequences required for transcription of the human α1 globin gene in a new SV40 host-vector system, Cell 27:279-288 (1981).
19. K. A. Jones, J. T. Kadonaga, P. J. Rosenfeld, T. J. Kelly, and R. Tjian, A cellular DNA binding protein that activates eukaryotic transcription and DNA replication, Cell 48:79-89 (1987).
20. M. Sawadogo, and R. G. Roeder, Factors involved in specific transcription by human RNA polymerase II: analysis by a rapid and quantitative in vitro assay, Proc. Natl. Acad. Sci. USA 82:4394-4398 (1985).
21. C. S. Parker, and J. Topol, A Drosophila RNA polymerae II transcription factor contains a promoter-region-specific DNA-binding activity, Cell 36:357-369 (1984).
22. D. J. Galas, and A. Schmitz, DNase footprinting: a simple method for the detection of protein-DNA binding specificity. Nucl. Acids Res. 5:3157-3170 (1978).
23. M. Sawadogo, and R. G. Roeder, Interaction of a gene specific transcription factor with the adenovirus major late promoter upstream of the TATA box region, Cell 43:165-175 (1985).
24. J. Lallane, C. Delarbre, G. Grachelin, and P. Kourilsky, A cDNA clone containing the entire coding sequence of a mouse H-2K^d histocompatibility antigen, Nucleic Acids Res. 1:1567-1577 (1983).
25. B. Arnold, H. G. Burgert, A. L. Archibald, and S. Kvist, Complete nucleotide seuqence of the murine H-2K^k gene. Comparison of three H-2K locus alleles. Nucl. Acids Res. 12:9473-9487 (1984).
26. S. Kvist, L. Roberts, and B. Doberstein, Mouse histocompatibility genes: structure and organization of a K^d gene, EMBO J. 2:245-254 (1983).
27. B. J. Graves, P. F. Johnson, and S. L. McKnight, Homologous recognition of a promoter domain common to the MSV LTR and the HSV tk gene, Cell 44:565-576 (1986).
28. K. A. Jones, K. R. Yamamoto and R. Tjian, Two distinct transcription factors bind to the HSV thymidine kinase promoter in vitro, Cell 42:559-572, (1985).
29. S. McKnight, R. Tjian, Transcriptional Selectivity of Viral Genes in Mammalian Cells, Cell 46:759-805.

MUTATION OF THE SPLICE ACCEPTOR SITES AT THE 5'END OF EXON 2 OF H-2K^d AND H-2D^d RESULTS IN THE EXPRESSION OF ALTERED CLASS I ANTIGENS EXPRESSED ON THE MEMBRANE OF L CELLS

Mary Lynne Hedley, Philip Tucker and James Forman

University of Texas Health Science Center at Dallas
5323 Harry Hines Boulevard
Dallas, Texas 75235-9048

INTRODUCTION

Major histocompatibility complex (MHC) class I antiens are highly polymorphic proteins expressed on the surface of most murine cells. These glycoproteins have a molecular weight of 37-45,000 daltons and are noncovalently associated with the nonpolymorphic β2-microglobulin light chain. The classical transplantation antigens H-2K, -D, and -L serve as restriction elements for viral and tumor antigens and thereby allow the specific recognition of target cells by cytotoxic T lymphocytes (CTL).

Recently, several examples of alternatively spliced class I mRNAs have been reported. The majority of the splices described occur at the 3' terminus of the mRNA transcript. cDNA clones representing *H-2K* have been found to have an exon 8 that is 27 nucleotides shorter than the normal exon 8 (Kress et al. 1983; Reddy and Pan 1985). However, H-2K pre-mRNA seems to be preferentially spliced to produce a longer exon 8 as compared to the shorter form more often represented by H-2D mRNAs (Kress et al. 1983). Proteins with a deleted exon 7 have been precipitated from the cell surface (Rogers et al. 1986; McCluskey et al. 1986) and are not phosphorylated due to the lack of the serine in exon 7. One study of 5' alternative splicing of a class I gene has been reported (Lalanne et al 1983). An *H-2K*^{d} cDNA with an abnormal α1 domain is generated by a complex double splicing event in which intronic nucleotides 5' of exon 2 are spliced into the mRNA and 96 nucleotides from within exon 2 are deleted. The transcript remains in an open reading frame and could generate a protein product.

One approach to identifying the products of alternatively spliced mRNAs has been to force splicing to proceed by a predicted route and thereby generate large quantities of aberrant message and its protein product. We have examined the H-2D^d genomic sequence for alternative splice sites which did not differ from the highly conserved GT/AG sequences bordering mammalian introns. We located an alternative acceptor site in the first intron. Alternative donor and acceptor sites are also present within exon 2. The utilization of these splice sites would generate a transcript similar to that of a *H-2K*^{d} cDNA clone previously reported.

We describe here the mutagenesis of normal acceptor sites bordering exon 2 of *H-2D*^{d} and *H-2K*^{d} and demonstrate altered cell surface proteins which are generated from the mutant genes.

MATERIALS AND METHODS

Antibodies

The α3 *H-2D*^{d} specific monoclonal antibody (mAb) 34-2-12 was kindly provided by Dr. T. Hansen (Washington University, St. Louis, MO). The α3 H-2K^d specific mAb K9-18 was provided by Dr. G. Hammerling (German Cancer Research Center, Heidelberg, Germany). 16-3-1 (anti-H-2K^k) was purchased as a culture supernatant from Bionetics, Inc.

DNA Clones

The pDd-1 plasmid containing *H-2D*^{d} cloned into PBR 327 was provided by Dr. J. Seidman (Harvard U. Boston, MA). The 16Kd construct containing the *H-2K*^{d} was cloned into pACYC and was provided by Dr. I. Stroynowski (Calif. Inst. Tech., Pasadena CA).

Construction of Mutagenized Class I Genes

A 704 base MstI/PstI fragment containing exons 1-3 of H-2-D^d was isolated from pDd-1 and cloned into M13 mp10 generating clone m18D. A 327 base SmaI fragment containing exon 1 of *H-2K*^{d} cloned into mp18 was provided by Dr. I. Stroynowski. Oligonucleotides (18b long) that were complimentary to sequences in *H-2K*^{d} or *H-2D*^{d} with the exception of single base differences at the conserved α1 donor splice sites were annealed to single stranded phage DNA from the m13 clones containing *H-2D*^{d} or *H-2K*^{d} fragments. Elongation reactions were performed using DNA polymerase I and followed by ligation with T4 DNA ligase. The resulting DNA was used to transform RR1 cells and positive clones were selected on the basis of hybridization to the mutant oligonucleotide probes. Single-stranded DNA from positive clones (m10D7C and m18K9G) was sequenced by the dideoxy chain termination technique (Sanger et al. 1980) to confirm that only a single base mutation had been created. A 345 base BssHII/AatII -D^d fragment from m10D7C was inserted back into the genomic DNA subclone pDd-1. This clone, Dmut7c, was used for transfection into L-cells. The 327 base XmaI H-2K^d fragment from M18K9G was shuffled back into the genomic DNA subclone 16Kd. This clone, 16KdmutG, was used for transfection into L-cells.

Transfection of Mouse L-cells

Mouse L-cells derived from C3H were used as recipients in transfection experiments. Ten million L-cells were seeded one day prior to transfection. Cells were transfected by the calcium phosphate technique using 1 μg of plasmid DNA, 20 ng of psv2neo (plasmid DNA containing the neomycin resistance gene), and 20 μg of carrier DNA (Goodenow et al. 1983). Transfectants were maintained in α-minimal essential medium containing 5% FCS, 0.2 μg/ml G418 antibiotic, glutamine, streptomycin and penicillin. For induction studies cells were cultured in the presence of 30% rat ConA supernatant for 72 hrs and subsequently tested for surface expression of H-2D^d or H-2K^d antigens on a fluorescence activated cell sorter.

Fluorescence Activated Cell Sorter (FACS) Analysis

Cells were harvested by trypsinization and washed once with HBSS containing 0.02% sodium azide. 5 x 10^5 cells were incubated for 15 min at 4° C with mAb, washed once, and incubated for 15 min with fluorescein isothiocyanate- $F(ab')_2$ goat anti-mouse IgG. Cells were washed twice and resuspended in 1 ml HBSS for FACS analysis.

Immunoprecipitation

Transfected cells were trypsinized and resuspended to 2 x 10^7 cells/ml. Cells were surface labeled with 2-2.5 mCi of ^{125}I by the lactoperoxidase method (Haustein 1975). Labeled cells were lysed and cell extracts were subjected to immunoprecipitation with formalin fixed *Staphylococcus aureus* Cowan 1 strain (SAC). Antibodies were added to the cell lysates and incubated 16-18 hrs at 4°C. After incubation, antigen-antibody complexes were isolated, eluted from SAC and analyzed by SDS-PAGE. The gels were fixed, dried and bands were visualized by autoradiography.

RESULTS

Mutation Strategy

It was reported that an alternative acceptor splice site is located 60 bases 5' of exon 2 in the H-2K^d gene (Lalanne et al. 1983). We examined the sequence of H-2D^d for alternative acceptor splice sites in the first intron. A splice site following the GT/AG consensus sequence was identified 51 bases 5' of exon 2. To generate large amounts of alternatively spliced mRNAs and the corresponding proteins, the acceptor splice sites bordering exon 2 of the *H-2D^d* or *H-2K^d* genes were mutated by site-directed mutagenesis (Figure 1). An M13 subclone containing exon 1 of *H-2K^d* and a subclone containing exons 1-3 of *H-2D^d* were used. Two oligonucleotides (18 bases long) were synthesized to construct the mutant genes. The oligonucleotides were complementary to the DNA bordering the splice sites but contained single nucleotide substitutions that replaced the codon CAG to CGG in the *H-2D^d* mutant and to CCG in the *H-2K^d* mutant (Figure 1). DNA from positive clones m10D7C and m18K9G was sequenced to verify the single base change. No unexpected base changes were detected in either mutant. Restriction enzyme fragments containing the mutated bases were isolated from m10D7C and m18K9G and inserted back into *H-2D^d* or *H-2K^d*. These genomic clones (16KdmutG and Ddmut7C) were isolated and co-transfected into C3H L-cells with the gene for neomycin resistance. G418 resistant cells were screened for the expression of H-2D^d or H-2K^d antigens by FACS analysis.

Detection of Mutant H-2K^d and H-2D^d Antigens on Transfected Cells

The monoclonal antibody 34-2-12 recognizes the α3 domain of H-2D^d (Ozato et al. 1985) and therefore should be capable of binding to an H-2D^d

molecule that has an altered $\alpha 1$ domain. Two independent Ddmut7c transfections were tested with this mAb and both contained a subpopulation of cells that stained with 34-2-12. This population was sorted on the FACS and the sorted cells were cloned by limiting dilution. The staining profile of one clone, Dmutsl.3, is shown in Figure 2. The normal *H-2D*^{d} gene was also transfected into L-cells and sorted cells expressing H-2D^d were cloned by limiting dilution. Cell surface expression of normal H-2D^d

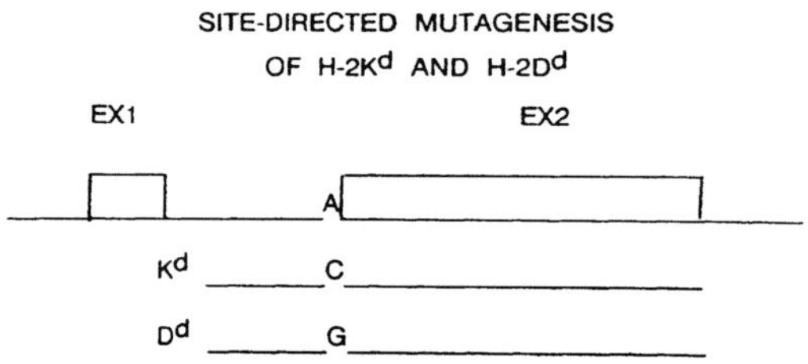

Figure 1. Strategy for mutation of splice acceptor sites at the 5' end of exon 2 for *H-2K*^{d} and *H-2D*^{d}. Alternative acceptor splice sites that follow the consensus sequence are located fifty-one bases upstream of the normal acceptor site bordering exon 2 of the H-2D^d gene and sixty bases upstream of exon 2 in the H-2K^d gene. To generate large quantities of pre-mRNA that follow the alternative pattern of splicing, the normal acceptor sites bordering exon 2 were mutated. M13 subclones containing exon 2 of the *H-2K*^{d} or *H-2D*^{d} genes were annealed to oligonucleotide primers complimentary to the genes but with single base mismatches. Annealing reactions were followed by elongation with DNA polymerase I and ligation with T4 DNA ligase. Phage DNA were screened with the mutagenic ologonucleotide using dot blot hybridization. Restriction enzyme fragments containing the mutated bases were isolated and inserted into the genomic DNA. DNA from these subclones were used in subsequent transfection experiments.

is approximately 10-fold higher than the mutant H-2D^d molecule (Fig. 2). However, if Dmutsl.3 cells are cultured in the presence of 30% Con A supernatant (containing γ interferon activity) for 72 hours, the level of H-2D^d mutant antigen increases to approximately that of normal H-2D^d on uninduced cells (Fig. 2).

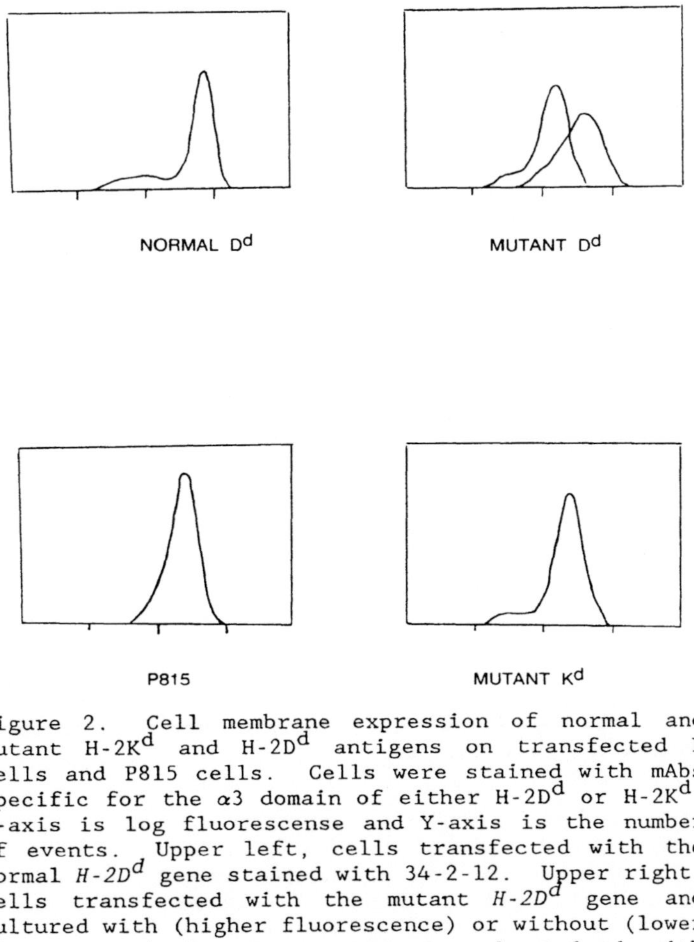

Figure 2. Cell membrane expression of normal and mutant H-2K^d and H-2D^d antigens on transfected L cells and P815 cells. Cells were stained with mAbs specific for the α3 domain of either H-2D^d or H-2K^d. X-axis is log fluorescense and Y-axis is the number of events. Upper left, cells transfected with the normal *H-2D^d* gene stained with 34-2-12. Upper right, cells transfected with the mutant *H-2D^d* gene and cultured with (higher fluorescence) or without (lower fluorescence) Con A supernatant and stained with 34-2-12. Lower left, P815 cells stained with K9-18; and lower right, cells transfected with the mutant *H-2K^d* gene stained with K9-18.

The monoclonal antibody K9-18 recognizes the α3 domain of the H-$2K^d$ (Arnold et al. 1985) and was used to study surface expression of the mutant H-$2K^d$ transfectants. Transfected cells were stained with K9-18 and the positive population was sorted on the FACS. The sorted cells were cloned by limiting dilution and the profile of one clone (Kmuts5) is shown in Figure 2. Since we do not presently have L-cells transfected with the normal *H-$2K^d$* gene, we compared the expression of the mutant H-$2K^d$ molecule with normal H-$2K^d$ on P815 cells. Although the level of total fluoresence from K9-18 binding on L cells transfected with the mutant H-$2K^d$ protein is similar to that of normal H-$2K^d$ on P815 cells, the former cells are larger. Thus, the cell membrane density of mutant H-$2K^d$ on L cells is less than that of normal H-$2K^d$ on P815.

Immunoprecipitation of the Mutant H-$2D^d$ Antigen

The mutation strategy described in Figure 1 should generate proteins with an elongated exon 2. We initiated the studies of these proteins by concentrating on *H-$2D^d$*. To demonstrate that the protein encoded by the mutant *H-$2D^d$* gene is different from normal H-$2D^d$, we immunoprecipitated the mutant molecule. Dmuts1.3 cells were harvested by trypsinization and surface labeled with ^{125}I. Cell lysates were precleared with SAC and normal mouse serum (NMS). The precleared lysates were subjected to immunoprecipitation with 34-2-12 mAb and then analyzed by SDS-PAGE. Since Dmuts1.3 has an altered splice acceptor site 5' of exon 2, we would predict it to use a cryptic splice site within the first intron. If the pre-RNA uses this cryptic splice site, the exon 1 -exon 2 reading frame remains the same, but the protein generated should be 17 amino acids larger than normal H-$2D^d$. Immunoprecipitates from Dmuts1.3 cells incubated with the 34-2-12 mAb gave a band running approximately 2 kd larger than the endogenous H-$2K^k$ protein precipitated from these same cells (Figure 3). In contrast, normal H-$2D^d$ protein precipitated from the surface of L-cells transfected with the unmutated *H-$2D^d$* gene gave rise to a band of the same size as *H-$2K^k$*.

We conclude that the mutation of a single base in the normal splice acceptor site from CAG to CCG or CGG renders the acceptor site nonfunctional and forces the cell to use cryptic splice sites located 5' of the mutated site. The mutant mRNA is functional and is translated into a protein with reaches the cell surface.

DISCUSSION

In this report we demonstrate the production of cell surface class I proteins from alternatively spliced mRNAs. Site-directed mutagenesis was utilized to change the normal acceptor splice sites at the 5' end of exon 2 from the consensus CAG to CCG (in *H-$2K^d$*) or CGG (in *H-$2D^d$*). The mutated genes were transfected into L-cells and cells expressing the transfected gene were isolated.

The protein products of the alternatively spliced transcripts were expressed on the cell surface as demonstrated by FACS analysis and immunoprecipitation. We used α3 directed anti-H-$2D^d$ or -K^d specific mAb to detect the mutant proteins on transfected L-cells. Thus, although the α1 domains were altered due by the addition of 17-20 amino acids, the α3 specific monoclonals still bound the mutant proteins. The mutant H-$2D^d$

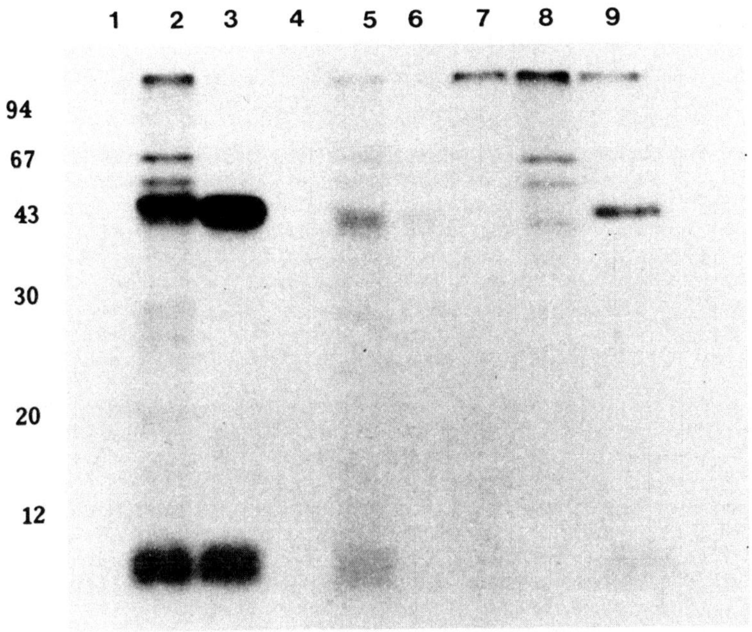

Figure 3. Immunoprecipitation of H-$2D^d$ from L cells transfected with normal and mutant *H-$2D^d$* genes. Lysates from radiolabeled cells were pre-cleared with SAC and NMS and precipitated. Lanes 1-3, L-cells transfected with the *H-$2D^d$* mutant gene. Lanes 4-6, L-cells transfected with the *H-$2D^d$* normal gene. Lanes 7-9, L-cells. Lanes 1,4 and 7, NMS; Lanes 2,5 and 8, 34-2-12; Lanes 3,6 and 9, 16-3-1.

protein was not expressed at a level similar to normal H-$2D^d$, but its expression could be induced to higher levels with a Con A supernatant. Immunoprecipitation of the H-$2D^d$ protein provided evidence that this mutant antigen was larger than its normal counterpart. Experiments are currently in progress to examine the size of the mutant H-$2K^d$ protein.

RNase mapping experiments demonstrated that the structure of RNA isolated from the mutant transfectants represented the predicted pattern of alternative splicing generated by use of the alternative acceptor sites (data not shown). Cells containing the normal *H-$2D^d$* or *H-$2K^d$* genes also express the mutant forms of mRNA albeit at a 10-20 fold lower level. Therefore, both the mutant and normally spliced transcripts can originate from the same pre-mRNA molecule and we have enriched for the alternatively spliced form by mutagenizing a single base in the *H-$2D^d$* or *H-$2K^d$* gene.

ACKNOWLEDGEMENT

Supported by NIH grant AI11851 and AI18016. MLH is supported by the Texas Department of the Ladies Auxillary, Veterans of Foreign Wars.

Evidence for heterogeneity of class I proteins exists at both protein and serological levels. When lysates from cells of mice bearing H-2K^d were immunoprecipitated with certain anti-H-2K^d mAbs, a second protein distinct from normal H-2K^d was also precipitated. The difference in size of these two proteins could not be attributed to glycosylation (Tryphonas et al. 1983). Data also exists for additional proteins that are encoded in the *D-region* of *H-2*^{d}. L2^d, H-2M^d, and H-2R^d proteins were identified by co-capping experiments with private and public specificity antisera and mAb (Hansen et al. 1981; Ivanyi and Demant 1982; Ivanyi and Demant 1979).

These proteins differ in their ability to react with specific alloantisera and their expression on cells of BALB/c derived mutant strains. For example, the L2^d and H-2R^d proteins are not found in BALB/c-H-2^{dm2}; whereas, H-2M^d antigens are found on in this strain. Genes encoding these proteins have not been identified although additional genes have been mapped to the *D-region* (Stephan et al. 1986). An explanation for the heterogeneity seen among class I proteins may be due to additional genes in this region and/or by alternative processing of class I transcripts generated from these genes.

Class I transcripts have been shown to utilize alternative processing and most examples represent splicing at the 3' terminus. For example, *H-2K* alleles can utilize two different splice acceptor sites to generate a long or shortened exon 8 (Kress et al. 1983). Both *H-2K* and *H-2D* alleles are capable of completely splicing out exon 7 (Rogers et al. 1986; Brickell et al. 1983). Proteins that lack exon 7 were immunoprecipitated from the cell surface and are not phosphorylated due to the absence of the serine (found in exon 7) (McCluskey et al. 1986; Rogers et al. 1986).

One example of alternative splicing at the 5' end of a class I gene has been reported (Lalanne et al. 1983). mRNA representing the alternative splice were found in normal tissues, although at lower levels than the normally spliced transcript (Transy et al. 1984). Recently, this cDNA has been cloned into an expression vector and transfected into L-cells. mRNA is found on polysomes but no protein was identified in the cytoplasm or on the cell surface (Cochet et al. 1986).

One possible function of proteins generated from alternatively spliced transcripts may be to create new determinants on class I molecules. The additional determinants may enable this protein to serve as a restricting element for a greater number of tumor or viral antigens. Alternatively, the novel proteins may down regulate the immune response by decreasing the level of cell surface class I and thereby protecting the cell from lysis by CTL. Thus, we noted an approximate 10-fold decrease in the level of mutant H-2D^d on transfected L-cells compared to normal H-2D^d. In addition, the new amino acids generated by an alternative splice may prevent the protein from serving as a restricting element by decreasing its affinity for immunogenic peptides. The combination of a low level of surface expression and decreased interaction with antigen would render the cell resistant to specific CTL. We are currently investigating the role of these mutant proteins in their ability to be recognized by both alloreactive and H-2 restricted CTL.

REFERENCES

Arnold, B., Horstmann, U., Kuon, W., Burgert, H-G., Hammerling, G.J., and Kvist, S., 1985, Alloreactive cytolytic T-cell clone preferentially recognize conformational determinants on histocompatibility antigens: Analysis with genetically engineered hybrid antigens. Proc. Natl. Acad. Sci. USA 82:7030.

Brickell, P.M., Latchman, D.S., Murphy, D.,Willison, K., and Rigby, P.W.J., 1983, Activation of a Qa/Tla class I major histocompatibility antigen gene is a general feature of oncogenesis in the mouse. Nature 306:756.

Cochet, M., Kast, W.M., Kummer, A.M., Transy, C., Melief, C.J.M., and Kourilsky, P., 1986, Alternative splicing in the mouse H-2K^{d} gene is not necessary for the classical K^{d} antigen function. Immunogen. 24:267.

Goodenow, R.S., Stroynowski, I., McMillan, M., Nicolson, M., Eakle, K., Sher, B.T., Davidson, N., and Hood, L., 1983, Expression of complete transplantation antigens by mammalian cells transformed with truncated class I genes. Nature 301:388.

Hansen, T.H., Ozato, K., Melino, M.R., Coligan, J.E., Kindt, T.J., Jandinski, J.J., and Sachs, D.H., 1981, Immunochemical evidence in two haplotypes for at least three D region-encoded molecules, D,L, and R. J. Immunol. 126:1713.

Haustein, D., 1975, Effective radioiodination by lactoperoxidase and solubilization of cell surface proteins of cultured murine T lymphoma cells. J. Immunol. Meth. 7:25.

Ivanyi, D. and Demant, P., 1979, Complex genetic effect of B10.D2 (M504) (H-2^{dm1}) mutation. Immuogen. 8:539.

Ivanyi, D. and Demant, P., 1982, Molecular heterogeneity of D-end products detected by anti-H-2.28 sera. Immunogen. 15:467.

Kress, M., Glaros, D., Khoury, G., and Jay, G., 1983, Alternative RNA splicing in expression of the H-2K gene. Nature 306:602.

Lalanne, J-L., Cochet, M., Kummer, A-M., Gachelin, G., and Kourilsky, P., 1983, Different exon-intron organization at the 5' part of a mouse class I gene is used to generate a novel H-2K^{d}-related mRNA. Proc. Natl. Acad. Sci. USA 80:7561.

McCluskey, J., Boyd, L.F., Maloy, W.L., Coligan, J.E., and Margulies, D.H., 1986, Alternative processing of H-2D^{d} pre-mRNAs results in membrane expression of differentially phosphorylated protein products. EMBO 5:2477.

Ozato, K., Takahashi, H., Appella, E., Sears, D.W., Murre, C., Seidman, J.G., Kimura, S., and Tada, N., 1985, Polymorphism of murine major histocompatibility class I antigen: Assignement of putative allodeterminants to distinct positions of the amino acid sequence within the first external domain of the antigen. J. Immunol. 134:1749.

Reddy, E.S.P. and Pan, J.Y., 1985, Molecular cloning and sequencing of H-2K^{k} cDNA: comparison with other H-2 genes and evidence for alternative splicing. Gene 38:239.

Rogers, M.J., Siwarski, D.F., Shacter, E., Maloy, W.L., Lillehoj, E.P., and Coligan, J.E., 1986, Three distinct H-2K^{s} molecules differing at the carboxy terminus are expressed on a tumor from SJL/J mice. J. Immunol. 137:3006.

Sanger, F., Coulson, A.R., Barrell, B.G., Smith, A.J.H., and Roe, D.A., 1980, Cloning in single-stranded bacteriophages as an aid to rapid DNA sequencing. J. Mol. Biol. 143:161.

Stephan, D., Sun, H., Fischer-Lindahl, K., Meyer, E.,Hammerling, G., Hood, L., and Steinmetz, M., 1986, Organization and evolution of D region class I genes in the mouse major histocompatibility complex. J. Exp. Med. 163:1227.

Transy, C., Lalanne, J.L., and Kourilsky, P., 1984, Alternative splicing in the 5' moiety of the H-2K^{d} gene transcript. EMBO 3:2383.

Tryphonan, M., King, D.P., and Jones, P.P., 1983, Identification of a second class I antigen controlled by the K end of the H-2 complex and its selective cellular expression. Proc. Natl. Acad. Sci. U.S.A. 80:1445.

COMPLEX EXPRESSION OF THE MOUSE H-2 CLASS I GENES

M. Cochet, B. David-Watine, A.-M. Dumont, C. Transy, S.R. Nash, C. Jacob*, G. Gachelin and P. Kourilsky

Unité de Biologie Moléculaire du Gène, INSERM U. 277 and CNRS UAC 115 - Institut Pasteur : 25 rue du Dr. Roux - 75724 Paris cédex 15 - France

* Medical Biology Department - Stanford University School of Medicine Stanford - California 94305 - U.S.A.

INTRODUCTION

Once molecular probes detecting mouse H-2 (Kvist et al., 1981) and human HLA (Ploegh et al., 1980 ; Sood et al., 1981) class I sequences had been isolated, it was quickly realized that the mouse class I H-2 multigene family was far more complex than initially anticipated (Cami et al., 1981 ; Steinmetz et al., 1981a). A considerable amount of cloning work performed in several laboratories has led to the isolation of almost the entire H-2 locus from both BALB/c (Steinmetz et al., 1982) and B10 mice (Weiss et al., 1984). These studies have established that there exists of the order of 26 to 36 class I H-2 genes, depending on the mouse strain. It has become usual to divide these genes into two major groups predominantly on the basis of serological data. The first group includes those genes which map to the K and D loci. They encode the quasi-ubiquitous and highly polymorphic class I major transplantation antigens, which serve as restriction elements in the recognition of target cells by cytotoxic T lymphocytes (Zinckernagel and Doherty, 1979 ; see also Kourilsky et al., 1987). The other group of genes (23 to 29 depending on the mouse strain) lie in the Qa-Tla region and includes the genes encoding the serologically detected Qa and Tla differentiation cell surface antigens. The latter are much less polymorphic than the class I molecules encoded in the K and D regions, and display a limited tissue distribution, being expressed mostly in B and/or T cells. Accordingly, it was believed for some time that the Qa-Tla region encoded only non-ubiquitous cell surface antigens.

This simple picture of the expression of class I genes has been challenged by a variety of observations :

1) The level of expression of K and D molecules in various tissues does in fact vary over a wide range from nothing in brain cells to high levels in spleen and lymph nodes cells (Mombrug et al., 1986), so that the dogma of their "ubiquity" is questionable. In fact, the term of "ubiquitous" could be misleading if it were to obscure these quantitative variations in expression.

2) Structural heterogeneity has been noted in cell surface proteins immunoprecipitated with antisera specific for K and D region products (Demant and Ivânyi, 1981 ; Hansen et al., 1983 ; Tryphonas et al., 1983 ; Lew et al., 1986a ; Rodgers et al., 1986).

3) Several class I genes give rise to more than one transcript by alternative splicing mechanisms. For instance this occurs at the 3' end of the K^b, K^k (Reyes et al., 1982a ; Archibald et al., 1986) and K^q genes (Kress et al., 1983a) as well as at the 5' end of the K^d and K^b genes (Lalanne et al., 1983a ; Transy et al., 1984). It was also found that the Q10 gene and the Q7 gene (initially named 27.1 by Steinmetz et al., 1981b) give rise to at least two distinct transcripts (Lalanne et al., 1985 ; Waneck et al., 1986).

4) The afore mentioned Q10 gene, which lies in the Qa region, was shown to be predominantly expressed in the liver where it is translated into a secreted class I molecule found in the serum of most adult mouse strains except $H\text{-}2^f$ haplotype (Cosman et al., 1982 ; Kress et al., 1983b ; Lew et al., 1986).

5) We identified a class I gene named "37" which, although poorly polymorphic and located in the Tla region, so far follows the pattern of expression of the K and D genes (Lalanne et al., 1985 ; Transy et al., 1987).

In more general terms, it may be emphasized that :

1) There exist many more class I genes than serologically identified products.

2) Serological reagents are limiting for the identification of new products. In addition, homologies within the gene family and the possible transfer of epitopes by conversion-like mechanisms may cast doubt on the specificity of well characterized reagents, such as monoclonal antibodies against individual transplantation antigens.

3) The use of genes rather than cDNAs (engineered into expression vectors) in many transfection experiments, could leave ambiguities with respect to the expressed product inasmuch as alternative splicing could generate several mRNAs.

4) The study of minor cell populations in adults as well as the analysis of cells generated during embryonic growth is hampered by the difficulty of gathering enough material. Accordingly, relatively little is known about such cell populations.

It is therefore not surprising that the previous simple picture of H-2 genes and their products has become obscured by observations which emphasized the complexity of the system. We review below some of the recent data obtained in our laboratory regarding the expression, both in the adult and during embryogenesis, of three class I genes (K^d, 37 and Q10) and the detection of two of their products.

RESULTS

1) Identification of the product of a K^d gene transcript alternatively spliced at its 5' end

We have previously shown that the cDNA 24 is nearly identical to the canonical $H\text{-}2K^d$ cDNA, except in the portion encoding the first half of the first domain of the protein (Lalanne et al., 1983a). This results from

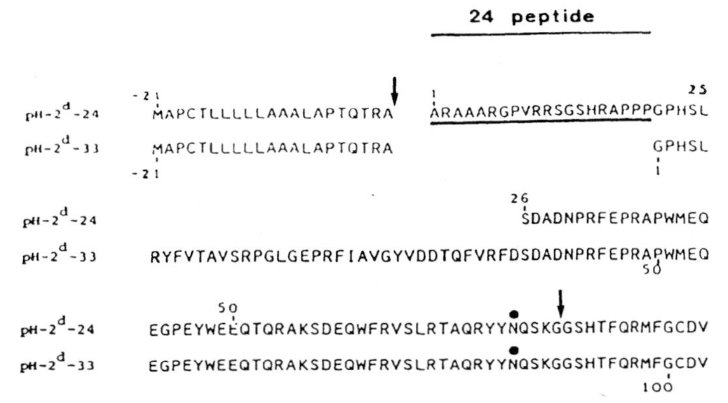

Fig. 1 : Amino acid sequence alignment of part of the 24 protein and of the H-2K^d antigen.
The sequence is deduced from the DNA clones pH-2^d-24 for the 24 protein and pH-2^d-33 for the H-2K^d antigen. The arrows delineate the different domains of the H-2K^d antigen and correspond to the position of the intron in the gene sequence. The closed circles represent the glycosylation sites of the K^d antigen. Amino acid + 1 refers to the first amino acid of the mature protein. The underlined amino acids 1 to 20 correspond to the synthetic 24 peptide.

a double alternative mode of splicing in the first intron and second exon of the H-2K^d gene. Only the canonical form is responsible for the known H-2K^d antigen functions (Cochet et al., 1986). No conventional sera detecting H-2K^d antigens were able to detect protein 24. However, using L cells transfected with cDNA 24, we have identified the protein encoded by cDNA 24. It has a molecular weight compatible with a glycosylated protein, but it is not found at the cell membrane despite its great homology with the H-2K^d antigen. It does not appear to be associated with beta-2-microglobulin either.

The cDNA 24 and its normal counterpart cDNA 33 (the canonical H-2K^d cDNA) had been previously engineered into a SV40 expression vector (Cochet et al., 1986). This has allowed the isolation of transfected L cells expressing one or the other of the cDNAs. These cells were called respectively LSV24 (clones 1 to 3) and LSV33 (clones 1 to 4). We used conventional H-2K^d monoclonal antibodies like 34.1.2, 31.3.4. (Ozato et al., 1982) which recognize epitopes respectively in the alpha-1 and alpha-2 domain of the K^d antigen (Arnold et al., 1985), as well as a panel of alloantisera. Whereas on LSV33 cells, the K^d specific sera were reactive, none of them were reactive on LSV24 cells (Cochet et al., 1986). Next, a 20 amino acids (AA) long peptide corresponding to the specific part of the molecule (Fig. 1), was chemically synthesized and a rabbit anti-24 peptide serum was prepared. LSV24-2 and LSV33-1 cells were metabolically labelled with ^{35}S-methionine, the cell lysates immunoprecipitated with this serum and analyzed by SDS-PAGE. As shown in figure 2, a 47 kDa protein is immunoprecipitated from LSV24-2 extracts (lane 1) which disappears when the serum is preincubated with the unlabelled peptide before the immunoprecipitation (lane 2). This protein is not present in L cells or LSV33-1 cells (not shown). It is 2 kDa lighter than the 49 kDa H-2K^d heavy chain (lane 4). This is in very good agreement with the expected molecular weight of the 24 protein devoid of its signal peptide. Only the

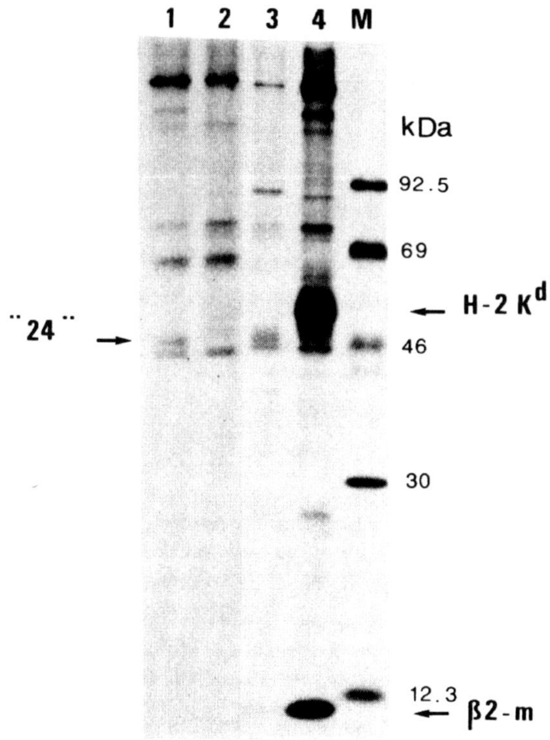

Fig. 2 : Detection of the 24 protein.
Immunoprecipitation of the 24 protein and H-2K^d polypeptide from L cells transformants LSV24-2 and LSV33-1. The cells were labelled with ^{35}S- methionine. LSV24-2 cell extracts (lane 1-3) were immunoprecipitated with the anti-24 alloantiserum either alone (lane 1), or after preincubation with unlabelled 24 peptide (lane 2). In lane 3, after preclearing with the anti-24 alloantiserum, the lysate was immunoprecipitated with an anti-H-2 alloantisera. In lane 5, LSV33-1 cell extracts were immunoprecipitated with the monoclonal antibody 34.1.2. The immune complexes were bound to fixed Staphyloccocus aureus Cowan I strain and extensively washed. The bound protein was solubilized and analyzed by electrophoresis on 7.5 to 15 % NaDodSO4-polyacrylamide gel, and subjected to fluorography. The molecular weight protein markers (lane M) are respectively from top to bottom : phosphorylase beta, bovin serum albumin, ovalbumin, anhydrase carbonic and cytochrome C.

heavy chain is detected, no beta-2m being found associated with the 24 protein. This is not due to a lack of beta-2m in these cells because it is present when the lysate previously precleared with the anti-24 serum is immunoprecipitated with a broad anti-H-2 xenoserum (lane 3).

Recently, using the same lysate, we have attempted to immunoprecipitate the 24 protein with the monoclonal antibody K9-18. This serum has been described to be specific for the alpha-3 domain of K^d (Arnold et al., 1985). Once again, this conventional antibody failed to detect the 24 protein.

Taken together, these results suggest that the addition of 20 AA coming from the first intron and the deletion of 30 AA of the first domain of H-2K^d antigen alter the structure of the molecule in such a way that it can neither associate with beta-2m, nor integrate into the plasma membrane, nor be detected by conventional anti-H-$2K^d$ sera.

2) Gene 37 and its product

The isolation of cDNA 37 has been described previously (Lalanne et al., 1985). The amino acids sequence corresponding to its two putative first domains is presented in figure 3 together with seven other class I molecules. The results illustrate clearly the divergence of the alpha-2 domain sequence of this molecule compared to other class I molecules. This property was used to derive a 37 cDNA specific probe which was then used to study the localisation and expression of the 37 gene.

a) Localisation of gene 37 - To localize gene 37 within the H-2 complex, we initially mapped it by restriction site polymorphism. Previous analysis had shown that DNA's from SJL/J (H-2^s) mice contain a single fragment which hybridizes to the second domain of cDNA 37. This pattern is easily distinguishable, in PvuII digests, from the two fragments present when using DNA's from mice of the b, d, k and q haplotypes (Lalanne et al., 1985). We found that DNA from A (H-2^a) or B10.M (H-2^f) mice display the same single band pattern as SJL/J mice DNA. We used this property to analyze several congenic strains made by crossing C57Bl/6 (B6) or C57Bl/10 (B10) (H-2^b) mice with A (H-2^a) mice. These congenics differ from each other in the parental origin of their respective MHC subregions. Their genomic DNAs and those of their parents was digested with PvuII and analyzed by Southern blotting with the 37 probe (Figure 4). The single band characteristic of A mice (2.1 kb) is observed for B6. Tla^a recombinant mice which have the Qa-Tla region from A mice and the K and D regions

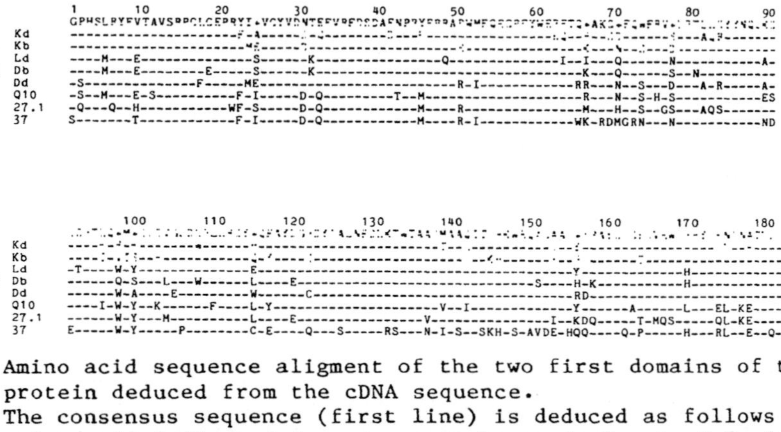

Fig. 3 : Amino acid sequence aligment of the two first domains of the 37 protein deduced from the cDNA sequence.
The consensus sequence (first line) is deduced as follows : the amino acid indicated is present at least in 3 out of 5 of the H-2 class I antigens : K^d (Lalanne et al., 1983b), K^b (Weiss et al., 1983), L^d (Moore et al., 1982), D^b (Reyes et al., 1982b), D^d (Sher et al., 1985). Q10 (Mellor et al., 1984), Q7 (or 27.1) (Steinmetz et al., 1981) and the 37 cDNA (Lalanne et al., 1985) are compared to this consensus sequence. The + sign indicates an absence of the consensus.

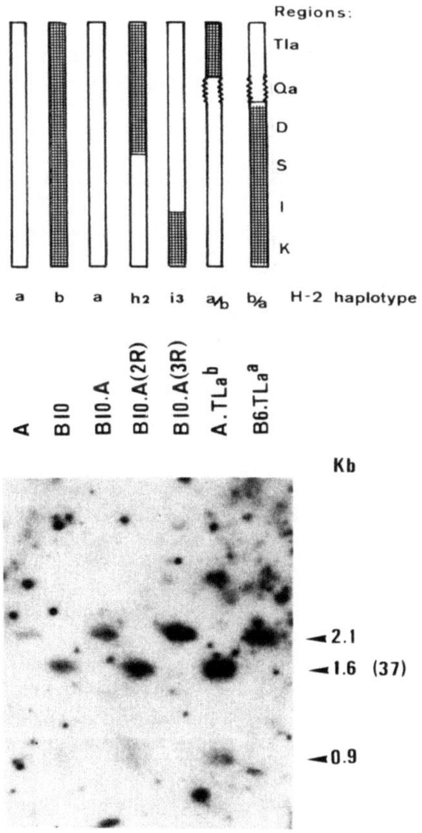

Fig. 4 : Assignment of the 37 gene to the Tla complex. Genomic DNA of H-2^b, H-2^a and of different recombinants H-2^b/H-2^a congenic mice were PvuII digested and analyzed by Southern blotting. The origin of the DNA is indicated above each lane. The Southern blotting and the hybridization condition with the 37 riboprobe are described by Transy et al. (1987). The size of the hybridizing fragments are indicated in kilobases on the right side; (37) indicates the fragment specific for the 37 gene. The size markers used were pBR322 plasmid DNA digested with HinfI and wild type lambda phage DNA digested with HindIII. Above the Southern blot, genetic maps of the mouse strains used are shown. Zig-zag lines correspond to region where the recombination point is unknown.

from B6 mice. An identical pattern is found in the two other recombinant strains which also have the Qa-Tla region derived from A mice (i.e. B10.A and B10.A(2R)). The two bands characteristic of B6 and B10 (1.6 and 0.9 kb) mice is observed for the A.Tla^b recombinant mice which have the Qa-Tla region from B6 mice and the K and D regions from A mice, as well as for B10.A(2R) which has the B10 mouse Qa-Tla region. These result imply that the 37 gene is located in the Qa-Tla region telomeric to the D region. As in the H-2^d haplotype, the D and Qa regions have been physically linked by chromosome walking (Stephan et al., 1986) without finding the 37 gene, so we can conclude that the 37 gene is in the Tla region rather than in the Qa region, like its counterpart $T10^c$ or $T11^b$ genes. In collaboration with Drs. S. Hunt and L. Hood, we have recently cloned the 37 gene, sequenced it and precisely mapped it adjacent to the $T17^c$ gene (Transy et al., 1987). This proves that it is indeed within the Tla region. Its precise localisation on the H-2 complex map is still unknown because even on the BALB/c MHC molecular map there are still some gaps between both the Qa and Tla region genes and within the Tla region genes.

Interestingly, the one band found with DNA's from B10.M and SJL/J mice is not restricted to laboratory mice. DNAs of other rodents like the wild mice Mus m. molossinus and Mus spretus and the Fisher rat strain present the same pattern (data not shown). After PvuII digestion, the fragment which is found in Mus m. molossinus and Mus spretus, is 2.1 kb long (as for A mice), whilst in the Fisher rat strain the fragment is 4 kb long. The two band profile which we know correspond to two different genes may have arisen by duplication of a unique ancestral gene.

b) Structure of gene 37 - The 37 gene was cloned from a lambda phage DNA library of BALB/c genomic DNA (Transy et al., 1987). Its sequence presents the same overall exon/intron organization as that of the other H-2 class I genes. The gene is divided in 7 exons, each exon coding for a putative protein domain. It contains a repetitive sequence of the B2 type which represents all 3' non coding regions. It may be recalled that the D, L and Q7 genes also contain B2 sequences in either the 3' untranslated region (D and L) or in the third intron (Q7).

This gene has no conventional TATA box and lacks upstream regulatory sequences identical to those found in the $H\text{-}2K^b$ gene (Kimura et al., 1986 ; Israël et al., 1986), although it has a CAAT box at the same position.

We have earlier discussed hypotheses according to which CpG's might play a role in the initiation of conversion events either in the donor or in the recipient gene (Jaulin et al., 1985 ; Kourilsky, 1986). It is striking to note that, along the 37 gene, the frequence of CpGs dinucleotides shows the same distribution as for the other H-2 class I genes previously analyzed (K, D, L, Q10, Q7), i.e. an under representation of CpG both in the 5' end of the gene and from the beginning of the third intron to the 3' end of the gene. This bias is not yet understood.

c) Expression at the mRNA level - The RNA probe corresponding to the second domain of the 37 cDNA (exon 3) and of the $T10^b$ and $T11^c$ genes, was used in an RNase mapping assay to study the expression of the respective genes. The results (Transy et al., 1987) show that the 37 mRNA is at least 10 times more expressed than the corresponding $T10^b$ and $T11^c$ mRNAs. A large variety of tissues (liver, kidney, thymus, spleen, heart, brain) and cell types (fibroblasts, thymomas, hepatoma) express the 37 mRNA. In A mice, the protected RNA-RNA hybrid size corresponds to $T10^b$ (or $T11^c$) mRNA. The level of expression of the 37 mRNA was compared to the level of expression of H-2 mRNA's in the liver and the spleen of mice of different haplotypes. The results show that in B10 or BALB/c mice, this level is quite high (1/4 th of all class I mRNA's) whereas in C3H mice the level is much lower. This could reflect mutations or rearrangements in the promotor region of the gene in C3H mice.

d) The 37 protein - In an attempt to identify the protein encoded by the 37 mRNA, we have engineered the full length cDNA into an SP6 driven transcription vector. The linearized vector was used in vitro to synthetise a capped 37 mRNA. The in vitro translation of this mRNA is shown in figure 5. A band corresponding to a protein of 40 kDa is clearly present in lane 2, the size of which is in good agreement with the expected size of the

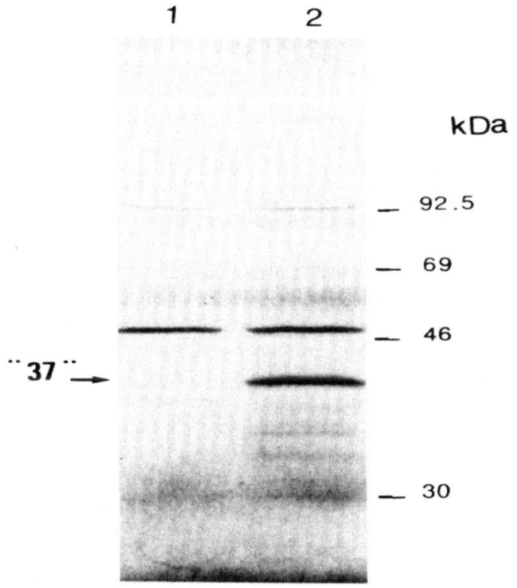

Fig. 5 : Cell free translation of in vitro synthetized 37 mRNA. SP6 transcripts of linearized plasmid psp37Δ9 containing the full length 37 cDNA were synthetized and capped according to Krieg and Melton (1984). After purification the RNA was translated in a rabbit reticulocyte lysate system with ^{35}S-methionine for 1 hr. The translated products were fractionated on a 10 % SDS-polyacrylamide gel.
Lane 1 : without mRNA ; lane 2 : with 100 ng of in vitro synthetized 37 mRNA. On the right side of the figure, molecular weight of protein standards are indicated.

primary product. The exact size and localization of the mature protein in vivo is however still unknown. Antibodies are being prepared to answer these questions.

3) Transcription of the K^d, 37 and Q10 genes in mouse embryos

The Q10 gene encodes at least one polypeptide with an altered COOH terminus, thus lacking the conventional intracytoplasmic domain and canonical membrane spanning region found in most class I molecules. This polypeptide has been detected as a soluble protein in the serum of most mouse strains (Kress et al., 1983), although not in that of the H-2^f haplotype (Lew et al., 1986b). Two mRNAs transcribed from the Q10 gene have been detected. They are produced by alternative splicing, one of them lacking the third exon, which encodes the second domain of class I molecules (Lalanne et al., 1985). During embryonic life, Q10 mRNA has also been detected in various amounts from day 12 to day 18 in the liver (where it increases) or in the visceral yolk sac (where it decreases) in the outbred CD1 mouse strain (Stein et al., 1986). We have independently made the same observation in a genetically better defined strain, namely DBA/2 (H-2^d), where we have studied the transcription of the K^d, 37 and Q10 genes during fetal life from day 12 on of embryogenesis.

RNA was extracted from fetal livers taken on days 12, 13, 14 and 18 of gestation, together with livers of 6 weeks old DBA/2 mice. RNAse mapping experiments with appropriate probes showed that both Q10 transcripts are detectable from day 12. Their level is then approximately 50 times lower than in adult liver, but subsequently this level increases 5 to 10 fold by day 18. Similarly, both the normal and 5' alternative transcripts of the K^d gene gradually increased in quantity over the same 12 to 18 day period, as do those of the 37 transcript. Interestingly, however, differences were found in fetal heart and placenta. K^d and 37 are both expressed after day 14 in these organs while Q10 is not. Q10 is however detectable on days 12 and 13 in these tissues. These and other data showing transcription of Q10 in fetal heart and adult kidney suggest that the expression of Q10 is probably not strictly associated with endodermal cells or tissues of endodermal origin. In addition, the time course of the expression of Q10 mRNA in embryonic organs as well as its tissue distribution might correlate with various stages of haematopoiesis in the developing embryo (David-Watine et al., submitted). This might be indicative of a role of the Q10 protein in embryonic haematopoiesis.

DISCUSSION

The above examples illustrate the increasing diversity of class I gene products and some of the complexities of their temporal expression.

1) The 24 protein, produced by an alternative spliced transcript of the K^d gene has been identified using an anti-peptide antiserum. In agreement with our previous data, which failed to detect it on the cell surface (Cochet et al., 1986), it is found within the cell. This rules out that the 24 protein corresponds to any of the identified K locus products, namely K' from Tryphonas et al. (1983), and $K1^d$ from Demant and Ivânyi (1981), which have been shown to be membrane-bound. We do not however know the precise localisation of the 24 protein in the cell except that it goes through the endoplasmic reticulum. An insertion of 20 AA of the intron followed by a deletion of 30 AA of the alpha-1 domain therefore changes completely the routing of the protein. Hedley et al. (this book) has introduced a mutation into the splicing acceptor site of the first intron of the K^d gene. This forces the use of the cryptic acceptor site located in the intron which serves partly to produce the 24 mRNA. The corresponding protein is now found at the cell surface. Therefore, it seems likely that the deletion of the 30 residues of K^d (position 6 to 37) in protein 24 is responsible for its intracellular localisation.

2) The "37" gene is peculiar in that it is "ubiquitously" transcribed like a gene coding for a major transplantation antigen, such as K^d, both in the adult and during embryonic development. The gene itself lies in the Tla region but displays more homologies with the H-2 and Qa region genes than with $T13^c$ (Transy et al., 1987). Like the D^d gene (Sher et al., 1985), the L^d gene (Moore et al., 1982) and the Q7 gene (Steinmetz et al., 1981), it contains a B2 sequence in the 3' non coding region. Several reports have shown that upon viral transformation, the expression of the B2 containing genes are stimulated (Brickell et al., 1983, 1985 ; Kress et al., 1984), contrary to K genes which do not contain any repetitive sequences.

In other respects, the regulation of expression of the 37 mRNA mimics classical class I gene expression (K, D, L). As we have already mentioned, the 37 mRNA is present in all tissues and cell lines analysed so far except teratocarcinoma cell lines such as PCC3 and F9. As for the K, D and L genes, the expression of the 37 gene is repressed in Adenovirus 12 transformed baby mouse kidney cells and stimulated in the presence of murine interferon (alpha + beta) (not shown). In this context, it is interesting that sequences 5' of the 37 gene display almost no detectable homology with those found 5' of the K, D and L genes, where important regulatory elements, including an interferon response sequence, have been shown to lie (Kimura et al., 1986 ; Miyazaki et al., 1986 ; Israël et al., 1987). The 37 gene is devoid of a conventional TATA box, like other Tla genes that have been cloned and sequenced (Fisher et al., 1985 ; Pontarotti et al., 1986).

The protein product of gene 37 has never been identified. A first step towards its identification is its in vitro synthesis, as shown here. The in vitro product is currently being used to test antibodies and obtain specific serological reagents.

3) Transcriptional studies during embryonic development have brought several pieces of information. First, they suggest, both for the K^d and the Q10 genes, that the processes of alternative splicing which operate in these two genes are not developmentally regulated -at least in the cells and tissues looked at. They also show that the regulation of expression of the Q10 gene is far more complicated than had been anticipated. Q10 is not solely expressed in adult liver and in the embryonic visceral yolk sac, but is also found in other fetal organs and in the adult kidney, and obeys a complex scheme of temporal expression.

Indeed, the most intriguing questions regarding these class I molecules relate to their biological functions.

1) What could be the function of the 24 protein ? It is encoded by an RNA which represents about 5 to 10 % of that coding for K^d in all the situations studied and represents, therefore, a minor cellular component. We suggest that it could be an accessory molecule which associates to other proteins and addresses them to different cellular compartments. Such associations have been shown between the E3/19K glycoprotein of Adenovirus 12 and the human classical class I antigens (Burgert and Kvist, 1985 ; Pääbo et al., 1986), between the invariant chain and class II antigens (Strubin et al., 1986) and between the BIP protein and immunoglobulin light chains (Haas and Wabl, 1983 ; Munro and Pelham, 1986). Nevertheless, we cannot rule out for the moment that the 24 protein has no biological function and that its existence is a consequence of a dysfunction in the splicing machinery of the cell.

2) The 37 product identified in vitro, but not yet in vivo, is likely to be a cell surface molecule. Like the major transplantation antigens, it could be involved in antigen presentation to cytotoxic T lymphocytes. One could argue that, if this is the case, it would create an exception to the rule of MHC restriction, but such exceptions have been reported (see in Transy et al., 1987). Alternatively, the 37 protein could participate in cellular interactions. Its partner could then be a non-polymorphic cell surface molecule, such as Lyt-2, which is known to play an important role in the interaction between cytotoxic T cells and their targets (Yakayama et al., 1979).

3) The function of the Q10 product(s) is, at present, as mysterious as that of the 24 and 37 proteins. It has been proposed that it is involved in self-tolerance (Cosman et al., 1982) or maternal tolerance to the fetus (Stein et al., 1986). We would like to suggest an additional or alternative hypothesis : we propose that Q10 expression is somehow associated with the differentiation of embryonic haematopoeitic stem cells, acting either as a growth factor, or as a mediator in cell-cell interactions.

One difficulty in understanding the function of class I molecules lies in the fact that many rearrangements have occurred in the H-2 multigene family as it is found in distinct haplotypes. For example, a large number of Qa genes are deleted in certain strains, and the Q10 gene seems not to be expressed in H-2^f mice (Lew et al., 1986). One is then faced with two possibilities : either the products of the deleted genes are not essential, or alternative genes can fulfil their function. Nevertheless, the on-going exploration of the expanding set of class I molecules raises the question of their participation in non immune phenomena. The findings that the 37 gene is transcribed in placenta and brain (alike several other immunological proteins) (Barclay et al., 1987) and that the Q10 gene is expressed in early embryonic stages suggests that this may be the case.

ACKNOWLEDGEMENTS

We are very grateful to our colleagues in the laboratory for helpful discussions and advices, particularly to J. Kanellopoulos and F. Rosa for handling immunoprecipitations, C. Jaulin for CpG's analysis, A. Casrouge for expert technical assisance and V. Caput for skilfull typing of the manuscript. We also thank G. Hämmerling for gift of K9-18 monoclonal antibody, P. Avner and M. Kieran for critical reading of the manuscript. B.D.-W. was recipient of a Ministère de la Recherche et de l'Industrie fellowship.

REFERENCES

Archibald, A.L., Thompson, N.A., and Kvist, S., 1986, A single nucleotide difference at the 3' end of an intron causes differential splicing of two histocompatibility genes, EMBO J, 5 : 957.

Arnold, B., Horstmann, U., Kuon, B., Burgert, H.G., Hämmerling, G.J., and Kvist, S., 1985, Alloreactive cytolytic T-cell clones preferentially recognize conformational determinants on histocompatibility antigens : analysis with genetically engineered hybrid antigens, Proc. Natl. Acad. Sci., USA, 82 : 7030.

Barclay, A.N., Johnson, P., McCaughan, G.W., and Williams, A.F., 1987, Immunoglobulin-related structures associated with vertebrates cell surfaces, in : "Ann. Rev. Immunol.", T. Mak, Ed., in press.

Brickell, P.M., Latchman, D.S., Murphy, D., Willison, K., and Rigby, P.W.J., 1983, Activation of a Qa/Tla class I major histocompatibility antigen gene is a general feature of oncogenesis in the mouse, Nature, 306 : 756.

Brickell, P.M., Latchman, D.S., Murphy, D., Willison, K., and Rigby, P.W.J., 1985, The class I major histocompatibility antigen gene activated in a line of SV40-transformed mouse cells in H-$2D^d$, not Qa/Tla, Nature, 316 : 162.

Burgert, H.-G., and Kvist, S., 1985, An adenovirus type 2 glycoprotein block cell surface expression of human histocompatibility class I antigens, Cell, 41 : 987.

Cami, B., Brégégère, F., Abastado, J.-P., and Kourilsky, P., 1981, Multiple sequences related to classical histocompatibility antigens in the mouse genome, Nature, 291 : 673.

Cochet, M., Kast, W.M., Kummer, A.-M., Transy, C., Melief, C.J.M., and Kourilsky, P., 1986, Alternative splicing in the mouse H-$2K^d$ gene is not necessary for the classical K^d antigen function, Immunogenetics, 24 : 267.

Cosman, D., Kress, M., Khoury, G., and Jay, G., 1982, Tissue specific expression of an unusual H-2 class I related gene, Proc. Natl. Acad. Sci., USA, 79 : 4947.

Démant, P., and Ivànyi, D., 1981, Further molecular complexities of H-2K- and D-regions antigens, Nature, 290 : 146.
Fisher, D.A., Hunt, S.W., III, and Hood, L.E., 1985, Structure of a gene encoding a murine thymus leukemia antigen and organization of Tla genes in the BALB/c mouse, J. Exp. Med., 162 : 528.
Haas, I.G., and Wabl, M., 1983, Immunoglobulin heavy chain binding protein, Nature, 306 : 387.
Hansen, T.H., Ozato, K., and Sachs, D., 1983, Heterogeneity of H-2D region associated genes and gene products, Adv. Immunol., 34 : 39.
Israël, A., Kimura, A., Fournier, A., Fellous, M., and Kourilsky, P., 1986; Interferon response sequence potentiates activity of an enhancer in the promotor region of a mouse H-2 gene, Nature, 322 : 743.
Israël, A., Kimura, A., Kieran, M., Yano, O., Kanellopoulos, J., Le Bail, O., and Kourilsky, P., 1987, A common positive trans-acting factor binds to enhancer-sequences in the promotors of mouse H-2 and beta-2-microglobulin genes, Proc. Natl. Acad. Sci., USA, 84 : 2653.
Jaulin, C., Perrin, A., Abastado, J.-P., Dumas, B., Papamatheakis, J., and Kourilsky, P., 1985, Polymorphism in mouse and human class I H-2 and HLA genes is not the result of random independent point mutations, Immunogenetics, 22 : 453.
Kimura, A., Israël, A., Le Bail, O., and Kourilsky, P., 1986, Detailed analysis of the mouse H-$2K^b$ promoter : enhancer-like sequences and their role in the regulation of class I gene expression, Cell, 44 : 261.
Kourilsky, P., 1986, Molecular mechanisms for gene conversion in higher cells, Tr. Gen., 2 : 60.
Kourilsky, P., Chaouat, G., Rabourdin-Combe, C., and Claverie, J.-M., 1987, Working principles in the immune system implied by the "peptidic self" model, Proc. Natl. Acad. Sci., USA, 84 : 3400.
Kress, M., Glaros, D., Khoury, G., and Jay, G., 1983a, Alternative RNA splicing in expression of the H-2K gene, Nature, 306 : 602.
Kress, M., Cosman, D., Khoury, G., and Jay, G., 1983b, Secretion of a transplantation-related antigen, Cell, 34 : 186.
Kress, M., Barra, Y., Seidman, J.G., Khoury, G., and Jay, G., 1984, Functional insertion of an alu type 2 (B2 SINE) repetitive sequence in murine class I genes, Science, 226 : 974.
Krieg, P.A., and Melton, D.A., 1984, Functional messenger RNAs are produced by SP6 in vitro transcription of cloned cDNAs, Nucl. Acids Res., 12 : 7057.
Kvist, S., Brégégère, F., Rask, L., Cami, B., Garoff, H., Daniel, F., Wiman, K., Larhamar, D., Abastado, J.P., Gachelin, G., Peterson, P.A., Dobberstein, B., and Kourilsky, P., 1981, A cDNA clone coding for part of a mouse H-2^d major histocompatibility antigen, Proc. Natl. Acad. Sci., USA, 78 : 2772.
Lalanne, J.L., Cochet, M., Kummer, A.M., Gachelin, G. and Kourilsky, P., 1983a, Different exon-intron organization at the 5' part of a mouse class I gene is used to generate a novel H-$2K^b$-related mRNA, Proc. Natl. Acad. Sci., USA, 80 : 7561.
Lalanne, J.L., Delarbre, C., Gachelin, G., and Kourilsky, P., 1983b, A cDNA clone containing the entire coding sequence of a mouse H-$2K^d$ histocompatibility antigen, Nucl. Acids Res., 11 : 1567.
Lalanne, J.L., Transy, C., Guérin, S., Darche, S., Meulien, P., and Kourilsky, P., 1985, Expression of class I genes in the major histocompatibility complex : identification of eight distinct mRNAs in DBA/2 mouse liver, Cell, 41 : 469.
Lew, A.M., Margulies, D.H., Maloy, W.L., Lillehoj, E.P., McCluskey, J., Coligan, J.E., 1986a, Alternative protein products with different carboxyl termini from a single class I gene H-$2K^b$, Proc. Natl. Acad. Sci., USA, 83 : 6084.

Lew, A.M., Maloy, W.L., and Coligan, J.E., 1986b, Characteristics of the expression of the murine soluble class I molecule (Q10), J. Immunol., 136 : 254.
Miyazaki, J.-I., Appella, E., and Ozato, K., 1986, Negative regulation of the major histocompatibility class I gene in undifferentiated embryonal carcinoma cells, Proc. Natl. Acad. Sci., USA, 83 : 9537.
Momburg, F., Koch, N., Möller, P., Moldenhauer, G., and Hämmerling, G.J., 1986, In vivo induction of H-2K/D antigens by recombinant interferon-gamma, Eur. J. Immunol., 16 : 551.
Moore, K.W., Sher, B.T., Sun, Y.H., Eakle, K.A., and Hood, L.E., 1982, DNA sequence of a gene encoding a BALB/c mouse L^d transplantation antigen, Science, 215 : 679.
Munro, S., and Pelham, H.R.B., 1986, An Hsp-70 like protein in the ER : identity with the 78 kd glucose regulated protein and immunoglobulin heavy chain binding protein, Cell, 46 : 291.
Ozato, K., Mayer, N.M., and Sachs, D.H., 1982, Monoclonal antibodies to mouse major histocompatibility complex antigens. IV A series of hybridoma clones producing anti-H-2^d antibodies and an estimation of expression of H-2^d antigens on the surface of these cells, Transplantation, 34 : 113.
Pääbo, S., Nilson, T., and Peterson, P.A., 1986, Adnovirus of subgeneria B, C, D and E modulate cell-surface expression of major histocompatibility complex class I antigens, Proc. Natl. Acad. Sci., USA, 83 : 9665.
Ploegh, H.L., Orr, H.T., and Strominger, J.L., 1980, Molecular cloning of a human histocompatibility antigen cDNA fragment, Proc. Natl. Acad. Sci., USA, 77 : 6081.
Pontarotti, P.A., Mashino, H., Zeff, R.A., Fisher, D.A., Hood, L., Mellor, A., Flavell, R.A., and Nathenson, S.G., 1986, Conservation and diversity in the class I genes of the major histocompatibility complex : sequence analysis of a Tla^b gene and comparison with a Tla^c gene, Proc. Natl. Acad. Sci., USA, 83 : 1782.
Reyes, A.A., Schöld, M., Itakura, K., and Wallace, B., 1982a, Isolation of a cDNA clone for the murine transplantation antigen H-$2K^b$, Proc. Natl. Acad. Sci., USA, 79 : 3270.
Reyes, A.A., Schöld, M., and Wallace, R.B., 1982b, The complete amino acid sequence of the murine transplantation antigen H-$2D^d$ as deduced by molecular cloning, Immunogenetics, 16 : 1.
Rodgers, M.J., Siwarski, D.F., Shacter, E., Maloy, W.L., Lillehoj, E.P., and Coligan, J.E., 1986, Three distinct H-$2K^s$ molecules differing at the carboxy terminus are expressed on a tumor from SJL/J mice, J. Immunol., 137 : 3006.
Sher, B.T., Nairn, R., Coligan, J.E., and Hood, L.E., 1985, DNA sequence of the mouse H-$2D^d$ transplantation antigen gene. Proc. Natl. Acad. Sci., USA, 82 : 1175.
Sood, A.K., Pereira, D., and Weissman, S.M., 1981, Isolation and partial nucleotide sequence of a cDNA clone for human histocompatibility antigen HLA-B by use of an oligodeoxynucleotide primer, Proc. Natl. Acad. Sci., USA, 78 : 616.
Stein, P., Barra, Y., Jay, G., and Strickland, S., 1986, Expression of a secreted transplantation antigen during murine embryogenesis, Mol. Cell. Biol., 6 : 3397.
Steinmetz, M., Frelinger, J.G., Fisher, G., Hunkapiller, T., Pereira, D., Weissman, S.M., Uehara, H., Nathenson, S., and Hood, L., 1981a, Three cDNA clones encoding mouse transplantation antigens : homology to immunoglobulin genes, Cell, 24 : 125.
Steinmetz, M., Moore, K.W., Frelinger, J.G., Sher, B.T., Shen, F.W., Boyse, E.A., and Hood, L., 1981b, A pseudogene homologous to mouse transplantation antigens : transplantation antigens are encoded by eight exons that correlate with protein domain, Cell, 25, 683.

Steinmetz, M., Moore, K.W., Frelinger, J.G., Sher, B.T., Shen, F.W., Boyse, E.A., and Hood, L., 1981b, A pseudogene homologous to mouse transplantation antigens : transplantation antigens are encoded by eight exons that correlate with protein domain, Cell, 25, 683.

Steinmetz, M., Winoto, A., Minard, K., and Hood, L.E., 1982, Clusters of genes encoding transplantation antigens, Cell, 28 : 489.

Stephan, D., Sun, H., Fisherlindahl, K., Meyer, E., Hämmerling, G., Hood, L., and Steinmetz, M., 1986, Organization and evolution of D region class I genes in the mouse major histocompatibility complex, J. Exp. Med., 163 : 1227.

Strubin, M., Long, E.O., and Mach, B., 1986, Two forms of the Ia antigens associated invariant chain result from alternative initiations at two in-phase AUGs, Cell, 47 : 619.

Transy, C., Lalanne, J.L., and Kourilsky, P., 1984, Alternative splicing in the 5' moiety of the H-2K^d gene transcript, EMBO J., 3 : 2383.

Transy, C., Nash, R.S., David-Watine, B., Cochet, M., Hunt, S.W., III, Hood, L.E., and Kourilsky, P., 1987, A low polymorphic mouse H-2 class I gene from the Tla complex is expressed in a broad variety of cell types, J. Exp. Med., 166 : 341.

Tryphonas, M., King, D.P., and Jones, P.P., 1983, Identification of a second class I antigen controlled by the K end of the H-2 complex and its selective cellular expression, Proc. Natl. Acad. Sci., USA, 80 : 1445.

Waneck, G.L., Sherman, D.H., Calvin, S., Allen, H., and Flavell, R.A., 1987, Tissue-specific expression of cell-surface Qa-2 antigen from a transfected Q7^b gene of C57Bl/10 mice, J. Exp. Med., 165 : 1358.

Weiss, E.M., Golden, L., Fahrner, K., Mellor, A.L., Devling, J.J., Bullman, H., Tiddens, H., Bud, H., and Flavell, R.A., 1984, Organization and evolution of class I gene family in the major histocompatibility complex of the C57Bl/10 mouse, Nature, 310 : 650.

Yakoyama, E., Shiku, H., Stockert, E., Oettgen, H.F., and Old, L.J., 1979, Cytotoxic T cells : Lyt phenotype and blocking of killing activity by Lyt antisera, Proc. Natl. Acad. Sci., USA, 76 : 1977.

Zinkernagel, R.M., and Doherty, P.C., 1979, MHC-restricted cytotoxic T cells : studies on the biological role of polymorphic major transplantation antigens determining T-cell restriction specificity, function, and responsiveness, Adv. Immunol., 27 : 52.

BIOCHEMICAL AND MOLECULAR CHARACTERIZATION OF Q-REGION CLASS I GENE PRODUCTS

Mark J. Soloski*, Gregory P. Einhorn*, Leroy Hood° and Iwona Stroynowski°

*Subdepartment of Immunology, Department of Molecular Biology and Genetics, Johns Hopkins School of Medicine Baltimore, Maryland 21205 and The Division of Biology, California Institute of Technology, Pasadena, Cal

INTRODUCTION

Telomeric to the H2D region is a chromosomal segment which encodes several serologically and/or biochemically defined class I molecules (1). These include the cell surface molecules Qa1, Qa2 and TL and the soluble proteins Qb1 and Q10 (2-4). Although related to H2-K, -D, -L molecules by subunit structure and primary sequence, the Qa/TL molecules are biologically distinct. For example, Qa/TL molecules display distinct tissue specific regulated expression, are relatively nonpolymorphic (conserved ?) and appear not to be utilized as restricting elements in T cell recognition. Although their class I counterparts H2-K, -D and -L have well defined roles in tissue/organ transplantation and T cell recognition of foreign antigens, the function(s) of the Qa/TL class I proteins remains obscure.

Studies on the genetic organization of the H2 complex has revealed that the Qa/TL region can contain up to 30 distinct class I genes (5,6). Structural analysis of several of these genes have shown them to be capable of encoding distinct protein products (2, 7, 8). Thus, in addition to Qa1, Qa2, TL, Qb1 and Q10 there is at least a genetic potential for additional class I polypeptides. In order to extend our understanding of the biology of the mammalian MHC, a study of the structure, expression and function of the Qa/TL region class I molecules is requisite. We have utilized gene transfection studies employing whole and exon-shuffled Q-region genes, in an effort to understand the relationship between the protein products of isolated Q-region genes and the serologically/biochemically defined Qa2 subregion polypeptides. These studies have revealed that the Q7 gene derived from Balb/c and C57BL/10 mice encodes a protein product that is biochemically and serologically identical to the lymphocyte Qa2 polypeptide. In addition, we will summarize some new information regarding the biochemical characterization of the Qa2 molecule expressed on the surface of T lymphocytes.

THE Q7 GENE ENCODES A 40K CELL SURFACE Qa2 MOLECULE

Previous studies from several laboratories have established that the Q-region genes from either the Balb/c ($H2^d$) or the C57BL/10 ($H2^b$) mouse do not express cell surface products reactive with Qa2 antibodies when transfected into L cell fibroblasts (7,9,10). Since the expression of the Qa2 antigen is tissue specific, we reasoned that cell lines derived from $Qa2^+$ tissue may be useful in Q-region gene transfection studies. Previous studies have determined that the Qa2 antigen is expressed in whole liver extracts (1). Therefore, we utilized a hepatoma cell line (Hepa-1) that was derived from a transplantable liver tumor of C57/J mice ($H2^b$ haplotype)(11). Initial studies revealed that the cell line expressed $H\text{-}2D^b$ but was negative for $H\text{-}2K^b$ and Qa2 proteins. Plasmid and cosmid clones containing Balb/c Qa2 region genes $Q1^d$-$Q10^d$ were transfected into Hepa-1 cells using the pSV 2-neo plasmid as a selectable marker. Only plasmids or cosmids containing the $Q7^d$ gene tested positive in these transfection studies employing a radioimmunoassay (RIA) with a specific Qa2 reactive monoclonal antibody 20-8-4, (anti-$H2K^b$, Qa2, ref 11). Parallel experiments were carried out with the $Q7^b$ gene, the allelic counterpart of the $Q7^d$ gene from C57BL/10 mice ($H2^b$)(8). Clones expressing high levels of $Q7^d$ and $Q7^b$ proteins were selected and utilized for subsequent biochemical and serological studies. Several criteria were used to evaluate the similarity between the Q7 products and the Qa2 antigens. First, the reactivity with a variety of anti-Qa2 subregion specific serological reagents was evaluated by both flow cytometry and immunoprecipitation. Secondly, the Q7 protein products on the liver transfectants as well as Qa2 molecules on lymphoid cells were compared using both one and two-dimensional gel electrophoresis. These studies demonstrated that the Q7 gene encodes a 40,000 mw cell surface polypeptide that is biochemically and serologically indistinguishable from the Qa2 protein expressed on the surface of lymphoid cells. Analysis utilizing an RIA, flow cytometry and immunoprecipitation data demonstrated that both the $Q7^b$ and the $Q7^d$ polypeptides were recognized by a battery of serological reagents that detect Qa2 subregion controlled determinants. These reagents include conventional anti-Qa2 serum (B6.K1 anti B6), monoclonal antibodies D3262, Qam2, Qam7, Qam8, Qam9, Y7, 34-1-2, and 20-8-4 (see Table I, ref 12,13). Biochemical analysis by both one- and two-dimensional gel electrophoresis demonstrated that the $Q7^b$ and $Q7^d$ polypeptides were identical by these criteria.

Further analysis of the reactivity of the serological reagents to $Q7^d$ as well as hybrid $Q7^d/L^d$ and $L^d/Q7^d$ gene products led us to conclude that the Q7 molecule expresses at least two spacially separate sets of determinants which are recognized by these antibodies (see Table I). One set of determinants is localized in the α_1 and/or α_2 regions (20-8-4, 34-1-2, and Y7) while the other set of determinants is dependent upon the presence of the α_3 region (Qam2, Qam7, Qam8 and D3262). It should be noted that several of the α_3 dependent reactivities were detected weekly or not at all on the $L^d/Q7^d$ hybrid molecules which suggests that these determinants require the presence of both α_1/α_2 and α_3 domains.

In summary, the above studies demonstrate that the Q7 gene encodes a 40,000 mw polypeptide that is expressed on the surface of hepatoma cells. The Q7 derived polypeptide is identical by both serological and biochemical criteria to the classically defined Qa2 polypeptide expressed on the surface of lymphoid cells.

TABLE I

Serological Characterization of Whole and Hybrid Q7 Molecules Expressed on Hepatoma Cells

	Transfected Gene			
Serological Reagent	$Q7^d$	$Q7^b$	$Q7^d$/Ld	$L^d/Q7^d$
Anti Qa2 serum	+	+	+	+
20-8-4	+	+	+	-
34-1-2	+	+	+	-
Y7	+	+	+	-
D3262	+	+	-	+/-
Qam2	+	+	-	+/-
Qam7	+	+	-	-
Qam8	+	+	-	-
Qam9	+	+	N.D.	N.D.

Reactivities were tested using flow cytometry, radioimmunoassay and immunoprecipitation. Designations: + = positive, - = negative, +/- = weak (clearly above negative). The negative control was untransfected Hepa-1 cells. Hybrid genes were constructed by exon shuffling 5' and 3'gene segments from $Q7^d$ and H2-L^d as described (10). The hybrid $Q7^d/L^d$ protein contains the leader, α-1, α-2 domains of $Q7^d$ and the α-3, transmembrane and cytoplasmic domains from H2-L^d. The $L^d/Q7^d$ molecule's leader, α-1, α-2 domains are derived from H2L^d while the α-3, transmembrane and cytoplasmic domains are derived from $Q7^d$.

Secretion of the Q7 polypeptide

Previous studies have demonstrated that activated T cells synthesize and express a secreted form of the Qa2 polypeptide (14,15). Based on these results, we wished to determine whether the Q7 gene likewise encoded a soluble secreted form of the Q7 polypeptide and whether this polypeptide was similar to the Qa2 polypeptide secreted from lymphoid cells. Hepatoma cells transfected with the Q7 gene were metabolically radiolabeled with ^{35}S-methionine and both cell lysates and cell free media were immunoprecipitated with anti-Qa2 reagents and analyzed by two-dimensional gels. Interestingly, both the $Q7^b$ and $Q7^d$ genes synthesized a soluble polypeptide which was indistinguishable by two-dimensional gel electrophoresis from the secreted soluble polypeptide synthesized by activated T cells. Further analysis of the $Q7^d/L^d$ and $L^d/Q7^d$ transfectants revealed that only the $L^d/Q7^d$ encoded a soluble secreted polypeptide.

Mouse L cells transfected with the Q7 gene fail to

express the Q7 polypeptide on the cell surface (7,9,10). Based on the observation that the Q7 polypeptide, as well as the Qa2 polypeptide, can be synthesized and expressed as a secreted soluble molecule, we evaluated whether Q7 gene transfected L cells encodes a secreted soluble polypeptide. L cells transfected with either $Q7^b$, $Q7^d$, $Q7^d/L^d$ or $L^d/Q7^d$ were metabolically radiolabeled with ^{35}S-methionine and both cell lysates and cell free media immunoprecipitated with anti-Qa2 serum and analyzed by two-dimensional gel electrophoresis. The results of this analysis is summarized in table II. Both the $Q7^b$ and $Q7^d$ genes, when expressed in L cells, encode a secreted soluble polypeptide of approximately 39,000 mw which is indistinguishable from the 39,000 mw Qa2 polypeptide synthesized and released from activated T cells. The hybrid gene $Q7^d/L^d$ synthesized and expressed only a cell associated polypeptide while the $L^d/Q7^d$ hybrid gene synthesized a secreted soluble polypeptide. The hybrid $L^d/Q7^d$ secreted molecule had a molecular weight of approximately 44,000 versus 39,000 mw for $Q7^d$. This difference is likely to be caused by the glycosylation of an additional site in the α_2 region which is predicted from the DNA sequence of the L^d gene, but is absent from the Q7 gene (16).

TABLE II. Summary of Q7 Transfection Studies

L Cell Fibroblasts

Gene	Cytoplasmic Polypeptide	Cell Surface Expression	Secreted Molecule
$Q7^b$	+	−	+
$Q7^d$	+	−	+
$L^d/Q7^d$	+	−	+
$Q7^d/L^d$	+	+	−

Hepa-1 Liver Cells

Gene	Cytoplasmic Polypeptide	Cell Surface Expression	Secreted Molecule	Lipase Sensitive
$Q7^b$	+	+	+	+
$Q7^d$	+	+	+	+
$L^d/Q7^d$	+	+	+	+
$Q7^d/L^d$	+	+	−	−

In summary, the Q7 gene when transfected into liver hepatoma cells encodes both a cell surface and a secreted polypeptide. The secreted polypeptide is biochemically and serologically indistinguishable from the secreted Qa2 polypeptide synthesized by activated T cells. Transfection of the Q7 gene into mouse L cells directs only the synthesis of the secreted soluble polypeptide. Analysis of exon shuffled genes reveals that the secretion and the membrane display of the Q7 polypeptides are genetically controlled by the sequence information located 3' to the third exon of the Q7 gene (see Table II and Figure 1).

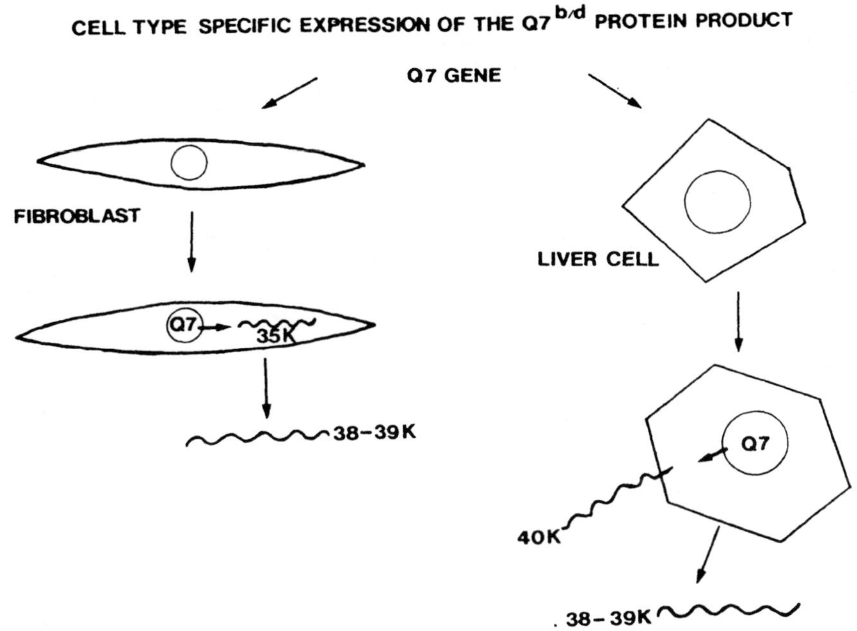

Figure 1. Tissue Specific Expression of Q7 Protein Isoforms.

THE CELL SURFACE Q7 POLYPEPTIDE IS ATTACHED TO THE CELL SURFACE BY A LIPASE SENSITIVE SRUCTURE

It has been recently demonstrated that several Qa2 subregion controlled serological determinants can be removed from the cell surface by the action of a purified phosphatidylinositol specific-phospholipase C (17). Several cell surface polypeptides have been shown to be attached to the surface by a phosphatidylinositol bearing anchor (e.g. Thy-1 TAP, DAF) (18-20). Interestingly, soluble forms of both Thy-1 and DAF have been found (19,21,22). Based on these observations, we tested the effects of a a phosphatidylinositol specific phospholipase C purified from S. aureus (PI-PLC) on the expression of the Q7 as well as the hybrid $L^d/Q7^d$ and $Q7^d/L^d$ polypeptides expressed on the surface of Hepa-1 cells. Hepa-1 transfectants were incubated with various concentrations of PI-PLC for two hours. Following incubation, the cells were washed and the expression of Q7 polypeptides was monitored by flow cytometry. The results of this analysis are summarized in table II. Interestingly, both the $Q7^{d/b}$ and the $L^d/Q7^d$ molecules were sensitive to the action of the PI-PLC. The endogenous $H2\text{-}D^b$ as well as the $Q7^d/L^d$ polypeptides were lipase insensitive. Furthermore, biochemical analysis of the lipase released Q7 protein revealed that its molecular weight was indistinguishable from the membrane bound form of the Q7 polypeptide and is associated with β_2-microglobulin.

These results indicate that the Q7 gene encodes a cell surface polypeptide that is attached to the cell membrane via a phospholipase C sensitive anchor. Analysis of exon shuffled genes reveal that the structural information required for lipid anchor attachment is encoded 3' to exon 3 in the Q7 gene.

LYMPHOCYTE Qa2 IS PHOSPHOLIPASE C SENSITIVE

Based on the observation that the Q7 polypeptide is lipase sensitive as well as the reports that Qa2 determinants can be removed by lipase treatment, we opted to re-examine the sensitivity of lymphocyte Qa2 expression to PI-PLC treatment. Treatment of whole spleen cells with PI-PLC removed approximately 90 to 95% of the Qa2 molecules. Since activated T cell populations synthesize and secrete a soluble form of the molecule, we evaluated whether the Qa2 molecules expressed on the surface of ConA activated cells were likewise sensitive to PI-PLC. Surprisingly, under conditions which removed 90 to 95% of the Qa2 molecules on resting spleen cells, approximately 40 to 50% of the activated T cells express PI-PLC resistant Qa2 molecules. It should be noted that under the conditions of these studies, the levels of endogenous $H2K^b$ or $-D^b$ expression is unchanged by lipase treatment. Further study examined the possibility that the lipase resistant Qa2 molecules expressed on activated T cells might represent a specific T cell subpopulation. Utilizing FITC-labeled anti Qa2 antibody and phycoerytherin labeled anti L3T4 or LyT-2 and two-color flow cytometric analysis we observed that $L3T4^+$ activated T cell populations displayed PI-PLC sensitive Qa2 molecules while $LyT-2^+$ activated T cells displayed PI-PLC insensitive Qa2 molecules.

LIPASE RELEASED AND SECRETED Qa2 MOLECULES ARE BIOCHEMICALLY DISTINCT

The soluble secreted Qa2 molecule synthesized by activated T cells may be generated by the release of membrane bound forms by an endogenous lymphocyte phospholipase C. To explore this possibility, we initiated a biochemical comparison of the Qa2 molecules released from the surface of lymphoid cells by PI-PLC and the secreted Qa2 molecule. In these experiments either resting spleenocytes or activated T cells were radiolabeled by lactoperoxidase catalyzed iodination and recultured in the presence of PI-PLC. Following digestion, both medium and cells are harvested and the presence of Qa2 molecules in cell free medium and cell lysates determined by immunoprecipitation. Paralleling the flow cytometric analysis, we observed that while 95% of the spleen cell surface Qa2 molecules were released into the medium following lipase treatment, only 40-50% of the cell surface Qa2 molecules expressed on activated T cells are released into the medium by lipase treatment. Lipase released and cell surface Qa2 molecules displayed apparent identical molecular weights of ≈40,000 kd. In contrast, the secreted Qa2 molecule has a molecular weight of 39,000 and clearly migrates differently in one-dimensional gel analysis from the lipase released Qa2 molecule. Thus, based on this analysis, the PI-PLC released and secreted Qa2 molecules are structurally distinct.

DETECTION OF SOLUBLE Qa2 (Q7) INTRACELLULAR PROTEINS

The finding that lipase released and secreted Qa2 molecules are biochemically distinct suggested that the secreted Qa2 molecule is not derived via simple release of cell surface forms by an endogenous PI-PLC. An alternative mechanism is the synthesis of a soluble intracellular Qa2 molecule which would be a precursor for the secreted Qa2 molecule. To address this possibility, we utilized the nonionic detergent Triton X-114 to detect intracellular membrane bound and/or soluble forms of the Qa2 polypeptide. Since Triton X-114 has two less ethoxy groups, it is soluble at 4°C and insoluble at 25°C (23). In these studies, cells are metabolically radiolabeled, lysed at 4°C with Triton X-114 and cell lysates partitioned into a detergent phase (membrane bound) and an aqueous phase (soluble molecules) after warming extracts to room temperature and centrifugation. The detergent phase is resolubilized at 4°C and the distribution of Qa2 molecules in both phases was monitored by immunoprecipitation and SDS-PAGE. This analysis revealed that the secreted Qa2 molecule partitions entirely into the aqueous phase. In contrast, the cell surface molecule detected by lactoperoxidase catalyzed iodination partitions exclusively into the detergent phase. When cell associated molecules isolated from cell lysates of ^{35}S-methionine labeled cells were analyzed, we observed two membrane bound forms at 38,000 and 40,000 mw. The 40,000 mw species corresponds to the cell surface Qa2 molecule while the 38,000 mw species is an intracellular biosynthetic intermediate. Interestingly, in the aqueous phase, a major species at about 35,000 mw and a minor species of 39,000 mw are found that specifically react with anti-Qa2 reagents. The 39,000 mw species appears identical to the secreted Qa2 molecule while the 35,000 mw molecule is a unique soluble intracellular form. Similar results were obtained when Q7 transfected Hepa-1 cells were analyzed. In brief, these studies have determined that a soluble intracellular 35,000 mw Qa2 polypeptide is synthesized by activated T cells. This observation supports the model that the secreted Qa2 molecule is derived from an intracellular precursor.

DISCUSSION OF RESULTS

In the past several years, numerous serological reagents have been developed which detect antigenic determinants controlled by the Qa2 subregion. Several of these epitopes have been distinguished based on tissue and/or strain distribution (12). Based on these properties, and the detection of multiple Qa2 subregion class I genes, it has been suggested that epitopes may define unique molecular species encoded by distinct class I genes (12). In our analysis, we have demonstrated that the Qa2 region gene, $Q7^b$ and its allelic counterpart $Q7^d$, encodes polypeptides that expresses all of the Qa2 subregion serological determinants defined by eight different serological reagents. Furthermore, the Q7 product expressed on the transfected murine hepatoma cells has been found to be biochemically indistinguishable from the membrane bound lymphoid Qa2 molecule. Thus, the Q7 gene encodes the serologically and biochemically defined Qa2 polypeptide.

However it is quite possible, as suggested by other results, that other class I genes from the Qa2 subregion may encode polypeptides that bear some Qa2 determinants (7). A likely candidate would be the $Q9^b$ gene since it has been shown to share >99% sequence homology with the $Q7^{b/d}$ gene and in L cells encodes a protein product related to the members of the Qa2 polypeptide family (8).

Previous studies have demonstrated that activated T cells synthesize and express both membrane bound as well as soluble Qa2 molecules (14,15). The mechanism by which these two polypeptides had been generated is not known. A possible mechanism was that distinct genes may encode serologically and biochemically related polypeptides, one which is membrane bound, the other which is soluble. However, the studies described above clearly show that a single gene, Q7, can encode both a membrane bound and a secreted soluble polypeptide. Moreover, the secreted soluble polypeptide is structurally and biochemically indistinguishable from the secreted Qa2 polypeptide synthesized by activated T cells. Therefore the generation of both a secreted and membrane bound Qa2 molecules must occur via a transcriptional(splicing) or post-translational pathway. This does not exclude the possibility that other class I genes may encode additional related secreted/soluble Qa polypeptides.

It has been observed that Qa2 determinants can be removed from spleen and lymph node cells by treatment with a phosphatidylinositol-specific phospholipase C (17). The observation that the Q7 protein is likewise sensitive to PI-PLC confirms these observations. Thus the Q7 gene (Qa2 polypeptide) is a new member of a growing family of cell surface proteins which are attached to the cell surface by a inositol bearing membrane anchor (24).

Studies utilizing exon shuffled genes clearly show that the structural information controlling both secretion and lipid anchor attachment is localized 3' to Q7 exon 3. We would propose that the ability of the Q7 gene to direct synthesis of secreted and/or cell surface forms of the Qa2 molecule may be a consequence of transcriptional and post-translational steps dependent upon the 3' information required for phospholipid attachment. Thus the failure to detect cell surface Q7 polypeptides in L cells transfected with the Q7 gene may relate to the failure to attach the glycolipid membrane anchor. The precise mechanism by which a secreted or cell surface form of the Qa2 polypeptide is generated is unclear. Studies on other glycolipid linked proteins have demonstrated that attachment of the phospholipid tail is preceded by cleavage of the normal transmembrane and cytoplasmic domain (24). Since the Q7 gene and a Q7 cDNA both contain a 25 amino acid long transmembrane region as well as a short 3 amino acid long cytoplasmic domain, it is reasonable to suggest that a similar cleavage and attachment step occurs for the Qa2 polypeptide (8,25,26). Failure to attach the glycolipid anchor would then generate a soluble molecule which may be secreted. Thus L cells, and to some extent activated T cells and Hepa-1 cells, may be defective in attachment of the glycolipid anchor to the transmembrane peptide-less Q7 polypeptide chain. Alternative possibilities are that Qa2 secreting cells may have very high concentrations of endogenous PI specific phospholipase C's or other phospholipases capable of degrading the lipid anchor structure. In this regard, the secreted Qa2(Q7) polypeptide (39,000) and the lipase generated soluble Qa2(Q7) polypeptides(40,000) are biochemically distinct, making it unlikely that a secreted polypeptide is simply derived by a PI-PLC cleavage. Alternative possibilities include post-transcriptional generation of a novel mRNA species or additional processing steps following removal of the glycolipid anchor. Further studies utilizing lipid tail specific biosynthetic markers are needed to establish the unique differences between the two pathways (destined for secretion or the cell membrane). In addition, direct chemical analysis of the COOH terminus amino acid sequence of the secreted and the membrane bound Qa2 molecule is necessary to determine whether in fact the cell surface molecules differ from the soluble polypeptides only by a phospholipid tail.

The biological significance of the identification of the Qa2 (Q7) polypeptide as a lipid anchor protein is unclear at present. It is interesting to note that the lymphocyte PI-linked polypeptides Thy-1 and TAP are known to participate in T cell activation pathways (27,28). Perhaps Qa2 molecules may also serve an analogous role in cell signaling. The observations that the Qa2 molecules are nonpolymorphic and are expressed in a tissue specific and regulated fashion are consistent with this possibility.

Flow cytometric, as well as immunoprecipitation studies, have demonstrated that while ~95% of the cell surface Qa2 molecules expressed by resting spleen cells are lipase sensitive, 40-50% of activated T cells express lipase insensitive Qa2 molecules. The activated T cells expressing lipase insensitive Qa2 molecules are LyT-2$^+$ while the lipase sensitive Qa2 molecules are expressed on L3T4$^+$ activated T cells. At present, the structural basis of lipase resistant vs sensitive Qa2 molecules awaits further structural analysis of the glycolipid anchor. The finding that Qa2 molecules may posses different transmembrane anchor structures dependent on LyT-2/L3T4 cell phenotype may suggest a role for Qa2 molecules in T cell subset functions.

In summary, by utilizing the hepatoma cell transfection system, we were to able to clearly identify the Q7 gene as encoding the lymphocyte Qa2 polypeptide. The utilization of this gene transfection system for the identification of the protein products of other Q-region genes is currently in progress and will greatly facilitate our understanding of the organization and function of genes encoded within the Qa2 and perhaps TL subregions. Biochemical characterization of the Qa2 (Q7) polypeptide has revealed unique structural features of the Qa2 molecule and has included it as a member of a new family of cell surface proteins which are attached to the lipid bilayer by a glycolipid anchor process.

Acknowledgements

The work described in this paper was supported by NIH

grant AI-20922 and American Cancer Society grant IM-378 to M.S. and NIH grant AI 19624 to L.H. We would like to thank Dr. Martin Low for his help in the phospholipase studies. The untiring assistance of Mrs. Dawn Schott and Mrs. Andrea Lulkowski during the preparation of this manuscript is gratefully acknowledged.

REFERENCES

1. Flaherty, L. (1981): The Tla region antigens. The Role of the Major Histocompatibility Complex in Immunobiology. M.E. Dorf (ed): Garland Press, New York, pp 33-57.

2. Lew, A., Lillehoj, E., Cowan, E., Maloy, W., VanSchravendijk, M., and J. Coligan. (1986). Class I genes and molecules: an update. Immunology 57:3.

3. Devlin, J., Lew, A., Flavell, R., and J. Coligan. (1985). Secretion of a soluble class I molecule encoded by the Q10 gene of the C57BL/10 mouse. The EMBO J. 4:369.

4. Robinson, P. (1985). Qb-1, a new class I polypeptide encoded by the Qa region of the mouse H-2 complex. Immunogenetics 22:285.

5. Winoto, A., Steinmetz, M., and L. Hood. (1983). Genetic mapping in the major histocompatibility complex by restriction enzyme site polymorphisms: most mouse class I genes map to the Tla complex. Proc. Natl. Acad. Sci. USA 80:3425.

6. Weiss, E.H., Golden, L., Fahrner, K., Mellor, A., Devlin, J.J., Bullman, H., Tidens, H., Bird, H., and R. Flavell. (1984). Organization and evolution of the class I gene family in the major histocompatibility complex of the C57BL/10 mouse. Nature 310:650.

7. Mellor, A.L., Antoniou, J., and Robinson, P. (1985). Structure and expression of genes encoding murine Qa-2 class I antigens. Proc. Natl. Acad. Sci. USA 82: 5920.

8. Devlin, J.J., Weiss, E.H., Paulson, M. and Flavell, R. (1985). Duplicated gene pairs and alleles of class I genes in the Qa-2 region of the murine major histocompatibility complex: a comparison. EMBO J. 4: 3203.

9. Goodenow, R.S., McMillan, M., Nicolson, M., Sher, B.T., Eakle, K., Davidson, N., and Hood, L. (1982). Identification of the class I genes of the mouse major histocompatibility complex by DNA-mediated gene transfer. Nature 300:231.

10. Stroynowski, I., Forman, J., Goodenow, R.S., Schiffer, S.G., McMillan, ,M., Sharrow, S. O., Sachs, D.H., and Hood, L. (1985). Expression and T-cell recognition of hybrid antigens with amino-terminal domains encoded by Qa-2 region of major histocompatibility complex and carboxyl termini of transplantation antigens. J. Exp. Med. 161,935-952.

11. Darlington, G.J., Bernhard, H.P., Miller, R.A., and

Ruddle, F.H. (1980). Expression of liver phenotypes in cultured mouse hepatoma cells. J. Natl. Cancer Inst. 64:809-819.

12. Sharrow, S.O., Flaherty, L., and Sachs, D.H. (1984). Serolgic cross-reactivity between class I MHC molecules and an H-2 linked differentiation antigen as detected by monoclonal antibodies. J. Exp. Med. 159:21-40.

13. Harris, R. A., Hogarth, P.M., Penington, D.G. and I.F.C. McKenzie. (1984). Qa Antigens and their Differential Distribution on Lymphoid, Myeloid and Stem Cells. J. Immunogenetics 11:265-281.

14. Soloski, M., Vernachio, J., Einhorn, G., and A. Lattimore. (1986). Qa gene expression: Biosynthesis and secretion of Qa2 molecules in activated T cells. Proc Natl Acad Sci (USA) 83:2949.

15. Robinson, P. (1987). Two different biosynthetic pathways for the secretion of Qa region-associated class I antigens by mouse lymphocytes. Proc. Natl. Acad. Sci. USA 84:527.

16. Moore, R.W., Sher, B.T., Sun, Y.H., Eakle, K.A. and Hood, L. (1982). DNA sequence of a gene encoding a Balb/c mouse L^d transplantation antigen. Science 215:679.

17. Stiernberg, J., Low, M.G., Flaherty, L., and P.W. Kincade. (1987). Removal of lymphocyte surface molecules with phosphatidyl inositol-specific phospholipase C. Effects on mitogen responses and evidence that ThB and certain Qa antigens are membrane-anchored via phosphatidylinositol. J. Immunol. 138:3877.

18. Low, M.G., and P.W. Kincade. (1985). Phosphatidylinositol is the membrane-anchoring domain of the Thy-1 glycoprotein. Nature 318:62.

19. Davitz, M.A., Low, M.G., and V. Nussenzweig (1986). Release of decay accelerating factor (DAF) from cell membranes by phosphatidylinositol-specific phospholipase C (PI-PLC): selective modification of a complement regulatory protein. J. Exp. Med. 163:1150.

20. Reiser, H., Oettgen, H., Yeh, E.T.H., Terhorst, C., Low, M.G., Benaceraf, .B, and K. Rock. (1986). Structural characterization of the TAP molecule: a phosphatidylinositol-linked glycoprotein distinct from the T-Cell receptor/T3 complex and Thy-1. Cell 47:365.

21. Freimuth, W.W., Miller, H.C., and W.J. Esselman. (1979). Soluble factors containing Thy-1 antigen shed from lymphoblastoid cells modulate in vitro plaque-forming cell response. J. Immunol. 123:201.

22. Fatemi, S.H., and A.M. Tartakoff. (1986). Hydrophobic anchor-deficient Thy-1 is secreted by a class E mutant T lymphoma. Cell 46:653.

23. Bordier, C. (1981). Phase separation of integral

membrane proteins in Triton X-114 solution. J. Bio. Chem. 256:1604.

24. Low, M.G. (1987). Biochemistry of the glycosyl-phosphatidylinositol membrane protein anchors. Biochem. J. 244 (in press).

25. Steinmetz, M., Moore, K.W., Frelinger, J.G., Sher, B.T., Shen, F.W., Boyse, E.A., and Hood, L. (1981). A pseudogene homologous to mouse transplantation antigens: Transplantation antigens are encoded by eight exons that correlate with protein domains. Cell 25:683-692.

26. Waneck, G.-L., Sherman, D.H., Calvin, S., Allen, H. and Flavell, R.A. (1987). Tissue-specific expression of cell-surface Qa2 antigen from a transfected Qa^b gene of C57BL/10 mice. J. Exp. Med. 165:1358.

27. Kroczek, R., Gunter, K., Germain, R., and E. Shevach. (1986). Thy-1 functions as a signal transduction molecule in T lymphocytes and transfected B lymphocytes. Nature 322:181.

28. Malek, T., Ortega, G., Chan, C., Kroczek, R., and E. Shevach. (1986). Role of Ly-6 in lymphocyte activation II. Induction of T cell activation by monoclonal anti Ly-6 antibodies. J. Exp. Med. 164:709.

STRUCTURAL AND FUNCTIONAL ANALYSIS OF MURINE CLASS II MOLECULES

Irwin J. Griffith* and Laurie H. Glimcher*,§

From the *Department of Cancer Biology, Harvard School of Public Health and the §Department of Medicine, Harvard Medical School, Boston, MA 02115

INTRODUCTION

Class II (Ia) major histocompatibility complex (MHC) molecules in the mouse are cell surface glycoproteins expressed on antigen presenting cells (APC; ref. 1). In the mouse two isotypic forms of Ia exist: the I-A and I-E molecules, each a heterodimer composed of noncovalently-associated α and β chains. The association of foreign antigen, Ia molecules and the clonally distributed antigen receptor on T cells is critical in the initiation and regulation of immune responses[1]. However, the exact nature of the interaction between T cell receptor, antigen and Ia molecule is still poorly understood at the molecular level.

Individual Ia polypeptides (A_α, A_β, E_α, and E_β) have similar protein structures. Each is composed of two extracellular domains of approximately 96 amino acids, a transmembrane domain and a short (12-15) amino acid cytoplasmic domain. The first, N-terminal (membrane distal), A_α, A_β, and E_β domains are polymorphic. That is, alleles from different inbred strains of mice contain multiple amino acid substitutions in the $\alpha 1$ and $\beta 1$ domains (see Figure 1). In contrast, the $E_{\alpha 1}$ domain is relatively nonpolymorphic. Similarly, the $\alpha 2$ and $\beta 2$ domains, which are membrane proximal, are much more conserved and are highly homologous to immunoglobulin constant region domains; Ia molecules are part of the immunoglobulin super gene family. Exon shuffling experiments have demonstrated that antigen associates with the $\alpha 1$ and $\beta 1$ domains[2,3]. It has been postulated that the clustering of polymorphic residues (see Figure 1) identifies regions of the Ia molecules that are critical in antigen presentation[4]. However, these allelic comparisons are not specific enough to identify precise relationships between Ia structure and function.

In contrast to the wealth of spontaneous class I mutants[5], only one naturally occurring class II mutant has been detected, the B6.CH-H-2^{bm12} strain of mouse, which contains 3 amino acid differences in its $A_{\beta 1}$ domain as the result of a gene conversion event from the $E_\beta{}^b$ gene[6]. The bm12 mutation has produced profound alterations in Ia-associated serology and function and has provided valuable insights into the structure/function relationship of the $A_\beta{}^b$ molecule. In order to determine more precisely the role of individual amino acids in the formation of serologically-defined determinants and T cell restriction sites, our laboratory has been analyzing Ia molecules in which limited mutations have been induced. This has been

```
      1        10        20        30        40        50        60        70        80        90
Aα^k  EDDIEADHVGSYGITVYQSPGDIGQYTFEFDGDELFYVDLDKKETVWMLPEFAQLRRFEPQGGLQNIATGKHNLEILTKRSNSTPATN
Aα^b  ----------T---S-------------------------------------G--AS-D---------VV----GV-----------
Aα^d  ----------F--T-------------H---------------K---R----G--IL-----------AE----G-------F-----
Aα^f  ----------F---S-------------------W------------R----G--TS-D------E--------G-------F-----
Aα^q              --V-----------H------W-----------------G--TS-D---------------GGW-----F-----
Aα^r  ----------V--T-----------F-H------W-----------------G--TS-D---------VV------------F---A-
Aα^s  ----------V--T-------------H------W----------I------G--TS-D------------YT-G-------------
Aα^u       ---------V------------------------------I----------S-D---------------GV-----------

Aβ^k  GNSERHFVHQFQPFCYFTNGTQRIRLVIRYIYNREEYVRFDSDVGEYRAVTELGRPDAEYWNKQ*Y*LERTRAELDTVCRHNYEKTETPTSLRRLE
Aβ^b  -D------Y--MGE-----------Y-T-----------Y------H---------------S-PEI-----------------GP--H-------
Aβ^d  --------V--KGE--Y----------T-----------Y----------------------S-PEI-------V--A------GP--S-------
Aβ^f  --------F--KGE-----------S-D---------L-----------------S----Y---*-*-----------------GV----------
Aβ^q  --------A-LKGE-----------S-N--------W-------------------------S-PEI-------V---------GV--H-------
Aβ^s  -D------F--KGE-----------S-D---------L---------------------Y---*-*--Q--------------GV--H-------
Aβ^u  -D-----LV----------------Y-T---------L---------------------Y---*-*-------------Y---E--V--------

Eβ^k  VRDSRPWFLEYCKSECHFYNGTQRVRLLVRYFYNLEENLRFDSDVGEFRAVTELGRPDAENWNSQPEFLEQKRAEVDTVCRHNYEIFDNFLVPRR
Eβ^b  ---------------------------E-----------------------------------------------------------S-K---R--
Eβ^d  ---T--R----VT----------H--F-E-FI--R------------Y-------------------I--DA--S---Y-------S-K---R--
Eβ^s        -----ST---------------E----------------------------------------R--A---Y-------L-K------
Eβ^u  RG----R--G-ST-------------F-D-----R--WV--------Y---------E---------I---T--A---Y-------S-K---R--
```

Figure 1. Allelic polymorphism in the first domain of the A_α, A_β, and E_β polypeptides. *, represents a break introduced for maximal alignment of the sequences. Amino acid sequences are predicted from the respective nucleotide sequences provided in references 4, 17-25.

accomplished in two ways. First, in vitro mutagenesis has been used to construct several distinct mutant A_β^b genes[7]. DNA-mediated gene transfer of these genes into a B lymphoma cell has resulted in the successful expression of these mutant class II antigens. Second, panels of cloned populations of APC that bear mutated $I\text{-}A^k$ and $I\text{-}E^k$ molecules have been produced by negative and positive immunoselection using anti-Ia monoclonal antibodies (mAbs; refs. 8-11). The appropriate genes from these serologically-selected mutants have then been isolated and sequenced to localize the mutation[10,12,13]. The results of these experiments and the conclusions that we have drawn from them will be discussed below.

RESULTS

Site-Directed Mutants

Site-directed mutagenesis permits the rapid introduction of specific alterations in a given gene. We used this technique to introduce mutations in the A_β^b gene[7]. We generated two mutations, 18.1 and 18.3, that resulted in single amino acid substitutions in the first domain of the A_β^b polypeptide (see Figure 2a). A third mutation, 23.1, resulted in the deletion of two amino acids and the substitution of a third. All mutations were selected to reflect polymorphic differences between the *b* and *k* haplotypes in the ß1 domain. Transfection of these mutant genes into an Ia-negative B cell lymphoma, M12.C3, permitted us to examine alterations in serology and effects on antigen presentation.

The 18.1 and 18.3 mutations do not alter the serology of their respective polypeptides[7]. That is, the 18.1 and 18.3 mutants are indistinguishable from wild-type with the monoclonal antibodies (mAbs) we used. In contrast, the 23.1 mutation causes a limited loss in mAb binding, eliminating binding of three of the twelve mAbs examined. This pattern is also

Table 1. Antigen presentation to a panel of $I\text{-}A^b$-restricted T cells by site-directed mutants.

		Antigen presenting cells				
T hybridoma	Specificity	Wild-type	18.1	18.3	23.1	bm12
4E3	Allo:$I\text{-}A^b$	+	+	+	+	-
RF13.35	GAT:$I\text{-}A^b$	+	+	+	+	-
3B8	Allo:$I\text{-}A^b$	+	+	+	+	-
4A4	Allo:$I\text{-}A^b$	+	+	+	-	+
AODH3.4	Allo:$I\text{-}A^b$	+	+	+	-	+
FS9.6.3	Allo:A_β^b:A_α^d	+	+	+	-	+
1C4.B2	Ova:$I\text{-}A^b$	+	+	-	+	-
1C4.B6	Ova:$I\text{-}A^b$	+	+	+	-	-
3G3	Allo:$I\text{-}A^b$	+	-	+	-	-
JB1C4	Allo:$I\text{-}A^b$	+	-	-	-	-

T hybridoma cells were co-cultured with antigen presenting cells (APC) and antigen as described in reference 7. Cell culture supernatants were assayed for the presence of IL-2 with an IL-2 dependent T cell line, HT-2. Results are presented schematically. Allo, alloreactive; GAT, poly($Glu^{60}Ala^{30}Tyr^{10}$); Ova, ovalbumin; +, wild-type response; -, background response.

A. SITE-DIRECTED MUTANTS

```
       1        10        20        30        40        50        60        70        80        90
Aβ^b   GDSERHFVYQFMGECYFTNGTQRIRLVTRYIYNREEYVRYDSDVGEHRAVTELGRPDAEYWNSQPEILERTRAELDTVCRHNYEGPETHTSLRRLE
18.1   --------H---------------------------------------------------------------------------------------
18.3   -------------F----------------------------------------------------------------------------------
23.1   ----------------------------------------------------------------*Y*-----------------------------
bm12   ------------------------------------------------------------------F--QM-------------------------
Aβ^k   -N------H--QPF-----------Y-I-----------F------Y---------------K-*Y*-----------------KT--P-------
```

B. SEROLOGIC MUTANTS

```
       1        10        20        30        40        50        60        70        80        90
Aα^k   EDDIEADHVGSYGITVYQSPGDIGQYTFEFDGDELFYVDLDKKETVWMLPEFAQLRRFEPQGGLQNIATGKHNLEILTKRSNSTPATN
3J9    --------------------------------------------------------------------------K-------------

Aβ^k   GNSERHFVHQFQPFCYFTNGTQRIRLVIRYIYNREEYVRFDSDVGEYRAVTELGRPDAEYWNKQ*Y*LERTRAELDTVCRHNYEKTETPTSLRRLE
B13    ----------------------------------------------------------------*-*-K---------------------------
JT1    ---------------------------------------------------------------R*-*-----------------------------
LD3    ---------------------------------------------------------------P*-*-----------------------------

Eβ^k   VRDSRPWFLEYCKSECHFYNGTQRVRLLVRYFYNLEENLRFDSDVGEFRAVTELGRPDAENWNSQPEFLEQKRAEVDTVCRHNYEIFDNFLVPRRV
2B1    ------------------------------------------------H-----------------------------------------------
```

Figure 2. Site-directed and serologically-selected mutations in the first domain of Ia polypeptides.

A. Sequences of site-directed mutants, bm12 mutant and A_{β}^{k} polypeptides relative to the wild-type A_{β}^{b} polypeptide. The sequences are from references 6, 7, 19 and 20. *, represents a break inserted for maximal alignment of the sequences.

B. Sequences of the serologically-selected mutants relative to wild-type sequences. Sequences are from references 4, 8, 12, 13, 20, 22, and unpublished data. *, represents a break inserted into the A_{β}^{k} sequence for maximal alignment with other A_{β} sequences.

reflected in the ability of the I-A^b molecules containing these mutant polypeptides to present antigen to a panel of alloreactive or antigen-specific, Ia-restricted T cell hybridomas: the 23.1 mutant has a more severe defect in antigen presentation than the 18.1 and 18.3 mutants (Table 1). Strikingly, the 23.1 and bm12 mutants have unique and distinctive patterns of antigen presentation, even though these mutations overlap each other (Table 1, Figure 2a).

Serologically-Selected Mutants

The serologically-selected mutants have been derived from a B cell hybridoma, TA3, that contains one copy of chromosome 17 of the *k* haplotype and three copies of the *d* haplotype[14]. Following chemical mutagenesis, the parent TA3 cells are negatively immunoselected with an anti-Ia^k mAb plus complement. The cells are then positively selected using a second Ia^k mAB that recognizes a separate epitope on the same Ia isotype as the first mAb. Therefore, the resulting clones have lost the epitope recognized by the first mAB, but continue to express the epitope (and Ia molecule) recognized by the second mAB. It has been possible to select variants that contain these serologically-defined mutations in their A_α, A_β and E_β polypetides (Figure 2b).

The mutations that have been examined are the result of single nucleotide changes that result in amino acid substitutions. The substitutions range from conservative (2B1) to full charge changes (3J9, B13). The type of substitution does not appear to correlate with the loss of mAb binding (see Table 2). For example, the JT1 and LD3 mutants both involve single base substitutions at amino acid 64. JT1 contains a Gln to Arg (polar to basic) substitution and involves the loss a single mAb binding site, while the LD3 mutant contains a Gln to Proline (polar to non-polar) substitution and involves the loss of several mAb binding sites (Figure 2b, Table 2). Further, the mutants B13 and LD3 have the same mAb binding pattern although their mutations involve amino acid substitutions three residues apart and entail different charge changes (acidic to basic and polar to non-polar, respectively)[11]. It is interesting to note that the LD3 mutation, which causes the loss of several distinct mAb binding sites on the $A_\beta{}^k$ chain, does not affect binding of several $A_\alpha{}^k$-reactive mAbs. The LD3 mutant was generated in the laboratory of Dr. D. J. McKean.

The $E_\beta{}^k$ mutant cell line 2B1 has a His substituted for an Arg at the non-polymorphic residue 49 and does not bind the $E_\beta{}^k$-specific mAb 17.3.3

Table 2. Phenotypes of the serologically-selected mutants

	$A_\alpha{}^k$ mAbs		$A_\beta{}^k$ mAbs			$E_\beta{}^k$ mAbs		
Cell	39J	1E9	10-2.16	39B	40L	17.3.3	Y17	39G
Wild-type	+	+	+	+	+	+	+	+
3J9	−	+	NT	NT	NT	NT	NT	NT
A19	NT	NT	−	−	+	NT	NT	NT
JT1	NT	NT	−	+	+	NT	NT	NT
LD3	+	+	−	−	+	NT	NT	NT
2B1	NT	NT	NT	NT	NT	−	+	+

Schematic of mAb binding to the specified cells in a FACS analysis. Data is from references 9-13, 26, and unpublished data.

Table 3. Antigen presentation by select serologic mutants.

Cell line	Wild-type	A_{β}^{k} A19	A_{β}^{k} LD3	A_{α}^{k} 3J9
C10	++	-	++	-
C4	++	-	++	-
C11	++	-	+	++
2A11	++	-	+	++
A4	++	-	+	++
19.47	++	-	+	++
3A9	++	++	-	++
A6	++	+	++	++
A2	++	++	++	++
18N	++	+	+	++
B14	++	++	++	++

T hybridoma cells were co-cultured with serologically selected mutant APC and hen egg-white lysozyme (HEL) antigen as described in reference 12. Cell culture supernatants were assayed for the presence of IL-2 with an IL-2 dependent T cell line, HT-2. Results are presented schematically. ++, wild-type response; +, intermediate response; -, background response.

(ref. 13, Table 2). However, other inbred strains lack reactivity with the 17.3.3 mAb even though they share the non-polymorphic Arg at residue 49. These 17.3.3⁻ strains differ from antibody binding strains at residue 48. There-fore the Arg at residue 49 is critical, to but not sufficient for, the formation of the 17.3.3 binding site. The 17.3.3 mAB binding site could be either a linear recognition sequence that includes residues 48 and 49 or a conformational determinant whose presence is disrupted by alteration at either residue 48 or 49. In the latter possibility, the conformational determinant could directly include one, both or neither of these residues.

In contrast, the amino acid (Glu_{75}) changed in the A_{α}^{k} mutant 3J9 appears to be a key residue in a conformational determinant recognized by the 39J mAb[12]. Glu_{75} is the only amino acid common to both the A_{α}^{k} and A_{α}^{r} polypeptides that is not shared by other haplotypes (see Figure 1); the *k* and *r* haplotypes are the only two haplotypes to share the 39J binding site. While it is possible that the 39J mAb binding site is formed as the result of a conformational effect generated at a distance by the presence of Glu at residue 75, it is more likely that the physical location of this epitope can be directly assigned to include residue 75.

We then used these mutant cell lines to ask whether a simple globular protein (hen egg-white lysozyeme [HEL]) can generate multiple T cell determinants. The effect their respective mutations have on the ability of three variant cell lines to present antigen is shown in Table 3. The A_{α}^{k} mutant 3J9 has lost a single mAb-defined epitope (Table 2) that results in a limited, specific, defect in antigen presentation. The loss of a single mAb binding site (39J mAb⁻) results in an inability to present HEL to the T cell hybridomas C10 and C4. The 3J9 mutant continues to present HEL to other T cell hybridomas, showing that the mutation has not abrogated the abiltiy of the 3J9 variant to specifically present HEL. The two A_{β}^{k}-specific mutants B13 and LD3 have very distinctive patterns of antigen presentation to the panel of HEL-specific, Ia^{k}-restricted T cells, even though both mutations are indistinguishable serologically[11]. These mutations affect polymorphic residues (3J9, B13) or non-polymorphic residues in a cluster of polymorphic residues (LD3). This provides support for the hypothesis of McDevitt and coworkers[4] that the polymorphic residues identify regions of the Ia molecule that are critical for antigen presentation. The 2B1 variant, whose mutation alters a non-polymorphic residue in a string of non-polymorphic residues, does not affect antigen presentation[13]. These results show that a single Ia molecule contains multiple domains critical for antigen presentation and T cell activation and that certain non-polymorphic residues are not involved in antigen presentation.

DISCUSSION

Both site-directed and serologically-selected mutagenesis demonstrate that there are multiple sites on the Ia molecule that can be critical for the presentation of antigen to T cells. For example, even though the bm12 and site-directed mutant 23.1 overlap at amino acid 67, the close proximity of these mutations in the primary protein sequence fails to predict how these mutant cells will function in T cell activation. This is analogous to the serologically-selected mutants LD3 and B13 that have very distinct patterns of antigen presentation although they are serologically indistinguishable. Further, one ovalbumin (OVA)-specific T cell hybridoma (1C4.B2) is not activated by the two mutants 18.3 and bm12, which lie 54 amino acids apart, but is activated by the other two site-directed mutants 18.1 and 23.1 whose alterations are adjacent to those in the 18.3 and bm12 (Table 2). Together, these observations suggest that the tertiary conformation of the Ia molecule is important in determining association with antigen and the T cell receptor.

It has recently been suggested that each Ia molecule possesses only one binding site for all peptides with which it normally associates[15]. Thus, peptides capable of being presented by a given class II molecule would compete with each other for T cell activation. Such peptides would bind to class II molecules through a region that shows homology to the class II molecule itself. The polymorphic regions, which distinguish the different Ia alleles, must therefore be involved in the binding of peptide to Ia.

If there is a single antigen binding site, then one might be able to account for the multiple domains that we have identified on the Ia molecule as being key contact sites for the T cell receptor. The tertiary conformation of these sites remains critical for T cell activation. Thus, the 18.3 and bm12 could fail to activate the T cell hybridoma 1C4.B2 if they are opposed in the tertiary structure of $I\text{-}A^b$ in the process of T cell recognition. It is as likely, however, that each of these mutations independently alters the T cel recognition site by affecting tertiary conformation. Therefore, although it is clear that there are multiple functional sites on an Ia molecule, it is not obvious that their exact number and physical location will be further localized until the crystallographic structure of Ia is known.

CONCLUSIONS

Attempts to localize sites on the class II molecules that interact with foreign antigen and T cell receptor have yielded much useful information. From this work it is possible to draw four major conclusions:

1. there are multiple determinants on a single Ia molecule,
2. a single class II molecule and a simple globular protein interact to form multiple T cell receptor ligands,
3. certain non-polymorphic residues are not involved in T cell recognition, and
4. the tertiary conformation is critical for the formation of serologic and T cell reactive sites on an Ia molecule.

Recent experiments by Germain and his coworkers have indicated that for an $A_\beta{}^b$ molecule, contributions from the ß2 and/or the paired $A_\alpha{}^k$ chain were necessary for antigen presentation to T cell hybridomas[17]. This highlights the importance of determining the crystallographic structure of an Ia molecule for pinpointing the key contact residues or conformations necessary for antigen presentation.

REFERENCES

1. R. H. Schwartz, T lymphocyte recognition of antigen in association with gene products of the major histocompatibility complex, Annu. Rev. Immunol. 3:237 (1985).
2. V. Folsom, D. Gay, and S. Tonegawa, The $ß_1$ domain of the mouse $E_ß$ chain is important for restricted antigen presentation to helper T-cell hybridomas, Proc. Natl. Acad. Sci. USA 82:1678 (1985).
3. R. N. Germain, J. D. Ashwell, R. I. Lechler, D. H. Margulies, K. M. Nickerson, G. Susuki, and J. Y. L. Tou, "Exon-shuffling" maps control of antibody- and T-cell-recognition sites to the NH_2-terminal domain of the class II major histocompatibility polypeptide $A_ß$, Proc. Natl. Acad. Sci. USA 82:2940 (1985).
4. C. O. Benoist, D. J. Mathis, M. R. Kanter, V. E. Williams II, and H. O. McDevitt, Regions of allelic hypervariability in the murine Aα immune response gene, Cell 34:169 (1983).
5. R. Nairn, K. Yamaga, and S. G. Nathenson, Biochemistry of the gene products from murine MHC mutants, Annu. Rev. Genet. 14:241 (1980).
6. K. R. McIntyre, and J. G. Seidman, Nucleotide sequence of mutant I-$Aß^{bm12}$ gene is evidence for genetic exchange between mouse immune response genes, Nature 308:551 (1984).
7. L. E. Cohn, L. H. Glimcher, R. A. Waldmann, J. A. Smith, A. Ben-Nun, J. G. Seidman, and E. Choi, Identification of functional regions on the I-A^b molecule by site-directed mutagenesis, Proc. Natl. Acad. Sci. USA 83:747 (1986).
8. M. A. Brown, L. H. Glimcher, E. A. Nielsen, W. E. Paul, and R. N. Germain, T-cell recognition of Ia molecules selectively altered by a single amino acid substitution, Science 231:255 (1986).
9. B. N. Beck, L. H. Glimcher, A. E. Nilson, M. Pierres, and D. J. McKean, The structure-function relationship of I-A molecules: correlation of serologic and functional phenotypes of four I-A^k mutant cell lines, J. Immunol. 133:3176 (1984).
10. H. Quill, R. H. Schwartz, and L. H. Glimcher, $Eß^k$ mutant antigen-presenting cell lines expressing altered $A_\alpha{}^k$ molecules. J. Immunol. 136:3351 (1986).
11. P. M. Allen, D. J. McKean, B. N. Beck, J. Sheffield, and L. H. Glimcher, Direct evidence that a class II molecule and a simple globular protein generate multiple determinants, J. Exp. Med. 162:1264 (1985).
12. I. J. Griffith, E. Choi, and L. H. Glimcher, A single base change in an I-A α-chain alters T-cell recognition. Proc. Natl. Acad. Sci. 84:1090 (1987).
13. I. J. Griffith, F. M. Carland, and L. H. Glimcher, Alteration of a non-polymorphic residue in a class II Eß gene eliminates an antibody-defined epitope without affecting T cell recognition, J. Immunol. 38:4480 (1987).
14. L. H. Glimcher, T. Hamano, R. Asofsky, D. H. Sachs, M. Pierres. L. E. Samelson, S. O. Sharrow, and W. E. Paul, I-A mutant functional antigen-presenting cell lines, J. Immunol. 130:2287 (1983).
15. L. G. Guillet, M.-Z. Lai, T. J. Briner, S. Buus, A. Sette, H. M. Grey, J. A. Smith, M. L. Gefter, Immunological self, nonself discrimination, Science 235:865 (1987).
16. R. N. Germain and B. Mallissen, Analysis of the expression and function of class-II major histocompatibility complex-encoded molecules by DNA-mediated gene transfer, Ann. Rev. Immunol. 4:281 (1986).

17. D. Landais, H. Matthes, C. Benoist, and D. Mathis, A molecular basis for the Ia.2 and Ia.19 antigenic determinants, Proc. Natl. Acad. Sci. USA 82:2930 (1985).
18. D. Larhammar, U. Hammerling, M. Denaro, T. Lund, R. A. Flavell, L. Rask, and P. A. Peterson, Structure of the murine immune response I-A_{β} locus: sequence of the I-A_{β} gene and an adjacent ß-chain second domain exon, Cell 34:179 (1983).
19. M. Malissen, T. Hunkapiller, and L. Hood, Nucleotide sequence of a light chain gene of the mouse I-A subregion: $Aß^{d}$, Science 221:750 (1983).
20. P. Estess, A. B. Begovich, M. Koo, P. P. Jones, and H. O. McDevitt, H.O. Sequence analysis and structure-function correlations of murine *q*, *k*, *u*, *s*, and *f* haplotype I-A_{β} cDNA clones, Proc. Natl. Acad. Sci. USA 83:3594 (1986).
21. G. Widera, and R. A. Flavell, The nucleotide sequence of the murine I-$Eß^{b}$ immune response gene: evidence for gene conversion events in class II genes of the major histocompatibility complex, EMBO J.
22. L. Mengle-Gaw, and H. O. McDevitt, Isolation and characterization of a cDNA clone for the murine I-E_{β} polypeptide chain, Proc. Natl. Acad. Sci. USA 80:7621 (1983).
23. H. Saito, R. A. Maki, L. K. Clauton, and S. Tonegawa, Complete primary structures of the Eß chain and gene of the mouse major histocompatibility complex, Proc. Natl. Acad. Sci. USA 80:5520 (1983).
24. L. Mengle-Gaw, and H. O. McDevitt, Predicted protein sequence of the murine I-$E_{\beta}{}^{s}$ polypeptide chain from CDNA and genomic clones, Proc. Natl. Acad. Sci. USA 82:2910 (1985).
25. L. Mengle-Gaw, and H.O. McDevitt, Allelic variation in the murine Ia ß chain genes, in: "Regulation of the immune system", H. Cantor, L. Chess, and E. Sercarz, eds., Alan R. Liss, Inc., NY, (1984).
26. G. G. Schlauder, M. P. Bell, B. N. Beck, A. Nilson, and D. J. McKean, The structure-function relationship of I-A molecules: a biochemical analysis of I-A polypeptides from mutant antigen-presenting cells and evidence of preferential association of allelic forms, J. Immunol. 135:1945 (1985).

STRUCTURE-FUNCTION ANALYSIS OF SEROLOGICALLY SELECTED CELL LINES EXPRESSING MUTANT A_{β}^{k} POLYPEPTIDES

B. N. Beck, M. Bell, L. R. Pease, A. Nilson, J.-M. Buerstedde, G. G. Schlauder and D. J. McKean

Department of Immunology
Mayo Clinic
Rochester, MN 55905

ABSTRACT

A panel of twleve mutant A_{β}^{k} expressing cell lines has been produced from a mutagenized B cell hybridoma using a protocol of negative and positive immunoselection. Each of the serologically-defined epitopes on the A_{β}^{k} polypeptide has been altered in one or more of the mutant cell lines. Immunoselection techniques have been used to select also for secondary mutations in some cell lines, resulting either in reversion to the wild-type or near wild-type phenotype or in the alteration of additional A_{β}^{k} serologic epitopes. Characterization of the ability of the mutant cell lines to stimulate antigen and alloantigen-reactive T cell hybridomas has shown that they display distinct functional phenotypes ranging from nearly wild-type to almost completely defective. DNA sequence analysis of the A_{β}^{k} gene cloned from each mutant cell line has revealed the structural basis for the mutant serologic and functional phenotypes. To date, each β chain mutant has been found to have a single amino acid substitution (resulting from a single nucleotide substitution) in the β1 domain. The substitutions are clustered in or near the third allelicly-defined variable region of the A_{β} polypeptide (residues 61-70). These results indicate that this region of the A_{β} polypeptide comprises multiple serologically defined epitopes. Furthermore, specific residues within this region appear to be important for effective T cell activation.

INTRODUCTION

The class II molecules encoded by the major histocompatibility complex are important cell-recognition molecules for the immune system. In the mouse, both the I-A and I-E subclasses of the class II molecules show extensive intraspecies polymorphism as detected by both serologic and biochemical techniques. Sequence analysis of several alleles of the I-A α and β polypeptides has revealed that the polymorphism is largely concentrated in the α_1 and β_1 N-terminal domains of these polypeptides (Choi et al., 1983; Estess et al., 1986; Benoist et al., 1983; Landais et al., 1985). Furthermore, exon-shuffling experiments have demonstrated that both the serologic epitopes and the sites recognized by T cells map to the N-terminal α_1 and β_1 domains (Germain et al., 1985). Examination of the sequence diversity reveals three clusters of variable residues in the $\alpha 1$ domain (Benoist et al., 1983) and four clusters in the $\beta 1$ domain (Estess et al., 1986). It seems reasonable to expect that the allelic series of I-A molecules will share overall three-dimensional structure and that the clusters of allelicly variable residues will be responsible for the sites recognized by alloantibodies and by T cells. In order to examine in detail the relationship between the sequence diversity and the sites recognized by alloantibodies and by T cells, we have isolated a number of I-A^k structural variants generated *in vitro* by ethylmethane-sulfonate (EMS) mutagenesis and subsequent selection with monoclonal antibodies (Beck et al., 1984). Several of these variants have now been characterized by DNA sequence analysis (Beck et al., 1987). This analysis has revealed that for the A^k_β polypeptide, the third of the four allelicly variable regions is serologically immunodominant.

MATERIALS AND METHODS

Cell lines. Mutants were obtained by a protocol of negative and positive selection using a panel of monoclonal anti-I-A^k antibodies after ethylmethane-sulfonate mutagenesis of the parental TA3 cells, as has been described (Beck et al., 1984). All cell lines have been cloned and subsequently maintained in RPMI 1640 supplemented with 10% fetal bovine serum, 2 mM glutamine, 10^{-4} M 2-mercaptoethanol, 10 mM HEPES, and antibiotics at 37°C in a humidified atmosphere of 5% CO_2 in air.

Serologic phenotypes. Serologic phenotypes of the cell lines were analyzed by indirect immunofluorescence on a flow cytometer (FACS IV) after staining under saturating conditions with various I-A^k reactive monoclonal antibodies (mAbs) as previously described (Beck et al., 1984). Fluorescence intensity was measured using a logarithmic amplifier and quantitated by the comparison of peak channel numbers. Antibodies 10-2.16 and 11-3.25 were derived by Oi et al. (1978), 4-2.1 and 4-2.3 by Harmon et al. (1983), and 39B, 39E, 30J, 40A, 40M, 40F, and 40L by Pierres et al. (1981).

Functional phenotypes. The ability of the various cell lines to present antigen to a panel of T hybridomas was assayed by quantitating antigen-specific IL-2 release. The panel of T hybridomas used included both I-A^k specific auto- and allo-reactive T cells and I-A^k restricted antigen-specific T cells. The antigen-reactive hybridomas recognized either keyhole limpet hemocyanin, hen egg lysozyme, or ovalbumin. Most of these data have been published previously (Beck et al., 1984). Additional functional studies have been carried out by Drs. E. Rosloniec and J. Freed, using lysozyme-reactive I-A^k restricted T hybridomas (unpublished data). In all cases, either the supernatants were titrated for IL-2 activity or supernatants from titrated numbers of stimulator cells were assayed for IL-2 activity.

I-A^k_β gene cloning and sequencing. A bacteriophage lambda clone of the 17 kb EcoRI fragment containing the A^k_β gene (Brown et al., 1986) from each mutant was isolated from a size-selected (16-20 kb) EcoRI genomic library prepared in either Charon 4 or EMBL4. The A_β insert-containing phage were identified by hybridization with either the pIAβ-1 (Robinson et al., 1983) or the pCA12 plasmid probe kindly provided by Dr. J. Seidman and Dr. L. Hood, respectively. The mutant A^k_β genes were digested with Pst I or Xma I or both and the fragments cloned into M13mp18 or 19 for nucleotide sequencing by the dideoxy chain termination method (Sanger et al., 1977). The desired recombinants were identified by hybridization with synthetic oligonucleotides complementary to intron sequences directly adjacent to the particular exons, based on published sequence (Choi et al., 1983). The same oligonucleotides subsequently were used as primers in the sequencing reactions. The exons encoding the β1 and β2 domains were sequenced in both directions and the leader exon sequenced only in the 3′ to 5′ direction.

RESULTS

The TA3 cell line, derived from the fusion of (BALB/c x A/J)F_1 spleen cells with the BALB/c B lymphoma cell line M12.4.1 (Glimcher et al., 1983a) and thus haploid for the I-A^k genes, was used as the parent for the isolation of cell lines expressing mutant I-A^k molecules (Beck et al., 1984). Several different A^k_α- and A^k_β-reactive monoclonal antibodies (mAbs) have been used for both the negative and positive selection steps, thus generating an extensive series of mutant cell lines expressing serologically altered I-A^k molecules (Table 1). This selection scheme favors the isolation of variant cell lines expressing A^k molecules with only limited alterations in either the A^k_β or A^k_α polypeptide (Schlauder et al., 1985). In addition, some of the original mutants have been subjected to a second round of mutagenesis and selection, resulting in the isolation of either revertants or double mutants. This was done in order to expand the number of sites that potentially could be identified by the mutagenesis and antibody-selection protocol.

Table 1 displays the serologic phenotypes of all twelve A^k_β mutant cell lines along with that of the parent TA3 cell line, using a panel of ten A^k_β-reactive mAbs. Reactivity with each of these antibodies has been eliminated in one or more of the mutant cell lines. Several cell lines have lost reactivity with antibodies from more than one epitope group. Several of the mutant cell lines have been extensively characterized for their ability to present antigen to a panel of antigen-reactive I-A^k restricted T hybridomas or to stimulate auto- or alloreactive T hybridomas (summarized in Table 2). Each mutant so far exhibits a unique phenotype.

The 17 kb Eco RI fragment containing the A^k_β gene has been cloned into either Charon 4 or EMBL4 as described (see Materials and Methods). Fragments containing exons 1, 2, and 3, encoding the β_1 and β_2 domains of A^k_β, have been subcloned into bacteriophage M13 for DNA sequence analysis. The sequences are reported in Figure 1. Each mutant so far sequenced has sustained a single nucleotide substitution resulting in a single amino acid substitution in the β_1 domain of the A^k_β polypeptide. The individual substitutions are indicated in Figure 1b.

Revertants were isolated from the LD3 mutant in an attempt to identify residues that might interact to form the serologic epitopes. The LD3 cell line was mutagenized with EMS and then selected for reexpression of the epitope recognized by mAb 10-2.16 by staining with the antibody and sorting

Table 1

Allospecificity	Ia.17			Ia.18	Ia.1				I-A^{k,f,u}	
mAb	10-2.16	11-3.25	4-2.1	4-2.3	39B	39E	40A	40M	40F	40L
Cell Line										
1. TA3 (parent)	++	++	++	++	++	++	++	++	++	++
2. LD3*	±	-	+	-	±	-	-	-	+	+
3. LD3.R2	++	++	++	++	++	++	++	++	++	++
4. LD3.R11	+	++	++	++	++	++	++	++	++	++
5. LD3.R220	++	++	++	++	++	++	++	++	++	++
6. SF14*	±	-	+	-	±	-	-	-	+	+
7. G1	±	++	++	++	++	++	++	++	++	++
8. G1.MF6	-	-	++	++	-	-	-	-	++	++
9. K5	++	++	++	++	+	-	-	-	++	++
10. K5.T15	-	-	++	-	+	-	-	-	++	++
11. F16	++	++	++	-	++	++	++	++	-	-
12. LM4	++	-	-	-	++	++	++	++	-	-
13. LM7	++	++	++	++	++	++	++	++	-	-

Reactivity with these A_{β}^{k}-reactive mAbs was analyzed by indirect immunofluorescence as previously described (Beck et al, 1984). Reactivity levels are designated as follows: - = no detectable reactivity above background; ± = weak reactivity (2-10% of control TA3 level); + = intermediate reactivity (10-30% of control TA3 level); ++ = parental-level reactivity (30-100% of control TA3 level).

*The LD3 and SF14 mutants appear to have lower overall expression of I-A^{k}, in addition to the indicated specific alterations in serologic reactivity, as evidenced by only an intermediate level of reactivity with all A_{α}^{k}-specific mAbs (data not shown).

A

```
          10        20        30        40        50        60        70        80        90

k   GNSERHFVHQFQPFCYFTNGTQRIRLVIRYIYNREEYVRFDSDVGEYRAVTELGRPDAEYWNKQ*Y*LERTRAELDTVCRHNYEKTETPTSLRRLE
b   -D------Y--MGE-----------Y-T-----------Y------H----------------S-PEI-----------------GP--H-------
d   --------V--KGE--Y----------T-----------Y----------------------S-PEI-------V--A------GP--S-------
f   --------F--KGE-----------S-D---------L-----------------S----Y----------------------GV----------
q   --------A-LKGE-----------S-N--------W-------------------------S-PEI-------V---------GV--H-------
s   -D------F--KGE-----------S-D---------L----------------------Y--------Q--------------GV--H-------
u   -D-----LV----------------Y-T---------L----------------------Y-------------------Y---E--V--------
```

B

```
LD3        ---------------------------------------------------------------P--------------------------------
LD3.R2     ------------------------------------------------------------------------------------------------
LD3.R11    ---------------------------------------------------------------L--------------------------------
LD3.R220   ------------------------------------------------------------------------------------------------
G1         ---------------------------------------------------------------R--------------------------------
K5         ---------------------------------------------------------------------Q--------------------------
F16        ---------------------------------------------------------D--------------------------------------
```

Fig. 1. A. Amino acid sequences of the $A_{\beta 1}$ domains of the seven sequenced alleles.

B. Amino acid sequences of seven A_{β}^{k} mutants compared with the parental k sequence.

Table 2. Functional Phenotypes of A^k Mutants

Cell line	Stimulation of A^k-reactive and A^k-restricted T hybridomas*	
	No. tested	No. positive
TA3 (parent)	36	36
LD3	35	20
G1	36	33
K5	23	2
F16	19	17
LM4	5	5
LM7	5	4

*The stimulatory capacity of the cell lines was determined as described in Materials and Methods. In almost all cases, the mutant cell lines were either clearly negative or virtually identical to the parent TA3 cell line in stimulatory capacity. The chief exception is the LD3 cell line which occasionally stimulated weak but clearly positive responses as described in the original report (Beck *et al.*, 1984).

for positive cells with a FACS IV flow cytometer. Three revertant cell lines were obtained in two independent experiments. Of these, two (LD3.R2 and LD3.R220) are true reversions to the parental amino acid at position 64 and one (LD3.R11) has undergone a Pro —> Leu substitution at position 64 in place of the Gln —> Pro substitution in LD3. Thus, none of the revertants has identified an additional residue involved in the formation of the serologic epitopes.

The SF14 mutant was isolated with a selection scheme similar to that used for the isolation of LD3 (Beck et. al., 1984) and B13 (Glimcher et al., 1983b). B13 also was derived from TA3 and differs from LD3 serologically only in reactivity with mAb 4-2.3 (unpublished data). The two mutants display different functional phenotypes (Beck et al., 1984) and have different amino acid substitutions, LD3 a Gln —> Pro at position 64, B13 a Glu —> Lys at position 69 (Brown et al., 1986). Thus, SF14 was isolated to probe further the range of mutations that could result in the basic serologic phenotype of LD3 and B13 (loss of or greatly reduced reactivity with Ia.1 and Ia.17 mAbs). However, despite its independent isolation, SF14 has exactly the same serologic phenotype as LD3 and exactly the same mutation as well.

Four mutants have not yet been sequenced. LM4 and LM7 have lost reactivity with mAbs 40F and 40L, similar to F16, but these two mutants differ from each other and from all others in reactivity with other mAbs. Mutants G1.MF6 and K5.T15 are presumably double mutants, isolated from G1 and K5 respectively, selected for the loss of reactivity with additional mAbs.

DISCUSSION

A comparison of the predicted amino acid sequences based on either gene or cDNA sequences (Choi et al., 1983; Estess et al., 1986) of seven A_β alleles reveals four clusters of variable residues in the β_1 domain (Figure 1a). The distribution among these clusters of the substitutions detected in the mutants so far sequenced is quite striking. All of the substitutions fall near or within the third of the four clusters of allelicly variable residues. The four mutants LD3, G1, K5, and F16 have among them sustained alterations such that reactivity with nine of the ten A_β^k-reactive mAbs has been altered. Thus, it was surprising to find that the mutations are clustered into only one of the four variable regions. This observation very strongly suggests that this region of the polypeptide is serologically dominant. Consistent with this observation are the results previously reported on the sequence analysis of the mutant B13 (Brown et al., 1986), which has a substitution at residue 69, and the A_β^b spontaneous *in vivo* mutant B6.C-H-2^{bm12}, which has substitutions at residues 67, 70, and 71 (McIntyre and Seidman, 1984). Furthermore, of three site-directed A_β^b mutants at positions 9, 13, or 65-67, only the 65-67 substitution altered the serology of the molecule (Cohn et al., 1986). Thus, all of the available data suggest that the region of the polypeptide encompassing the variable residues 61-70 is the major determinant of the serologic alloantigenicity.

While the mutation carried by each cell line appears to have some effect on the functional capacity of the A^k molecule, the magnitude of the effect varies considerably. The F16 cell line is nearly wild-type in function whereas the K5 cell line is nearly completely defective in ability to stimulate A^k-restricted and reactive T hybridomas. As yet no pattern of reactivities has emerged that correlates with either the structural data or the serologic phenotypes. Because these mutants have been isolated in a selection scheme dependent on reactivity with mAbs, the contribution to T cell recognition of the A^k molecule of variable regions not detectable with mAbs cannot be determined by analysis of these mutants. Thus, while substitutions in the serologically dominant, third allellicly variable region of the A^k_β polypeptide can have dramatic effects on the ability of the molecule to be recognized by T cells, studies of cell lines carrying alterations (generated by site-directed mutagenesis and DNA-mediated gene transfer) in the other allelicly variable regions will be needed to examine to what extent these other regions are involved in determining functionally important sites on the I-A molecule.

ACKNOWLEDGEMENTS

This work was supported by NSF grant DCB8417369 (to B.N.B.), NIH grants AI22420 and AI00706 (L.R.P) and NIH grant CA26297 (D.J.M.).

REFERENCES

Beck, B. N., Glimcher, L. H., Nilson, A. E., Pierres, M., and McKean, D. J., 1984, The structure-function relationship of I-A molecules: Correlation of serologic and functional phenotypes of four I-A^k mutant cell lines. J. Immunol., 133:3176.

Beck, B. N., Pease, L. R., Bell, M. P., Buerstedde, J.-M., Nilson, A. E., Schlauder, G. G., and McKean, D. J., 1987, DNA sequence analysis of I-A^k_β mutants reveals serologically immunodominant region. J. Exp. Med., in press.

Benoist, C. O., Mathis, D. J., Kanter, M. R., Williams, V. E., II, McDevitt, H. O., 1983, Regions of allelic hypervariability in the murina A_α immune response gene. Cell, 34:169.

Brown, M. A., Glimcher, L. H., Nielsen, E. A., Paul, W. E., and Germain, R. N., 1986, T-cell recognition of Ia molecules selectively altered by a single amino acid substitution. Science, 231:255.

Choi, E., McIntyre, K., Germain, R. N., and Seidman, J. G., 1983, Murine I-A_β chain polymorphism: Nucleotide sequences of three allelic I-A_β genes. Science, 221:283.

Cohn, L. E., Glimcher, L. H., Waldmann, R. A., Smith, J. A., Ben-Nun, A., Seidman, J. G., and Choi E., 1986, Identification of functional regions on the I-A^b molecule by site-directed mutagenesis. Proc. Natl. Acad. Sci. USA, 83:747.

Estess, P., Begovich, A. B., Koo, M., Jones, P. P., and McDevitt, H. O., 1986, Sequence analysis and structure-function correlations of murine q, k, u, s, and f haplotype I-A$_\beta$ cDNA clones. Proc. Natl. Acad. Sci. USA, 83:3594.

Germain, R. N., Ashwell, J. D., Lechler, R. I., Margulies, D. H., Nickerson, K. M., Suzuki, G., and Tou, J. Y. L., 1985, "Exon-shuffling" maps control of antibody and T-cell-recognition sites to the NH_2-terminal domain of the class II major histocompatibility polypeptide A$_\beta$. Proc. Natl. Acad. Sci. USA, 82:2940.

Glimcher, L. H., Hamano, T., Asofsky, R., Sachs, D. H., Pierres, M., Samelson, L. E., Sharrow, S. O., and Paul, W. E., 1983a, I-A mutant functional antigen-presenting cell lines. J. Immunol., 130:2287.

Glimcher, L. H., Sharrow, S. O., and Paul, W. E., 1983b, Serologic and functional characterization of a panel of antigen-presenting cell lines expressing mutant I-A class II molecules. J. Exp. Med., 158:1523.

Harmon, R. C., Stein, N., and Frelinger, J. A., 1983, Monoclonal antibodies reactive with H-2 determinants. Immunogenetics, 18:541.

Landais, D., Matthes, H., Benoist, C., and Mathis, D., 1985, A molecular basis for the Ia.2 and Ia.19 antigenic determinants. Proc. Natl. Acad. Sci. USA, 83, 747.

McIntyre, K. R., and Seidman, J. G., 1984, Nucleotide sequence of mutant I-A^{bm12} gene is evidence for genetic exchange between mouse immune response genes. Nature, 308, 551.

Oi, V. T., Jones, P. P., Goding, J. W., Herzenberg, L. A., and Herzenberg, L. A., 1978, Properties of monoclonal antibodies to mouse Ig allotypes, H-2, and Ia antigens. Curr. Top. Microbiol. Immunol., 81:115.

Pierres, M., Devaux, C., Dosseto, N., and Marchetto, S., 1981, Clonal analysis of B- and T-cell responses to Ia antigens. I. Topology of epitope regions on I-A^k and I-E^k molecules analyzed with 35 monoclonal antibodies. Immunogenetics, 14:481.

Robinson, R. R., Germain, R. N., McKean, D. J., Mescher, M., and Seidman, J. G., 1983, Extensive polymorphism surrounding the murine Ia A_β chain gene. J. Immunol., 131:2025.

Sanger, F., Nicklen, S., Coulson, A. R., 1977, DNA sequencing with chain-terminating inhibitors. Proc. Natl. Acad. Sci. USA, 74:5463.

Schlauder, G. G., Bell, M. P., Beck, B. N., Nilson, A., and McKean, D. J., 1985, The structure-function relationship of I-A molecules: A biochemical analysis of I-A polypeptides from mutant antigen-presenting cells and evidence of preferential association of allelic forms. J. Immunol., 135:1945.

TRANSGENIC MICE: NEW SYSTEMS FOR STUDYING THE FUNCTION OF MHC CLASS II MOLECULES

Gabrielle Lang, Philippe Gerber, Jan Bohme, Beatrice Durand, Jorg Fehling, Marianne Le Meur, Corinne Marfing, Christophe Benoist and Diane Mathis

Institut de Chimie Biologique - Faculte de Medicine
11, rue Human
67085 Strasbourg (France)

ABSTRACT

Transgenic mice have great potential as systems for studying the function of major histocompatibility complex class II molecules. Several mouse lines that bear a wild-type E alpha transgene have been created and characterized. The transgene is expressed efficiently, accurately, and with tissue- and cell type-specificity. The recipient (E alpha negative) strain is endowed with new immunological capabilities ; namely, it can now respond to E-restricted antigens. Other transgenic lines have been created by injecting E alpha clones that harbor promoter deletions. These mice display novel patterns of E alpha expression eg absent on B cells, but present on peripheral macrophages and in the thymus ; or absent in the thymic cortex but present in the medulla. These mice may provide new insights into tolerance induction, MHC restriction etc.

INTRODUCTION

Transgenic mice are produced by injecting a cloned gene into fertilized mouse eggs and reimplanting the embryos into foster mothers. Amongst the offspring are some that have incorporated the injected gene into the germline and transmit it to subsequent generations in a stable fashion. These offspring can serve as founders for transgenic lines. In many transgenic lines, the incorporated gene is expressed efficiently, accurately, and with tissue- and developmental stage- specificity (Brinster and Palmiter, 1986 ; Palmiter and Brinster, 1986).

The list of injected DNAs has grown beyond easy enumeration, but it includes genes expressed in divergent cell-types, several oncogenes, and loci involved in the workings of various systems of the body. (Palmiter and Brinster, 1986). In particular, several genes that operate in the immune system have been injected into mouse eggs, and transgenic lines with novel immune capabilities derived. (for reviews, see Alt et al, 1985 ; Benoist et al, 1986 ; Storb, 1987).

New systems for studying the function of major histocompatibility complex (MHC) class II molecules can be created using transgenic mice. Our progress in this direction is summarized below. Some of the transgenic lines have already been described (Le Meur et al, 1985 ; Flood et al, 1986 ; Dorn et al, 1987a) ; others will be presented in more detail elsewhere (eg. Dorn et al, in preparation).

Creation of Eα transgenic lines

It was first necessary to demonstrate tnat an MHC class II transgene can function correctly. An excellent system for establishing this point is provided by mice of the H-2^b and H-2^s haplotypes (Jones et al, 1981 ; Mathis et al, 1983 ; Dembic et al, 1985). These mice have a 627 base pair (bp) deletion that encompasses the promoter region and first exon of the E_α gene. Consequently, they make no E_α mRNA or protein, they display nc E_α:E_β complex at the cell surface even though the E_β gene functions normally, and they are unable to make an antibody response to E-restricted antigens like GLØ and moth cytochrome C. We decided, then, to inject a cloned E_α^k gene into C57B16 x SJL (H-2^b x H-2^s) eggs and develop transgenic lines from them.

To date, we have established four such lines (Le Meur et al, 1985 and unpublished data ; see Table I for details). As far as we can tell, transcription of the E_α^k transgene faithfully mimics normal class II gene expression. Northern blotting and S1 mapping experiments on spleen RNA established that transcription from the transgene is efficient and accurate. It is also tissue- and cell type- specific, according to four lines of evidence : 1) S1 analysis of RNA from various tissues shows that the E_α transgene is transcribed concomitantly with the endogenous A_α gene (Le Meur et al, 1985).

2) S1 analysis of "panned" B and T cell RNAs shows an enrichment of transcripts from both $A_\alpha$and the E_α transgene in B cell fractions, and a depletion in T cell fractions.

3) Two-dimensional cytoflourimetric analysis of splenocytes simultaneously stained with an anti-E and an anti-A or an anti-E and an anti-IgM reagent demonstrates that essentially all A^+ cells and all IgM^+ cells are also E^+ (Le Meur et al, 1985).

4) Flourescence microscopy of thymic sections stained with anti-A and anti-E reagents shows that the E_α transgene is expressed normally in the thymic cortex and medulla.

Transgene expression can be induced in macrophages by treatment with gamma interferon (γIFN) and in B cells by interleukin-4. Two other groups have produced E_α transgenic lines and they also have documentated the fidelity of transcription from the injected gene (Yamamura et al, 1985 ; Pinkert et al, 1985).

Can the E_α transgene endow new immunological capabilities on the recipient strain ? Quite clearly, the answer is yes. Spleen cells from E_α transgenics, but not from the H-2^{bxs} recipients, can act as antigen presenting cells for T hybridomas specific for a herpes simplex glycopeptide seen in the context of E (Pinkert et al, 1985). Also, GLØ-primed E_α transgenics yield lymph node cells that proliferate in response to this E-restricted antigen, whereas lymph nodes from identically primed H-2^b haplotype controls are unreactive (Yamamura et al, 1985). As the ultimate test of immune response gene function, the blood of E_α transgenics was titred for anti-GLØ antibodies after two challenges with the antigen (Le Meur et al, 1985). These mice make a healthy anti-GLØ response, but the recipient strain does not. Finally, H-2^b and H-2^s haplotype mice do not express the I-J^k determinant ; E_α^k transgenic mice become I-J^k positive (Flood et al, 1986).

TABLE I LINES CARRYING A WILD-TYPE E^k_α TRANSGENE

Transgenic line	DNA injected	Amount of 5' flanking sequence	Transgene copy number[1]	Expression in				Anti GLØ response[4]	Reference[5]
				splenic B cells[2]	peritoneal macrophages (+γIFN)[2]	thymic cortex[3]	thymic medulla[3]		
E_α 16	BglI fragment from λA/Jp34.13	2 kb	8-12	+++	+++	+++	+++	+++	Le Meur et al, 1985
E_α 23	λA/Jp34.13 - entire clone, with λ arms	5 kb	4	+++	+++	ND	ND	+++	Le Meur et al, 1985
WE32.25	BglI fragment from WE32	2 kb	~4	+++	+++	+++	+++	+++	Dorn et al 1987a
WE32.29	BglI fragment from WE32	2 kb	~4	+++	+++	ND	ND	ND	Dorn et al 1987b

(1) Estimated from Southern blots of tail DNA.

(2) Evaluated by S1 analysis of RNA and by cytoflourimetric analysis of stained cells

(3) Evaluated by microscopic analysis of stained tissue sections.

(4) Quantitated by ELISA on blood drawn after a secondary challange.

(5) Some of the data are published as indicated ; some remains unpublished.

(6) WE32 is a plasmid carrying the 9 kb XbaI fragment from λA/Jp34.13. It has three minor modifications that are detailed in Dorn et al, 1987a.

Thus by all criteria we (and others) have considered, the E_α transgene functions normally : it is transcribed efficiently and specifically, and its product functions normally within the immune system.

Compartmentalizing Eα transgene expression

MHC class II molecules, or Ia antigens as they are known in the mouse, function in various compartments of the immune system :

1) They occur on the surface of macrophages and other antigen presenting cells. Ample evidence now exists that antigen (or a processed derivative) binds directly to class II molecules ; it is the specificity of this antigen:Ia interaction that "restricts" T_H cell recognition and subsequent activation (Buus et al, 1987 ; Guillet et al, 1987).

2) Ia antigens are expressed at high levels on B cells. Class II molecules seem to be involved in regulating T-B cell cooperation during the antibody response. They also function in antigen presentation by B cells *in vitro*, but it is not yet clear whether B cell presentation has significance *in vivo*. (Ron and Sprent, 1987 and references therein).

3) Ia antigens occur in the thymic cortex on epithelial cells, and in the medulla on macrophages and dendritic cells. Class II molecules on the cortical epithelium have been implicated in imprinting MHC restriction ; molecules on the medulla are thought to function in tolerance induction, particularly to "self" MHC antigens (Lo et al, 1986 and references therein).

It is clear, then, that class II molecules play a multi-faceted role in regulating the immune response. However, the mechanisms involved remain largely obscure. As one approach to elucidating these mechanisms we have sought to compartmentalize class II gene expression in transgenic mice. More specifically, we attempted to create transgenic lines that have a particular Ia molecule expressed on the thymic epithelium but not the cortex and *vice versa*, or in B cells but not macrophages and *vice versa*.

Experiments on the original E_α^k transgenic mice indicated that correct expression of the transgene can be achieved in all compartments by injecting an 8.4 kilobase (kb) genomic fragment bearing only 2 kb of 5' flanking DNA. In order to produce altered patterns of expression, we made various deletions at the 5' end of the E_α^k clone and injected these mutant constructs into embryos. The points of deletion were chosen primarily on the basis of DNA sequence comparisons, assuming that segments important for expression would be conserved amongst all of the class II genes. In addition, we considered preliminary functional data on the delineation of sequences required for E_α transcription. Several transgenic lines that exhibit novel patterns of E_α expression have now been created (see Table II for details). These are :

WEΔY301.54 This line originates from an embryo that was injected with an E_α^k fragment bearing a clean deletion of the 14 bp Y box. The Y box is situated about 50 bp upstream from the startsite of E_α RNA initiation, and its position and sequence is conserved amongst all MHC class II genes. It is the recognition site for a sequence-specific DNA-binding protein, NF-Y (Dorn et al, 1987a,b ; Hooft van Huijsduijnen et al, 1987). Thus, it is not surprising that most mice carrying this construct transcribe E_α weakly and inaccurately, and express no detectable cell-surface E complex. However, WEΔY301.54 mice have about 60 copies of the mutant trangene, and express readily detectable E complex in the thymus and in the periphery. In the thymus, E_α occurs on cortical epithelial cells, but not on the medullary macrophages ; in the periphery, E_α is expressed essentially on B cells. Thus, the WEΔY301.54 line seems to lack E_α expresssion on macrophages, whether thymic or peripheral. Furthermore, macrophage expression can not be induced by treatment with γIFN. WEΔY301.54 mice are not able to make an effective antibody response against GLØ after a secondary challenge with this E-restricted antigen.

TABLE II LINES WITH ABERRANT PATTERNS OF E_{α}^{k} TRANSGENE EXPRESSION

Transgenic line	DNA injected	Transgene copy number[1]	Expression in				anti GLØ response[1]	Reference
			splenic B cells[1]	peritoneal macrophages (+γIFN)[1]	thymic cortex[1]	thymic medulla[1]		
WEΔY301.54	BglI fragment of E_{α}^{k} mutant bearing a Y box deletion	∿ 60	++	-	+++	-	+/-	Dorn et al, 1987a
WEΔX21.16	BglI fragment of E_{α}^{k} mutant bearing an X box deletion	∿ 20	+++	++	-	+++	-	Dorn et al, 1987a
Sma 58	SmaI-BglI fragment of E_{α}^{k} [2]	∿ 4	- (< 4%)	++	+++	+++	+++	Dorn et al, in preparation
Sma 65	SmaI-BglI fragment of E_{α}^{k} [2]	∿ 3	- (< 4%)	++	+++	+++	+++	Dorn et al, in preparation

(1) Explained in Table I.

(2) This fragment has only 1 kb of 5' flanking sequence, rather than the usual 2 kb (as with the BglI fragment).

WEΔX21.16 These mice derive from an embryo injected with an E_{α}^{k} fragment bearing a clean X box deletion. The 14 bp X box is situated 17 or 18 bp uptream from the Y box, ie about 70 bp upstream from the mRNA initiation site. It, too, is conserved amongst all MHC class II genes and serves as the recognition sequence for a DNA-binding protein, in this case NF-X (Dorn et al, 1987a). Most of the mice carrying this mutant trangene transcribe it feebly and inaccurately. But one line, WEΔX21.16, expresses E_{α} RNA at essentially normal levels in the periphery ; the E complex is detected both on B cells and on γIFN-treated peritoneal macrophages. It was surprising, then, to find that WEΔX21.16 mice are incapable of mounting an antibody response to GLØ after two injections of this antigen. A careful analysis of stained tissue sections revealed that the defect lies in thymic expression of E_{α} ; although E complex is expressed in the medulla, it is absent from the cortical epithelium.

Sma 58 and Sma 65 Two lines were developed from embryos injected with an E_{α}^{k} fragment bearing only 1 kb of 5' flanking sequence instead of the usual 2 kb. The stretch of DNA between one and two kilobases upstream from the RNA initiation site harbors several interesting sequence motifs (Dorn et al, in preparation) : 1) another X and Y box 2) W, a segment that serves as the recognition site for a B cell-specific DNA-binding protein 3) E_{α} κB, a sequence that bears a striking resemblance to an important segment of the Igκ gene enhancer (Sen and Baltimore, 1986a,b). The absence of any or all of these sequence motifs might explain the fact that Sma 58 and Sma 65 mice are essentially devoid of E complex on B cells. Furthermore, expression can not be induced by treatment of splenocytes with either interleukin-4 or rabbit anti-mouse immunoglobulin. In contrast, expression of E_{α} is detected on the peritoneal macrophages of Sma 58 and Sma 65 mice as is expression in the thymic cortex and medulla. Despite the apparent absence of E complex on B cells, these mice are able to mount an effective antibody response to injected GLØ antigen.

Thus, we have been able to create transgenic lines with novel patterns of MHC class II gene expression. Analysis of the immunological capabilities of these mice are as yet only preliminary. We hope that more extensive analyses will reveal much about the role of class II molecules in immunological phenomena such as MHC restriction, tolerance induction and B cell presentation.

ACKNOWLEDGEMENTS

This work was supported by institutional grants from the INSERM and the CNRS, and by grants to DM and CB from the Association pour la Recherche contre le Cancer, la Fondation de France, the Juvenile Diabetes Foundation and the National Multiple Sclerosis Society. J.B. received a fellowship from the European Molecular Biology Organization and J.F. had fellowships from the Deutscher Akademischer Austauschdienst, the Dr. Carl Duisberg Stiffung and the Boehringer Ingelheim Foundation.

REFERENCES

Alt, F.W., Blackwell, T.K., and Yancopoulos, G.D.: Immunoglobulin genes in transgenic mice. Trends in Genetics 1:231-236,1985

Benoist, B., Gerlinger, P., LeMeur, M., and Mathis, D.: Transgenic mice: "new wave" immunogenetics. Immunology Today 7:138-141,1986

Brinster, R.L., and Palmiter, R.D.: Introduction of genes into the germ line of animals. The Harvey Lectures, series 80:1-38,1986

Buus, S., Sette, A., Colon, S.M., Miles, C., Grey, H.M.: The relation between major histocompatibility complex (MHC) restriction and the capacity of Ia to bind immunogenic peptides. Science 235:1353-1358, 1987

Dembic, Zlatko, Ayane, M., Klein, J., Steinmetz, M., Benoist, C.O., and Mathis, D.J.: Inbred and wild mice carry identical deletions in their E_α MHC genes. EMBO J. 4:127-131,1985

Dorn, A., Durand, B., Marfing, C., Le Meur, M., Benoist, C., Mathis, D.: The conserved MHC class II boxes -X and Y- are transcriptional control elements and specifically bind nuclear proteins. Proc. Natl. Acad. Sci. USA in press 1987a

Dorn, A., Bollekens, J., Staub, A., Benoist, C., and Mathis, D.: A multiplicity of CCAAT box-binding proteins. Cell, in press 1987b

Flood, P.M., Benoist, C., Mathis, D., and Murphy, D.B.: Altered I-J phenotype in E_α transgenic mice. Proc. Natl. Acad. Sci. USA 83:8308-8312, 1986

Guillet, J.G., Lai, M.Z., Briner, T.J., Buus, S., Sette, A., Grey, H.M., Smith, J.A., Gefter, M.L.: Immunological self, nonself discrimination. Science 235:865-870,1987

Hooft Van Huijsduijnen, R., Bollekens, J., Dorn, A., Benoist, C., and Mathis, D.: Properties of a CCAAT box-binding protein. Nucl. Acids. Res. submitted, 1987.

Jones, P.P., Murphy. D.B., and McDevitt, H.O.: Variable synthesis and expression of E_α and A_e (E_β)Ia polypeptide chains in mice of different H-2 haplotypes. Immunogenetics 12:321-337,1981

Le Meur, M., Gerlinger, P., Benoist, C., and Mathis, D.: Correcting an immune-response deficiency by creating E_α gene transgenic mice. Nature 316:38-42,1985

Lo, D., Ron, Y., Sprent, J.: Induction of MHC-restricted specificity and tolerance in the thymus. Immunol. Res. 5:221-232,1986

Mathis, D.J., Benoist, C.O., Williams, V.E., Kanter, M., and McDevitt, H.O: Several mechanisms can account for E_α gene expression in different mouse haplotypes. Proc. Natl. Acad. Sci. U.S.A. 80:273-277, 1983

Palmiter, R.D., and Brinster, R.L.: Germ-line transformation of mice. Ann. Rev. Genet. 20:465-499,1986

Pinkert, C.A., Widera, G., Cowing, C., Heber-Katz, E., Palmiter, R.D., Flavell, R.A., and Brinster, R.L.:Tissue-specific, inducible and functional expression of the E_α^d MHC class II gene in transgenic mice. EMBO J. 4:2225-2230,1985

Ron, Y., and Sprent, J.:T cell priming in vivo: a major role for B cells in presenting antigen to T cells in lymph nodes. J. Immunology 138: 2848-2856,1987

Sen, R., and Baltimore, D.:Multiple nuclear factors interact with the immunoglobulin enhancer sequences. Cell 46:000-000,1986

Sen, R., and Baltimore, D.:Inducibility of κ immunoglobulin enhancer-binding protein NF-κB by a posttranslational mechanism. Cell 47: 921-928,1986

Storb, U.:Transgenic mice with immunoglobulin genes. Ann. Rev. Immunol. 5:151-174,1987

Yamamura, K.I., Kikutani, H., Folsom, V., Clayton, L.K., Kimoto, M., Akira, S., Kashiwamura, S.I., Tonegwa, S., and Kishimoto, T.:Functional expression of a microinjected E_α^d gene in C57BL/6 transgenic mice. Nature 316, 67-69,1985.

ACTIVATION OF I-A GENE PRODUCTS BY A_β GENE TRANSFECTION USING BOVINE PAPILLOMA VIRUS - VECTOR SYSTEMS

Kenji Okuda, Jun Fukushima, Susumu Kawamoto, Ichiro Aoki* and Toyozoh Takahashi

Departments of Bacteriology and *Pathology, Yokohama City University School of Medicine, Yokohama, Japan

SUMMARY

The bovine papilloma virus (BPV) recombinant which carried class II MHC (A_β^d) gene (pBPA$_\beta$-d) has been constructed at first. The recombinant plasmid was introduced into the mouse B cell hybridoma by co-transfection method with neomycin resistance gene. Using this method we could impose into B cell hybridomas many copies of A_β^d genes extrachromosomally. The several transfectants which had been introduced only beta chain gene of I-A^d have been revealed to expressed the I-A^d proteins on the cell surface by direct immunofluorescent technique. Moreover, these I-A^d molecules could induce the IL-2 production of the I-A^d restricted autoreactive T cell hybridoma. So I-A^d molecules which express on the cell surface of the transfectants are fully functional to the T-cell response. RNA dot-blot analysis has revealed that the cells express not only A_β^d gene but also A_α^d gene. Thus, A_β^d gene transfection induced the expression of internally latent A_α^d gene by trans gene effect.

INTRODUCTION

The class II major histocompatibility (MHC) antigens have been elucidated to play some important roles in cell-cell interactions of the immune system[1-3]. T cells recognize antigen with the association of appropriate class II antigens on the surface of antigen presenting cells with the altered or dual recognition system[4]. Efficient membrane expression of Ia molecules appears to require assembly of α:β pairs[5-10], and individual chains have generally not been detected on the cell surface[7,11]. To analyze more detail of the function and regulation of MHC gene, we employ the gene transfer experiments into the mammalian cultured cells using bovine papilloma virus shuttle vector system. Bovine papilloma virus replicates extrachromosomally in the rodent cells and its copy number is high, so gene can be introduced into the cells efficiently and its function could be analyzed easier[12].

In the previous study, we reported that the bovine papilloma-virus vector system was far more efficient and could inject over 5-10 times more copies of gene into the fibroblastic cells by the co-transfection with neomycin resistance gene (Fukushima et al. submitted). Using this method, we could introduce the class II MHC, A_β^d gene into the non-fibroblastic cells, i.e. B cell hybridoma or fibroblast.

To clarify the molecular interaction of antigen and MHC antigen, we transfected A_β^d gene into B cell hybridomas, which did not express both A_α^d and A_β^d gene products. Our results revealed that these transfected cells were detected to express A^d gene product by immunofluorescent test and these A^d gene product induced IL-2 production using autoreactive T cell hybridomas.

MATERIALS AND METHODS

Cultured mice cell and bacterial strain. The B cell hybridomas that produced anti-thyloglobulin antibody (hybridoma A) and antibody non-producer (hybridoma B) were used in the DNA transfection experiment. These hybridomas were obtained from fusions of the NS-1 cell line with spleen of BALB/c mice. The *Escherichia coli* HB101 was used as the host of DNA recombination experiments.

Plasmids. Plasmid pdBPV-1 containing the entire bovine papilloma-virus sequense was kindly provided by P.M.Howly. That plasmid works as vector in both *E. coli* and rodent cultured cells in which this plasmid replicates at episomal state and the multi copy number. This plasmid was recombinated with the A_β gene, the class II major histcompatibility complex gene, at the region of the bacterial vector with replacement of the smallest fragment of EcoRI-BamHI digestion, that is called pBA_β-d plasmid.

Transfection. Transfection experiment of B-cell hybridoma was performed by the calcium phosphate method as described by elsewhere[13]. Briefly, 10 ug of each pBAbeta-d and pSV2neo DNA were used to co-transfect 2 x 10^6 hybridoma cells. After 15 hours incubation with the calcium phosphate-DNA precipitate, the cells were washed with serum-free medium and cultured with normal medium containing antibiotics G418 (Gibco Co.) at 200 ug/ml. After 3 weeks G418 resistrant colonies were isolated, propagated and analyzed the existance of A_β sequence in the low molecular weight DNA fraction. Low molecular weight, extrachromosomal DNA was prepared according the method of Hirt[14], and analyzed the standard hybridization experiment.

RNA preparation and blot hybridization analysis. Total RNA was isolated by the method of Manser and Gefter[15]. RNA samples were blotted to the nitrocellulose filter using blotting chamber (Bio-Rad). Then the filter was dried and hybridized with various ^{32}P labeled probes according to standard hybridization technique. And the filter was washed at high stringent conditions.

Monoclonal antibodies. Monoclonal antibodies were obtained from American Type Culture Association.

T cell hybridoma. Mouse splenocytes from (NZB/NZE)F mice were incubated in anti-mouse Ig-coated plate for 60 min at room temparature. Unbound cells were collected and reincubated with the above plates. These partially purified T cells were then hybridized with AKR derived BW5147 thymomas. Detailed hybridization techniques and cloning methods will be described elsewhere (Yanoma et al. submitted).

Cell cultures. Both IL-2 stimulation and IL-2 assay were described previously[5]. In brief, 3 x 10^4 T cell hybridomas were cultured with or without varying numbers (1-3 x 10^6) of mitomycin C (MMC)-treated stimulator cells. Cultures were incubated at 37 C for 18 to 24 hr, at which time 100 ul of culture supernatant were harvested. The IL-2 content of culture supernatants were measured with an IL-2 dependent T cell line, CTLL.

Table 1. Copy Number of Episomal Circular DNA in Transfected Cell Lines

Cell lines	AB1	AB2	BB1	AV-1	BV-1	A
Copy number per cell	45	33	52	81	92	0

The copy number of extrachromosomal DNA was determined by the dot blot hybridization experiment and scanning densitometry. Low molecular weight, extrachromosomal DNA was prepared by the method of Hirt as described in Materials and Methods.

Immunofluorescent test. Specimens of glass smeared hybridomas were studied by immunoflurorescence.

Data analysis. Statistical analysis of the experimental data as compared to controls was calculated using two-tailed Student's t-test.

RESULTS

Establishment of transfected B cell hybridomas. In the present study we chose Ia B cell hybridomas for our purpose. Four cell lines which incorporated pBA_{β}-d gene were selected among these transfected B cell hybridomas. The methods to construct the pBA_{β}-d plasmid in details have been described in Materials and Methods. The pBA_{β}-d and pSV2 neo DNA were co-transfected into B cell hybridomas. After 3 weeks of continuous medium exchange, neomycin-resistant hybridomas were collected. These established cell lines were recloned with a single cell manupilation method. The first experiment was designed to see whether or not these established cell hybridomas contain extrachromosomal A_{β}^{d} gene. DNA from low molecular weight fraction from various hybridomas was isolated and hybridized with ^{32}P labeled probes. Table 1 show these data. All of the pBA_{β}-d transfected hybridomas contained extrachromosomal A_{β}^{d} gene, while control non-transfected hybridomas displayed no A_{β}^{d} gene.

Surface phenotypes and $I\text{-}A^{d}$ gene product on the surface of transfected hybridoma. Surface phenotypes of the transfected hybridoma were tested with both the immunofluorescent and microcytotoxic test. Interestingly, both AB1 and AB2 were positive of $I\text{-}A^{d}$ gene products (Table 2), since both hybridoma lines were only A_{β}^{d} injected cells. While BB1, AV-1, A, and B were negative for it. Both AB1 and AB2 were still immunoglobulin secreting cells. Cytoplasmic chain were detected in both B and BB1. Of course all cells were negative for Thy 1 antigen. These results suggest that these hybridomas are in the B cell lineage.

IL-2 activation by autoreactive T cell hybridoma. The next experiment was designed to see whether these activated $I\text{-}A^{d}$ gene products were able to induce IL-2 production into $I\text{-}A^{d}$ specific autoreactive T cell hybridomas. Each B cell hybridoma treated by mitomycin C was incubated with autoreactive T cell hybridomas. As another control we employed both BALB/c($H\text{-}2^{d}$) and B10.BR ($H\text{-}2^{k}$) spleen cells. In addition, in certain experiments the final concentration of 1ng/ml of monoclonal

Table 2. Expression of Surface Antigens of DNA-Transfected Cells

Cells		Antibodies		
Strains	Transfected DNA	Anti-cyt-μ	Anti-I-A^d (MDK6)	Anti-I-A^d (17-227)
AB1	pBA_β-d	–	+++	+
AB2	"	–	+	+
BB1	"	+[a]	–	–
AV-1	pdBPV-1	–	–	–
A	---	–	–	–
B	---	+	–	–

Except Thy-1 antigen, all of the other tests were done with immunofluorescent techniques. [a]+ means over the 60% of these cells were positive by these tests. [b]+++ means the titer of over 128 times. In addition, all cell lines were Thy 1(-).

antibody was added in these reaction systems. After 18-24 hrs, IL-2 production of each of these cultured supernatnat was assayed using IL-2 dependent CTLL cell lines. As shown in Table 3, both AB1 and AB2 could stimulate autoreactive T cell hybridoma to induce IL-2 production. These IL-2 production was inhibited by addition of monoclonal anti-I-A^d antibody. However, BB1 or BB2 could not induce IL-2 production into T cell hybridomas.

Transcription of I-A^d transfected hybridoma. The last experiment was designed to study whether or not these A_β^d gene-transfected hybridoma could also transcribe A_α^d gene. Messenger RNA was purified as described in Materials and Methods, and dot hybridization was performed using A_α^d probe. Figure 1 shows the results of these experiments. Messenger RNA of A_α^d gene was confirmed in both AB1 and AB2. But A, AV-1, and BB1 hybridomas were not shown to have A_α^d messenger RNA in their cells. Thus our present experiment clearly demonstrated that only one gene transfection can activate other related gene by trans gene effect.

DISCUSSION

Our present study clearly demonstrated that pBA_β-d transfected B cell hybridoma was activated not only A_β^d gene but also A_α^d gene. This activation was observed by both immunofluorescent test and dot hybridization technique. In addition, this A^d product was biologically detected by IL-2 production using autoreactive T cell hybridoma.

In the present study A_β^d gene transfection could also induce A_α^d gene expression in some B cell hybridomas. But most of the previous reports[6,7,11,16] of class II gene transfection have revealed that the

Table 3. Response of I-A^d Restricted T cell Hybridoma to to A_β^d Transfected B cell

Stimulaor	Transfected DNA	IL-2 production ($x10^2$ cpm)		
		No antibody	Anti-I-A^k	Anti-I-A^d
BALB/c spleen cell	---	97.6 ± 11.3	95.4 ± 5.6	18.3 ± 4.3
B10.BR spleen cell	---	3.1 ± 1.0	N.T.	N.T.
AB1	pB_β^d	61.2 ± 6.7	57.9 ± 6.2	16.7 ± 2.3
AB2	pB_β^d	66.9 ± 9.6	63.6 ± 9.0	6.4 ± 1.2
BB1	pB_β^d	4.3 ± 0.6	5.2 ± 1.0	4.9 ± 0.4
AV-1	pdBPV-1	3.0 ± 0.5	N.T.	N.T.
A	---	4.1 ± 1.1	N.T.	N.T.

N.T. : Not tested

MMC-treated stimulator cells ($1-3 \times 10^6$) were co-cultured with 3×10^4 autoreactive (I-A^d) T cell hybridomas for 18-24 hours in the presence or absence of anti-Ia antibodies. The released IL-2 was assayed with CTLL cell line.

reports [6,7,11,16] of class II gene transfection have revealed that the only injected one gene makes only one gene produced in the transfected cells. These experiments were observed by Ca phosphate co-transfection or spheroplast fusion methods using fibroblast (L cells) as the host cell. But the methods that we used and those previous observations were different. In the present study we used bovine-papilloma virus as the vector system. This system has a good point to inject many genes into one host cell. But these imposed DNA exist extrachromosomally.

In the present study A^d gene products were observed only in some hybridomas. Thus, various types of B cell hybridomas exist in our present exteriment. The data of DNA dot hybridization reveals pBA_β-d gene was incorporated equally in each hybridoma. In the normal B cell differentiation, cytoplasmic µ chain appears in the immature stage and both class II and Ig secretion were observed in mature stage. From the present data we are now considering that in some hybridoma might not have enough enzymes to activate class II antigen, because of its immaturity. To confirm this idea we are now making a vast series of B cell hybridomas, which display various steps of B cell differentiation. The host cells that have been reported elsewhere [6,7,11,16] were mostly L cells. Only a few reports are studied with B cells [4,17]. We have not enough data to compare these cells using BPV-vector system. However, none of the report have mentioned one (A_β chain) gene activates another A_α chain gene. These previous reports are also indirectly suggesting the A gene activation is resulting from the host cell enzymes or some factors.

This is the first report to observe only A_β^d gene transfection could

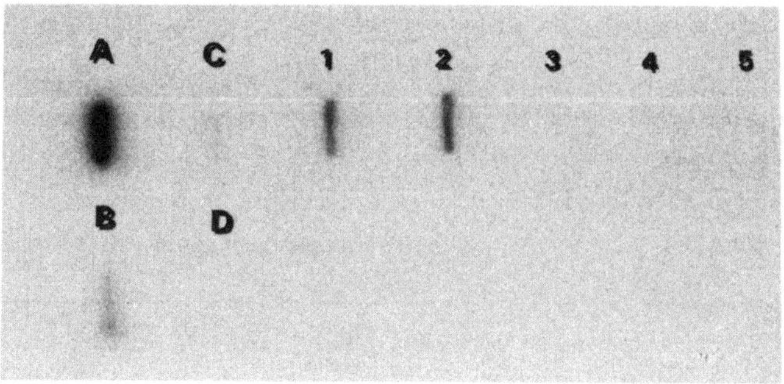

Fig. 1. Analysis of A-alpha mRNA Sequence in The Transfected or Nontransfected Cells by Dot Blot Hybridization.

Total cytoplasmic mRNA was prepared from the cells of AB1 (1), AB2 (2), BB1 (3), A (4), and B (5) by the method of White and Bancroft (J.B.C., 1982). Hybridization with the ^{32}P labeled probe of A-alpha fragment at the high stringent conditions and autoradiography were performed. 100 pg, 10 pg, 1 pg, and 0 pg of probe DNA was dotted at A,B,C, and D, respectively as controls.

induce resting A_{α}^{d} gene activation. These results were obtained with the BPV-vector and B cell hybridoma as host system. In the present study several new findings were obtained using these systems. However, more detailed analysis is necessary to explain these new issues.

ACKNOWLEDGEMENTS

We would like to express our thanks to Misses K. Saito and K. Chiba for their technical and secretarial assistances.

REFERENCES

1. Benacerraf, B. and H.O. McDevitt. Histocompatibility-linked immune response genes : A new class of genes that controls the formation of specific immune responses has been identified. Science 175 : 273 (1972).

2. Klein, J., A. Juretic, C.N. Baxevanis, and Z.A. Nagy. The traditional and a new version of the mouse H-2 complex. Nature (London) 291 : 455 (1981).

3. Hammerling, G., B. Deak, G. Mauve, U. Hammerling, and H.O. McDevitt. B lymphocyte alloantigens controlled by the I region of the major histocompatibility complex in mice. Immunogenetics 1 : 68 (1974).

4. Schwartz, R. H. T lymphocyte recognition of antigen in association with gene products of the major histocompatibility complex. Ann. Rev. Immunol. 3 : 262 (1985).

5. Kappler, J., B. Skidmore, J. White, and P. Marrack. Antigen-inducible, H-2 restricted, interleukin-2 producing T cell hybridomas. Lack of independent antigen and H-2 recognition. J. Exp. Med. 153 : 1198 (1981).

6. Rabourdin-Combe, C., and B. Mach. Expression of HLA-DR antigens at the surface of mouse L cells co-transfected with cloned human genes. Nature 303 : 670 (1983).

7. Norcross, M. A., D. M. Bentley, D. H. Margulies, and R. N. Germain. Membrane Ia expression and antigen-presenting accessory cell funtion of L cells transfectecd with class II major histocompatibility complex genes. J. Exp. Med. 160 : 1316 (1984).

8. Jones, P. P., D. B. Murphy, and H. O. McDevitt. Two gene control of the expression of a murine Ia antigen. J. Exp. Med. 148 : 925 (1978).

9. Shackelford, D. A., L. Lampson, and J. L. Strominger. Separation of three class II antigens from a homozygous human B cell line. J. Immunol. 130 : 289 (1983).

10. Kaufman, J. F., C. Auffray, A. J. Korman, D. A. Shackelford, and J. Strominger. The class II molecules of the human and murine major histocompatibility complex. Cell 36 : 1 (1984).

11. Malissen, B., M. Steinmetz, M. McMillan, M. Pierres, and L. Hood. Expression of $I\text{-}A^{k}$ molecules in mouse L cells after DNA-mediated gene transfer. Nature 305 : 440 (1983).

12. Law, M. F., D. R. Lowy, I. Dvoretzky, and P. M. Howly. Mouse cells transformed by bovine papilloma virus contain only extrachromosomal viral DNA sequences. Proc. Natl. Acad. Sci. USA 78 : 2727 (1981).

13. Karin. M., G. Cathala, and M. C. Nguyen-Huu. Expression and regulation of a human metallothionein gene carried on an autonomously replicating shuttle vector. Proc. Natl. Acad. Sci. USA 80 : 4040 (1983).

14. Hirt, B. Selective extraction of polyoma DNA from infected mouse cell cultures. J. Mol. Bilo. 26 : 365 (1967).

15. Manser, T., and M. L. Gefter. Isolation of hybridomas expressing a specific heavy chain variable region gene segment by using a screening technique that detects mRNA sequences in whole cell lysates. Proc. Natl. Acad. Sci. USA 81 : 2470 (1984).

16. Germain, R. N., and H. Quill. Unexpected expression by L cell transfectants of a unique mixed isotype (A_{β} : E) class II MHC molecule. Nature 320 : 72 (1986).

17. Ben-Nun, A., L. H. Glimcher, J. Weiss, and J. G. Seidman. Functional expression of a cloned $I\text{-}A_{\beta}^{k}$ gene in B lymphoma cells. Science 223 : 825 (1984).

18. Nir, U., M. D. Walker, and W. J. Rutter. Regulation of insulin I gene expression : Evidence for negative regulation in nonpancreatic cells. Proc. Natl. Acad. Sci. USA 83 : 3180 (1986).

REGULATION OF MHC CLASS II AND INTERLEUKIN-1 GENE EXPRESSION IN DIFFERENTIATING MACROPHAGES

Lawrence B. Schook, Jeffrey K. Pullen,[1] Michael J. Myers, Elizabeth P. Eustis-Turf and Xiu-Mei Wang[2]

Laboratory of Molecular Immunology, Department of Animal Sciences, University of Illinois, Urbana, IL 61801

ABSTRACT

The expression and regulation of the MHC class II and interleukin-1 genes was studied during the differentiation of bone marrow stem cells into macrophages. Bone marrow cells were cultured in the presence of CSF-1 and allowed to differentiate for 3, 5, 7, and 9 d. Cells were stimulated with either medium, endotoxin (1 μg/ml) or interferon-γ (IFN-γ, 100 U/ml) 24 hr prior to the end of the culture period. Upon completion of culture, total cytoplasmic RNA was isolated from the adherent bone marrow-derived macrophages (BMDM) and subjected to Northern blot analysis. The A_α and E_α mRNA was constitutively expressed by medium treated BMDM after 3, 5, and 7 d, but by 9 d the mRNA had declined to values lower than those observed on d 3. IFN-γ treatment augmented A_α and E_α mRNA at each time point, whereas endotoxin treatment decreased values after 5 and 7 d. Additional studies demonstrated that IFN-γ was not being produced by either the non-adherent or adherent cells nor was the production of PGE responsible for the decline in MHC class II gene expression. IL-1 mRNA was only detected in those cultures stimulated with endotoxin; medium alone or IFN-γ treatment did not induce IL-1 mRNA transcription. Antigen-primed lymph node T cells and T cell hybridomas demonstrated that the ability of BMDM to function as antigen presenting cells was limited by the differentiation-specific regulation of both class II and IL-1 gene products. Exogenous E_α and A_β genes were inserted into bone marrow stem cells using either a modified calcium phosphate transfection or an electroporation procedure and their expression was monitored using Northern blot and immunofluorescence analysis. However, there was no alteration in the expression of membrane IL-1 following transfection. We currently are examining the expression of regulatory factors which are responsible for the differentiation-specific regulation of MHC class II and IL-1 gene expression.

---

[1]Current address: Laboratory of Immunology, Mayo Clinic, Rochester, MN 55905.

[2]Current address: Department of Microbiology, Inner Mongolian Medical School, Huhehoute, Inner Mongolia, PRC.

INTRODUCTION

The past several years have witnessed the identification and cloning of many cytokines that are responsible for the intricate regulatory network of the immune system (Bender *et al.* 1986, Ihle and Weinstein 1987, Kawasaki *et al.* 1985, Metcalf 1984, Old 1987). These cytokines are responsible for cell growth, differentiation, and the activation of phenotypic characteristics and functions ascribed to specific cell lineages (e.g., B cells, T_h, CTL and macrophages) (Collart *et al.* 1986, Grabstein *et al.* 1986, Ihle and Weinstein 1987, Warren and Ralph 1986, Unanue and Allen 1987). Our previous efforts have focused on the differentiation of macrophage from bone marrow cells as a model of "differentiation-specific" gene regulation (Pullen and Schook 1986). In particular, we and others have demonstrated the expression of class II MHC gene products (Ia antigens) on these bone marrow-derived macrophages (BMDM) without the addition of exogenous interferon-γ (IFN-γ) (Eustis-Turf *et al.* 1987b, Lee and Wong 1982, Mottram and Miller 1980, Schook *et al.* 1984, Stern *et al.* 1979).

Recently several laboratories using severely combined immunodeficient (SCID) and athymic mice have demonstrated that Ia-bearing macrophages are generated in vivo in the absence of T cells (Bancroft *et al.* 1986, Wentworth and Ziegler 1987). These results clearly support our in vitro findings and raise many new questions that must be addressed regarding the role of T cells and their products during macrophage differentiation into affector and effector cells of the immune system. Other studies have suggested that non-T cell-derived cytokines may be responsible for the "differentiation-specific" expression of Ia antigens on BMDM, whereas peripheral regulation of mature macrophage function is via T cell-derived cytokines (Tripp *et al.* 1986b, Wentworth and Ziegler 1987).

In this study we have analyzed the expression and regulation of MHC class II and IL-1 genes during the differentiation of macrophage from bone marrow stem cells. Using this model we have compared the kinetics of gene transcription with the acquisition of antigen presenting cell functions. Furthermore, this model has allowed the development of gene transfer procedures which permit examination of the regulatory factors responsible for the "differentiation-specific" transcription of MHC class II genes.

MATERIALS AND METHODS

Mice

The experiments were conducted using female, virus free C3H/HeN, (C57Bl/6 x C3H)F1 [(B6C3)F1], (Balb/c x C57Bl/6)F1 [(CB6)F1], and C57Bl/6 mice obtained from Charles River. Mice used in each experiment were matched for age (8-12 wks) and maintained in virus free conditions.

Preparation of BMDM

The BMDM were obtained from cultures of bone marrow stem cells. The marrow was flushed from femurs using supplemented DMEM containing 5% fetal calf serum (FCS). The marrow plugs were disrupted into single-cell suspensions, gravity sedimented for 5 min, washed, and cultured at a cell density of 1.0×10^6 nucleated cells/ml in 100-mm polystyrene tissue culture dishes containing 20 mls of DMEM supplemented with 10% L-cell-conditioned medium, 10% FCS, and 10% horse serum. Following various periods of incubation at 37^oC in 7.5% CO_2, the non-adherent cells were decanted, and the remaining adherent monolayers were washed by the addition of fresh media and harvested using cold 1 mM EDTA in HBSS (Ca^{++} and Mg^{++} free).

Preparation of Colony-Stimulating Activity

Mouse L-cell (strain 929) conditioned medium was used as a source of colony-stimulating activity (CSF-1). The L-cells were grown in DMEM supplemented with 10% FCS and fed every 3 d with fresh medium (50% v/v). After 7 d, the culture medium was removed, centrifuged at 300 x g for 10 min, filter-sterilized, aliquoted, and frozen until needed.

Lymphokine and IFN-γ Treatment

Recombinant IFN-γ used in this study was generously supplied by Patrick W. Gray (Genentech). Purified murine IFN-γ was kindly provided by S. Grossberg (Medical College of Wisconsin). Endotoxin (*E. coli* 055:B5) was obtained from Difco Laboratories.

RNA Isolation

Adherent macrophages were harvested from culture plates using cold HBSS-EDTA and were washed twice with ice-cold PBS, pH 7.2. Guanidine thiocyanate (4 M) was added to the cell pellet and the suspension was disrupted using a 23 gauge needle. The disrupted cell suspension was mixed with 20% sarkosyl and passed twice through a 23 gauge needle. The suspension (8 ml) was then pipetted into a 15 ml sterile quick seal tube and 4.5 ml of CsCl solution was pipetted underneath. The samples were then centrifuged for 16 h at 41,000 rpm. After centrifugation, the RNA was resuspended in 2.0 ml of sterile distilled H_2O. The RNA was purified by ethanol precipitation, resuspended in 100 μl of sterile distilled water and quantitated by spectrophotometry.

Electrophoresis and Transfer of RNA

The gel was prepared by melting agarose in sterile distilled water, cooling to 60°C, and adding 5x gel buffer [0.2 M morpholinopropanesulfonic acid (MOPS) pH 7.0, 50 mM sodium acetate, 5 mM EDTA (pH 8.0)] and formaldehyde to give 1x and 2.2 M final concentrations, respectively. RNA (10-20 μg in 1x MOPS, 2.2 M formaldehyde and 50% formamide) was placed into one of the wells of the formaldehyde-agarose gel and electrophoresed at 15 volts for 24 h. The RNA was then electrophoretically transferred from the formaldehyde-agarose gels to Genatran 45 (Plasco, Inc.), a positively charged, nylon membrane. Upon completion of the electrophoretic transfer, the membrane was washed for 30 min at room temperature in 2x SSC, air dried and then baked for 2 h under vacuum at 80°C.

Prehybridization-Hybridization

The membranes were incubated overnight at 42°C in prehybridization solution containing 100 mM Tris-HCl at pH 7.5, 6x SSC, 2 mM EDTA, 10x Denharts (0.2% ficoll, 0.2% polyvinyl pyrrolidone, 0.2% bovine serum albumin), 200 μg/ml salmon sperm DNA and 1% (w/v) SDS). At the end of the incubation, the membrane was removed from the prehybridization solution and placed in the hybridization mixture which consisted of the prehybridization solution containing 10% dextran sulfate and 2 x 10^6 cpm/ml of the denatured [^{32}P]-labeled insert. The membranes were incubated in this mixture for 12-24 h at 42°C and then washed for 1 h at room temperature in a high salt solution (2x SSC and 0.1% SDS) followed by a 2 h wash at 55°C in a low salt solution (0.1x SSC and 1% SDS). The membranes were allowed to air dry and then exposed to XAR-5 film with the aid of intensifying screens. Autoradiograms were analyzed with a Zeinen scanning laser densitometer.

Antibody Reagents

A number of hybridoma cell lines were used as a source of monoclonal antibodies (mAbs). These lines included 10-2.16 (anti-I-A^k, γ2b), 11-5.2 (anti-I-A^k, γ2b), and BP107 (anti-I-A^b, γ1) which were obtained from ATCC. Additional antisera were purchased from Southern Biotechnology, Inc., Birmingham, AL (mouse isotype controls γ1, γ2a and γ2b). A hamster mAb (H22.1) directed against murine IFN-γ was kindly provided by R. Schreiber, Washington University, St. Louis, MO.

Flow Cytometry

The stained bone marrow cells were analyzed on a Coulter Epics 751 flow cytometer using a 515 long pass filter. The mean fluorescence intensity of control and test samples were compared using the Coulter "Immuno" software program.

DNA Reagents

The murine MHC class II genes A_β^b and E_α^d (cosmid 17.2) were kindly provided by E. Choi and L. Hood, respectively. The DNA inserts used in the experiments were: a cDNA insert encoding mouse IL-1β that was excised from the plasmid pIL-1-1301 with Bam HI; a cDNA insert encoding the class II MHC E_α^k chain (E_α) that was excised from the plasmid pEAC II with EcoR1; a cDNA insert encoding the class II A_α^k chain, excised from the plasmid pAAC6 with EcoR1; a cDNA insert encoding murine IFN-γ excised from the plasmid pmc14 with EcoR1; and a human rRNA DNA fragment, inserted into the EcoRI site of the plasmid pAD-19.IIa, which was used to demonstrate that equivalent amounts of total RNA had been added to each lane. The DNA fragments were nick translated using an Amersham Nick Translation Kit.

Antigen Presentation Assay

C57Bl/6 bone marrow cells were obtained and cultured in the presence of CSF-1 for 3, 5, 7 and 9 d, and treated with additional medium, *E. coli* endotoxin (1 μg/ml), recombinant interferon-γ (rIFN-γ, 100 U/ml) or both endotoxin and rIFN-γ 24 hr before their use in the antigen presentation assay. Macrophages (5 x 10^3 in 100 μl) were harvested and placed in a 96 well culture plate. Indomethacin was added to some wells, at a final concentration of 1 x 10^{-7} M, to block prostaglandin synthesis. Purified keyhole limpet hemocyanin (KLH, 200 μg) was added. The macrophages were allowed to process the antigen for 2 hr at 37°C and were washed with HBSS to remove free antigen. Then 1 x 10^5 BDK-11.1 T-hybridoma cells were added in 200 μl of RPMI 1640 with 10% FCS. BDK-11.1 is a T-lymphocyte hybridoma that responds to the antigen KLH when it is presented in the context of I-A^b. This hybridoma was a gift from Dr. John Kappler. The cultures were incubated at 37°C for 24 hr, and at the end of the culture period the 96 well plates were spun at 2000 rpms for 30 min. Supernatant (150 μl) from each well was transferred to a well of a duplicate plate containing 1 x 10^4 CTLL-2 (IL-2 dependent cell line) in 50 μl of RPMI. The cultures were incubated at 37°C for 24 hr and, during the last 4 hr of the culture period, the cells (CTLL-2) were pulsed with 1 μCi of [^{3}H]-thymidine, and proliferation was determined by scintillation spectrophotometry.

Preparation of Immune T Cells

Mice were immunized with poly-L-glutamic-L-alanine-L-tyrosine (GAT) emulsified in complete Freund's adjuvant containing *Mycobacterium butyricum* to a final antigen concentration of 500 μg GAT/ml of emulsion. Each animal received 0.2 ml of emulsion divided between injection sites in both hind footpads and the base of the tail. The popliteal, inguinal, and periaortic lymph nodes were harvested 14 to 21 d after immunization with GAT. Lymph nodes were minced into single cell suspensions and cells were washed twice and then resuspended in supplemented HEPES-buffered Hanks' minimal essential medium (MEM) with 3% human AB serum. The cell suspension (5×10^7 cells) was added to a nylon wool column, incubated at 37^oC for 40 min, and the nonadherent cells were eluted with the slow addition of fresh medium.

Calcium Phosphate Transfection Procedure

Bone marrow cells were obtained from the femurs of C57Bl/6 mice, washed, and placed in 20 ml of bone marrow culture medium at 1×10^6 cells/ml. The cells were incubated for various time periods from 0 to 48 hr in 10 ml of bone marrow culture medium. Cosmid 17.2 DNA (20 μg gave optimal results) was ethanol precipitated and resuspended in 100 μl of 2.5 M $CaCl_2$ and 900 μl sterile distilled H_2O. This DNA-$CaCl_2$ solution was added dropwise to an equal volume of 1.4 mM HEPES-PO_4 while vigorously bubbling the solution. After a 30-min incubation at room temperature, this mixture was added to the 20×10^6 cells and incubated from 6 to 24 hr at 37^oC. Some cultures were shocked with polyethylene glycol (PEG) and then washed 2x in HBSS, resuspended in fresh bone marrow culture medium, plated, and incubated in 7.5% CO_2 at 37^oC for the indicated period of time. Duplicate cultures were transfected with the thymidine kinase (TK) gene and designated "mock transfected" controls.

Electroporation Transfection Procedure

The DNA was transfected into bone marrow cells by electroporation using a Bio-Rad Gene Pulser equipped with a capacitance extender. Approximately 6×10^8 bone marrow cells were placed in a sterile cuvette along with 10 μg of super-coiled DNA and placed on ice for 15 min. The cell-DNA mixture was subjected to an electrical pulse and again left on ice for 15 min before being cultured.

RESULTS

Expression of MHC Class II and IL-1 Genes During Macrophage Differentiation

Previous work in our laboratory has phenotypically characterized BMDM during their differentiation in vitro. Current efforts are focused on examining the relationship between the initiation of MHC class II transcription and Ia expression on BMDM. We have previously been unable to detect secreted IL-1 under a wide range of culturing conditions and so wished to determine whether this inability to detect secreted IL-1 was due to transcriptional or translational regulation. Bone marrow cells (C3H/HeN) were cultured in the presence of CSF-1 and allowed to differentiate for 3, 5, 7, and 9 d. During this culture period, cells were stimulated with either medium alone, endotoxin or recombinant IFN-γ 24 hr prior to the end of the culture period. Total cytoplasmic RNA was then isolated from the adherent BMDM and analyzed for A_α, E_α and IL-1 transcription by Northern blot analysis (Fig. 1, upper panel).

The A_α and E_α genes were constitutively expressed by medium-treated BMDM after 3, 5 and 7 d, but by 9 d the mRNA levels had declined to values less than those at 3 d of culture. IFN-γ treatment augmented A_α and E_α transcription at each point in time, whereas endotoxin treatment decreased values after 5 and 7 d (data not shown). The kinetics of transcription closely followed those of Ia antigen expression (Fig. 1, middle panel). IL-1 mRNA was only detected in those cultures stimulated with endotoxin and followed the same kinetics as A_α and E_α expression (Fig. 1, upper panel).

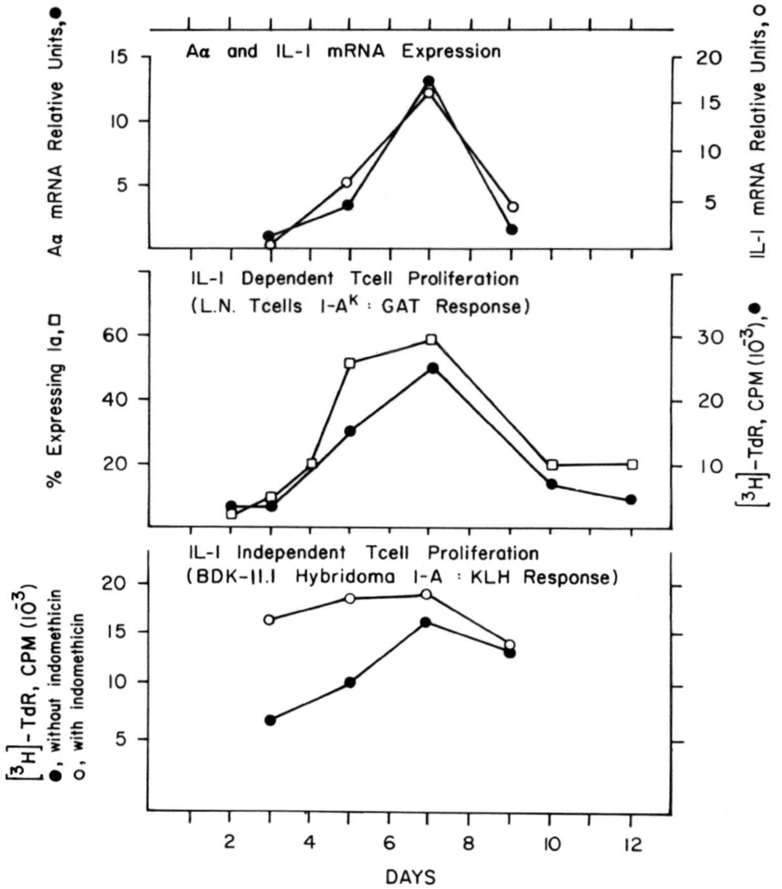

Fig. 1. Kinetics of macrophage MHC class II and IL-1 gene expression and activity during differentiation. Upper panel: Northern blot analysis was performed using RNA obtained from C3H BMDM after various days of culture. The blots were probed with either a cDNA to A_α, IL-1β or rRNA. RNA used for the A_α Northern blot was obtained from unstimulated BMDM and that used for the IL-1 analysis, from endotoxin stimulated BMDM. Values were determined by laser densitometry readings of the autoradiographs and are expressed as relative units using the rRNA value as the baseline standard. Middle panel: Illustrates the Ia antigen expression (% of cells positive using immunofluorescence) and ability of BMDM to function in IL-1 dependent T cell proliferation. T cells were purified from lymph nodes of C3H mice immunized with GAT and cultured with paraformaldehyde-fixed GAT-pulsed BMDM obtained after various days of differentiation. T cell proliferation was measured by the incorporation of [^{3}H]-thymidine (TdR). Lower panel: Demonstrates that the ability of C57Bl/6 BMDM, obtained after various periods of culture, to present KLH to the T cell hybri doma BDK-11.1 is an IL-1 independent response. Values shown represent the production of IL-2, with or without the addition of indomethacin, as determined using the IL-2-dependent cell line CTLL.

The treatment of cultures with medium containing CSF-1 or IFN-γ did not stimulate IL-1 transcription.

Additional studies were performed to determine whether the ability of BMDM to function as antigen presenting cells (APC) paralleled the kinetics of A_α and IL-1 transcriptional regulation. BMDM from medium treated cultures were used as APC. Two approaches were used; the first used $I\text{-}A^k$-restricted T cells obtained from GAT-primed lymph nodes and the second, the T cell hybridoma BDK-11.1 which responds to the $I\text{-}A^b$:KLH restriction element. The former T cell population requires the presence of IL-1 to permit clonal expansion (Fig. 1, middle panel), whereas the latter hybridoma responds independently of IL-1 (Fig. 1, lower panel). As shown, the IL-1 dependent T cell population of GAT-primed T cells followed the kinetics of A_α and IL-1 transcription shown in Fig. 1, upper panel. The kinetics of the T cell responses of both populations correlated with the Ia expression by BMDM.

<u>Production of MHC Class II and IL-1 Regulators During Macrophage Differentiation</u>

During the past several years a number of potential regulatory products have been shown to be produced during an immune response. Two factors, IFN-γ and prostaglandins have been shown to be strong up- and down-regulators, respectively, of MHC class II and IL-1 gene expression in peripheral macrophage (Steeg *et al.* 1982, Tripp *et al.* 1986a). The above results suggested a differentiation-specific regulation of MHC class II gene expression by BMDM. Previous work in our laboratory had shown that the addition of anti-IFN-γ did not affect Ia expression during macrophage differentiation (Eustis-Turf *et al.* 1987b). Therefore, we wished to expand on these studies to determine whether IFN-γ was being produced and utilized perhaps intracellularly by non-adherent and adherent cells in our culture system or whether the affinity of IFN-γ for the cell receptor was higher than that for the monoclonal antibody used to block activity. RNA was isolated from both non-adherent and adherent cells of our culture system and probed by Northern blot analysis with a cDNA insert to IFN-γ. As shown in Fig. 2, no IFN-γ mRNA was observed in either the non-adherent or adherent cell populations whether these cells were cultured in the presence of exogenous IFN-γ or with added anti-IFN-γ. These findings corroborate our previous efforts in demonstrating that MHC class II gene expression during macrophage differentiation is independent of IFN-γ.

The production of PGE_2 by macrophage has been shown to down-regulate both macrophage and T cell functions. We wished to determine what role PGE_2 played during macrophage differentiation and how PGE_2 affected the ability of macrophages to function as APC. Using the previously described culture system, we harvested supernatants during various stages of macrophage differentiation and analyzed them for the production of prostaglandins E_1 and E_2. As shown in Table 1, there was no detectable production of PGEs in medium-stimulated cultures or in cultures treated with indomethacin (10^{-7} M). Stimulation of the BMDM with endotoxin resulted in the production of PGEs by cells following 7 and 9 d of culture. The addition of IFN-γ resulted in a different kinetic pattern of PGE synthesis from endotoxin. In those cultures receiving IFN-γ, PGE synthesis was observed at 5 d and 7 d of culture but not at 9 d of culture.

Additional experiments were done using the BDK-11.1 T cell hybridoma. As shown in Fig. 1, lower panel, the addition of indomethacin to the culture increased the production of IL-2 at the earlier time points but had little effect following 7 and 9 d of differentiation. Clearly, PGE synthesis by BMDM has an effect on their ability to function as APC.

Table 1. PGE Synthesis During Macrophage Differentiation

Treatment of BMDM[a]	PGE_{1+2} (pg/100 μl) Produced[b]			
	3 Day	5 Day	7 Day	9 Day
Medium	25*	11*	26*	30*
Indomethacin (10^{-7} M)	30*	28*	37	46
Endotoxin (*E. coli* 055:B5, 1 μg/ml)	52	31*	127	130
Interferon-γ (recombinant, 100 U/ml)	31*	62	250	34

[a]Cultures were treated 18 hr prior to assay.

[b]After indicated period of culture, supernatants from the various conditions were collected and assayed using a Seragen RIA kit.

*Values below sensitivity range of assay (linear range, 32-500 pg PGE/100 μl).

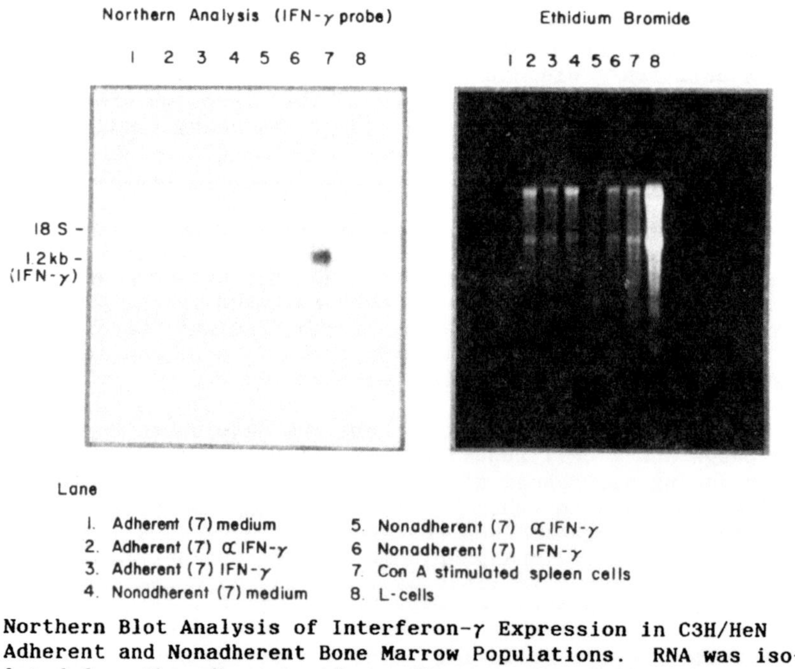

Fig. 2. Northern Blot Analysis of Interferon-γ Expression in C3H/HeN Adherent and Nonadherent Bone Marrow Populations. RNA was isolated from the adherent and nonadherent cells following 7 d of culture. The cell populations were treated with: fresh medium (Lanes 1 and 4), fresh medium containing a monoclonal anti-IFN-γ (neutralizing capacity of 7500 IFN-γ U/ml) (Lanes 2 and 5), or fresh medium followed by the addition of IFN-γ (25 U/ml) (Lanes 3 and 7) 18 hr prior to isolation of the RNA. Lane 7 contains RNA isolated from spleen cells after 48 hr of Con A stimulation. Lane 8 contains RNA isolated from L-cells. The Northern blot analysis was performed on 5 μg of RNA in Lanes 1-7 and 50 μg of RNA in Lane 8.

Table 2. Summary of Calcium Phosphate Transfection Parameters

Time of Transfection (days in culture)	Length of[a] Transfection (hours)	Amount[b] of DNA (μg)	Length of PEG Shock (seconds)	Expression[c] of I-E by Adherent BMDM (relative units)
1	18	10	0	117±25
	18	20	0	215±125
	18	30	0	405±27
2	18	10	0	1201±200
	18	20	0	1920±255
	18	30	0	2175±327

[a]Transfection was conducted in the presence of $CaPO_4$.

[b]DNA was cosmid 17.2.

[c]Expression of I-E was determined using a radiobinding assay with anti-Ia.7 (14-4-4).

Regulation of Exogenous and Endogenous MHC Class II Genes During Macrophage Differentiation

One approach to augmenting the immune response is through the insertion of genes into the bone marrow of animals. Cells derived from such gene transfers may have new phenotypes and functions. Our laboratory has been successful in developing a modified calcium phosphate procedure and an electroporation technique which permit the insertion of MHC class II genes into marrow cells with their subsequent expression on BMDM (Pullen and Schook 1986). We have used this approach to study the transient expression of exogenous MHC class II genes in differentiating BMDM and to determine whether exogenous genes will be regulated as endogenous MHC class II genes. Exogenous E_α^d and A_α^b genes were inserted into bone marrow stem cells using either our modified calcium phosphate or electroporation transfection procedure (Pullen and Schook 1986, Eustis-Turf *et al.* 1987) and their expression monitored using Northern blot and immunofluorescence analysis, respectively.

A summary of the modified calcium phosphate procedure parameters which were used is shown in Table 2. Using these conditions, we have shown that the insertion of E_α^d into C57Bl/6 marrow cells resulted in maximal expression of I-E at 5 d of differentiation with subsequent decline (Pullen and Schook, 1986). However, in contrast to endogenous I-A^b expression, expression of the exogenous I-E was undetectable without the addition of IFN-γ. RNA obtained from these BMDM was probed with both the endogenous A_α^b and the exogenous E_α^d to further understand this differential expression. As shown in Fig. 3, A_α^b transcripts are observed during the differentiation of macrophage. However, it is clear that this procedure results in decline of the endogenous A_α^b RNA levels when exogenous MHC class II genes are inserted. Note that there is no change in mock transfected cells indicating that this procedure does not affect A_α^b levels.

In order to determine whether the above findings were related to the insertion of the gene or perturbation of macrophage differentiation by the procedure, we also determined the effect of transfection on membrane IL-1 expression by BMDM. As shown in Table 3, the expression of mIL-1 is detected following 5 d of culture and increases after 7 d of differentiation

Table 3. Effect of Transfection on Membrane IL-1 (mIL-1) Expression by Bone Marrow Derived Macrophage

Treatment of Bone Marrow Cells (C57Bl/6)	BMDM Accessory Cells (Days of Culture)[a]	Membrane IL-1 Activity[b]		
		Without Con A	With Con A	Δ Activity
No treatment	5	2252	4338	2386
	7	2313	11138	7926
Mock (TK) transfection	5	1517	9385	7868
	7	4234	16245	12011
E_{α}^{d} transfection	5	7531	14936	7405
	7	4624	16516	11891
———	None	384	2303	1919

[a]Days in culture in the presence of CSF-1 after treatment of bone marrow cells.

[b]Membrane IL-1 was determined using the D10.G4.1 cell line.

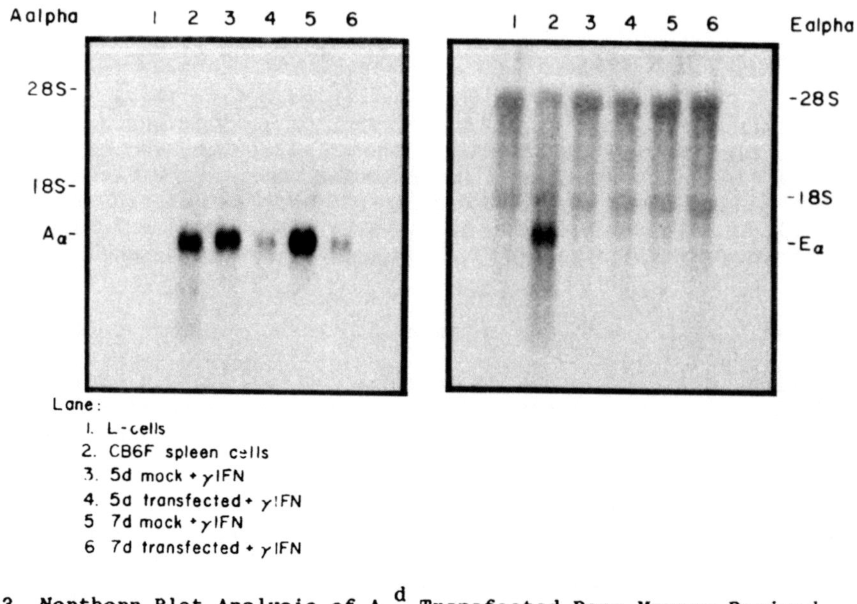

Fig. 3. Northern Blot Analysis of A_{α}^{d} Transfected Bone Marrow Derived Macrophage. RNA was isolated from L-cells (Lane 1), spleen cells (Lane 2), and BMDM (Lanes 3-6), and analyzed for the expression of A_{α} and E_{α} RNA. The RNA was obtained from either 5 d or 7 d BMDM following transfection with the E_{α}^{d} gene from cells that received IFN-γ 18 hr previously. Cells were transfected with the TK (Mock) gene on the 8.5 Kb insert from cosmid 17.2 which contains the E_{α}^{d} gene.

Table 4. Parameters for Electroporation: Adherent vs. Non-adherent Cells

	L-929 Cells	Bone Marrow Cells
Buffer	phosphate/sucrose	PBS
Capacitance (μFd)	25 μFd	500 μFd
Voltage (V)	250 V	250-300 V
Pulse time (msec)	7-10 msec	8-11 msec

in untreated controls. There was no difference between the mock (TK) transfected or E_{α}^{d} transfected mIL-1 activity at either 5 or 7 d of culture; in fact there may actually be an increase in mIL-1 activity following the calcium phosphate transfection. However, no difference was apparent in mIL-1 activity whether the gene product remained cytosolic (TK) or membrane-associated (E_{α}).

One negative aspect of the calcium phosphate transfection procedure was poor cell recovery. In order to overcome that, we developed an alternative gene transfer method. Table 4 summarizes the parameters for the electroporation of adherent and non-adherent cells which we have established (Eustis-Turf *et al.* 1986a). Using electroporation, we have transferred

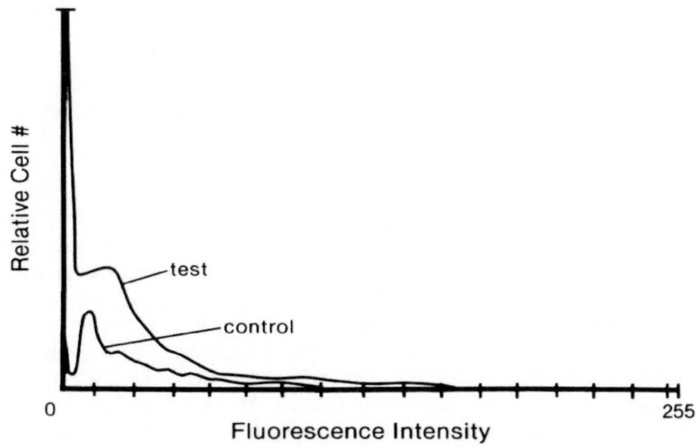

Fig. 4. Electroporation of MHC class II genes into bone marrow cells. Bone marrow cells from C3H/HeN mice were transfected with the A_{β}^{b} gene using electroporation. After 7 d in culture, transfected BMDM and control BMDM were stained with the monoclonal antibody BP.107 (anti-A_{β}^{b}). Stained BMDM were then analyzed by flow cytometry to determine expression of the A_{β}^{b} chain. Test values refer to the BP.107 staining pattern of C3H BMDM transfected with the A_{β}^{b} gene and Control refers to the staining pattern of mock transfected BMDM using the BP.107 antibody. Both test and control cultures were treated with IFN-γ (25 U/ml) 24 hr before staining.

the MHC class II gene A_β^b into C3H bone marrow cells. The transient expression of this gene was then monitored by staining BMDM (7 d) with an A_β^b gene product-specific monoclonal antibody BP.107 (Fig. 4). The results shown represent expression of the $A_\alpha^k A_\beta^b$ gene product after treatment of the bone marrow culture 24 hr prior to staining with IFN-γ.

DISCUSSION

These studies have addressed the mechanisms responsible for controlling the regulation of MHC class II and IL-1 gene products during macrophage hematopoiesis. The kinetics and differential requirements for expression of these two macrophage gene products suggest that, while both are expressed at the same stage of differentiation, each has a unique regulatory mechanism.

The expression of MHC class II genes occurs independently of the addition of IFN-γ. We have not been able to demonstrate either the presence of cells known to produce IFN-γ or IFN-γ itself in our culture. Broxmeyer and Dupont (1985) have suggested that the expression of class II genes may be associated with regulation of myelopoiesis; in particular they have shown that the production of Ia-expressing colonies is specifically inhibited by isoferritans. While the reason for the expression of MHC class II genes is still unresolved, it is clear that they are expressed. Moreover, they are expressed independently of T cell-derived IFN-γ, although the addition of IFN-γ does augment MHC class II transcription by BMDM (Eustis-Turf *et al.* 1987).

The expression of IL-1 by BMDM clearly is regulated in a different manner. Unlike the expression of MHC class II genes, transcription of IL-1 is not seen in unstimulated (cultured with CSF-1) cells. IL-1 induction was also not stimulated by IFN-γ but rather only by endotoxin, under our culture conditions. These findings are in agreement with recent work by Weaver and Unanue (1986) in which they showed the inability of IL-2, IFN-γ, BSF-1 or CSF-1 to induce membrane IL-1. Also, in agreement with their findings, it appears that T cell-macrophage interactions can induce IL-1 synthesis since BMDM were able to function as APC to IL-1-requiring antigen-primed lymph node T cells.

These studies also demonstrate that down-regulation of these gene products is under control of different mechanisms. As shown, BMDM after 5 and 7 d of culture express MHC class II transcripts and membrane Ia antigen without requiring IFN-γ. However, the addition of endotoxin down-regulates the level of transcription detected in these BMDM. Similar observations were made by Steeg *et al.* (1982) and Ziegler *et al.* (1984). The latter study demonstrated that the modulation of macrophage Ia expression by endotoxin _in vivo_ had two effects. First, there was an initial decline in Ia-expressing macrophage following the endotoxin injection with a subsequent increase in the number of Ia-expressing macrophage. We interpret these results to indicate that differentiating macrophage leaving the bone marrow compartment are sensitive to endotoxin downregulation of MHC class II transcription, whereas alternative regulation may exist in the peripheral tissue, most likely the induction by endotoxin of up-regulators such as TNF-α (Old 1987).

Our findings also show that BMDM can be induced by IFN-γ and endotoxin to produce PGE; however, we could not demonstrate the production of PGE in unstimulated cultures. PGE has been implicated as a down regulator of class II expression, yet we observed maximal A_α transcription and Ia expression following IFN-γ stimulation of BMDM after 7 d of culture. This was also when maximal PGE synthesis was observed. Broxmeyer and Dupont

(1985) have reported that immature BMDM are stimulated by the addition of PGE to express Ia antigens. This point again reflects the difference in gene regulation of the differentiating macrophage from the peripheral tissue-associated progeny.

Finally, the transfer of MHC class II genes into bone marrow stem cells has provided exciting information regarding the regulation of these genes. Although the kinetics of expression for both endogenous and exogenous genes are identical, the latter are sometimes detectable following IFN-γ stimulation. Furthermore, it appears that these two forms of genes (chromosomal vs. extra-chromosomal) may actually compete for transacting factors since we observed a decrease in endogenous transcripts following insertion of the exogenous gene. This decrease seems specific since insertion of the TK gene had no effect on endogenous MHC class II levels and mIL-1 expression was unaffected by the transfection procedure. We currently are examining the regulatory factors that are responsible for the differentiation-specific regulation of MHC class II and IL-1 gene expression.

ACKNOWLEDGMENTS

The authors wish to extend their appreciation to Drs. D. Landais, C. Benoist, D. Mathis, E. Choi and L. Hood for their generosity in providing genetic material for these studies. We also thank Genentech and Hoffman-LaRoche for their kindness in providing the interferon-γ and IL-1 containing plasmids, respectively. The generosity of Drs. P. Gray, S. Grossberg and J. Kappler is also greatly appreciated. A special thanks is extended to J. Monaco, J. A. Frelinger, and E. Westin for their comments and support. Finally, the authors wish to recognize the dedication of M. Sweetser to the completion of this work. This work was supported in part by NIH grants ES-04348 and CA-09210.

REFERENCES

Bancroft, G. J., Bosma, M. J., Bosma, G. C., and Unanue, E. R.: Regulation of macrophage Ia expression in mice with severe combined immunodeficiency: induction of Ia expression by a T cell-independent mechanism. J. Immunol. 137:4-9, 1986.

Bender, J. G., Van Epps, D. E., and Stewart, C. C.: A model for the regulation of myelopoiesis by specific factors. J. Leuk. Biol. 39:101-111, 1986.

Broxmeyer, H. E., and Dupont, B.: A role for class-II major histocompatibility complex antigens in the reguiation of myelopoiesis. Prog. Allergy 36:203-221, 1985.

Collart, M. A., Belin, D., Vassalli, J.-D., de Kossodo, S., and Vassalli, P.: γ-Interferon enhances macrophage transcription of the tumor necrosis factor/cachectin, interleukin 1, and urokinase genes, which are controlled by short-lived repressors. J. Exp. Med. 164:2113-2118, 1986.

Eustis-Turf, E. P., Wang, X.-M., and Schook, L. B.: Electroporation of bone marrow cells: parameters and applications. Bio-Radiation, in press, 1987a.

Eustis-Turf, E. P., Pullen, J. K., Myers, M. J., Wang, X.-M., and Schook, L. B.: Regulation of class II MHC gene expression during macrophage differentiation. In, L. B. Schook and J. G. Tew (ed.), Antigen Presenting Cells: Diversity, Differentiation, and Regulation. Alan R. Liss Publications, Inc., (in press), 1987b.

Grabstein, K., Mochizaki, D., Kronheim, S., Price, V., Cosman, D., Urdal, D., Gillis, S., and Conlow, P.: Regulation of antibody production in

vitro by granulocyte-macrophage colony stimulating factor. J. Mol. Cell. Immunol. 2:199-207, 1986.
Ihle, J. N., and Weinstein, Y.: Immunological regulation of hematopoietic/lymphoid stem cell differentiation by interleukin-3. Adv. Immunol. 39:1-50, 1986.
Kawasaki, E. S., Ladner, M. B., Wang, A. M., Van Arsdell, J., Warren, M. K., Coyne, M. Y., Schweickart, V. L., Lee, M.-T., Wilson, K. J., Boosman, A., Stanley, E. R., and David, D. F.: Molecular cloning of a complementary DNA encoding human macrophage-specific colony-stimulating factor (CSF-1). Science 230:291-296, 1985.
Lee, K. C., and Wong, M.: Functional heterogeneity of culture-grown bone marrow-derived macrophages. II. Lymphokine stimulation of antigen-presenting function. J. Immunol. 128:2487-2494, 1982.
Metcalf, D.: The granulocyte-macrophage colony stimulating factors. Science 229:16-22, 1985.
Mottram, P. L., and Miller, J. F. A. P.: Delayed-type hypersensitivity induced by antigen-pulsed, bone marrow-derived macrophages. Eur. J. Immunol. 10:165-170, 1980.
Old, L. J.: Tumour necrosis factor. Polypeptide mediator network. Nature 326:330-331, 1987.
Pullen, J. K., and Schook, L. B.: Bone marrow derived macrophage: Expression of endogenous and transfected class II MHC genes during differentiation. J. Immunol. 137:1359-1365, 1986.
Schook, L. B., Allen, P. M., and Niederhuber, J. E.: Bone marrow-derived macrophage as accessory cells in antigen-induced T cell proliferation: *H-2*I region requirements for L-glutamic acid^{60}-L-alanine^{30}-L-tyrosine^{10} response. J. Immunol. 130:661-664, 1983.
Schook, L. B., Bingham, E. L., Gutmann, D. H., and Niederhuber, J. E.: Characterization and expression of *H-2*I region gene products on bone marrow-derived macrophages. Eur. J. Immunol. 12:991-997, 1982.
Schook, L. B., Gutmann, D. H., Marlin, L. E., and Niederhuber, J. E.: *In vitro* derived bone marrow C57BL/6: expression of Ia antigens during macrophages differentiation. Transplantation 37:585-590, 1984.
Stern, A. A., Erb, P., and Gisler, R. H.: Ia-bearing bone marrow-cultured macrophages induce antigen-specific helper T cells for antibody synthesis. J. Immunol. 123:612-615, 1979.
Steeg, P. S., Johnson, H. M., and Oppenheim, J. J.: Regulation of murine macrophage Ia antigen expression by an immune interferon-like lymphokine: inhibitory effect of endotoxin. J. Immunol. 129:2402-2406, 1982.
Tripp, C. S., Wyche, A., Unanue, E. R., and Needleman, P.: The functional significance of the regulation of macrophage Ia expression by endogenous arachidonate metabolites in vitro. J. Immunol. 137:3915-3920, 1986a.
Tripp, C. S., Unanue, E. R., and Needleman, P.: Monocyte migration explains the changes in macrophage arachidonate metabolism during the immune response. Proc. Natl. Acad. Sci., U.S.A. 83:9655-9659, 1986b.
Unanue, E. R., and Allen, P. M.: The basis for the immunoregulatory role of macrophage and other accessory cells. Science 236:551-557, 1987.
Warren, M. K., and Ralph, P.: Macrophage growth factor CSF-1 stimulates human monocyte production of interferon, tumor necrosis factor, and colony stimulating activity. J. Immunol. 137:2281-2285, 1986.
Weaver, C. T., and Unanue, E. R.: T cell induction of membrane IL-1 on macrophages. J. Immunol. 137:3868-3873, 1986.
Wentworth, P. A., and Ziegler, H. K.: Induction of macrophage Ia expression by lipopolysaccharide and *Listeria monocytogenes* in congenitally athymic nude mice. J. Immunol. 138:3167-3173, 1987.
Ziegler, H. K., Staffileno, L. K., and Wentworth, P. Modulation of macrophage Ia-expression by lipopolysaccharide. I. Induction of Ia expression in vivo. J. Immunol. 133:1825-1835, 1984.

MACROPHAGE IA HYBRID MOLECULE AS PRODUCT OF THE

Ir-Thy-1 GENES

P. Zhou, L.J. Quackenbush, B. Albini and M.B. Zaleski

Department of Microbiology
State University of New York at Buffalo
Buffalo, NY 14214

INTRODUCTION

A primary anti-Thy-1 response in mice is under complex genetic control (Zaleski et al. 1986). This control has been shown to involve either class I or class II H-2 molecules depending on the form in which the Thy-1 antigen is presented to a responder. Briefly, when thymocytes from an H-2-compatible donor are used, the cell-bound Thy-1 antigen seems to be presented directly to the responder's T cells. The latter are believed to require simultaneous stimulation by the carrier-like or helper determinants (Lake and Douglas 1978) or acolytes (Klein and Zaleski 1987). In contrast, when thymocytes from H-2-incompatible donors are used, the cell-free Thy-1 antigen, which is shed from the immunizing thymocytes, appears to be presented by the responder's macrophages. This presentation most likely involves associative recognition of the Thy-1 antigen and the product of the two complementary Ir-Thy-1 genes (Zaleski and Klein 1978). Recently, it was demonstrated that the product of these genes is identical with a hybrid IA molecule (Quackenbush et al. 1985, Zaleski et al. 1985). The working hypothesis outlined above is based on two crucial observations. First, a good anti-Thy-1 response to the cell-free antigen is demonstrable only in F1 hybrids that express a particular hybrid IA molecule (Quackenbush et al. 1985). Second, *in vivo* administration of monoclonal antibodies specific for a particular class II molecule inhibits the response to the cell-free, but not to the cell-bound antigen (Zaleski et al. 1985, Quackenbush et al. 1987).

In this paper, the earlier findings on the role of hybrid IA molecules will be reiterated and expanded and evidence for the involvement of macrophages that bear these molecules will be presented.

MATERIALS AND METHODS

Mice used in the experiments reported were bred in the mouse colony maintained in this laboratory or received from the colony of Dr. C.S. David (Mayo Clinic, Rochester, MN). In all experiments, adult (6-10 weeks) mice of both sexes were used. They were immunized by a single i.v. or i.p. injection of 4×10^7 thymocytes from either an H-2-compatible or H-2-incompatible donor.

Monoclonal antibodies, MK-S4, 25-9-17S, 25-9-3S, and MK-D6 (Kappler et al. 1981, Ozato et al. 1981) were produced as tissue culture supernatant fluids according to the procedure described earlier (Quackenbush et al. 1985). Mice received i.p. 1 ml of antibody, with immunofluorescent titer of at least 2^4, 4 hr before and 20 hr after immunization. Control animals received MK-S4 antibody, specific for IA molecules not expressed by these individuals, while experimental animals received one of the remaining three antibodies.

To study the requirements for macrophages, mice were treated with lambda carrageenan (Sigma, St. Louis, MO) or chloroquine diphosphate (Sigma, St. Louis, MO). Carrageenan (0.1-1.0 mg) was injected i.v. 24 hr before immunization (Bice et al. 1972), while chloroquine was administered s.c. in five doses of 1 or 2 mg injected in 24 hr intervals beginning 24 hr before immunization (Shoemaker 1978).

The immune response to the Thy-1 antigen was assessed on day 6 after immunization using the plaque assay described elsewhere (Fuji et al. 1971). Although the specificity of this assay has been well documented (Zaleski and Klein 1978), thymocytes from mice Thy-1-congenic or at least H-2-identical with responders were used whenever possible.

The phagocytic function of macrophages was ascertained by i.v. injection of 0.1 ml of a 10% suspension of India ink (Pelikan, F.R.G.). The India ink suspension was injected 15-20 min before killing and paraffin sections of the spleens were stained with Nuclear Fast Red and examined under a light microscope for the presence of India ink-containing cells (Pittaluga 1935).

Percent of inhibition was calculated from the formula: Control PFC - Experimental PFC/Control PFC; negative values are shown as < 0. The quantitative data were analyzed statistically using the Student's t-test with $\alpha = 0.05$. All statistical calculations were performed using Macintosh 512 computer and Statworks™ software.

RESULTS

Table 1 summarizes the results of experiments in which the effects of the anti-IA antibodies on anti-Thy-1 responses of (C57BL/6Kh x BALB/cKh)F1 hybrids were tested. As can be seen, administration of anti-IA antibodies had no appreciable effect on the responses elicited by the cell-bound antigen presented by the H-2-compatible AKR.B6 thymocytes. In contrast, two antibodies significantly ($p < 0.01$) inhibited the responses elicited by the cell-free antigen derived from the H-2-incompatible AKR thymocytes. Specifically, antibodies directed to the epitopes on IA^b chain, i.e., 25-9-17S and 25-9-3S, resulted in 69% and 56% inhibition of responses. The observed inhibition was true inhibition and not merely a delay of the response since testing for the response through day 13 after immunization did not reveal an increased number of plaque-forming cells in spleens of treated animals.

A cursory histological examination of spleens showed that the phagocytic function of splenic macrophages had not been affected by treatment with inhibiting as compared to non-inhibiting antibodies. In both instances, India ink-containing cells, characteristically located in the marginal zones could be clearly discerned.

Table 2 presents the results of an experiment in which the effect of the two anti-macrophage agents were studied. Again, neither

Table 1. Effect of the anti-IA monoclonal antibodies on the anti-Thy-1 response (x PFC/spleen ± SE) of (C57BL/6Kh x BALB/cKh)F1 hybrids immunized i.v. with either cell-bound (AKR.B6) or cell-free (AKR) antigen. Number of animals tested, in parenthesis.

Treatment	IA_{β} chain specificity	Response to AKR.B6	% Inhibition	Response to AKR	% Inhibition
None	--	16550± 362 (8)	<0	2090±422 (10)	<0
MK-S4	s,f	20508±3144 (12)	<0	1845±307 (20)	12
25-9-17S	b,d,p,q	21509±2941 (11)	<0	650± 71 (20)	69
MK-D6	d	n.t.		2140±421 (15)	<0
25-9-3S	b	21600± 391 (6)	<0	929±169 (7)	56

carrageenan nor chloroquine affected the responses of (C57BL/6Kh x BALB/cKh)F1 hybrids to the cell-bound antigen. In contrast, both carrageenan and chloroquine significantly ($p < 0.01$) reduced the responses to the cell-free antigen and produced 47% and 43% inhibition, respectively.

Table 2. Effect of anti-macrophage agents on the primary response (x PFC/spleen ± SE) of (C57/BL/6Kh x BALB/cKh)F1 hybrids immunized i.p. with cell-bound (AKR.B6) or cell-free (AKR) Thy-1 antigen. Number of animals tested, in parenthesis.

Treatment and dose	Response to AKR.B6	% Inhibition	Response to AKR	% Inhibition
None	6860± 880 (10)	<0	3750±464 (20)	<0
Carrageenan 0.1 mg	7143±1004 (7)	<0	2000±316 (10)	47
Chloroquine 5 x 1 mg	8017±2086 (6)	<0	2239±242 (13)	43

While the degree of inhibition elicited by the two agents was similar, histological examination (Fig. 1) revealed that the mechanism underlaying the inhibition was quite different. Administration of carrageenan resulted in an almost total disappearance of India ink-containing cells, whereas after injection of chloroquine, these cells were as numerous as in control animals.

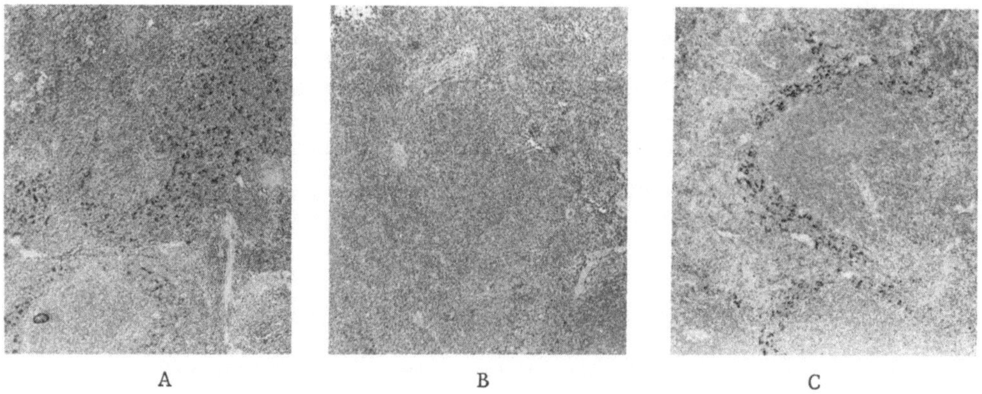

Figure 1. Histological pictures of spleens from control animals (A) and animals treated with carrageenan (B) or chloroquine (C). Animals received i.v. injection of India ink 15-20 min before killing. India ink-containing cells located in the marginal zones are visible in normal and chloroquine-treated animals. These cells are almost totally absent in animals treated with carrageenan. Nuclear Red Fast staining. Magnification 400x.

Fig. 2 illustrates an experiment in which the effect of increasing doses of carrageenan on anti-Thy-1 responses was tested. As can be seen, increased doses of carrageenan produced progressive inhibition of responses to both forms of antigen until almost total inhibition (95%) was induced by injection of 1 mg of carrageenan. Interestingly, doubling the dose of chloroquine (from 5 x 1 mg to 5 x 2 mg) resulted in the increased inhibition of the response to the cell-free antigen without any significant change in the response to the cell-bound antigen.

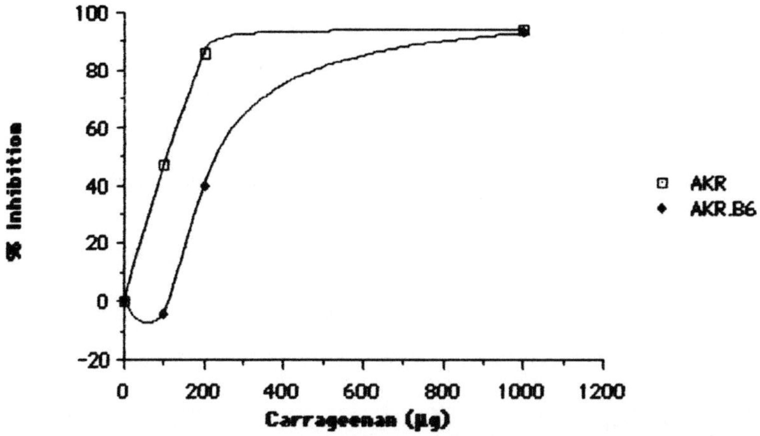

Figure 2. Relationship between the dose of carrageenan (single i.v. injection) and percent inhibition of the response elicited by cell-bound (AKR.B6) or cell-free (AKR) Thy-1 antigen.

In inbred strains (Table 3), which recognize only the cell-bound Thy-1 antigen, the effects of carrageenan and chloroquine were similar to those described above. Briefly, even a relatively small dose of carrageenan (0.1 mg) produced partial, but still significant, inhibition, whereas a relatively high dose of chloroquine (5 x 2 mg) was ineffective except in one case (C57BL/6).

Table 3. Effect of anti-macrophage agents on the responses (x PFC/spleen±SE) of the inbred strains immunized with cell-bound Thy-1 antigen. Number of animals tested, in parenthesis.

Responder	Donor	Responses after treatment with: None	Carrageenan 0.1 mg	Chloroquine 5 x 2 mg
C57BL/6Kh	AKR.B6	9433±1822 (12)	4178±692 (9)	4545± 561 (11)
BALB/cKh	AKR.D2	3700± 311 (4)	n.t.	5700±1145 (6)
B10.PL	PL	4791± 923 (12)	2567±419 (6)	4020±1198 (5)

DISCUSSION

The experiments reported above were designed to test some elements of the working hypothesis advanced in this laboratory (Zaleski et al. 1986). Specifically, the answers to the following interrelated questions were sought. (1) Are the class II molecules on antigen-presenting cells involved in recognition of the cell-free Thy-1 antigen, and are they indeed products of the complementary Ir-Thy-1 genes? (2) Are the antigen-presenting cells required for recognition of the cell-free, but not the cell-bound Thy-1 antigen? and (3) Does the cell-free antigen require processing prior to its presentation? The results obtained provided at least important clues, if not definitive answers, to the posed questions.

Selective inhibition of the responses to cell-free but not to the cell-bound antigen by anti-IA antibodies clearly demonstrated involvement of the class II molecules. Indeed, one may confidently identify a specific hybrid molecule $IA^{d}_{\alpha}:IA^{b}_{\beta}$ as being predominantly, if not exclusively involved (Quackenbush et al. 1987). The selectivity of the antibody effect, i.e., the same antibody in a given animal inhibiting the response to one but not the other form of the Thy-1 antigen, leads to the conclusion that the antibodies employed did not impair the function of B cells. This conclusion suggests that the inhibitory effect of the antibodies is exerted on the other category of class II-bearing cells, i.e., the antigen-presenting cells (Unanue 1984). Furthermore, histological examination clearly indicated that the antibodies did not physically eliminate splenic macrophages. Thus, it seems reasonable to postulate that the inhibition was caused by either blocking or modulating class II molecules on the surface of the antigen-presenting cells (Kruisbeek et al. 1985). Consequently, one is tempted to propose that the hybrid $IA^{d}_{\alpha}:IA^{b}_{\beta}$ molecule expressed on the antigen-presenting cells indeed serves as the product of the complementary Ir-Thy-1 genes that influences the magnitude of the anti-Thy-1 response by serving as the associative element (Ogasawara et al. 1987).

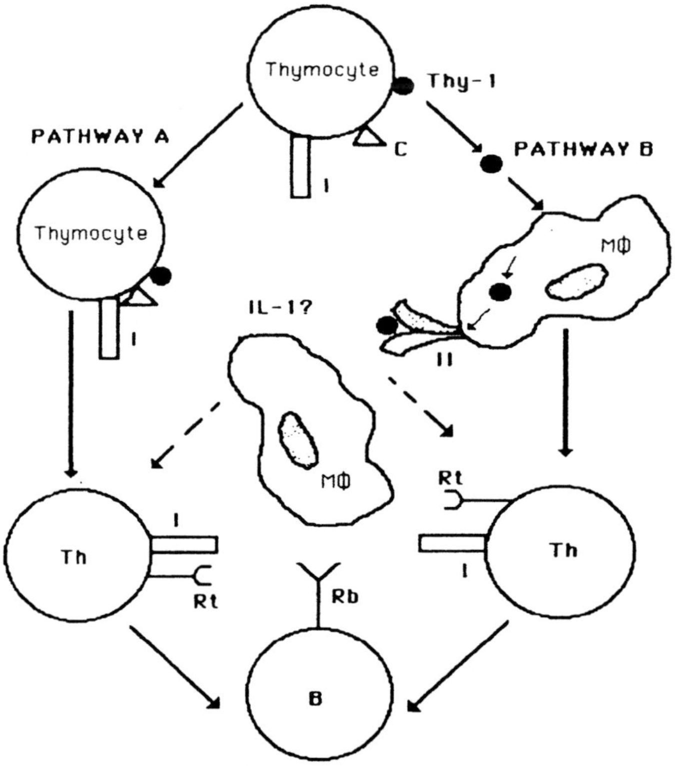

Figure 3. Schematic representation of a working hypothesis for the mechanism of anti-Thy-1 response in mice. Pathway A: the cell-bound Thy-1 antigen ( ) that forms a complex with carrier-like (C) and class I H-2 molecules (1) is presented by the donor thymocytes to T helper (Th) cells via the T-cell receptor (Rt). Pathway B: the cell-free Thy-1 antigen ( ) shed from donor thymocytes is processed and then presented by the recipient macrophages (MØ) in association with their class II H-2 molecules (11) to T halper (Th) cells. In both pathways Th cells interact with B-cell receptors (Rb) in B cells that ultimately produce antibodies to Thy-1 antigen.

The above conclusion provided, in turn, a strong indication that macrophages are important elements of the anti-Thy-1 response. This indication has been convincingly confirmed by experiments in which two anti-macrophage agents selectively, like anti-IA antibodies, inhibited the response to the cell-free antigen. While the inhibition elicited by carrageenan could be attributed to a physical destruction of macrophages (Cantanzaro et al. 1971), such an explanation could not be applied to the inhibition that followed the administration of chloroquine. Indeed, available data suggest that chloroquine interfers with antigen processing by exerting a stabilizing effect on the lyosomal membranes (Weissman et al. 1967, de Duve et al. 1974) or by increasing lysosomal pH (Gerson et al. 1981). Thus, it seems reasonable to assume that the inhibitory effect of chloroquine indicates the need for processing of the cell-free Thy-1 antigen before it is presented by macrophages. As in the case of anti-IA antibodies, the selectivity of inhibition by anti-macrophage agents rules out a possible effect on B cells or on antibodies.

The experiments in which the dose effect of carrageenan was studied provided further indication of the role played by macrophages in anti-Thy-1 responsiveness. The fact that treatment with low doses inhibited only response to the cell-free antigen, whereas high doses inhibited responses to both forms of the antigen suggests that macrophages may be involved at two distinct levels. First, macrophages, to be precise their antigen-processing and -presenting functions, may be required for recognition of the cell-free antigen in the context of or in association with class II molecules. Second, some minimal function of macrophages may be required to initiate the response of T cells, regardless of the form of the antigen. This latter function may reflect the need for certain soluble factors, e.g., IL-1, produced and secreted by macrophages (Oppenheim et al. 1986). The plausibility of such a proposition is strengthened by finding that chloroquine, which should not affect the synthetic or secretory function of macrophages, even in relatively large doses did not interfere with the responses to the cell-bound antigen. However, to confirm this notion further experiments are needed. Prominent among such experiments are attempts to reverse the carrageenan-induced inhibition by *in vivo* administration of IL-1.

Preliminary experiments with inbred strains essentially confirmed the results obtained with F1 hybrids, even though it appears that both inbred strains tested are more susceptible to carrageenan, which in a dose of 0.1 mg produced significant inhibition. The unexpected inhibition elicited by a relatively high dose of chloroquine in C57BL/6Kh mice cannot be explained at this time. While it may reflect an unusual susceptibility of the macrophages of this strain, it is still possible that it merely reflects a sampling error.

In summary, the results presented above seem to provide convincing support for the working hypothesis that accounts for the complex mechanism of the anti-Thy-1 response in mice (Fig. 3). Specifically, it was demonstrated that availability of specific hybrid IA molecules expressed on the responder's macrophages is required for recognition of the cell-free Thy-1 antigen. Furthermore, it appears that the cell-free Thy-1 antigen must undergo processing before being presented. Finally, preliminary data indicate that in addition to the antigen-processing and -presentation of cell-free antigen, macrophages may be needed as a source of soluble factor(s) required for initiation of the responses to both forms of the antigen.

ACKNOWLEDGEMENTS

This work was supported by NIH, NIAID grant AI-13628 and by the Genetics Graduate Group at the State University of New York at Buffalo.

REFERENCES

Bice, D.E., Gruwell, D.G., Salvagio, J.E. and Hoffmann, E.O. 1972. Suppression of primary immunization by carrageenan - a macrophage toxic agent. Immunol. Communic., 1: 615.

Cantanzaro, P.J., Schwartz, H.J. and Graham, R.C. 1984. Spectrum and possible mechanism of carrageenan cytotoxicity. Am. J. Pathol., 64: 387.

de Duve, C., de Barsy, T., Poole, B., Trovet, A., Tulkens, P. and van Hoff, F. 1974. Lysosomotropic agents. Biochem. Pharmacol., 23: 249.

Fuji, H., Zaleski, M.B. and Milgrom, F. 1971. Immune response to alloantigens of thymus studied in mice with plaque assay. J. Immunol., 106: 56.

Gerson, M.J., D'Arcy Hart, P. and Young, M.R. 1981. Temporal changes of lysosome and phagosome pH during phagolysosome formation in macrophages studied by fluorescence spectroscopy. J. Cell. Biol., 89: 645.

Kappler, J.W., Skidmore, B., White, J. and Marrack, P. 1981. Antigen inducible, H-2 restricted, interleukin-2-producing T-cell hybridomas. J. exp. Med. 153, 1198.

Klein, J. and Zaleski, M.B. 1987. Genetic control of immune responses to Thy-1. In: Thy-1 Immunology, Neurology, and Therapeutic Applications. A.E. Reif and M. Sclesinger, eds., Marcel Dekker, New York.

Kruisbeek, A.M., Titus, J.A., Stephany, D.A. Gause, B.L. and Longo, D.D. 1985. In vivo treatment with monoclonal anti-IA antibodies. Disappearance of splenic antigen-presenting cell function concommitant with modulation of splenic cell-surface IA and IE antigens. J. exp. Med., 134: 3605.

Lake, P. and Douglas, T.C. 1978. Recognition and control of helper determinants for cell-surface antigen Thy-1. Nature, 275: 430.

Ogasawara, K., Maloy, W.L. and Schwartz, R.H. 1987. Failure to find holes in the T-cell repertoire. Nature 325: 450.

Oppenheim, J.J., Kovacs, E.J., Matsushimo, K. and Durum, S.K. 1986. There is more than one interleukin 1. Immunol. Today 7: 45.

Ozato, K., Epstein, S.L., Hemkart, P., Hansen, T.H. and Sachs, D.H. 1981. Studies on monoclonal antibodies to mouse MHC products. Transpl. Proc., 13: 958.

Pittaluga, G. 1935. Las infermidades del sistema reticulo-endotelial. Calpe, Madrid.

Quackenbush, L.J., Dowjat, W.K. and Zaleski, M.B. 1985. IA mutation affects anti-Thy-1 response in mice. Immunogenetics, 21: 617.

Quackenbush, L.J., Dowjat, W.K. and Zaleski, M.B. 1985. Search for IA trans-complementation affecting the anti-Thy-1 response in mice: A final report. Immunol. Inv., 14: 379.

Quackenbush, L.J., Dowjat, W.K., Gorzynski, T.J. and Zaleski, M.B. 1987. Identification of the IA hybrid molecule affecting anti-Thy-1 responsiveness. Transplantation 43: (in press).

Shoemaker, J.P. 1978. Fifty-five percent complete remission of mammary carcinoma in mice with 5-fluorouracil and chloroquine. Cancer Res., 38: 2700.

Unanue, E.R. 1984. Antigen-presenting function of the macrophage. Ann. Rev. Immunol., 2: 395.

Weissman, G., Sessa, G. and Bevans, V. 1967. Effect of DMSO on the stabilization of lysosomes by cortisone and chloroquine in vitro. Ann N.Y. Acad. Sci., 141: 326.

Zaleski, M.B., Gorzynski, T.J., Quackenbush, L.J. and Dowjat, W.K. 1985. In vivo inhibition of anti-Thy-1 response by monoclonal antibody to the IA molecules of the responder. Immunogenetics 22: 673.

Zaleski, M.B., Quackenbush, L.J., Gorzynski, T.J. and Reichner, J.S. 1986. The Ir-Thy-1 concept: Continuing saga. Immunol. Res., 5: 79.

PROBING MHC DNA IN SEARCH OF CODING SEQUENCES : DETECTION OF A NOVEL GENE LOCATED BETWEEN C4 AND Bf IN MOUSE AND MAN

Matthieu Lévi-Strauss*, Michael Carroll+, Michael Steinmetz▽ and Tommaso Meo*

* INSERM U 276 and Unité d'Immunogénétique, Institut Pasteur, 25 rue du Docteur Roux, 75724 Paris Cedex 15 France
+ Harvard Medical School, 300 Longwood Av., Boston, MA 02115, USA
▽ Basel Institute for Immunology, Grenzacherstrasse 487 CH-4058 Basel, Switzerland

INTRODUCTION

The search for specific genes in chromosomal regions implicated in particular diseases or associated with certain functions is one of the approaches that may lead to a molecular analysis of inherited albeit biochemically ill defined traits. This strategy is presently pursued to understand the mechanism of some genetically determined diseases such as the Duchenne Muscular Dystrophy (Monaco et al., 1986).

The large physical size of the major histocompatibility complex stands in contrast with the scarcity of its actually known gene content and suggests that this chromosomal region harbors indeed a number of genes yet to be discovered. The detection of such genes would be valuable in many respects.

First, the precise molecular characterization of this complex locus would provide an ideal model for studying the organization, evolution and gene interrelations over a long and best studied chromosomal fragment. Moreover, the knowledge of new genes should open the way to the molecular bases of those MHC-linked diseases which, as narcolepsy (Juji et al., 1984) or hemochromatosis (Simon et al., 1984), cannot be satisfactorily explained on the basis of the genes presently known to be located in this region. Last, the characterization of genes, possibly submitted to hiterto overlooked selective pressures which could influence the transmission of the whole region, might help to understand certain observed idiosyncrasies (i.e. segregation distorsions, linkage disequilibria, etc.) in the genetics of some haplotypes.

So far, four main methodologies can be in general implemented for the discovery of new genes.

One method that has been reported very recently is based on the finding that peculiar sequences (HTF-islands) surround the transcription start site of many animal genes (Bird, 1986). These sequences can be detected by their unusual high content in restriction endonuclease sites recognizing two C-G dinucleotides (Lindsay and Bird, 1987).

The second method involves the transfection of cultured cells with genomic clones characterized only for their location in a chromosomal region of genetic interest. This method has been successfully used for the isolation of previously unsuspected MHC class I genes (Lemonnier et al., 1982) but suffers of some limitations. First, the detection of proteins encoded by the transfected cosmids can be performed only if an antibody or a biological assay are available for the gene whose presence has already been suspected within the region under study. In the case of unknown genes, however, the detection can be carried out at the mRNA level using the whole cosmid as probe in hybridization experiments with the RNA of the transfected cells. Second, such method stands better chance with relatively short-sized genes which can be assumed to be entirely contained within the chosen cosmid clones. Third, the gene introduced by DNA transfer must be expressable by the particular cell line selected for the transfection experiment. For example, among the class III products of the murine major histocompatibility complex neither the C4-Slp gene nor the 21-hydroxylase genes are expressed in L-cells (Tosi et al. 1985, Parker et al. 1985) commonly used for DNA transfer experiments.

The third approach involves hybridization of cosmid clones DNA with RNA extracted from various organs. This method has been for example successfully used for the detection of the 21-hydroxylase genes. Amor et al. (1985) hybridized radio-active cDNA made from liver mRNA on filters carrying DNA from H-2S region cosmid clones. Repetitive sequences, present in essentially all cosmid clones and possibly expressed in several messengers are hard to be removed quantitatively from the hybridization probe and therefore represent an important pitfall of this strategy. In addition, if in this method one fails to use RNA from the appropriate tissue, the new gene can easily go undetected.

The last approach is the most inclusive and is based on the fact that coding sequences are usually more conserved between species than the non coding ones. The first step of this method involves generation of several probes for the cloned region under study. These probes are subsequently hybridized at high stringency on blots of genomic DNA from different, although evolutionary not too distant, species. The conserved, and thus potentially coding sequences, are likely to be the only ones for which the hybridization signal remains detectable on all the DNA samples under these conditions. This method, recently referred to as the "zoo blot", has been used in the case of Duchenne Muscular Dystrophy (Monaco et al., 1986) retinoblastoma (Friend et al., 1986) and cystic fibrosis (Estivill et al., 1987) and has lead to the detection of interesting genes within regions corresponding to the genetic location of the disease. A major advantage offered by this method is that it can be used even with DNA containing repetitive sequences which, owing to their poor evolutionary conservation, fail to crosshybridize at high stringency between different species. Of course, strong interspecies DNA hybridizations may also be found for non coding sequences such as the minisatellite elements of Jeffreys et al. (1985) (Burke and Bruford, 1987). Conversely, some genes may have no direct counterpart in another species. Nevertheless, the general applicability and rapidity of this method in screening a large number of cosmid clones outweigh these possible shortcomings.

We describe in this paper the application of this strategy to the search of new genes within the H-2S region which, due to its size (Tosi et al., 1985, Müller et al., 1987), must still hide several.

RESULTS AND DISCUSSION

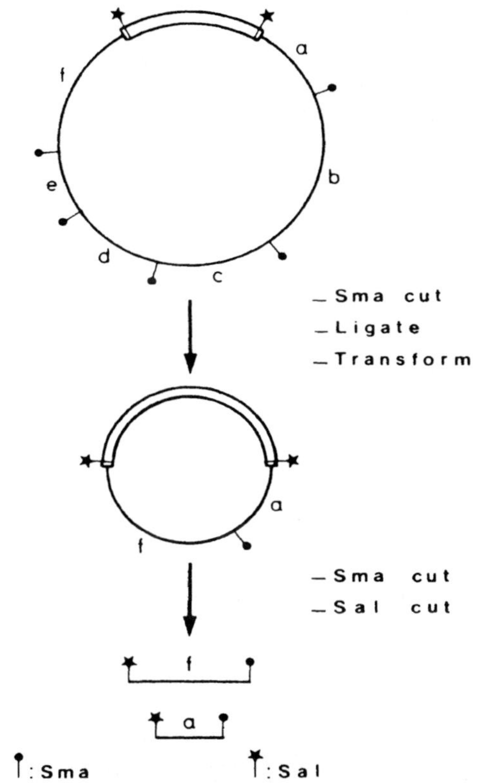

Fig. 1. Preparation of evenly spaced genomic probes for the H-2S region : Supercoiled DNA was prepared from a collection of cosmid clones characterized for their genetic location within the H-2S region. Each of these DNA preparations was restricted with the Sma I endonuclease which doesn't cut within the pNNL5 vector (Grosveld et al., 1982) but which usually cleaves the genomic DNA insert in multiple fragments. 10 ng of this cleaved DNA preparation were then self-ligated in 10 μl of the appropriate buffer and were subsequently used to transform competent HB101 bacteria. Supercoiled DNA was prepared from ampicilline-resistant clones and was restricted with the Sma I and Sal I endonucleases. The latter enzyme recognizes two cleavage sites located on both sides of the Bam HI restriction site used for inserting the Sau 3A -cleaved genomic DNA. The two genomic DNA fragments corresponding to both ends of each cosmid clone were then prepared by agarose gel electrophoresis.

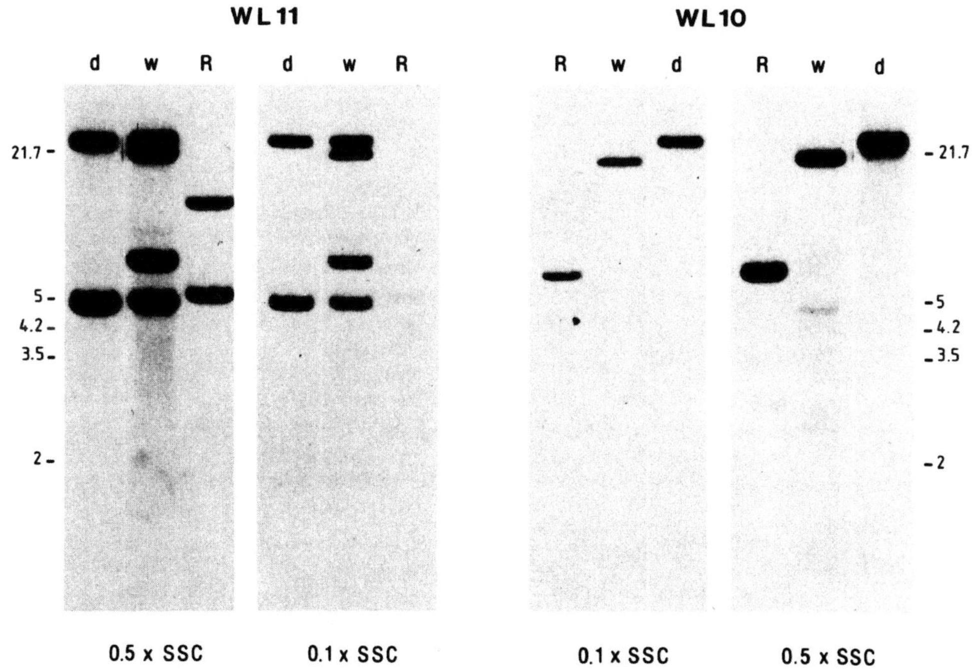

Fig. 2. Probes WL10 (1300 bp) and WL11 (1200 bp) corresponding to the two extremities of cosmid 2.1 (Steinmetz et al., 1984) were prepared according to the procedure summarized in Fig. 1 and labelled using the random-priming technique (Feinberg and Vogelstein, 1983). These two probes were hybridized on Southern Blot filters bearing Hind III - restricted genomic DNAs. Lanes R : 15 μg of rat DNA (Lou strain), lanes d : 15 μg of $\underline{H\text{-}2^{d}}$ mouse DNA (BALB/c strain), lanes w : 15 μg of $\underline{H\text{-}2^{w16}}$ mouse DNA (B10.BUA1 strain). The hybridization was performed at 42°C during 40 hours in the following solution : 30% formamide, 5 x SSC, 50 mM sodium phosphate pH 6.5, 0.4% SDS, 200 μg/ml denatured salmon sperm DNA, 200 μg/ml Yeast RNA.

Filters were washed extensively at room temperature and finally four times 20 minutes at 65°C in the following solution : 0.5 x SSC, 0.1% SDS, 16 mM Sodium Phosphate pH 7.5, 1 mM Sodium Pyrophosphate. Sealed plastic bags containing the wet filters were then exposed overnight at -80°C for autoradiography (panels : 0.5 x SSC). After exposure the same filters were washed four times 20 minutes at 65°C in the following solution : 0.1 x SSC, 0.1% SDS, 16 mM Sodium Phosphate ph 7.5, 1 mM Sodium Pyrophosphate, and were dryed for autoradiography (panels 0.1 x SSC).

Selection of the probes

In order to prepare evenly spaced probes within the H-2S region, different cosmid clones from a BALB/c library were cut with the Sma I restriction endonuclease (which doesn´t cut into the pNNL5 vector) and ligated at low DNA concentration to increase the rate of recircularization. In order to purify the vector molecules still linked to fragments corresponding to both ends of the DNA insert, bacteria were transformed with the ligated DNA and the deleted "mini-cosmids" grown to prepare supercoiled DNA. The fragments corresponding to the two ends of the original cosmids were then prepared with a Sal I (which cuts just on both sides of the Bam HI cloning site of the pNNL5 cosmid vector) - Sma I double digestion (Fig.1).

Figure 2 shows the hybridization on genomic Southern blots of the probes corresponding to the ends of the H-2S cosmid 2.1 (Steinmetz et al., 1984) which contains almost the whole C4-Slp gene and extends approximatively 20 kb on its 5´ end. Probe WL11 corresponds to the C4-Slp end of the cosmid and displays an hybridization pattern characteristic for a C4 or C4-Slp 3´ probe (Lévi-Strauss et al., 1985a). Indeed, the two Hind III bands of the BALB/c DNA (lanes d) identify the single C4 and C4-Slp genes typical of the $H-2^d$ haplotype (Lévi-Strauss et al., 1985a, Chaplin et al., 1983). The four Hind III bands of the $H-2^{w16}$ haplotype (lanes w) correspond to its three C4-Slp and to its single C4 gene (Lévi-Strauss et al., 1985b). Probe WL10 corresponds to the other end of the cosmid which is located between the C4-Slp and the Bf genes.

While probe WL11 is clearly part of a duplicated ($H-2^d$) or of a quadruplicated ($H-2^{w16}$) DNA segment, probe WL10 detects a single Hind III fragment in both haplotypes. One of the boundaries of the amplified segment must therefore be located between the WL10 probe and the 5´ end of the C4-Slp gene.

Stringent washes (0.1 x SSC) of the blots result in an almost complete disappearance of the hybridization signal of the WL11 probe on rat DNA (lanes R) suggesting that this probe, although probably located within the 3´ part of the C4-Slp gene, doesn´t contain exonic sequences. In contrast, the hybridization of the WL10 probe on rat DNA is, even at high strigency, as strong as the hybridization on mouse DNA suggesting that this probe might contain a coding sequence.

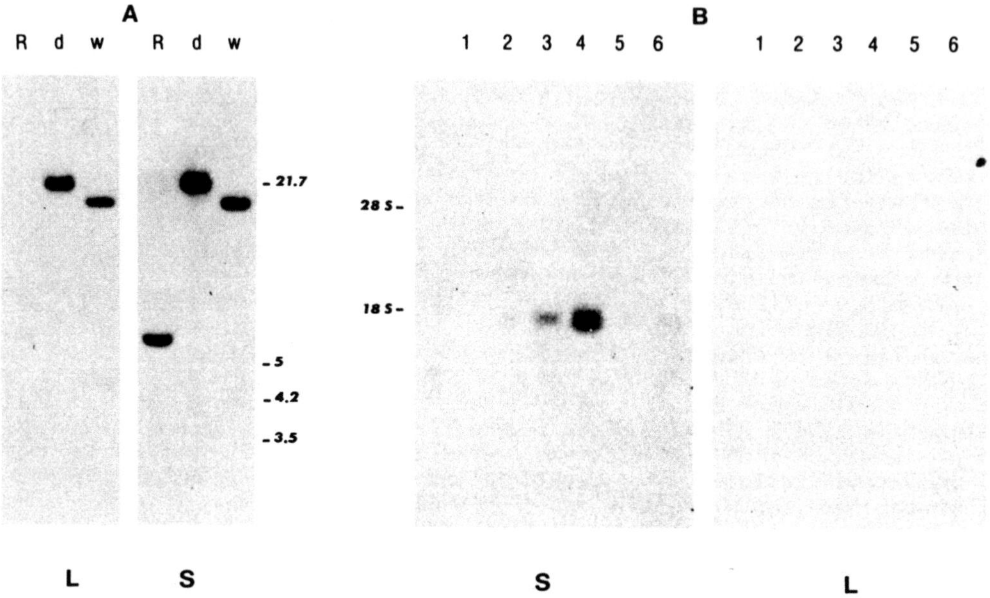

Fig. 3. Probe WL10 was cut in two subfragments with the Pst I endonuclease; these two subprobes (WL10 L : panels L, and WL10 S : panels S) were labelled and hybridized in the solution described in the legend of Fig. 2 on DNA(panel A) or on RNA blots (panel B). These filters were subsequently washed etensively at room temperature and finally four times 20 minutes at 65°C in the following solution : 0.1 x SSC, 0.1% SDS, 16 mM Sodium phosphate pH 7.5, 1 mM Sodium Pyrophosphate. Dryed filters were then exposed overnight (Southern blot experiments) or during a week (Northern blot experiments) at -80°C for autoradiography.

Panel A : lanes R : 15 μg of Hind III - restricted rat DNA (Lou strain), lanes d : 15 μg of Hind III - restricted $H\text{-}2^d$ mouse DNA (BALB/c strain), lanes w : 15 μg of Hind III - restricted $H\text{-}2^{w16}$ mouse DNA (B10.BUA1 strain).

Panel B : lanes 1 : 20 μg of rat brain total RNA, lanes 2 : 20 μg of mouse LPS blasts total RNA, lanes 3 : 20 μg of total RNA from the F12 (Mallat et al., 1986) mouse astroblastic cell line, lanes 4 : 10 μg of mouse liver poly A+ RNA, lanes 5 : 20 μg of mouse liver total RNA, lanes 6 : 20 μg of mouse spleen total RNA.

Refinement of the WL10 probe

Probe WL10 was submitted to a more detailed study. This DNA segment was cut in two fragments with Pst I in order to select a putatively more exon-rich region.
The contiguous subfragments WL10 L (750 bp) and WL10 S (550 bp) were used as probes at high stringency in Southern blots and Northern blots experiments. Fig. 3 shows that the WL10 L sequences are not conserved between rat and mouse and that the probe fails to detect a RNA species. In contrast, the WL10 S probe, which recognizes strongly an homologous sequence in the rat genome is also able to hybridize to a slightly smaller than 18S RNA species. These observations appear thus to validate

the efficiency of the method to uncover new expressed sequences. Comparisons of lanes 4 and 5, corresponding respectively to poly A+ and to total mouse liver RNA show that the hybridizing RNA, highly enriched in the poly A+ fraction is indeed polyadenylated. Fig. 3 and other unpublished data show that the RNA species is expressed at very low levels in many tissues or cultured cell lines.

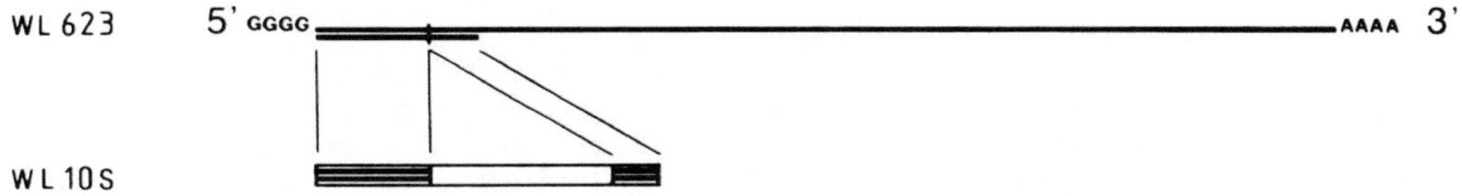

Fig. 4. Schematic alignment of the sequences of the WL623 cDNA clone and of the WL10 S genomic clone. AAAA at the 3′ end of clone WL623 represents the poly A tail of the corresponding messenger, GGGG at the 5′ end of the clone represents the artificial polydG sequence which was used for the initiation of the synthesis of the cDNA second strand.

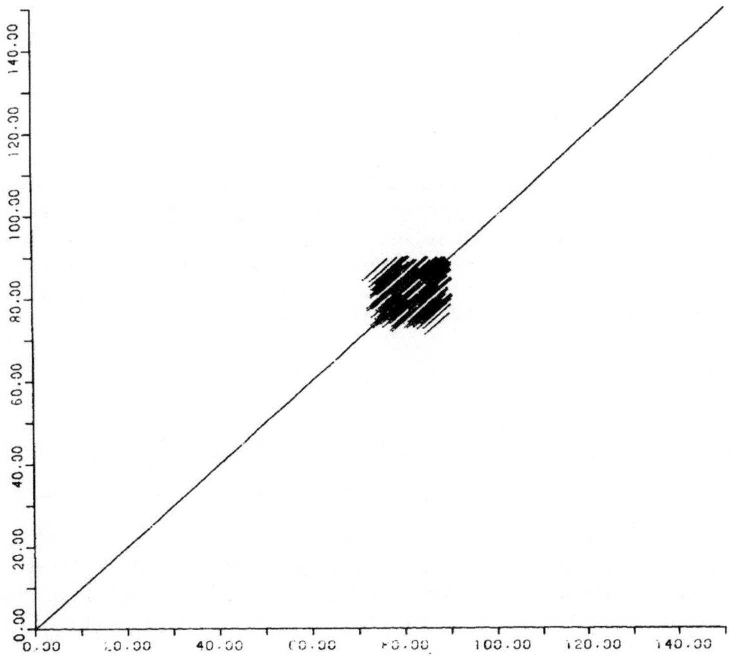

Fig. 5. Dot matrix analysis of the sequence of the WL623 cDNA clone. WL623 sequence was compared to itself, the window stringency corresponds to a 80% homology on 10 bp, the filter stringency corresponds to a 55% homology on 40 bp.

cDNA cloning

In order to give information on the coding potential of the polyadenylated RNA, we decided to isolate cDNA clones hybridizing with WL10 S. We constructed, in the λgt10 vector a mouse liver cDNA library of large complexity. Taking into account the level of expression of the sought RNA, we screened approximatively 1.5×10^6 independent clones. Clones WL623 and WL691 were isolated in the first screening whereas 10 additional positive clones were obtained in a second screening using clone WL623 as a probe.
Clones WL10 S and WL623 were then sequenced, Fig. 4 shows that the WL10 S genomic probe corresponds to the 5′ end of the WL623 cDNA clone. This 550 bp genomic probe contains in fact two exonic segments separated by an intron of approximately 250 bp. The sequence of the 1500 bp long WL623 cDNA clone reveals a very peculiar central region, made of approximately 8 imperfect repeats of 15 nucleotides, which is noticeable on the dot matrix analysis shown in Fig. 5. This region is included in the longest open reading frame which, in phase with the first ATG of the sequence, corresponds to a methionine-initiated 42 kDa polypeptide. The deduced amino acid sequence failed to show significant homology with any known protein family.

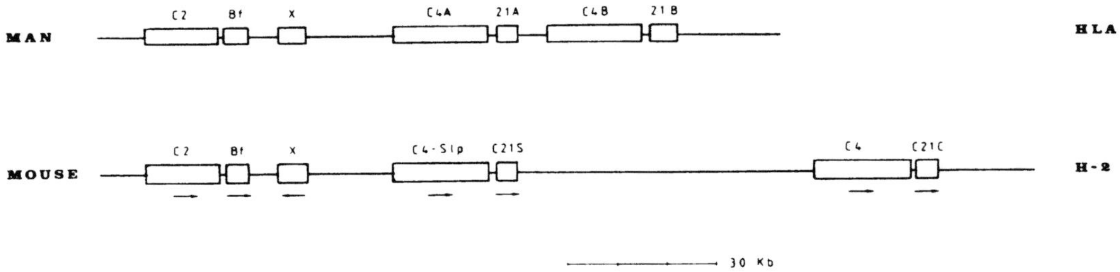

Fig. 6. Schematic representation of the organization of the class III genes of the human and murine major histocompatibility complex showing the localization, the approximate size and the transcriptional orientation of the new "X" gene. The original data used to construct these maps are from the volume 87 of Immunological Reviews (1985) "Molecular Genetics of Class III MHC antigenes" (Munksgaard, Copenhagen).

Genomic localization in man and in mouse of the WL623 sequences

The localization of the murine gene corresponding to the WL623 cDNA clone was confirmed and its transcriptional orientation was determined using cosmids from another genomic library (B10.W7R, H-2^{w7}). In this haplotype, the gene corresponding to the WL623 cDNA clone is also situated (data not shown) between the Bf gene and one of the four C4-Slp gene copies characteristically amplified in this strain (Lévi-Strauss et al., 1985b).
The 3′ end of the gene was found to be very close to the Bf gene whereas

its 5′ end is some 20 kb away from C4-Slp (not shown). Surprigsingly, this new gene has a transcriptional orientation unlike the other class III genes.
In man, the gene is also located in the corresponding genetic region (Fig. 6). Indeed, the WL623 cDNA clone, when used as a probe on Southern blots of human DNA detects a unique sequence in the genome present in the human cosmid clone 1a (Carroll et al., 1984) covering the region situated between the C4A and Bf genes in the human major histocompatibility complex.
In summary, our work has brought to light a new gene, expressed as a 18 S polyadenylated RNA, transcribed ubiquitously and located in H-2 and HLA, between the C4 and Bf genes. The sequence derived from liver cDNA clones indicates that this new gene may encode a 42 kDa polypeptide which can not so far be assigned to a known protein family.

REFERENCES

Amor, M., Tosi, M., Duponchel, C., Steinmetz, M., and Meo, T. : Liver mRNA probes disclose two cytochrome P-450 genes duplicated in tandem with the complement C4 loci of the mouse H-2S region. Proc. Natl. Acad. Sci. USA 82 : 4453, 1985

Bird, A.P. : CpG-rich islands and the function of DNA methylation. Nature 321 : 209, 1986

Burke, T., and Bruford, M.W. : DNA fingerprinting in birds. Nature 327 : 149, 1987

Carroll, M.C., Campbell, R.D., Bentley, D.R., and Porter, R.R. : A molecular map of the human major histocompatibility complex class III region linking complement genes C4, C2 and factor B. Nature 307 : 237, 1984

Chaplin, D., Woods, D., Whitehead, A., Goldberger, G., Colten, H.R., and Seidman, J.G. : Molecular map of the murine S region. Proc. Natl. Acad. Sci. USA 80 : 6947, 1983

Estivill, X., Farrall, M., Scambler, P.J., Bell, G.M., Hawley, K.M.F., Lench, N.J., Bates, G.P., Kruger, H.C., Frederick, P.A., Stanier, P., Watson, E.K., Williamson, R., and Wainwright, B.S. : A candidate for the cystic fibrosis locus isolated by selection for methylation-free islands. Nature 326 : 840, 1987

Feinberg, A.P., and Vogelstein, B. : A technique for radiolabelling DNA restriction endonuclease fragments to high specific activity. Analytical Biochemistry 132 : 6, 1983

Friend, S.H., Bernards, R., Rogelj, S., Weinberg, R.A., Rappaport, J.M., Albert, D.M., and Dryja, T.P. : A human DNA segment with properties of the gene that predisposes to retinoblastoma and oasteosarcoma. Nature 323 : 643, 1986

Grosveld, F.G., Lund, T., Murray, E.J., Mellor, A.L., Dahl, H.H.M., and Flavell, R.A. : The construction of cosmid libraries which can be used to transform eukaryotic cells. Nucl. Ac. Res. 10 : 6715, 1982

Jeffreys, A.J., Wilson, V., and Thein, S.L. : Hypervariable "minisatellite" regions in human DNA. Nature 314 : 67, 1985

Juji, T., Satake, M., Honda, Y., and Doi, Y. : HLA antigens in Japanese patients with narcolepsy. Tissue Antigens 24 : 316, 1984

Lemonnier, F.A., Malissen, M., Goldstein, P., Le Bouteiller, P., Rebai, N., Damotte, M., Birnbaum, D., Caillol, D., Trucy, J., and Jordan, B.R. : Expression of human class I histocompatibility antigens at the surface of DNA transformed mouse L cells. Immunogenetics 16 : 355, 1982

Lévi-Strauss, M., Tosi, M., Steinmetz, M., Klein, J., and Meo, T. : Multiple duplications of complement C4 gene correlate with H-2 controlled testosterone-independent expression of its sex-limited isoform, C4-Slp. Proc. Natl. Acad. Sci. USA 82 : 1746, 1985a

Lévi-Strauss, M., Georgatsou, E., Tosi, M., and Meo, T. : Gene-specific probes demonstrate selective duplications of the C4-Slp gene. Immunogenetics 21 : 397, 1985b

Lindsay, S., and Bird, A.P. : Use of restriction enzymes to detect potential gene sequences in mammalian DNA. Nature 327 : 336, 1987

Mallat, M., Moura Neto, V., Gros, F., Glowinski, J., and Prochiantz, A. : Two simian virus 40 (SV40) transformed cell lines from the mouse striatum and mesencephalon presenting astrocytes characters. II : Interaction with mesencephalic neurons. Dev. Brain Res. 26 : 23, 1986

Monaco, A.P., Neve, R.L., Colletti-Feener, C., Bertelson, C.J., Kurnit, D.M., and Kunkel, L.M. : Isolation of candidate cDNAs for portions of the Duchenne muscular dystrophy gene. Nature 323 : 646, 1986

Müller, U., Stephan, D., Philippsen, P., and Steinmetz, M. : Orientation and molecular map position of the complement genes in the mouse MHC. EMBO J. 6 : 369, 1987

Parker, K.L., Chaplin, D.D., Wong, M., Seidman, J.G., Smith, J.A., and Schimmer, B.P. : Expression of murine 21-hydroxylase in mouse adrenal glands and in transfected Y1 adrenocortical tumor cells. Proc. Natl. Acad. Sci. USA 82 : 7860, 1985

Simon, M., Fauchet, R., Hespel, J.P., Beaumont, C., Brissot, P., Hita de Nercy, Y., Genetet, B., and Bourel, M. : Idiopathic homochromatosis, a study of biochemical expression in 247 heterozygous members of 63 families. Evidence for a single major HLA-linked gene. Gastroenterology 78 : 703, 1980

Steimetz, M., Malissen, M., Hood, L., Orn, A., Maki, R.A., Reza-Dastoornikoo, G., Stephan, D., Gibb., E., and Romaniuk, R. : Tracts of high or low sequence divergence in the mouse major histocompatibility complex. EMBO J. 3 : 2995, 1984

Tosi, M., Lévi-Strauss, M., Georgatsou, E., Amor, M., and Meo, T. : Duplications of complement and non complement genes of the H-2S region : evolutionary aspects of C4 isotypes and molecular analysis of their expression variants. Immunological Reviews 87 : 151, 1985

MUTATION IN THE A_β GENE OF B6.C-H-2^{bm12}. ANTIBODY BINDING SITE VS. T CELL RECOGNITION SITES

Kathleen A. Donovan, Sujay K. Singh* and Chella S. David

Department of Immunology, Mayo Clinic and Medical School
Rochester, MN 55905

Four functional Ia genes are coded within the I (immune response) region of mouse, e.g., A_α, A_β, E_α, and E_β (Jones et al. 1978; Klein et al. 1981). In recent years using congenic inbred and recombinant strains of mice, several investigators have demonstrated a relationship between Ia molecules and immune response. The I-A mutant mouse strain, B6.C-H-2^{bm12} is to date the only known example of a mutant involving the class II genes. This strain was originally identified by Melvold and Kohn from a (B6 x BALB/c)F_1 by reciprocal skin graft rejection. The findings on this mutant, B6.H-2^{bm12}, have helped in further characterization of fine specificities on an Ia molecule. In analyzing this mutant strain, McKenzie and co-workers were able to map the mutation to the I-A subregion using complementation studies with recombinant strains. Tryptic peptide maps revealed a limited number of differences between B6 and bm12, mapping the mutation to the I-A beta polypeptide chain (McKean et al. 1981). The tryptic peptide studies showed that this mutation is not due to a single point mutation, but involves a minimum of three different amino acid substitutions. Recently, McIntyre and Seidman (1984) have cloned and sequenced a gene coding for the bm12 A-beta polypeptide chain. Three nucleotide substitutions result in three amino acid substitutions within a span of five amino acids; isoleucine at position 67, arginine at position 70 and threonine at position 71, are being substituted by phenylalanine, glutamine and lysine respectively (Fig. 1). Two of these amino acid substitutions (arginine- glutamine and threonine-lysine) are non-conservative changes in the tertiary structure of the beta polypeptide chain, resulting in the observed alterations in the serology and function of the bm12 I-A molecule. Amino acid sequence comparison also shows that two of the amino acid substitutions found in the bm12 A_β chain are found at the same positions in several human class II beta chains (McIntyre and Seidman, 1984). These comparisons suggest that the bm12 mutation in the I-A beta gene arose from a gene-conversion type event in which another class II beta chain gene acted as a donor sequence.

*Present address: Howard Hughes Medical Institute, Vanderbilt University, Nashville, TN 37232.

Comparison of the bm12 nucleotide substitutions to the sequence of a cosmid clone for the I-E^b gene has suggested that the I-E^b served as this donor sequence (Widera and Flavell, 1984), where a minimum of 14 nucleotides of the A_β gene are replaced by homologous information from the E_β gene.

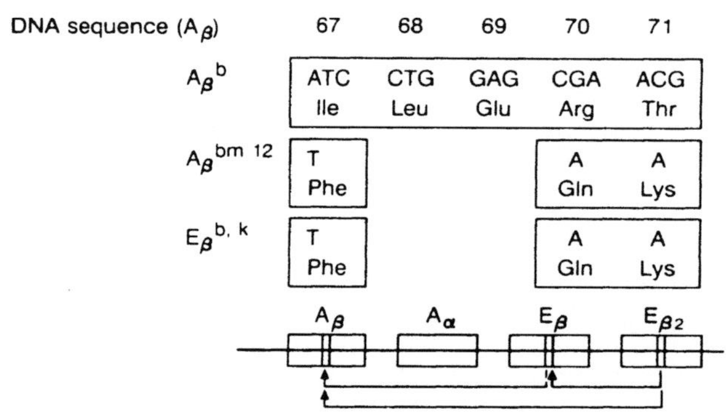

<u>Figure 1:</u> Depicts the sequence alterations in the bm12 mutant from the parent A_β^b chain with a comparison of potential donor sequences from E_β^b for the gene conversion-like event.

This gene conversion event may have been generated by the donating of sequences from an alternate gene or the E_β to A_β or a prior donation from an alternate gene to E_β with subsequent donation to the A_β gene.

Analysis of the bm12 mutant from a serological viewpoint has shown the loss of 2 Ia specificities, Ia.8 (Lafuse et al. 1981) and Ia.39 (Huber et al. 1982). The Ia.8 is expressed in the b, q and d haplotypes. In comparing the nucleotide sequences of the A_β chains of these haplotypes in the region of 55-70, these sequences are very similar. This includes the region of mutation in the bm12 lacking this specificity and suggests this region may code for this determinant. Additional serologic work done in our laboratory by David et al. using A.BY anti-bm12 antisera absorbed against B6 splenocytes shows the existence of a determinant called Ia.51. As shown by Table 1, the % cytotoxicity indicates this determinant is present on B6.bm12 as well as B10.A(5R) and B10.A both of which contain the linear determinant in amino acids 67 through 71 donated to the bm12 mutant. This determinant is also present on the B10.S(9R) cells with an E_β^s gene, whose sequence is the same as the donating sequence with the exception of amino acid number 71 which has an arginine in place of lysine. This suggests the antibodies may be recognizing the linear determinant in the E_β gene.

Table 1. Microcytotoxicity assay of A.BY anti-bml2 sera absorbed with B6 cells. 100 µl antiserum diluted 1/10 was absorbed with 100 x 10^6 B6 spleen cells.

A.BY Anti-bml2
(absorbed with B6)

	A_α	A_β	E_β	E_α	E Molecule	% Cytotoxicity
B6	b	b	b	-	-	10
B6.bml2	b	bml2	b	-	-	75
B10.A(5R)	b	b	b	k	+	35
B10.S(9R)	s	s	s	k	+	30
B10.A	k	k	k	k	+	45

The I-A mutant, bml2 has been used by several investigators to define structure-function relationship of the I-A molecule. Hochman and Huber (1985) and Mengle-Gaw et al. (1984) have shown that functional determinants are shared between A_β^{bml2} and E_β^b polypeptides. This is based upon responsiveness of bml2 to sheep insulin. B6, the parental strain of bml2 is a non-responder to sheep insulin. Studies by Lin et al. (1981) have shown that the lymph node proliferation response to beef insulin in the bml2 mutant is greatly reduced compared to parent B6, while response to other antigens (T,G)-A--L, DNP-OVA, PPD, and pork insulin is unaffected. Using bml2, Mengle-Gaw et al. (1984) have demonstrated that the I-A subregion is responsible for Ir gene phenomenon and mixed lymhocyte reaction. They have also shown that alloreactive T cell clones recognize a determinant shared by A_β^{bml2} and E_β^b molecules. Based upon the above findings it was proposed that, the segment of gene donated by E_β^b maintains its functional determinants in bml2. However, this notion has been challenged by Tse et al. (1985), who used a number of alloreactive clones generated against Ia^{bml2} antigens. If bml2 inherits a functional E_β^b unit, these B6-anti-bml2 alloreactive T cells should be stimulated by E_β^b positive cells. However, in their study B10.A(5R) (E_β^b, E_β^k) failed to stimulate B6-anti-bml2 T cell clones. Recently, Hansen et al (1986) have shown that responses of B6.C-H-2^{bml2} to heterologous insulins show no correlation with the putative gene conversion but define Ia^{bml2} as functionally unique. Since activation of T cells depends on the concommitant recognition of Ia and antigen on the surface of antigen presenting cells, any change in the primary or tertiary structure of the Ia molecule might affect the immune response.

In the present study, we have used a different approach. We have used (B6 x A.TFR5)F_1 mice to characterize the Ia recognition by T cells. B6, being a nonexpressor of the I-E molecule does not express E_β^b on the cell surface. A.TFR5 has an E^f gene which fails to make a protein product. However, A.TFR5 synthesizes a functional E_α^k polypeptide chain. The (B6 x A.TFR5)F_1 expresses a functional I-E molecule, which is comprised of E_β^b and E_α^k. This molecule carries the linear determinant which is expressed on the surface of bml2 lymphocytes (Fig. 2). So, one would predict that if T cells recognize only the altered region of the A_β^{bml2} chain, bml2 skin grafts would be accepted by (B6 x A.TFR5)F_1s. However, this is not the case. These F_1s reject the bml2 skin grafts as readily as B6 strains (Table 2). This suggests that the T cells recognize either new conformational determinants on the I-A^{bml2} molecule or new recognition sites generated by the stretches on the class II molecule which comprise the borders of the sequence shared between A_β^{bml2} and E_β^b. To further characterize the T cell recognition sites, we also tested the (B6 x A.TFR5)F_1 anti-bml2 proliferative response. B6 anti-bml2 cells respond strongly to each other in a primary mixed lymphocyte response. If new T cell recognition sites are not generated in the I-A^{bm12} molecule, one would not expect a (B6 x A.TFR5)F_1-anti-bm12 response. However, as demonstrated in Table 3, a strong mixed lymphocyte response is observed, confirming the skin graft experiments.

Skin Graft/MLR

Recipient/Responder	Donor/Stimulator
(B6 x A.TFR5)F_1	B6.C-H-2^{bm12}
$\dfrac{A^b_\beta\ A^b_\alpha\ E^b_\beta\ -}{A^f_\beta\ A^f_\alpha\ -\ E^k_\beta}$	$A^{bm12}_\beta\ A^b_\alpha\ E^b_\beta\ -$

Figure 2. In these experiments we have chosen to use the (B6 x A.TFR5)F_1 as the recipient/responder. This mouse expresses a functional I-E molecule composed of E^b_β and E^k_α. This molecule carries the linear determinant found on A^{bm12}_β.

Table 2. bm12 tail skin was grafted according to the method published elsewhere (Steinmuller, 1984).

The accepted skin grafts were for a period of greater than 35 days.

Skin Grafting

Recipient*	Donor	Days of bm12 Graft Survival
B6	bm12	10-16
A.TFR5	bm12	10-16
(B6 x A.TFR5)F_1	bm12	10-16
bm12	bm12	Accepted

* 7 mice were used as recipients per group

Table 3. Mixed lymphocyte reactions were performed according to Johnson et al. (1982) Briefly, 1 x 10^6 splenocytes from responder strains were stimulated with 1 x 10^6 (irradiated) splenocytes from stimulator strains for 3 days. The lymphocyte proliferation was measured by the incorporation of ^{3}H-thymidine added on day 3 of culture.

Mixed Lymphocyte Reaction

Stimulators	Responders					
	B6		bm12		(B6 x A.TFR5)F_1	
	cpm*	SI+	cpm*	SI+	cpm*	SI+
B6	-	-	33.0	3.0	-	-
bm12	14.1	2.4	-	-	30.3	3.0
(B6 x A.TFR5)F_1	20.0	3.0	28.3	2.8	-	-

* cpm in thousands over syngeneic controls.
\+ SI = stimulation index

In summary, the data presented here strongly supports the idea that T cells recognize predominantly the tertiary structure of Ia in allogeneic responses. In the bm12 mice, the sequences from E_β gene is flanked by the sequences from A_β. This results in a different tertiary structure than the E molecule in F_1 mice, where E_β is represented in its normal conformation. Further, there is evidence that the association of E^b_β and E^k_α chains generate new functional determinants. Thus, the combinatorial structure of $E^b_\beta E^k_\alpha$ in (B6 x A.TFR5)F_1 may be different from $A^{bm12}_\beta A^b_\alpha$ which would be seen as non-self. So, "gene conversion" like events would create entirely new restricting elements. This could explain why the F_1 mice see Ia bm12 as alloantigen and mount both mixed lymphocyte response and skin graft rejection.

Acknowledgements

The authors would like to thank Mrs. Mary Brandt for secretarial assistance. The work was supported by grants AI-14764 and CA-24473 from the National Institutes of Health.

References

David, C.S., McCormick, J.F., Lafuse, W.P. and Hirose, S.: Serological confirmation in I-A mutant B6.C-H-2^{bm12} of gene conversion. Transplantation 42:429-433, 1986.

Hansen, T.H., Walsh, W.D., Rubocki, R.J. and Kapp, J.A.: Responses of B6.C-H-2^{bm12} to heterologous insulins show no correlation with the putative gene conversion but define Ia^{bm12} as functionally unique. J. Mol. Cell. Immunology 2:359-368, 1986.

Hochman, P.S., and Huber, B.T.: A class II gene-conversion event defines an antigen-specific Ir gene epitope. J. Exp. Med. 160:1925-1930, 1984.

Huber, B.T., Hansen, T.H., Skelly, R.R. and Thorley-Lawson, D.A.: Ia.W39 expression correlated with a specific Ir Function. J. Immunology 128:2349-2352, 1982.

Johnson, E.D., Krco, C.J. and David, C.S.: Ia antigens are the stimulating determinants in the syngeneic mixed lymphocyte reaction. Transplantation 33:552-555, 1982.

Jones, P.P., Murphy, D.B. and McDevitt, H.O.: Two-gene control of the expression of murine Ia antigens. J. Exp. Med. 148:925-939, 1978.

Klein, J., Juretic, A., Baxevanis, C.N. and Nagy, Z.A.: The traditional and a new version of the mouse H-2 complex. Nature (Lond.) 291:455-460, 1981.

Lafuse, W.P., McCormick, J.F., Melvold, R.N. and David, C.S.: Serological and biochemical analysis of Ia molecules in the I-A mutant B6.C-H-2^{bm12}. Transplantation 31:434-438, 1981.

Lin, C.S., Rosenthal, A.S., Passmore, H.C. and Hansen, T.H.: Selective loss of antigen-specific Ir gene function in Ia mutant B6.C-H-2^{bm12} is an antigen-presenting cell defect. Proc. Natl. Acad. Sci. USA 78:6406-6410, 1981.

McIntyre, K.R. and Seidman, J.G.: Nucleotide sequence of the mutant I-A^{bm12} genes is evidence for genetic exchange between mouse immune response genes. Nature 308:551-553, 1984.

McKean, D.J., Melvold, R.W. and David, C.S.: Tryptic peptide comparison of Ia antigen and polypeptides from the I-A mutant B6.C-H-2^{bm12} and its congenic parental strain B6. Immunogenetics 14:41-51, 1981.

McKenzie, I.F.C., Morgan, G.M., Sandrin, M.S., Michaelides, M.M., Melvold, R.W. and Kohn, H.I.: B6.C-H-2^{bm12} a new H-2 mutation in the I region in the mouse. J. Exp. Med. 150:1323-1338, 1979.

Melvold, R.N. and Kohn, H.I.: Eight new histocompatibility mutations associated with the H-2 complex. Immunogenetics 3:185-191, 1976.

Mengle-Gaw, L., Conner, S., McDevitt, H.O. and Fathman, C.G.: Gene conversion between murine class II major-histocompatibility complex loci. Functional and molecular evidence from the bm12 mutant. J. Exp. Med. 160:1184-1194, 1984.

Steinmuller, D.: Skin grafting. Methods in Immunology 108:20-28, 1984.

Tse, H.Y., Kanamori, S., Walsh, W.D. and Hansen, T.H.: The murine bm12 gene conversion provides evidence that T cells recognize predominantly Ia conformation. Proc. Natl. Acad. Sci. USA 82:7058-7062, 1985.

Widera, G. and Flavell, R.A.: The nucleotide sequence of the murine I-E$^{b}_{\beta}$ immune response gene: Evidence for gene conversion events in class II genes of the major histocompatibility complex. EMBO Journal 3:1221-1225, 1984.

CLONING OF A TESTIS-SPECIFIC GENE LOCATED BETWEEN *Qa-2* AND *Upg-1* ON MOUSE CHROMOSOME 17

Masanori Kasahara[1], Felipe Figueroa[2] and Jan Klein[1,2]

1. Department of Microbiology and Immunology
University of Miami School of Medicine
Miami, FL 33101

2. Department of Immunogenetics
Max Planck Institute for Biology
D-7400 Tubingen 1, Federal Republic of Germany

INTRODUCTION

The *t* complex of the mouse is a large genetic region occupying proximal one third of chromosome 17. Mutant forms of this region, known as *t* haplotypes, show several unique properties such as segregation distortion, male sterility, embryonic lethality, and suppression of crossing-over (for review, see Silver 1985, Klein 1986). Recently, several investigators have demonstrated that *t* haplotypes have two non-overlapping inversions relative to their non-*t* counterparts, thus accounting for the observed suppression of crossing-over between *t* and non-*t* haplotypes (Artzt et al. 1982, Pla and Condamine 1984, Herrmann et al. 1986). However, precise mechanisms underlying segregation distortion, male sterility, and embryonic lethality remain poorly understood because of lack of available information at the molecular level.

With an aim to isolate *t* complex genes, we have constructed a cosmid library from a mouse x Chinese hamster hybrid cell line that contains only one mouse chromosome--a metacentric, the p arm of which is chromosome 17--on a Chinese hamster background. This library was screened with a mouse-specific repetitive sequence probe, and the mouse-derived cosmid clones thus identified were tested at random for the presence of testicular transcripts (Kasahara et al. 1987a). Using this approach, a testis-specific gene was cloned from mouse chromosome 17 (Kasahara et al. 1987a,b).

We describe here initial characterizations of this gene, which we call *Tpx-1* (a gene coding for an unknown testicular protein), including its regional mapping on mouse chromosome 17.

MATERIALS AND METHODS

Cell lines

R4 4-1 is a mouse x Chinese hamster hybrid cell line that contains only one mouse chromosome, termed M1, on a Chinese hamster background (Smiley et al. 1978). The p arm of M1 is chromosome 17, whereas its q arm consists of chromosome 18 and some additional unidentified material (Richards et al. 1985). JS17 is a mouse x Syrian hamster hybrid containing all mouse chromosomes except chromosome 17 on a Syrian hamster background (Szymura et al. 1981).

Construction and screening of a cosmid library

A cosmid library was constructed from high molecular mass DNA isolated from R4 4-1, as previously described (Kasahara et al. 1987a). To isolate mouse-derived cosmid clones, the library was screened with a BAM5 (now referred to as L1) family repetitive sequence probe pMBA14 (Fanning 1982), which hybridizes with mouse, but not with Chinese hamster DNA.

RNA isolation and cDNA synthesis

Cytoplasmic RNA was isolated from various mouse organs according to the method of Chirgwin and his co-workers (1979). Mouse-derived cosmid clones containing testicular transcripts were identified using ^{32}P-labeled cDNA synthesized from BALB/c testis poly $(A)^+$ RNA as a probe (Kasahara et al. 1987a).

Southern and Northern blot hybridizations

They were done as described (Kasahara et al. 1987a) using probes radiolabeled by the hexamer-priming method (Feinberg and Vogelstein 1984).

RESULTS

Isolation of a testis-specific gene *Tpx-1* from a cosmid library

Screening of the R4 4-1 library with pMBA14 has yielded approximately 3000 pMBA14-positive, and hence mouse-derived, cosmid clones. Since the *t* complex is believed to affect sperm differentiation, these cosmid clones were then tested at random for the presence of testicular transcripts. In short, cosmid DNA was digested with one or two restriction enzymes, blotted to duplicates of nitrocellulose filters, and probed with (i) total mouse DNA and (ii) cDNA synthesized from BALB/c testis poly$(A)^+$ RNA. Restriction fragments, which were negative with total mouse DNA (and thus free of highly repetitive sequences) but positive with testicular cDNA, were isolated and subjected to Northern blotting analyses.

One cosmid clone, designated 1-1-1, was found to contain a repetitive sequence-free *Hind*III fragment (0.95 kb) hybridizing strongly with testicular cDNA. This fragment (1-1-1H4) was used as a probe for Northern blots of RNA isolated from various organs of BALB/c or CBA mice. Among the nine tissues examined (testis, ovary, brain, liver, kidney, spleen, lung, heart, and thymus), only testis RNA showed positive hybridization (Fig. 1B; data for thymus, not shown), indicating that 1-1-1 contains a gene specifically transcribed in the testis.

We next examined the expression of the 1-1-1H4 transcript in testes of mice of various ages. Under the experimental conditions we used (10 µg of total cellular RNA, overnight exposure with an intensifying screen), no testicular transcript was detectable in 7 and 13 day old mice; however, it was clearly detectable in 20 day old mice and increased dramatically in 27 day old mice (data not shown).

Thus, *Tpx-1* is a testis-specific gene whose expression is developmentally regulated.

Mapping of *Tpx-1* between *Qa-2* and *Upg-1* on mouse chromosome 17

1-1-1H4 was used as a probe for Southern blots of DNA isolated from BALB/c, Syrian hamster, Chinese hamster, JS17, and R4 4-1. Positive hybridizations were found only with BALB/c and R4 4-1 (Fig. 1A). Since JS17 contains all mouse chromosomes except 17, lack of hybridization in JS17 localizes *Tpx-1* to mouse chromosome 17.

Further regional mapping of *Tpx-1* within chromosome 17 was performed using *Tla*-region congenic and B10 congenic mice, shown in Table 1. The fact that B6 and B6.K1 (or B6.K2) share regions proximal to *H-2D*, but differ in *Pst*I fragments detected with 1-1-1H4, places *Tpx-1* distal to *H-2D*. Similarly, comparison of B6.K2 with B6-*Tla*^{a} places *Tpx-1* distal to *Qa-2*. Finally, the observation that B10 and B10.TFR1, which share regions distal to *Upg-1* (urinary pepsinogen-1), differ in *Pst*I fragments detected with 1-1-1H4, localizes *Tpx-1* proximal to *Upg-1*.

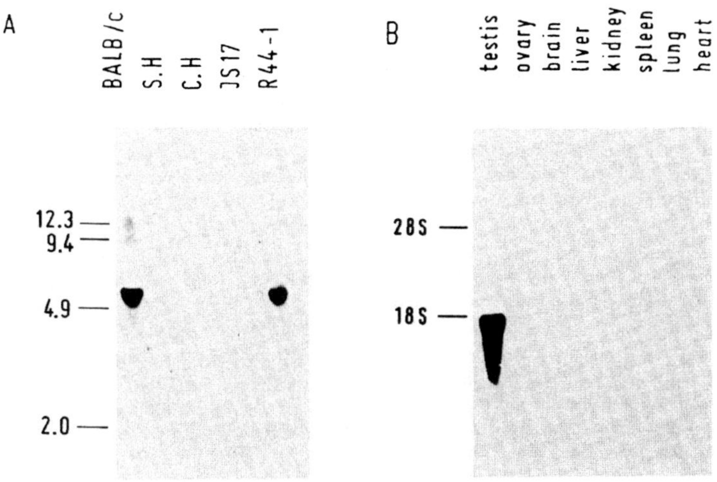

Figure 1. Southern and Northern blot hybridization analyses of cosmid clone 1-1-1. (A) Localization of cosmid clone 1-1-1 to mouse chromosome 17. A 0.95 kb *Hind*III fragment (1-1-1H4), isolated from 1-1-1, was subcloned into pUC18 and used as a probe for Southern blots of *Bam*HI-digested DNA from BALB/c, Syrian hamster (SH), Chinese hamster (CH), JS17, and R4 4-1; (B) Tissue distribution of the 1-1-1 transcript. 1-1-1H4 was used as a probe for Northern blots of total cellular RNA (20 μg) from the indicated sources. RNA was obtained from BALB/c mice, with the exception of ovary RNA that was isolated from CBA mice. The film was developed after overnight exposure with a Kodak intensifying screen. Even after a 5-day exposure, no bands showed up in the lanes other than testes (data not shown). From Kasahara et al. (1987a).

Table 1. Mapping of *Tpx-1* between *Qa-2* and *Upg-1*[a]

Line	Alleles at Loci[b]							Length of the *Pst*I Fragment Detected with 1-1-1 H4 (kb)[c]
	K	*D*	*Qa-2*	*Tla*	*Qa-1*	*Pgk-2*	*Upg-1*	
A	*k*	*d*	a^{A}	a^{A}	a^{A}	a^{A}	f^{A}	~13
B6	*b*	*b*	a^{B6}	b^{B6}	b^{B6}	a^{B6}	s^{B6}	~13
AKR	*k*	*k*	b^{AKR}	b^{AKR}	b^{AKR}	b^{AKR}	f^{AKR}	~20
B6.K1	*b*	*b*	b^{AKR}	b^{AKR}	b^{AKR}	b^{AKR}	f^{AKR}	~20
B6.K2	*b*	*b*	$a^{A\ or\ B6}$	b^{AKR}	b^{AKR}	b^{AKR}	f^{AKR}	~20
B6-*Tla*[a]	*b*	*b*	$a^{A\ or\ B6}$	a^{A}	a^{A}	$a^{A\ or\ B6}$	s^{B6}	~13
B10	*b*	*b*	a^{B10}	b^{B10}	b^{B10}	a^{B10}	s^{B10}	~13
B10.TFR1	*s*	*f*	$b^{A.CA}$	$d^{A.CA}$	$b^{A.CA}$	$b^{A.CA}$	s^{B10}	~12
A.CA	*f*	*f*	b^{CA}	d^{CA}	b^{CA}	b^{CA}	$f^{A\ or\ CA}$	~12

[a]Part of the data in this table was taken from Kasahara et al. (1987b).
[b]Index symbols at allelic designation indicate strains of origin of allele.
[c]Because of high molecular masses, molecular size given is only approximate.

Thus, we conclude that *Tpx-1* is located between *Qa-2* and *Upg-1*.

Polymorphism of *Tpx-1* in *t* mice

Since the exact extent of the distal inversion in *t* haplotypes is not known, it is not clear whether or not *Tpx-1* is located within this inversion. One indirect way to address this question is to examine polymorphisms of *Tpx-1* in *t* mice. Since *t* haplotypes most likely arose from one or a few ancestors (Klein et al. 1986), genes and non-coding sequences located on the proximal and distal inversions show a greatly reduced polymorphism compared to that normally found in non-*t* haplotypes. In addition, genes located within the inversions often show distinct alleles in *t* mice that are rarely found in non-*t* counterparts.

We digested DNA isolated from a total of 25 *t*-bearing mice captured at various locations in Europe with *Pst*I, and Southern-hybridized using 1-1-1H4 as a probe. At least five distinct restriction fragment length polymorphism (RFLP) patterns were obtained, of which three were common and two rare (data not shown). The three RFLP patterns commonly found in *t* mice were also common in non-*t* laboratory mice (data not shown). Furthermore, a survey of non-*t* laboratory mice revealed no extra RFLP patterns absent in *t* mice, suggesting that *Tpx-1* is equally polymorphic in *t* and non-*t* mice. These observations, together with the fact that some *t* mice with the identical *H-2* haplotype differ in their *Tpx-1* RFLP patterns, suggest that *Tpx-1* is located outside of the distal inversion of the *t* complex, and hence outside of the *t* complex.

DISCUSSION

A testis-specific gene located between *Qa-2* and *Upg-1* was cloned from mouse chromosome 17. We initially suggested a possibility that this gene might encode an autosomal phosphoglycerate kinase-2 (Pgk-2) isozyme (Kasahara et al. 1987b), since (i) its tissue specificity and chromosomal location is consistent with that of *Pgk-2* (Eicher et al. 1978), and (ii) its transcription, like that of *Pgk-2* (Kramer 1981), is developmentally regulated. However, the fact that *Tpx-1* cDNA clones show no significant DNA sequence homology to human *PGK-1* (Michelson et al. 1983) or *PGK-2* (McCarrey and Thomas 1987) rules out this possibility (M. Kasahara and J. Klein; unpublished observations). Since analyses of the EMBO nucleotide sequence data base revealed no known sequences homologous to *Tpx-1*, *Tpx-1* appears to be a novel gene. Furthermore, we recently found a second gene on the cosmid from which *Tpx-1* was isolated. This second gene is transcribed specifically in the testis and brain (V. Vincek, M. Ayane, F. Figueroa, and J. Klein; unpublished observations). Thus, including *Pgk-2*, at least three genes transcribed in the testis are located in an interval between *Qa-2* and *Upg-1*.

The distribution of *Tpx-1* RFLP patterns in *t* mice suggests that *Tpx-1* is located outside of the distal inversion of the *t* complex. This notion is also supported by analyses of *t* congenic mice, which indicate that *Tpx-1* is exempt from suppression of crossing-over (J.-Y. Tsai and L.M. Silver; personal communication). Precise location of *Tpx-1* relative to *Pgk-2* still remains to be determined.

Acknowledgements

We thank Ms. M.S. Newman and Dr. F.H. Ruddle, Department of Biology and Human Genetics, Yale University, New Haven, Connecticut, for the cell line R4 4-1; Dr. L.A. Leinwand, Department of Microbiology and Immunology, Albert Einstein College of Yeshiva University, Bronx, New York, for pMBA14; and Dr. J. Wayne Streilein, Department of Microbiology and Immunology, University of Miami School of Medicine, Miami, Florida, for encouragement. We also thank Ms. Angela Hilton for technical assistance, and Ms. Wynn Howard for typing the manuscript. This work was supported by a grant from the National Institutes of Health, Bethesda, Maryland (AI23667-1).

REFERENCES

Artzt, K., Shin, H.-S., and Bennett, D.: Gene mapping within the T/t complex of the mouse. II. Anomalous position of the *H-2* complex in *t* haplotypes. Cell 28: 471-476, 1982.

Chirgwin, J.M., Przybyla, A.E., MacDonald, R.J., and Rutter, W.J.: Isolation of biologically active ribonucleic acid from sources enriched in ribonuclease. Biochemistry 18: 5294-5299, 1979.

Eicher, E.M., Cherry, M., and Flaherty, L.: Autosomal phosphoglycerate kinase linked to mouse major histocompatibility complex. Mol. Gen. Genet. 158: 225-228, 1978.

Fanning, T.G.: Characterization of a highly repetitive family of DNA sequences in the mouse. Nucl. Acids Res. 10: 5003-5013, 1982.

Feinberg, A.P. and Vogelstein, B.: A technique for radiolabeling DNA restriction endonuclease fragments to high specific activity. Anal. Biochem. 137: 266-267, 1984.

Herrmann, B., Bucan, M., Mains, P.E., Frischauf, A.-M., Silver, L.M., and Lehrach, H.: Genetic analysis of the proximal portion of the mouse *t* complex: Evidence for a second inversion within *t* haplotypes. Cell 44: 469-476, 1986.

Kasahara, M., Figueroa, F., and Klein, J.: Random cloning of genes from mouse chromosome 17. Proc. Natl. Acad. Sci. USA. 84: 3325-3328, 1987a.

Kasahara, M., Figueroa, F., and Klein, J.: Molecular cloning of a testis-specific gene from mouse chromosome 17. Transplant. Proc. 19: 815-816, 1987b.

Klein, J., Golubic, M., Budimir, O., Schoepfer, R., Kasahara, M., and Figueroa, F.: On the origin of *t* chromosomes. Curr. Top. Microbiol. Immunol. 127: 239-246, 1986.

Klein, J.: Natural History of the Major Histocompatibility Complex. John Wiley and Sons, New York, 1986.

Kramer, J.M.: Immunofluorescent localization of PGK-1 and PGK-2 isozymes within specific cells of the mouse testis. Dev. Biol. 87: 30-36, 1981.

McCarrey, J.R. and Thomas, K.: Human testis-specific PGK gene lacks introns and possesses characteristics of a processed gene. Nature 326: 501-505, 1987.

Michelson, A.M., Markham, A.F., and Orkin, S.H.: Isolation and DNA sequence of a full-length cDNA clone for human X chromosome-encoded phosphoglycerate kinase. Proc. Natl. Acad. Sci. USA. 80: 472-476, 1983.

Pla, M. and Condamine, H.: Recombination between two mouse *t* haplotypes ($t^{w12}tf$ and t^{Lub-1}): Mapping of the *H-2* complex relative to centromere and tufted (*tf*) locus. Immunogenetics 20: 277-285, 1984.

Richards, J.E., Pravtcheva, D.D., Day, C., Ruddle, F.H., and Jones, P.P.: Murine invariant chain gene: Chromosomal assignment and segregation in recombinant inbred strains. Immunogenetics 22: 193-199, 1985.

Silver, L.M.: Mouse *t* haplotypes. Ann. Rev. Genet. 19: 179-208, 1985.

Smiley, J.R., Steege, D.A., Juricek, D.K., Summers, W.P., and Ruddle, F.H.: A herpes simplex virus 1 integration site in the mouse genome defined by somatic cell genetic analysis. Cell 15: 455-468, 1978.

Szymura, J.M., Wabl, M.R., and Klein, J.: Mouse mitochondrial superoxide dismutase locus is on chromosome 17. Immunogenetics 14: 231-240, 1981.

THE END OF H-2

Kirsten Fischer Lindahl, Bruce E. Loveland and C. Sue Richards

Howard Hughes Medical Institute and Departments of Microbiology and Biochemistry, University of Texas Health Science Center at Dallas, Dallas, Texas 75235-9050

THE MATERNALLY TRANSMITTED ANTIGEN

Mta, the maternally transmitted antigen of mice, was discovered and its analysis was pursued because it seemingly had nothing to do with H-2. Immunization of NZB/BlNJ mice with H-2-compatible BALB/c cells gave rise to cytotoxic T lymphocytes (CTL) that killed target cells of more than eighty strains of mice, independent of their H-2 type. Cold target competition showed that they all shared one antigen, and it was hard to find a strain whose cells were not lysed (Fischer Lindahl et al. 1980). Mta was thus a clear exception to the rule that CTL are H-2-restricted, i.e. recognize their target antigens in association with one of the class I major histocompatibility antigens (MHC I), H-2K, H-2D and H-2L. Obviously, we were not dealing with a rare case of MHC II-restricted CTL either.

Crosses with NZB mice showed that the antigen was strictly maternally transmitted - hence its name (Fischer Lindahl et al. 1980). Mta could not be influenced by foster-nursing (Fischer Lindahl and Hausmann 1983), by transfer of single-cell embryos to surrogate mothers or by extensive cell contact in bone marrow chimeras (Fischer Lindahl and Bürki 1982). We therefore postulated the existence of an extra-chromosomal, maternally transmitted factor, Mtf, that is present in the oocyte and can be stably inherited through the maternal line for at least twenty generations of backcrossing.

THE MATERNALLY TRANSMITTED FACTOR

Mitochondrial DNA (mtDNA) has all the properties of Mtf described above (reviewed by Fischer Lindahl 1985a), and it is therefore the obvious candidate for Mtf. From time to time, the isolation of small circular DNA molecules from mammalian cells has been reported. These are most likely excised transposons or "left-overs" from rearrangements of T cell receptor genes (Fujimoto and Yamagishi 1987, Okazaki et al. 1987), and mtDNA remains the only stably inherited extrachromosomal genetic element in mouse cells.

All mice have an immunogenic form of Mtf, and to date we have identified four alleles of Mtf, each of which determines unique epitopes of Mta (Hirama and Fischer Lindahl 1985, Smith and Rich 1985, Fischer Lindahl et al. 1987). To distinguish these alleles from nuclear genes, we designate them by Greek letters. By far the most common is the α type found in nearly all strains of inbred mice. MtDNA is easily characterized by restriction enzyme analysis, and the finding that all mice with Mtf^{β}, such as NZB/BlNJ, share a unique form of mtDNA was the first support for the notion that Mtf is a mitochondrial gene (Ferris et al. 1983, Huston et al. 1983).

It could be argued that since both Mtf and mtDNA are maternally transmitted, one would expect such correlation of alleles with RFLPs, even if Mtf resides elsewhere. With current reports of differential imprinting of paternal and maternal chromosomes (McGrath and Solter 1984, Barton et al. 1984) and failure of males to transmit a particular transgene (Palmiter et al. 1983), it was therefore important to obtain more direct evidence for the involvement of mtDNA in expression of Mta. This came from analysis of somatic cell hybrids.

When BALB/c myeloma cells (Mtf^{α}) are fused with NZB lymphocytes (Mtf^{β}), most hybrid clones retain only the mtDNA from BALB/c and express only Mta epitopes associated with Mtf^{α}. If the myeloma cells are treated before the fusion with the mitochondrial poison, rhodamine-6G, their mtDNA is eliminated, and the hybrids survive only if they retain the NZB mtDNA. Such clones now express the Mta associated with Mtf^{β}. The exceptional clones that retained BALB/c mtDNA prove the rule in that they express the corresponding form of Mta (Smith et al. 1983, Huston et al. 1985). By fusing fibroblast cell lines with different drug resistance markers in their mtDNA and selecting with both drugs, Rodgers et al. (1987) obtained lines that retained both types of mtDNA and stably expressed both forms of Mta.

We have found that fusion of BALB/c myeloma cells with Mtf^{γ} lymphocytes, unlike Mtf^{β}, yields hybrids with relatively stable co-expression of the two corresponding forms of Mta. One can then apply CTL of appropriate specificity to select segregants that have lost one or the other form of the surface antigen (Hirama and Fischer Lindahl 1985), and then determine what mtDNA these clones contain.

BACK TO H-2

Given only a mitochondrial gene, it was hard to imagine how Mta could be a target antigen for unrestricted CTL, expressed on the cell surface. It seemed possible that all the mice we had analyzed so far were identical for a chromosomal gene involved in Mta, and we therefore continued to screen wild mice in the hope of detecting a new polymorphism (Fischer Lindahl and Hausmann 1983) . Any mouse with a variant form of Mta would be bred to determine its mode of inheritance.

A stock of Mus musculus castaneus mice, descended from wild mice caught in Thailand, were the first Hmt variants. These mice had a normal Mtf^{α}, but carried a null allele (b) at a chromosomal gene, Hmt, and therefore did not express any Mta. Not unexpectedly, Hmt was found to be closely linked to the H-2 complex, distal to H-2D (Fischer Lindahl et al. 1983). We have isolated two castaneus haplotypes, CAS3 or c3 and CAS4 or c4, by backcrossing for ten generations and are now establishing the first congenic strains, C3H.CAS3 and B10.CAS4. Jan Klein's congenic strains B10.CAS1 and B10.CAS2 are descended from the same Thai mice; B10.CAS2 is also Hmt^{b} and is identical to CAS3 and CAS4 at the H-2D locus (Fischer Lindahl et al. 1983 and to be published).

All spretus mice we have studied have a third allele, c, of Hmt. The products of the a and c alleles crossreact, but we could make CTL that were specific for the Mta[α,c] (Fischer Lindahl et al. 1986). Other variant forms of Hmt are under analysis, but they have so far been found together with only a single H-2 haplotype. Until they can be separated by recombination from the strongly immunogenic H-2 loci, we cannot prove that we have CTL reagents specific for the new variants and must rely on their crossreactions to characterize them. A d allele has tentatively been assigned to a bactrianus haplotype (Fischer Lindahl 1986), and almost every t haplotype we have analyzed promises to be a new variant (Fischer Lindahl 1984 and 1985b).

$BETA_2$-MICROGLOBULIN

We believe that Hmt encodes a class I heavy chain that associates with β2m. Mta cannot be detected on cells that make no β2m. The R1 cell line is Mta positive; the $R1(TL^-)$ variant has defective B2m genes (Parnes and Seidman 1982), it makes class I heavy chains but does not express them on the cell surface, and it is not lysed by Mta-specific CTL, unless PHA is added to glue the killers and targets together nonspecifically (Fischer Lindahl and Langhorne 1981).

Table 1. Failure of a $\beta 2m^-$ variant of the EARAD1 cell line to express Mta.

Target cells	Lysis by anti-Mta[α,a] CTL: Range for eight TL	Lysis by anti-Mta[α,a] CTL: In presence of PHA	Binding (cpm) of ^3H-labeled monoclonal antibodies specific for: K^k	D^d	K^b	D^b
Cell lines						
EARAD1	44.8 - 57.0	56.4	206	133	86	12
$H\text{-}2^{a-}$ variant	31.0 - 53.7	47.7	15	21	222	168
$\beta 2m^-$ variant	-0.9 - 0.6	15.5	0	24	49	13
Thymocytes						
$H\text{-}2^b$	21.7 - 42.4	n.d.	4	11	131	162
$H\text{-}2^a$	22.5 - 36.0	n.d.	94	14	18	5
ConA blasts						
Mta[α,a]	31.0 - 50.5	n.d.	n.d.	n.d.	n.d.	n.d.
Mta[β,a]	-6.6 - 1.5	n.d.	n.d.	n.d.	n.d.	n.d.

Results are given at 30:1 effector: target ratio, and, unless otherwise noted, target cells are genetically Mta[α,a]. Antibody binding was measured as described (Fischer Lindahl 1985c), and counter background of 19 cpm subtracted.

More recently, we have obtained similar results with another set of cell lines from Dr. F.W. Shen. The EARAD1 thymoma from a (B6 x A)F1 mouse expresses a very low level of H-2, but it is killed very well by anti-Mta CTL, as is the $\underline{H\text{-}2}^b$ homozygous variant (Shen et al. 1984). The $\beta 2m^-$ variant, on the other hand, which expresses no detectable class I antigen (Table 1), is not lysed at all by anti-Mta CTL. As can also be gleaned from Table 1, Mta is very well expressed on thymocytes, in contrast to H-2; this may perhaps be useful in distinguishing killing specific for Mta from reactions specific for or restricted by H-2 when dealing with the new Hmt alleles.

The lysis of $\underline{B2m}^b$ target cells by anti-Mta CTL can be inhibited effectively by the monoclonal antibody S19.8 that is specific for $\beta 2m^b$, whether the target expresses Mta[α,a] (Fischer Lindahl et al. 1983), Mta[β,a] (Han et al. 1987) or Mta[γ,a] (Fischer Lindahl et al. 1987). The same reactions are not affected at all by a mixture of monoclonal antibodies specific for H-2 antigens that completely block H-2 specific killing, and the anti-β2m antibody is actually very poor at inhibiting H-2 specific lysis. The fact that Mta-specific killing is not inhibited completely is probably due to exchange of endogenous mouse $\beta 2m^b$ with bovine β2m from the culture medium (Hyafil and Strominger 1979).

MAJOR, MEDIAL OR MINOR?

The term medial was coined to describe the properties of antigens, such as Qa-1, Qa-2 and Mta, that resemble major MHC antigens in being recognized "on their own" by T cells that are not H-2-restricted, but differ by being weak transplantation antigens and by not in turn restricting the T cell recognition of other antigens (Fischer Lindahl and Langhorne 1981).

There can be no question that recognition of Mta is independent of H-2 (Fischer Lindahl et al. 1980, 1983, 1986, Fischer Lindahl and Hausmann 1983), and Mta is indeed a weak transplantation antigen: on the high responder background, a skin graft is rejected only after five weeks, and a low responder may accept it permanently (Chan and Fischer Lindahl 1985).

We may have to revise our view of the inability of medial antigens to act as restriction elements. At this meeting, Murphy and Homer (1987) have presented evidence that a Qa-2 molecule may present a ligand encoded in the H-2I region to CTL, and we are now working on the assumption that Hmt acts as a class I restriction element, presenting a mitochondrially encoded ligand (Fig. 1). There are now several examples that a virally encoded antigen recognized by class I restricted CTL is a short peptide that can be added to the medium of the target cells (Townsend et al. 1986, Gotch et al. 1987). The pathway for processing antigens to be presented with class I may be different than for class II restriction elements (Morrison et al. 1986), but there is as yet no indication that the end product is not a peptide.

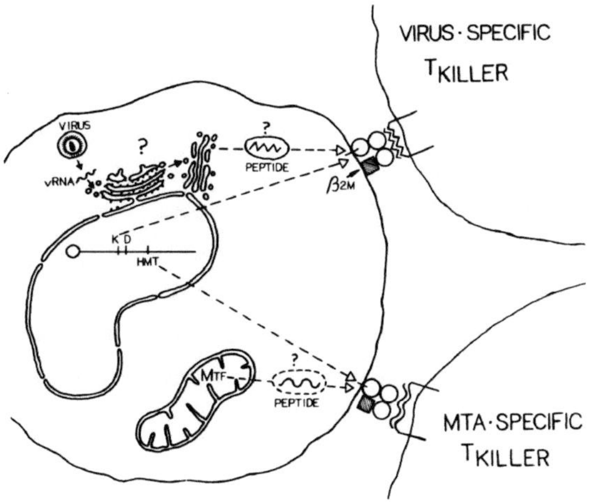

Figure 1. An artist's view of Mta. By analogy to T cell recognition of viral antigens, a peptide encoded by the mitochondrial gene Mtf is presented on the cell surface by Hmt that functions as an MHC class I restriction element (courtesy of Dr. Laurie Roman).

The epitopes of Mta are determined jointly by Hmt and Mtf (Fischer Lindahl et al. 1986), and we have prepared CTL specific for five of the sixteen possible combinations of four alleles of Mtf with four alleles of Hmt. We have no reason to suspect that an intact mitochondrially encoded protein is exported to the cell surface, but a peptide may well be, perhaps as a result of autophagy. A receptor-ligand complex accounts more easily for the distinct effects of at least four different mitochondrial types and for the co-dominant expression of Mta in heteroplasmic cells than do many other models (Rodgers et al. 1986).

To identify the mitochondrial gene that is Mtf and characterize its product, we are comparing the sequences of mtDNA from mice of α, β, γ, and δ types of Mtf (Yonekawa and Fischer Lindahl, 1987). The amino acid divergence between the allelic forms of the mitochondrial proteins is on the order of one percent, and some do not differ at all.

CLONING Hmt

To test our model and rule out alternatives (Fischer Lindahl 1985a), we must isolate the Hmt gene, show that its product is an MHC class I heavy chain protein and demonstrate that this molecule differs between Hmt alleles but is unaffected by the Mtf type of the cell. A variety of immunization schemes have failed to yield an antibody specific for Mta that could be used for biochemical characterization, and we have therefore chosen a genetic and molecular approach.

We have a number of recombinant haplotypes that separate Hmt from H-2D (Fischer Lindahl 1986). Of these, CAS(R4) has been the most useful so far, because it has the entire H-2 complex, from H-2K to Tla and Qa-1, from strain C3H/HeJ, and only Hmt from CAS3. New recombinants are being uncovered as we establish homozygous congenic lines after ten generations of backcrossing castaneus or recombinant haplotypes, and we are collecting DNA probes for the H-2D to Upg-1 interval of chromosome 17 to establish a detailed molecular map of the distal end of H-2.

Probing blots of genomic DNA from R4 and the C3H and CAS3 parental strains with clones that mark the ends of the class I gene clusters from the Tla region revealed that Hmt is distal to all hitherto defined class I genes in the MHC (Kiefer et al. 1985). We therefore reasoned that if we probed the same blots with the conserved fourth exon of a class I gene, nearly all the bands we see in the C3H lane should be shared with R4, and most would differ from those in the CAS3 lane. Any class I gene distal to the crossover breakpoint in R4 might show up as a band unique to C3H or shared between R4 and CAS3. As Fig. 2 shows, such bands are revealed by several different enzymes, suggesting that there is at least one class I gene in the Hmt region. We are now cloning and characterizing these bands with the aim of transfecting full length candidates for Hmt^{a} into an $Hmt^{b/b}$ cell line, which should start to express Mta and become susceptible to lysis.

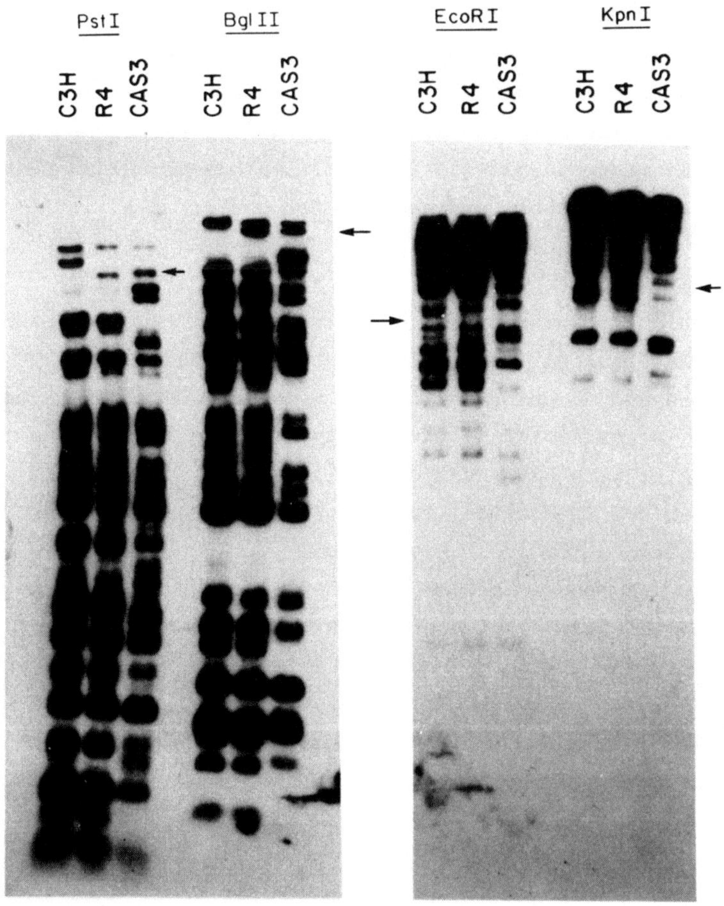

Figure 2. MHC class I restriction fragment length polymorphisms associated with the Hmt region. Liver DNA (20 μg) was digested with restriction endonucleases, electrophoresed on a 0.6% agarose gel in Tris-borate buffer overnight, and transfered to nitrocellulose using 10 x SSC. After a 12 hour prehybridization, the filter was hybridized overnight at 42°C in a solution of 50% formamide, 5 x SSC, 5 x Denhardt's, 0.1% SDS, 0.2% pyrophosphate, and 0.1 μg/ml salmon sperm DNA to the ^{32}P-labeled (>10^9 cpm/μg) probe pH-2IIa (Steinmetz et al. 1981). The filter was washed in 2 x SSC, 0.1% SDS at 68°C and then exposed to XAR-5 film overnight. The arrows indicate Hmt candidates for cloning.

CURRENT QUESTIONS

In our current model of Mta, Mtf plays the role of a minor histocompatibility antigen as the ligand that is presented to the immune system by an MHC class I restriction element, in this case Hmt. Mtf may be the first minor H antigen to be understood in molecular terms. As the rules that govern the binding and presentation of peptides by MHC molecules are uncovered, they may explain the privileged association of Mtf and Hmt. We have seen no evidence to suggest that Hmt can present any other ligand. As an alloantigen Hmt can be recognized in two modes: some CTL are specific for the complex of Hmt with Mtf and others ignore Mtf.

We do not know whether Mta has a function nor what it might be. Once Mtf and Hmt are identified, we should be able to work out how Mta is created. We hope to follow the path of the Mtf product from mitochondria to the cell surface and will know whether it proceeds via the nucleus. Conversely, Hmt might be found in mitochondria, as the presence of TL antigens on mitochondrial membranes has been reported (Jeng et al. 1978).

The unique involvement of Hmt in Mta, rather than one of the usual MHC class I restriction elements, and the high degree of conservation of Hmt would suggest a special and conserved function. It is therefore important to determine whether Hmt^b is truly a null allele or whether the product is merely immunologically silent, perhaps because it represents the most junior form of a fairly conserved molecule (Fazekas de St.Groth 1981). Once probes are available, it should be simple to determine whether homologues of Hmt and Mtf are expressed in other vertebrates.

REFERENCES

Barton, S.C., Surani, M.A.H., and Norris, M.L., 1984. Roles of paternal and maternal genomes in mouse development. Nature, 311:374.

Chan, T., and Fischer Lindahl, K., 1985. Skin graft rejection due to a maternally transmitted antigen, Mta. Transplantation, 39:477.

Fazekas de St.Groth, S., 1981. The joint evolution of antigens and antibodies, in: "The Immune System. Vol. I: Past and Future," C.M. Steinberg and I. Lefkovits, eds., Karger, Basel, pp. 155.

Ferris, S.D., Ritte, U., Fischer Lindahl, K., Prager, E.M., and Wilson, A.C., 1983. Unusual type of mitochondrial DNA in mice lacking a maternally transmitted antigen. Nucleic Acids Res., 11:2917.

Fischer Lindahl, K., 1984. The Mta of spretus mice and new alleles of Hmt and Mtf. Ann. Rep. Basel Inst. Immunol., 13:90.

Fischer Lindahl, K., 1985a. Mitochondrial inheritance in mice. Trends Genet., 1:135.

Fischer Lindahl, K., 1985b. The Hmt alleles of t haplotypes. Ann. Rep. Basel Inst. Immunol., 14:64.

Fischer Lindahl, K., 1985c. Tissue typing using biosynthetically labeled monoclonal antibodies, in: "Immunological Methods, Vol. III," I. Lefkovits and B. Pernis, eds., Academic Press, New York, pp. 187.

Fischer Lindahl, K., 1986. Genetic variants of histocompatibility antigens from wild mice. Curr. Top. Microbiol. Immunol., 127:272.

Fischer Lindahl, K., and Bürki, K., 1982. Mta, a maternally inherited cell surface antigen of the mouse, is transmitted in the egg. Proc. Natl. Acad. Sci. U.S.A., 79:5362.

Fischer Lindahl, K., and Hausmann, B., 1983. Cytoplasmic inheritance of a cell surface antigen in the mouse. Genetics, 103:483.

Fischer Lindahl, K., and Langhorne, J., 1981. Medial histocompatibility antigens. Scand. J. Immunol., 14:643.

Fischer Lindahl, K., Bocchieri, M., and Riblet, R., 1980. Maternally transmitted target antigen for unrestricted killing by NZB T lymphocytes. J. Exp. Med., 152:1583.

Fischer Lindahl, K., Hausmann, B., and Chapman, V.M., 1983. A new H-2-linked class I gene whose expression depends on a maternally transmitted factor. Nature, 306:383.

Fischer Lindahl, K., Hausmann, B., Robinson, P.J., Guénet, J.-L., Wharton, D.C., and Winking, H., 1986. Mta, the maternally transmitted antigen, is determined jointly by the chromosomal Hmt and the extrachromosomal Mtf genes. J. Exp. Med., 163:334.

Fischer Lindahl, K., Hausmann, B., and Guénet, J.-L., 1987. Distinct epitopes of the maternally transmitted antigen, Mta, determined by three allelic forms of the cytoplasmic gene Mtf. Submitted for publication.

Fujimoto, S., and Yamagishi, H., 1987. Isolation of an excision product of T-cell receptor α-chain gene rearrangements. Nature, 327:242.

Gotch, F., Rothbard, J., Howland, K., Towsend, A., and McMichael, A., 1987. Cytotoxic T lymphocytes recognize a fragment of influenza virus matrix protein in association with HLA-A2. Nature, 326:881.

Han, A.C., Rodgers, J.R., and Rich, R.R., 1987. Unglycosylated Mta^a expressed an Mta^b-like determinant. Immunogenetics, 25:234.

Hirama, M., and Fischer Lindahl, K., 1985. Mouse mitochondria and the cell surface, in: "Achievements and perspectives of mitochondrial research, Vol. II: Biogenesis," E. Quagliariello, E.C. Slater, F. Palmieri, C. Saccone, and A.M. Kroon, eds., Elsevier, Amsterdam, pp. 445.

Huston, M.M., Smith, R., III, Huston, D.P., and Rich, R.R., 1983. Differences in maternal lineages of New Zealand black mice defined by restriction endonuclease analysis of mitochondrial DNA and by expression of maternally transmitted antigen. J. Exp. Med., 157:2154.

Huston, M.M., Smith, R., III, Hull, R., Huston, D.P., and Rich, R.R., 1985. Mitochondrial modulation of maternally transmitted antigen: analysis of cell hybrids. Proc. Natl. Acad. Sci. U.S.A., 82:3286.

Hyafil, F. and Strominger, J.L., 1979. Dissociation and exchange of the β_2-microglobulin subunit of HLA-A and HLA-B antigens. Proc. Natl. Acad. Sci. U.S.A., 76:5834.

Jeng, M.W., Finegold, M.J., Basch, R.S., and Lamm, M.E., 1978. Demonstration of thymus-leukemia (TL) antigens on mitochondria of lymphoid cells by immunoelectron microscopy. Lab. Invest., 38:41.

Kiefer, M.C., Steinmetz, M., and Fischer Lindahl, K., 1985. Genetic mapping in the Tla:Qa-1 region of the mouse MHC by restriction enzyme site polymorphisms. Ann. Rep. Basel Inst. Immunol., 14:51.

McGrath, J., and Solter, D., 1984. Completion of mouse embryogenesis requires both the maternal and paternal genomes. Cell, 37:179.

Morrison, L.A., Lukacher, A.E., Braciale, V.L., Fan, D.P., and Braciale, T.J., 1986. Differences in antigen presentation to MHC class I- and II-restricted influenza virus-specific cytolytic T lymphocyte clones. J. Exp. Med., 163:903.

Murphy, D.B., and Homer, R.H., 1987. A Q region product as a restriction element, in: "Major Histocompatibility Genes and their Roles in Immune Function," C.S. David, ed., Plenum, New York.

Okazaki, K., Davis, D.D., and Sakano, H., 1987. T cell receptor β gene sequences in the circular DNA of thymocyte nuclei: direct evidence for intramolecular DNA deletion in V-D-J joining. Cell, 49:477.

Palmiter, R.D., Wilkie, T.M., Chen, H.Y., Brinster, R.L., 1983. Transmission distortion and mosaicism in an unusual transgenic mouse pedigree. Cell, 36:869.

Parnes, J.R., and Seidman, J.G., 1982. Structure of wild type and mutant mouse β_2-microglobulin genes. Cell, 29:661.

Rodgers, J.R., Smith, R., III, Huston, M.M., and Rich, R.R., 1986. Maternally transmitted antigen. Adv. Immunol., 38:313.

Rodgers, J.R., Smith, R., III, and Rich, R.R., 1987. Maternally transmitted antigens are codominantly expressed by mouse cells containing two kinds of mitochondrial DNA. J. Exp. Med., 165:560.

Shen, F.W., Chaganti, R.S.K., Doucette, L.A., Litman, G.W., Steinmetz, M., Hood, L., and Boyse, E.A., 1984. Genomic constitution of an H-2:Tla variant leukemia. Proc. Natl. Acad. Sci. U.S.A., 81:6447.

Smith, R., III, and Rich, R.R., 1985. Polymorphism and tissue distribution of maternally transmitted antigen defined by cytotoxic T lymphocyte lines. J. Immunol., 134:2191.

Smith, R., III, Huston, M.M., Jenkins, R.N., Huston, D.P., and Rich, R.R., 1983. Mitochondria control expression of a murine cell surface antigen. Nature, 306:599.

Steinmetz, M., Frelinger, J.G., Fisher, D., Hunkapillar, T., Pereira, D., Weissman, S.M., Uehara, H., Nathenson, S., and Hood, L., 1981. Three cDNA clones encoding mouse transplantation antigens: homology to immunoglobulin genes. Cell, 24:125.

Townsend, A.R.M., Rothbard, J., Gotch, F.M., Bahadur, G., Wraith, D., and McMichael, A.J., 1986. The epitopes of influenza nucleoprotein recognized by cytotoxic T lymphocytes can be defined with short synthetic peptides. Cell, 44:959.

Yonekawa, H., and Fischer Lindahl, K., 1987. Searching for the molecular basis of a mitochondrial transplantation antigen. Genetics, 116:s41.

SECTION IV

FUNCTION OF H-2 GENES AND GENE PRODUCTS

HISTORICAL DEVELOPMENTS IN UNDERSTANDING THE FUNCTION OF CLASS I MHC GENES

Peter C. Doherty*

Department of Experimental Pathology, The John Curtin School Medical Research, Canberra ACT 2601 Australia

INTRODUCTION

It is reasonable to state that, as late as 1973, the reason for the existence and extraordinary polymorphism of the strong transplantation antigens (now known as the class I MHC glycoproteins) was not understood (Amos *et al.*, 1971; Bodmer, 1972). Two sets of facts were undisputed: that the allograft response was extremely potent, and that the frequency of effector T cells specific for foreign transplantation antigens was very high (Simonsen, 1967; Wilson, *et al.*, 1968). This had led to a variety of speculations, a few of the more perceptive of which are listed in Table 1.

TABLE 1

Transfer Factor is receptors for "self + x", with self being the strong transplantation antigens.	Lawrence 1959, reviewed in Lawrence, 1973
Polymorphism of MHC prevents molecular mimicry by viruses from eliminating the species.	Snell 1968
Transplanted skin from mice persistently infected with lymphocytic choriomeningitis virus is rejected like an allograft by syngeneic mice.	Holterman and Majde 1971
Histoincompatibility prevents horizontal transmission of malignancy between individuals of the same species. Somatic mutation of H-2 will lead to rejection of tumor cells.	Burnet 1972

*Present address: Department of Immunology
St. Jude Children's Research Hospital
Memphis, Tennessee 38101

The geneticists had also developed a very powerful technology in the form of the H-2 recombinant and H-2 mutant mouse strains (David and Shreffler, 1975; Kohn and Melvold, 1976), which was to facilitate greatly the subsequent analysis of the interaction between virus-immune T cells and virus infected target cells (Zinkernagel and Doherty, 1979).

The function of the immune response (Ir) gene products (since shown to be the class II MHC glycoproteins) in T cell recognition had received considerable attention, with the dominant concept being that the Ir genes encoded recognition structures expressed on the T lymphocyte (Katz and Benacerraf, 1975). Matching of Ir genes was found to be necessary for effective collaboration between T and B lymphocytes (Shreffler and Kindred, 1974; Katz, *et al.*, 1973) and the interaction between specifically-sensitized T cells and antigen-pulsed macrophages (Shevach and Rosenthal, 1973). The speculations concerning the Ir genes were not extended to the strong transplantation antigens, obviously because the two systems were being considered in quiet different intellectual contexts.

Thus, the class I MHC glycoproteins were thought of as target antigens for alloreactive T cells involved in graft rejection, but were not known to be important for other aspects of cell-mediated immunity (CMI). Antigen-specific T cell responses had been clearly demonstrated for both viruses and bacteria (Langman and Blanden, 1972; Blanden, 1974), and shown to be responsible for, for instance, elimination of ectromelia virus from mouse liver (Blanden, 1974). However, the difference between B cells and T cells in viral immunity was thought to rest on the fact that the former secreted antibody, while the latter did not, and the T cells were part of the recirculating pool and could readily invade into tissue sites of virus growth. There was no *a priori* thinking that the T cells were specific for other than viral or bacterial antigen as such. However, it had to be that the strong transplantation antigens were not present simply to "confuse surgeons and employ geneticists" (D.B. Wilson, personal communication).

The discovery of Class I MHC restriction: The right deed for the wrong reason

The initial finding was that cytotoxic T lymphocytes (CTL) primed with antigen in a syngeneic environment interact only with H-2 compatible, antigen modified target cells. This phenomenon was called "H-2 restriction." The discovery was made simultaneously in Washington (Shearer, 1974) and Canberra (Doherty and Zinkernagel, 1974; Zinkernagel and Doherty, 1974a) and was serendipitous. Gene Shearer (Shearer, 1974) was working with CTL responses to haptenated cells and was, as I recall from an early discussion with him, trying to escape from the H-2 field which had led him into such painful topics as the analysis of hybrid resistance effects with Gustavo Cudcowicz. Rolf Zinkernagel and I had been working on the cellular immunology of the immunopathological disease murine lymphocytic choriomeningitis (LCM), caused by the T cell-mediated elimination of LCM virus (LCMV)-infected cells in the central nervous system (Doherty and Zinkernagel, 1974; Cole, *et al.*, 1972). Both of us had backgrounds in the experimental analysis of infectious disease, and had not been directly involved in the transplantation area. However, Kevin Lafferty was an established figure in alloreactivity, and the work on T cell-B cell collaboration (14) had been discussed among the local group of cellular immunologists. This included Goron Ada, Bob Blanden, Peter Bretscher, Alastair Cunningham, Wendy Davidson, Malcolm Dunlop, Ian Gardner, Andrew Hapel, Rod Langman, Chris Parish, Linda Pilarski; Peter McCullagh, Ian Ramshaw, Yvonne Rosenberg, Pam Russell, and Karen Walker, some of whom were then graduate students. It was a congenial environment, in which speculation and open discussion of ideas were important.

Zinkernagel and I had earlier demonstrated the presence of virus-specific CTL in the cerebrospinal fluid of mice with clinical LCM (Zinkernagel and Doherty, 1973). We then set out to determine whether a reported Ir gene effect governing susceptibility to disease induction by LCMV (Oldstone, *et al.*, 1973) might be correlated with levels of CTL activity in the spleens of different mouse strains. We found, however, that the CTL effectors that were generated could lyse only H-2 identical LCMV-infected cells, a phenomenon that looked superficially similar to the effect described for T-B collaboration by Katz, Benacerraf and colleagues (Katz, *et al.*, 1973). One possibility was that, along the lines suggested by them, the H-2 gene products were contributing to the physiological interaction between sensitized T cell and virus-infected target (Zinkernagel and Doherty, 1974b). This "intimacy" model is shown in the upper segment of Figure 1, which is the diagram used in the original paper (Zinkernagel and Doherty, 1974b). We were soon to discard "intimacy" as a viable hypothesis (Doherty, *et al.*, 1976), though various other formulations (Doherty, *et al.*, 1976), of "two-receptor" models were discussed later (Figure 2) and in turn rejected (Bennink and Doherty, 1979).

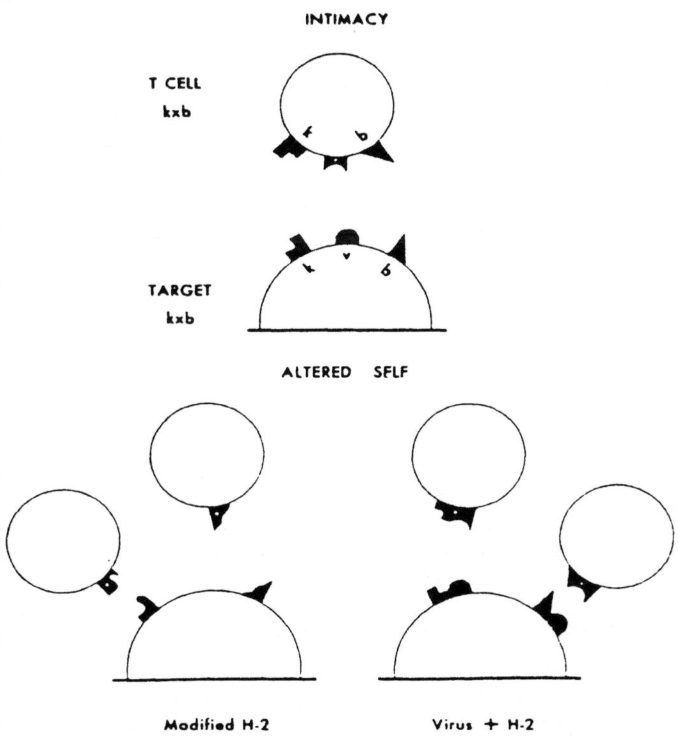

Fig. 1 Capacity of sensitised F_1 (H-$2^{k/b}$) T cells to interact only with histocompatible virus-infected target cells may be considered to reflect any one of the models shown. The intimacy concept **proposes a single immunologically specific T cell receptor for viral** (v) antigen, additional to a requirement for physiological interaction coded for by the H-2 gene complex (mutuality between either H-2^k or H-2^b). The two models proposed for altered self postulate that, in each case, there are at least two T cell populations with receptors of different immunological specificities recognising modified H-2, or virus + H-2 of either parent type.

Figure 1. Figure and legend, reproduced directly from Zinkernagel and Doherty, 1974b.

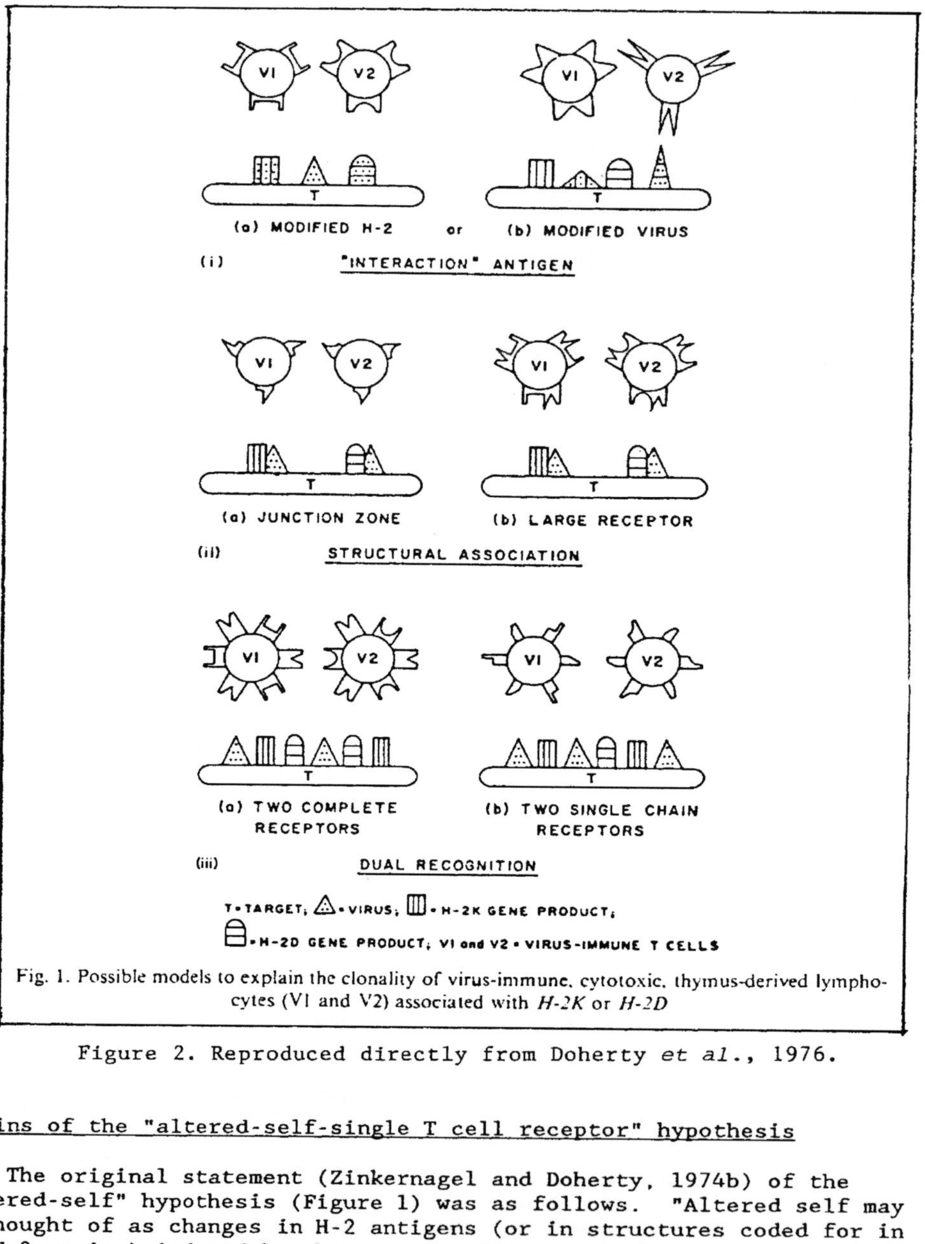

Fig. 1. Possible models to explain the clonality of virus-immune, cytotoxic, thymus-derived lymphocytes (VI and V2) associated with *H-2K* or *H-2D*

Figure 2. Reproduced directly from Doherty *et al.*, 1976.

Origins of the "altered-self-single T cell receptor" hypothesis

The original statement (Zinkernagel and Doherty, 1974b) of the "altered-self" hypothesis (Figure 1) was as follows. "Altered self may be thought of as changes in H-2 antigens (or in structures coded for in the H-2 region) induced by the process of virus synthesis, or as some complex of viral and H-2 antigens." This was not inconceivable in the context of then current thinking about virus infections, as discussed in the first description that we wrote of the H-2 restriction phenomenon (Doherty and Zinkernagel, 1974). Viruses were, for instance, thought to cause derepression of genes coding for "onco-foetal" antigens (Coggin and Anderson, 1972) and there was data that budding vesicular stomatitis virus could incorporate H-2 antigen (Summers and Hecht, 1972).

Evidence that T cell recognition of minor H antigens was restricted in the same way (which emerged in the following year; Bevan, 1975; Gordon, *et al.*, 1975) might have made the "altered self" model less attractive, though it now seems likely that at least some antigens that act as minor H determinants are products of endogenous retroviruses (Columbo, *et al.*, 1987). Also, subsequent claims that T cells and B cells were using the same V^H gene products to see a single antigen (Wigzell and Binz, 1977; Eichmann, 1978) would have greatly obscured the issue, and did cause us to develop a later variant of the "two-receptor" model (Figure 2).

It was obvious from the outset that the "altered self" hypothesis had a number of attractive features (Doherty and Zinkernagel, 1975a). The first was that recognition of modified syngeneic and allogeneic cells could be accommodated within the same conceptual framework if self + x is simply equivalent to alloantigen (Zinkernagel and Doherty, 1974b). An explanation was also provided for class I MHC polymorphism via "some pathogens (or oncogenic processes) may not cause an immunogenic modification of self associated with a particular H allele, and existence of multiple polymorphisms thus minimizes the risk of there being general unresponsiveness throughout the population (Doherty and Zinkernagel, 1975a)." The more recent idea that H-2 polymorphism has to do with pheromones, sexual preference, territorial marking and so forth (Singh, *et al.*, 1987) is a good deal more entertaining.

Preliminary evidence for differential induction of CTL effector function associated with various class I alleles was found early on in the analysis of the phenomenon (Blanden, *et al.*, 1975), though the topic was somewhat left in abeyance for several years until we ran into some very complex interactions between class I molecules that were determining levels of responsiveness (Doherty, *et al.*, 1978; Zinkernagel, *et al.*, 1978). We hesitated, at least initially, to describe these as "Ir gene effects", though the topic was debated at some length. The reason was that the term "Ir gene" was the province of those working with class II, who were then operating in a very different conceptual framework (Katz and Benacerraf, 1975). This was to change over the next few years (Benacerraf, 1978).

We did, however, speculate that "modification of Ia may thus lead to T cell helper activity and to a more effective antibody response, whereas changes in H antigen structure lead to immune elimination mediated by surveillance T cells (Doherty and Zinkernagel, 1975a)." The recent evidence that the antigenic entity seen by class I and class I restricted T cells may be peptide + MHC glycoprotein has, of course, provided a very satisfactory convergent model for the two systems (Townsend, *et al.*, 1986; Buus, *et al.*, 1987, Bjorkman *et al.*, 1987) which is in accord with the rather crude, early speculation of the altered self hypothesis. We can now talk of class I and class II Ir genes, with the operational difference between the two systems apparently begin in the nature of antigen processing (Buus, *et al.*, 1987).

Early analysis of class I MHC restriction

The first experiments (Doherty and Zinkernagel, 1974; Zinkernagel and Doherty, 1974a) established restriction of T cell mediated cytotoxicity at the level of the H-2 haplotype. This was soon confirmed for the ectromelia poxvirus by Ian Gardner and Bob Blanden (Gardner, *et al.*, 1975). Furthermore, we showed quickly that the same constraint applies for the induction of T cell-mediated inflammatory process in the brains of mice infected with LCMV (Zinkernagel and Doherty, 1975b), and for clearance of ectromelia virus from mouse liver (Blanden, *et al.*, 1975). We thus knew early on that we were dealing with a biologically relevant phenomenon that could, especially as we were working with mice and mouse pathogens, have been important during evolution. The *in vivo* studies were only possible because the systems used (Doherty and Zinkernagel, 1975b; Blanden, *et al.*, 1975) operated to show effector function in 48-72 hours, so there was no obvious modifying influence of alloreactivity. We were also fortunate in that sufficiently large doses of cells were used so that we did not have problems due to hybrid histocompatibility effects, which were encountered later (Doherty and Allan, 1986) and could have caused considerable confusion at that time.

The further analysis of H-2 restriction *in vitro* proceeded rapidly because of two factors: the availability of H-2 recombinant mice (mostly provided via Don Shreffler and Chella David); and the obvious advantages of working with a simple, two-component system - T cell and target. We were also helped by the fact that both LCMV and ectromelia generate very potent, primary CTL responses *in vivo*, the effector population used in all these early studies.

The next big surprise was when the first intrahaplotype mapping experiment, done with LCMV in A/J mice (Doherty and Zinkernagel, 1975c), showed that lysis was associated with compatibility between T cell and target for both the H-2K and H-2D ends of the MHC, which tended to rule out H-2I as the sole restricting element. The phenomenon was thus not identical to that being studied by Katz, Benacerraf and colleagues (Katz, *et al.*, 1973), who were hampered by the need to work with a very complex model. The *in vitro* mapping studies were quickly extended using a variety of H-2 recombinants (Blanden, *et al.*, 1975), and the same constraint was again shown to apply *in vivo* (Doherty, *et al.*, 1976).

The basic conceptual problem was to distinguish between the "like-like" interaction model ("intimacy", Figure 1) and the "single T cell receptor-altered self" hypothesis ("altered self", Figure 1). This was done by selective proliferation of (A x B) F_1 immune T cells in LCMV-infected, cyclophosphamide-suppressed A and B parental mice for 72 hours (Zinkernagel and Doherty, 1974b; Zinkernagel and Doherty, 1975). The starting population of (A x B)F_1 CTL effectors killed both LCMV-infected A and B targets, while further exposure to A + LCMV or B + LCMV generated CTL specific only for the self + x present in the stimulator environment: simple presence of B on the (A x B)F_1 $\rightarrow$ A population did not allow lysis of the B + LCMV targets. Apparently the (A x B)F_1 contained different "clones" of T cells specific for A + LCMV and B + LCMV. This excluded the intimacy model, and provided support for the "altered-self-single T cell receptor hypothesis" (altered self, Figure 1). Later experiments with cloned T cell lines (Weiss, *et al.*, 1980) were to demonstrate this in a much more rigorous way.

The first experiment showing MHC-restricted recognition of LCMV-infected targets was done in October 1973. By July 1974, we had mapped the effect to H-2D as well as to K-IA, eliminated the like-like interaction model and were strongly oriented to the "single T cell receptor-altered self" hypothesis. The emphasis on the essential site for MHC expression had thus been switched conceptually from the T cell to the target cell, a realization which was to have some influence on the subsequent direction of T cell immunobiology.

Only the initial, descriptive papers (Doherty and Zinkernagel, 1974; Zinkernagel and Doherty, 1974a) had been published by the time of the second International Immunology Congress in Brighton in late 1974. We thus had a very interesting, and completely novel, tale to tell. Rolf Zinkernagel visited several institutes in Europe prior to the Brighton meeting, and put the story forward at every possible opportunity during the Congress: a colleague dubbed him "hyper-Zink". I gave seminars at a great number of venues in the USA en route, including NIH and Harvard where Alan Rosenthal and David Katz were my hosts. The "one receptor-altered self" model was greeted with surprise and, in some cases, a degree of hostility (as I heard later). We had been very fortunate indeed to be isolated from the bandwagon that was rolling at the time in the east coast immunology establishment.

Some key events in the subsequent analysis of class I MHC restriction

The above (summarized in Table II) is a somewhat personal account of the events surrounding the early analysis of class I MHC restriction as they seemed to use in the relative isolation of the Australian National University. The more specifically scientific aspects of these, and subsequent experiments, have been reviewed *as nauseam* by us (Zinkernagel and Doherty, 1979; Doherty, *et al.*, 1976; Doherty, *et al.*, 1984; Doherty, 1985; Doherty, 1986) and by others (Burakoff, *et al.*, 1984; Schwartz, 1986). There is no point in repeating a further, abbreviated version of this here. Instead, I have summarized my impression of some major events that occurred (or were published) after 1975 in Tables II to VI. This is a highly selective, and admittedly eclectic, account which misses some important experiments that have been reviewed by us previously. I apologize in advance to any of my colleagues who may feel slighted, and would be grateful for correction of priorities that have been wrongly assigned. Also, as this is a history, I have not attempted to review the very latest findings: history requires some hindsight.

TABLE II
SEQUENCE OF EARLY EVENTS IN THE ANALYSIS OF CLASS I MHC RESTRICTION

Discovery of MHC restriction of virus-immune and hapten-specific CTL.	Shearer* 1974 Doherty and Zinkernagel, 1974a; Zinkernagel and Doherty, 1974a
Demonstration of "clonality" of virus-immune CTL effectors for class I MHC gene products: statement of the "single T cell receptor-altered self hypothesis" and concepts arising from this model.	Zinkernagel and Doherty, 1974b Doherty and Zinkernagel, 1975a
Mapping of CTL effector function to H-2K and H-2D. Preliminary evidence for class I MHC Ir gene effects.	Doherty and Zinkernagel, 1975c Blanden *et al.*, 1975
T cell effector function *in vivo* is MHC restricted.	Doherty and Zinkernagel, 1975b Gardner *et al.*, 1975
Discovery that CTL specific for "minor" H antigens are class I MHC restricted.	Bevan 1975 Gordon *et al.*, 1975

*Some of the experiments listed below were paralleled by studies with TNP in Gene Shearer's laboratory (Shearer, *et al.*, 1977). I have not covered this work because both the high frequency of TNP-specific CTL precursors in unprimed mice and the fact that the H-2 antigen is directly derivatized (Schwartz, 1986) make TNP-self seem more like alloantigen.

TABLE III
SOME KEY BIOLOGICAL EXPERIMENTS IN THE SUBSEQUENT ANALYSIS OF CLASS I MHC RESTRICTION

Discrimination of virus-immune CTL effectors in H-2K^b mutant mice.	Blanden *et al.*, 1976 Zinkernagel, 1976
Lysis of allogeneic cells by self-MHC restricted CTL at the population level.	Bevan 1977
Confirmation of MHC restriction in other species: demonstration for influenza in man and the rat.	McMichael *et al.*, 1977 Marshak *et al.* 1977
Radiation-resistant thymus cells confer the MHC restriction phenotype on T cells in [(A x B)F1/A] chimeras.	Zinkernagel 1978 Fink and Bevan 1978
Negatively selected (to B) A T cells can sometimes be sensitized to B + virus. A very few A T cell clones lytic for A + virus may also show a lower level of killing of B + virus when stimulated with A + virus.	Bennink and Doherty 1979 Weiss *et al.* 1980
Self MHC-restricted CTL clones may also be alloreactive	Von Boehmer *et al.*, 1979 Braciale *et al.*, 1981
An (A x B)F_1 T cell clone may recognize both A + x and B + y.	Bevan and Hunig 1982

TABLE IV
MOLECULES AND MHC RESTRICTION*

CD4 and CD8 define the MHC restriction phenotype, not the function of T cells, and may be involved in binding to constant regions of the MHC molecules.	Swain 1983 Reinherz *et al.*, 1983
Transfection of H-2L^d into L cells demonstrates that this is the Ir gene coding for the MHC glycoprotein targeting virus-immune effector T cells in LCM.	Orn *et al.*, 1982
"Exon-shuffling" protocols define the need for the α_1 and α_2 domains of the MHC glycoproteins for targeting CTL.	Murre *et al.*, 1984 Allen *et al.*, 1984
CTL lyse-MHC-negative target cells coated with an antibody which is anti-idiotypic for the receptor of the effector T cells. Hybrid antibodies binding to a component of the T-cell receptor and to the MHC glycoprotein on the target overcome T cell specificity. The MHC molecule does not seem to be a "channel" for delivering the cytotoxic signal.	Kranz *et al.*, 1984 Staerz *et al.*, 1985

*I have not attempted to review the advances in understanding the protein and DNA structure of the MHC (Nathenson, *et al.*, Hood and Steinmetz, 1983) or the work on the T cell receptor (Davis, 1985; Hood, *et al.*, 1985), as these topics will be covered by others at this symposium who have been closely involved.

TABLE V
A VIRAL ANTIGEN IN CLASS I MHC RESTRICTION: THE INFLUENZA NUCLEOPROTEIN (NP)

CTL generated in influenza primed mice are highly cross-reactive and do not follow the specificity pattern predicted for the major surface hemagglutinin glycoprotein.	Effros *et al.*, 1977 Zwerink *et al.*, 1977
The explanation for the above is that many cross-reactive* influenza-immune CTL recognize targets transfected with the viral NP gene, or infected with vaccinia virus carrying NP.	Townsend *et al., 1984* *Yewdell et al.*, 1985
CTL recognize NP peptides associated with class I MHC glycoproteins. The immunogenic peptide varies for different class I MHC molecules.	Townsend *et al.*, 1986

*Other viral determinants are also recognized by CTL, in particular the viral matrix (M) protein, a fragment of which (peptide 55-73) associates with HLA-A2 (Gotch, *et al.*, 1987).

TABLE VI
IMMUNOLOGICAL SURVEILLANCE OF TUMORS AND CLASS I MHC GLYCOPROTEIN EXPRESSION*

Thymocytes transformed by radiation leukemia virus down-regulate MHC glycoprotein expression in susceptible, but not resistant, strains of mice†.	Meruelo 1979
SV40-transformed tumor cells that grow in mice do so by modulating the expression of the class I MHC Ir gene H-$2K^k$.	Gooding 1982
Adenovirus 12 down-regulates class I MHC gene expression and the resultant tumors grow in immunologically intact rats. Adenovirus 5 does not have this effect and cells transformed with this virus are rejected.	Schrier *et al.*, 1983 Bernards *et al.*, 1983
Tumor specific transplantation antigens on a UV-transformed fibrosarcoma are modified class I MHC glycoproteins.	Phillips *et al.*, 1985

*Early work is reviewed in greater detail in Doherty, *et al.*, 1984.

†Down regulation is associated with increased methylation and altered restriction enzyme patterns of MHC DNA (Meruelo, *et al.*, 1986).

CONCLUSIONS

This short, historical account has concentrated on early events in the analysis of class I MHC restriction, in which I was involved directly, and is unashamedly skewed towards supporting the "single T cell receptor-altered self" hypothesis that Zinkernagel and I developed to explain T cell recognition (Zinkernagel and Doherty, 1974b; Doherty and Zinkernagel, 1975a). The latter at last makes sense in the light of recent evidence that T cells see peptide fragments bound to MHC molecules (Townsend, *et al.*, 1986; Buus, *et al.*, 1987; Gotch, *et al.*, 1987, Bjorkman, *et al.*, 1987). "Altered self" was problematic when we had to think of two glycoproteins (the "clash of titans" model) getting together on cell surface.

Even so, viral glycoproteins may bind to MHC molecules (Doherty, 1985). The best characterized example is an immunosuppressive system, where the adenovirus E19 early glycoprotein interacts with nascent class I in the endoplasmic reticulum and prevents transport to cell surface (Paabo, *et al.*, 1986). It may thus be premature to reject completely the possibility that separate molecules can associate at the plasma membrane in an antigenic mode (Finberg, *et al.*, 1978). However, the peptide model is obviously easier to deal with conceptually, and also offers a ready explanation for the fact that "internal" viral components often seem to be the major targets in cell-mediated immunity (Townsend, *et al.*, 1984; Yewdall, *et al.*, 1985; Gotch, *et al.*, 1987).

The likelihood that the active site on the T cell receptor is equivalent to that on the Ig molecule (Goverman, 1986), together with the findings from the recent crystallographic analysis (Colman, *et al.*, 1987) of Ig bound to the influenza neuraminidase (the "flexible-handshake" model) point to the possibility that the peptide and self MHC components are seen together in an integral way. It may thus be the case that the T cell receptor has some affinity for unmodified, self class I MHC glycoprotein (Benacerraf and Rock, 1984). The latter postulate, or the concept that MHC restriction phenotype is determined during late thymic ontogeny (perhaps selected from the CD4+ CD8+ population, Smith, 1987) by binding of CD4 or CD8 (Swain, 1983; Reinherz, *et al.*, 1983), or both ideas together, seems currently to offer the most reasonable way of developing an MHC-restricted T cell repertoire. The big questions in MHC restriction still concern the nature of the T cell repertoire, and the characteristics of receptor binding.

ACKNOWLEDGEMENTS

This was written while a visitor at the Medical Biology Institute, La Jolla, California. I thank Darcy Wilson, Matt Mescher, Carol Cowing, Dan Gold and Nancy Johnson for helpful discussion, and Annemarie Reid for typing the manuscript.

REFERENCES

Allen, H., Wraith, D., Pala, P., Askonas, B. and Flavell, R.A. Domain interactions of H-2 class I antigens alter cytotoxic T-cell recognition sites. Nature (London) 309:279 (1984).

Amos, D.B., Bodmer, W.F., Ceppellini, R., Condliffe, P.G., Dausset, J., Fahey, M.L., Goodman, H.C., Klein, J., Lilly, F., Mann, D.L., McDevitt, H., Nathenson, S., Palm, J., Reisfeld, R.A., Rogentine, H.G., Sanderson, A.R., Shreffler, D.C., Simonsen, M., and Van Rood, J.J. Biological significance of histocompatibility antigens. Fed Proc. 31:1087 (1971).

Benacerraf, B. A hypothesis to relate the specificity of T lymphocytes and the activity of I region-specific Ir genes in macrophages and B lymphocytes. J. Immunol. 20:1809 (1978).

Benacerraf, B. and Rock, K.L. Thymic T cells are driven to expand upon interaction with self class II major histocompatibility gene products on accessory cell. Proc. Natl. Acad. Sci. USA 81:1221 (1984).

Bennink, J.R. and Doherty, P.C. Vaccinia specific cytotoxic T cell responses in the context of H-2 antigens not encountered in thymus may reflect aberrant recognition of a virus-H-2 complex. J. Exp. Med. 149:150 (1979).

Bernards, R., Schrier, P.I., Houwelling, A., Bos, J.L., van der Eb, A.J., Zijlstra, M., and Melief, C.J.M. Tumorigenicity of cells transformed by adenovirus type 12 by evasion of T cell immunity. Nature 305:776 (1883).

Bevan, M.J. Interaction antigens detected by cytotoxic T cells with the major histocompatibility complex as modifier. Nature 256:419 (1975).

Bevan, M.J. Killer cells reactive to altered self antigens can also be alloreactive. Proc. Natl. Acad. Sci. USA 74:2094 (1977).

Bevan, M.J. and Hunig, T.R. Antigen recognition by cloned cytotoxic T lymphocytes follows rules predicted by the altered self hypothesis. J. Exp. Med. 155:111 (1982).

Bjorkman, P.J., Saper, M.A., Samraoui, B., Bennett, W.S., Strominger, J.L. and Wiley, D.C. The foreign antigen-binding site and T cell recognition regions of class I histocompatibility antigens. Nature 329:512 (1987).

Blanden, R.V. T cell response to viral and bacterial infection. Transplant. Rev. 19:56 (1974).

Blanden, R.V., Doherty, P.C., Dunlop, M.B.C., Gardner, I.D., Zinkernagel, R.M. and David, C.S. Genes required for T cell mediated cytotoxicity against virus infected target cells are in the K or D regions of the H-2 gene complex. Nature 254:269 (1975).

Blanden, R.V., Bowern, N.A., Pang, T.E., Gardner, J.D. and Parish, C.R. Effects of thymus-independent (B) cells and the H-2 gene complex or antiviral function of immune thymus-derived (T) cells. Aust. J. Exp. Biol. Med. Sci. 53:187 (1975).

Blanden, R.V., Dunlop, M.B.C., Doherty, P.C., Kohn, H.I. and McKenzie, I.F.C. Effects of four H-2K mutants on virus-induced antigens recognized by cytotoxic T cells. Immunogenetics 3:541 (1976).

Bodmer, W.F. Evolutionary significance of the HL-A system. Nature 237:139 (1972).

Braciale, T.J., Andrew, M.E. and Braciale, V.L. Simultaneous expression of H-2 restricted and alloreactive recognition by a cloned line of influenza virus-specific cytotoxic T lymphocytes. J. Exp. Med. 153:1371 (1981).

Burakoff, S.J., Weinberger, O., Krensky, A.M., and Reiss, C.S. A molecular analysis of the cytolytic T lymphocyte response. Adv. Immunol. 36:45, (1984).

Burnet, F.M. Multiple polymorphism in relationship to histocompatibility antigens. Nature 245:359 (1972).

Buus, S., Sette, A., Colon, S.M., Miles, C., and Grey, H.M. The relation between major histocompatibility complex (MHC) restriction and the capacity of Ia to bind. Science 235:1353 (1987).

Coggin, J.H. and Anderson, N.G. Embryonic antigens in virally transformed cells. In "Membranes and Viruses in Immunopathology", S.B. Day and R.A. Good, eds., pp. 217-247, Academic Press, New York and London (1972).

Cole, G.A., Nathanson, N. and Prendergast, R.A. Requirement for θ-bearing lymphocytes in lymphocytic choriomeningitis virus-induced central nervous system disease. Nature 238:355 (1972).

Colman, P.M., Laver, W.G., Varghese, J.N., Baker, A.T., Tullock, P.A., Air, G.M. and Webster, R.G. Three dimensional structure of a complex of antibody with influenza virus neuraminidase. Nature 326:358 (1987).

Colombo, M.P., Jaenisch, R. and Wettstein, P.J. Endogenous retrovirus leads to the expression of a histocompatibility antigen detectable by skin graft rejection. Proc. Natl. Acad. Sci. USA 84:189 (1987).

David, C.S. and Shreffler, D.C. The H-2 major histocompatibility complex and the I immune response region: Genetic variation, function and organization. Adv. Immunol. 20:125 (1975).

Davis, M.M. Molecular genetics of the T cell receptor β chain. Ann. Rev. Immunol. 3:357 (1985).

Doherty, P.C. and Zinkernagel, R.M. T cell mediated immunopathology in viral infections. Transplant. Rev. 19:89 (1974).

Doherty, P.C. and Zinkernagel, R.M. A biological role for the major histocompatibility antigens. Lancet June 38, 1406 (1975a).

Doherty, P.C. and Zinkernagel, R.M. Capacity of sensitized thymus derived lymphocytes to induce fatal lymphocyte choriomeningitis is restricted by the H-2 gene complex. J. Immunol. 114:30 (1975b).

Doherty, P.C. and Zinkernagel, R.M. H-2 compatibility is required for T cell-mediated lysis of target cells infected with lymphocytic choriomeningitis. J. Exp. Med. 141:502 (1975c).

Doherty, P.C., Blanden, R.V., and Zinkernagel, R.M. Specificity of virus-immune effector T cells for H-2K or H-2D compatible interactions: Implications for H antigen diversity. Transplant. Rev. 29:89 (1976).

Doherty, P.C., Gotze, D., Trinchieri, G. and Zinkernagel, R.M. Models for recognition of virally modified cells by immune thymus derived lymphocytes. Immunogenetics 3:517 (1976).

Doherty, P.C., Biddison, W.E., Bennink, J.R. and Knowles, B.B. Cytotoxic T cell responses in mice infected with influenza and vaccinia viruses vary in magnitude with H-2 genotype. J. Exp. Med. 148:534 (1978).

Doherty, P.C., Knowles, B.B. and Wettstein, P.J. Immunological surveillance of tumors in the context of major histocompatibility complex restriction of T cell function. Adv. Cancer Res. 42:1 (1984).

Doherty, P.C. T cells and viral infections. Brit. Med. Bull. 41:7 (1985).

Doherty, P.C. Virus-immune T cells and the major histocompatibility complex: Evolution of some basic concepts over the past two years. Experientia 42:972 (1986).

Doherty, P.C. and Allen, J.E. Differential effect of hybrid resistance on the targeting of virus-immune effector T cells to spleen and brain. Immunogenetics 24:409 (1986).

Effros, R.B., Doherty, P.C., Gerhard, W. and Bennink, J. Generation of both cross-reactive and virus-specific T cell populations after immunization with serologically distinct influenza A viruses. J. Exp. Med. 145:557 (1977).

Eichman, K. Expression and function of idiotypes on lymphocytes. Adv. Immunol. 26:195 (1978).

Finberg, R., Mescher, M., and Burakoff, S.J. The induction of virus-specific cytotoxic T lymphocytes with solubilized viral and membrane proteins. J. Exp. Med. 148:1620 (1978).

Fink, P.J. and Bevan, M.J. The influence of thymus H-2 antigens on the specificity of maturing killer and helper cells. Immunol. Rev. 42:4 (1978).

Forman, J., Vitetta, E.S., Hart, D.A., and Klein, J. Relationship between trinitrophenyl and H-2 antigens on trinitrophenyl-modified spleen cells. I. H-2 antigens on cells treated with trinitrobenzene sulfonic acid are derivatized. J. Immunol. 118:797 (1987).

Gardner, I.D., Bowern, N.A., and Blanden, R.V. Cell-mediated cytotoxicity against ectromelia virus-infected target cells. III. Role of the H-2 gene complex. Eur. J. Immunol. 118:797 (1977).

Gooding, L.R. Characterization of a progressive tumor from C3H fibroblasts transformed *in vitro* with SV40 virus. Immunoresistance *in vivo* correlates with phenotypic loss of H-2K^k. J. Immunol. 129:1306 (1982).

Gordon, R.D., Simpson, E., and Samelson, L.E. *In vitro* cell-mediated immune responses to the male specific (H-Y) antigen in mice. J. Exp. Med. 142:1108 (1975).

Gotch, F., Rothbard, J., Howland, K., Townsend, A. and McMichael, A. Cytotoxic T lymphocytes recognize a fragment of influenza virus matrix protein in association with HLA-A2. Nature 326:881 (1987).

Goverman, J., Hunkapiller, T. and Hood, L. A speculative view of the multicomponent nature of T cell antigen recognition. Cell 45:475 (1986).

Hood, L. and Steinmetz, M. Genes of the major histocompatibility complex in mouse and man. Science 222:727 (1983).

Hood, L., Kronenberg, M. and Hunkapiller, T. T cell antigen receptors and the immunoglobulin supergene family. Cell 40:225 (1985).

Katz, D.H., Hamaoka, T., Dorf, M.E., Maurer, P.H. and Benacerraf. B. Cell interactions between histoincompatible T and B lymphocytes. VII. Cooperative responses between lymphocytes are controlled by genes in the I region of the H-2 complex. J. Exp. Med. 138:734 (1973).

Katz, D.H. and Benacerraf, B. The histocompatibility-linked immune response genes. Adv. Cancer Res. 21:121 (1975).

Kohn, H.I. and Melvold, R.W. Eight new histocompatibility mutations associated with the H-2 complex. Immunogenetics 3:185 (1976).

Kranz, D.M., Tonegawa, S. and Eisen, H.N. Attachment of an anticeptor antibody to non-target cells renders them susceptible to lysis by a clone of cytotoxic T cells. Proc. Natl. Acad. Sci. USA 81:7922 (1984).

Langman, R.E. and Blanden, R.V. Cell-mediated immunity to bacterial infection in the mouse. Thymus-derived cells as effectors of acquired resistance to Listeria monocytogenes. Scand. J. Immunol. 1:379 (1972).

Lawrence, H.S. Transfer factor in cellular immunity. Harvey Lectures 68:239 (1973).

Majde, J.A. and Holterman, O.A. An apparent histoincompatibility between mice chronically infected with lymphocytic choriomeningitis virus and their uninfected syngeneic counterparts. Transplantation 11:20 (1971).

Marshak, A., Doherty, P.c. and Wilson, D.B. The control of specificity of cytotoxic T lymphocytes by the major histocompatibility complex (Ag-B) in rats and identification of a new alloantigen system showing no Ag-B restriction. J. Exp. Med. 146:1773 (1977).

McMichael, A.J., Ting, A., Zweerink, H.J. and Askonas, B.A. HLA-restriction of cell-mediated lysis of influenza virus-infected human cells. Nature 270:524 (1977).

Meruelo, D. A role for elevated H-2 antigen expression in resistance to neoplasia caused by radiation-induced leukemia virus. J. Exp. Med. 149:898 (1979).

Meruelo, D., Kornreich, R., Rossomando, A., Pampeno, C., Boral, A., Silver, J.L., Buxbaum, J., Weiss, E.H., Devlin, J.J., Mellor, A.L., Flavell, R.A. and Pellicer, A. Lack of class I H-2 antigens in cells transformed by radiation leukemia virus is associated with methylation and rearrangement of H-2 DNA. Proc. Natl. Acad. Sci. USA 83:4504 (1986).

Murre, C., Choi, E., Weis, J., Seidman, J.G., Ozato, K., Liu, L., Burakoff, S.J. and Reiss, C.S. Dissection of serological and cytolytic T lymphocyte epitopes on murien major histocompatibility antigens by a recombinant H-2 gene separating the first two external domains. J. Exp. Med. 160:167 (1984).

Nathenson, S.G., Uehara, H., Ewenstein, B.M., Kindt, T.J. and Goligan, J.E. Primary structural analysis of the transplantation antigens of the murine H-2 major histocompatibility complex. Ann. Rev. Biochem. 50:1025 (1981).

Oldstone, M.B.A., Dixon, F.J., Mitchell, G.F. and McDevitt, H.O. Histocompatibility linked genetic control of disease susceptibility. Murine lymphocytic choriomeningitis virus infection. J. Exp. Med. 137:1201 (1973).

Orn, A., Goodenow, R.S., Hood, L., Brayton, P.R., Woodward, J.G. and Harmon, R.C. Product of a transfected H-2L^d gene acts as a restriction element for LCMV-specific killer T cells. Nature 298:529 (1982).

Paabo, S., Nilsson, T. and Peterson, P.A. Adenoviruses of subgenera B,C,D and E modulate cell-surface expression of major histocompatibility complex class I antigens. Proc. Natl. Acad. Sci. USA 83:9665 (1986).

Philips, C., McMillan, M., Flood, P.M., Murphy, D.B., Forman, J., Lancki, D., Womack, J.E., Goodenow, R.S. and Schreiber, H. Identification of a unique tumor specific antigen as a novel class I major histocompatibility molecule. Proc. Natl. Acad. Sci. USA 85:5140 (1985).

Reinherz, E.L., Meuer, S.C. and Schlossman, S.F. The human T cell receptor: analysis with cytotoxic T cell clones. Immunol. Rev. 74:83 (1983).

Schrier, P.I., Bernards, R., Vaessen, R.T.M.J., Houweling, A., and van der Eb, A.J. Expression of class I major histocompatibility antigens switched off by highly oncogenic adenovirus 12 in transformed rat cells. Nature 305:771 (1983).

Schwartz, R.H. Immune response (Ir) genes of the murine major histocompatibility complex. Adv. Immunol. 38:31, (1986).

Shearer, G.M. Cell-mediated cytotoxicity to trinitrophenyl modified syngeneic lymphocytes. Eur. J. Immunol. 4:527 (1974).

Shearer, G.M., Schmitt-Verhulst, A-M. and Rehn, T.G. Significance of the major histocompatibility complex as assessed by T cell-mediated lympholysis involving syngeneic stimulating cells. Contemp. Top. Immunobiol. 7:221 (1977).

Shevach, E.M. and Rosenthal, A.S. Function of macrophages in antigen recognition by guinea pig T lymphocytes. II. Role of the macrophage in the regulation of genetic control of the immune response. J. Exp. Med. 138:1213 (1973).

Shreffler, D.C. and Kindred, B. H-2 dependence of co-operation between T and B cells *in vivo*. J. Immunol. 109:940 (1974).

Simonsen, M. The clonal selection hypothesis evaluated by grafted cells reacting against their hosts. Cold Spring Harbor Symp. Quant. Biol. 32:519 (1967).

Singh, P.B., Brown, R.E. and Roser, B. MHC antigens in urine as olfactory recognition cues. Nature 327:161 (1987).

Smith, L. $CD4^+$ murine T cells develop from $CD8^+$ precursors *in vivo*. Nature 326:798 (1987).

Snell, G.D. The H-2 locus of the mouse. Observations and speculations concerning its comparative genetics and its polymorphism. Folia Biol. 14:335 (1968).

Staerz, U.D., Kanaganwa, O. and Bevan, M.J. Hybrid antibodies on target sites are attached by T cells. Nature 314:628 (1985).

Summers, D.F. and Hecht, T.T. Effect of vesicular stomatitis virus infection on the histocompatibility antigen of L cells. J. Virol. 10:578 (1972).

Swain, S.L. T cell subsets and the recognition of MHC class. Immunol. Rev. 74:129 (1983).

Townsend, A.R.M., McMichael, A.J., Carter, N.P., Huddleston, J.A. and Brownlee, G.C. Cytotoxic T cell recognition of the influenza nucleoprotein recognized by cytotoxic T lymphocytes can be defined with short synthetic peptides. Cell 44:959 (1986).

Townsend, A.R.M., Rothbard, J., Gotch, F.M., Bahadur, G., Wraith, D., and McMichael, A.J. The epitopes of influenza nucleoprotein recognized by cytotoxic T lymphocytes can be defined with short synthetic peptides. Cell 44:959 (1986).

vonBoehmer, H., Hengartner, H., Nabholz, M., Lenhardt, W., Schreier, M. and Haas, W. Fine specificity of a continuously growing killer cell clone specific for H-y antigen. Eur. J. Immunol. 9:592 (1979).

Weiss, A., Brunner, K.T., MacDonald, H.R., and Cerottini, J-C. Antigen specificity of the cytolytic T lymphocyte response to murine sarcoma virus-induced tumors. III. Characterization of cytolytic T lymphocyte clones specific for Moloney leukemia associated cell-surface antigens. J. Exp. Med. 152:1210 (1980).

Wigzell, H. and Binz, H. Antigen-binding, idiotypic T-lymphocyte receptors. Contemp. Top. Immunobiol. 7:113 (1977).

Wilson, D.B., Blyth, J.L. and Nowell, P.C. Quantitative studies on the mixed lymphocyte interaction in rats. III. Kinetics of the response. J. Exp. Med. 128:1157 (1968).

Yewdall, J.W., Bennink, J.R., Smith, G.L. and Moss, B. Influenza A virus nucleoprotein is a major target antigen for cross-reactive anti-influenza A virus cytotoxic T lymphocytes. Proc. Natl. Acad. Sci. USA 82:1785 (1985).

Zinkernagel, R.M. and Doherty, P.C. Cytotoxic thymus-derived lymphocytes in cerebrospinal fluid of mice with lymphocytic choriomeningitis. J. Exp. Med. 138:1266 (1973).

Zinkernagel, R.M. and Doherty, P.C. Restriction of *in vitro* T cell mediated cytotoxicity in lymphocytic choriomeningitis within a syngeneic or seminallogenic system. Nature 251:547 (1974b).

Zinkernagel, R.M. and Doherty, P.C. Immunological surveillance against altered self components by sensitized T lymphocytes in lymphocytic choriomeningitis. Nature 251:547 (1974b).

Zinkernagel, R.M. and Doherty, P.C. H-2 compatibility requirement for T cell-mediated lysis of targets infected with lymphocytic choriomeningitis virus. Different cytotoxic T cell specificities are associated with structures coded in H-2K or H-2D. J. Exp. Med. 141:1427 (1975).

Zinkernagel, R.M. H-2 compatibility requirement for virus-specific T cell-mediated cytolysis. The H-2K structure is coded by a single citron defined by H-2K^{b} mutant mice. J. Exp. Med. 143:437 (1976).

Zinkernagel, R.M. Thymus and lymphohemopoietic cells: Their role in T cell maturation in selection of T cells H-2 restriction specificity and in H-2 linked Ir gene control. Immunol. Rev. 42:202 (1978).

Zinkernagel, R.M., Althage, A., Cooper, S., Kreeb, G., Klein, P.A., Sefton, B., Flaherty, L., Stimpfling, J., Shreffler, D., and Klein, J. Ir genes in H-2 regulate generation of anti-viral cytotoxic T cells: Mapping to K or D and dominance of unresponsiveness. J. Exp. Med. 148:592 (1978).

Zinkernagel, R.M. and Doherty, P.C. MHC-restricted cytotoxic T cells: Studies on the biological role of polymorphic major transplantation antigens determining T-cell restriction-specificity, function, and responsiveness. Adv. Immunol. 27:51 (1979).

Zweerink, H.J., Courtneidge, S.A., Skehel, J.J., Crumpton, M.J. and Askonas, B.A. Cytotoxic T cells kill influenza virus-infected cells but do not distinguish between serologically distinct type A viruses. Nature 267:354 (1977).

A Q REGION PRODUCT AS A CTL RESTRICTION ELEMENT?

Donal B. Murphy and Robert J. Homer

Section of Immunobiology and
Department of Pathology
Yale University School of Medicine
New Haven, Connecticut 06510

ABSTRACT

The function of class I genes mapping in the Q and TL regions of the MHC is unknown. Data presented in this study will show that two genes control a determinant (Qc-1) recognized by cloned cytotoxic T lymphocytes (CTL). One gene is a class I gene and maps in the Q region. The second gene maps in the K-end of the MHC and has tentatively been mapped between $\underline{A}_{\beta 3}$ and $\underline{A}_{\beta 2}$ with recombinant strains. Monoclonal antibody reactive with Q region encoded class I molecules blocks CTL recognition of the Qc-1 determinant at the target cell level. An attractive interpretation of these data is that the Q region class I molecule serves as a CTL restriction element for the recognition of a K-end encoded peptide.

INTRODUCTION

Class I genes mapping in the K (H-2K) and D (H-2D, H-2L) regions of the MHC are highly polymorphic and are expressed on most cells of the body. Products of these genes function as restriction elements for cytotoxic T lymphocytes (CTL), and play an important role in host immunity against virus infected cells (Klein 1986). In contrast, class I genes mapping in the Q (Q1-Q10) and TL (T1-T17) regions display limited polymorphism. Some of these genes are pseudogenes, while others encode molecules with restricted cellular distribution. The function of these latter class I genes is unknown (Flaherty et al 1985, Flavell et al 1986, Mellor 1986).

Recently, we set out to study the expression and function of Q region genes utilizing cloned CTL (Homer and Murphy 1987). Our study showed that a novel Q region controlled determinant, Qc-1, was expressed on B lymphocytes. In the present study, we will show that two genes control the Qc-1 determinant. One gene maps in the Q region and encodes a class I molecule bearing a Qa-2-like determinant. The second gene, which has not yet been identified, maps in the K-end of the complex. Our working hypothesis is that the Q region class I molecule serves as a CTL restriction element and is recognized together with a K-end encoded peptide.

MATERIALS AND METHODS

Mice. Inbred, H-2 congenic, and H-2 recombinant strains were obtained from our mouse breeding facility at Yale, from The Jackson Laboratory, Bar Harbor, Maine, or from other investigators (Dr. Chella David, Mayo Clinic, Rochester, Minnesota and Dr. L. Flaherty, Albany, New York). We are particularly indebted to Dr. Chella David for providing many of the H-2 recombinant strains utilized in this study.

Antibody. Monoclonal antibodies utilized in this study include: 34-1-2 and 20-8-4 (Ozato and Sachs 1981), D3.262 (Lynes et al 1982), and Qa-7 and Qa-8 (Sandrin et al 1983). All of these antibodies react with Qa-2 bearing molecules (Sharrow et al 1984, Stroynowski et al 1987). 34-1-2 and 20-8-4 also react with other class I products.

T cell clones. Details of the production and properties of the CTL clones utilized in this study have been published (Homer and Murphy 1987). Briefly, following the protocol of Forman et al (1982), B6.K1 mice were immunized in vivo with A.BY lymphocytes and their spleen cells restimulated four weeks later in vitro with B6.K2 lymphocytes in the presence of T cell growth factor (Con A activated rat spleen cell culture supernatants). T cell lines were established and maintained on B6 feeder cells, and later cloned by limiting dilution.

Cytolytic assay. A ^{51}Cr cytolytic assay was conducted as previously described (Homer and Murphy, 1987). Since the CTL effector cells utilized in this study crossreact with H-2K^k determinants, radiolabelled AKR derived BW5147 thymoma cells were utilized as target cells. Cold target inhibition analysis was conducted by titrating unlabelled normal spleen cells into cultures containing effector and target cells (E:T, 2:1). Percent specific lysis was calculated as $(cpm_{exp} - cpm_{spon}/cpm_{max} - cpm_{spon}) \times 100$, where spontaneous lysis was determined by culturing target cells in medium, and maximum lysis was determined by culturing target cells in water containing 1% NP-40.

RESULTS

Previously, we showed that cloned L3T4$^-$, Ly-2$^+$ CTL produced by cross-immunizing in Q region incompatible strains recognize a novel determinant, designated Qc-1 (Homer and Murphy 1987). The Qc-1 determinant is crossreactive with an H-2K^k determinant, and, among lymphocytes, is preferentially (exclusively ?) expressed on B lymphocytes. Three phenotypes were identified (illustrated in Fig 1). Some strains (eg B10, B6, B6.K2) express high levels of the antigen (Qc-1^{++} strains). Other strains (eg B10.D2, BALB/cJ, BALB/cByJ) express intermediate levels of the antigen (Qc-1$^+$ strains). Finally, several strains (eg B6.K1) do not express the antigen (Qc-1$^-$ strains). The Qc-1 phenotypes of inbred, congenic, and recombinant strains are listed in Table 1.

Monoclonal Q region class I antibodies block CTL recognition of Qc-1 determinants

The observed cross-reactivity between the Q region controlled CTL determinant and the H-2K^k product raised the possibility that the

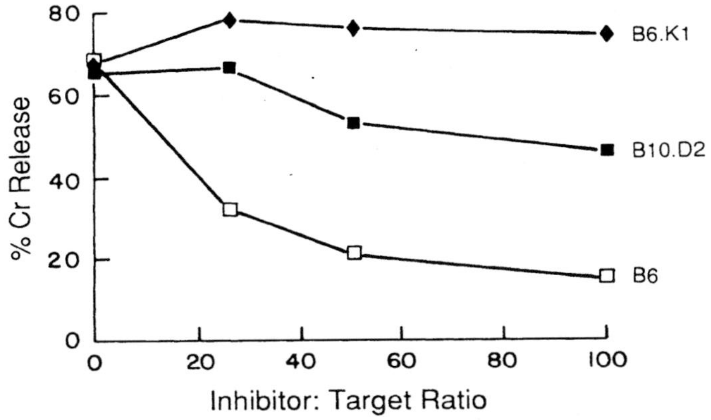

Fig. 1. Competitive inhibition analysis of CTL activity. Unlabelled normal spleen cells were titrated into cultures containing cloned CTL effector cells and radiolabelled BW5147 target cells. The strains included are representative of high expressor (Qc-1^{++}, B6), intermediate expressor (Qc-1^{+}, B10.D2), and negative (Qc-1^{-}, B6.K1) strains.

Table 1. Qc-1 phenotypes of inbred, congenic, and recombinant mouse strains.

Qc-1^{++} strains*

A.BY, B6, B6-*Tla*^{a}, B6.AC1, B6.AC2, B6.K2, B10, B10.GD, B10.HIR1, B10(R297)-*Tla*^{a}, B10(R310)-*Tla*^{a}, B10.RFB2, B10.RFB3, BALB.B, CWB

Qc-1^{+} strains

A.TFR5, B10.A(3R), B10.A(5R). B10.A(18R), B10.D2, B10.DSR1, B10.DSR2, B10.DSR3, B10.RBQ1, B10.RFD1, B10.SBR, BALB/cJ, BALB/cByJ, DBA/2

Qc-1^{-} strains

A.CA, A.SW, A.TH, A.TL, B6.AK1, B6.K1, B10.AQR, B10.DSR4, B10.DSR6, B10.DSR7, B10.F(13R), B10.F(14R), B10.G, B10.HTT, B10.M, B10.MBR, B10.P, B10.RIII, B10.RBF, B10.RPD1, B10.RPF1, B10.RQB1, B10.RQB3, B10.RSB7, B10.RSF4, B10.S, B10.S(7R), B10.S(9R), B10.SM, B10.T(6R), BALB.S, C3H.OH, C3H.OL, P, TBR2, TBR3

---

* Since Qc-1 crossreacts with H-2K^{k}, the following strains also type strongly positive with the CTL: A,A.AL, AKR, B6-*H-2*^{k}, B10.A, B10.A(2R), B10.A(4R), B10.AKM, B10.A(R149)-*Tla*^{b}, B10.A(R410)-*Tla*^{b}, B10.S(8R), BALB.K, C3H.

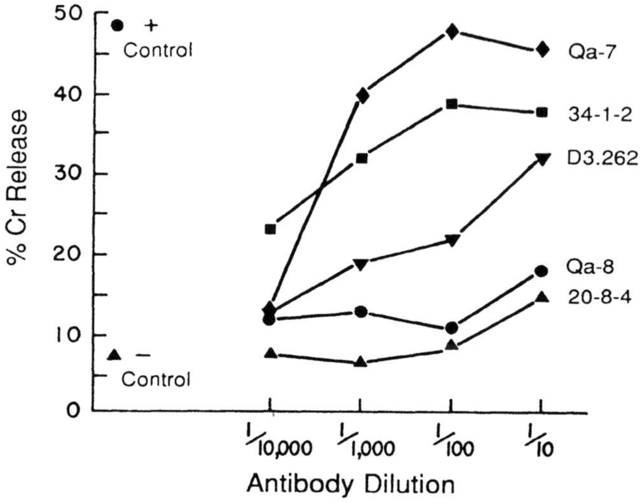

Fig. 2. Monoclonal Q region class I antibodies block CTL recognition of the Qc-1 determinant. Antibodies were tested for their ability to block the competitive inhibition by Qc-1^{++} B6 spleen cells in cultures containing cloned CTL effector cells and radiolabelled BW5147 target cells. Positive (+) control = no competitive inhibitor spleen cells or antibody added. Negative (-) control = competitive inhibitor spleen cells but no antibody added. None of the monoclonal antibodies used block CTL lysis of BW5147 target cells (data not shown).

Qc-1 determinant resides on a Q region encoded class I molecule. In order to test this possibility, blocking studies were conducted with monoclonal antibodies which had previously been shown to react with Q region controlled molecules which bear the Qa-2 determinant. Some (Qa-7, 34-1-2, D3.262) but not all (Qa-8, 20-8-4) of these antibodies blocked the ability of Qc-1^{+} cells to inhibit CTL activity (Fig 2). We conclude from these data that the Qc-1 determinant resides on a Q region encoded class I molecule which also bears a Qa-2-like determinant.

Two genes control the Qc-1 determinant

Previously, we showed that $\underline{H\text{-}2}^b$ (Q^b) and $\underline{H\text{-}2}^d$ (Q^d) strains express the Qc-1 determinant (Homer and Murphy 1987). $\underline{H\text{-}2}^b$ strains express high levels of the antigen (phenotype Qc-1^{++}), while $\underline{H\text{-}2}^d$ strains express intermediate levels of the antigen (phenotype Qc-1^{+}). The first clue that control of the Qc-1 determinant was more complicated than we originally thought came from the observation that several MHC recombinant strains carrying Q^b (Fig 3) or Q^d (Fig 4) typed Qc-1^{-}. In addition, we observed that while strains carrying $\underline{H\text{-}2}^q$ or $\underline{H\text{-}2}^s$ typed Qc-1^{-}, several recombinant strains carrying Q^q or Q^s typed Qc-1^{+} (data not shown). This raised the possibility that a second gene, mapping in the K-end of the MHC, also controlled the Qc-1 determinant.

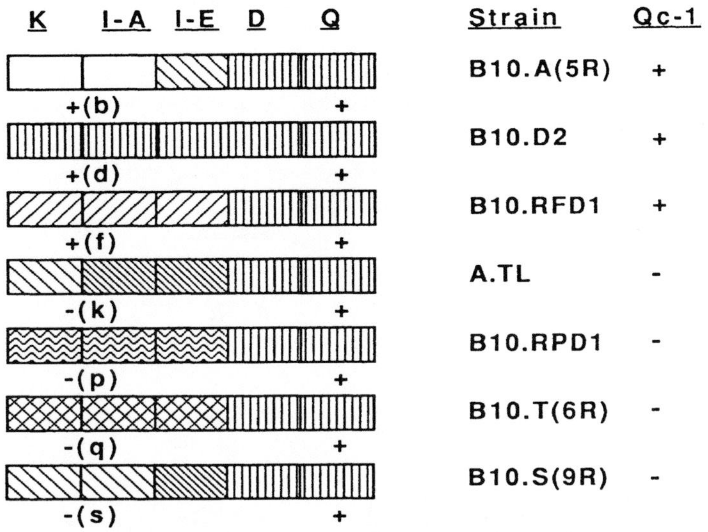

Fig. 3. Two genes control the Qc-1 determinant (recombinant strains carrying Q^b).

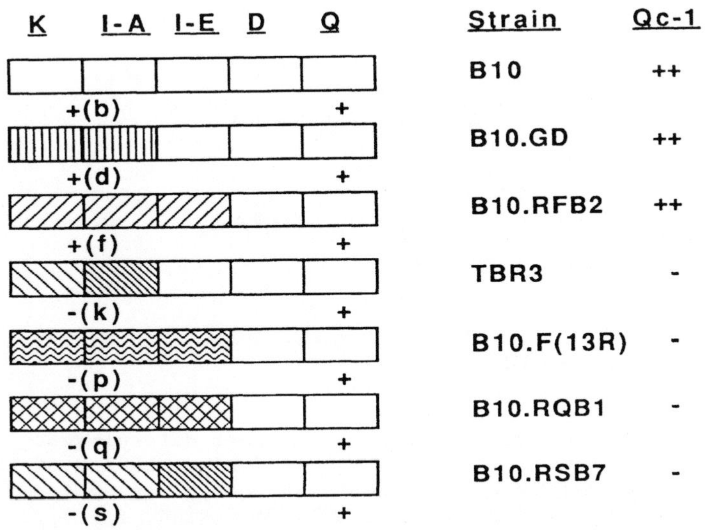

Fig. 4. Two genes control the Qc-1 determinant (recombinant strains carrying Q^d).

Evidence supporting this interpretation comes from several sources. First, recombinant strain A.TFR5, which was derived from $Qc\text{-}1^-$ progenitor strains A.TL and A.CA, types $Qc\text{-}1^+$ (Fig 5). The crossover in A.TFR5 positions the second gene centromeric to $\underline{E}_\beta$. Second, an F1 hybrid between two $Qc\text{-}1^-$ strains types $Qc\text{-}1^+$ (Fig 6). This result formally rules out mutation in the Q region gene as a possible explanation for the $Qc\text{-}1^-$ status of Q^b strains. Finally, control of the Qc-1 determinant segregates with the MHC in (B10 x B10.G)F1 x B10.G backcross mice, thus formally proving that the second gene is linked to the MHC (data not shown).

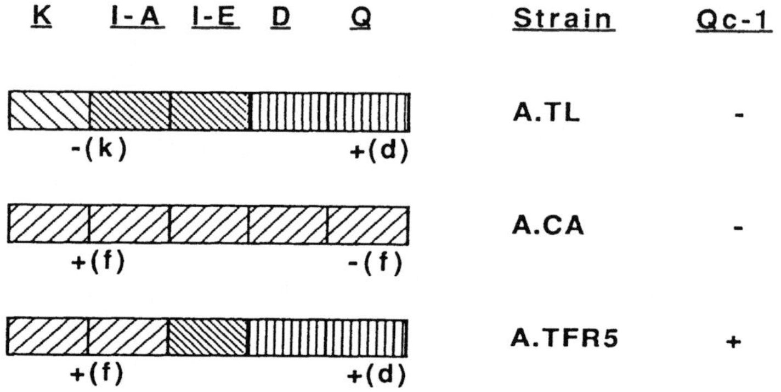

Fig. 5. Two genes control the Qc-1 determinant. A recombinant derived from two $Qc\text{-}1^-$ strains types $Qc\text{-}1^+$.

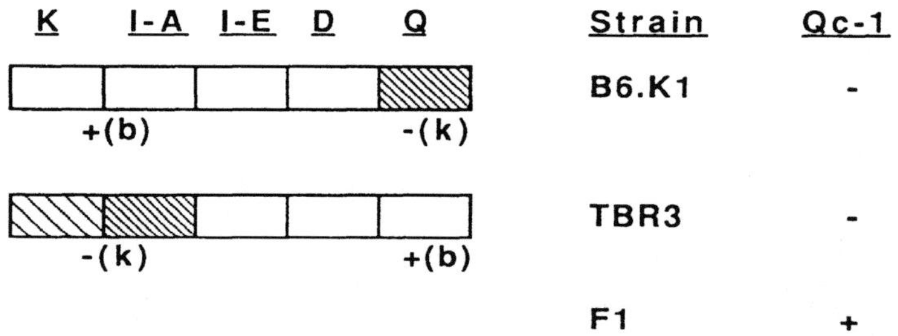

Fig. 6. Two genes control the Qc-1 determinant. An F1 hybrid between two $Qc\text{-}1^-$ strains types $Qc\text{-}1^+$.

In sum, two genes interact to control the Qc-1 determinant. Appropriate alleles at both loci are required for expression of the Qc-1 determinant. Appropriate (+) alleles at the Q region locus include b,d,q,s while inappropriate (-) alleles include f,k,p,v. Appropriate (+) alleles at the K-end locus include b,d,f while inappropriate (-) alleles include k,p,q,s.. Any + allele at the K-end locus appears to interact with any + allele at the Q region locus to generate the Qc-1 determinant. The Q region allele determines the $Qc\text{-}1^{++}$ (b) or $Qc\text{-}1^+$ (d,q,s) phenotype.

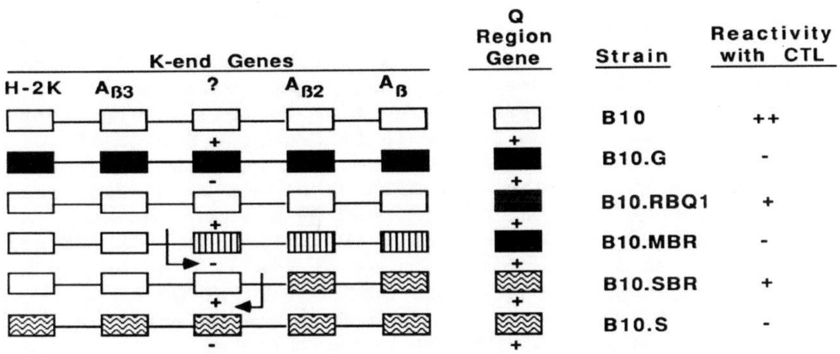

Fig. 7. The K-end gene appears to map between $\underline{A}_{\beta 3}$ and $\underline{A}_{\beta 2}$. The crossover in strain B10.MBR occurred to the right of $\underline{A}_{\beta 3}$ (Steinmetz et al 1986) while the crossover in B10.SBR occurred to the left of $\underline{A}_{\beta 2}$ (M. Steinmetz, personal communication).

The K-end gene appears to map between $\underline{A}_{\beta 3}$ and $\underline{A}_{\beta 2}$

In an attempt to identify the K-end gene, additional recombinant strains were tested (Fig 7). The crossover in strain B10.MBR appears to position the K-end locus inside the complex, to the right of the $\underline{A}_{\beta 3}$ locus. In addition, the crossover in strain B10.SBR appears to position the K-end locus to the left of the $\underline{A}_{\beta 2}$ locus. This mapping assumes that 1) single, equal crossovers occurred in the generation of the recombinant strains, 2) the number and position of MHC loci in the progenitor haplotypes is invariant, and 3) no mutation occurred during or subsequent to the derivation of the recombinant strains. Clearly, analysis of additional recombinants together with molecular genetic analysis is required to confirm this map position.

DISCUSSION

Three major questions concerning the Qc-1 system remain to be resolved. First, what MHC genes control this determinant? Second, what is the nature of the interaction between the two genes? Third, what is the biological significance of this system?

We have attempted to address the first question in several ways. Studies with recombinants clearly show that one gene maps in the Q region. Blocking studies with monoclonal antibodies provide strong evidence that the Q region gene is a class I gene which encodes a Qa-2 bearing molecule. The one apparent exception to this interpretation is the observation that the Qa-2^{-} strain BALB/cByJ types Qc-1^{+}. Possibly, the CTL crossreact with a determinant residing on another class I molecule in this strain. Studies by others with transfected cells provide evidence that Q6, Q7, Q8, and Q9 all may encode molecules bearing Qa-2-like determinants (Mellor et al 1985, Straus et al 1985, Waneck et al 1987, Stroynowski et al 1987). Any one or all of these genes are possible candidates for control of Qc-1, particularly Q6 which appears to encode a molecule detected by monoclonal antibody 34-1-2 (blocks CTL recognition of Qc-1) but not monoclonal antibody 20-8-4 (does not block CTL recognition of Qc-1) (Stroynowski et al 1985). Studies with recombinant strains B10.MBR and B10.SBR provide tentative evidence that the K-end gene maps between $\underline{A}_{\beta 3}$ and $\underline{A}_{\beta 2}$. At present, no gene has been identified which maps in this interval. However, the same two recombinants have been used to map control of a set of low molecular weight proteins (LMP) to this chromosomal segment (Monaco and McDevitt 1986). Molecular analyses, including transfection studies, are currently in progress to identify the genes involved.

Numerous studies have shown that cytotoxic T lymphocytes recognize foreign antigen together with self class I restriction elements (H-2K, H-2D, H-2L) (Klein 1986). Evidence is also accumulating that the antigen is usually processed and presented as a peptide (Watts and McConnell 1987). A straight forward interpretation of our data is that the CTL recognize a Q region class I restriction element together with a K-end encoded peptide (LMP?). Compatible with this interpretation is the observation that antibody reactive with a Q region controlled class I determinant blocks CTL activity.

If this interpretation is correct, it is the first example of a Q region product serving as a restriction element. Since the Q region restriction element is foreign and the K-end controlled antigen is a self antigen, this would also be the first example of a Matzinger-Bevin cloned T cell which recognizes a non-self MHC determinant as a restriction element together with a self MHC determinant as nominal antigen (Matzinger and Bevin 1977). Data in the maternally transmitted antigen (mta) system are also compatible with the interpretation that a TL region encoded class I molecule may serve as a restriction element which is recognized together with a mitochondrial antigen (Fischer-Lindahl et al 1987). Thus, the species may have evolved numerous forms of class I molecules which restrict CTL interaction.

Other interpretations of the data are possible. For example, the K-end gene may post-translationally modify the Q region class I product. Possible precedent for this type of model can be drawn from the serologically defined Qa-6 and Qa-11 determinants, where a TL region gene and a Q region gene both appear to control the determinant (Widacki et al 1985, van de Meugheuvel 1985). However, the molecular basis for control of these determinants is unknown. We have looked at molecules precipitated by antibodies which block Qc-1 CTL activity, and find no difference in the one dimensional or two dimensional gel patterns between molecules from Qc-1^+ and Qc-1^- strains or between T cells and B cells (unpublished data). This, of course, does not rule out a possible qualitative difference in the molecules. If a difference does exist, the methods we have used simply do not detect the difference.

In sum, one of the mysteries surrounding the MHC centers on the function of class I genes mapping in the Q and TL regions. Data presented in this study are compatible with the possibility that at least one of these genes mapping in the Q region may function as a restriction element for cytotoxic T lymphocytes. The data also provide evidence for the expression of a novel K-end gene. Identification of the two genes involved, coupled with an understanding of the interaction between these genes, should provide further clues to MHC gene expression and function.

ACKNOWLEDGMENTS

This work was supported by NIH grants AI-14349 and CA-16359. R. Homer was also supported by NIH training grants AI-07019 and T32GM 07205. The authors would like to thank Charlie Janeway for critical and invaluable discussions of the work, and Lisa Messner for excellent secretarial assistance.

REFERENCES

Fischer-Lindahl, K., Loveland, B.E., and Richards, C.S.: The end of "H-2"? In C.S. David (ed): Major Histocompatibility Genes and Their Role in Immune Function, Plenum Publishing Corp, New York, in press.

Flaherty, L., Karl, M., and DiBiase, K.: The Qa series of antigens. In B. Pernis and H.J. Vogel (eds): Cell Biology of the Major Histocompatibility Complex, pp229-237, Academic Press, New York, 1985.

Flavell, R.A., Allen, H., Burkly, L.C., Sherman, D.H., Waneck, G.L., and Widera, G.: Molecular biology of the H-2 histocompatibility complex. Science 233:437-443, 1986.

Forman, J., Trial, J., Tonkonogy, S., and Flaherty, L.: The Qa-2 subregion controls the expression of two antigens recognized by H-2 unrestricted cytotoxic T cells. J. Exp. Med. 155:749-767, 1982.

Homer, R.J. and Murphy, D.B.: Qc-1, a novel Q region controlled CTL determinant expressed on B lymphocytes. J. Immunol. 138:4322-4328, 1987.

Klein, J.: Natural History of the Major Histocompatibility Complex, John Wiley & Sons, New York, 1986.

Lynes, M.A., Tonkonogy, S., and Flaherty, L.: Qa-1 and Qa-2 expression on CFU-s. J. Immunol. 129:928-930, 1982.

Matzinger, R. and Bevan, M.: Why do so many lymphocytes respond to major histocompatibility antigens? Cell. Immunol. 29:1-5, 1977.

Mellor, A.: The class I MHC gene family in mice. Immunology Today 7:19-24, 1986.

Mellor, A., Antoniou, J., and Robinson, P.: Structure and expression of genes encoding murine Qa-2 class I antigens. Proc. Natl. Acad. Sci. U.S.A. 82:5920-5924, 1985.

Monaco, J.J. and McDevitt, H.O.: The LMP antigens: a stable MHC-controlled multisubunit protein complex. Human Immunology 15:416-426, 1986.

Ozato, K. and Sachs, D.H.: Monoclonal antibodies to mouse MHC antigens. III. Hybridoma antibodies reacting to antigens of the $H\text{-}2^b$ haplotype reveal genetic control of isotype expression. J. Immunol. 126:317-321, 1981.

Sandrin, M., Hogarth, P., and McKenzie, I: Two "Qa" specificities Qa-m7 and Qa-m8 defined by monoclonal antibodies. J. Immunol. 131:546-547, 1983.

Sharrow, S.O., Flaherty, L., and Sachs, D.H.: Serologic cross-reactivity between class I MHC molecules and an H-2-linked differentiation antigen as detected by monoclonal antibodies. J. Exp. Med. 159:21-40, 1984.

Steinmetz, M., Stephan, D., and Fischer-Lindahl, K: Gene organization and recombinational hot spots in the murine histocompatibility complex. Cell 44:895-904, 1986.

Straus, D., Stroynowski, I., Schiffer, S., and Hood, L.: Expression of hybrid class I genes of the major histocompatibility complex of the mouse in L cells. Proc. Natl. Acad. Sci. U.S.A. 82:6245-6249, 1985.

Stroynowski, I., Forman, J., Goodenow, R., Schiffer, S., McMillian, M., Sharrow, S., Sachs, D., and Hood, L.: Expression and T cell recognition of hybrid antigens with amino terminal domains encoded by Qa-2 region of major histocompatibility complex and carboxyl termini of transplantation antigens. J. Exp. Med. 161:835-952, 1985.

Stroynowski, I., Soloski, M., Low, M., and Hood, L.: A single gene encodes soluble and membrane bound forms of the major histocompatibility Qa-2 antigen: Anchoring of the product by a phospholipid tail. Cell, in press.

van de Meugheuvel, W., van Seventer, G., and Demant, P.: A new Tla region antigen, Qa-11, similar to Qa-2 and associated with B type ß2-microglobulin. J. Immunol. 134:2507-2512, 1985.

Waneck, G.L., Sherman, D.H., Calvin, S., Allen, H., and Flavell, R.A.: Tissue-specific expression of cell-surface Qa-2 antigen from a transfected $Q7^b$ gene of C57BL/10 mice. J. Exp. Med. 165:1358-1370, 1987.

Watts, T.H. and McConnell, H.M.: Biophysical aspects of antigen recognition by T cells. Ann. Rev. Immunol. 5:461-475, 1987.

Widacki, S.M., Flaherty, L., and Cook, R.G.: Biochemical characterization of the molecules reactive with Qa-6 antiserum and the monoclonal antibody 20-8-4: Evidence for structural similarity with the Qa-2 molecule. J. Immunol. 135:3333-3339, 1985.

AN H-2 LINKED GENE, PED, INFLUENCES THE TIMING OF EARLY MOUSE EMBRYO DEVELOPMENT

Carol M. Warner

Department of Biochemistry and Biophysics
Iowa State University
Ames, Iowa 50011

ABSTRACT

The preimplantation period of development is crucial for the survival of mammalian species. During this time the fertilized egg goes through a series of cleavage divisions and cell differentiation events leading to blastocyst formation. Only then can the embryo implant in the uterus and continue its development. We have discovered a gene, Ped, Preimplantation embryo development, linked to the H-2 complex, which influences the rate of early mouse embryo development. The Ped gene maps to the Q region of the H-2 complex. Moreover, concordance of expression of the fast Ped allele with the presence of Qa-2 antigens on preimplantation embryos, and concordance of expression of the slow Ped allele with the absence of Qa-2 antigens on preimplantation embryos, have been found. On the basis of these results we have hypothesized that the Ped gene product may be the Qa-2 antigen.

INTRODUCTION

In mice, preimplantation development encompasses about five days of a 21 day gestation period. During this time the single cell of the fertilized egg undergoes a series of cleavage divisions and cell differentiation events leading to the late blastocyst embryo which contains about 120 cells. From 1971 to 1978 our laboratory was engaged in the collection of preimplantation embryos from inbred strains of mice for the purpose of producing allophenic chimeras to study cell-cell interactions in the immune response. In the course of collecting over 50,000 embryos, we noticed that embryos from mice of the $H\text{-}2^k$ haplotype were slower in their rate of preimplantation development than mice of the other haplotypes with which we were working (b,d,q,s) (Goldbard et al. 1982a). We hypothesized that there was a gene, Ped, (Preimplantation embryo development), associated with the H-2 complex, which was responsible for controlling the rate of embryonic cleavage divisions.

LINKAGE OF THE PED GENE TO THE H-2 COMPLEX

The availability of inbred strains of mice congenic at the H-2 complex, which had been developed by George Shell, allowed us to test our hypothesis. We examined the rate of development of preimplantation mouse embryos from several sets of congenic strains (Goldbard and Warner, 1982; Goldbard et al. 1982a; Goldbard et al. 1982b). Our most extensive study of congenic strains was the analysis of six congenic strains on the C57BL/10Sn background (Goldbard and Warner, 1982). From this study we concluded that the fast Ped allele was associated with the b, d, q, s, and u haplotypes, whereas the slow Ped allele was associated with the k and r haplotypes. A summary of the data collected on embryos from congenic mice with B10 background genes is shown in Table 1. The data are for embryos collected 89 hours post hCG (human chorionic gonadotropin) injection. This time point is about 75 hours after fertilization. The number of cells per embryo was determined by the Tarkowski (1966) procedure. These data show that seven of the 11 classical H-2 haplotypes of laboratory strains of *Mus musculus*, described by Klein (1986), have been analyzed for Ped gene phenotype. The Ped gene phenotype of the f, p, v, and z haplotypes remains to be determined.

The genetic analyses described above were based on the use of congenic strains. To truly prove linkage of two traits one must do segregation analyses in backcross or F_2 generations. We have recently completed a set of experiments which have shown linkage of the Ped gene to the H-2 complex (Warner et al., 1987b). In these experiments, C57BL/10Sn (H-2^b,Ped^{fast}) mice were crossed with B10.BR (H-2^k,Ped^{slow}) mice to produce an F_1 generation. Because H-2 antigens are expressed codominantly and because the fast Ped allele is dominant, the phenotype of the F_1 mice was H-2^{bk}, Ped^{fast}. These mice were then backcrossed to the B10.BR strain. The prediction was that half of the resulting embryos would show the fast Ped phenotype and half of the embryos would show the slow Ped phenotype. The embryos could then be separated and tested for the presence of H-2^b or H-2^k antigens.

In this study, backcross embryos were collected 96 hours post-hCG injection. At this time point about half of the embryos were morulae and half were blastocysts. In two separate experiments, the morulae and blastocysts were tested for the presence or absence of H-2 b and k antigens using monoclonal antibodies and an enzyme linked immunosorbent assay (ELISA) procedure which has been described previously (Goldbard et al., 1984). The results, shown in Figures 1 and 2, demonstrate linkage of the fast Ped allele to the b haplotype and the slow Ped allele to the k haplotype.

MAPPING THE PED GENE TO THE Q REGION OF THE H-2 COMPLEX

After linkage of the Ped gene to the H-2 complex was proven, we sought to locate the Ped gene within the H-2 complex. First, we examined four recombinant congenic strains on the B10 background with the results shown in Table 1. It was immediately obvious that the fast Ped allele mapped to the telomeric end of the H-2 complex. The report by Winoto et al. in 1983 that most MHC Class I genes were found in the Q/TL region of the H-2 complex prompted us to consider the possible location of the Ped gene in the Q/TL region. Table 2 shows the Class I MHC alleles and the Ped gene phenotype of all the strains we had examined on the B10 background. The only concordance between Ped gene phenotype and Class I alleles is for the Qa-2 antigen. All strains expressing the fast Ped allele are Qa-2^a whereas all strains expressing the slow Ped allele are Qa-2^b. Qa-2^a denotes the presence of the Qa-2 antigen and Qa-2^b denotes the absence of the Qa-2 antigen on adult cells.

Our next experiment was to test the Ped gene phenotype of congenic mice on the C57BL/6 background which we obtained from Dr. Lorraine Flaherty, New York State Department of Health, Albany, NY. These mice,

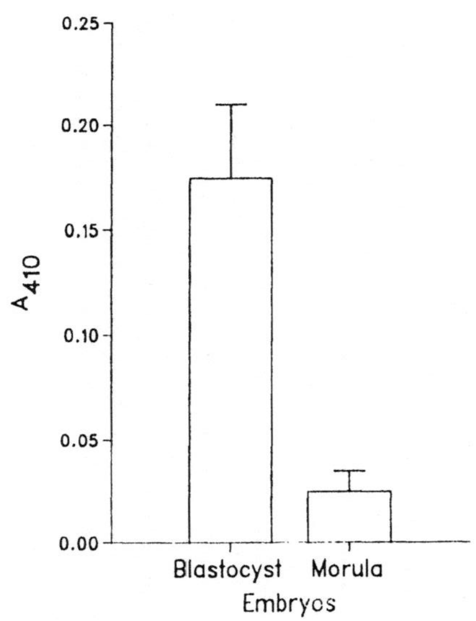

Figure 1. Detection of H-2^b antigens on backcross embryos. Embryos from a (B10 x B10.BR)F_1 x B10.BR backcross were collected 96 h post-hCG injection and separated into morulae and blastocysts. H-2^b antigens were assayed with an ELISA procedure. Data are from Warner et al. (1987b).

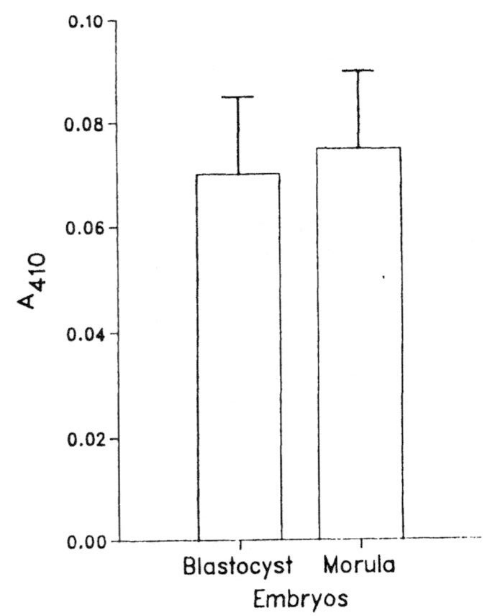

Figure 2. Detection of H-2^k antigens on backcross embryos. Embryos from a (B10 x B10.BR)F_1 x B10.BR backcross were collected 96 h post-hCG injection and separated into morulae and blastocysts. H-2^k antigens were assayed with an ELISA procedure. Data are from Warner et al. (1987b).

Table 1. Number of cells per embryo and *Ped* gene phenotype of B10 congenic mouse strains.[a]

Mouse Strain	H-2 haplotype	No. embryos scored	Mean cell no. per embryo (S.E.M.)	*Ped* gene phenotype
C57BL/10Sn	b	48	33.1 (2.1)	FAST
B10.D2	d	47	39.1 (1.5)	FAST
B10.BR	k	50	22.8 (1.3)[b]	SLOW
B10.III	r	46	25.4 (0.9)[b]	SLOW
B10.S	s	28	33.8 (2.4)	FAST
B10.Q	q	34	30.2 (1.3)	FAST
B10.PL	u	35	30.4 (1.7)	FAST
B10.A	a	65	32.0 (1.1)	FAST
B10.A(4R)	h4	35	30.7 (1.9)	FAST
B10.A(5R)	i5	36	31.1 (1.5)	FAST
B10.AM	h3	34	29.6 (1.7)	FAST

[a]Data from Goldbard and Warner (1982) and Warner (unpublished) for embryos collected 89 h post-hCG.
[b]Significantly lower than C57BL/10Sn ($P < 0.05$).

as shown in Table 3, differ at only the Qa-2 region of the H-2 complex. The results suggest that the *Ped* gene is located in the Qa-2 region of the H-2 complex. Testing of linkage of the *Ped* gene to the Qa-2 subregion of the H-2 complex, through the use of backcross mice, is currently underway in our laboratory.

EXPRESSION OF QA-2 ANTIGENS ON PREIMPLANTATION MOUSE EMBRYOS

The tentative mapping of the *Ped* gene to the Qa-2 region of the H-2 complex prompted us to examine expression of Qa-2 antigens on early mouse embyros. For these studies we used an IgM monoclonal antibody (D3.262) which was prepared in Dr. L. Flaherty's laboratory. We tested for the presence or absence of Qa-2 antigens on mouse blastocysts by using the ELISA procedure (Warner et al., 1987a). The results are shown in Figure 3. It is seen that there is complete concordance of Qa-2 antigen expression on embryos when compared to Qa-2 antigen expression by adult mice. Moreover, all embryos expressing the *fast Ped* gene phenotype expressed Qa-2 antigens whereas all embryos expressing the *slow Ped* gene phenotype showed the absence of detectable Qa-2 antigens.

These results suggest that cell division in embryos may be at least partly controlled by the presence or absence of a particular MHC antigen, namely the Qa-2 antigen. Goodenow et al. (1985) have suggested that the presence or absence of MHC antigens might affect the metastatic potential of cancer cells. Perhaps the principle of cell surface proteins controlling cell division applies to all cells, including embryos. The molecular mechanisms by which cell surface proteins influence the rate of cell division remain to be determined.

Table 2. Class I MHC alleles and Ped gene phenotype of B10 congenic mouse strains.

Mouse Strain	Class I MHC alleles					Ped gene phenotype
	K	D	Qa-2	Tla	Qa-1	
C57BL/10Sn (B10)	b	b	a	b	b	FAST
B10.D2	d	d	a	c	b	FAST
B10.BR	k	k	b	a	a	SLOW
B10.RIII	r	r	b	b	b	SLOW
B10.S	s	s	a	b	b	FAST
B10.Q	q	q	a	b	b	FAST
B10.PL	u	u	a	a	a	FAST
B10.A	k	d	a	b	b	FAST
B10.A(4R)	k	b	a	b	b	FAST
B10.A(5R)	b	d	a	a	a	FAST
B10.AM	k	b	a	b	b	FAST

Table 3. Number of cells per embryo and Ped gene phenotype of B6 congenic mouse strains.[a]

Mouse Strain	Class I MHC Alleles					Number embryos scored	Mean cell number per embryo (S.E.M.)	Ped gene phenotype
	K	D	Qa-2	Tla	Qa-1			
C57BL/6	b	b	a	b	b	56	29.6 (1.7)	FAST
B6.K1	b	b	b	b	b	33	20.4 (1.1)[b]	SLOW
B6.K2	b	b	a	b	b	78	31.0 (1.4)	FAST

[a]Data from Warner (1986) and Warner (unpublished) for embryos collected 89 h post-hCG.
[b]Significantly lower than C57BL/6 ($P < 0.05$).

BIOLOGICAL IMPORTANCE OF THE PED GENE

The discovery of the H-2 linked *Ped* gene suggests an important biological role for the MHC in development and reproduction. First of all, the presence of MHC antigens on early embryos presents an interesting immunological problem. Why aren't the allogeneic embryos rejected by the mother? There has been mounting evidence over the past few years that recognition of an allogeneic pregnancy may be beneficial for the survival of the fetus (reviewed in Toder and Beer, 1985; Lewis et al., 1986; Rodger and Drake, 1987). Still controversial are observations that recurrent spontaneous abortion is associated with homogeneity of certain human HLA types (Gill, 1983; Balasch et al., 1986; McIntyre and Faulk, 1986). Immunization with allogeneic lymphocytes often leads to a successful pregnancy where none was possible before (Beer et al., 1985).

Second, the idea that timing of early development is at least partly controlled by a gene linked to the MHC has some interesting biological implications. The embryo and the uterus must have coordinated timing so that the uterus is physiologically prepared for the embryo when it is ready to implant. In mice, embryos surgically transferred to a uterus too early in a pseudopregnancy will wait for the uterus to catch up before implanting, but embryos transplanted to a uterus too advanced in a pseudopregnancy will die (Rafferty, 1970). Likewise, human embryos fertilized *in vitro* must be reimplanted in the mother at exactly the correct time to achieve a successful pregnancy (Edwards et al., 1980; Steptoe et al., 1980). A small amount of data is beginning to accumulate

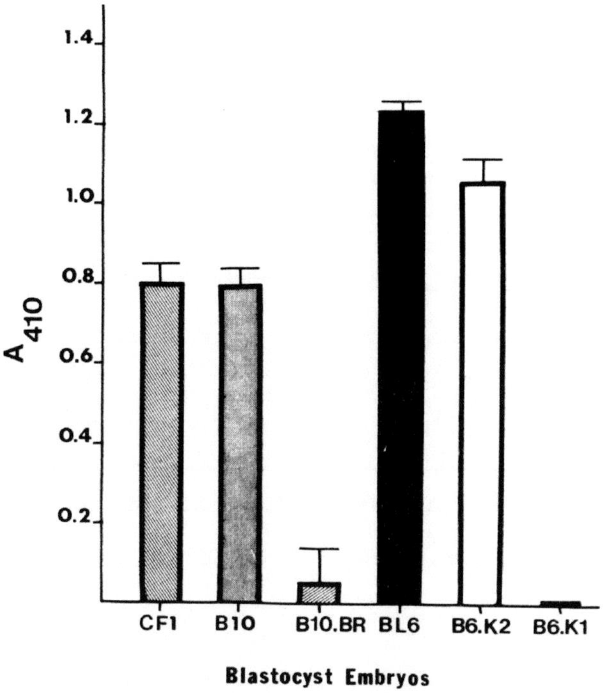

Figure 3. Detection of Qa-2 antigens on mouse blastocysts. Data, from an ELISA procedure, are from Warner et al. (1987a).

on preimplantation human embryos due to the establishment of many *in vitro* fertilization and embryo transfer clinics. One interesting recent observation on human embryos is that among embryos fertilized at the same time, some embryos had reached the blastoyst stage by day 5, whereas others were still morulae or in earlier cleavage stages (Buster et al., 1985). Moreover, there is evidence both in mice (C. Warner, unpublished), and in humans (Buster et al., 1985), that those embryos most advanced in their development are the ones most likely to survive after embryo transfer. Thus, it is appealing to speculate that there may be a *Ped* gene in humans as well as in mice, and that this gene and the MHC in general are important for the survival of preimplantation mammalian embryos.

REFERENCES

Balasch, J., Pastor, M., Martorell, J., Vanrell, J. A., Cuturi, C., Gonzalez-Merlo, J. (1986). Shared HLA antigens between parents and recurrent spontaneous abortion. *Int. J. Fert.* *31*, 213-217.

Beer, A. E., Quebbeman, J. F., Semprini, A. E., McGaw, T. G., and Jijon, A. (1985). Survival and rejection of the fetal allograft. *Contrib. Gynec. Obstet.* *14*, 114-130.

Buster, J. E., Busillo, M., Rodi, I. A., Cohen, S. W., Hamilton, M., Simon, J. A., Thorneycroft, I. H., and Marshall, S. R. (1985). Biologic and morphologic development of donated human ova recovered by nonsurgical uterine lavage. *Amer. J. Obs. Gyn.* *153*, 211-223.

Edwards, R. G., Steptoe, P. C., and Purdy, J. M. (1980). Establishing full-term human pregnancies using cleaving embryos grown *in vitro*. *Brit. J. Obs. and Gyn.* *87*, 737-757.

Gill, T. J. III (1983). Immunogenetics of spontaneous abortions in humans. *Transplantation* *35*, 1-6.

Goldbard, S. B., Gollnick, S. O., and Warner, C. M. (1984). A highly sensitive method for the detection of cell surface antigens on preimplantation mouse embryos. *J. Immunol. Methods* *68*, 137-146.

Goldbard, S. B., Verbanac, K. M., and Warner, C. M. (1982a). Role of the H-2 complex in preimplantation mouse embryo development. *Biol. Reprod.* *26*, 591-596.

Goldbard, S. B., Verbanac, K. M., and Warner, C. M. (1982b). Genetic analysis of *H-2* linked gene(s) affecting early mouse embryo development. *J. Immunogenetics* *9*, 77-82.

Goldbard, S. B. and Warner, C. M. (1982). Genes affect the timing of early mouse embryo development. *Biol. Reprod.* *27*, 419-424.

Goodenow, R. S., Vogel, S. M., and Linsk, R. L. (1985). Histocompatibility antigens on murine tumors. *Science* *30*, 777-783.

Klein, J. (1986). "Natural History of the Major Histocompatibility Complex," John Wiley & Sons, New York, p. 286.

Lewis, J. E., Doulam, C. B., and Moore, S. B. (1986). Immunologic mechanisms in the maternal-fetal relationship. *Mayo Clin. Proc.* *61*, 655-665.

McIntyre, J. A. and Faulk, W. P. (1986). Clinical value of research in chronic spontaneous abortion. *Amer. J. Reprod. Immunol. and Microbiology* *10*, 121-126.

Rafferty, K. A. (1970). "Methods in Experimental Embryology of the Mouse," The Johns Hopkins Press, Baltimore, 94 pps.

Rodger, J. C. and Drake, B. L. (1987). The enigma of the fetal graft. *Amer. Scientist* *75*, 51-57.

Steptoe, P. C., Edwards, R. G., and Purdy, J. M. (1980). Clinical aspects of pregnancies established with cleaving embryos grown *in vitro*. *Brit. J. Obs. and Gyn.* *87*, 757-768.

Tarkowski, A. K. (1966). An air-drying method for chromosome preparations from mouse eggs. *Cytogenetics* *5*, 394-400.

Toder, V. and Beer, A. E. (eds.)(1985). "Immunopathology of Reproduction," Karger, Basel, 212 pps.

Warner, C. M. (1986). Genetic manipulation of the major histocompatibility complex. J. Anim. Sci. 63, 279-287.

Warner, C. M., Gollnick, S. O., Flaherty, L., and Goldbard, S. B. (1987a). Analysis of Qa-2 antigen expression by preimplantation mouse embryos: Possible relationship to the Ped gene product. Biol. Reprod. 36, 611-616.

Warner, C. M., Gollnick, S. O., and Goldbard, S. B. (1987b). Linkage of the Ped gene to the mouse major histocompatibility complex (MHC). Biol. Reprod. 36, 606-610.

Winoto, A. M., Steinmetz, M., and Hood, L. (1983). Genetic mapping in the major histocompatibility complex by restriction enzyme site polymorphisms: most mouse class I genes map to the Tla complex. Proc. Natl. Acad. Sci. USA 80, 3425-3429.

ASSOCIATIONS BETWEEN CLASS I MHC ANTIGENS AND VIRAL GLYCOPROTEINS DETECTED BY FLUORESCENCE RESONANCE ENERGY TRANSFER

Jerome H. Hochman and Michael Edidin

Department of Biology
The Johns Hopkins University
Charles and 34th Streets
Baltimore, MD 21218

Cytotoxic T lymphocytes, CTL, recognize viral antigens of infected cells in the context of the cells' class I MHC antigens (Zinkernagel and Doherty, 1979). The basis of this MHC restriction is not defined. The weight of the evidence favors recognition of some complex of all or part of viral antigen with the class I antigen. The route of formation of this complex and its stability are still unclear. In some instances, influenza virus infection (Townsend et al., 1984; Yewdell et al., 1985) and SV40 transformation (Gooding and O'Connell, 1983) it is evident that the CTL are primarily directed against internal viral proteins, the nucleocapsid protein of the influenza virus or the T antigen of SV40. This, together with the demonstration that peptides derived from these proteins (Townsend, et al., 1986) can sensitise target cells, strongly implies that these antigens are partly digested, and associated with class I MHC antigens before appearing at the cell surface. Such a mechanism of association parallels that mechanism for the formation of nominal antigen/class II MHC antigen complexes for presentation to helper T cells (Buus et al., 1987; Unanue and Allen, 1987) and unifies our view of antigen presentation to T cells. However, the generality of this scheme is still not clear. Some virus antigens, even the influenza virus nucleocapsid, can be presented to cells under conditions in which processing is blocked (Wraith and Vessey, 1986), suggesting that they associate with class I antigens without internalization and processing.

Whatever the mechansim, it would be useful to demonstrate directly the association of viral antigens with class I MHC antigens in the membrane of intact cells. Previous attempts to do so in terms of co-capping or cross-linking have yielded equivocal results (summarized in Klein, 1986). The resolution of viral antigen/MHC antigen complex is poor with these techniques and they greatly perturb the cell surface. In order to overcome these difficulties we have turned to a purely physical technique for detecting the proximity of two molecules, fluorescence resonance energy transfer. The technique depends upon the fact that energy may be transfered from an excited state fluorophore, the donor, to a neighboring, acceptor, fluorophore by a non-radiative resonance process (Lakowicz, 1983). Energy transfer is detected both in terms of increased fluorescence, sensitized emission, of the fluorescent acceptor and in terms of decreased fluorescence, quenching, of the fluorescent donor. The expression for sensitized fluorescence, k_T due to energy transfer between a pair of fluorophores, donor and acceptor, is:

Equation 1

$$k_T = [r^{-6}J(\kappa)^2 \lambda_d] \times 8.71 \times 10^{23} sec^{-1}$$

For a given donor/acceptor pair all the terms of the equation are constant, except for r, the intermolecular distance. Since k_T is a function of r^{-6}, fluorescence due to energy transfer falls off rapidly with increasing intermolecular distance (Stryer, 1987). Practically, this means that the donor and acceptor fluorophore must be within 80 A of one-another if transfer is to occur at all. This is the distance scale of protein/protein interactions and hence appropriate to the study of associations between viral antigens and class I MHC antigens.

Here we present our initial results on energy transfer between class I MHC antigens and Sendai virus Hemagglutinin/neuraminidase and fusion glycoproteins. The principal CTL response to Sendai virus is against these membrane glycoproteins, rather than against internal viral proteins (Al-Ahldal et al., 1985). This response can be triggered with fusigenic, non-infectious Sendai virus or Sendai virus envelopes; active infection is not necessary for CTL killing of sensitized target cells. On the other hand, target cells must be sensitized to Sendai-specific CTL by fusion of the virus to the target membrane, rather than by coating with non-fusigenic virus (which is never-the-less internalized) (Sugamura et al., 1977). Killing of newly sensitized targets is not inhibited by inhibitors of internalization and antigen processing (J. Forman, personal communication). Thus, it seems likely that the target structure recognized by anti-Sendai CTL is a complex of intact viral glycoproteins with class I MHC antigens.

Energy transfer is detected both in terms of increased fluorescence, sensitized emission, of the fluorescent acceptor and in terms of decreased fluorescence, quenching, of fluorescent donor. We labeled the class I MHC antigens of living cells with fluorescent donor, a fluorescein derivative of their endogenous light chain, beta-2-microglobulin, b-2m. This derivative, subsituted with 1 fluorescein molecule per b-2m, can be exchanged for endogenous b-2m (Hochman and Edidin, 1987). The Sendai virus glycoproteins were labeled with the fluorescent acceptor, a sulforhodamine, Texas Red (Titus et al., 1982). Preparation of the labeled viral glycoproteins and their constitution into viral envelopes, TRSVE, (Vainstein et al., 1984) is diagrammed in Figure 1.

Class I MHC antigens of mouse fibroblasts are labeled by overnight incubation with micromolar Fl-b-2m in serum-free medium. The half-time for exchange of endogenous beta-2-m with the labeled b-2m is approximately 3 hours, with equilbrium reached at 10 hours (Hochman and Edidin, 1987). TRSVE are added to cells in suspension either as intact envelopes or after brief treatment with trypsin, which damages the fusion protein (Sugamura et al., 1977). 1) cell plus intact evelopes incubated at 37°C, 2) cells plus intact envelopes incubated at 4°C, 3) cells plus trypsin-treated envelopes incubated at 37°C. Only the first treatment results in fusion of TRSVE with the target cell surface and integration of the viral glycoproteins into the membrane bilayer. Other controls include cells labeled withe Fl-b-2m and unlabeled viral envelopes, cells labeled only with TRSVE, and unlabeled cells.

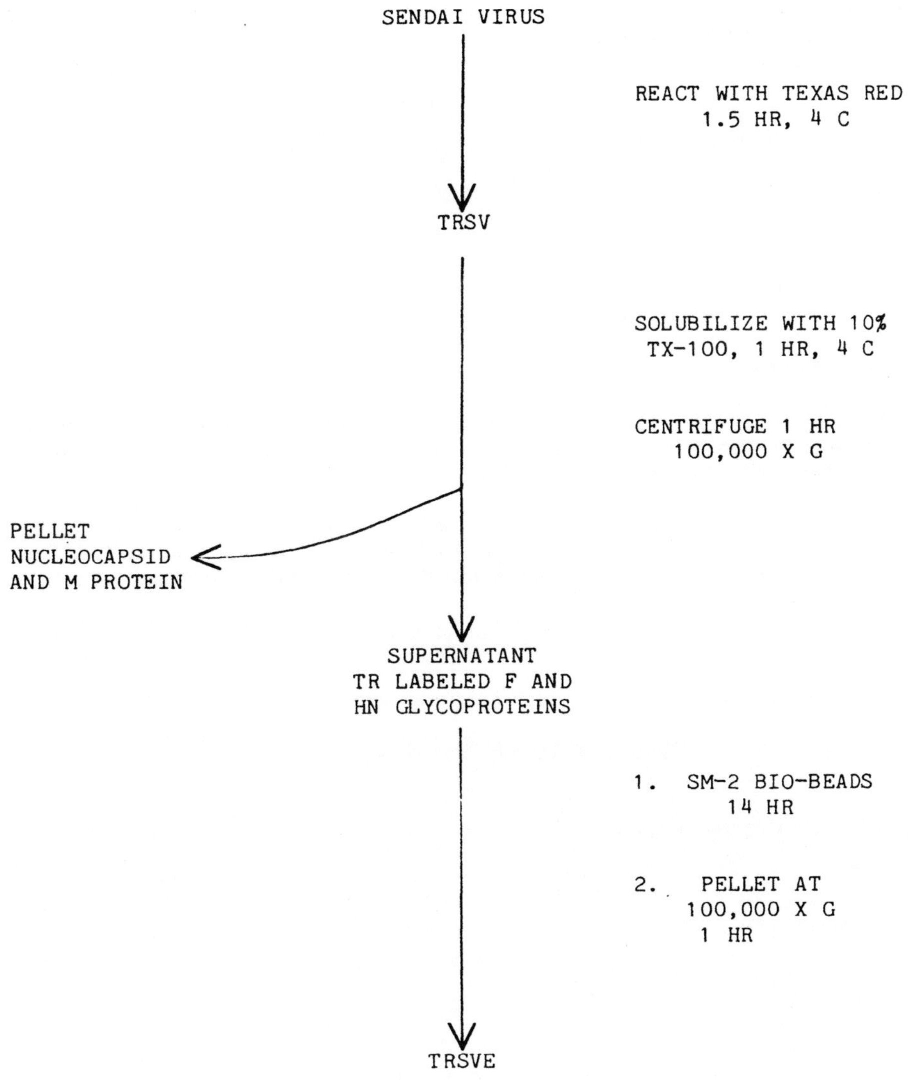

Figure 1

Preparation of Labeled Sendai Virus Envelopes

Measurement of fluorescence from labeled cell populations is quite difficult in conventional spectrofluorimeters due to light scattering from the cells. Hence we measured cell fluorescence in an EPICS 752 flow cytometer (Coulter Instruments). The signal/noise is greatly improved in this way at the cost of lost spectral resolution. We excited Fl-b-2m with the 488nm line of an argon laser, which does not significantly excite TRSVE, and excited TRSVE with the 600nm emission from a rhodamine 6G dye laser. The pattern of fluorescence expected from control cells, from cells labeled with only one label, and from double-labeled cells in which energy transfer occurs is shown in Table 1.

Table 1

Fluorescence expected exciting with 488nm, blue, light

Cell Label	Fluorescein Fluorescence	Texas Red Fluorescence
Fl-beta-2m	++++	-
TRSVE	-	-
Fl-beta-2m + TRSVE	++	++

Note that when exciting with 488nm light only double-labeled cells in which energy transfer takes place significant TRSVE (red) fluorescence, and that fluorescein (green) fluorescence of these cells will be reduced.

In over twenty experiments we found that this was indeed the case when $H\text{-}2^b$ fibroblasts, TIB 88 (American Type Culture Collection) were labeled. The quenching of fluorescein fluorescence in a typical experiment is summarized in Table 2.

Table 2

Quenching of Fluorescence of Fl-b-2m by Texas Red-

Labeled Sendai Virus Proteins

Sendai Virus Envelopes Added	% Quenching
None	0
Texas Red/50µl	14
Texas Red/25µl	5
Texas Red/10µl	1

This quenching was specific to the extent that another fluorescein-labeled membrane protein-Fl-ribonuclease, tailed with palmitic acid to secure its integration into the bilayer (Ho, Hochman, and Edidin, in preparation), is not quenched by the added TRSVE. Trypsin-treated TRSVE or TRSVE added to cells at 4°C also failed to quench fluorescein fluorescence. Thus it appeared that only fusion of the envelope glycoporteins resulted in their proximity to MHC antigens, and that this proximity was specific to the extent that the fluorescence of another membrane-integrated protein, presented at about the same level as the class I MHC was not quenched by TRSVE.

Quenching of donor fluorescence may occur due to other processes than energy transfer. However, enhanced emission of the fluorescent acceptor is certainly due to energy transfer, if concentrations of acceptor are kept constant. Since this constancy was hard to maintain, we normalized our results in terms of the amount of acceptor fluorescence emitted when cells were illuminated by 488nm light (strong excitation of the fluorescent donor, little or no weak excitation of the fluorescent acceptor) versus acceptor fluorescence emitted when cells were illuminated withd 600nm light (no excitation of the fluorescent donor, direct excitation of the fluorescent acceptor). Representative normalized results are presented in Table 3, for H-2^b TIB 88 fibroblasts and for the H-2^k c1ld fibroblasts.

Table 3

Sensitized emission of Texas Red-Labeled Sendai Virus Proteins

Sample Peak Channel - Blank Peak Channel

Sample	Red Emission Excite 488nm	Red Emission Excite 600nm	Red ex 488/ Red ex 600
TIB88			
F1-b2-m + TRSVE	19	22	.86
B2-m + TRSVE	6	36	.17
c11d			
F1-b2-m + TRSVE	13	21	.62
b2-m + TRSVE	13	25	.52

Note that the ratio of red fluorescence intensities excited by 488/600 nm light is 5-fold higher for H-2^b cells bearing both donor and acceptor than for H-2^b cells bearing only acceptor. In contrast, there is no difference in this ratio between double-labeled and single-labeled H-2^k cells. The large value of the ratio for b2-m + TRSVE c11d, 0.52, versus that for TIB 88, 0.17, is not significant and reflects varying levels of overall labeling and of laser power in the two experiments. Again, there was no sensitized acceptor emission if cells were treated with trypsinized TRSVE, or were never brought to 37° to induce virus fusion.

The combined results of donor, fluorescein, fluorescence quenching and enhanced, Texas Red, acceptor fluorescence strongly indicate the proximity of Sendai virus glycoproteins and class I MHC antigens on doubly-labeled cells. Uncertainties about the location of the acceptor prevent us from quantitating the association, either in terms of average proximity or in terms of fraction of all viral antigens associated with class I MHC antigens. However the data make it clear that a subsstantial fraction of viral antigen molecules, 10% or more, are within 10's of A of class I MHC antigens.

The specificity of our results is indicated 1) by the failure of TRSVE antigens to quench fluorescence of a biologically irrelevant membrane protein, F1-palmitoylribonuclease, 2) by the absence of energy transfer if TRSVE are merely adherent, rather than fused, to the cell surface, and 3) by the failure to detect energy transfer in any experiment using H-2^k fibroblasts. Though primary responses to Sendai virus plus H-2^k have been described (Zinkernagel et. al., 1978), Shapiro and co workers (Shapiro et al., 1981) found that H-2^K mice were defective in secondary responses to Sendai antigens. Perhaps this failure was due to defective association of viral and class I MHC antigens in the cell membranes. The idea that failure to associate viral and class I MHC antigens may be further tested by measuring associations between mutants H-$2K^b$ antigens, some of which do and other of which do not provide a context for responses to Sendai virus antigens (De Waal et al., 1983).

Though our experiments involve a viral antigen that may not be processed before association with class I antigen, it ought to be possible to apply the techniques used here to labeled peptides, for example from influenza virus nucleoprotein (Townsend et al., 1986). These peptides may bind to intact cells with low overall specificity but their specific associations with class I MHC antigens ought to be detectable in terms of sensitized emission of fluorescence. This approach will provide further data on the physical associations between viral antigens and class I MHC antiges. It may also be useful in elucidating the structural features of these antigens which are important in forming these associations.

Acknowledgements

We thank Mrs. Taiyin Wei for skilled flow cytometry. J.H.H. is a fellow of the Damon Runyon/Walter Winchell Cancer Society. This work was supported by a grant, AI-14584, from the National Institutes of Health. It is contribution 1370 from the Department of Biology.

References

Al-Ahldal, M.N., I. NaKamura and T.D. Flanagan. 1985. J. Virol., 54:53-57.

Buus, S., A. Sette, S. M. Colon, C. Miles, H. M. Grey. 1987. Science 235:1353-1358.

De Waal, L. P., W. M. Kast, R. W. Melvold and C. J. M. Melief. 1983. J. Immunol. 130:1090-1096.

Gooding, L. R. and K. A. O'Connell. 1983. J. Immunol. 131:2580.

Hochman, J. H. and M. Edidin. 1987. J. Immunol. in the press.

Klein, J. 1986. "Natural History of the Major Histocompatibility Complex". John Wiley and Sons, New York, pp. 455-461.

Kurrle, R., M. Rollinghoff and H. Wagner. 1978. Eur. J. Immunol. 8:910-912.

Lakowicz, J. R. 1983. "Principles of Fluorescence Spectroscopy". Plenum Press, New York and London, ch. 10.

Shapiro, M. W., S. J. Burakoff, B. Benacerraf and R. W. Finberg. 1981. J. Immunol. 127:2571-2574.

Stryer, L.. 1978. Ann. Rev. Biochem. 47:819-846.

Sugamura, K., K. Shimizu, D. A. Zarling and F. H. Bach. 1977. Nature 270:251-253.

Titus, J. A., R. Haugland, S. O. Sharrow and D. M. Segal. 1982. J. Immunol. Methods 50:193-.

Townsend, A. R. M., A. J. McMichael, H. P. Carter, J. A. Huddleston, and G. G. Brownlee. 1984. Cell 39:13-25.

Townsend, A. R. M., J. Rothbard, F. M. Gotch, G. Bahdur, D. Wraith and A. J. McMichael. 1986. Cell 44:951-968.

Unanue, E. R. and P. M. Allen. 1987. Science 236:551-557.

Vainstein, A., M. Hershkovitz, S. Israel, S. Rabin and A. Loyter. 1984. Biochim Biophys. Acta 773:181-188.

Wraith, D. C., and A. E. Vessey. 1986. Immunology 59:173-180.

Yewdell, J. W., J. R. Bennink, G. L. Smith and B. Moss. 1985. Proc. Natl. Acad. Sci. USA 82:1785-1789.

Zinkernagel, R. and P. Doherty. 1979. Adv. Immunol., 27:51-177.

Zinkernagel, R., A. Althage, S. Cooper, G. Kreeb, P. A. Klein, B. Sefton, L. Flaherty, J. Stimpfling, D. Shreffler and J. Klein. 1978. J. Exp. Med. 148:592-606.

MIXED BONE MARROW CHIMERAS AS AN APPROACH TO TRANSPLANTATION TOLERANCE

Megan Sykes, Caroline H. Chester, and David H. Sachs

Transplantation Biology Section
Immunology Branch, DCBD
National Cancer Institute
Bethesda, Maryland 20892

INTRODUCTION

Transplantation tolerance across a complete MHC barrier can be achieved in mice using lethal irradiation followed by reconstitution with a mixture of T-cell-depleted (TCD) syngeneic and allogeneic bone marrow cells.[1,2] Such animals repopulate as stable mixed lymphohematopoietic chimeras, and enjoy improved survival compared with recipients of allogeneic TCD marrow alone,[3] probably due, in part, to the improved immunocompetence they demonstrate.[3] In addition, such animals are free from any clinical sign of graft-versus-host disease (GVHD), and this is also the case even if T-cells are not removed from the allogeneic marrow.[4] Experiments in which allogeneic spleen cells were added to the donor inoculum to intentionally produce GVHD indicated that the syngeneic TCD component of the bone marrow inoculum improved the survival of such animals, presumably due to protection from GVHD.[4] The data presented in this paper address the possible mechanism of this protective effect. We show that the syngeneic marrow inoculum provides a source of precursor cells which, in recipient spleens, develop the ability to suppress the generation of cytolytic activity by mature T-lymphocytes. We also demonstrate an enhanced protection from GVHD when the syngeneic TCD inoculum is allowed to develop its suppressive activity spontaneously in the recipient before the allogeneic inoculum is given. Such protection could have potential clinical applications.

RESULTS AND DISCUSSION

Several forms of suppression of alloresponses have been described in various animal models, including specific suppression of responses against donor or host antigen,[5-8] veto cells, which suppress anti-self responses,[9-11] and non-specific suppression.[12-17] In order to distinguish among these possibilities, we studied the ability of splenocytes from mixed allogeneic chimeras to suppress a panel of six different alloresponses in a CML coculture system. The results obtained from mixed allogeneic chimeras in the early weeks after BMT are summarized in Fig. 1 and the data will be presented in detail elsewhere (manuscript in preparation). The data obtained

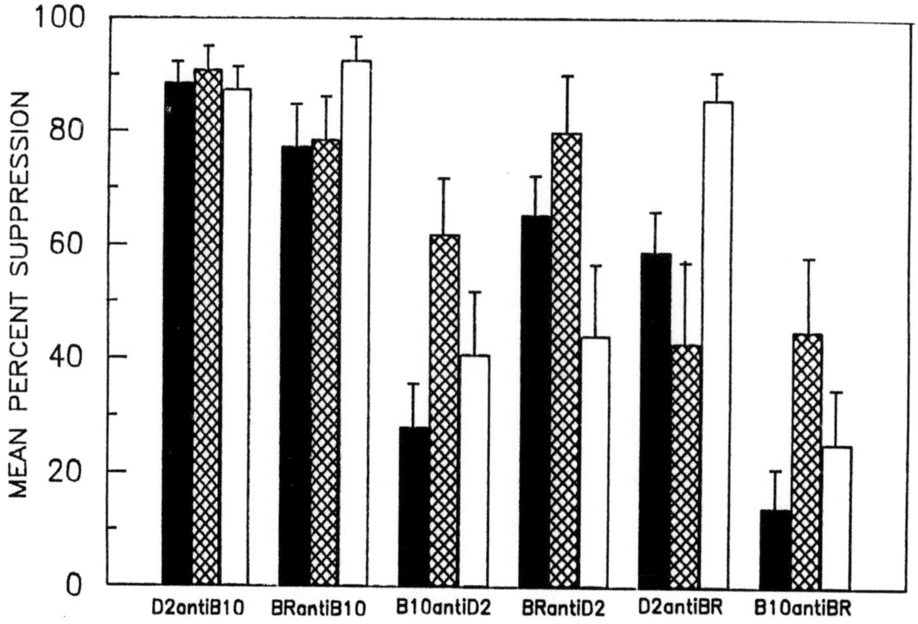

Fig. 1 Summary of experiments examining ability of splenocytes from bone marrow transplant (BMT) recipients 8 to 22 days after BMT to suppress six different CML responses: (solid bars) suppression by splenocytes from B10+B10.D2 -->B10 chimeras, n=18-27; (hatched bars) suppression by splenocytes from B10+B10.D2-->B10.D2 chimeras, n=19-11; (open bars) suppression by splenocytes from B10-->B10 syngeneic BMT recipients, n=7-15. (Variation in "n" values due to the fact that not all responses were examined in every experiment, depending on response tested.) "BR"=B10.BR; "D2"=B10.D2. Error bars indicate standard error of the mean.

from B10 recipients indicated predominant suppression of responses directed against host (in this case C57BL/10, $H-2^b$) antigen, suggesting that suppression might be mediated by veto cells syngeneic to the recipient. However, when similar studies were performed using B10.D2 ($H-2^d$) recipients, the pattern of suppression was not dramatically different from that observed for B10 recipients (Figure 1, hatched bars). Additional experiments indicated that suppression of all responses in both recipient strains was mediated exclusively by cells which were syngeneic to the recipient. Therefore, suppression of the B10.D2αB10 responses in B10.D2 recipients was mediated by $H-2^d$-bearing cells (data not shown), which could not, by definition, be due to veto activity. Thus, the observed patterns of suppression are most readily interpreted as antigen non-specific, although some responses, such as the B10.D2αB10 response, appeared to be more suppressible than others.

The observed suppression did not appear to result from subclinical GVHD, as evidenced by the fact that recipients of TCD syngeneic marrow alone, rather than mixed marrow inocula, exhibited an identical pattern and frequency of suppression (data not shown) as did recipients given mixed marrow inocula.

Phenotypic analysis of the suppressor cells in spleens of early chimeras indicated that they were "null" cells, i.e. they were non-T cells, non-B cells, and non-macrophages, as indicated by the inability to remove suppression using anti-theta serum, anti-Ia monoclonal antibody, and passage over Sephadex-G10 columns (Table 1). Furthermore, treatment with anti-asialo GM_1,

Table 1. Effects of Selective Depletions on Suppression

Chimera	Treatment of cells	% Suppression of Response[1]				
		D2αB10	BRαB10	B10αD2	BRαD2	D2αBR
Mix-->B10[2]	C'	85	88	0	>94	ND[3]
	RAMB/C'	85	88	0	>94	ND
Mix-->B10	C'	>94	>94	50	ND	>94
	$\alpha ASGM_1$/C'[4]	88	>94	32	ND	85
B10-->B10	C'	>94	>94	70	67	84
	αIa[5]	>94	>94	71	95	81
Mix-->B10	No treatment	50	ND	ND	ND	ND
	G10 passage[6]	70	ND	ND	ND	ND

[1]Percent suppression as determined by comparing lytic units in cultures to which chimeric spleen cells were added with lytic units in control cultures.
[2]Mixed allogeneic chimeras {(B10+D2)(-T)-->B10} 12 and 14 days after BMT.
[3]Not done.
[4]Splenocytes from chimeras were treated with anti-asialo GM_1 and rabbit complement.
[5]Splenocytes from BMT recipients were treated with Y3P (anti-Ia^b) and rabbit complement. This treatment was found, using an indirect staining technique and FACS analysis, to remove 93% of Ia-positive cells.
[6]Passage through Sephadex G10 column. Depletion of adherent cells was confirmed by demonstrating loss of APC function of G10-passed cell populations.

while sufficient to remove lymphokine activated killer (LAK) cell precursors, did not remove suppressive activity (Table 1). Thus, the suppressor cells did not resemble classical natural killer (NK) or LAK cells. Overall, the non-specificity of suppression of alloresponses, as well as the "null" cell phenotype of these suppressor cells, suggest that they may be similar to the natural suppressor cells described in several other models.[14-17]

The observations that the cells responsible for suppression in early mixed allogeneic chimeras are exclusively of recipient phenotype, and that syngeneic marrow confers protection from a GVHD-inducing inoculum,[4] are consistent with the possibility that cells derived from syngeneic bone marrow protect recipients from the activity of allogeneic GVHD-inducing T-lymphocytes. We have developed an additional model based on the suppressor phenomenon which was designed to optimize the anti-GVH effects of such suppressor cells within the recipient prior to exposure to allogeneic T-cells. In this model, lethally irradiated mice were reconstituted with TCD syngeneic marrow, and eight days later, allogeneic marrow was administered intravenously (Table 2). Such animals reconstituted as fully allogeneic chimeras,[18] similar to mice given non-TCD allogeneic marrow and

Table 2. Delayed Allo Protocol

{B10(TCD)+B10.D2-->B10}

Group	Day -8	Day 0	Median Survival Time (day)
No Delay		Irradiation B10(TCD)+B10.D2	12
8-Day Delay	Irradiation B10(TCD)	B10.D2	47

syngeneic marrow simultaneously. Since potent suppressive activity is present in whole body irradiated (WBI) syngeneic BMT recipients by 8 days after BMT, an attempt was made to determine whether such suppression might confer increased protection from a GVHD-inducing inoculum compared with animals given the same allogeneic inoculum on the day of irradiation and syngeneic BMT. Animals were irradiated and reconstituted with $5x10^6$ syngeneic TCD bone marrow cells and 8 days later $15x10^6$ allogeneic spleen cells plus $15x10^6$ allogeneic bone marrow cells were administered. Survival of these animals was compared to that of control mice which received irradiation and syngeneic BMT on the same day as the allogeneic inoculum. As reported in detail elsewhere,[18] the 8-day delay led to marked protection from the lethal effects of the GVHD-inducing inoculum. In a subsequent experiment, we followed white blood cell counts as an indicator of hematopoietic recovery, and found that WBC counts were equivalent in the two groups by 8 days after allogeneic BMT.[18] Thus, the 8-day delay in administration of the allogeneic inoculum probably led to improved survival by protecting the animals from GVHD, rather than by a mechanism related to earlier hematopoietic recovery. This is consistent with the possibility that allowing suppressive activity to develop in the spleens of such recipients before exposure to the GVHD-inducing inoculum may have resulted in the observed protection. Regardless of the mechanism of protection, this approach may provide a means of protecting BMT recipients from the GVHD associated with allogeneic marrow administration without necessitating the depletion of T-cells from the inoculum. This would be desirable in clinical situations, since there is increasing evidence that allogeneic T-cells have a beneficial effect on alloengraftment.[19,20]

SUMMARY

Null cells with the ability to non-specifically suppress CML responses have been found in the spleens of lethally irradiated mice reconstituted with mixed syngeneic and allogeneic marrow or syngeneic marrow alone. The finding that only cells syngeneic to recipients developed this activity when mixed marrow inocula were given, suggests that such suppressor cells, derived from syngeneic marrow, may be responsible for the protection from GVHD previously observed when syngeneic marrow was added to an allogeneic spleen cell/marrow inoculum. Consistent with this hypothesis is the observation that a delay of 8 days after syngeneic BMT, which allows sufficient time for suppressor activity to develop, results in increased protection from GVHD compared with syngeneic marrow given simultaneously with the allogeneic inoculum. These results suggest that allogeneic T-cells, possibly helpful for attaining alloengraftment, can be administered as part of a BMT inoculum if autologous TCD marrow is also given in order to protect from GVHD.

REFERENCES

1. A. Singer, K. S. Hathcock, and R. J. Hodes, Self recognition in allogeneic radiation bone marrow chimeras: A radiation-resistant host element dictates the self specificity and immune response gene phenotype, J. Exp. Med. 153:1286 (1981).
2. S. T. Ilstad, and D. H. Sachs, Reconstitution with syngeneic plus allogeneic or xenogeneic bone marrow leads to specific acceptance of allografts or xenografts, Nature (Lond.) 307:168 (1984).
3. S. T. Ildstad, S. M. Wren, S. A. Barbieri, and D. H. Sachs, Characterization of mixed allogeneic chimeras: Immunocompetence, in vitro reactivity, and genetic specificity of tolerance, J. Exp. Med. 162:231 (1985).
4. S. T. Ildstad, S. M. Wren, J. A. Bluestone, S. A. Barbieri, D. Stephany, and D. H. Sachs, Effect of selective depletion of host and/or donor bone marrow on lymphopoietic repopulation, tolerance, and graft-vs-host disease in mixed allogeneic chimeras (B10+B10.D2-->B10), J. Immunol. 136:28 (1986).
5. P. J. Tutschka, P. F. Ki, W. E. Beschorner, A. D. Hess, and G. W. Santos, Suppressor cells in transplantation tolerance. 2. Maturation of suppressor cells in the bone marrow chimera, Transplantation (Baltimore) 32:321 (1981).
6. M. L. Wood, and A. P. Monaco, Suppressor cells in specific unresponsiveness to skin allografts in ALS-treated, marrow-injected mice. Transplantation 29:196 (1980).
7. T. Maki, R. Gottschalk, M. L. Wood, and A. P. Monaco, Specific unresponsiveness to skin allografts in antilymphocyte serum-treated, marrow-injected mice: Participation of donor marrow-derived T cells, J. Immunol. 127:1433, (1981).
8. S. Dorsch, and B. Roser, Suppressor cells in transplantation tolerance. 2. Identification and probable mode of action of chimeric suppressor cells. Transplantation 33:525 (1982).
9. R. G. Miller, An immunological suppresor cell inactivating cytotoxic T-lymphocyte precursor cells recognizing it, Nature (Lond.) 287:544 (1980).
10. S. Muraoka, and R. G. Miller, Cells in bone marrow and in T cell colonies grown from bone marrow can suppress generation of cytotoxic T lymphocytes directed against their self antigens, J. Exp. Med. 152:54 (1980).
11. S. Muraoka, and R. G. Miller, Cells in murine fetal liver and in lymphoid colonies grown from fetal liver can suppress generation of cytotoxic T lymphocytes directed against their self antigens, J. Immunol. 131:45 (1983).

12. D. P. King, S. Strober, and H. S. Kaplan, Suppression of the mixed lymphocyte response and of graft-vs-host disease by spleen cells following total lymphoid irradiation (TLI), J. Immunol. 126:1140 (1981).

13. S. Okada, and S. Strober, Spleen cells from adult mice given total lymphoid irradiation or from newborn mice have similar regulatory effects in the mixed lymphocyte reaction. 1. Generation of antigen-specific suppressor cells in the mixed lymphocyte reaction after the addition of spleen cells from adult mice given total lymphoid irradiation, J. Exp. Med. 156:522 (1982).

14. M. Weigensberg, S. Morecki, L. Weiss, Z. Fuks, and S. Slavin, Suppression of cell-mediated immune responses after total lymphoid irradiation (TLI). 1. Characterization of suppressor cells of the mixed lymphocyte reaction, J. Immunol. 132:971 (1984).

15. A. Oseroff, S. Okada, and S. Strober, Natural suppressor (NS) cells found in the spleen of neonatal mice and adult mice given total lymphoid irradiation (TLI) express the null surface phenotype. J. Immunol. 132:101 (1984).

16. T. Maier, J. H. Holda, and H. N. Claman, Graft-vs-host reactions (GVHR) across minor murine histocompatibility barriers. 2. Development of natural suppressor cell activity, J. Immunol. 135:1644 (1985).

17. K. Dorshkind, and C. Rosse, Physical, biologic and phenotypic properties of natural regulatory cells in murine bone marrow, Am. J. Anatomy 164:1 (1982).

18. M. Sykes, C. H. Chester, and D. H. Sachs, submitted for publication.

19. P. J. Martin, J. A. Hansen, C. D. Buckner, J. E. Sanders, H. J. Deeg, P. Stewart, F. R. Appelbaum, R. Clift, A. Fefer, R. P. Witherspoon, M. S. Kennedy, K. M. Sullivan, N. Flournoy, R. Storb, and E. D. Thomas, Effects of in vitro depletion of T cells in HLA-identical allogeneic marrow grafts, Blood 66:664 (1985).

20. C. C. B. Soderling, C. W. Song, B. R. Blazar, and D. A. Vallera, A correlation between conditioning and engraftment in MHC-mismatched T cell-depleted murine bone marrow transplants, J. Immunol. 135:941 (1985).

ROLE OF H-2 ANTIGEN INDUCTION IN THE REJECTION OF THYROID AND PANCREATIC ISLET ALLOGRAFTS

Francisco G. La Rosa and David W. Talmage

Department of Microbiology and Immunology, School of Medicine and
Webb-Waring Lung Institute
University of Colorado Health Science Center
Denver, Colorado 80262

ABSTRACT

Three basic observations on the rejection of mouse endocrine allografts are used to support a model of graft rejection in which the induction of the expression of H-2 major histocompatibility complex (MHC) antigens is required. First, we found a close spatial relationship between the foci of T cell infiltration and the areas of the graft expressing allo-MHC antigens during rejection. Second, cultured endocrine allografts disparate from the recipient in MHC antigens were rejected only when they were associated with inflamatory processes mediated by minor histocompatibility antigens. And third, immunization of B6 mice to bml antigens was required for the rejection of uncultured bml thyroids, but this immunization had no effect on cultured bml grafts.

INTRODUCTION

Since the discovery of the H-2 locus in 1936 by Gorer, considerable information has been obtained about the organization and structure of the genes and molecules of this complex system. Simultaneously, there have been several demonstrations of a relationship between this MHC locus and the overall function of the immune system. Most importantly, there is an evident association of particular MHC alleles with specific immune-related diseases. However, the real function of the MHC in mice (H-2) and humans (HLA) is just beginning to be understood (refer to other articles in this publication).

There is considerable evidence that quantitative and qualitative changes in MHC antigen expression play a major role in many different immunological events such as the immune response to viruses, autoimmunity, tumor immunity, and allograft rejection (Harris and Gill, 1986). It seems that a very complex but unique mechanism is common to all these events. The difference in their manifestation may be based on the different antigenic stimuli that activate such a response. The expression of MHC antigens in all these instances could be related to the same molecular processes at the level of cell to cell interaction.

MATERIAL AND METHODS

Mice

The B6.C-H-2^d, BALB/c(H-2^d), C57Bl/6(H-2^b), C57Bl/10(H-2^b), BALB.B(H-2^b), C3H.SW(H-2^b), C3H(H-2^k), B10.BR(H-2^k), B6.C-H-2^{bml}, and (B10.BRxC3H.SW)F1 mice used in these experiments were all bred at the Webb-Waring Lung Institute, University of Colorado HSC. Mice were used at 10-15 weeks of age for recipients, and 10-30 weeks for donors.

Thyroid culture

Thyroids were removed from donors that were treated on days -4 and -2 before sacrifice with 300 µg/g of cyclophosphamide (Nosar by Adria Labs. Columbus, OH). The organs were cultured as previously described (La Rosa and Talmage, 1983), during 48 hours in MEM media containing 1.1 g/L $NaHCO_3$ (pH 6.9), 2% fetal calf serum, sodium pyruvate and antibiotics, and in a mixture of 95% O_2 + 5% CO_2 at 25 psi.

Isolation of pancreatic islets

Donor mice were injected with pilocarpine (Isoptocarpine by Alcon) 40mg/Kg body weight. 30 minutes later the pancreata were removed, and in groups of four they were transferred to siliconized vials filled with 5 ml of Hanks Balanced Salt Solution (HBSS) containing 1.5 mg/ml fresh collagenase (Boehringer, W. Germany, #103586), 10 µg/ml DNAse I (Sigma, St. Louis, MO, #D-4527), and 1.5 mg/ml bovine serum albumine (BSA). After 20 minutes incubation at 37°C in a water shaking bath (250 oscillations per minute), the digestion was stopped with cold HBSS containing 1.5 mg/ml BSA. After allowing the tissue to settle on ice for 5 minutes, the supernatant was removed and the digestion was continued in similar conditions but using 0.75 mg/ml collagenase. This last step was repeated two more times. Islets were isolated by picking them up with a siliconized glass pipet, under a dissector microscope, and in HBSS containing 10% fetal bovine serum plus antibiotics. Islet clusters were produced by incubating for 72 hours 50-60 islets in 96 well round-bottom plates (Flow 76-213-05), in RPMI1640 medium (Gibco #380-2400) supplemented with 10% fetal bovine serum plus antibiotics, at 37°C, and 1 atmosphere pressure of humidified 5%CO_2 + 95% O_2. This time of culture did not remove the allo-stimulating capacity of the clusters to induce rejection. In some experiments the donors were treated with cyclophosphamide (300 µg/g) on days -4, -2 and -1 before sacrifice. Then, after clustering the islets for 3 days, they were cultured for 7 more days under similar conditions, in 1.5 ml RPMI medium plus supplements, in 6-well flat-bottom plates (Flow 76-258-05), and placing one cluster per well.

Transplantation

Working under a dissector microscope, thyroids and pancreatic islet clusters were grafted under one or both kidney capsules of the recipient mice. In some experiments we grafted two thyroids in close contact under the same kidney capsule. Skin grafts were performed transplanting 1.5x2 cm pieces of donor skin on the back of the recipient mice.

Assay of graft function and viability

3 or 5 weeks after grafting, the thyroid graft function was evaluated by the uptake of 0.25 uC carrier free ^{125}I injected 24 hours before the sacrifice of the animals. Then, the isolated kidneys were counted in a gamma counter (Beckman, Gamma 5500), and histological examination of the grafts were made using parafin sections processed with hematoxilyne-eosine (H-E) staining. Grafts were evaluated according to their degree of lymphocytic infiltration in syngeneic (S), focal minus (F-), focal plus (F+), general (G), and destruction (D), as previously described (La Rosa and Talmage, 1983, 1985).

Pancreatic islets grafts were studied only by histology. We have found that there was a very good correlation between the histological appearance of these grafts and their insulin production.

Incubation with gamma interferon

Individual thyroids or pancreatic islet clusters were incubated in 24 well plates (COSTAR 3524) for 24 hours, in 1 ml RPMI1640 medium (10% fetal bovine serum plus antibiotic), containing 50 U/ml recombinant gamma interferon (DNAX Labs. Palo Alto, CA), at 37°C, and 1 atmosphere pressure of 5% CO_2 + 95% O_2.

Immunofluorescent staining

Frozen tissue sections were placed in gelatin coated slides, air dried and then fixed in acetone for 10 minutes. Next, they were incubated with biotinilated monoclonal antibodies 30-H12 (anti-Thy 1.2, Becton Dickinson # 1331), MKD6 (anti-IA^d) or 34-5-8S (anti-D^d). The last two antibodies were prepared in our laboratory from hybridomas provided by P. Marrack (National Jewish Hospital at Denver, CO). After washing with Dulbecco PBS (0.01M, pH 7.4), the sections were incubated with fluorescein-labeled avidin (Vector Laboratories, Burlingame, CA #A-2011), followed by washing in PBS and mounting with buffered glycerin (pH 8). In some sections, a two color staining was performed by using rhodamine-labeled avidin (Cooper Biomedical, Malvern, PA #2000-0470) after the first antibody, followed by incubation in biotin 100 ug/ml in PBS to block the nonreactive sites of the avidin. Then a second antibody was used followed by fluorescein-labeled avidin. The observations were made in a Zeiss microscope with epifluorescent ilumination and filter sets for fluorescein and rhodamine. Two-color pictures were obtained by a double exposure of the same film to the same microscopic field, and using two different filters. Photographs were made using 400 ASA Kodak Ektachrome film. For a better reproduction in this publication we prepared black and white prints using the slides as negatives; the dark areas in the **Figures** 1, 2 and 3 represent positive fluorescence.

RESULTS

Graft H-2 antigen induction correlates with foci of lymphocytic infiltration

We grafted fresh B6.C-H-2^d thyroids under the kidney capsule of C57Bl/6 (B6) recipients (H-2 antigenic difference only). Eight days later, the kidneys carrying the grafts undergoing rejection were removed, and frozen sections were made. The sections were treated with a double immunofluorescent staining which identified cells carrying Thy 1.2 antigen (T cells), and either class I (D^d) or class II (IA^d) H-2 antigens. The results showed high expression of D^d antigen on the thyroid follicular cells throughout the grafts, in contrast with the low expression they had before grafting. The IA^d antigen was also induced on the grafted tissues (**Figure** 1), but showing a gradient effect. Only the thyroid follicular cells that were in close contact to the T cell infiltrates showed high expression of this class II MHC antigen, whereas cells from the same follicles that were further away from the T cell infiltrate remained weakly positive or negative. Areas of the grafts that were not infiltrated were negative for the IA^d antigen, similar to fresh thyroids before grafting. Fresh thyroids showed expression of IA^d antigen only on the passenger leuckocytes normally present in these tissues.

These in vivo findings were reproduced in vitro by incubating B6.C-H-2^d thyroids in 50 U/ml recombinant gamma interferon. The D^d antigen was induced throughout the thyroid tissue (**Figure** 2) whereas the IA^d antigen was expressed only on the surface of the thyroid that was in close contact with the gamma interferon present in the culture medium (**Figure** 3). Control thyroids incubated under the same conditions but without gamma interferon showed some increased expression of D^d antigen but were negative for IA^d.

Using the same mouse strains we had similar in vivo observations in pancreatic islets undergoing graft rejection or after in vitro gamma interferon induction. The difference was that in both situations, the pancreatic islets did not show induction of the IA^d antigen. The islets used in this case were cultured in vitro during 72 hours for cluster formation. This time of incubation did not affect the allo-stimulating capacity of the islets to induce rejection. **Table** 1 shows a summary of our observations about H-2^d antigen expression in thyroids and pancreatic islets from B6.C-H-2^d mice.

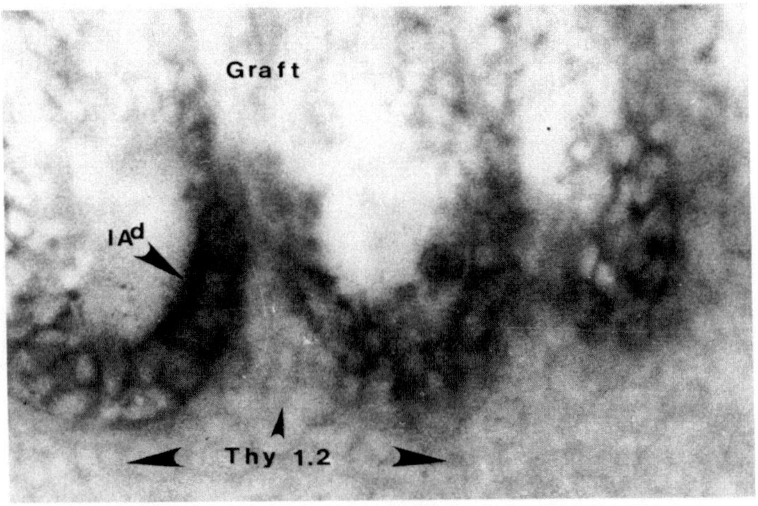

Figure 1. Frozen section of a fresh B6.C-H-2d thyroid grafted under the kidney capsule of a B6 recipient, 8 days after grafting. This section was processed with a double immunofluorescent staining using first a biotinilated monoclonal antibody (b-MAb) anti-Thy1.2 (30-H12), followed by rhodamine-labeled avidin. After that, the section was incubated in a biotin solution to block the nonreactive sites of the avidin-rhodamine, and then the section was treated by a second b-MAb anti-IA^d (MKD6) followed by fluorescein-labeled avidin. T: area of T cell infiltration (red in the original color picture). IA^d: follicular cells of the graft expressing the class II MHC antigen (yellow-green in the original color picture). Notice the gradient effect in the expression of this antigen. Dark areas show positive fluorescence. 100X objective.

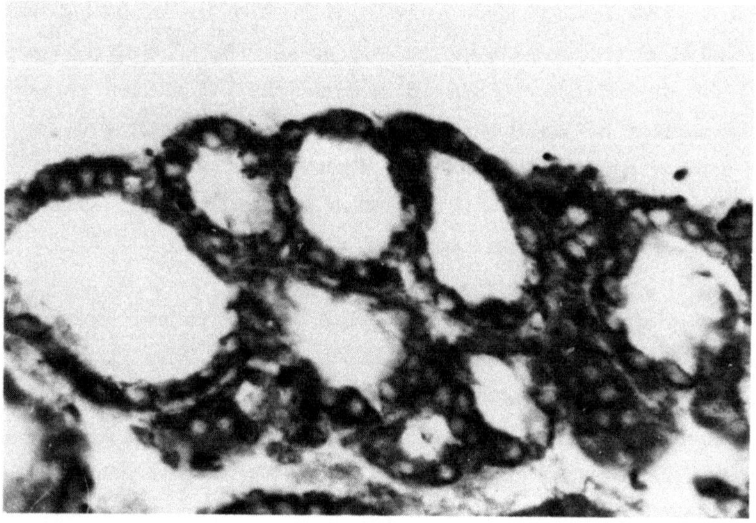

Figure 2. B6.C-H-2d thyroid incubated for 24 hours in 50 U/ml of gamma interferon. A frozen section has been treated with b-MAb anti-D^d followed by fluorescein-labeled avidin. Notice the high expression of the class I MHC antigen throughout the tissue. Similar expression was present during allograft rejection.

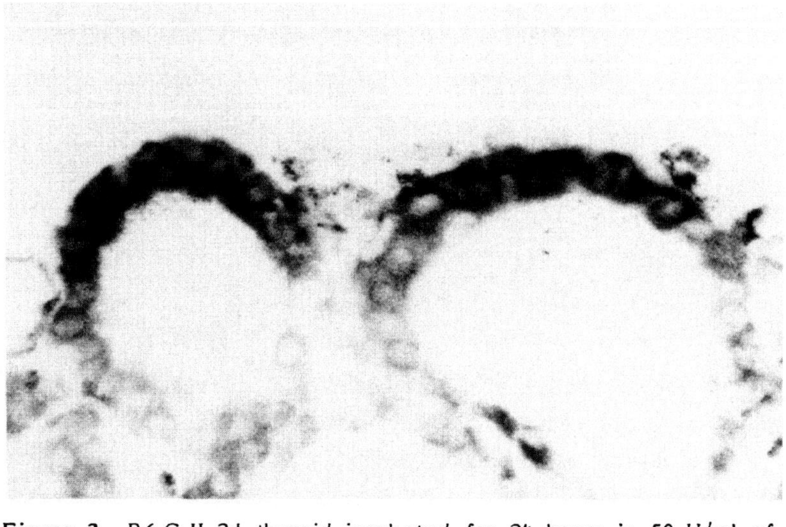

Figure 3. B6.C-H-2d thyroid incubated for 24 hours in 50 U/ml of gamma interferon. A frozen section has been treated with b-MAb anti-IA^d followed by fluorescein-labeled avidin. Notice the high expression of the class II MHC antigen only on the cells in close contact with the culture medium. Compare this image with the IA^d expression during allograft rejection (Figure 1).

TABLE 1

H-2^d ANTIGEN EXPRESSION ON THE PARENCHYMAL CELLS OF B6.C-H-2^d THYROIDS AND PANCREATIC ISLETS

	Control		Gamma IFN cultured		7 days after allograft	
	Class I	Class II	Class I	Class II	Class I	Class II
THYROIDS	+	-	+++	++	+++	++
PANC. ISLETS	+	-	+++	-	+++	-

Synergism between minor and MHC antigens in the rejection of oxygen cultured allografts

Abrogation of rejection of thyroids and pancreatic islet allografts has been accomplished by culturing these organs before grafting in high concentrations of oxygen (La Rosa and Talmage, 1983, 1985, and Lafferty et al, 1983). This treatment produces a selective inactivation or destruction of the allo-stimulating passenger leukocytes of the graft. The injection of these leukocytes at the time of grafting reverses the effect of culture and causes a rapid rejection (Vesole, Dart and Talmage, 1982). The remaining parenchymal cells of the cultured allografts are not able to activate an allo-immune response (Lafferty el al, 1983).

Cultured thyroid allografts with only H-2 antigenic differences were always accepted, and the histological examination of these tissues after grafting showed no lymphocytic infiltration. Allografts that differed from the recipient in minor histocompatibility antigens alone were nearly always accepted after hyperbaric oxygen treatment. But, most of these grafts showed different degrees of lymphocytic infiltration which usually persisted for several months after grafting without destroying the tissues (La Rosa and Talmage, 1983). However, when cultured allografts carried a combination of minor-plus-MHC antigenic differences, a significant number of spontaneous rejections and a stronger degree of lymphocytic infiltration were seen. The rate of rejection in these cases depended on the strain combination used, and was very variable as to time of occurrence, showing either acute or chronic rejections (La Rosa and Talmage, 1985).

Recently, we have made a similar observation in pancreatic islets cultured in 95% oxygen for 10 days, and grafted in allogeneic recipients. Table 2 shows the histological evaluation of these islets 5 weeks after grafting into B6 recipients. BALB/c grafts carrying minor-plus-H-2 antigenic differences showed 2 rejections out of 14, and different degrees of lymphocytic infiltration. Whereas B6.C-H-2^d (H-2 difference) and BALB.B (minor difference) grafts showed no rejection (0/12 and 0/7) and less infiltration.

TABLE 2

HISTOLOGICAL EVALUATION OF PANCREATIC ISLETS AT 5 WEEKS AFTER GRAFTING INTO C57BL/6 RECIPIENTS

	GRAFTS		
INFILTRATION[a]	BALB/C	B6.C-H-2^d	BALB.B
Syngeneic	7	9	6
Focal minus	3	3	0
Focal plus	2	0	1
General	0	0	0
Destruction	2	0	0
Rejection/Total	2/14	0/12	0/7

[a]See material and methods.

In **Table 3** we present the results of thyroid allograft rejection in a group of related strain combinations where a very clear synergistic effect between minor and H-2 antigens could be seen. In Group A, C3H cultured grafts showed a very high degree of spontaneous rejection by male C57Bl/10 (B10) recipients. This is the most reactive strain combination we have found with minor and H-2 antigenic differences, and female recipients were even more effective rejectors than males. In Group B, we used the congenic strain C3H.SW that carries the same minor antigenic differences as C3H, but has the same MHC as the recipients (H-2^b); in this case a significant ($p=2x10^{-4}$) reduction in the rejection rate was seen. A more striking difference ($p=8x10^{-8}$) was observed when only the H-2 difference from the C3H (B10.BR, H-2^k into H-2^b) was used (Group C). However, when the minor plus MHC differences of the C3H were reconstituted in the (B1O.BRxC3H.SW)F1 (Group D), a significant rate of rejection was seen (B vs D, p=0.01, and C vs D, $p=2x10^{-5}$), similar to Group A (A vs D, p=0.1).

Also in **Table 3,** Groups E and F show the results of an experiment in which two thyroids were grafted in close contact under the kidney capsule of B10 recipients. Group E had a cultured B1O.BR graft together with an uncultured C3H.SW graft. Group F had a cultured C3H.SW together with an uncultured B1O.BR graft. The uncultured grafts were always rejected similar to previous control experiments in which only uncultured allografts were used (data not shown in the table). The cultured grafts were only rejected in a significant rate (C vs E $p=3x10^{-4}$) in Group E where cultured B10.BR thyroids carrying H-2 antigenic difference alone were associated with the strong inflamatory reaction of the rejection of the uncultured C3H.SW grafts. However, the inflammatory reaction of the rejection of the uncultured B10.BR graft (Group F) did not affect the survival of the minor antigen incompatible cultured C3H.SW thyroids. Five weeks after the first graft, the Group E recipients were regrafted with new cultured B10.BR thyroids. Three weeks later the same 6 mice that had rejected the first B10.BR graft had also rejected the second graft, whereas the other mice had not.

TABLE 3

SYNERGISM BETWEEN MINOR AND MHC ANTIGENS IN THE REJECTION OF CULTURED ALLOGRAFTS[a]

GROUP	DONOR	Ag DIFFERENCE	REJEC/TOTAL
A	C3H	(MHC + minor)	16/20
B	C3H.SW	(minor)	4/20
C	B10.BR	(MHC)	0/20
D	(B10.BRxC3H.SW)F1	(MHC + minor)	12/20
E	(cB10.BR)+(uncC3H.SW)	(MHC)+(minor)	6/10[b]
F	(cC3H.SW)+(uncB10.BR)	(minor)+(MHC)	0/ 9[b]

[a] 5 weeks after grafting in C57Bl/10 recipients.

[b] Rejection of cultured (c) grafts. Uncultured (unc) grafs were all rejected.

A vs B: $p= 2x10^{-4}$ B vs D: p= 0.01 A vs C: $p= 8x10^{-8}$

C vs E: $p= 3x10^{-4}$ A vs D: p= 0.1 C vs D: $p= 2x10^{-5}$

E vs F: $p= 8x10^{-3}$

Difference in the rejection of cultured and uncultured bml thyroid grafts by B6 recipients

B6.C-H-2bml (bml) mice are different from B6 mice in three aminoacids at the level of the H-2K molecule. In this strain combination skin grafts are rejected promptly and strong in vitro CTL responses are generated. However, when we grafted fresh bml thyroids under the kidney capsule of B6 recipients, only 1/10 grafts were rejected (Group A **Table 4**). Also in **Table 4**, significant rates of rejection were seen only when the recipients were immunized with donor spleen cells (17/25, Group B, p= 0.002) or skin grafts (7/10, Group C, p= 0.009). The thyroids that were not rejected showed different degrees of lymphocytic infiltration. However no rejection was seen when the grafts were cultured in hyperbaric oxygen, even after immunization of the recipients with donor spleen cells or skin grafts (only one rejection was seen after immunization with bml skin graft, Group F). The histological examination of these grafts showed no infiltration or a focal minor infiltration.

In order to overcome individual variability in the immune response, we grafted another group of 10 B6 mice with uncultured bml thyroids in the right kidney, and cultured bml thyroids in the left kidney. At time of grafting they were all injected in the peritoneal cavity with $2x10^6$ bml spleen cells (**Figure 4**). 3 weeks later the recipients were injected with ^{125}I, and 24 hours later the isolated kidneys were counted in a gammacounter. The results are also shown in **Figure 4**; uncultured grafts were mostly rejected (1173 $\pm$413 counts per minute) or had heavy lymphocytic infiltration, whereas cultured grafts showed no rejection (13560 $\pm$1870 cpm) nor infiltration. **Figure 5** shows the histological appearence of two grafts from one of the mice in this experiment; even though this recipient was able to develop a good immune response that destroyed the uncultured bml thyroid, the cultured graft was not affected. Using other strain combinations with more antigenic differences at the level of the MHC locus, we always found rejection of both cultured and uncultured grafts when placed in the same recipient; although there was some delay in the rejection of the cultured grafts.

TABLE 4

REJECTION OF bml THYROIDS BY B6 RECIPIENTS

GROUP	CULTURE	SPLEEN CELLS	SKIN GRAFT	REJEC/TOTAL
A	-	-	-	1/10
B	-	+	-	17/25
C	-	-	+	7/10
D	+	-	-	0/10
E	+	+	-	0/20
F	+	-	+	1/10

A vs B: p= 0.002; A vs C: p= 0.009; B+C vs E+F: p= $2x10^{-8}$

Lack of correlation in the rejection of uncultured and cultured bm1 thyroid grafts by B6 recipients

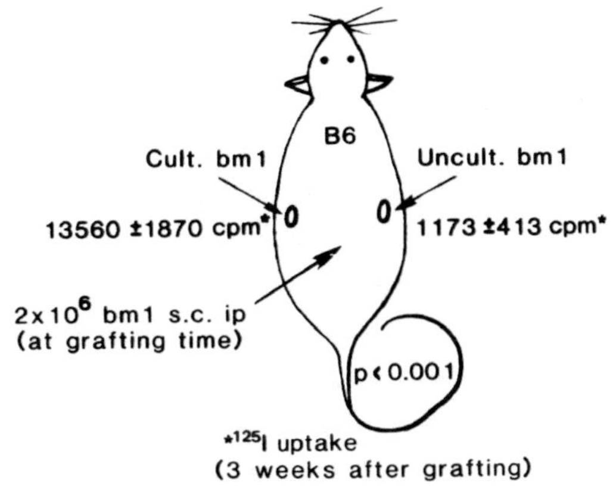

Figure 4. See text for explanation.

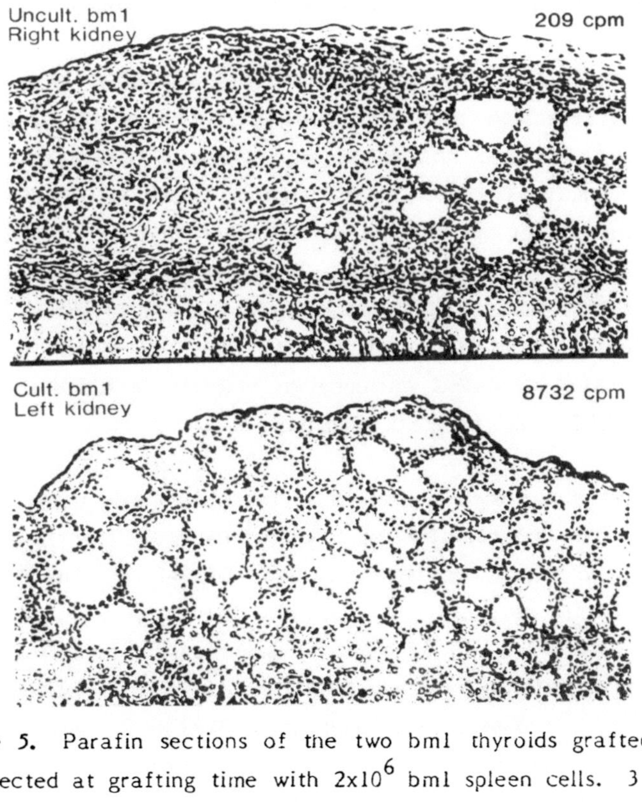

Figure 5. Parafin sections of the two bm1 thyroids grafted in one B6 recipient injected at grafting time with $2x10^6$ bm1 spleen cells. 3 weeks after grafting the uncultured graft (above) was almost completely destroyed showing a very heavy lymphocytic infiltration, whereas the cultured graft (below) was not affected showing the appearance of a syngeneic graft. H-E, 100X.

DISCUSSION

The three basic findings reported here show a direct correlation between the expression of H-2 antigens and the phenomenon of graft rejection. Our first observation demonstrates a very close spatial relationship between the areas of induction of H-2 antigens on the endocrine grafts and the foci of T cell infiltration. The high degree of expression of the D^d antigen throughout the graft, and the gradient effect observed in the induction of the IA^d antigen (**Figure 1**) suggest that the substance responsible for this phenomenon is being secreted by the T cells in the foci. This substance could be gamma interferon since the in vitro experiments in which we incubated thyroids and pancreatic islets in recombinant gamma interferon showed a very similar pattern in MHC antigen induction (**Figures 2** and **3**, and **Table 1**). Undetectable expression of IA antigen on pancreatic islet cells after gamma interferon incubation correlates with a previous report (Campbell et al, 1985). The low induction of D^d antigen that was observed in the control thyroids incubated without gamma interferon could be explained by the presence of some stimulating factor(s) in the culture medium that can affect the class I MHC antigen expression but not the class II.

Other investigators have already reported allo-MHC antigen induction on grafts undergoing rejection, such as kidneys (Henny et al, 1986), and livers (Gouw et al, 1987), but we have not found any previous observation in which this induction is so closely associated to the foci of T cell infiltration. We consider that the unique follicular morphology of the thyroid tissues has been a significant advantage for our study. It is relevant to mention that this relationship between MHC antigen induction and graft rejection is so important that some of these authors (Henny et al, 1986) have suggested that the finding of expression of class II allo-MHC antigens on biopsies of kidneys grafts could be used as an early indication of graft rejection.

The second observation is related to the synergistic effect between minor and MHC antigens in the rejection of oxygen cultured allografts. Similar to our previous report, in which we used BALB/c, B6.C-H-2^d and BALB.B cultured thyroid grafts into B6 recipients (La Rosa and Talmage, 1985), we are presenting here some observations made in cultured pancreatic islet allografts. **Table 2** shows that graft rejection (2/14) and stronger lymphocytic infiltration were seen in grafts bearing minor-plus-H-2 differences (BALB/c), whereas no rejection (0/19) and less infiltration were seen in pancreatic islets carrying H-2 (B6.C-H-2^d) or minor (BALB.B) antigenic differences alone. More clear evidence about this synergism is presented in the experiments in **Table 3**, in which C3H cultured thyroids grafted into allogeneic B10 recipients (Group A) showed a high degree of rejection (16/20). However, when grafts from congenic strains that differed from the recipient in minor (C3H.SW) or H-2 (B10.BR) antigens were used, low (4/20, A vs B: $p= 2x10^{-4}$) or no rejection (0/20, A vs C: $p= 8x10^{-8}$) was seen. A direct demonstration of this synergism was observed when the (B10.BRxC3H.SW)F1 mice were used as donors for B10 recipients. This strain combination carried the same minor-plus-MHC antigenic differences as the C3H into B10 combination, but with less concentration of these antigens. Nevertheless, Group D showed a similar rate of rejection as Group A (p= 0.1), and significantly higher rate than Group B (p= 0.01) and Group C ($p= 2x10^{-5}$). A further demonstration of this synergism was seen in Group E (**Table 3**), in which 6 out of 10 cultured allografts with H-2 antigenic differences (B10.BR) were rejected when in close contact with the inflamatory reaction from the rejection of an uncultured graft carrying minor antigenic differences (C3H.SW). Group F (**Table 3**) showed that this synergism did not work in the opposite direction, and that there was no cross-reaction between minor and H-2 antigens. That is, cultured minor antigen grafts (C3H.SW) were not rejected (0/9) when in close contact with uncultured allo-MHC grafts (B10.BR) (Groups E vs F: $p= 8x10^{-3}$). The rejection of a second cultured B10.BR graft by the same rejectors from Group E showed that these animals were systemically immunized to the $H\text{-}2^k$ antigen. Similar observations have been previously reported (La Rosa and Talmage, 1985); the only difference in the results was in the rate of rejection which varied according to the strain combinations used.

The evidence reported here may suggest that, in a cultured allograft with minor-plus-MHC antigenic differences, minor antigens shed from the graft (see **Figure 6**) are processed by host macrophages, inducing a delayed type hypersensitivity (DTH) reaction. In this type of immune response, T cells always appear to be aggregated into small or large foci, rather than being evenly distributed throughout the tissues. This could be required for some lymphokines to reach threshold concentrations and induce activation in other cells. In our proposed synergistic model (**Figure 6**) a consequence of this focal lymphokine production (i.e. gamma interferon) would be the induction in the expression of MHC antigens on the adjacent parenchymal cells of the graft. Another action could be mediated by growth factors (i.e. IL-2) on cytotoxic T lymphocytes (CTL) which in the presence of IL-2 and allo-MHC antigen can become activated, proliferate, and destroy the graft. It has been reported by Talmage et al in 1977 that activation of CTLs can be achieved in the presence of lymphokines in vitro by nonstimulating tumor cells carrying allo-MHC antigens.

Since all cultured allografts carrying minor-plus-MHC antigenic differences are not destroyed, the acceptance of several of them could be explained by a weak DTH reaction to minor antigens in some recipients, or by a smaller T cell clone size reactive to allo-MHC antigens. Variabilities in the response to cultured allografts between individuals of the same strain, and between different strain combinations have been previously observed (La Rosa and Talmage, 1983, 1985).

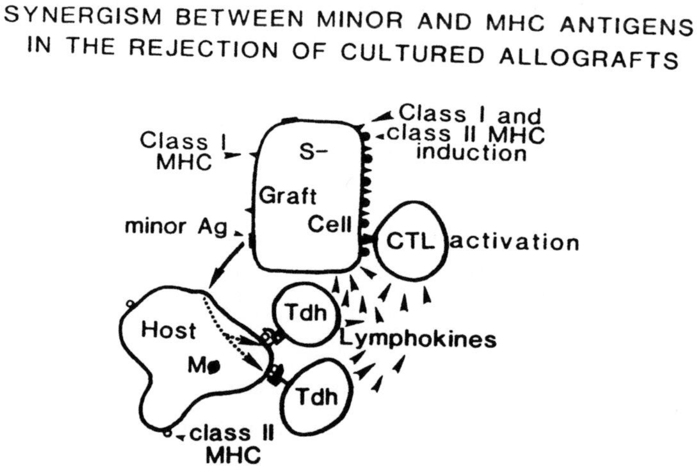

Figure 6: See text for explanation.

The rejection induced by the synergism between minor and MHC antigens in grafts free of allostimulating cells seems to be less effective than the rejection induced by passenger leukocytes. Nevertheless, with the evidence reported here, the presence of minor antigens on the parenchymal cells of any graft should be taken in consideration as a potential factor in graft rejection, mainly when allo-MHC antigens are also present. Thus, this synergism could account for the strong rejection of MHC incompatible cultured pancreatic islets grafted into individuals with Type I diabetes mellitus (Prowse, Bellgrau, and Lafferty, 1986), where a strong autoimmune T cell reaction to beta cell antigens is most likely present.

The third observation was the marked difference in the rejection of cultured and uncultured bml thyroids by immune B6 recipients. As mentioned before, oxygen cultured tissues are considered free of the stimulating cells that induce specific immune reaction to the allo-antigens they carry. We had previously observed that cultured thyroid allografts, followed by the immediate intraperitoneal injection of the recipients with donor leukocytes, were always rejected (Vesole, Dart, and Talmage, 1982). But they suffered a process of rejection that was slower by a few days than the time required for rejection of uncultured thyroids grafted into unimmunized recipients (La Rosa, unpublished data). Rejection of cultured thyroids or pancreatic islets grafted in one kidney of the recipient could also be accomplished by an uncultured graft from the same donor placed in the opposite kidney. Thus, the immune cells generated in the regional lymph nodes of the peritoneal cavity, or of the kidney carrying the uncultured graft, were able to travel to the cultured graft and destroy it. However, in the results reported in **Table 4**, this correlation of rejection was not present. B6 mice immunized with bml spleen cells or skin grafts were able to destroy most of the uncultured bml thyroid grafts (Groups B and C), whereas similar recipients did not reject nor infiltrate their oxygen cultured bml grafts (Groups E and F; $p = 2x10^{-8}$).

A more convincing evidence of this phenomenon was seen when we grafted in the same B6 mice both cultured and uncultured bml thyroids, and at the same time the recipients were immunized with bml spleen cells. As we show in **Figures 4** and **5** there was an evident difference in the immune response to each one of these grafts, despite the fact they shared the same antigenic origin. The most attractive explanation for these results is that there was a failure in the induction of MHC antigens on the cultured bml grafts. We think that in this particular strain combination, in order to get graft rejection, it is first necessary to immunize the recipients to the bml antigen(s), and second to have the presence of stimulating cells inside the grafts, as in the case of the uncultured tissues. These two factors are important in order to produce adequate foci of lymphocytic infiltration that could induce sufficient allo-MHC antigens on the parenchymal cells of the grafts, so that the CTLs can recognize and destroy the foreign tissue.

A Model for Graft Rejection

The transplantation of tissues in genetically incompatible recipients is an artificial event that obviously has not affected the evolution of the immune system. Nevertheless, the rejection of allografts is a highly efficient response that activates very specific mechanisms of immunity. It seems likely that the immune response that has evolved to deal with viral infections and tumor antigens is the same one that is activated for allograft rejection.

In order to explain the three basic observations discussed above, we are proposing a model of graft rejection in which the presence of allostimulatory cells in the graft (i.e. macrophages), and an immune competent host are required. The high level of allo-MHC antigens expressed on the membrane of the stimulating cells (1) could be compared to self-MHC antigens associated with viral or tumor antigens (self-MHC+x). In either case, specific T helper lymphocytes are activated around the stimulatory cells, proliferating, and attracting more lymphocytes and macrophages to produce foci of infiltration (2). Within these foci, the activated T lymphocytes produce threshold concentrations of a great variety of lymphokines which can induce activation in other cells. One of these substances is gamma interferon that can induce hyperexpression of MHC molecules on the membrane of non stimulating cells (S-) (3), and many other parenchymal cells (Rosa and Fellous, 1984), and can also induce macrophage activation (Unanue, 1983). Another important lymphokine is interleukin-2 (IL-2) which is a very important T cell growth factor. IL-2 and high concentrations of allo-MHC or self-MHC+x antigens can activate specific CTL (Talmage et al, 1977) that would eventually destroy target cells expressing such antigens (4).

In this model, the induction of hyperexpression of MHC antigens on the parenchymal cells of the affected tissue is of relevant importance. In the case of a viral infection, or the presence of a tumor, it is necessary that high concentrations of MHC molecules are expressed on the surface of the cells in order to associate effectively with the viral or tumor antigens. These antigens may have to compete with many other self antigens for MHC association. Thus, the greater the availability of MHC molecules, the greater the chance of viral and tumor antigens to produce self-MHC+x complexes. This event would allow the effector immune cells to distinguish viral infected cells, or tumor cells, from normal cells. In the case of allograft rejection, this same mechanism is activated, inducing high expression of allo-MHC molecules on the parenchymal cell of the graft. In a similar fashion to the self-MHC+x response, hyperexpression of allo-MHC antigens would produce a positive feedback mechanism to keep active the foci of lymphocytic infiltration until the foreign tissue is totally destroyed.

A MODEL OF GRAFT REJECTION

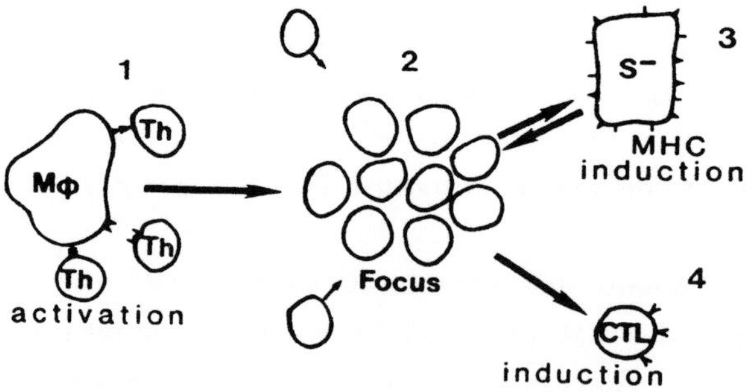

Figure 7: See text for explanation.

REFERENCES

Campbell, I.L., Wong, G.H.W., Schrader, J.W., and Harrison, L.C.: Interferon-Y enhances the expression of the major histocompatibility class I antigens on mouse pancreatic beta cells. Diabetes, 34:1205, 1985.

Gorer, P.A.: The detection of a hereditary antigenic difference in the blood of mice by means of human group A serum. J. Genet. 32:17-31, 1936.

Harris, H.W. and Gill III, T.J.: Expression of class I transplantation antigens. Transplantation 42:479, 1986.

Lafferty, K.J., Prowse, S.J., Simeonovic, C.J., and Waren, H.J.: Immunobiology of tissue transplantation: areturn to the passenger leukocyte concept. Ann. Rev. Immunol. 1:143, 1983.

La Rosa, F.G., and Talmage D.W.: The failure of a major histocompatibility antigen to stimulate a thyroid allograft reaction after culture in oxygen. J. Exp. Med. 157:898, 1983.

La Rosa, F.G., and Talmage, D.W.: Synergism between minor and major histocompatibility antigens in the rejection of cultured allografts. Transplantation 39:480, 1985.

Mason, D.W., and Morris, P.J.: Effector mechanisms in allograft rejection. Ann. Rev. Immunol. 4:119, 1986.

Prowse, S.J., Bellgrau, D., and Lafferty, K.J.: Islet allografts are destroyed by disease occurrence in the spontaneously diabetic BB rat. Diabetes 35:110, 1986.

Rosa, F., and Fellous, M.: The effect of gamma interferon on MHC antigens. Immunol. Today 5:261, 1984.

Talmage, D.W., Woolnough, J.A., Hemmingsen, H., Lopez, L., and Lafferty, K.J.: Activation of cytotoxic T cells by nonstimulating tumor cells and spleen cell factor(s). Proc. Natl. Acad. Sci, U.S.A., 74:4610, 1977.

Unanue, E.R.: Antigen presenting function of the macrophage. Ann. Rev. Immunol. 2:395, 1984.

Vesole, D.H., Dart, G.A., and Talmage, D.W.: Rejection of stable cultured allografts by active or passive (adoptive) immunization. Proc. Natl. Acad. Sci. U.S.A., 79:1626, 1982.

Acknowledgements: We thank Mrs. Marlyce George for the preparation of the parafin sections, and Mrs. Cathy Balliu for her assistance breeding and taking care of the mice. We also thank Dr. Donald Bellgrau and Dr. Rick Duke for their helpful revision and discussion of the manuscript.

Supported by NIH Grant AM-30836, and The Juvenile Diabetes Foundation International Fellowship.

CONTROL OF SELF REACTIVE CTL INDEPENDENT OF THYMIC SELECTION

Hans-Georg Rammensee

Basel Institute for Immunology
Grenzacherstrasse 487
CH-4058 Basel, Switzerland

ABSTRACT

Normal mice are extemely resistant to experimentally introduced CTL reactive against self MHC: B-reactive CTL could not be recovered from (A X B)F_1 mice injected i.p. with 2 x 10^8 strain A spleen cells, whereas third party reactive CTL of donor origin were found. Irradiation (600 rad) of F_1 mice before injection abolished this resistance, and B reactive CTL could be readily recovered. In nude mice of strain A, which carried a grafted thymus of strain B and are therefore tolerant of B by thymic negative selection, B-reactive CTL were recovered after injection of as few as 10^7 normal strain A spleen cells.

Thus self-class I reactive CTL are vigorously eliminated in normal mice. This mechanism is dependent on radiosensitive, antigen expressing peripheral cells, presumably of bone marrow origin.

The vigorous elimination of self class I reactive CTL is in contrast to the fate of self class II reactive T helper cells: A → (A x B)F_1 injections can lead to T helper mediated "lymphoproliferative", but usually nonlethal GVH. The lethality in this situation may be avoided by the buffer system described above. Whether the buffer system is required to maintain normal self tolerance is not known.

INTRODUCTION

T cell tolerance to self antigens is induced by negative selection of self reactive cells in the thymus (Kappler et al. 1987). In the present work it was investigated how an organism might eliminate self reactive T cells arising in peripheral immune organs by somatic variation of T cell receptor genes, or by extrathymic differentiation of T cells, or by expansion of self reactive clones escaping intrathymic negative selection.

The approach is to introduce T cells reacting to self MHC into a) naturally tolerant F_1 mice and b) thymus grafted nude mice tolerant by thymic negative selection only and to compare the fate of these self reactive T cells.

RESULTS AND DISCUSSION

To construct mice tolerant to one MHC haplotype by negative thymic selection only, athymic BALB/c nu/nu mice were grafted with day 14 C57BL/6 (B6) fetal thymus. Such mice develop a normal T cell compartment and are tolerant to BALB/c as well as to B6 MHC ($H-2^d$ and $H-2^b$, respectively) (Ready et al. 1984; von Boehmer and Schubiger 1984). As controls for "natural tolerance", normal (BALB/c x B6)F_1 mice ($CB6F_1$) were used. Individuals from both groups were injected i.v. with 10^8 spleen cells of normal BALB/c, containing a substantial number of $H-2^b$-reactive CTL precursors. Six days later, recipient splenocytes were stimulated in vitro with $H-2^b$ and third party $H-2^k$ antigens. CTL arising in the cultures were tested in a ^{51}Cr release assay on 3d-Con A blasts, which are mostly Class II negative. Whereas the noninjected BALB/c nu/nu with B6 thymus do not respond to $H-2^b$, but well to third party, cells from the injected nude lyse $H-2^b$-targets as well (Fig. 1a,b). The $H-2^b$ reactive CTL are presumably derived from the injected cells. In contrast, no $H-2^b$ reactive cells could be recovered from normal F_1 mice (Fig. 1a). Injection of 10^7 BALB/c spleen cells into BALB/c nudes with B6 thymus did not result in the emergence of $H-2^b$ reactive CTL in these recipients (not shown). However, injection of 10^8 irradiated (3,300 rad) B6 spleen cells as a source of antigen in vivo along with 10^7 BALB/c spleen cells allowed recovery of almost as many $H-2^b$ reactive CTL (Fig. 2b) as after injection of 10^8 BALB/c spleen cells (Fig. 2c). In contrast again was the absence of $H-2^b$ reactive CTL in $CB6F_1$ mice injected with the same mixture (Figure 2d).

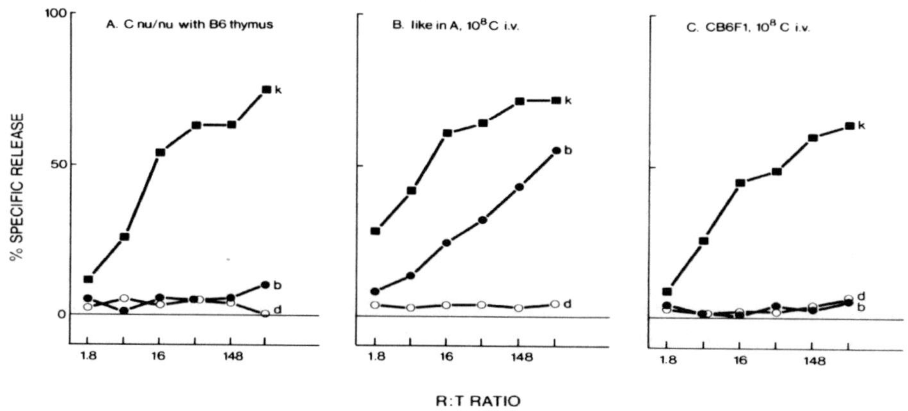

FIGURE 1. Thymus grafted nude mice are not resistant to thymus reactive CTL injected i.v.
BALB/c nu/nu were grafted with B6 fetal thymus taken at day 14 of gestation. Nine weeks after grafting, a thymus grafted nude (b) and a normal $CB6F_1$ (c) were each injected with 10^8 BALB/c spleen cells. After another 6 days, splenocytes of these mice and of an uninjected thymus grafted nude (a) were stimulated in MLC against a mixture of irradiated $H-2^k$ and $H-2^b$ cells in Il-2 rich medium and tested in a ^{51}Cr release assay. ○ , $H-2^d$; ■ , $H-2^k$; ● , $H-2^b$ targets (ConA induced blast cells).

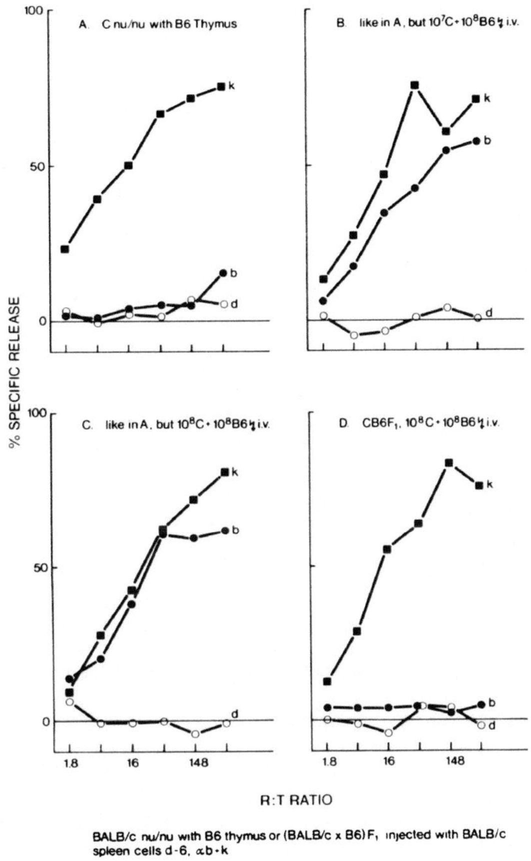

FIGURE 2. Coinjection of H-2^b antigen improves the recovery of H-2^b reactive CTL in H-2^b-thymus grafted H-2^d nudes.
Thymus grafted nudes as in Figure 1 were injected with 10^8 irradiated (3300 rad) B6 spleen cells plus 10^7 (b) or 10^8 (c) nonirradiated BALB/c spleen cells. A CB6F_1 mouse was injected with 10^8 irradiated B6 + 10^8 nonirradiated BALB/c spleen cells (d). Splenocytes from these mice as well as from an uninjected, thymus grafted nude (a) were stimulated and tested as in Figure 1. o, H-2^d; ■, H-2^k; ● H-2^b targets.

At this point, it was not clear, whether donor derived CTL might be eliminated nonspecifically in the CB6F_1 recipients. Therefore, we sought to test whether donor derived CTL could be recovered from A→ (A X B)F_1 mice. CB6F_1 mice were injected with 10^8 B6.PL.Thy-1^a spleen cells, which express the Thy1.1 antigen on T cells, in contrast to the recipients, which are Thy1.2. Six days later, splenocytes were treated with recipient specific antibody (Thy1.2) as well as CD4 specific antibody (to enrich for $CD4^-$ CTL) and C and stimulated against H-2^d and H-2^k in Il-2-rich medium. Only small donor derived activity could be found in those mice (Figure 3). The recovery of donor-derived, third party reactive CTL could be improved by coinjection of either irradiated third party antigen or CD4 specific antibodies. This result may be explained as follows. Parental donor cells react against F_1 antigen. All $CD4^-$ T cells reactive to recipient class I are inhibited by the control mechanism described in this paper. The class II reactive $CD4^+$ T cells expand, and they dilute the $CD8^+$ cells specific for third party antigen. If third party antigen is included in the inoculum, those third party reactive $CD8^+$ cells also expand, which - as well as inhibition with CD4 antibodies - would lead to a relative

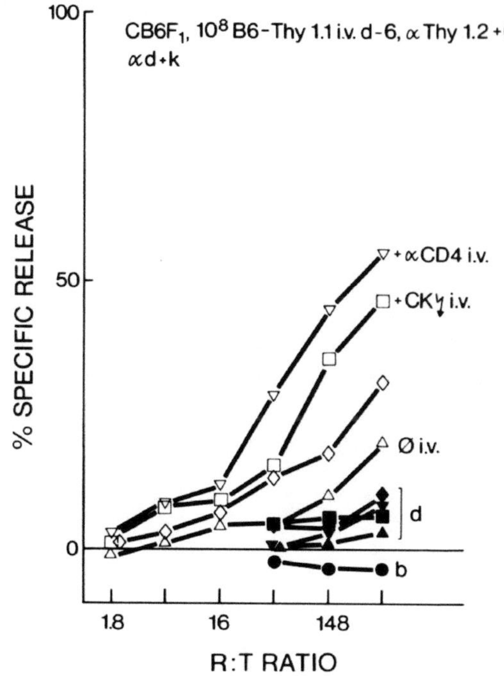

FIGURE 3. Recovery of 3rd party reactive, donor derived CTL from parent-cell injected F_1 mice.
$CB6F_1$ mice were either left untreated (Δ,▲) or were injected with 10^8 B6.PL-$Thy1^a$ spleen cells. Together with this injection mice received 10^8 irradiated (3300 rad) BALB.K cells (□,■) or CD4 specific antibody GK1.5 (Dialynas et al. 1983) (▽,▼) at a dose eliminating T helper activity, or nothing additional (◆,◇). Six days after injection, splenocytes were treated with a cocktail of recipient-specific Thy1.2 antibodies HO-13-4 (MarshakRothstein, et al. 1979) and CD4 specific antibodies and complement, stimulated against $H\text{-}2^d$ and $H\text{-}2^k$ in Il-2 rich medium, and tested in a ^{51}Cr release assay. Empty symbols: $H\text{-}2^k$ targets; full symbols: $H\text{-}2^b$ and $H\text{-}2^d$ targets.

increase of $CD8^+$ cells. More importantly, however, is here that none of the donor derived CTL reacted against recipient MHC, $H\text{-}2^d$. Donor origin in the group injected with CD4 antibodies from Fig. 3 was verified by another round of treatment with both recipient and donor-specific antibodies after restimulation.

The fact that A-donor derived anti B CTL can be recovered from the spleens of A-thymus grafted B nude mice injected with A-donor cells, but not from (A x B)F_1 mice injected in the same way may simply be due to trapping of B-reactive CTL in the body of F_1 mice. To test this, F_1 mice were irradiated with 600 rad before injection of donor cells. The combination used in this experiment was (B6 x B6.C $H\text{-}2^{bm1}$)F_1 injected with 5 x 10^7 B6 spleen cells. CTL reactive against bm1 could be readily detected in those mice (not shown). This experiment provides evidence, that the disappearance of recipient reactive CTL in unirradiated F_1 mice is not due to trapping.

In conclusion, CTL reactive to self MHC Class I are eliminated vigorously in normal mice, but not in mice tolerant by thymic selection only. The control system responsible for the elimination of self reactive CTL is a) independent of thymic MHC, b) sensitive to 600 rad irradiation,

c) dependent on MHC expressing cells in the periphery and d) independent of $CD4^+$ T cells. Based on earlier in vitro and in vivo studies showing essentially that bone marrow derived cells, predominantly CTL, can inhibit CTLp recognizing them (Miller 1980; for review see Rammensee et al. 1985), it is assumed, that the peripheral MHC expressing cells responsible for the control system are of hemopoeitic lineage. The control system described here seems not to work for Class II reactive T helper cells: $A \rightarrow (A \times B)F_1$ injections result in the persistence of T helper cells, but not CTL reactive to F_1 antigens, causing a "lymphoproliferative", but usually nonlethal GVHD (Pals et al. 1984). We conclude that lethality in this situation is avoided by the buffer system eliminating recipient-reactive CTL, because the latter have shown to be responsible for lethality of GVHD in irradiated mice (Thiele et al. 1987).

Acknowledgements

I thank D. Hügin and K. Hafen for technical and J. Hossmann for secretarial assistance, and B. Stockinger and M. Flajnik for reading the manuscript. The Basel Institute for Immunology was founded and is supported by F. Hoffmann-La Roche and Co., Basel, Switzerland.

REFERENCES

Dialynas, D.P., Wilde, D.B., Marrack, P., Pierres, A., Wall, K.A., Havran, W., Otten, G., Loken, M.R., Pierres, M., Kappler, J. and Fitch, F.W. 1983, Characterization of the murine antigenic determinant designated L3T4a, recognized by monoclonal antibody GK1.5: Expression of L3T4a by functional T cell clones appears to correlate primarily with class II MHC antigen-reactivity. Immunol. Rev. 74:29.

Kappler, J.W., Roehm, N. and Marrack, P. 1987, T cell tolerance by clonal elimination in the thymus. Cell 49:273.

Marshak-Rothstein, A., Fink, P., Gridley, T., Raulet, D.H., Bevan, M.J. and Gefter, M.L. 1979, Properties and application of monoclonal antibodies directed against determinants of the Thy-1 locus. J. Immunol. 122:2491.

Miller, R.G. 1980, An immunological suppressor cell inactivating cytotoxic T lymphocyte precursor cells recognizing it. Nature 287:544.

Pals, S.T., Gleichmann, H. and Gleichmann, E. 1984, Allosuppressor and allohelper T cells in acute and chronic graft vs. host disease. V. F_1 mice with secondary chronic GvHD contains F_1 reactive allohelper but no allosuppressor T cells. J. Exp. Med. 159: 508.

Rammensee, H.-G., Bevan, M.J. and Fink, P.J. 1985, Antigen specific suppression of T cell responses - the veto concept. Immunol. Today 6:41.

Ready, A.R., Jenkinson, E.J., Kingston, R. and Owen, J.J.T. 1984, Successful transplantation accross major histocompatibility barrier of deoxyguanomine treated embryonic thymus expressing class II antigen. Nature 310:231.

Thiele, D.L., Charley, M.R., Calomaki, J.A. and Lipsky, P.L. 1987, Lethal graft-vs-host disease across major histocompatibility barries: requirement for leucyl leucine methyl ester sensitive cytotoxic T cells. J. Immunol. 138:51.

Von Boehmer, H. and Schubiger, K. Thymocytes appear to ignore class I major histocompatibility complex antigens expressed on thymus epithelial cells. Eur. J. Immunol. 14:1048.

ROLE OF MHC CLASS I ANTIGENS IN TUMOR REJECTION

Suzanne Ostrand-Rosenberg*, Geoffrey A. Cole*, Gerald A. Cole+, Michael Nishimura*, Virginia Clements*, Hilde Cheroutre#, Stephen Hunt III# and Iwona Stroynowski#

*Department of Biological Sciences
University of Maryland Baltimore County
Catonsville, Maryland 21228

+Department of Microbiology
University of Maryland at Baltimore
Baltimore, MD 21201

#Division of Biology
California Institute of Technology
Pasadena, CA 91125

INTRODUCTION

The mouse H-2 or major histocompatibility complex (MHC) encodes a series of antigens that are centrally involved in immune responses. The K and D MHC class I antigens are highly polymorphic glycoproteins expressed on the surface of most nucleated cells, and consist of a 45 KD heavy chain noncovalently associated with a 12 KD protein, beta-2-microglobulin (B2m). Genetic differences between MHC class I antigens of graft donor and recipient result in allogeneic graft rejection. MHC class I antigens are also required for T cell mediated recognition of virally infected (Zinkernagel and Doherty 1979) or modified self cells (Shearer 1974).

A number of observations indicate that MHC class I antigen expression is also important in recognition and rejection of allogeneic or syngeneic neoplastic cells. Some studies suggest that the absence of class I molecules correlates with increased malignancy, presumably due to the inability of host lymphoid cells to recognize the tumor. For example, serologically MHC antigen negative tumors, such as teratocarcinomas, can often be transplanted across allogeneic barriers (Avner et al. 1978, Siegler et al. 1979, Ostrand-Rosenberg et al. 1980). The absence of tumor cell class I antigen expression is frequently associated with enhanced malignancy (Schrier et al. 1983, Schmidt and Festenstein 1982, Isakov et al. 1983, Gooding 1982), while increased MHC class I antigen expression can be associated with decreased malignancy (Ostrand-Rosenberg and Cohan 1981, Meruelo 1979). Novel tumor cell class I antigens can also be specifically immunogenic and presumably contribute to decreased malignancy, as in the case of certain UV-induced fibrosarcomas (Linsk et al. 1986). Other studies, however, suggest that tumor cells expressing low levels of class I antigens are particularly susceptible to natural killer (NK) cells and hence are readily cleared from a host. Tumor cells expressing high levels of class I antigens are more malignant because they are not targets for NK effectors (Karre et al. 1986).

While these observations suggest a role for tumor cell MHC class I antigen expression in tumor rejection, their precise role is unclear. Additional studies have therefore been undertaken in this laboratory to define the role of class I molecules in immunologically mediated tumor recognition and rejection. The present experiments are aimed at elucidating 1) The role of allogeneic class I antigens in tumor rejection. 2) The relationship between tumor cell class I antigen expression and NK cell susceptibility *in vivo* and *in vitro*. 3) The identity of class I molecules expressed in teratocarcinoma cells that do not express classical K or D encoded MHC antigens. The results presented demonstrate that 1) Allogeneic class I antigen expression on a sarcoma tumor is insufficient for tumor rejection. 2) There is no correlation between NK cell susceptibility and level of class I antigen expression in hepatoma cells. 3) mRNA that encodes non-K or D class I antigens is expressed in MHC antigen negative teratocarcinoma cells. These transcripts may encode class I molecules (presumably Qa or TLA antigens) involved in rejection of this tumor.

RESULTS AND DISCUSSION

Expression of an Allogeneic MHC Class I Gene (H-2K^b) on SaI Sarcoma Cells is Insufficient for Tumor Rejection

Because of their important role in T cell mediated MHC restriction and allograft rejection, MHC class I antigens are thought to play a critical role in T cell mediated tumor rejection. This hypothesis can readily be tested by assessing the tumorigenicity of malignant cells transfected with MHC class I genes. In those tumors studied to date, re-expression of an absent class I antigen results in the reduction or abrogation of *in vivo* tumorigenicity and metastatic properties (Tanaka et al. 1985, Hui et al. 1984, Bahler et al. 1987). In the present studies, a dibenzanthrene induced sarcoma (SaI) of A (*H-2K^{k}D^d*) strain origin has been transfected with the *H-2K^b* gene in order to determine the effect of expression of an allogeneic MHC class I antigen on tumorigenicity.

SaI sarcoma cells have been transfected by protoplast fusion (Rasoulzadegan et al. 1982) with a pSV2.gpt/H-2K^b gene (Schulze et al. 1983) construct. As shown in figure 1, 2 transfectant clones (SKB3.1L and SKB3.1M) are strong expressors of the K^b alloantigen as measured by flow cytometry using the 20-8-4 (anti-H-2K^b) monoclonal antibody. Three additional SKB clones (SKB3.1D, SKB3.1E, and SKB3.10) show similar fluorescence profiles (not shown). Untransfected SaI cells do not express H-2K^b antigen. Immunoprecipitations of SKB cells with an anti-H-2K^b specific monoclonal antibody (20-8-4), demonstrate that the product of the transfected H-2K^b gene is a 45 KD protein non-covalently associated with B2m, that comigrates with H-2K^b antigen from EL-4 (*H-2^b*) thymoma cells (not shown). L929 cells transfected with the same *H-2K^b* gene construct are readily lysed by H-2K^b specific bulk or cloned CTL (not shown). Therefore, the *H-2K^b* gene used in the SaI transfection studies encodes a class I molecule that is biochemically and functionally indistinguishable from H-2K^b antigen found on other cells.

To determine the effect of the expression of the allogeneic H-2K^b antigen on SaI tumorigenicity, A/J and B10.*A* (both *K^{k}K^d*) mice were challenged intraperitoneally (ip.) with 1 X 10^5 SaI, SKB3.1L, or SKB3.1M cells, and followed for survival. As shown in figure 2, 4 of the 5 SKB

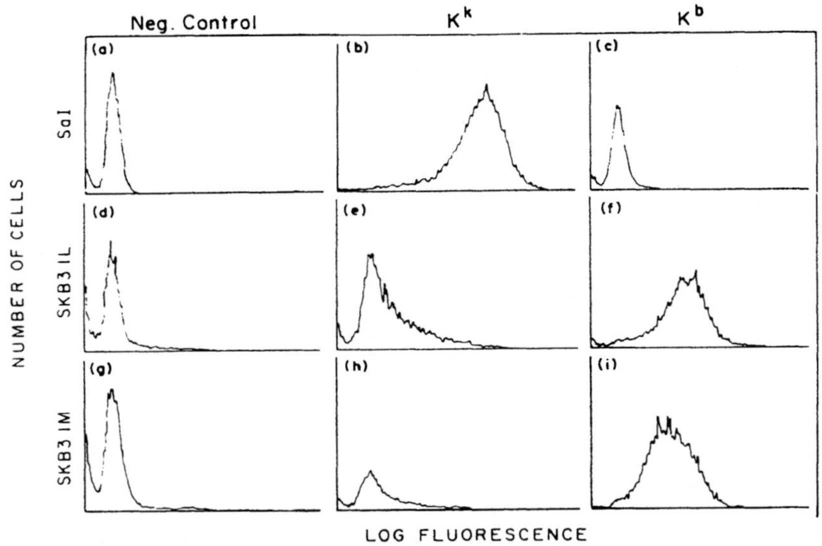

Figure 1. Flow cytometry profiles of SaI and $\underline{H\text{-}2K^b}$ gene transfected SKB3.1M and SKB3.1L cells labelled by indirect immunofluorescence with goat-anti-mouse-IgG for $H\text{-}2K^k$ (11-4-1 monoclonal), $H\text{-}2K^b$ (20-8-4 monoclonal), and a negative control (19/178, anti-Lyt 2.2 monoclonal). Each panel shows 5 X 10^3 cells.

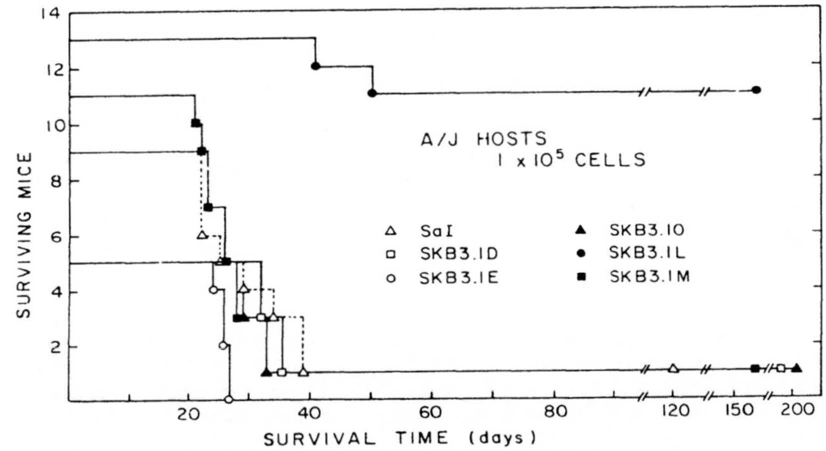

Figure 2. Survival times of A/J mice challenged i.p. with 1 X10^5 SaI and $\underline{H\text{-}2K^b}$ transfected SKB clones 3.1D, 3.1E, 3.1O, 3.1L, and 3.1M. All mice had demonstrable ascities tumor at time of death.

clones show equivalent tumorigenicity to the untransfected SaI line. One clone (SKB3.1L) shows reduced tumorigenicity compared to SaI cells. Analagous experiments with B10.A mice demonstrate similar survival kinetics (not shown). To ensure that H-2K^b antigen expression is stable in vivo, tumor cells have been removed from the peritoneal cavity of A/J mice 5 days after tumor challenge, and stained by indirect immunofluoresence with the anti-H-2 monoclonal antibodies used in figure 1. The fluorescence profiles of these cells are very similar to the fluorescence profiles shown in figure 1 for the in vitro cultured cells, demonstrating that the H-2K^b antigen is expressed on in vivo proliferating cells. To ascertain that A/J mice are capable of responding to H-2^b antigens on tumor cells, A/J hosts have been challenged i.p. with 1 X 10^5 EL-4 (H-2^b) thymoma cells. A/J mice are completely resistant to the EL-4 tumor challenge. Therefore, despite the strong cell surface expression of an allogeneic MHC class I molecule, the majority of these sarcoma cells are not rejected by immunologically competent hosts, suggesting that the expression of an allogeneic class I antigen is insufficient for tumor rejection.

Previous studies (North and Kirstein 1977) demonstrated that syngeneic immunity to the SaI sarcoma is accomplished by T cells, and that allogeneic immunity is mediated by Lyt 2$^+$ T cells (Smith et al. 1987). Resistance in allogeneic hosts is probably directed against allogeneic MHC antigens (Duc et al. 1978). Untransfected SaI and H-2K^b transfected SKB3.1L and SKB3.1M cells have therefore been tested to determine their susceptibility to cytotoxic T lympholysis (CTL). As shown in table 1, SaI, SKB3.1M, and SKB3.1L cells are not lysed by anti-K^b specific bulk effectors [A/J anti-B10.A(5R); K^{k}D^d anti-K^{b}D^d] or a K^b specific T cell clone (BM11-41, Bluestone et al. 1984). SaI and SKB transfectant clones are also not lysed by lymphocytic choriomeningitis virus (LCMV) specific H-2K^b restricted bulk effector cells (data not shown). These results suggest that the sarcoma cells are inherently resistant to CTL mediated lysis and that CTL effectors are probably not the in vivo population of cells responsible for rejection of the SaI tumor.

Table 1. CTL Lysis of Sa I and SKB cells.

		% specific lysis of					
Effector Cells	E:T ratio	EL-4	Sa I	SKB3.IL	SKB3.1M	L929-K^b	L929
A/J anti-BIO.A (5R)	12:1	77	3	3	0	54	8
BM11-41	5:1	83	0	0	0	59	0

Cr-51 labelled untransfected SaI and H-2K^b gene transfected SKB cells were incubated with anti-H-2K^b specific bulk effectors [A/J anti-B10.A(5R); K^{k}D^d anti-K^{b}K^d] and cloned T cell line (BM11-41) in a 4 hour release assay. % specific lysis =

$$100 \text{ X } \frac{\text{(experimental release - spontaneous release)}}{\text{(total release - spontaneous release)}}$$

Target cell labelling and effector cells were prepared as described (Ostrand-Rosenberg and Clements 1987). Each number represents the average of 3 replicates.

Although rejection of SaI cells by immunocompetent hosts is mediated by T lymphocytes, MHC class I antigen recognition is not obviously important in this system. Clearly, MHC class I antigen expression is critical in other tumor systems in which class I restricted effector cells are the mediators of tumor rejection (Hui et al. 1984, Schrier et al. 1983, Tanaka et al. 1985, Wallich et al. 1985). However, non-class I restricted T cells may be important in rejection of other tumors such as the SaI sarcoma. It will probably be necessary to study a variety of tumor systems to determine the relative importance of MHC class I restricted T effector cells versus non-class I restricted T cells in tumor rejection. Studies are in progress to isolate and characterize the effector T cell population(s) in the sarcoma system.

Expression of MHC Class I Antigens on Tumor Cells Does Not Determine Susceptibility to Natural Killer (NK) Cells

In addition to serving as target moieties for MHC restricted CTL, it has been suggested that tumor cell MHC class I antigen expression is inversely proportional to NK cell susceptibility (Ljunggren and Karre 1986). According to this hypothesis, tumor cells that express low or negligible amounts of MHC class I antigen are eliminated *in vivo* by NK cells, while tumor cells expressing high levels of class I molecules escape NK mediated surveillence and can proliferate and/or metastasize *in vivo*. In the following experiments, this hypothesis has been tested using the BW7756 derived hepatoma, Hepa Ova (Darlington et al. 1980). *In* vitro adapted lines of this tumor do not express serologically or biochemically detectable H-2K^b class I molecules (figure 3c), and therefore serve as a model system for an H-2K^b antigen negative tumor. Hepa Ova cells have been cotransfected by the calcium phosphate method with *H-2K^b* and neomycin resistance genes, and selected for growth in the antibiotic G418. The resulting transfected cells were cloned by limiting dilution, stained by indirect immunofluorescence, and analyzed by flow cytometry for H-2K^b antigen expression. As shown in figure 3 for one clone, K78-1.16, the transfected cells express H-2K^b antigen (panel 3f versus 3c). One dimensional gels of immunoprecipitates of H-2K^b antigen from Hepa Ova, K78-1.16, and positive control EL-4 (*H-2^b*) cells demonstrate that the transfected cells express a 45 KD protein that comigrates with the H-2K^b antigen immunoprecipitated from EL-4 cells (not shown). In order to determine that the transfected cells express a functional H-2K^b antigen, K78-1.16 cells have been used as CTL targets for the anti-K^b specific CTL clone BM11-41. At a 4:1 effector: target ratio, specific lysis of K78-1.16 and hepa ova is 11% and 1% respectively, compared to 43% specific lysis of positive control K^b transfected L929 cells. Therefore, the transfected hepatoma K78-1.16 cells express a molecule that is serologically, biochemically, and functionally identical to H-2K^b antigen.

The H-2K^b negative Hepa Ova and the H-2K^b positive K78-1.16 cells have been tested for their *in vivo* and *in vitro* susceptibility to NK cells to determine the role of H-2K^b antigen expression in NK mediated lysis. Splenocytes were removed from Tilerone treated (Orn et al. 1981) CBA/J (high NK strain) mice and used as effector cells against Cr-51 labelled Hepa Ova, K78-1.16, P815 (*H-2^d* mastocytoma), and YAC (*H-2^a* lymphoma) targets in a 10-hour release assay. Nine independent NK assays have been performed under identical experimental conditions. In all 9 experiments the highly NK susceptible YAC cells are readily killed, and the NK resistant P815 line is not significantly killed. The killing is mediated by NK effector cells as shown by the absence of killing in anti-asialo-GM1 antibody treated mice. Two types of results were observed for CBA/J NK effectors on Hepa Ova target cells. Table 2 shows 2 representative experiments. In experiment #1, Hepa Ova and K78-1.16 are equival-

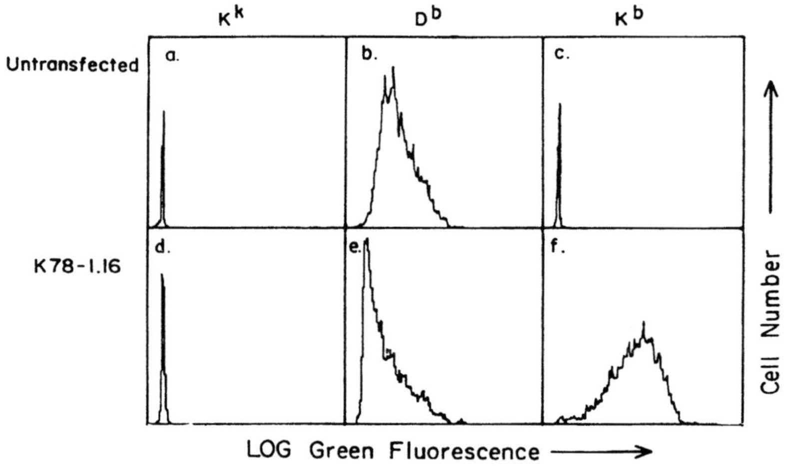

Figure 3. Flow cytometry profiles of untransfected Hepa Ova and H-$2K^b$ transfected hepa ova clone K78-1.16 labelled by indirect immunofluorescence for H-$2K^b$ (20-8-4 monoclonal), H-$2D^b$ (28-14-8 monoclonal), and a negative control (11-4-1, H-$2K^k$ monoclonal). Each panel shows 5×10^3 cells.

ently killed (22% vs. 18% specific release at 80:1 E:T ratio; $p > 0.05$), while in experiment #2 Hepa Ova cells are lysed to a greater extent than are K78-1.16 cells (18% vs. 2% specific release at 80:1 E:T ratio; $p < 0.05$). Results similar to those of experiment 1 were observed in 5 of the independent experiments. Results similar to those of experiment 2 were observed in 4 of the independent experiments. Hepatoma cells have also been assayed for their in vitro susceptibility to syngeneic C57L/J derived NK effectors. As shown in Table 2, experiment #3, the syngeneic host shows a low NK response to Hepa Ova cells. Therefore, CBA/J mice show varying levels of NK effector cells from experiment to experiment, and syngeneic mice demonstrate a marginal, but reproducible, level of NK lysis.

Hepa Ova and K78-1.16 cells have been monitored regularly for MHC class I antigen expression by indirect immunofluorescence. The observed levels of H-$2K^b$ antigen are routinely those shown in figure 3. Therefore, the variation in specific lysis of H-$2K^b$ antigen positive vs. H-$2K^b$ antigen negative hepatoma cells seen in approximately half of the experiments represented in Table 2 cannot be due to variation in tumor cell H-$2K^b$ antigen expression. Given the heterogeneity of NK cell phenotype and function, (Ortaldo and Herberman 1984) it is probable that the variability in target cell lysis seen in Table 2 reflects NK effector cell variation rather than target cell variation.

In order to test the effect of H-$2K^b$ antigen expression on in vivo tumorigenicity, syngeneic C57L/J, 650 Rad irradiated C57L/J, NK deficient C57BL/6J-beige, T cell deficient CByB6F1/J-nude, and normal F1-nude mice have been challenged intramuscularly (i.m.) with 1×10^7 Hepa Ova or K78-1.16 cells and followed for tumor development. Hosts were considered to be tumor bearing if they developed a minimum 1 cm. diameter tumor that was retained or increased in size during the 1-12 week observation

Table 2. CBA/J and C57L/J NK cell mediated lysis of Hepa Ova and H-$2K^b$ transfected Hepa Ova cells in a 10 Hour ^{51}Cr release assay.

				% Specific Release			
Experiment	Effector	Treatment	E:T Ratio	Yac 1	P815	Hepa Ova	K78-1.16
1	CBA/J	Tilerone	80:1	64	5	22	18
			40:1	50	0	12	9
2	CBA/J	Tilerone	80:1	58	1	18	2
			40:1	51	0	14	3
	CBA/J	anti-asialo GM1	80:1	3	0	1	2
			40:1	0	0	1	1
3	C57L/J	Tilerone	80:1	33	0	5	5
			40:1	24	0	3	2
	C57L/J	anti-asialo GM1	80:1	7	0	3	2
			40:1	4	0	3	2

CBA/J and C57L/J NK cell mediated lysis of Hepa Ova and H-$2K^b$ transfected Hepa Ova cells in a 10 hour Cr-51 release assay as described in table 1. Tilerone treated mice received 2-3 mg tilerone orally 48 hours prior to assay. Anti-asialo GM1 treated donors were injected i.v. in the tail vein with 0.1 ml of a 1/10 dilution of rabbit antibody 3-5 days prior to assay to remove NK cells.

period. As shown in Table 3, fully immunocompetent mice (C57L/J, CByB6F1/J-nu/+) as well as NK deficient mice (C57BL/6J-bg) are capable of rejecting the hepatoma. T cell deficient (CByB6F1/J-nu) and immunocompromised (sublethally irradiated C57L/J) mice do not reject the tumor. There is no difference in response to the transfected versus the untransfected tumor cells. These results indicate that rejection of this tumor is T cell mediated, and that H-$2K^b$ antigen expression and NK effector cells are not critical for tumor rejection.

The in vitro NK assays and the in vivo tumor studies demonstrate that in the BW7756 tumor system, H-$2K^b$ MHC class I antigen expression does not correlate with NK cell susceptibility. Therefore, the hypothesis that tumor cell MHC class I antigen expression governs NK cell activity is not applicable to all tumor systems. Further studies with other tumor systems and other MHC class I antigens are necessary to determine whether the BW7756 tumor is unique in its NK cell susceptibility. Additional studies are currently in progress to determine whether H-$2D^b$ negative and double negative (H-$2K^b$ and H-$2D^b$ negative) Hepa Ova cells show similar NK cell susceptibility.

cDNA Libraries of Teratocarcinoma PCC4 Cells Contain a Variety of MHC Class I Clones

Teratocarcinomas are malignant tumors derived from sperm, ova, or preimplantation stage embryos. They consist of undifferentiated embryonal carcinoma (EC) cells that have the ability to differentiate in vitro and in vivo into a variety of differentiated cell types. EC cells are serologically and biochemically negative for MHC class I antigens, presumably due to their undifferentiated stem cell status. A number of indirect studies, however, suggest that EC cells express MHC class I-like antigens. Immunization of genetically susceptible mice with L cells expressing transfected MHC class I genes of the tumor MHC genotype, protects against a subsequent EC cell challenge (Moser et al. 1985).

Table 3. Tumorigenicity of Hepa Ova cell lines.

Strain	# of mice with tumors / total mice challenged	
	Hepa Ova	K78-1.16
C57L/J	1/5	0/5
CByB6F$_1$/J-nu/+	0/5	0/5
C57L/J, 650 Rads	5/5	5/5
CByB6F$_1$/J-nu	5/5	5/5
C57BL/6J-bg^J	0/9	0/9

Syngeneic (C57L/J, 650 Rad), T cell deficient nude (CByB6F1/J-nu), normal nude/+ littermates (CByB6F1/J-nu/+), and NK cell deficient (C57BL/6J-bg) mice were challenged i.m. with 1 X 10^7 H-2K^b antigen negative Hepa Ova or H-2K^b antigen positive K78-1.18 tumor cells. Susceptible mice developed and maintained a tumor of 1 cm in diameter within 10 days of tumor challenge.

Likewise, immunization of susceptible mice with spleen cells of tumor cell class I genotype, but not class I mutant spleen cells protects against an EC cell challenge (Demant and Oudshoorn-Snoek, 1985). These experiments indicate that EC cells express MHC class I antigens that function as recognition molecules in tumor rejection. EC cells are also capable of specific cold target inhibition of CTL's directed against tumor genotype minor histocompatibility (Hm) antigens (Ostrand-Rosenberg and Clements 1987). Since recognition of Hm antigens is MHC class I restricted (Bevan 1975), this result also indicates that EC cells express MHC class I-like molecules. Therefore, although EC cells do not biochemically and serologically express class I antigens, they functionally express molecules that are MHC class I-like. The present studies were undertaken to define the class I-like genes expressed in PCC4 teratocarcinoma cells (129, H-2^b derived; Jakob et al. 1973), and to reconcile the apparent inconsistencies between the serological, biochemical, and tumor rejection data.

Poly A+ RNA was isolated from extremely sparse (undifferentiated, "PCC4") and retinoic acid and dibutyrl cyclic AMP induced confluent (differentiated, "dPCC4") PCC4 cultures (Strickland et al. 1980). Double stranded cDNA's were prepared from the poly A+ RNA using reverse transcriptase, size selected on Agarose A1.5 for greater than 1.5 kb, and ligated into the EcoR1 site of lambda gt10 phage. Recombinant phage were selected on the delta HFL strain (Huynh et al. 1985). The resulting libraries were screened by hybridization with a twice gel purified 200 base pair sequence corresponding to the 4th exon (alpha 3 domain) of an MHC class I gene (AC-14; Sher et al. 1985). Positive plaques were 4 times plaque purified and hybridized with a second class I probe corresponding to the fourth exon through the 3' untranslated region (pH2IIa; Steinmetz et al. 1981).

As shown in Table 4, the undifferentiated PCC4 and differentiated PCC4 libraries contain MHC class I clones at low frequencies. DNA from class I positive clones was EcoR1 digested, electrophoresed on 1% agarose gels, blotted onto nitrocellulose and hybridized with the 200 bp fourth exon probe AC-14. As shown in Table 5, the large majority of class I clones are 1.5, 2.5, or 3.0 KB in size. The frequency of the different sized inserts varies between the undifferentiated and differentiated libraries.

Table 4. Frequency of MHC class I CDNA clones in undifferentiated (PCC4) and differentiated (dPCC4) libraries.

cDNA library	size of library (plaques)	frequency of class I clones	# of 4x plaque purified clones
PCC4	1.8×10^6	.008 %	136
differentiated PCC4	2.5×10^6	.02 %	98[a]

a) An additional 325 clones screened positive, but have not been 4x plaque purified.

DNA from class I positive clones EcoR1 digested, electrophoresed on 1% agarose gels, blotted onto nitrocellulose, and baked for 2 hours at 80°C. Filters were prehybridized for 1 hour at 68°C with 5X SSC, 10% dextran sulfate, 300 ug/ml sonicated salmon sperm DNA, 0.1% SDS, 0.005M EDTA, and 5X Denhardts. Hybridization was in prehybridization fluid plus 1-5 X 10^5 cpm/ml alpha-P-32 labelled nick-translated AC-14 probe at 68°C overnight. Filters were washed twice at 68°C in 2X SSC, 0.1% SDS.

Table 5: Sizes and frequencies of PCC4 and dPCC4 clones

Library	# of Clones	% Clones	Insert Size (kb)
PCC4	52	41%	1.5
PCC4	28	22%	2.5
PCC4	44	34%	3.0
PCC4	4	3%	4.4, 5.0, 8.3
dPCC4	17*	18%	1.5
dPCC4	53*	55%	2.5
dPCC4	29	31%	3.0

*3 clones have inserts of 1.5 and 2.5kb

DNA from class I positive clones was Eco R1 digested, electrophoresed on 1% agarose gels, blotted onto nitrocellulose and hybridized with the AC-14 probe as described in Table 4.

In order to begin identifying and characterizing the class I clones, they have been hybridized with several cDNA MHC class I specific probes. The probes include TLA gene specific probes (T9, T18), a Q6,Q8,Q9 specific probe (381), a K,D,L specific probe (121), "37" gene probe (Lalanne et al. 1985), a cytoplasmic to 3' untranslated region probe (pH2I) and an alpha 1, alpha 2 region probe (pH2III) (Steinmetz et al. 1981). For controls, all probes were hybridized under identical conditions to control dot blots of 0.25-0.5 ug m13, pBR322, K^b-genomic, K^d-genomic, Q7-genomic, and Q8-genomic DNA's. Intensity of hybridization is defined relative to the positive control hybridization, where +++ is the strongest signal. Table 6 shows the intensity of hybridization, insert sizes and percent of clones hybridizing with the various class I probes. Hybridization of all of the purified clones with the pH2IIa and AC-14 probes indicates that these teratocarcinoma libraries contain class I-related clones. The 121, pH2I, and pH2III probes should react with any K,D, or L related class I cDNA. Because there are very few clones that hybridize with these probes, the PCC4 and dPCC4 libraries contain very few K, D, or L encoded class I clones. Since most of the PCC4 undifferentiated clones show a moderate reactivity with 381 probe, they

Table 6: Hybridization of PCC4 and dPCC4 clones to MHC class I probes

Library	Probe	% Reactive Clones	Insert Size of Reactive Clones	Reactivity
PCC4	AC.14	100%	all sizes	+++
	pH-2IIa	100%	all sizes	+++
	pH-2I	1%	1.5 kb	++
	pH-2III	2%	1.5, 5 kb	++
	121	0%		
	381	100%	all sizes	+
	T9	1%	2.0 kb	++
	T18	1%		
	"37"	22%	2.5 kb	++
dPCC4	AC-14	100%	all sizes	+++
	pH-2IIa	100%	all sizes	+++
	pH-2I	6%	all sizes	+
	pH-2III	30%	all sizes	+
	121	0%		
	381	0%		
	T9	0%		++
	T18	0%		
	"37"	52%	2.5 kb	++

Individual probes are described in the text. All hybridizations used probes at 1-5 X 10^5 cpm/ml hybridization fluid. Hybridizations and wash conditions for AC-14, pH-2IIa, pH-2I, pH-2III were as described in Table 4. Filters for 121 and 381 probe hybridizations were prehybridized 1-2 hours at 37°C in 6XSSC, 40% foramide, 0.5% Carnation Instant non-fat dry milk, 1% SDS, 100 ug/ml sonicated, boiled salmon sperm DNA. Hybridization was in prehybridization buffer plus 10% dextran sulfate at 37°C overnight. Washes were prehybridization buffer for 30 minutes at 68°C followed by 3 30 minute washes in 0.1X SSC at 68°C. Filters for "37" oligonucleotide hybridization were prehybridized at 37°C in the same solution as for the AC-14 probe, hybridized at 37°C overnight, and washed twice at 45°C for 1 hour with 0.1X SSC, 0.1% SDS. Hybridizations with the T9 and T18 probes were under the same conditions as AC-14, except the washes were in 0.1X SSC, 0.1% SDS.

are probably Q-related. 22% and 52% of the cDNAs of the undifferentiated and differentiated libraries, respectively, are 2.5 KB in size and hybridize to a second domain (third exon) specific "37" gene oligonucleotide. The "37" gene is a TLA region gene described by (Lalanne et al. 1985) and based on a 1.5 KB cDNA clone isolated from a DBA/2 liver library. It is expressed in a wide variety of cell types, however, no protein or function has been associated with a product of this gene. The hybridization results shown in Table 6 suggest that PCC4 and differentiated PCC4 cells express a "37" gene related message. The significance of the difference in size between the PCC4, dPCC4, and liver "37" cDNAs (2.5 KB vs. 1.5 KB) is unclear.

With the exception of the "37" gene clones, the majority of the clones do not correspond to known MHC class I genes. Therefore, if teratocarcinoma cells express MHC class I antigens, it is likely that they express "37"-gene related and previously undescribed class I molecules. It is tempting to speculate that these presumably Q and/or TLA region gene products are important in immune mediated tumor recognition and rejection.

CONCLUSIONS

Immune mediated tumor rejection is presumably dependent on the ability of the immune system to recognize a tumor as foreign, generate effector cells against the tumor, and remove the tumor cells from the host. MHC class I antigens are therefore potentially important as recognition or priming molecules for the host's immune system, and as target antigens recognized by lymphoid effector cells.The experiments presented here were designed to determine whether MHC class I antigens can function in these roles. The results of the 3 tumor systems presented here demonstrate that the function of MHC class I antigens in tumor rejection varies from tumor to tumor.In the sarcoma and hepatoma systems described, MHC class I antigens do not appear to be directly involved in T cell-mediated or NK-mediated lysis respectively. In the teratocarcinoma system, however, MHC class I antigens do seem to be critical for immunological rejection, although the precise identity of the relevant class I antigens is unknown. Therefore, the significance of MHC class I antigen expression for immune mediated tumor rejection must be assessed for individual tumors.

ACKNOWLEDGEMENTS

The authors thank Drs. D. Schulze and S. Nathenson for the H-$2K^b$ genomic DNA, Dr. J. Bluestone for the BM11-41 CTL clone, Dr. T. Hecht for the anti-VSV G antibody, and the Eli Lilly Co. for the mycophenolic acid. These studies were supported by Maryland Cancer Program/ACS Institutional Grants IN-147D and IN-174C, NIH R01CA34368, and American Cancer Society FRA #251.

REFERENCES

Avner, P.R., Dove, W.F., Dubois, P., Gaillard, J.A., Guenet, J.L., Jacob, F., Jakob, H., and Shedlovsky, A., 1978, The genetics of teratocarcinoma transplantation: tumor formation in allogeneic hosts by the embryonal carcinoma cell lines F9 and PCC3, Immunogenetics, 7:103.

Bahler, D., Frelinger, J., Harwell, L., and Lord, E., 1987, Reduced tumorigenicity of a spontaneous mouse lung carcinoma following H-2 gene transfection, Proc. Natl. Acad. Sci., USA 84:4562.

Bevan, M., 1975, The major histocompatibility complex determines susceptibility to cytotoxic T cells directed against minor histocompatibility antigens, J. Exp. Med. 142: 1349.

Bluestone, J., Palman, C., Foo, M.,Geier, S., and Nathenson, S., 1984, In Regulation of the Immune System, UCLA Ortho Meeting, eds. Sercarz, E., Cantor, H., and Citess, E., 89.

Darlington, G., Bernhard, H., Miller, R., and Ruddle, F., 1980, Expression of liver phenotypes in cultured mouse hepatoma cells, JNCI 64: 809.

Demant, P. and Oudshoorn-Snoek, M., 1985, H-2 class i antigen expression on mouse teratocarcinoma cell lines, Immunogenetics 22: 543.

Duc, H., Kinsky, R., and Voisin, G., 1978, Ia versus K/D antigens in immunological enhancement of tumor allografts, Transplan., 25: 182.

Gooding, L., 1982, Characterization of a progressive tumor from C3H fibroblasts transformed in vitro with SV40 virus. Immunoresistance in vivo correlates with phenotypic loss of H-$2K^k$, J. Immunol., 129: 1306.

Hui, K., Grosveld, F., and Festenstein, H., 1984, Rejection of transplantable AKR leukemia cells following MHC DNA-mediated cell transformation, Nature, 311: 750.

Huynh, T., Young, R., and Davis, R., 1985, Constructing and screening cDNA libraries in lambda gt10 and lambda gt11. In DNA cloning, vol. I, Glover (eds.), IRL Press, p. 49.

Isakov, N., Katzav, S., Feldman, M. and Segal, A., 1983, JNCI, 71: 139.

Jakob, H., Boon, T., Gaillard, J., Nicolas, J., and Jacob, F., 1973, Teratocarcinome de la souris, Isolement, culture et proprietes de cellules a potentialites multiples, Ann Microbiol. Inst. Pasteur, 124B: 269.

Karre, K., Ljunggren, H.G., Piontek, G., and Kiessling, R., 1986, Selective rejection of H-2-deficient lymphoma variants suggests alternative immune defence strategy, Nature, 319: 675.

Lalanne, J., Transy, C., Guerin, S., Darche, S., Meulin, P., and Kourilsky, P., 1985, Expression of class I genes in the major histocompatibility complex: identification of eight distinct mRNAs in DBA/2 mouse liver, Cell 41: 469.

Linsk, R., Vogel, J., Strauss, H., Forman, J., and Goodenow, R., 1986, Structure and function of three novel MHC class I antigens derived from a C3H ultraviolet-induced fibrosarcoma, J. Exp. Med. 164: 794.

Ljunggren, H., and Karre, K., 1985, Host resistance directed selectively against H-2 deficient lymphoma variants, J. Exp. Med. 162, 1745.

Meruelo, D., 1979, A role for elevated H-2 antigen expression in resistance to neoplasia caused by radiation-induced leukemia virus, J. Exp. Med., 149: 898.

Moser, A., Johnson, L., and Dove, W., 1985, Mice coisogenically immunized against H-2 class I antigens on transfected L cells reject transplanted embryonal carcinoma cells, Immunogenetics 22: 533.

North, R. and Kirstein, D., 1977, T cell mediated concomitant immunity to syngeneic tumors, J. Exp. Med. 145: 275.

Orn, A., Gidlund, M., Wigzell, H., and Gresser, I., 1981, Variation of interferon induction at the bone marrow level. Studies on interferon induction in relation to natural cell-mediated cytotoxic mechanisms, Eur. J. Immunol. 11, 795.

Ortaldo, J. and Herberman, R., 1984, Heterogeneity of natural killer cells, Ann. Rev. Immunol. 2, 359.

Ostrand-Rosenberg, S., Rider, T.M., and Twarowski, A., 1980, Susceptibility of allogeneic mice to teratocarcinoma 402AX, Immunogenetics, 10: 607.

Ostrand-Rosenberg, S. and Cohan, V., 1981, H-2 negative teratocarcinoma cells become H-2 positive when passaged in genetically resistant host mice, J. Immunol., 126: 2190.

Ostrand-Rosenberg, S. and Clements, V., 1987, Resistance to 402AX teratocarcinoma involves immunity to minor histocompatibility antigens, Immunogenetics, in press.

Rasoulzadegan, M., Binetruy, B., and Cuzin, F., 1982, High frequency of gene transfer after fusion between bacteria and eukaryotic cells, Nature 295: 257.

Schmidt, W. and Festenstein, H., 1982, Resistance to cell-mediated cytotoxicity is correlated with reduction of H-2K gene products in AKR leukemia, Immunogenetics, 16: 257.

Schrier, P., Bernards, R., Vaessen, R., Houweling, A., and van der Eb, A., 1983, Expression of class I major histocompatibility antigens switched off by highly oncogenic adenovirus 12 in transformed rat cells, Nature, 305: 771.

Schulze, D., Pease, L., Obata, Y., Nathenson, S., Reyes, A., Ikuta, S., and Wallace, R., 1983, Identification of the cloned gene for the murine transplantation antigen H-2K^{b} by hybridization with synthetic oligonucleotides, Mol. Cell. Biol., 3: 750.

Shearer, G.M., 1974, Cell-mediated cytOtoxicity to trinitrophenyl-modified syngeneic lymphocytes, Eur. J. Immunol. 4: 527.

Sher, B., Nairn, R., Coligan, J., and Hood, L., 1985, DNA sequence of the mouse H-2D^d transplantation antigen gene, Proc. Natl. Acad. Sci. USA 82: 1175.

Siegler, E.L., Tick, N., Teresky, A.K., Rosenstraus, M., and Levine, A.J., 1979, Teratocarcinoma transplantation rejection loci: an H-2 linked tumor rejection locus, Immunogenetics, 9: 207.

Smith, D., Stuart, F., and Fitch, F., 1987, Cellular pathway for rejection of class I MHC disparate skin and tumor allografts, Fed. Proc., 46: 756.

Steinmetz, M., Frelinger, J., Fisher, D., Hunkapiller, T., Pereira, D., Weissman, S., Uehara, H., Nathenson, S., and Hood, L., 1981, Three cDNA clones encoding mouse transplantation antigens: homology to immunoglobulin genes, Cell, 24: 125.

Strickland, S., Smith K., and Marotti, K., 1980, Hormonal induction of differentiation in teratocarcinoma stem cells: generation of parietal endoderm by retinoic acid and dibutyryl cAMP, Cell 21: 347.

Tanaka, K., Isselbacher, K., Khoury, G., and Jay, G., 1985, Reversal of oncogenesis by the expression of a major histocompatibility complex class I gene, Science 228: 26.

Wallich, R., Bulbuc, N., Hammerling, G., Katzav, S., Segal, S., and Feldman, M., 1985, Abrogation of metastatic properties of tumour cells by de novo expression of H-2K antigens following H-2 gene transfection, Nature, 315, 301.

Zinkernagel, R. and Doherty, P., 1979, MHC restricted cytotoxic T cells: Studies on the biological role of polymorphic major transplantation antigens determining T cell restriction-specificity, function, and responsiveness, Adv. Immunol. 27: 51.

GENETIC CONTROL OF INTERACTION BETWEEN CLASS I AND CLASS II ANTIGENS IN MURINE ISLET REJECTION

Vera Hauptfeld[1], Denise Faustman[2], Reiji Terasaka[2], Paul E. Lacy[2] and Donald C. Shreffler[1]

Departments of Genetics[1] and Pathology[2], Washington University School of Medicine, St. Louis, Missouri 63110

Abstract

Successfully implanted islets of Langerhans between two H-2 disparate strains are rejected following injection of cells bearing class I antigens syngeneic to the graft, together with either syngeneic or allogeneic class II antigens. Such rejection does not occur if class II syngeneic to the graft, but class I antigens are not.

Beta cells of islets of Langerhans bear class I but not class II antigens (Faustman et al. 1980 and Baekkeskov et al. 1980). Allografts of these islets, when depleted of Ia-bearing cells, by either long-term culture (Lafferty et al. 1975; Sollinger et al. 1977; and Lacy et al. 1979a), anti-Ia sera and complement treatment (Faustman et al. 1981) or anti-dendritic antibody and complement treatment (Faustman et al. 1984) are successfully transplanted across an MHC barrier. Such a successfully transplanted graft is rejected if immunocompetent cells of donor origin are injected. This can be achieved in the mouse-to-mouse allograft system with splenocytes (Faustman et al. 1981), PEC (Bowen et al. 1981) and dendritic cells (Faustman et al. 1984), in as well as in rat-to-rat (Lacy et al. 1979b) and rat-to-mouse (Lacy et al. 1979a) systems. The dose required for initiation of rejection is positively correlated with the time the graft is residing in the recipient. When challenged at 100 days, 10^5 PEC cause rejection of only half of accepted transplants (Bowen et al. 1981) and at 200 days more than 50 x 10^6 splenocytes are required (Faustman et al. 1981). On the first day after blood glucose levels were determined to be normal however, even 10^3 splenic macrophages or 10^4 nylon-wool purified splenic T cells or anti-Thy-1 plus complement-purified B cells, is sufficient (Table 1).

The immunological status of recipients with successfully transplanted islet allografts is different at various intervals after the transplantation, as measured by the fate of skin grafts. At 100 days after islet transplantation, skin grafts of the same haplotype as the islet transplant not only are rejected, but cause rejection of some of the accepted islet allografts (Morrow et al. 1983a). When challenged at 200 days, haplotype-specific tolerance is observed (Faustman et al. 1985).

The intriguing finding that B lymphocytes are more efficient in initiating the rejection in small rather than large doses (Table 1) is in concordance with results previously obtained on rats (Zitron et al. 1981), where the large dose (60 x 10^6) B lymphocytes did not lead into islet graft rejection.

Since Lauchart et al. (1980) have shown that B lymphocytes can induce allograft enhancement, one can postulate that with large doses one induces tolerance, presumably through active suppression (Zitron et al. 1981), as is the case with tolerance induced by large doses of erythrocytes (Faustman et al. 1985 and Fuastman et al. 1982).

The importance of the presence of a graft in initiating or maintaining tolerance is also clear from other sets of experiments. Mice can be made to accept a fresh islet allograft by large injections (more than 50 x 10^6) of erythrocytes of donor origin (Faustman et al. 1982). However, only those mice that receive an islet allograft after the erythrocytes also accept a skin allograft of the same origin, showing haplotype-specific tolerance. Mice which receive only the injection of erythrocytes without the islet graft reject skin grafts with the same speed as untreated animals (Faustmen et al. 1985). The fact that the continuous presence of the graft is crucial in maintaining tolerance was also observed by Donohue et al. (1983). They explain the mechanism as one of continuous leakage of the alloantigen.

As mentioned above, islet allografts are accepted across an *H-2* barrier if Ia-bearing cells are eliminated, for example by anti-Ia plus complement treatment. On the other hand, islet allografts between strains compatible in the *I*-region, but differing in *H-2K* and/or *H-2D* (by selection of appropriate intra-*H-2* recombinants), are rejected (Morrow et al. 1983b).

These two sets of results are not really discrepant if one postulates that, in the first case, where anti-Ia serum and complement were used, the Ia-bearing cells are either eliminated or reduced below threshold levels, whereas, in the second case, where *I* regions are matched, but *K* or *D* differ, Ia-bearing cells are plentiful and thus available to mediate a reaction.

Since antisera directed against *I* region determinants inhibit MLR reactions (Minami et al. 1980) and generation of class II-restricted CTL cells against incompatible class I antigens (Mizuochi et al. 1985), it seems to imply that donor class II is important, if not totally responsible, for presentation of class I antigens on the same cell. In the anti-Ia plus complement model, there would be none or too few of the class II-bearing cells to present class I antigens.

To investigate the genetic requirements for interactions between class I and class II molecules in inititation of islet allograft rejection, we used the first model, *i.e.* elimination of Ia-bearing cells with anti-Ia plus complement. Donor B10.BR (*H-2*^{k}) islets were isolated by the collagenase technique (Lacy and Kostianovsky 1967) separated on a Ficoll gradient (Lindall et al. 1969), and then meticulously handpicked with the use of a Pasteur pipette under a dissecting microscope with a green filter. 550-750 islets that had been treated with anti-Ia^k serum (A.TH anti A.TL) plus complement were implanted into the portal vein of C57BL/6J (*H-2*^{b}) recipients that had previously been made diabetic by treatment with streptozotocin. At 21 days, normoglycemic, allograft-bearing mice were challenged with splenocytes from various intra-*H-2* recombinant haplotypes selected in such a way as to share different regions of the *H-2* complex with the *H-2*^{k} islet allografts. The challenge dose which would be sufficient to cause rejection of the islet grafts at 21 days was determined with B10.BR cells. The dose chosen was 10 x 10^6, although 5 x 10^6 B10.BR cells was sufficient to initiate rejection (Table 2, Group 1). Cells from the B10.BR (H-2^k) strain and from H-2^k recombinant strains B10.AM (K^k A^k E^k D^b), B10.A(4R) (K^k A^k E^b D^b) and B10.OL (K^d I^d D^k) all initiated rejection of previously accepted B10.BR islet allografts (Table 2, Groups 1,4,5,8). Cells from B10.MBR (K^b I^k D^q) and B10.TBR3 (K^s A^k E^b D^b) had no effect on the survival of the graft (Table 2, Groups 6,7).

The findings in this and some previous studies (Faustman et al. 1980 and Faustman et al. 1981) allow us to draw several conclusions. First, beta cells of Langerhans, which lack class II antigens, do not alone initiate a cellular response against the class I (K/D) antigens which they carry. Secondly, to supply cells bearing donor class II antigens without the proper (donor) class I antigens is not sufficient to initiate a response. This is clearly demonstrated by the inability of B10.MBR (K^b I^k D^q) and B10.TBR3 (K^s A^k E^b D^b) cells to initiate rejection of H-2-K^k or H-2-D^k target cells (Table 2, Groups 6,7). Thirdly, cells bearing *any* class II antigens with appropriate (graft donor) class I will initiate an anti-class I-specific response as seen with B10.OL cells (K^d I^d D^k) (Table 2, Group 8).

Thus class I antigens are the molecules which serve as targets in this system. The question remains, what is the target molecule in the case in which intra-*H-2* recombinants differing only in the *I*-region are chosen as the recipient-donor combination? Results obtained from such experiments vary greatly, depending on the organ chosen, as well as the haplotype combination. These differences might be explained by varying tissue distributions of class I antigens (perhaps including class I other than classical K/D) in different organs. The involvement of class I antigens other than K/D would explain results by Okazaki et al. (1981), in which they were unable to induce tolerance to skin grafts across *KI*-region differences with purified erythrocyte populations. Erythrocytes carrying K/D antigens could induce tolerance to K/D antigens, but not to any other antigens involved in the skin graft rejections.

On the other hand, the successful induction of tolerance for β cells of Langerhans by erythrocytes (Faustman et al. 1982) or UV-irradiated splenocytes (Agostino et al. 1984) indicates that β cells do not carry any additional class I antigens that erythrocytes do not. Faustman et al. (1982) also showed that injection of whole blood sensitizes the recipient, leading to second-set type rejections of islets of Langerhans.

Okazaki et al. (1981) induced tolerance toward skin grafts by injecting whole blood. Their success in initiating tolerance might be another proof that, in the case of whole blood-skin graft combinations, only one of two required antigens was present (Ia^+ K/D^-) to initiate an immune response. Recent data by Coughman et al. (1986), showing that murine epidermal dendritic (Langerhans) cells are quite deficient in K/D expression, support this notion and suggest that we should look more broadly at the mechanisms involved in interactions between class II and class I antigens, e.g. Qa, that lead to immune response or tolerance.

Acknowledgement

We wish to thank Mrs. Evelyne Dye, Susan Bassett-Chu and Pat Talley for their excellent technical assistance and Mrs. Karen Perks for expert typing of the manuscript. The work was supported by NIH grants AI 12734 and AM 01226.

TABLE 1. REJECTION OF ESTABLISHED B10.BR ISLET ALLOGRAFTS INITIATED BY VARIOUS CELL TYPES OF DONOR HAPLOTYPE[a]

Cell Type	Dose	Rejected (days)
Macrophages[b]	1×10^6	7, 9, 10
	1×10^4	8, 12, 14
	1×10^3	26, 29, >400, >400
B cells[c]	1×10^6	10, 13, 30, 35
	1×10^5	7, 8, 14
	1×10^4	6, 7, 8, 9
T cells[d]	1×10^4	2, 4, 7

[a]Recipients were B6 mice which had received anti-Ia+C'-treated B10.BR islets. On the first day after blood glucose levels were determined to be normal, they were injected with the cells indicated.

[b]24h glass-adherent.

[c]anti-BAT+C' and Ficoll treatment.

[d]nylon wool and glass adherent.

TABLE 2. EFFECT OF SPLENOCYTE INJECTIONS 21-24 DAYS AFTER SUCCESSFUL ISLET TRANSPLANTATION ON SUBSEQUENT ISLET ALLOGRAFT SURVIVAL: (B10.BR [$H-2^k$] to B6 [$H-2^b$])

Group	Splenocyte Injection	Individual Survival After Challenge (days)
1	5×10^6 B10.BR	21, 24, 30, 31, 35
2	1×10^7 B10.BR	14, 14, 17, 21, 49
3	No Splenocytes	>200, >200, >200 >200, >200, >200 >200
4	B10.AM (K^k, A^k, E^k, D^b)	14, 14, 14, 23, 36
5	B10.A(4R) (K^k, A^k, E^b, D^b)	6, 15, 20, 35, 37
6	B10.MBR (K^b, A^k, E^k, D^q)	>150, >150, >150 >150, >150
7	B10.TBR3 (K^s, A^k, E^b, D^b)	>100, >100
8	B10.OL (K^d, A^d, E^d, D^k)	45, 48, 89, 140
9	Control mice transplanted with untreated allogeneic islets	5, 6, 8, 10, 22, 38 >100, >100

In groups 4-8, recipients received 1×10^7 cells.

Reference

Agostino, M., Prowse, S.J., and Lafferty, K.J. Induction of tolerance using ultraviolet-irradiated cells. Transplantation Proceedings, Vol. XVI: 959-960, 1984.

Baekkeskov, S., Lernmark, A., Klareskog, L. Presence of transplantation antigens in pancreatic islets. Diabetologia 19: 255, 1980.

Bowen, K., Prowse, S., Lafferty, K. Reversal of diabetes by islet transplantation: Vulnerability of the established allograft. Science 213: 1261-1262, 1981.

Caughman, S.W., Sharrow, S.O., Shimada, S., Stephany, D., Mizuochi, T., Rosenberg, A.S., Katz, S.I. and Singer, A. Ia^+ murine epidermal Langerhans cells are deficient in surface expression of the class I major histocompatibility complex. Proc. Natl. Acad. Sci. USA 83: 7438-7442, 1986.

Donohoe, J.A., Andrus, L., Bowen, K.M., Simeonovic, C., Prowse, S.J., Lafferty, K.J. Cultured thyroid allografts induce a state of partial tolerance in adult recipient mice. Transplantation 35: 62-67, 1983.

Faustman, D., Hauptfeld, V., Davie, J.M., Lacy, P.E. and Shreffler, D.C. Murine pancreatic β-cells express H-2K and H-2D but not Ia antigens. J. Exp. Med. 151: 1563-1568, 1980.

Faustman, D., Hauptfeld, V., Lacy, P.E. and Davie, J.M. Prolongation of murine islet allograft survival by pretreatment of islets with antibody directed to Ia determinants. Proc. Natl. Acad. Sci. USA 78: 5156-5159, 1981.

Faustman, D.L., Steinman, R.M., Gebel, H.M., Hauptfeld, V., Davie, J.M., and Lacy, P. Prevention of rejection of murine islet allografts by pretreatment with anti-dendritic cell antibody. Proc. Natl. Acad. Sci. USA 81: 3864-3868, 1984.

Faustman, D.L., Hauptfeld, V., Davie, J.M., and Lacy, P.E. Prolonged survival of donor skin grafts on mice bearing established islet of Langerhans transplants. Transplantation 40: 216-218, 1985.

Faustman, D., Lacy, P., Davie, J., and Hauptfeld, V. Prevention of allograft rejection by immunization with donor blood depleted of Ia-bearing cells. Science 217: 1570158, 1982.

Lacy, P., Davie, J., Finke, E. Prolongation of islet allograft survival following in vitro culture (24°C) and a single injection of ALS. Science 204: 312-313, 1979.

Lacy, P., Davie, J., Finke, E. Induction of rejection of successful allograft of rat islets by donor peritoneal exudate cells. Transplantation 28: 415-420, 1979.

Lacy, P.L. and Kostianovsky, M. Method for the isolation of intact islets of Langerhans from the rat pancreas. Diabetes 16: 35-39, 1967.

Lafferty, K., Cooley, M., Woolnough, J., Walker, K. Thyroid allograft immunogenicity is reduced after a period in organ culture. Science 188: 259-261, 1975.

Lauchart, W., Alkins, B.J., Davies, D.A.L. Only B lymphocytes induce active enhancement of rat cardial allografts. Transplantation 29: 259-261, 1980.

Lindall, A., Steffes, M., Sorenson, R. Immunoassayable insulin content of sùbcellular fractions of rat islets. Endocrinology 85: 218, 1969.

Minami, M., Shreffler, D.C. and Cowing, C. Characterization of the stimulator cell in the murine primary mixed leucocyte response. J. Immunology 124: 1314-1321, 1980.

Mizuochi, T., Golding, H., Rosenberg, A.S., Glimcher, L.H., Malek, T.R., and Singer, A. Both $L3T4^+$ and $Lyt\text{-}2^+$ helper T cells initiate cytotoxic T lymphocyte responses against allogeneic major histocompatibility antigens but not against trinitrophenyl-modified self. J. Exp. Med. 162: 427-443, 1985.

Morrow, C.E., Sutherland, D.E.R., Steffers, M.W., Najarian, J.S. and Bach, F.H. Lack of donor-specific tolerance in mice with established anti-Ia-treated islet allografts. Transplantation 36: 691-694, 1983.

Morrow, C.E., Sutherland, D.E.R., Steffes, M.W., Najarian, J.S. and Bach, F.H. H-2 antigen class: Effect on mouse islet allograft rejection. Science 219: 1337-1339, 1983.

Okazaki, H., Maki, T., Wood, M.L., Jones, S. and Monaco, A.P. Prolongation of skin allograft survival in H-2 K and I region-incompatibile mice by pretransplant blood transfusion. Transplantation 32: 111-115, 1981.

Sollinger, H., Burkholder, P., Rasmus, W., Bach, F. Prolonged survival of xenografts after organ culture. Surgery 81: 74-79, 1977.

Zitron, I.M., Ono, J., Lacy, P.E. and Davie, J.M. The cellular stimuli for the rejection of established islet allografts. Diabetes 30: 242-246, 1981.

I-J: AN INDUCIBLE ISOMORPHIC RECEPTOR INVOLVED IN THE H-2-RESTRICTED CELL INTERACTION AND INHIBITION

Tomio Tada, Yoshihiro Asano, Toshinori Nakayama and Isao Fujisawa

Department of Immunology, Faculty of Medicine
University of Tokyo, Tokyo

INTRODUCTION

I-J still remains to be a premium grade paradox in H-2 genetics. Although it is not a direct product of H-2 genes, its polymorphism is clearly influenced by the intra H-2 genes. Recent functional data suggested that I-J is associated with the inducible T cells receptor for self class II antigens (1,2). It has been found that some of the anti-I-J monoclonal antibodies (mAb) could block the syngeneic and allogeneic mixed lymphocyte reactions (MLR) by reacting with the responder but not with stimulator cells (1). The I-J epitopes on responder cells were inducible in allogeneic bone marrow chimeras (2). Since some of the anti-I-J mAb were able to inhibit the H-2-restricted T helper cell (Th) function, we have recently tested their effect on Th and T cell clones derived from various intra H-2 recombinant mice and their bone marrow chimeras (3). The following are the summary of experimental results which suggest that I-J is an inducible isomorphic marker different from both class II products and conventional class II restricted T cell receptors.

EXPRESSION OF $I\text{-}J^k$ ON H-2-RESTRICTED Th

We have examined the $I\text{-}J^k$ expression on Th cells derived from various H-2 haplotypes, intra-H-2 recombinant strains and their F_1, and radiation bone marrow chimeras constructed by combinations of recombinant mice (3). Table 1 summarizes the results of vast experiments: when Th cells of $H\text{-}2^k$ strains were treated with anti-$I\text{-}J^k$ and complement (C) before cocultivation with hapten-primed B cells, the resulting antibody response was greatly inhibited. The same treatment of $H\text{-}2^b$ (B10) Th cells did not show any alterations suggesting that the I-J epitopes on Th are controlled by H-2 genes.

$I\text{-}J^k$ epitopes are also found on Th cells of $H\text{-}2^{kxb}F_1$ mice restricted to help the $H\text{-}2^k$ B cells. This was demonstrated by both the elimination of $H\text{-}2^k$-restricted Th with anti-$I\text{-}J^k$ and C and the blocking of $H\text{-}2^k$-restricted Th activity without C. The same treatments of F_1 Th cells with anti-$I\text{-}J^k$ did not alter the helper activity for $H\text{-}2^b$ B cells indicating that $I\text{-}J^k$ is exclusively expressed on $H\text{-}2^k$-restricted Th of the F_1 spleen cells. The limiting dilution analysis of $I\text{-}J^k$

Table 1. Expression of the I-J epitope on MHC-restricted T helper cells

Origin of Th[a]		H-2 restriction[b] specificity	$I-J^k$ on Th[c]
B10.A		A^k	+
B10		A^b	–
$(B10xB10.A)F_1$		A^b	–
		A^k	+
$(4Rx5R)F_1$		A^b	+
		A^k	–
B10.A(4R)		A^k	–
B10.A(3R)		A^b	–
B10.A(5R)		A^b	+
B10.A(3R)	→ B10	A^b	–
B10.A(5R)	→ B10	A^b	–
B10.A(3R)	→ B10.A	A^k	+
B10.A(5R)	→ B10.A	A^k	+
$B6AF_1$	→ B10	A^b	–
$B6AF_1$	→ B10.A(3R)	A^b	–
$B6AF_1$	→ B10.A(5R)	A^b	+
$B6AF_1$	→ B10.A(4R)	A^k	–
$B6AF_1$	→ B10.A	A^k	+

[a] T cells from KLH-primed animals. Chimeras are designated as bone marrow donor → irradiated host.

[b] Tested by the helper function to TNP-primed B cells of appropriate haplotype.

[c] Determined by the cytotoxic treatment of Th fraction with anti-$I-J^k$ and C.

positive Th cells in $(B10 \times B10.A)F_1$ capable of helping 4R B cells indicated that virtually all $I-A^k$-restricted Th cells carry the $I-J^k$ epitope. This suggested that $I-J^k$ epitopes are associated with the $H-2^k$ restriction site of Th cells.

However, there was no absolute association between the I-J phenotype and the $H-2^k$ restriction specificity. $I-J^k$ was found on Th of B10.BR and B10.A having the $H-2^k$ restriction specificity, whereas Th from 4R having the same $H-2^k$ restriction specificity was not inhibitable by the same anti-$I-J^k$. Furthermore, Th cells of 5R were shown to be positive for $I-J^k$ regardless of the fact that they are $H-2^b$-restricted. The same $H-2^b$-restricted Th of both 3R and B10 were always negative for $I-J^k$. The results bring us back to the original mapping study of I-J in between I-A and I-E based on the genetic analyses (4,5).

All above findings were verified in radiation bone marrow chimeras where these recombinant mice were used as recipients of bone marrow stem cells of different genotypes. Th cells from chimeras were treated with anti-$I-J^k$ and C to examine whether the I-J phenotype of Th is determined by the H-2 haplotype of the bone marrow donor or of the recipient.

Without any exceptions, the restriction specificity of Th cells was found to follow the host MHC type, and the I-J expression on Th was exactly the same as that expected for the host haplotype (Table 1). By examining the I-J expression of Th cells of $F_1 \rightarrow$ recombinant chimeras, where Th cells were primed in the presence of the identical F_1 type antigen-presenting cells (APC), it was concluded that the I-J expression of at least Th cells is solely determined by the selection in the thymic environment rather than at the priming with APC.

The most striking finding is the linked expression of the parental H-2 restriction specificity and the I-J phenotype in the F_1 Th cell population (see Table 1). This was best exemplified in Th cells in (4R x 5R)F_1, where Th cells were either $H-2^k$- or $H-2^b$-restricted. $I-J^k$ was found only on $H-2^b$-restricted but not on $H-2^k$-restricted Th cells. As the $H-2^b$ restriction specificity was a trait possessed by 5R, the strain with $I-J^k$, there was an absolute linkage between the restriction specificity and the I-J phenotype in F_1 Th cells. If we refer to the original mapping of I-J, the results obtained here indicate that there is only a <u>cis</u>-expression of the restriction specificity and I-J phenotype in the F_1 (e.g., 5R has the linked expression of $I-A^b$ and $I-J^k$, and 4R, $I-A^k$ and $I-J^b$). The experiments with chimeras also support the notion that there is no case where an expression of $I-J^k$ is associated with MHC restriction other than that originally possessed by the host.

EXPRESSION OF $I-J^k$ ON $I-A^k$- AND $I-E^k$-RESTRICTED T CELL CLONES

$I-J^k$ expression on T cell clones has also been studied. These clones have been established from splenic T cells of different H-2 haplotypes, their F_1 and chimeric mice primed with keyhole limpet hemocyanin (KLH) or fowl gamma globulin (FGG). Clones were maintained by occasional stimulation with the homologous antigen on relevant APC followed by the addition of IL-2-containing medium. Some were found to be Th clones, while others were H-2-restricted Ts, as the latters showed a strong inhibitory effect on the secondary antibody response mounted by the syngeneic Th and B cells. Both Th and Ts clones are strictly H-2-restricted in terms of the antigen-induced proliferation and of their ultimate effects in the secondary antibody response. The origins of these clones are also diverse; some are from $H-2^{kxb}$ F_1 and selected by parental APC, and some are of chimeric mouse origin. The nature and properties of these clones are depicted in the left part of Table 2.

All the $H-2^k$-restricted Th clones were found to be positive for the $I-J^k$ expression as determined by the inhibition with anti-$I-J^k$ of the helper function in the secondary antibody response, and blocking of their antigen-induced proliferation. Two $H-2^k$-restricted Ts clones were also found to be $I-J^k$ positive as their proliferative response to the antigen and APC was strongly inhibited by anti-$I-J^k$. Functions of the $H-2^b$-restricted T cell clones were not inhibited by the same anti-$I-J^k$ mAb.

The inhibition of T cell responses by anti-$I-J^k$ was regardless of their haplotype origins and antigen-specificity. For example, a clone MS202 is an auto-I-A-reactive Th cell which produces IL-4. This clone is persistently $I-J^k$ positive as determined by both above responses. Both A^k- and E^k-restricted clones either from F_1 or chimeric mice were also positive for $I-J^k$. $H-2^b$-restricted clones established from the same cell sources were all negative for $I-J^k$.

More recently, we have studied the effect of anti-$I-J^k$ on the Ca^{++} influx induced by the stimulation with antigen and APC. The pretreatment of the $H-2^k$-restricted T cell clones with anti-$I-J^k$ inhibited the movement of Ca^{++} which was associated with the early signal transduction. Again, the same anti-$I-J^k$ had no effect on the Ca^{++} influx of $H-2^b$-restricted T cell clones. The Ca^{++} influx of

Table 2. Expression of I-J^k on H-2^k-restricted Th and Ts Clones

Clones	Origin	Specificity	Function	Effect of anti-I-J^k		
				Ab response[a]	Proliferation[b]	IF[c]
MS202	C3H	A^k	Th	+	+	+
28-4	F_1	A^k + KLH	Th	+	+	+
23-1-8	$F_1 \rightarrow$C3H	A^k + KLH	Th	+	+	−
9-16	F_1	E^k + KLH	Th	+	+	−
23-2	$F_1 \rightarrow$C3H	E^k + KLH	Th	+	+	−
9-5	F_1	A^k + KLH	Ts	—[d]	+	−
25-18	B6$\rightarrow F_1$	E^k + KLH	Ts	—	+	+
8-5	F_1	A^b + KLH	Th	−	−	−
2-19-2	B10	A^b + FGG	Th	−	−	−
24-15-1	$F_1 \rightarrow$B6	A^b	Th	−	−	−
8-4	F_1	A^b + KLH	Ts	—	−	−

[a] DNP-primed B cells were cocultured with Th clones to induce the in vitro secondary antibody response, and anti-I-J^k (JK10-23) was added to the culture. + means the response was inhibited by anti-I-J^k.

[b] Anti-I-J^k (JK10-23) was added to the in vitro stimulation of T cell clones with relevant APC and antigen. + means the positive inhibition of proliferation.

[c] Immunofluorescence staining.

[d] No helper function.

H-2^k-restricted Ts clones was also inhibited.

Some of the T cell clones were positively stained with anti-I-J^k in immunofluorescence (Figure 1), while the fluorescence intensity was always one log scale lower than the staining with anti-T3. Furthermore, anti-T3 at a concentration sufficient to comodulate the the T cell receptor heterodimer did not comodulate the I-J^k molecules. The results indicate that I-J is an inducible receptor for a self component being dictated by H-2 genes while being different from conventional T cell receptor heterodimers.

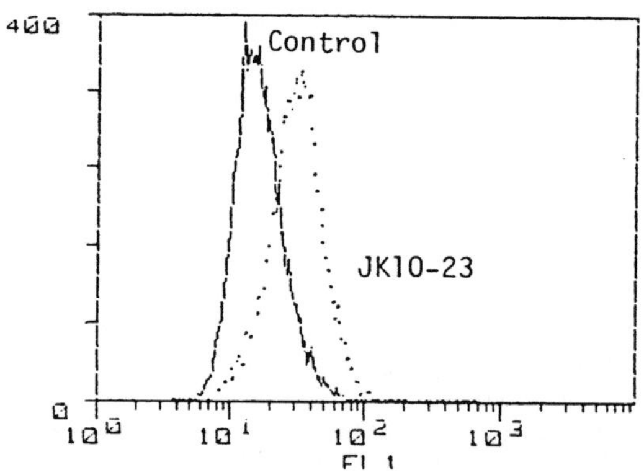

Fig. 1. Fluorescence staining of MS202 with anti-I-J^k

DISCUSSION AND SPECULATION

The above results indicate that I-J is not a product of H-2 genes, but is an inducible isomorphic structure on T cells. It undergoes a systematic adaptive changes during the ontogeny of T cells being influenced by the H-2 genes. I-J seems to be involved in the inhibition of early signal transduction induced by antigen and APC.

If I-J is an inducible receptor for self, is it associated with the T cell receptor heterodimer? The present results do not support this postulate. I-J epitope does not correlate with the restriction specificity both in recombinant mice and in T cell clones. The exclusive <u>cis</u>-expression of I-J and restriction specificity in recombinant F_1 is also hard to explain. The failure to comodulate the I-J with T3 indicates that I-J is not associated with conventional T cell receptor. Finally, it is difficult to explain that I-J is expressed on virtually all the $H\text{-}2^k$-restricted Th cells which utilize a variety of T cell receptor V_α and V_β genes.

What, then, does the I-J represent? The prevalence of the I-J among class II-restricted population of T cells indicates that I-J is an isomorphic structure shared by a large population of T cells having class II MHC-restricted functions involved either in help or suppression. Our more recent results indicated that the generation of both suppressor and augmenting regulatory T cells was inhibitable by the administration of the anti-I-J mAb into the in vitro culture of primed lymphocytes. Since these regulatory T cells are selectively interacting with specified target cells, the isomorphism of I-J should be an ideal device to direct their cell interactions. Thus, one of the roles of I-J appears to be involved in the construction of MHC-restricted regulatory circuits.

The other possibility is that I-J is indeed the second T cell receptor for self, which plays a role to transmit a negative signal in the cell activation. All T cells are known to be selected to recognize self MHC antigens in the thymus. However, it is not known why these T cells do not respond to self MHC in peripheral lymphoid tissues. It has been argued that such T cells with a high affinity for self MHC are negatively selected. No compelling evidence for it has been presented. If I-J is the second receptor for self, the activation of T cells by self MHC can always be inhibited by the negative signal given through the I-J receptor that recognizes the similar but not identical self determinants on APC. The I-J interacting molecule (IJIM) suggested by Dorf and his colleagues (6) may have such a role in educating Th and Ts for this negative signalling.

The low density of I-J on cloned Th has prevented the biochemical and molecular analyses. However, we think that the I-J issue discussed here would encourage further studies on the specialized MHC restriction site for the negative signal transduction in addition to known T cell receptor molecules.

REFERENCE

1. W. Uracz, R. Abe, and T. Tada, Involvement of I-J epitopes in the self- and allo-recognition sites of T cells: blocking of syngenic and allogeneic mixed lymphocyte reaction-responder cells by monoclonal anti-I-J antibodies. <u>Proc. Natl. Acad. Sci. USA</u> 82:2905 (1985).
2. W. Uracz, Y. Asano, R. Abe, and T. Tada, I-J epitopes are adaptively acquired by T cells differentiated in the chimeric condition. <u>Nature</u> 316:741 (1985).

3. Y. Asano, T. Nakayama, M. Kubo, J. Yagi, and T. Tada, Epitopes associated with MHC restriction site of T cells. III. I-J epitope on MHC-restricted T helper cells. (submitted).
4. D.B. Murphy, L.A. Herzenberg, K. Okumura, L.A. Herzenberg, and H.O. McDevitt, A new I subregion (I-J) marked by a locus (Ia-4) controlling surface determinants on suppressor T lymphocytes. J. Exp. Med. 144:699 (1976).
5. T. Tada, M. Taniguchi, and C.S. David, Properties of the antigen-specific suppressive T-cell factor in the regulation of antibody responses in the mouse. IV. Special subregion assignment of the gene(s) that codes for the suppressive T cell factor in the H-2 histocompatibility complex. J. Exp. Med. 144:713 (1976).
6. H. Kawasaki, K. Zupko, B. Diamond, M. Minami, and M.E. Dorf, Antibody inhibition of suppressor cell induction. J. Immunol. 138: 2063 (1987).

RECOGNITION OF MHC CLASS II ANTIGENS BY THE CD4: T CELL RECEPTOR COMPLEX

Charles A. Janeway, Jr, Pilar Portoles, John P. Tite,
Jose Rojo, Kaj Saizawa, and Barry Jones

Section of Immunobiology and Department of Pathology
Howard Hughes Medical Institute at Yale University
School of Medicine, New Haven, CT 06510, USA

ABSTRACT

T lymphocytes that express CD4 respond to foreign antigens presented in the context of syngeneic class II MHC molecules. T cells responding to allogeneic class II MHC molecules generally express CD4, but exceptions are observed. We show that the same receptor on a cloned T cell line recognizes both foreign antigen associated with self-class II MHC and nonself-class II MHC molecules. The role of CD4 in these recognition responses appears to be to bind to class II MHC molecules and, through association with the T cell receptor recognizing the same class II MHC molecule, to effectively activate the T cell. It is proposed on the basis of these two findings that the high ligand multiplicity of alloantigens recognized in unmodified form by high affinity anti-nonself-MHC receptors can explain the finding of $CD8^+$ T cells responding to nonself-class II MHC molecules, as well as the inability of anti-CD4 to inhibit such nonself-class II MHC recognition completely. Finally, data will be presented to suggest that class II may also play a role in selecting the functional activity elicited in response to a protein antigen in vivo. These data show that the CD4:T cell receptor complex interaction with the complex of foreign antigen and self-MHC is the critical event in initiating most immune responses and may also play a role in controlling their functional outcome.

INTRODUCTION

T lymphocytes bearing heterodimeric receptors made up of α and ß T cell receptor chains associated with the molecules of the CD3 complex can be subdivided into two major populations on the basis of the mutually exclusive expression of the molecules CD4 and CD8 (Swain 1983). Conventionally, $CD4^+$ T cells are referred to as helper cells. While helper function is found predominantly in the $CD4^+$ subset, $CD4^+$ T cells have also been shown to suppress antibody responses (Bottomly et al. 1983, Asano and Hodes 1983), to kill activated B cells (Tite et al. 1984, Tite et al. 1985) and to mediate delayed-type hypersensitivity reactions (Cher and Mosmann 1987, Ratzlaff et al. unpublished). Thus, the $CD4^+$ subset of T cells is functionally heterogeneous. Analyses of cloned $CD4^+$ T cell lines suggest that such cells fall into two major categories (Kim et al. 1985, Mosmann et al. 1986), both of which activate B cells to produce polyclonal immunoglobulin, but only one of which, termed the helper $CD4^+$ T cell subset, can help antigen specific B cells synthesize specific antibody (Kim et al. 1985). The other subset contains cells that kill, suppress, and mediate delayed-type hypersensitivity reactions; we term this subset the inflammatory $CD4^+$ T cell subset.

Expression of CD4 molecules correlates most strongly with the recognition of foreign antigens in the context of self-class II MHC molecules (Swain 1983). A somewhat weaker correlation exists between the expression of CD4 and the recognition of allogeneic or nonself-class II MHC molecules (Golding and Singer 1985). Anti-CD4 antibodies are highly effective at inhibiting the recognition of antigen in the context of self-class II MHC molecules, and significantly less effective at inhibiting the recognition of nonself-class II MHC molecules (Janeway and Katz 1985). Taken together, these results suggest that CD4 might be directly involved in the recognition of class II MHC molecules, and that such class II MHC recognition would be directed at nonpolymorphic portions of class II MHC molecules. Based on an analysis of a rare cloned line that recognizes class I MHC molecules but expresses CD4, it has been suggested that the function of CD4 is to bind class II MHC molecules independently of the T cell receptor, and to stabilze the interaction between $CD4^+$ T cells and class II MHC bearing antigen presenting cells (Greenstein et al. 1985, Gay et al. 1987). This is consistent with the finding that CD4 molecules migrate on the cell surface independently of the T cell receptor:CD3 complex.

Our studies have examined several of the issues mentioned above. Here, the results of several such studies will be summarized. First, we will examine the question of whether a single receptor on a cloned T cell line recognizes both antigen in association with self-MHC molecules and nonself-MHC molecules on a cloned T cell line. Second, experiments suggesting the physical association of CD4 with the α and β chains of the T cell receptor will be described. Third, these studies will be used to suggest that the finding of cloned lines of T cells responding to unmodified class I molecules and expressing CD4, or unmodified class II molecules and expressing CD8 can be predicted on the basis of these two sets of findings. Finally, we will summarize data suggesting that class II MHC molecules also play a role in selecting the functional subset of $CD4^+$ T cells activated in the response to a defined protein antigen. Taken together, these studies demonstrate that the critical events of an immune response, involving activation to effector function of $CD4^+$ T cells, involves the interaction between antigen associated with class II MHC with the CD4:T cell receptor complex.

MATERIALS AND METHODS

Details of materials and methods in all of the experiments described in this manuscript can be found in the appropriate primary publication of these data, and will be designated by references.

RESULTS AND DISCUSSION

A Single Receptor on a $CD4^+$ $CD8^-$ Cloned T Cell Line Can Recognize Foreign Protein Antigen Associated with Self-MHC Molecules and Nonself-MHC Molecules.

One of the more surprising attributes of the immune system is the extremely high frequency of T cells responsive to particular nonself-MHC molecules (Wilson 1974). Indeed, this high frequency of recognition of allogeneic MHC molecules suggested to some early observers that the clonal selection theory could not apply. Subsequent studies suggested that populations of cells selected for alloreactivity could in addition respond to antigen in the context of self-class II MHC molecules (Heber-Katz and Wilson 1976, Bottomly and Janeway 1981). This has now been confirmed at the level of individual cloned T cell lines (Sredni and Schwartz 1981, Janeway et al. 1982), and the frequency of alloreactivity directed at a particular nonself-class II MHC molecule is comparable to that seen in an unselected population of T cells from an animal of the same strain. This observation left open the possibility that T cells express two distinct receptors, one recognizing antigen in the context of self-class II MHC, and the other recognizing nonself-class II MHC molecules. The advent of monoclonal anti-T cell receptor antibodies allowed a direct examination of this question. As originally demonstrated by Kaye and Janeway (1984), monoclonal antibodies directed at a single α:ß heterodimeric T cell receptor could inhibit the response of the cloned line expressing that receptor to both the foreign protein antigen conalbumin presented in the context of syngeneic class II MHC molecules, and the response to allogeneic class II MHC molecules. Recently, we have extended these findings in several ways. First, we have demonstrated that the cloned T cell line responds to five different nonself-I-A molecules. Secondly, we have shown that all of these recognition events involve the same α:ß heterodimeric T cell receptor. Third, we have shown that the more potent an allogeneic class II MHC molecule is at stimulating this cloned T cell line, the higher the affinity of the receptor for the nonself-I-A molecule. As originally described by Kaye and Janeway, the recognition of nonself-class II MHC molecules by this cloned T cell line represents a lower affinity binding event than that involving the recognition of conalbumin in the context of syngeneic class II MHC molecules. Thus, for this cloned T cell line, the recognition of nonself-class II MHC molecules represents the low affinity interaction of a receptor having a high affinity for specifically modified self-class II MHC molecules with apparently unmodified nonself-class II MHC molecules presented at a high ligand multiplicity on the surface of an allogeneic antigen presenting cell. This could account for a good deal of nonself-class II MHC recognition on the basis of two principles. First, that T cell receptors are inherently biased towards MHC recognition, either through evolutionary or ontogenetic selection, and secondly, that nonself-MHC molecules are presented at very high ligand multiplicity, and therefore require significantly lower affinity to generate sufficient T cell receptor cross-linking for T cell activation. This interpretation will be significantly augmented in a subsequent section of this paper.

CD4 is Part of the Receptor for Antigen:Self-Class II MHC

As mentioned in the introdution, a number of findings have suggested that CD4 recognizes class II MHC molecules independently of the T cell receptor, and contributes to class II MHC recognition by promoting the interaction between $CD4^+$ T cells and class II MHC.

molecules. Unfortunately, such hypotheses can not explain the absolute association of CD4 expression and the recognition of foreign protein antigen in the context of self-class II MHC molecules. This follows because class II MHC-bearing cells also express class I MHC, the putative target of CD8 molecules. Thus, independent recognition of MHC molecules by the receptor and CD4 or CD8 could not explain the association of CD4 with self-class II MHC recognition. In analyzing the response of cloned T cell lines to antigen in the context of syngeneic class II MHC molecules, allogeneic MHC molecules, and anti-T cell receptor antibodies, we have come to a different conclusion. Our findings, summarized in Table 1, strongly suggests that CD4 is an essential part of the receptor for antigen:class II MHC recognition.

Table 1

Evidence that CD4 is Part of the T Cell Receptor for Antigen:Class II MHC

1. The effect of anti-CD4 on the response of a cloned T cell line to anti-receptor antibodies is determined by the epitope recognized on the T cell receptor V region (Janeway et al. 1987, Rojo and Janeway submitted for publication).

2. Fab fragments of anti-CD4 can block responses induced by antibodies directed at a particular T cell receptor V region epitope, but do not negative signal (Haque et al. submitted for publication, Tite et al. 1986).

3. Some anti-receptor antibodies are 30 - 100 fold more potent in T cell activation than others, depending on the V region epitope recognized; high potency antibodies co-modulate CD4 and the receptor, while low potency antibodies do not (Rojo and Janeway submitted for publication, Saizawa et al. in press).

4. The Fab fragment of a high potency anti-T cell receptor antibody allows activation of T cells in the presence of bivalent, but not monovalent, anti-CD4 (Haque et al. submitted for publication, Saizawa et al. in press).

5. On T cells expressing both CD4 and CD8 and recognizing antigen plus self-class II MHC, anti-CD4 is 25 - 100 fold more active at inhibiting activation than anti-CD8 (Fazekas de St. Groth et al. 1986, Jones et al. in press).

6. During antigen:class II MHC recognition, CD4 colocalizes with the T cell receptor in the contact site (Kupfer et al. in press).

During physiological antigen:class II MHC recognition, we propose that CD4 molecules bind to the same class II MHC molecule being recognized by the T cell receptor, albeit to a nonpolymorphic portion of that molecule. This joint recognition of class II MHC molecules by CD4 and the T cell receptor brings them into close proximity, which in some way not yet defined, greatly increases the potency of transmembrane signalling via the receptor. We have estimated the increase in sensitivity for T cell activation that results from the co-localization of CD4 and the T cell receptor. Two distinct approaches show that cross-linking CD4 and the T cell receptor is 30 to 100 times as effective as cross-linking the T cell receptor alone. That is to say, comparable levels of T cell activation are obtained by the cross-linking of 100 T cell receptor:CD4 complexes or 3,000 to 10,000 T cell receptor complexes alone. Given that CD4 and CD8 behave in what appears to be an analogous manner, these findings make it extremely unlikely though not impossible that cloned T cells expressing only CD8 will respond to antigen + self-class II MHC.

The High Ligand Multipicity of Unmodified MHC Molecules and the Role of CD4 and CD8 in T cell Triggering Suggests that Recognition of Class II MHC Molecules Independent of CD4 Will Involve Recognition of Alloantigen Predominantly

In the first two sections of this paper, we have presented our findings on nonself-class II MHC recognition by a $CD4^+$ cloned T cell line, and on the importance of co-localization of CD4 and the T cell receptor in T cell activation. Basically, the results of these experiments suggest that recognition of nonself-class II MHC molecules involves the direct recognition of MHC molecules by the T cell receptor at high ligand multiplicity. As the cloned T cell line used in these experiments was selected by immunization and culture for high affinity recognition of antigen:self-class II MHC molecules, it is perhaps not suprising that recognition of nonself-MHC molecules involves a lower affinity interaction of the receptor with its ligand. However, direct stimulation of T cells with nonself-MHC molecules could easily reveal cloned T cell lines whose affinity for unmodified nonself-class II MHC molecules could be quite high. Under such conditions, very extensive cross-linking of the T cell receptor would be predicted to occur. As discussed in the second section of this paper, such high multiplicity cross-linking of the T cell receptor can apparently lead to activation of T cells in the absence of CD4 co-localization. Thus, one would predict that T cells recognizing nonself-class II MHC might in some cases not express CD4. Indeed, at the present time all reported responses of $CD8^+$ T cells to class II MHC molecules involve the recognition of allogeneic or autologous unmodified MHC molecules (Greenstein et al. 1985, Schilham et al. 1986, Aparicio et al. 1987). Furthermore, anti-CD4 antibodies inhibit nonself-class II MHC recognition in unfractionated T cell responses far less effectively than they inhibit the response to antigen plus self-class II MHC molecules. Interestingly, when T cells from animals partially tolerized to nonself-class II MHC molecules, a procedure that would be predicted to deplete clones with high affinity receptors for nonself-MHC, are stimulated in mixed lymphocyte culture, the response becomes readily inhibitable by anti-CD4 antibodies (Sprent personal communication). Likewise, we have examined the effect of anti-CD4 on the response of T cells to various stimulating ligands, and find that anti-CD4 most readily inhibits those responses to class II MHC molecules which interact with the T cell receptor at lowest affinity. Thus, our model of CD4 as an essential component of the receptor for recognition of antigen:class II MHC molecules explains not only the association of CD4 with antigen:class II MHC recognition, but also those exceptional cases in which class II recognition is not associated with CD4 expression.

Class II MHC Molecule Polymorphism Appears to Play a Role in the Selective Activation of Functionally Distinct $CD4^+$ T Cells

As described in the Introduction, $CD4^+$ T cells have recently been shown to consist of two major subpoplations (Kim et al. 1985, Mosmann et al 1986), termed helper T cells and inflammatory T cells (Tite et al. submitted for publication). As the functional outcome of an immune response will depend critically upon which of these two $CD4^+$ T cell subsets is activated by exposure to antigen, the control of this process is critical to manipulation of the immune response. Because function appears to be independent of the specificity of antigen recognition, one might not expect to find that the functional outcome of an immune response would be determined by polymorphism in class II MHC molecules. Thus, we were surprised to observe that immunization of inbred strains of mice with human basement membrane collagen type IV gave rise to two reciprocal immune response patterns, both under the control of MHC class II genes. Mice expressing the $I\text{-}A^s$ molecule give potent lymph node proliferative responses, but produce no anti-type IV collagen antibody. Inbred mice not expressing $I\text{-}A^s$ produce T cell dependent antibody responses to basement membrane collagen, but do not show lymph node proliferative responses. We have independently shown that the lymph node proliferative response reflects largely or entirely the activation of inflammatory type $CD4^+$ T cells, while the generation of antibody reflects the activation of $CD4^+$ helper T cells. Thus, in this system, the particular antigen:MHC complex generated appears to determine which functional subset of T cells becomes activated. Finally, it should be noted that F1 hybrids between $I\text{-}A^s$ and $I\text{-}A^{non\text{-}s}$ mice give rise to offspring that make potent lymph node proliferative responses but fail to synthesize significant levels of anti-collagen antibody. This result is consistent with our earlier observation that activated inflammatory type $CD4^+$ T cells can suppress the helper activity of $CD4^+$ helper T cells in antibody responses. While these experiments have not definitively been shown to depend upon selective activation of the two $CD4^+$ T cell subsets, they may well provide a clue as to the mechanism by which these two subsets are selectively activated. We are currently analyzing this system in detail to find the answer to these two questions.

In summary, the present findings demonstrate that the activation of $CD4^+$ T cells involves the α:β heterodimeric T cell receptor working together with the CD4 molecule in the recognition of class II MHC molecules. The coordinate recognition of class II MHC by these two molecules enhances signalling by approximately 100 fold, allowing the T cell receptor to respond to ligands presented at very low multiplicity, such as one might expect to be generated by the association of antigenic peptides with self-class II MHC molecules. Indeed, the functions of CD4 and CD8 may be centrally involved in the preoccupation of T cells with MHC molecules. While CD4 does not appear to be directly involved in functional determination, our results in the immune response to human basement membrane collagen suggests that the overall functional phenotype of an immune response can also be determined by class II MHC molecules through the selective activation of functionally distinct $CD4^+$ T cell subsets. These results provide further evidence for the central importance of the interplay between $CD4^+$ T cells and class II MHC molecules.

ACKNOWLEDGEMENTS

These studies were supported in part by NIH grants AI-14579 and CA-29606, the Howard Hughes Medical Institute, and a gift from the Johnson & Johnson Company. P.P. is the recipient of a postdoctoral fellowship of the Spanish Research Council (CSIC) and J.R. is the recipient of a Fulbright award. The authors would like to thank Pat Conrad, Nancy Lindberg and Barbara Broughton for technical help in their studies, John Tite, Harald Foellmer and Joe Madri for assistance in some of the studies, and Don Murphy and Kim Bottomly for invaluable discussions. The manuscript was kindly prepared by Liza Cluggish.

REFERENCES

Aparicio, P., Jaraquemada, D., and Lopez de Castro, J.A.: Alloreactive cytolytic T cell clones with dual recognition of HLA-B27 and HLA-DR2 antigens. Selective involvement of CD8 in their class I directed cytotoxicity. J. Exp. Med. 165:428, 1987.

Asano, Y., and Hodes, R.J.: T cell regulation of B cell activation. Cloned Lyt-1^{+}2^{-} suppressor cells inhibit the major histocompatibility complex restricted interactions of T helper cells with B cells and/or accessory cells. J. Exp. Med. 158:1178, 1983.

Bottomly, K., Kaye, J., Jones, F., III, Jones, B., and Janeway, C.A., Jr.: A cloned antigen-specific Ia-restricted Lyt-1^{+}, 2^{-} T cell with suppressive activity. J. Mol. Cell. Immunol. 1:42, 1983.

Bottomly, K., and Janeway, C.A.: Selected populations of alloreactive T cells contain helper T cells but lack ThId, an antigen-specific helper T cell required for dominant production of the T15 idiotype. Eur. J. Immunol. 11:270, 1981.

Cher, D.J., and Mosmann, T.R.: Two types of murine helper T cell clone. II. Delayed-type hypersensitivity is mediated by Th 1 clones. J. Immunol. 138:3688, 1987.

Fazekas de St. Groth, B., Gallagher, P.F., and Miller, J.F.A.P.: Involvement of Lyt-2 and L3T4 in activation of hatpen-specific Lyt-2^{+}, L3T4^{+} T cell clones. Proc. Nat. Acad. Sci. (USA) 83:2584, 1986.

Gay, D., Kappler, J., and Marrack, P.: L3T4 interacts with class II molecules on target cells. Ann. Inst. Pasteur (Immunology) 138:127, 1987.

Golding, H., and Singer, A.: Specificity, phenotype and precursor frequency of primary cytolytic T lymphocytes specific for class II major histocompatibility antigens. J. Immunol. 135:1610, 1985.

Greenstein, J.L., Malissen, B., and Burakoff, S.F.: Role of L3T4 in antigen-driven activation of a class I-specific T cell hybridoma. J. Exp. Med. 162:369, 1985.

Haque, S., Saizawa, K., Rojo, J., and Janeway, C.A., Jr.: The influence of valence on the functional activities of monoclonal anti-L3T4 antibodies: discrimination of signaling from other effects. Submitted for publication.

Heber-Katz, E., and Wilson, D.B.: Sheep red blood cell-specific helper activity in rat thoracic duct lymphocyte populations positively selected for reactivity to strong specific histocompatibiltiy alloantigens. J. Exp. Med. 143:701, 1976.

Janeway, C.A., Jr., and Katz, M.E.: The immunobiology of the T cell response to Mls-locus disparate stimulator cells. I. Unidirectionality, new strain combinations, and the role of Ia antigens. J. Immunol. 134:2057, 1985.

Janeway, C.A., Jr., Lerner, E.A., Conrad, P.J., and Jones, B.: The precision of self and nonself major histocompatibility complex encoded antigen recognition by cloned T cells. Behring Inst. Mitteilungen 70:200, 1982.

Janeway, C.A., Jr., Haque, S., Smith, L.A., and Saizawa, K.: The role of the murine L3T4 molecule in T cell activation: Differential effects of anti-L3T4 on activation by monoclonal anti-receptor antibodies: J. Mol. Cell. Immunol. 3:121, 1987.

Jones, B., Khavari, P.A., Conrad, P.J., and Janeway, C.A., Jr.: Differential effects of antibodies to Lyt-2 and L3T4 on cytolysis by cloned, Ia-restricted T cells expressing both proteins. J. Immunol. In press.

Kaye, J., and Janeway, C.A., Jr.: The Fab fragment of a directly activating monoclonal antibody that precipitates a disulfide-lined heterodimer from a helper T cell clone blocks activation by either allogeneic-Ia or antigen and self-Ia. J. Exp. Med. 159:1397, 1984.

Kim, J., Woods, A., Becker-Dunn, E., and Bottomly, K. Distinct functional phenotypes of cloned Ia-restricted helper T cells. J. Exp. Med. 162:188, 1985.

Kupfer, A., Singer, S.J., Janeway, C.A., Jr., and Swain, S.L.: Co-clustering of CD4 (L3T4) with the T cell receptor is induced by specific direct interaction of helper T cells and antigen presenting cells. Proc. Nat. Acad. Sci. (USA). In press.

Mosmann, T.R., Cherwinski, H., Bond, M.W., Giedlin, M.A., and Coffman, R.L.: Two types of murine helper T cell clone. I. Definition according to profiles of lymphokine activities and secreted proteins. J. Immunol. 136:2340, 1986.

Ratzlaff, R., Porcelli, S., Bottomly, K., Askenase, P.W., and Janeway, C.A., Jr. Unpublished observations.

Rojo, J., and Janeway, C.A., Jr.: The biological activity of anti-T cell receptor variable region antibodies is determined by the epitope recognized. Submitted for publication.

Saizawa, K., Rojo, J., Janeway, C.A., Jr.: Physical association of CD4 and the CD3:α:ß T cell receptor. Nature (Lond). In press.

Schilham, M.W., Lang, R., Benner, R., Zinkernagel, R.M., and Hengartner, H.: Characterization of an Lyt-2^+ alloreactive cytotoxic T cell clone specific for H-$2D^b$ that cross-reacts with I-E^k. J. Immunol. 137:2748, 1986.

Sredni, B, and Schwartz, H.: Antigen-specific, proliferating T lymphocyte clones. Methodology, specificity, MHC restriction and alloreactivity. Immunol. Rev. 54:187, 1981.

Swain, S.A.: T cell subsets and the recognition of MHC class. Immunol. Rev. 74:129, 1983.

Tite, J.P., and Janeway, C.J., Jr.: Cloned helper T cells can kill B lymphoma cells in the presence of specific antigen: Ia restriction and cognate vs. non-cognate interactions in cytolysis. Eur. J. Immunol. 14:878, 1984.

Tite, J.P., Powell, M.B., and Ruddle, N.H.: Protein-antigen specific Ia-restricted cytolytic T cells: Analysis of frequency, target cell susceptibility and mechanism of cytolysis. J. Immunol. 135:25, 1985.

Tite, J.P., Sloan, A, and Janeway, C.A., Jr.: The role of L3T4 in T cell activation: L3T4 may be both an Ia-binding protein and a receptor that transduces a negative signal. J. Mol. Cell. Immunol. 2:179, 1986.

Tite, J.P., H.G. Foellmer, J.A. Madri, and C.A. Janeway, Jr. 1987. Inverse Ir gene control of the antibody and T cell proliferative responses to human basement membrane collagen. Submitted for publication.

Wilson, D.B.: Immunologic reactivity to major histocompatibility alloantigens: HARC, effector cells and the problem of memory. Prog. Immunol. 2:45, 1974.

EPITOPES OF I-A^k INVOLVED IN ANTIGEN PRESENTATION TO T-CELL HYBRIDOMAS

John H. Freed,[1] Edward F. Rosloniec,[1] Denise Gay,[1] Laura J. Vitez,[1] David J. McKean [2] and Diane Mathis[3]

[1]National Jewish Center for Immunology and Respiratory Medicine, Denver, CO

[2]Department of Immunology, Mayo Clinic, Rochester, MN; and

[3]Laboratoire de Génétique Moléculaire des Eucaryotes du CNRS, INSERM, Strasbourg, Cédex, France

INTRODUCTION

The discovery of MHC-restricted recognition of foreign antigens by cytotoxic and helper T lymphocytes marked a fundamental breakthrough in our understanding of antigen recognition by T cells and simultaneously provided the first convincing explanation for the physiologic function of MHC Class I and Class II molecules. However, fourteen years after the first description of MHC-restricted antigen recognition, the molecular details of the implied ternary complex involved in that recognition, i.e. processed antigen, MHC product, and T cell receptor, have yet to be described in depth. Primarily due to technical complexities of the system, it is only in the last two to three years that the problem has been examined at the biochemical level. Three basic approaches have been taken thus far. The first has been an examination of how the structure of the antigen itself influences the antigen presentation process, specifically which residues contact the T cell receptor or the Ia molecule (Ashwell et al. 1986, Guillet et al. 1986, Sette et al. 1987). The second approach has been to carry out molecular modelling of the T cell receptor in order to predict its potential binding sites (Novotny et al. 1986). The third approach has been to examine what effect Ia structure has on antigen presentation (Allen et al. 1985, Beck et al. 1986, Cohn et al. 1986, and Lechler et al. 1986) and specifically on the interaction of Ia with processed antigen (Buus et al. 1987) and with the T cell receptor. Our laboratories have recently adopted the third approach to dissecting the ternary complex of Ia, processed antigen and T cell receptor.

RESULTS

The experiments described here make use of an *in vitro* antigen presentation system originally described by Kappler and Marrack (Kappler et al. 1982) in which Ia positive B cell lymphomas (or other culture-adapted Ia positive cells) are used to present antigen to antigen-specific, MHC-restricted T-cell hybridomas. Upon activation the T-cell hybridomas release IL-2 which is measured by titrating the culture supernatant with the IL-2-dependent indicator cell line HT-2. This assay provides a semi-quantitative measure of T cell activation which is assumed to be proportional to IL-2 secretion.

The particular system chosen for study employs a panel of I-A^k-restricted T-cell hybridomas specific for processed hen eggwhite lysozyme (HEL) and which, in all but one case, may be stimulated by a tryptic fragment of HEL even when fixed cells are used as the antigen presenting cells (APC) suggesting that the tryptic fragment contains the epitope(s) required for T-cell activation. This basic read-out system has allowed us to use two separate, but essentially complementary, methods to probe the role of Ia structure on antigen presentation. The first of these is to use APC expressing I-A^k with mutant or chimeric α or β chains to determine the impact that these alterations have on antigen presentation. The second method is to treat wild type I-A^k with monoclonal antibodies to determine the effect that these potential inhibitors have on antigen presentation and/or antigen binding by the I-A^k molecule.

Antigen Presentation by I-A^k Molecules with Alpha or Beta Chain Mutations

Cells expressing altered I-A^k molecules were used as antigen presenting cells for the HEL-specific T-cell hybridomas in our panel. All of the mutants were produced by treating the H-2^k/H-2^d heterozygous B-cell hybridoma TA3 with ethyl methanesulfonate (EMS) in culture. A protocol employing sequential negative and positive selection with monoclonal antibodies allowed isolation of surviving cells expressing mutant I-A^k molecules that had lost some antibody-defined determinants while retaining others (Beck et al. 1984). Some of the mutants were selected and their I-A molecules were further characterized by biochemical methods. Both α and β chain mutants were obtained and for several of the mutants the site of mutation was localized by sequencing of cDNA. This revealed that the two A_α chain mutants JE50 and JE67 (Table 1), had two and one amino acid interchanges respectively, in the third hypervariable region of the α1 domain (Landais et al. 1986). The A_β chain mutants, G1, K2, LD3, A19 and F16.3, all had single amino acid interchanges in the region of positions 59 to 68 in the β1 domain (Beck et al. 1987).

Each of the lymphomas with mutant $I\text{-}A^k$ was used to present lysozyme (or lysozyme peptides) to the panel of T-cell hybridomas. The results shown in Table 1 allow several conclusions to be drawn. First, each of the T cell hybridomas had a unique response phenotype as measured by the mutant $I\text{-}A^k$ molecules. This statement, most significantly, is true for the three hybridomas which respond to the HEL peptide containing lysozyme residues 46-61, denoted HEL(46-61). Second, each of the lymphomas bearing mutant $I\text{-}A^k$ molecules shows a unique antigen presentation pattern although the phenotypes (but not the mutations) of F16.3 and JE67 are highly similar. Third, there is a partial correlation between the nature of the mutation and the effect it has on the function of the $I\text{-}A^k$ molecule. For example, mutant F16.3 which has the conservative glutamic acid to aspartic acid interchange in a position (#59) that lies somewhat outside of the allelic hypervariable regions of the β chain, demonstrates a wild-type antigen-presenting phenotype. Conversely, K2 and A19 which have non-conservative interchanges within the apparently key region of the ᵅ chain between position #65 and #68 (A^k_β numbering), are able to present to very few of the T-cell hybridomas in our panel. The data in Table 1 suggests that some substitutions at the neighboring position #64 do not produce significant disruption of antigen presentation capability, at least as measured by the T-cell hybrids in our panel. Similarly, the A^k_α mutants show two discrete phenotypes with JE50 displaying a highly disrupted antigen presentation profile while JE67 shows a nearly wild type antigen presentation phenotype.

<u>Antigen Presentation by $I\text{-}A^k$ Molecules with Chimeric A_α Chains</u>

The second set of variant $I\text{-}A^k$ molecules tested for antigen presentation capacity were produced using the method of "cassette shuffling". Using this technique chimeric α chains were produced in which the first, second or third allelic hypervariable regions of the α1 domain (Landais et al. 1986) were switched between the "b" and"k" alleles giving rise to chimeric chains. For example, if the first

Table 1. T-Cell Hybridoma Responses to HEL Peptides Presented by Cells Bearing EMS-Generated Mutant I-A^k Molecules

		IL-2, U/ml							
		A_β^k Mutant APC (Position of Mutation; Amino Acid Interchange)					A_α^k Mutant APC (Pos.; Change)		Wild Type APC
T-Hybrid	HEL Peptide Specificity	G1 (64 Q→R)	K2 (68 R→Q)	LD3 (64 Q→P)	A19 (67 E→K)	F16.3 (59 E→D)	JE50 (69 T→I) (79 K→Q)	JE67 (75 E→K)	TA3
h4Ly7.5	34-45	1280	-[a]	-	-	320	-	160	80
kLy7.4	46-61	640	-	1280	-	640	-	640	640
h4Ly50.5	46-61	2565	-	1536	770	250	-	1020	1448
kLy4.10	46-61	-	-	-	-	212	-	80	80
kLy1.3	74-96?[b]	640	320	320	640	320	40	40	320
kLy6.10	74-96?	-	-	160	-	160	-	80	80
h4Ly18.2	?	535	784	182	-	1750	398	747	702

[a] "-" = Less than 20 U/ml of IL-2

[b] Antigen peptide specificity not yet confirmed by synthetic peptide.

Table 2. T-Cell Hybridoma Responses to HEL Peptides Presented by Cells Bearing I-A with Chimeric A_α Chains

	IL-2, U/ml						
	Antigen Presenting Cell						
T-hybrid	kkk[a]	bkk	kbk	bbk	kbb	bkb	kkb
h4Ly50.5	160	320	-[b]	40	-	-	-
kLy18.4	80	80	-	-	-	-	-
kLy1.1	1280	80	80	-	-	-	-
kLy7.4	640	640	-	-	-	-	-
kLy1.2	160	160	160	20	-	-	-
kLy4.3	40	40	40	-	-	-	-
kLy17.5	320	320	-	-	-	-	-
kLy11.3	80	80	160	160	-	-	-

[a] The three letters represent the allelic form of each of the three hypervariable regions of the A_α chain.

[b] "-" = Less than 20 U/ml of IL-2.

allelic hypervariable region of the b allele was added to a molecule which contains the sequence of the k allele in the second and third allelic hypervariable regions this gives rise to a molecule which would be denoted "bkk" in the short-hand notation used in Table 2. Although the constructs were prepared in such a way that the α2, transmembrane and cytoplasmic domains were derived from the donor of the third allelic hypervariable region, this should cause little difficulty as there is only a single amino acid difference between the chains outside the hypervariable regions of the α1 domain, viz., a Thr to Ala interchange between the k and b alleles at position #133.

Each of the "parental type" mixed molecules, e.g., $A_\alpha^k A_\beta^b$ or $A_\alpha^b A_\beta^k$, were typed and the responses of our panel of hybrids were found to be specific for the $A_\alpha^k A_\beta^k$ molecule (data not shown). Each of the constructs bearing a chimeric A_α chain, associated with the A_β^k chain, was tested for its capacity to present HEL fragments to our panel of T-cell hybridomas. The results, which are summarized in Table 2, indicate that the major influence on antigen presentation is exerted by the third allelic hypervariable region (positions #69 to #79), with a lesser influence being produced by the second (positions #53 to #59). Thus the I-A molecule in which the b allele has been substituted for the first allelic hypervariable region (bkk) displays a nearly wild type (kkk) phenotype, showing a diminished antigen presentation capacity only with the kLy1.1 T-cell hybridoma. Substitution of the b allele for the second allelic hypervariable region (kbk) causes a more pronounced loss of wild type presentation phenotype. These effects appear to be additive as the substitution of the b allele in both the first and second regions (bbk) further reduces the number of responding T-cell hybridomas. However, the substitution of the b allele in the third allelic hypervariable region (kkb, bkb, or kbb) has the most profound effect on antigen presentation: none of the APCs expressing these chimeric α chains present HEL peptides to any of the T-cell hybridomas in our panel.

While these results are striking, one must exercise caution about over-generalizing the role of the third allelic hypervariable region of the A_α chain in antigen presentation. Other studies (Landais et al. 1986) employing I-A^k-specific, alloreactive T-cell hybridomas have demonstrated that the second allelic hypervariable region exerts an influence roughly comparable to that seen here for the third region.

Anti-I-A^k Monoclonal Antibodies as Probes of Ia Function

In this, the second general method for understanding the role of the Ia molecule in antigen presentation, we have employed anti-I-A^k monoclonal antibodies to inhibit antigen presentation by APC expressing wild type I-A^k. The presentation cultures consisted of equal numbers of a given T-cell hybridoma and the B cell lymphoma, CH12, which expresses I-A^k. An amount of antigen known to be in excess of the minimum required for maximal response was used and monoclonal antibodies were added at concentrations ranging from 10 µg/well to 0.1 µg/well. In most cases an antibody dose-dependent inhibition of T-cell hybridoma stimulation was observed although in a few cases a particular antibody failed to inhibit antigen presentation to one of the T-cell hybridomas (Fig. 1). Relative to the control antibody, 14-4-4S (anti-I-E^k), some antibodies were always inhibitory as exemplified by antibodies 10-2.16 and 40M in this figure. On the other hand, the antibody 17/227 failed to inhibit the presentation of HEL to the T-cell hybridoma h4Ly7.5 while inhibiting presentation to h4Ly18.2. Conversely, the antibody 10-3.6 failed to inhibit presentation to h4Ly18.2 but not to h4Ly7.5. Finally,

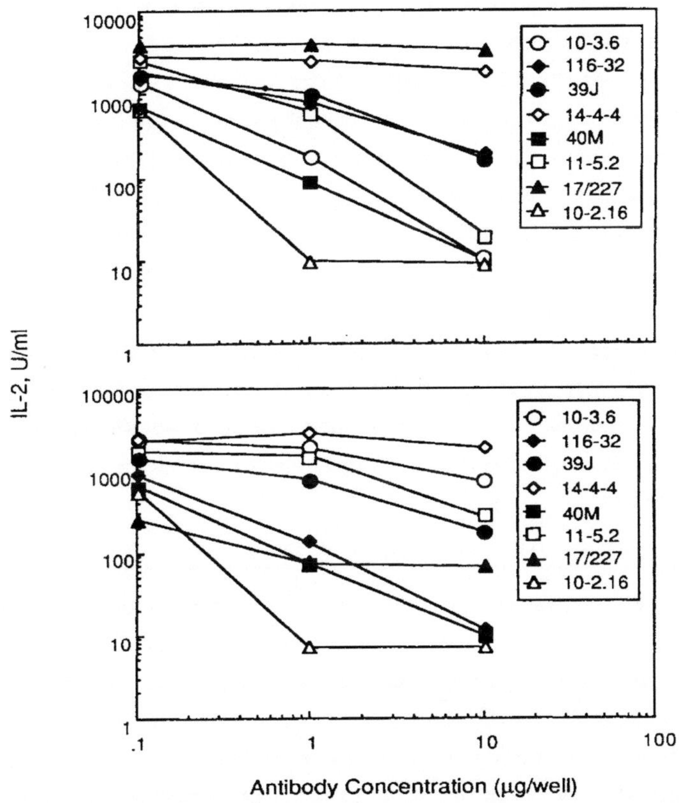

Fig. 1. Inhibition of antigen presentation by monoclonal antibodies. The I-A^k-positive B-cell lymphoma (10^5 cells), CH-12, was combined with 10^5 T-cell hybridomas, h4Ly7.5 (top) or h4Ly18.2 (bottom) in the presence of excess lysozyme. Various doses of monoclonal antibodies were added as shown. The y axis indicates the units of IL-2 produced in the antigen presentation cultures as measured by the HT-2 assays.

a number of monoclonal antibodies were moderately inhibitory with both cell lines shown as exemplified by antibodies 39J. 11-5.2 and H116-32.

When the entire panel of T-cell hybridomas was probed with the entire battery of monoclonal antibodies, it was found that inhibition was far more common than non-inhibition. This suggested that "non-specific" steric hinderance by the 150 kilodalton monoclonal antibodies may explain many of the inhibitions observed. A number of the studies were repeated using Fab' fragments of the antibodies. Except for the fact that certain weakly inhibitory antibodies were non-inhibitory when used as Fab' fragments, the pattern of inhibition produced by the Fab' fragments matched that obtained using whole antibodies (data not shown). These results suggest that most of the inhibitions observed were not due to "non-specific" steric hinderance but were the result of the antibody or its Fab' fragment interfering with Ia/antigen or Ia/T-cell receptor interactions. The failure of Fab' fragments from weakly-inhibitory antibodies to inhibit antigen presentation may be interpreted as indicating that the binding sites for these antibodies are somewhat peripheral to the central contact region(s) mentioned above and that the decreased steric bulk of the Fab' fragments results in loss of a "non-specific" inhibition.

Anti-I-A^k Monoclonal Antibodies Disrupt Binding of Antigen to I-A^k

An alterantive explanation for the high frequency of inhibition observed with the battery of monoclonal antibodies is that the antibodies can interfere either with antigen/I-A binding or with I-A/T-cell receptor binding (or with both). In order to begin to dissect this possibility, we have employed the peptide/Ia direct binding assay originally described by Buus et al. (1986) to examine the role of the antibodies in modulating the interaction between the immunodominant lysozyme peptide, HEL(46-61), and the I-A^k molecule. The results obtained thus far are summarized in Table 3. It should be apparent from Table 3 that while all monoclonal antibodies block antigen presentation of HEL to some of the hybridomas in the panel there is a nearly perfect correlation between the effect that a monoclonal antibody has on presentation to HEL(46-61)-specific hybridomas and the effect it has on disrupting the direct binding of HEL(46-61) to I-A^k. Specifically, with the exception of the 11-5.2 antibody, every monoclonal antibody which blocked binding of HEL(46-61) to I-A^k was inhibitory for all of the HEL(46-61)-specific T-cell hybridomas tested, i.e., h4Ly50.5, kLy7.11 and kLy4.10. We interpret this result to mean that these antibodies

Table 3. Effects of Monoclonal Antibodies on Antigen Presentation and Binding of HEL(46-61) to I-A^k

		Blocks Antigen Presentation?		
Anti-I-A^k Antibody	Nominal Ia Specificity	All HEL Specific T-hybrids	T-hybrids Specific for HEL (46-61)	Blocks I-A-Antigen Binding?
40M	1	5/5	3/3	Yes
11-5.2	2	2/5	1/2	Yes
17/227	15	2/4	1/3	No
10-3.6	17	4/5	3/3	Yes
10-2.16	17	4/4	2/2	Yes
H116-32	19	1/5	0/3	No
39J	19	3/5	1/3	No

exert their inhibitory effect on antigen presentation by disrupting peptide/I-A interaction (and, perhaps, also I-A/T-cell receptor interaction) while the other monoclonal antibodies inhibit antigen presentation by disrupting the I-A/T-cell receptor interaction exclusively.

DISCUSSION

The experiments summarized here allow several conclusions to be drawn about the nature of the site by which the Ia molecule interacts with peptide antigen and the T-cell receptor. First, the ability of some but not other monoclonal antibodies to disrupt the binding of the HEL(46-61) peptide to I-A^k suggests that it is possible to separate, at least in a functional sense, the interaction of Ia with peptide from the interaction between Ia and T cell receptor.

Second, given this functional dissection, the loss in antigen presenting function in the EMS-induced mutants appears to be due primarily to the mutation interfering with the T-cell receptor/Ia interaction. This is demonstrated by the fact that, with the exception of K2 and JE50, all of the mutants are capable of presenting HEL(46-61) to at least one of the HEL(46-61)-specific hybridomas. Furthermore, mutant I-A^k isolated from JE50 has been tested in the direct binding assay and binds HEL(46-61) within the normal range of binding (E.F. Rosloniec, unpublished data). This result implies that even though JE50 fails to present HEL(46-61) to any of the T-cell hybridomas in our panel, the lesion lies in the interaction between the I-A^k of JE50 and the T-cell receptor. One may presume a similar situation for the K2 mutant.

There is an alternate possibility that the EMS-induced mutations lower the binding affinity of Ia for peptide to such an extent that only T-cell receptors with high affinity for Ia/peptide are capable of binding the mutant Ia/peptide complex. While the data presently available cannot formally exclude this possibility, it appears to be less likely than the explanation that the mutations disrupt Ia/T-cell receptor interactions.

Third, it would appear that the carboxy-terminal portions of the $\alpha 1$ and $\beta 1$ domains play a predominant role in determining the antigen presentation phenotype of the I-A^k molecule at least as far as the HEL-specific hybridomas used in this study are concerned. This conclusion follows directly from the data for the chimeric A_α chains presented in Table 2 and it is based, indirectly, on the following observations about the A_β chains. 1) All of the EMS-induced A_β^k mutations which have an effect on antigen presentation occur in positions #64, 67 and 68 in the carboxy-terminal portion of the β1 domain. 2) The use of site-directed mutagenesis to produce chimeric A_β chains in which amino acids found in the d allele are put en bloc into each of the four hypervariable regions of the A_β^k chain has shown that the specificity of all tested anti-A_β^k monoclonal antibodies is determined by the residues #63-67 (A_β^d numbering) (D.J. McKean, unpublished observations). Thus, the majority of the anti-A_β^k antibodies used in this study to inhibit antigen presentation most likely are directed against the carboxy-terminal portion of the β1 domain.

Each of the experimental approaches used in the present study to elucidate the structure-function relationships of the I-A^k molecule has its own inherent limitations and/or requires that assumptions be made in interpreting the results obtained. For the mutants or molecules possessing chimeric chains one must assume that the amino acid interchanges that have produced the mutant or chimeric molecule exert their major effect in the area in which they occur or in the areas linearly adjacent to them. Likewise, for the mapping of the specificities of the monoclonal antibodies one must assume that the amino acid interchanges which give rise to loss of specificity most likely are the contact residues for the monoclonal antibodies. While formal proof that these assumptions are indeed valid is lacking at the present time a mounting body of correlative evidence supports the idea that the assumptions are true, at least as a first approximation. An additional concern with the use of monoclonal antibodies is that they, and even their Fab' fragments, are quite bulky as probes of structure and function. Thus, there may be an element of "non-specific" inhibition even in the inhibitions which are interpreted as "specific". The observation that certain monoclonal antibodies fail to inhibit antigen presentation to T-cell hybridomas or to disrupt antigen binding by Ia argues that this concern may not need to be given too much weight. In spite of these caveats, it seems significant that all of the experimental approaches produce data which appear to be mutually consistant and which can be used in the construction of a unified model of the functional region of the Ia molecule.

Based on the data presented here and on results obtained by others (Buus et al. 1987), we propose the following model for the functional site of the I-A molecule: There is a single antigen binding site on the I-A molecule which is composed of segments from both the α and the β chain. While the allelic hypervariable regions of the carboxy-terminal portions of the α1 and β1 domains appear to play the dominant role in determining the specificity of this interaction, it is likely that other parts of the α1 and β1 domains (especially the other hypervariable regions) are involved in providing contact residues for this interaction.

Although the data from the monoclonal antibody inhibitions of antigen presentation and of antigen binding allow the functional separation of the Ia/antigen interaction from the Ia/T cell receptor interaction, we do not postulate that these interactions necessarily occur at distinct sites on the Ia molecule. Rather, we envisage a situation in which the peptide antigen lies in a shallow cleft, formed by the α1 and β1 domains of Ia, which is part of the contact surface between Ia and the T cell receptor. Recent modelling of the T cell receptor (Novotny et al. 1986) suggests that the T cell receptor's antigen combining region should be analogous to that of immunoglobulin. Thus, the T cell receptor/Ia contact surface could be quite large, possibly on the order of the 20 x 30 Å contact surface recently reported by Amit et al. (1986) for the contact surface between lysozyme and a monoclonal antibody directed against it. Such a large contact surface clearly could accomodate a peptide antigen lying in a shallow groove. This arrangement would allow the peptide to contact the Ia molecule and the T cell receptor simultaneously as implied by studies (Sette et al. 1987) in which homologues of the antigen have been employed to measure Ia binding and antigenicity.

While this model lacks the kind of high resolution that X-ray diffraction of the ternary complex will provide, it does begin to focus attention to a relatively small region of the molecule. Further studies are in progress in our laboratories to test the details of the proposed model.

ACKNOWLEDGEMENTS

These studies were supported in part by a grant from the Kroc Foundation (to J.H.F.), by USPHS grants CA 37600 (to J.H.F.), and CA 26297 (to D.J.M.) and by CNRS grant ATP 3285 (to D.M.).

REFERENCES

Allen, P. M., McKean, D. J., Beck, B. N., Sheffield, J., and Glimcher, L. H.: Direct evidence that a class II molecule and a simple globular protein generate multiple determinants. J. Exp. Med. 162:1264-1274, 1985

Amit, A. G., Mariuzza, R. A., Phillips, S. E. V., and Poljak, R. J.: Three-dimensional structure of an antigen-antibody complex at 2.8 A resolution. Science 233:747-753, 1986.

Ashwell, J. D., Fox, B. S., and Schwartz, R. H.: Functional analysis of the interaction of the antigen-specific T cell receptor with its ligands. J. Immunol. 136:757-768, 1986.

Beck, B. N., Glimcher, L. H., Nilson, A. E., Pierres, M., and McKean, D. J.: The structure-function relationship of I-A molecules: Correlation of serologic and functional phenotypes of four $I\text{-}A^k$ mutant cell lines. J. Immunol. 133:3176-3182, 1984.

Beck, B. N., Pease, L. R., Bell, M. P., Buerstedde, J. M., Nilson, A. E., Schlander, G. G., and McKean, D. J.: DNA sequence analysis of $I\text{-}A^k_\beta$ mutants reveals serologically immunodominant region. J. Exp. Med. In press, 1987.

Buus, S., Sette, A., Colon, S. M., Jenis, D. M., and Grey, H. M.: Isolation and characterization of antigen-Ia complexes involved in T cell recognition. Cell 47:1071-1077, 1986.

Buus, S., Sette, A., Colon, S. M., Miles, C., and Grey, H. M.: The relationship between MHC restriction and the capacity of Ia to bind immunogenic peptides. Science 235:1353-1358, 1987.

Cohn, L. E., Glimcher, L. H., Waldmann, R. A., Smith, J. A., Ben-Nun, A., Seidman, J. G., and Choi, E.: Identification of functional regions on the $I\text{-}A^b$ molecule by site-directed mutagenesis. Proc. Natl. Acad. Sci. U.S.A. 83:747-751, 1986.

Guillet, J. G., Lai, M. Z., Briner, T. J., Smith, J. A., and Gefter, M. L.: Interaction of peptide antigens and class II major histocompatibility complex antigens. Nature 324:260-262, 1986.

Kappler, J., White, J., Wegmann, D., Mustain, E., and Marrack, P.: Antigen presentation by Ia^+ B cell hybridomas to H-2-restricted T cell hybridomas. Proc. Natl. Acad. Sci. U.S.A. 79:3604-3607, 1982.

Lechler, R. I., Ronchese, F., Braunstein, N. S., and Germain, R. N.: I-A-restricted T cell antigen recognition. Analysis of the roles of $A\alpha$ and $A\beta$ using DNA-mediated gene transfer. J. Exp. Med. 163:678-696, 1986.

Landais, D., Waltzinger, C., Beck, B. N., Staub, A., McKean, D. H., Benoist, C., and Mathis, D.: Functional sites on Ia molecules: A molecular dissection of $A\alpha$ immunogenicity. Cell 47:173-181, 1986.

Novotny, J., Tonegawa, S., Saito, H., Kranz, D. M., and Eisen, H. N.: Secondary, tertiary and quaternary structure of T-cell-specific immunoglobulin-like polypeptide chains. Proc. Natl. Acad. Sci. U.S.A. 83:742-746, 1986.

Sette, A., Buus, S., Colon, S., Smith, J. A., Miles, C., and Grey, H. M.: Structural characteristics of an antigen that are required for its interaction with Ia and recognition by T cells. Nature In press, 1987.

MOLECULAR ANALYSIS OF MAJOR HISTOCOMPATIBILITY COMPLEX (MHC) MOLECULE RECOGNITION BY THE T CELL RECEPTOR ALPHA-BETA (α-β) HETERODIMER

Louis A. Matis,* Simona B. Sorger,† Pamela J. Fink,†
David L. McElligot† and Stephen M. Hedrick†

*Molecular Immunology Laboratory, Division of Biochemistry and Biophysics, Center for Drugs and Biologics, Food and Drug Administration, Bethesda, MD 20892
†Department of Biology and the Cancer Center, University of California, San Diego, La Jolla, CA 92093

ABSTRACT

We have examined the molecular basis of MHC-restricted antigen recognition and alloreactivity by the T cell receptor (TCR) α-β heterodimer in murine T cell clones specific for the peptide antigen pigeon cytochrome c. The T cell proliferative response to this antigen has been extensively characterized with regard to the fine specificity of both antigen and MHC molecule recognition. All T cell clones derived from B10.A strain mice share specificity for an antigenic determinant on the COOH-terminal peptide in association with the self E_α^k:E_β^k Ia molecule. However, distinct clonotypes can be identified based upon differences in the fine specificity of both antigen and MHC recognition, or concomitant alloreactivity. Structure-function analysis of TCR gene expression was performed by cDNA cloning and sequencing of productively rearranged α and β TCR genes from T cell clones representative of each clonotype, and by Southern blot analysis of a series of T cell clones of defined specificity using V segment probes derived from the cDNA clones.

This analysis demonstrated definite correlations between sequence changes in particular regions of the TCR and functional specificity. A single V_α subfamily gene segment was predominantly expressed by all the B10.A T cell clones. In association with this V_α gene, a limited set of V_β genes were expressed, each correlating exactly with a unique response phenotype. A striking selection of both J_α and J_β gene segments was also observed within each clonotype. Thus, V_α-V_β combinatorial association, V-J combinatorial joining, and junctional diversity were shown to affect both antigen and MHC specificities of the cytochrome c-specific T cell clones. These represent the predominant mechanisms for the generation of diversity in the TCR repertoire.

In addition, the data revealed significant homologies between TCR that recognize Ia molecules as restriction elements in association with antigen and TCR that recognize the same Ia molecules as alloantigens. This suggests that MHC-restricted recognition and alloreactivity may simply reflect differences in the affinity of the interaction between the TCR and the MHC molecule.

INTRODUCTION

Selection of the T cell receptor repertoire for the recognition of MHC-encoded molecules is manifested by the phenomena of MHC-restriction (Shevach et al., 1973; Katz et al., 1973) and alloreactivity (Bevan et al., 1976; Fischer-Lindahl et al., 1977). MHC-restricted recognition, the obligate co-recognition of foreign antigens in association with MHC-encoded molecules expressed on the surface of antigen-presenting cells (APC) has been definitively demonstrated by gene transfection analysis to be mediated by the TCR_{α}-β heterodimer (Dembic et al., 1986; Saito et al., 1987). Another striking aspect of the relationship between the T cell repertoire and the MHC is the high frequency of alloreactive T cells, namely T cells specific for intraspecies allelic variants of self MHC molecules (Bevan et al., 1976).

The molecular basis of MHC recognition has not been determined. Both TCR α and β proteins are encoded by distinct genetic elements (V, (D), J, and C) which recombine during differentiation to form mature functional genes in a fashion analogous to that of the immunoglobulin (Ig) genes (Hedrick et al., 1984; Yanagi et al., 1984; Chien et al., 1984). Analysis of key sequence homologies between TCR and Ig genes has led to the proposal that the TCR heterodimer very likely constitutes a multiple domain protein with overall structure quite similar to that of Ig (Barth et al., 1985; Novotny et al., 1986). Thus, the MHC specificity of the TCR repertoire may be directly encoded in germline sequences (Blackman et al., 1986), or may reflect selection during intrathymic maturation (Jerne, 1971; Zinkernagel et al., 1978; Schwartz, 1984).

One approach to understanding the structural basis of MHC molecule recognition is to examine TCR α and β chain expression in T cells with well-defined specificity for both antigen and restricting MHC molecules. For example, the murine immune response to pigeon cytochrome c has been extensively characterized (Hedrick et al., 1982; Heber-Katz et al., 1982; Matis et al., 1983; Schwartz et al., 1985). $CD4^{+}$ pigeon cytochrome c-specific proliferative T cells almost invariably recognize a COOH-terminal antigenic determinant in association with I-E subregion encoded $E_{\alpha}:E_{\beta}$ class II (Ia) molecules. Thus, in B10.A ($H\text{-}2^{k}$) mice, all pigeon cytochrome c-specific T cell clones recognize an epitope on the COOH-terminal fragment 81-104 in association with the self $E_{\alpha}{}^{k}:E_{\beta}{}^{k}$ (E^{k}) molecule. However, among such closely related clones, distinct phenotypes can be identified based upon differences in the fine specificity of antigen recognition (defined on the basis of patterns of responsiveness to a variety of species variant (and synthetic) cytochrome c peptides) and the fine specificity of MHC restriction molecule recognition (based upon the ability to recognize cytochrome c in association with non-self allelic E region encoded Ia molecules such as $E_{\alpha}{}^{k}:E_{\beta}{}^{b}$ (E^{b}) and $E_{\alpha}{}^{k}:E_{\beta}{}^{s}$ (E^{s})).

This systematic analysis of the B10.A cytochrome c response has revealed the expression of a limited number of germline TCR gene elements, thus allowing definite correlations to be made between TCR gene expression and T cell specificity (Fink et al., 1986; Sorger et al., 1987; Matis et al., 1987). These studies have provided valuable insights with regard to the mechanisms for the generation of T cell receptor diversity, the contribution of distinct genetic elements to T cell specificity , and the relationship between MHC restriction and alloreactivity.

MATERIALS AND METHODS

Animals

B10.A, B10.A(5R), and B10 mice were obtained from the Jackson Laboratory, Bar Harbor, ME. B10.S and B10.S(9R) mice were bred at the National Institutes of Health (NIH), Bethesda, MD. Mice of either sex from 6 to 12 weeks of age were used for experiments.

T Cell Lines and Clones

The derivation of T cell lines and clones, the analysis of their specifictity by proliferation assays, their in vitro selection for distinct specificities, and their expansion to large numbers of cells for the preparation of DNA and RNA, have been described in detail previously (Sorger et al., 1987).

Preparation of High Molecular Weight DNA and Southern Hybridization Analysis

These procedures have been thoroughly described in previous publications (Sorger et al., 1987).

Preparation of cDNA Libraries and DNA Sequencing of T Cell Receptor Genes

The methodology for preparation of poly $(A)^+$ RNA, synthesis of oligo (dT)-primed double-stranded cDNA, cloning of cDNA into plasmid vectors, and cDNA sequencing by the method of Maxam and Gilbert have all been previously published (Fink et al., 1986).

DNA Probes

The V_β2B4 probe was a 550 bp fragment subcloned into pGEM (Chien et al., 1984). The V_α2B4.2 probe was subcloned as a 400 bp BamHI-PstI fragment derived from a full length cDNA clone as previously described (Sorger et al., 1987). The V_βB10 probe was subcloned as 450 bp BamHI-AvaII fragment from the β chain cDNA of clone 4C3 (Fink et al., 1986). The V_βC8 probe was isolated as a 380 bp fragment by an EcoRI-XmnI digest from the β chain cDNA clone of the T cell clone C8. The 86T1V_β probe was a 350 bp EcoRI-BamHI fragment previously subcloned into the puC9 plasmid. The V_αD6 probe was a 550 bp EcoI-HindIII fragment isolated from a full length cDNA clone (D.L.M., unpublished data).

V_β2B4 is alternatively referred to as V_β3 (Barth et al., 1985), V_α2B4.2 as V_α11.1 (Winoto et al., 1986), and $V_\beta 86T_1$ as V_β1 (Barth et al.,

1985). $V_\alpha D6$ has not been reported previously, but appears to be in the same V_α subfamily as V_α FN1-18 (Becker et al., 1985) as well as $V_\alpha 10$ reported by Arden et al., 1985.

RESULTS

T cell receptor gene expression was examined through a combination of DNA sequencing and Southern hybridization analyses using V segment DNA probes. Thus, cDNA clones were derived representing the productively rearranged and expressed α and β genes from a number of representative pigeon cytochrone c-specific E^k-restricted B10.A T cell clones (Fink et al., 1986; Sorger et al., 1987). V segment subclones were derived from these cDNA clones and were used as DNA probes of genomic Southern blots to examine a larger series of pigeon cytochrome c-specific T cell clones and lines (Sorger et al., 1987). Expression of functional T cell receptor polypeptides requires the complete in-frame rearrangement of all the gene elements comprising the V region exon. Using a V segment probe, it can be determined whether that V gene segment is rearranged in a T cell clone. The particular V_α-J_α and V_β-D_β-J_β rearrangements of the T cell clone can be determined from the size of the rearranged restriction fragment hybridizing to the V segment probe (Sorger et al., 1987). Our studies to date have demonstrated a strict correlation between the antigen/MHC proliferative specificity of a T cell clone and the expression of a particular V_α-J_α and V_β-D_β-J_β gene elements (Fink et al., 1986; Sorger et al., 1987). These observations indicate that by both DNA sequencing and Southern hybridization analysis we are in fact examining the relevant, productively rearranged TCR α and β genes.

TCR Gene Expression and T Cell Specificity

A number of independently derived T cell clones were examined for specificity and for α and β TCR gene expression. All the clones displayed in TABLE 1 share specificity for pigeon cytochrome c fragment 81-104 in association with the self E^k Ia molecule. However, they could be categorized into one of three distinct subsets based upon differences in antigen and/or MHC specificity. Thus, T cell clones of the first subset, represented by C.F6, respond to moth cytochrome c as well as pigeon cytochrome c in association with E^k, and to moth cytochrome c presented by E^b-expressing (B10.A(5R)) APC. Clones of the second subset, illustratd by 3.G8, also respond to moth and pigeon cytochromes c presented by syngeneic E^k-bearing APC, and also to cytochrome c in the presence of E^s (B10.S(9R))-expressing APC. These clones could be further subdivided based upon an antigen fine specificity difference, such that clones 3.G8, B10, and C12 respond preferentially to pigeon cytochrome c in the presence of E^s, whereas clones D2 and 4.C3 manifest a stronger response to the moth peptide presented by E^s APC. Finally, the third group of clones, represented by C8, respond to pigeon but not significantly to moth cytochrome c in the presence of E^k, E^s, and E^b APC.

Analysis of TCR gene expression in these B10.A T cell clones revealed that all expressed a member of a single V_α gene subfamily, $V_\alpha 2B4$ ($V_\alpha 2B4$ is otherwise designated $V_\alpha 11$ by Winoto et al., 1986). Clones specific for cytochrome c plus E^k,E^b expressed $V_\beta 2B4$ (designated

Table 1. Relationship between TCR α and β gene expression and specificity in cytochrome c-specific B10.A T cell clones [a]

T Cell Clone	MHC restriction[b]	Antigen specificity[c]	V2B4[d] (HindIII)	V_β2B4 (HindIII)	V_βB10 (EcoRI)	V_βC8 (HindIII)	V_α/J_α	V_β/J_β
C.F6*	E^k	M,P	2.4 Kb	9.2 Kb	-	-	2B4.2/84	2B4/1.2
	E^b	M						
D4			2.4 Kb	4.3 Kb	-	-	2B4.2/84	2B4/2.5
6.AE1			8.4 Kb	4.3 Kb	-	-	2B4.2/28	2B4/1.2
E2			3.7 Kb	4.3 Kb	-	-	?	2B4/2.5
2C2			3.6 Kb	4.3 Kb	-	-	?	2B4/2.5
2B4*			2.6 Kb	4.3 Kb	-	-	2B4.1/2B4	2B4/2.5
3.G8	E^k	M,P	2.4 Kb	-	6.0 Kb	-	2B4.2/84	B10/2.1
	E^s	P>M						
B10*			2.4 Kb	-	6.0 Kb	-	2B4.2/84	B10/2.1
C12			2.4 Kb	-	6.0 Kb	-	2B4.2/84	B10/2.1
D2	E^k	M,P	2.4 Kb	-	6.0 Kb	-	2B4.2/84	B10/2.1
	E^s	M>P						
4.C3*			2.4 Kb	-	6.0 Kb	-	2B4.2/84	B10/2.1
C8*	E^k	P	8.4 Kb	-	-	3.1 Kb	2B4.2/28	C8/2.4
	E^s	P						
	E^b	P						
A9			8.4 Kb	-	-	3.1 Kb	2B4.2/28	C8/2.4
A6			8.4 Kb	-	-	3.1 Kb	2B4.2/28	C8/2.4
C10			8.4 Kb	-	-	8.5 Kb	2B4.2/28	C8/1.?

a. Pigeon cytochrome c-specific B10.A T cell clones, derived by limiting dilution, were analyzed for antigen and MHC specificity as well as TCR α and β gene expression by DNA sequencing and Southern hybridization analysis. Clones for which complete DNA sequence data has been derived are denoted by an asterisk.

b. The MHC restriction was determined using APC from B10.A(E^k), B10.A(5R)(E^b), and B10.S(9R)(E^s) mice.

c. Specificity was examined by proliferation in response to moth (M) versus pigeon (P) cytochrome c.

d. The data represent the sizes of the rearranged restriction fragments which hybridize to the indicated variable segment probes. The restriction endonucleases generating the fragments are shown in parentheses.

$V_\beta 3$ by Winoto et al., 1986), clones specific for cytochrome c plus E^k,E^s all rearranged a V_β segment termed $V_\beta B10$, and clones such as C8, specific for only pigeon cytochrome c in the context of E^k,E^s, or E^b, expressed a V_β segment termed $V_\beta C8$. Thus, the manifestation of distinct response phenotypes correlated with $V_\alpha 2B4$ expression in association with unique V_β gene products.

Analysis of the J segment expression in this group of clones revealed a striking selection of these gene elements. For example, although the 5 distinct V_α/J_α rearrangements displayed by the first group of clones (TABLE 1) imply little if any selection, subsequent analysis of multiple independently-derived T cell clones of this response phenotype has revealed the reproducible expression of the same J_α elements (data not shown). In consideration of the likelihood that greater than 50-60 J_α elements are encoded in the germline (Kronenberg et al., 1986), this degree of J_α selection is striking. Selection of J_α elements is even more readily apparent in the analysis of clones representing the other two response phenotypes. Thus, the clones shown that recognize E^k and E^s as restriction molecules (3.G8, B10, C12, D2, and 4.C3), although derived from 4 separate immunizations, invariably express a single J_α, $J_\alpha 84$ ($J_\alpha 84$ is from Winoto et al., 1985). Similarly, all the clones of the third subset display the same 8.4 Kb HindIII $V_\alpha 2B4$ rearrangement and were shown to express $J_\alpha 28$ ($J_\alpha 28$ is from Arden et al., 1985).

A similar selection of J_β elements was noted (TABLE 1). The $V_\beta 2B4$-expressing clones all concurrently expressed one of two J_β elements, either $J_\beta 1.2$ (9.2 Kb Hind III rearrangement) or $J_\beta 2.5$ (4.3 Kb Hind III rearrangement). The $V_\beta B10$-expressing clones invariably co-expressed $J_\beta 2.1$ (6.0 Kb EcoRI rearrangement), and the third group of clones expressed either $V_\beta C8/J_\beta 2.4$ (3.1 Kb Hind III band) or $V_\beta C8$ rearranged to a J_β element in the first (upstream) J segment cluster (8.5 Kb Hind III rearrangement) (Kronenberg et al., 1986). Thus, analysis of cytochrome c-specific T cell clones based upon categorization into particular response phenotypes revealed a striking selection of all the TCR_α and β gene elements comprising the receptor heterodimer. Finally, although the cytochrome c-specific B10.A T cell clones responding in the presence of E^k or E^s restriction molecules displayed an antigen fine specificity difference with regard to the response to the moth peptide presented by E^s, all such clones expressed the same V_α/J_α and V_β/J_β elements (TABLE I). These data indicate that the difference in specificity must be a consequence of junctional diversity in the α and/or β chains resulting from inexact V-(D)-J joining and the addition of N-region nucleotides.

Molecular Analysis of Cytochrome c-Specific T Cell Clones Displaying Concomitant Alloreactivity

Insight into the origin of the extensive alloreactive T cell repertoire has emerged from studies showing that individual T cell clones can be both antigen-specific and alloreactive (Sredni et al., 1980; Braciale et al., 1981). Independent analyses of multiple cloned T cell populations have demonstrated that a high proportion (20-60%) of antigen-specific, MHC-restricted T cell clones display concomitant alloreactivity (Janeway et al., 1982; Ashwell et al., 1986). We

Table 2. TCR Gene Rearrangements in I-E Restricted Pigeon Cytochrome c-Specific T Cell Clones Expressing Distinct Alloreactive Specificities

T Cell Clone	Strain of Origin	V_α2B4.2 (HindIII)	V_β2B4 (HindIII)	V_αD6 (BamHI)	$V_\beta 86T_1$ (HindIII)	Alloreactivity	V_α/J_α	V_β/J_β
1.C8	B10.A(E^k)	2.4 Kb	9.2 Kb	-	-	none	2B4.2/84	2B4/1.2
5C.C6	B10.A	3.5 Kb	9.2 Kb	-	-	A^s	2B4.2/C7	2B4/1.2
1.C2	B10.A	3.5 Kb	9.2 Kb	-	-	A^s	2B4.2/C7	2B4/1.2
B3	B10.A	3.5 Kb	9.2 Kb	-	-	A^s	2B4.2/C7	2B4/1.2
F7	B10.A	3.5 Kb	9.2 Kb	-	-	A^s	2B4.2/C7	2B4/1.2
6.AE1	B10.A	8.4 Kb	9.2 Kb	-	-	none	2B4.2/28	2B4/1.2
2.C2	B10.A	8.4 Kb	4.6 Kb	-	-	A^b	2B4.2/28	2B4/2.3
1.C5	B10.A	8.4 Kb	4.6 Kb	-	-	A^b	2B4.2/28	2B4/2.3
D10	B10.A	8.4 Kb	4.3 Kb	-	-	A^b	2B4.2/28	2B4/2.5
G5	B10.A	8.4 Kb	4.3 Kb	-	-	A^b	2B4.2/28	2B4/2.5
D4	B10.A	2.4 Kb	4.3 Kb	-	-	none	2B4.2/28	2B4/2.5
E2	B10.A	3.7 Kb	4.3 Kb	-	-	none	2B4?	2B4/2.5
3.D3	B10.A	2.6 Kb	4.3 Kb	-	-	none	2B4.1/2B4	2B4/2.5
5.D11	B10.A	2.3 Kb	9.2 Kb	-	-	E^b	2B4?	2B4/1.2
5.G3	B10.A	2.3 Kb	9.2 Kb	-	-	E^b	2B4?	2B4/1.2
5.G10	B10.A	2.3 Kb	9.2 Kb	-	-	E^b	2B4?	2B4/1.2
3.3	B10.A	-	-	7.0 Kb	7.6 Kb	E^s	D6/C7	$86T_1$/2.?
1B	B10.A	-	-	7.0 Kb	7.6 Kb	E^s	D6/C7	$86T_1$/2.?
.3H	B10.A	-	-	7.0 Kb	7.6 Kb	E^s	D6/C7	$86T_1$/2.?
9R.D6	B10.S(9R)(E^s)	-	-	7.0 Kb	14.0 Kb	E^k	D6/C7	$86T_1$/1.2

The data are presented as in TABLE 1. In addition, the alloreactive specificity of each antigen-specific clone is also shown. A and E refer to the major classes of murine class II MHC molecules encoded by genes within the I-A and I-E subregions, respectively, of the murine H-2 gene complex.

explored the molecular basis for the generation of multiple distinct alloreactive specificities among T cell clones sharing the same antigen and MHC-restriction specificities by examing TCR α and β gene expression in a series of pigeon cytochrome c-specific clones crossreactive for four different allogeneic class II MHC molecules (A^s, A^b, E^b, E^s). The data are presented in TABLE 2. As in the antigen and MHC-restriction specificity analysis of the previous set of clones, TCR gene rearrangements were examined using V segment probes derived from productively rearranged full length α and β cDNA clones. Again, particular V and J segment usage could be determined from the size of the rearranged bands, based upon direct comparison to the Southern analyses of the T cell clones from which the sequenced cDNA clones were originally derived.

Alloreactive specificity was assessed by the determination of proliferation in the presence of allogenic APC from four H-2 congenic strains: B10.S, B10, B10.S(9R) and B10.A(5R). B10 and B10.A(5R) APC express the same I-A subregion-encoded molecule (A^b); B10.S and B10.S(9R) APC both express A^s. However, in contrast to B10.A(5R) and B10.S(9R) APC, neither B10 nor B10.S APC express an E_α:E_β Ia molecule. Therefore, APC from these strains can be used to distinguish between I-A and I-E subregion-specific alloreactivity.

A series of independently derived B10.A T cell clones alloreactive for the A^s_α:A^s_β (A^s) molecule were analyzed. The alloreactive specificity of the clones was assessed by clonal proliferation in response to allogeneic APC in the absence of cytochrome c (data not shown). All 4 clones alloreactive to A^s expressed the same $V\alpha/J\alpha$ and $V\beta/J\beta$ gene elements (TABLE 2). In particular, alloreactivity to A^s in these clones correlated with the expression of $J\alpha C7$ (Fink et al., 1986), insofar as clone 1.C8 (TABLE 2), which is not alloreactive to A^s, expresses the same $V\beta 2B4/J\beta 1.2$ β chain as the A^s alloreactive clones.

The 4 cytochrome c-specific B10.A clones alloreactive to A^b_α:A^b_β (A^b) all expressed $V\alpha 2B4.2/J\alpha 28$ paired with either $V\beta 2B4/J\beta 2.3$ or $V\beta 2B4/J\beta 2.5$. These data suggested that the acquisition of this cross-reactive allospecificity required the combinatorial association of selected $J\alpha$ and $J\beta$ gene segments. This conclusion follows from the fact that clone 6.AE.1 expresses $V\alpha 2B4.2/J\alpha 28$ and $V\beta 2B4/J\beta 1.2$ and is not A^b alloreactive, while clones D4, E2, and 3.D3 express $V\beta 2B4/J\beta 2.5$ and a $V\alpha 2B4$ subfamily gene different from $V\alpha 2B4.2/J\alpha 28$ and are also not A^b alloreactive (TABLE 2). Thus, it appears that A^b alloreactivity results from the specific pairing of the $V\alpha 2B4.2/J\alpha 28$ and $V\beta 2B4/J\beta 2.5$ (or $J\beta 2.3$) polypeptides.

Alloreactivity to the E^b and E^s Ia Molecules

Analysis of B10.A T cell clones alloreactive against the E^b and E^s molecules was of particular interest because, as previously noted, both E^b and E^s can function as restriction molecules for cytochrome c recognition by some E^k-restricted B10.A T cell clones (see TABLE 1).

Analysis of three E^b-alloreactive B10.A T cell clones (5.D11, 5.G3, 5.G10) demonstrated that all expressed the same $V\beta 2B4$-$J\beta 1.2$ 9.2 Kb

HindIII rearrangement as observed in the nonalloreactive clone 1.C8 as well as the A^s alloreactive clones (TABLE 2). However, hybridization of HindIII-digested DNA from these clones to the V_α2B4.2 probe revealed a 2.3 Kb rearranged band in all three cases. As this rearrangement has not been observed in any clone from which sequence data are available, this novel rearrangement may reflect the expression of a distinct 2B4V_α subfamily gene segment, a unique J_α element, or both. Nonetheless, it appears from these results that E^b alloreactivity is conferred by the expression of this unique V_α2B4 gene family-encoded polypeptide. In addition, proliferation data (not shown) demonstrated that these E^b-alloreactive B10.A clones manifested additional antigen-specific proliferation in response to moth cytochrome c and E^b-expressing APC. Thus, for these T cell clones the E^b molecule functioned both as an alloantigen and as a restriction molecule for cytochrome c recognition.

In summary, E^k-restricted cytochrome c-specific T cell clones cross-reactive for three distinct allospecificities (A^s, A^b, E^b) all expressed the same V_α and V_β gene segments. Each different pattern of alloreactivity correlated with unique rearrangements of these V gene segments and, therefore, with the expression of a limited set of selected J_α and J_β gene segments.

Three cytochrome c-specific E^k-restricted B10.A T cell clones alloreactive against the allelic E^s molecule were shown not to express either V_α2B4 or V_β2B4 genes (TABLE 2, clones 3.3, 1B, and .3H). However, TCR α and β cDNA clones were isolated and sequenced from a related B10.S(9R) strain-derived T cell clone 9R.D6 that recognized cytochrome c in association with the syngeneic E^s molecule and that displayed concomitant alloreactivity to the E^k molecule (D.L.M., manuscript in preparation). This E^s-restricted, E^k-alloreactive clone expressed a V_α termed V_αD6 (a member of the FN-1 family, Becker et al., 1985), rearranged to J_αC7, and $V_\beta 86T_1$ (otherwise designated V_β1 by Barth et al., 1985) rearranged to J_β1.2. Analysis of the three E^k-restricted, E^s-alloreactive B10.A T cell clones, 3.3, 1B, and .3H, revealed that they also expressed V_αD6-J_αC7 (identical 7.0 Kb BamHI rearrangement) and $V_\beta 86T_1$, but rearranged the latter to a different D_β-J_β element (7.6 Kb versus 14.0 Kb HindIII rearrangement, TABLE 2). Thus, we conclude that the expression of different D_β-J_β elements by T cell clones that express the same V_α, J_α, and V_β segments accounts for the alternate recognition of the E^k and E^s molecules as restriction elements versus alloantigens.

DISCUSSION

Generation of T Cell Receptor Diversity

We have examined the molecular basis for the generation of distinct patterns of antigen fine specificity, MHC-restriction specificity, and alloreactivity among cytochrome c-specific E^k-restricted T cell clones. The results show that the mechanisms which generate sequence diversity can in each instance be shown to correlate with significant changes in functional specificity.

Germline Diversity

A limited number of germline V and J elements are expressed in cytochrome c-specific, E^k-restricted B10.A T cells. Thus, all the gene elements encoding the antigen and MHC ligand are selected, implying perhaps that complementarity-determining regions of the TCR might encompass a significant proportion of the primary sequence of the V, D, and J regions. The data presented here do not necessarily imply that only a very limited set of variable gene elements can assemble to encode a receptor capable of binding the ligand formed by cytochrome c and the E^k molecule, but rather that certain elements are preferentially expressed. For example, there is little sequence homology between V_α2B4-V_β2B4 and V_αD6-V_β86T_1 encoded heterodimers, yet both are specific for the COOH-terminal cytochrome c antigenic determinant in association with the E^k Ia molecule.

Combinatorial Association

This mechanism was most strikingly illustrated by the data in TABLE 1, and was shown to influence both MHC restriction and antigen specificity. Thus, clones expressing V_α2B4-V_β2B4 recognize cytochrome c in association with both E^k and E^b, clones expressing V_α2B4-V_βB10 recognize the antigen presented by E^k and E^s, and clones rearranging V_α2B4 and V_βC8 recognize pigeon but not moth cytochrome c in association with E^k, E^s, and E^b. Moreover, combinatorial association of selected J elements also appeared to determine certain cross-reactions for alloantigens among cytochrome c-specific T cell clones. Specifically, both J_αC7 and J_β1.2 were selected in A^s alloreactive clones (TABLE 2), and the expression of both J_α28 and J_β2.5 was required in association with the appropriate V gene segments (V_α2B4 and V_β2B4) in order to confer A^b alloreactivity.

Combinatorial Joining

As implied by the foregoing, rearrangement of the same V elements to distinct J elements resulted in the acquisition of new MHC alloreactive specificities. Several conclusions can be drawn from these observations. First, they provide evidence that the J elements encode sequences critical to TCR-mediated recognition, a notion consistent with the considerable germline repertoires that have evolved for both the J_α and J_β regions (Kronenberg et al., 1986). Second, they demonstrate significant sequence homology between TCR that recognize Ia molecules in MHC-restricted recognition of antigen and TCR that recognize the same Ia molecules as alloantigens, in that such receptors may differ significantly only in sequences encoded by a single J region. Thus, the B10.A clone 3.3 described in this report (TABLE 2) is E^k-restricted for cytochrome c recognition, whereas the B10.S(9R) clone 9R.D6 is E^k-alloreactive. Yet 3.3 and 9R.D6 express the same V_α, J_α and V_β gene elements, differing only in D_β-J_β expression. We would conclude that the TCR on 3.3 has some affinity for the self-E^k molecule alone, and that substitution of the J_β1.2 element (which is expressed by 9R.D6) enhances this affinity for E^k such that the reactivity observed only in the presence of antigen is now apparent in the presence of the E^k Ia molecule alone. These data thus support the concept that the T cell repertoire is selected for low affinity self MHC recognition.

Does one α-β Heterodimer Mediate Both MHC-Restricted Antigen Recognition and Alloreactivity?

Recently, the successful transfection by Saito et al. (1987) of complete V_α2B4 and V_β2B4 genes, derived from the 2B4 hybridoma (Hedrick et al., 1982), into the human T cell tumor JURKAT (Weiss et al., 1984) was shown to result in the expression of the murine TCR heterodimer and in the acquisition of both pigeon cytochrome c specificity and E^k MHC restriction. The evidence available to date further indicates that for a given T cell clone, one α-β heterodimer mediates both MHC-restricted antigen recognition and alloreactivity. For instance, a clonotypic anti-TCR monoclonal antibody has been shown to block both the antigen-specific and alloreactive responses of a single dual specific T cell clone (Kaye et al., 1984). In addition, the pattern of alloreactivity observed in several antigen-specific responses has been shown not to be random but rather to correlate with the antigen and MHC restriction specificity of the responding T cells (Abromson-Leeman et al., 1983; Ashwell et al., 1986). The participation of a third α or β chain in association with one of the chains of the antigen receptor in the formation of a separate alloreactive receptor is not ruled out by the above evidence, and has indeed been demonstrated as a mechanism for generating alloreactivity in several antigen-specific T cell hybridomas (Blackman et al., 1986). However, the rules of allelic exclusion appear to apply in most diploid nontransformed T lymphocytes. Thus, the majority of T cells studied have been shown to possess only one productive β chain gene rearrangement (Kronenberg et al., 1986). In this regard, we have demonstrated that the productive V_β2B4 rearrangement is the only complete V_β-D_β-J_β rearrangement in several cytochrome c-specific T cell clones (Sorger et al., 1987). Allelic exclusion is more difficult to demonstrate for the α chain genes, but there is no direct evidence for the expression of two distinct α polypeptides in any T cell clone. Furthermore, a cDNA clone encoding a second V_α-J_α rearrangement was isolated from the 9R.D6 T cell clone described in this report. DNA sequencing revealed this V_α-J_α rearrangement to be out-of-frame, establishing V_αD6-J_αC7 as the only productive α rearrangement in this clone (D.L.M., unpublished data). Moreover, we have never isolated an antigen-specific T cell clone with both V_α and V_β rearrangements identical to those of an alloreactive clone which failed to also manifest the same alloreactivity. Thus, the expression of more than one α or β chain is unlikely to represent a common mechanism for amplification of the T cell repertoire in normal T lymphocytes. Finally, the data presented here, demonstrating that multiple, independently-derived antigen-specific T cell clones and lines with the same alloreactive specificity displayed identical V_α-J_α as well as V_β-D_β-J_β rearrangements, provide the firmest evidence to date that, in general, one receptor mediates both antigen-specific and alloreactive recognition.

ACKNOWLEDGMENTS

The authors wish to thank Ms. Ellen Kirshbaum for preparation of the manuscript.

This work was supported in part by U.S. Public Health Service (USPHS) grants AI 21372, GM 35880, and NSF DCB-8452023 (to S. M. Hedrick). S. B. Sorger is supported by USPHS training grant CA 09174 and S. M. Hedrick is supported by Research Career Development Award AI 00662. P. J. Fink is a senior fellow of the California Division of the American Cancer Society (Ordway Fellowship S-14).

REFERENCES

Abromson-Leeman, S. R. and Cantor H., 1983, Specificity of T cell clones for antigen and autologous major histocompatibility complex products determines specificity for foreign major histocompatibility complex product, J. Exp. Med., 158:428.

Arden, B., Klotz, J. L., Siu, G., and Hood, L. E., 1985, Diversity and structure of genes of the α family of mouse T cell antigen receptor, Nature, 316:783.

Ashwell, J. D., Chen, C., and Schwartz, R. H., 1986, High frequency and non-random distribution of alloreactivity in T cell clones selected for recognition of foreign antigen in association with self class II molecules, J. Immunol., 136:389.

Barth, R., Kim, B., Lan, N., Hunkapiller, T., Sobieck, N., Winoto, A., Gershenfeld, H., Okada, C., Hansburg, D., Weissman, I., and Hood, L., 1985, The murine T cell receptor employs a limited repertoire of expressed V_β gene segments, Nature, 316: 517.

Becker, D. M., Patten, P., Chien, Y.-H., Yokota, T., Eshhar, Z., Giedlin, M., Gascoigne, N. R. J., Goodnow, C., Wolf, R., Arai, K., and Davis, M. M., 1985, Variability and repertoire size of T cell receptor V_α segments, Nature, 317:430.

Bevan, M. J., Langman, R. E., Cohn, M., 1976, H-2 antigen-specific cytotoxic T cells induced by Concanavalin A: Estimation of their relative frequency, Eur. J. Immunol., 6:150.

Blackman, M., Yague, J., Kubo, R., Gay, D., Coleclough, C., Palmer, E., Kappler, J., and Marack, P., 1986, The T cell repertoire may be biased in favor of MHC recognition, Cell 47:349.

Braciale, T., Andrew, M., and Braciale, V., 1981, Simultaneous expression of H-2-restricted and alloreactive recognition by a cloned line of influenza virus-specific cytotoxic T lymphocytes, J. Exp. Med., 153:1371.

Chien, Y. H., Gascoigne, N. R. J., Kavaler, J., Lee, N. E., and Davis, M. M., 1984, Somatic recombination in a murine T cell receptor gene, Nature, 309:322.

Dembic, Z., Haas, W., Weiss, S., McCubrey, J., Kiefer, H., von Boehmer, H., and Steinmetz, M., 1986, Transfer of specificity by murine α and β T cell receptor genes, Nature, 320:232.

Fink, P., Matis, L., McElligott, D., Bookman, M., and Hedrick, S., 1986, Correlations between T cell specificity and the structure of the antigen receptor, Nature, 321:219.

Fischer-Lindahl, K. and Wilson, D. B., 1977, Histocompatibility antigen-activated cytotoxic T lymphocytes. II. Estimates of the frequency and specificity of precursors, J. Exp. Med., 145:508.

Heber-Katz, E., Schwartz, R. H., Matis, L. A., Hannum, C., Fairwell, T., Apella, E., 1982, Contribution of antigen-presenting cell major histocompatibility complex gene products to the specificity of antigen-induced T cell activation, J. Exp. Med., 155:1086.

Hedrick, S. M., Matis, L. A., Hecht, T. T., Samelson, L. E., Longo, D. L., Heber-Katz, E., and Schwartz, R. H., 1982, The fine specificity of antigen and Ia determinant recognition by T cell hybridoma clones specific for pigeon cytochrome c, Cell, 30:141.

Hedrick, S. M., Cohen, D. I., Nielson, E. A., and Davis, M. M., 1984, Isolation of cDNA clones encoding T cell-specific membrane-associated proteins, Nature 308:149.

Janeway, C.A., Jr., Lerner, E. A., Conrad, P. J., and Jones, B., 1982, The precision of self and non-self major histocompatibility complex encoded antigen recognition by cloned T cells, Behring Inst. Mitt. 70:200.

Jerne, N., 1971, The somatic generation of immune recognition, Eur. J. Immunol., 1:1.

Katz, D. H., Hamaoka, T., and Benacerraf, B., 1973, Cell interactions between histoincompatible T and B lymphocytes. II. Failure of physiologic cooperative interactions between T and B lymphocytes from allogeneic donor strains in humoral response to hapten-protein conjugates, J. Exp. Med., 137:1405.

Kaye, J. and Janeway, C. A., Jr., 1984, The Fab fragment of a directly activating monoclonal antibody that precipitates a disulfide-linked heterodimer from a helper T cell clone blocks activation by either allogeneic Ia or antigen and self-Ia, J. Exp. Med., 159:1397.

Kronenberg, M., Siu, G., Hood, L. E., and Shastri, N., The molecular genetics of the T cell antigen receptor and T cell antigen recognition, Ann. Rev. Immunol., 4:529.

Matis, L. A., Longo, D. L., Hedrick, S. M., Hannum, C., Margoliash, E., and Schwartz, R. H., 1983, Clonal analysis of the major histocompatibility complex restriction and the fine specificity of antigen recognition in the T cell proliferative response to cytochrome c, J. Immunol., 130:1527.

Matis, L. A., Sorger, S. B., McElligot, D. L., Fink, P. J., and Hedrick, S. M., 1987, The molecular basis of alloreactivity in antigen-specific, major histocompatibility complex restricted T cell clones, Cell, in press.

Novotny, J., Tonegawa, S., Saito, H., Kranz, D. M., and Eisen, H. N., 1986, Secondary, tertiary, and quaternary structure of T cell-specific immunoglobulin-like polypeptide chains, Proc. Natl. Acad. Sci. USA 83:742.

Saito, T., Weiss, A., Miller, J., Norcross, M. A., and Germain, R. N., 1987, Specific antigen-Ia activation of transfected human T cells expressing murine Ti $\alpha\beta$-human T3 receptor complexes, Nature 325:125.

Schwartz, R. H., The role of gene products of the major histocompatibility complex in T cell activation, in: "Fundamental Immunology," W. E. Paul ed., Raven Press, New York (1984).

Schwartz, R. H., Fox, B. S., Fraga, E., Chen, C., and Singh, B., 1985, The T lymphocyte response to cytochrome c. V. Determination of the minimal peptide size required for stimulation of T cell clones and assessment of the contribution of each residue beyond this size to antigenic potency, J. Immunol., 135:2598.

Shevach, E. M. and Rosenthal, A. S., 1973, Function of macrophages in antigen recognition by guinea pig T lymphocytes. II., J. Exp. Med., 138:1213.

Sorger, S. B., Hedrick, S. M., Fink, P. J., Bookman, M. A., and Matis, L. A., 1987, Generation of diversity in the T cell receptor repertoire specific for pigeon cytochrome c, J. Exp. Med. 165:279.

Sredni, B. and Schwartz, R. H., 1980, Alloreactivity of an antigen-specific T cell clone, Nature 287, 855.

Weiss, A. and Stobo, J., 1984, Requirement for the coexpression of T3 and the T cell antigen receptor on a malignant human T cell line, J. Exp. Med., 160:1284.

Winoto, A., Mjolsness, S., and Hood, L., 1985, Genomic organization of the genes encoding the mouse T cell receptor α chain: 18 J segments map over 60 kilobases of DNA, Nature, 316:832.

Winoto, A., Urban, J. L., Lan, N. C., Goverman, J., Hood, L., and Hansburg, D., 1986, Predominant use of a V_α gene segment in mouse T cell receptors for cytochrome c, Nature, 324:679.

Yanagi, Y., Yoshikai, Y., Leggett, K., Clark, S. P., Aleksander, I., and Mak, T. W., 1984, A human T cell-specific cDNA clone encodes a protein having extensive homology to immunoglobulin chains, Nature, 308:145.

Zinkernagel, R. M., Callahan, G. N., Althage, A., Cooper, S., Klein, P.A., and Klein, J., 1978, On the thymus in the differentiation of H-2 self-recognition by T ells: Evidence for dual recognition, J. Exp. Med., 147:882.

THE MAJOR HISTOCOMPATIBILITY COMPLEX AND THE T CELL REPERTOIRE

Guy Gammon, Nilabh Shastri, Stanley Wilbur, Shahrzad Sadegh-Nasseri, John Cogswell, Alexander Miller and Eli Sercarz

UCLA Department of Microbiology
405 Hilgard Avenue
Los Angeles, California 90024-1489

ABSTRACT

We examined the ability of peptides corresponding to different regions of hen eggwhite lysozyme to stimulate proliferative T-cell responses in several mouse strains. The relationship of the major histocompatibility complex (MHC) and other non-MHC genes to the T cell repertoire was studied. It was found that the MHC was the major influence on the specificity of the T cell repertoire. The T cell response following immunization with native hen eggwhite lysozyme was also investigated. Challenge with the whole protein preferentially induces responses to some determinants compared to others. Hence, some regions of the protein appear to be immunodominant while other determinants are sub-dominant.

INTRODUCTION

The antigenic determinants on a protein molecule recognized by T cells can be investigated using peptides corresponding to different regions of the immunogen (Benjamin et al., 1984, Livingstone and Fathman, 1987). We have examined the proliferative T cell response in different mouse strains to peptides corresponding to several regions of hen egg-white lysozyme (HEL). Mice were immunized with different HEL peptides to define individual determinants on the molecule, and with native HEL to examine which determinants predominated in the anti-HEL response.

Several questions can be answered using this approach. First the specificity of the response in different mouse strains and the different determinants for each strain can be shown. The relationship of the MHC and other gene loci to the specificity of the T cell response can be compared using congenic strains. Second, an overlapping panel of peptides can be tested to define the boundaries of individual determinants and show how different MHC gene products influence the way the same peptide is recognized. Thirdly, utilization of potential determinants on the HEL molecule and competition between different determinants, following immunization with native HEL, can be examined.

RESULTS

The proliferative response to immunization with 4 HEL peptides corresponding to amino acid residues 30-53, 46-61, 74-96 and 106-129 was tested in three mouse strains, B10.A, C57BL/6(B6) and BALB/c. These peptides were chosen because they have been found to contain determinants recognized by T cells from B10.A mice (Maizels et al., 1980, Bixler et al., 1985, Allen et al., 1985). The peptides 30-53, 46-61 and 74-96 were prepared by solid phase peptide synthesis. Peptide 106-129 was prepared by reduction and carboxymethylation of HEL followed by cleavage with cyanogen bromide. Responsiveness was assayed by a T cell proliferation assay (Maizels et al., 1980). Each mouse was immunized with 3.5 nanomoles of peptide in complete Freund's adjuvant and the draining lymph nodes were removed 10 days later. The in vitro proliferative response to HEL or peptides at 7μM concentration was measured by ^{3}H-thymidine incorporation.

The data from several experiments is summarized in Table 1. It is clear from these results that the immunogenicity of a peptide depends on the strain tested; although all the peptides tested were immunogenic, none stimulated responses in all three strains. The responses to individual peptides were highly crossreactive in vitro with native HEL, except for the 74-96 induced response in B10.A mice. Although immunization with 74-96 induces a good response to itself, little or no proliferation is observed to HEL. This is a surprising result since the B6 response to 74-96 can be recalled by native HEL and it would seem unlikely that antigen processing would differ between the B10.A and B6 strains. Possible explanations have been discussed elsewhere (Gammon et al. 1987). It is apparent also, that the number of determinants which can induce a response in a particular strain is very variable. B10.A mice can respond to each of the four peptides tested and possibly others. BALB/c mice only respond to one, 106-129, and previous work has suggested that this is the only determinant on HEL for this strain (Katz et al., 1982).

In addition to comparing MHC disparate strains, different strains sharing H-2^b were also tested (Table 2). The data show that the response to peptides is almost identical in different H-2^b strains, a pattern quite different than that between MHC disparate strains. All the H-2^b strains tested responded to peptide 30-53 and 74-96, but not to 106-129. Interestingly, they were not identical in that 2 strains, B6 and A.BY, responded very poorly to 46-61. Most mice from these two strains did not show any response; while a few did respond significantly

TABLE 1. Proliferative Response to Immunization with HEL Peptides

Strain	Ia	30-53	46-61	74-96	106-129
B10.A	A^kE^k	+	+	+*	+
B6	A^b	+	-	+	-
Balb/c	A^dE^d	-	-	-	+

*not recalled by HEL

TABLE 2. Proliferative Response to Immunization with HEL Peptides in Different H-2^b Strains

Strain	30-53	46-61	74-96	106-129
B6	+	±	+	-
BALB.B	+	+	+	-
C57L	+	+	+	-
C3H.SW	+	+	+	-
A.BY	+	±	+	-
bm12	-	-	+	-

above background, the response in the other strains was significantly better. The dominant effect of the MHC on the response repertoire was confirmed by testing the B6.C-H-2^{bm12}(bm12) strain. Although bm12 differs at only 3 amino acid residues in the I-A^b molecule the pattern of responsiveness is quite different from H-2^b mice. The bm12 mice respond to 74-96 only and not to 30-53, 46-61 or 106-129.

The data in Table 1 show that B10.A and B6 mice respond to the peptide 74-96. These responses were examined in detail to define the boundaries of the minimal determinant and compare the determinants recognized by the MHC-disparate strains. The response of 74-96-specific T cell clones from each strain, as well as primed lymph node cells, was examined (Shastri et al. 1986). Both strains recognized 2 distinct determinants on 74-96 but the minimal peptides recognized were different (Table 3). T cell clones from B6 mice responded to 74-90, but not to 74-86; or to 81-96, but not 85-96. B10.A mice responded to 74-86 and 85-96. Thus, even when the same peptide region is recognized, the MHC affects the way in which it is seen. The response to 74-96 was examined also in the bm12 mouse. This strain responded to the determinant within 74-90, but not to the determinant within 81-96, again confirming the major role of the MHC in deciding the specificity of responses.

Table 3. T Cell Determinants Within Peptide 74-96.

Strain	Ia	74-96	74-90	74-86	81-96	85-96
B10.A	A^kE^k	+	+	+	+	+
B6	A^b	+	+	-	+	-
bm12	A^{bm12}	+	+	-	-	-

Table 4. Utilization of Determinants Following Immunization With Native HEL

Strain	1-18	13-35	30-53	46-61	74-96	106-129
B10.A	-	++	+	++	-	+
B6	-	++	-	-	++	-
BALB/c	-	-	-	-	-	

Finally, the T cell proliferative response of different mouse strains to immunization with HEL was tested. The results from 3 strains (B10.A, B6 and BALB/c) are summarized in Table 4. The most striking finding is that although a strain may show approximately equal responsiveness to peptides, after priming with each peptide, immunization with the whole protein preferentially stimulates responses to some determinants at the expense of others. For example, the peptides 30-53 and 46-61 both induce strong proliferative responses, which are highly cross-reactive with native HEL, in B10.A mice. However, immunization with HEL appears to induce a much stronger response to 46-61 than to 30-53. A similar result has been show by other laboratories (Bixler et al., 1985, Allen et al., 1985). B6 mice respond to 30-53 and 74-96 following immunization with each peptide. However, priming with HEL induces a good 74-96 response _in vitro_ but only a minimal response to 30-53. These results demonstrate that the response to some determinants is much greater than the response to others, and that a hierarchy of immunodominant and sub-dominant determinants can occur in the response to a multi-determinant antigen.

DISCUSSION

Examination of the proliferative response to HEL and several HEL peptides, clearly shows the dominant role of the MHC in determining the repertoire of T cell responses. Even when the same peptide is recognized in association with different Ia molecules, detailed analysis shows that the actual determinant recognized is different. This finding has important implications for predicting the site of T cell determinants. Recently 2 algorithms have been proposed for use in predicting T cell sites, but neither take MHC differences into account (Margalit et al. 1987, Rothbard et al., 1986). Furthermore, our data combined with others indicates that T cell determinants are situated on all parts of the HEL molecule.

The finding that there is differential utilization of determinants in the immune response to proteins requires the reinterpretation of data relating to the extent of the T cell repertoire. A limited T cell response to one or a few determinants has been found in the T cell response to several proteins, e.g., sperm whale myoglobin (Berkower, et al, 1984) cytochrome c (Solinger et al., 1979), β-galactosidase (Krzych et al., 1982) and staphylococcal nuclease (Finnegan et al, 1986). This has been thought to reflect either a restricted T cell receptor repertoire, due to self-tolerance, or the requirement for peptides to bind Ia molecules. However our data suggest that the potential number of determinants may be quite large in some strains, but that a choice is made between determinants. This choice could be decided on the basis of T cell precursor frequency or the binding affinity of a peptide for Ia, but other factors (Gammon et al, 1987) such as availability of specific determinants after antigen processing, competition between determinants in binding Ia or regulation by other lymphocyte sub-populations, e.g., suppressor T cells, may be important.

ACKNOWLEDGEMENTS

We wish to thank Bonnie Hechinger for secretarial services. This work was supported in part by NIH grants AI-11183 and CA-24442. Nilabh Shastri was a Fellow of the Leukaemia Society. John Cogswell and Stanley Wilbur were supported by training grant NCI-09120.

REFERENCES

Allen, P.M., McKean, D.J., Beck, B.N., Sheffield, J. and Glimcher, L.H. (1985), Direct evidence that a class II molecule and a simple globular protein generate multiple determinants. J Exp Med 162:1264.

Benjamin, C.D., Berzofsky, J.A., East, I.J., Gurd, F.R.N., Hannum, C., Leach, S.J, Margoliash, E., Michael, J.G., Miller, A., Prager, E.M. Reichlin, M., Sercarz, E.E., Smith-Gill, S.J., Todd, P.E. and Wilson, A.C., (1984), The antigenic structure of proteins: A reappraisal. Ann. Rev. Immunol. 2:67-101.

Berkower, I., Matis, L.A., Buckenmeyer, G.K., Gurd, F.R.N., Longo, D.L. and Berzofsky, J.A., (1984), Identification of distinct predominant epitopes recognized by myoglobin-specific T-cells under the control of different Ir genes and characterization of representative T-cell clones. J. Immunol. 132:1370.

Bixler, G.S., Yoshida, T. and Atassi, M.Z., (1985), Antigen presentation of lysozyme: T cell recognition of peptide and intact protein after priming with synthetic overlapping peptides comprising the entire protein chain. Immunology 56:103.

Finnegan, A., Smith, M.A., Smith, J.A., Berzofsky, J.A., Sachs, D.M. and Hodes, R.J., (1986), The T cell repertoire for recognition of a phylogenetically distant protein antigen. Peptide specificity and MHC restriction of Staphylococcal nuclease-specific T cell clones. J. Exp. Med. 164:897.

Gammon, G., Shastri, N., Cogswell, J., Wilbur, S., Sadegh-Nasseri, S., Krzych, U., Miller, A., and Sercarz, E., (1987), The choice of T cell epitopes utilized on a protein antigen depends on factors distant from, as well as at, the determinant site. Immunol. Reviews. 98, In press.

Katz, M., Maizels, R., Wicker, L., Miller, A., and Sercarz, E.E., (1982), Immunological focussing by the mouse MHC: mouse strains confronted with distantly related lysozymes confine their attention to very few epitopes. Eur. J. Immunol. 12:535-540.

Livingstone, A.M. and Fathman, C.G., (1987), The structure of T-cell epitopes. Ann. Rev. Immunol. 5:477.

Maizels, R., Clarke, J., Harvey, M., Miller, A. and Sercarz, E.E., (1980), Epitope specificity of the T cell proliferative response to lysozyme: T proliferative cells react predominantly to different determinants from those recognized by B cells. Eur. J. Immunol. 10:509-515.

Margalit, M., Spouge, J., Cornette, J., Cease, K., DeLisi, C. and Berzofsky, J.A., (1987), Prediction of immunodominant helper T cell antigenic sites from the primary sequence. J. Immunol. 138:2213.

Rothbard, J., Townsend, A., Edwards, M., and Taylor W., (1986), Pattern recognition among T cell epitopes, in: "Modern Trends in Human Leukemia VII".

Shastri, N., Gammon, G., Miller, A. and Sercarz, E.E., (1986), Ia molecule associated selectivity in T-cell recognition of a 23 amino acid peptide of lysozyme. J. Exp. Med. 164:882-896.

Solinger, A.M., Ultee, M.E., Margoliash, E. and Schwartz, R.H., (1979), Lymphocyte response to cytochrome c. Demonstration of a T-cell heteroclitic proliferative response and identification of a topographic antigenic determinant on pigeon cytochrome c whose immune recognition requires two complementary immune response genes. J. Exp. Med. 150:830.

THE PRESENTATION OF PROCESSED, Ia RESTRICTED, T CELL ANTIGENIC PEPTIDES ON ANTIGEN PRESENTING CELL SURFACES

Susan K. Pierce, Ellen K, Lakey, Emanuel Margoliash, Lori A. Smolenski and Lisa A. Casten

Department of Biochemistry, Molecular Biology and Cell Biology, Northwestern University, Evanston, Illinois 60201, USA

INTRODUCTION

The helper T cell response to a soluble protein requires the processing of the native antigen by an antigen presenting cell (APC) to a peptide containing an antigenic determinant, which is transported to and held on the APC surface, where it is recognized by the specific T cell in the context of the appropriate Ia molecule[1]. The requirement for processing and presentation of antigens for T cell recognition would not appear to apply only to T cells of the helper subset, in that recent studies have indicated that cytolytic T cells may also recognize processed forms of their antigens in the context of the MHC class I molecules. Thus, Townsend *et al.*[2] demonstrated that cytolytic T cells specific for influenza virus infected cells recognize peptides of the nucleocapsid protein which is not normally expressed in its native form on the cell surface. Furthermore, cells transfected with genes encoding a truncated soluble form of influenza virus hemagglutinin which lacks a membrane anchoring domain and consequently is not expressed on cell surfaces are, all the same, targets of hemagglutinin specific cytolytic T cells[3]. Thus, the ability to process and present both extracellular and intracellular proteins appears to be a general function of all cells which presumably have the machinery to anchor T cell antigenic peptides on their surfaces.

At present, little is known concerning the mechanisms by which peptides are displayed on cell surfaces. For Ia expressing APC, it has been suggested that T cell antigenic peptides bind to Ia, and that Ia may transport peptides from their site of cleavage within acidic vesicles to the cell surface. Indeed, Babbitt *et al.*[4] demonstrated, using equilibrium dialysis, that an antigenic peptide of hen lysozyme binds to a purified preparation of a responder Ia, with a Kd of 10^{-6} M, but not to that of a nonresponder Ia. Buus *et al.*[5-7] report similar findings measuring the binding of several antigenic peptides to a variety of Ia's.

A second approach to determining the nature of the association of T cell antigenic peptides with the APC surface, is to attempt to compete the stimulatory peptide from binding sites on the APC surface using non-stimulatory peptide analogs. There are several cases in which peptides incapable of activating specific T cells, namely non-stimulatory peptides, have been demonstrated to block T cell activation by their specific antigen as presented by APC[8-12], presumably by competing with the stimulatory peptides for binding sites on the APC surface. Thus, Rock and

Benacerraf[8] showed that the stimulation of T cells specific for a synthetic amino acid polymer was blocked by structurally related but non-stimulatory amino acid polymers. Similarly, when we studied the I-E^k restricted mouse T cell response to pigeon cytochrome c (Pc), it was found that peptides representing the C-terminus of cytochromes c from a variety of species, which do not activate Pc-specific T cells, block their recognition of Pc as processed and presented by APC[9]. Because APC pulsed with Pc in the presence of a blocking peptide were unable to activate the specific T cells, even after excess peptide was washed away, the blocking effect appeared to be the result of the competition at the APC surface for a peptide binding site[9]. Babbitt *et al.*[10] showed that the T cell response to an antigenic peptide from hen lysozyme is blocked by the corresponding peptide of the very similar mouse lysozyme. In all these cases, the competing peptides were highly homologous to the stimulatory peptides. However, Guillet *et al.*[11,12] recently showed that the T cell responses to antigenic peptides of the bacteriophage cI protein and of OVA can be blocked by immunodominant peptide fragments from unrelated proteins which share no obvious primary sequence similarity with the T cell antigenic peptides, but which display the same MHC restriction. Moreover, competing peptides were demonstrated to bind to the appropriate Ia, with which the stimulatory peptides were recognized by the T cells[12], leading these authors to conclude that blocking was the result of competition for a peptide binding site on Ia. However, such a correlation would not appear to hold in all cases, in that recent results from our laboratory[13] indicate that peptides with no obvious primary amino acid sequence homology, and which are not capable of being recognized in the context of the same Ia, compete with one another for the sites on the APC necessary for presentation of processed antigen to T cells. These results suggest that there are structures on the APC surface, in addition to Ia, which are necessary for effective antigen presentation following processing. A suitable candidate for such a cell surface material is the recently identified peptide binding protein, PBP 72/74[14]. In this report, the results from our laboratory which support this conclusion will be reviewed.

RESULTS AND DISCUSSION

To examine what structural features of peptides allow them to function as T cell antigens, and to further investigate the role of Ia in anchoring antigenic peptides produced during processing on the APC surface, the T cell response to a well characterized, soluble globular protein antigen, cytochrome c, was studied. Mouse T cell hybrids were generated which recognize an antigenic determinant in the C-terminus of Pc and show a characteristic higher affinity heteroclitic response to tobacco hornworm moth cytochrome c (THMc)[15]. As is the case for the majority of helper T cell responses to the soluble globular antigen studied to date, Pc-specific T cells require that the native Pc antigen be processed and presented by an APC. This is shown by the inability of APC, treated to block processing functions, to present the native protein, while retaining the ability to present a processed form of Pc, namely a C-terminal cyanogen bromide peptide fragment residues 81-104 (Pc 81-104)[16]. The minimum size peptide fragment sufficient for T cell activation was determined by synthesizing peptides of increasing length representing the C-terminus of THMc. Peptides of less than 10 residues failed to function as T cell antigens even though these contain residues previously determined[17] to be involved in the specific T cell recognition of THMc (Table 1). However, none of the peptides shorter than 24 amino acids in length functioned to induce the high affinity heteroclitic response. Interestingly, the addition of a cysteinyl residue to the N-terminus of the 12 amino acid peptide, THMc 92-103, conferred on it the ability to stimulate the heteroclitic response, inducing a half maximal T cell response with 1/300*th* the peptide concentration required for Pc 81-104.

This may reflect the ability of the cysteine-containing peptide to stably associate at the APC surface through disulfide binding to APC surface structures.

Table 1. The Minimal Size Peptide Fragment Required to Stimulate Pigeon Cytochrome c Specific T Cells*

	Sequence (residues 81, 85, 90, 95, 100, 104)	Concentration (μM) Required for 50% Max. IL-2 Response
Mc 81-104	IFAGIKKKGERADLIAYLKKATNE	>1000
Pc 81-104	--------A----------Q--AK	3.0
THMc 81-103	V---L--AN----------Q--KΔ	0.05
THMc 86-103	--AN----------Q--KΔ	2.5
THMc 91-103	---------Q--KΔ	2.8
THMc 92-103	--------Q--KΔ	2.5
THMc Cys 92-103	C--------Q--KΔ	0.01
THMc 93-103	-------Q--KΔ	2.7
THMc 94-103	------Q--KΔ	1.5
THMc 96-103	----Q--KΔ	>1000
THMc 97-103	---Q--KΔ	>1000

*T cell activation was measured by incubating 5 X 10^4 B cells as APC with 5 X 10^4 irradiated TPc9.1 cells, an I-E^k restricted Pc-specific T cell hybrid, in 0.2 ml culture media in the presence of increasing concentrations of the peptides listed, for 24 hours at which time the culture supernatants are tested for their IL-2 content as described[15]. The peptide concentration yielding 50% maximal IL-2 response is given. Mc is mouse cytochrome c.

Previous results[9] showed that peptides of the cytochromes c of a variety of species which do not activate Pc-specific T cells, block their recognition of Pc as processed and presented by APC (Table 2). There is a minimal length required for blocking, in that peptides of 8 residues or less, THMc 96-103 and THMc 97-103, which do not stimulate, also do not block. In addition, the tyrosine at position 97 appears to be important in both blocking and stimulation, as iodination of this residue eliminates both activities. Lastly, the C-terminal 5 residues of the blocking mouse peptide can be deleted, as in Mc 81-99, and the blocking activity is retained even though this region is critical to the activity of the stimulatory cytochrome c peptides.

The range of peptides capable of competing with the processed stimulatory Pc peptide for binding sites on the APC was investigated. A series of fourteen, 20-amino acid overlapping peptides, representing the entire length of staphylococcal nuclease (Nase), were tested for their ability to block the Pc-specific T cell response to Pc, as processed and presented by APC. These peptides are of particular interest as they have been characterized as to their antigenicity and MHC restriction for Nase-specific T cells[18]. As summarized in Table 3, three of the Nase peptides, namely Nase 61-80, Nase 91-110 and Nase 101-120, block the I-E^k-restricted T cells response to Pc. Two of these three, Nase 61-80 and Nase 91-110, have been identified as antigens for T cells from Nase immunized mice, and are recognized in the context of I-A^d and I-A^b, respectively. The third has not been identified as a T cell antigen. In contrast, the I-E^k-restricted Nase peptides, Nase 51-70 and Nase 81-100, have no effect.

Table 2. The Ability of Cytochrome c Peptides to Block the Pc-specific T Cell Response*

	81 85 90 95 100 104	Stimulates	Blocks
Mc 81-104	IFAGIKKKGERADLIAYLKKATNE	–	+
Mc 81-99	-------------------	–	+
Pc 81-104	--------A----------Q--AK	+	
	I		
Idiotyr 97 Pc 81-104	--------A-------Y--Q--KK	–	–
THMc 81-103	V---L--AN----------Q--KΔ	+	
THMc 96-103	----Q--KΔ	–	–
THMc 97-103	---Q--KΔ	–	–
Duck c 81-104	--------S----------D--AK	–	+
Chicken c 81-104	--------S--V-------D--SK	–	+
Screw worm c 81-104	----L--PN--G-------AS-KΔ	+	
Hippopotamus c 81-104	--------G----------Q----	–	+
Rabbit c 81-104	--------D---------------	–	+
Horse c 81-104	--------T--E------------	–	+
Drosophila c 81-103	----L--PD--G-------S--KΔ	+	
Samia c 81-103	V---L--AN----------ES-KΔ	+	

*Taken from Lakey *et al.*[9]. Blocking is determined by incubating TPc9.1 cells (5 X 10^4) with 4 X 10^5 Pc-pulsed B cells, in the presence of increasing concentrations of the competitor peptide, as described[9], and by measuring the IL-2 response 24 hours later. For blocking, a plus "+" indicates that the complete blocking of the TPc9.1 response was observed requiring 30-100μM competitor peptide; a minus "–" indicates that no blocking was observed with concentrations of 150-300 μM competitor. Stimulatory ability was measured as described in Table 1 and a plus "+" indicates T cells were activated at peptide concentrations of 1-10 μM; a minus "–" indicates no activation was observed at peptide concentrations >360 μM.

Table 3. Blocking Effect of Peptides Derived From Staphlococcal Nuclease on The T cell Responses to Pc*

Peptide	MHC Restriction	Blocks T cell Response to Pc
Nase 1-20	u	-
Nase 11-30	u	-
Nase 21-40	u	nt
Nase 31-50	u	nt
Nase 41-60	u	-
Nase 51-70	I-E^k	-
Nase 61-80	I-A^d	+(41 μM)
Nase 71-90	u	-
Nase 81-100	I-E^k	-
Nase 91-110	I-A^b	+(52 μM)
Nase 101-120	u	+(43 μM)
Nase 111-130	u	-
Nase 121-140	u	-
Nase 131-149	u	-

*Taken from Lakey *et al.*[13]. The blocking studies are carried out as described in Table 2. The MHC restriction of the peptides is shown; a "u" indicates that T cells which recognize these peptides have not been identified. Two peptides were not tested "nt" due to their poor solubility (Nase 21-40) or toxicity on B cells (Nase 31-50). The concentration of peptide required to reduce the TPc9.1 cell response by 50% is shown in parentheses.

That these peptides are not nonspecifically toxic to the T cell response could be shown by their inability to block the higher affinity heteroclitic response to THMc[9,13]. Moreover, the I-E^k-restricted C-terminal peptides of pigeon cytochrome c (Pc 81-104) and tobacco hornworm moth cytochrome c (THMc 81-103) block the I-A^d-restricted T cell response to OVA as do the I-A^d and I-A^b-restricted Nase peptides, Nase 61-80 and Nase 91-110, but not the I-E^k-restricted Nase 81-100 (Table 4)[13]. Thus, peptides which share no obvious primary sequence similarity and are not recognized in the context of the same Ia, appear to compete with one another for peptide binding sites on the APC.

If these blocking phenomena are indeed a consequence of competition at the APC surface for peptide binding sites, our results indicate that peptides bind to structures which particpate in antigen presentation other than, or in addition to, Ia. Even though an apparent correlation between the ability of a peptide to be recognized in association with a given Ia and its ability to block an Ia-restricted T cell response has been reported[5-7,10-12], the present results indicate that such a correlation

Table 4. Ability of Peptides to Block the I-A^k Restricted OVA-specific T Cell Response*

Competitor Peptide	MHC Restriction	Blocks T Cell Response to OVA α
Pc 81-104	I-E^k	+ (20)
Mc 81-104		+ (30)
Mc 81-99		+ (160)
THMc 81-103	I-E^k	+ (60)
THMc 90-103	I-E^k	+ (225)
THMc 91-103	I-E^k	+ (21)
THMc 92-103	I-E^k	+ (145)
THMc Cys 92-103	I-E^k	+ (90)
Nase 61-80	I-A^d	+ (32)
Nase 91-110	I-A^b	+ (32)
Nase 81-100	I-E^k	–

*Taken from Lakey *et al.*[13]. Blocking was measured by incubating 5 X 10^4 OVA-pulsed B cells with 5 X 10^4 AODH 3.4 cells, I-A^k restricted, OVA-specific T cell hybrid, in the presence of graded concentrations of competitor peptides. Supernatants were collected 24 hours later and their IL-2 content determined. A plus "+" indicates complete blocking was observed and the concentration of competitor peptide required to reduce the T cell response by 50% is shown in parentheses. The MHC restriction of the peptides is given.

does not always hold. These discrepancies could be explained if there are peptide binding sites on the APC surface, in addition to Ia, and if the contributions of these binding sites to the stabilization of the interaction between the antigenic peptide, Ia and the T cell receptor, are different for different antigenic peptides. Thus, if a peptide is anchored on an APC surface solely through its attachment to Ia, then only peptides with the same Ia restriction could block. If, however, a second APC protein such as the recently described PBP 72/74[4] binds the peptide and stabilizes its interaction with Ia or the T cell receptor, then there may be no correlation between a peptide's ability to block and its Ia restriction. In fact, structures other than Ia may play a more pivotal role in the presentation of antigen that has been processed in the presenting cells as was investigated in the studies reviewed here. By contrast, Ia may play a greater role in the presentation of exogenously added peptides, as investigated by others[5-7,10-12]. These are provided in large excess as compared to the quantity of peptides produced from native proteins and present on the APC surface. As more detail will be forthcoming concerning the mechanisms of antigen presentation and the molecules which participate in the process, the structural basis for the observed blocking phenomenon should become clearer.

This work is supported by grants from the National Institutes of Health AI. SKP is a recipient of an American Cancer Society Faculty Research Award FRA .

REFERENCES

1. E.R. Unanue, Antigen-presenting function of the macrophage, Ann. Rev. Immunol. 2:395-428 (1984).
2. A.R.M. Townsend, J. Rothbard, F.M. Gotch, G. Bahadur, D. Wraith and J.J. McMichael, The epitopes of influenza nucleoprotein recognized by cytolytic T lymphocytes can be defined with short synthetic peptides, Cell 44:959 (1986).
3. A.R.M. Townsend, I. Bastin, K. Gould and G.G. Brownlee, Cytotoxic T lymphocytes recognize influenza hemagglutinin that lacks a signal sequence, Nature 234:575.
4. B.R. Babbitt, P.M. Allen, G. Matsueda, E. Haber and E.R. Unanue, Binding of immunogenic peptides to Ia histocompatibility molecules, Nature 317:359-361 (1985).
5. S. Buus, S. Colon, C. Smith, J.H. Freed, C. Miles and H.M. Grey, Interaction between a "processed" ovalbumin peptide and Ia molecules, Proc. Natl.Acd. Sci. USA 83:3968-3971 (1986).
6. S. Buus, A. Sette, S.M. Colon, D.M. Jenis and H.M. Grey, Isolation and characterization of antigen-Ia complexes involved in T Cell recognition, Cell 47:1071-1077 (1986).
7. S. Buus, A. Sette, S.M. Colon, C. Miles and H.M. Grey, The relationsip between Major Histocompatibility Complex (MHC) restriction and the capacity of Ia to bind to immunogenic peptides, Science 235:1353-1358 (1987).
8. K.L. Rock and B. Benacerraf, Inhibition of antigen-specific T lymphocyte activation by structurally related Ir gene controlled polymers, J. Exp. Med. 160:1864-1879 (1984).
9. E.K. Lakey, E. Margoliash, G. Flouret and S.K. Pierce, Peptides related to the antigenic determinant block T cell recognition of the native protein as processed by antigen-presenting cells, Eur. J. Immunol. 16:721-727 (1986).
10. B.R. Babbitt, G. Matsueda, E. Haber, E. Unanue and P.M. Allen, Antigenic competition at the level of peptide-Ia binding, Proc. Natl. Acad. Sci. USA 83:4509-4513 (1986).
11. J.G. Guillet, M.Z. Lai, T.J. Briner, J.A. Smith and M.L. Gefter, The interaction of peptide antigens and class II major histocompatibility complex antigens as studies by T cell activation, Nature 423:260-262 (1986).
12. J.G. Guillet, M.Z. Lai, T.J. Briner, S. Buus, A. Sette, H.M. Grey, J.A. Smith and M.L. Gefter, Immunological self, nonself discrimination, Science 235:865-870 (1987).
13. E.K. Lakey, L.A. Casten, M.S. Anderson, L. Smolenski, J.A. Smith, E. Margoliash and S.K. Pierce, T. cell activation by processed antigen is equally blocked by I-E and I-A restricted peptides. (submitted for publication) (1987).
14. E.K. Lakey, E. Margoliash and S.K. Pierce, A peptide binding protein which plays a role in antigen presentation, Proc. Natl. Acad. Sci. USA 84:1659-1663 (1987).
15. E.K. Lakey, F.W. Fitch, E. Margoliash and S.K. Pierce, Role of L3T4 and Ia in the heteroclitic response of T cells to cytochrome c, J. Immunol. 136:3933-3938 (1986).
16. L.A. Casten, E.K. Lakey, M.L. Jelachich, E. Margoliash and S.K. Pierce, Anti-immunoglobulin augments B cell antigen-presentation function independently of internalization of receptor antigen complex, Proc. Natl. Acad. Sci. USA 81:6831-6835 (1985).

17. A.M. Solinger, M.E. Ultee, E. Margoliash and R.W. Schwartz, I. Demonstration of a T cell heteroclitic proliferative response and identification of a topographic antigenic determinant on pigeon cytochrome c whose immune recognition requires two complementary Major histocompatibility complex-linked immune response genes, J. Exp. Med. 150:830-848 (1979).
18. A. Finnegan, M.A. Smith, J.A. Smith, J. Berzofsky, D.H. Sachs and R.J. Hodes, The T cell repetoire for recognition of a phylogenetically distinct protein antigen. Peptide specificity and MHC restriction of staphylococcal nuclease-specific T cell clones, J. Exp. Med. 164:897-910 (1986).

VISUALIZATION OF DIRECT T-B CELL INTERACTION

Susan L. Swain

Department of Biology and
Cancer Center, Q-063
University of California, San Diego
La Jolla, CA 92093

INTRODUCTION

The concept that an antigen-specific helper T cell directly binds to a B cell stimulated by the same antigen and that this direct interaction is essential for B cell antibody production is well accepted. The most convincing evidence until recently that such cell-cell contact was necessary came from studies of Mitchison (1971) and his colleagues, subsequently repeated in numerous permutations, which showed that the epitopes recognized by both the T cell and B cell must be present on the same molecule. The current picture we have of the events in this interaction is that the specific immunoglobulin on the B cell binds determinants on the antigen, that the antigen is internalized and processed into fragments, and that these fragments are somehow presented on the B cell surface in association with class II. A helper T cell then recognizes the antigen fragment-class II complex by virtue of its specific receptor and thus a direct interaction of the two cells occurs. The recognition of antigen/class II activates the T cells and stimulates the T cell to synthesize and secrete lymphokines. Both the direct interaction of the T cell with the B cell and the soluble lymphokines secreted by the helper T cell are considered essential for B cell activation and subsequent proliferation and differentiation to antibody secretion. Despite the wide acceptance of this scenario actual T-B cell interactions have not been directly visualized until recently, and the details of the interaction and its consequences are largely unknown. In this report, I will review several recent studies we have done in collaboration with our colleagues, Dr. Abraham Kupfer, Dr. Charles Janeway and Dr. Jonanthan Singer. These studies reveal several striking events which occur during specific T cell-B cell interaction.

OBSERVATIONS

The binding of cytotoxic T lymphocytes to their effectors is easily visualized and has been studied for some years (Berke, 1983). Our colleagues Abraham Kupfer and Jonathon Singer had collaborated with Gunther Dennert (Kupfer et al., 1985; Kupfer et al., 1986a) to use fluorescence microscopy to examine some of the intracellular events which occur during the T cell effector-target interaction. They found that the microtubule organizing center (MTOC) which is associated with the golgi secretory apparatus invariably became reoriented to face the target cell during specific interaction (Kupfer et al., 1985; Kupfer et al., 1986a). They also found that a submembranal protein, talin, which is associated with the cytoskeleton of all cells become redistributed within the T effector cell so that it was concentrated beneath the area of effector-target cell contact (Kupfer et al., 1986a). In these studies, the dramatic T cell events required specific recognition and appeared to be a consequence of the binding event (Kupfer et al., 1985).

During effector-target interaction, granules containing cytotoxins appear to be directly deposited onto the target cell surface (Podack and Konigsberg, 1984) and the polar events in the T cell which involve the secretory apparatus were postulated to be part of the mechanism to carry out granular exocytosis.

Recently, we undertook similar studies to see if we could visualize helper T cell-B cell interactions and study, using immunofluorescence, the intracellular and membrane events that would be involved in this interaction. Our strategy was to use homogeneous T cell lines specific for antigen and also homogeneous B cell sources with the ability to present antigen to T cells. In most of our studies, we have used the D10.G4.1 T cell line (D10) developed by Drs. Jonathan Kaye and Charles Janeway (Kaye et al., 1983) which is specific for egg white protein, Conalbumin, with IA^k and we have used the LK (IA^k/IA^d) hybridoma (Kappler et al., 1982) as an antigen-presenting B cell source (APC). The APC are preincubated with specific or nonspecific antigen and then mixed one to one with the T cells. Such cells are incubated briefly at 37°C and spun onto slides, followed by fixation and permeabilization. Monoclonal antibodies to structures or molecules of interest are added and secondary antibodies, labelled with fluorescein or rhodamine and specific for the primary antibodies are used to visualize molecules in the T and B cells. Couples of T-B cells are identified by staining with a B cell specific reagent and a large number of couples are examined. Negative controls include B hybridomas mixed with inappropriate antigen or antigen added just before T-B mixing, B cell hybridomas or lymphomas with APC ability but inappropriate class II and other T cell lines or hybridomas with distinct specificity (Kupfer et al., 1986b).

We first examined the cell couples for the orientation of the MTOC, using antibody to tubulin. We found a very dramatic effect. In virtually all the cell couples between D10 T cells and Conalbumin pulsed LK B cells, the MTOC was oriented to face the B cell. The MTOC orientation in B cells in this instance and of both T and B cells in negative controls was random. Thus, it appears that one consequence of specific helper T cell recognition of antigen on B cells is a polarization of the golgi apparatus like that which occurs during cytotoxic T cell target interaction. We have seen this effect with other helper T cell lines and hybridomas and with other B cell hybridomas and lymphomas, and with alloantigen as well as soluble antigen recognition (Kupfer et al., 1987a). This event occurs rapidly (<15 minutes) requires extracellular Ca^{++} and antigen processing in the case of soluble but not alloantigen.

We have also examined talin distribution in the interacting T-B cell couples. We observe that talin but not two other cytoskeleton associated proteins (vinculin and α-actinin) becomes concentrated in the T cell under the span of T cell-B cell contact. This redistribution of talin occurs only in the T cell and is antigen and class II specific (Kupfer et al., 1987a). It requires antigen processing by the B cell. The talin redistribution is a particularly useful marker because it occurs in virtually all T-B cell couples under optimum conditions of interaction but T cell-B cell couples formed without potential recognition show no talin redistribution. T-B cell couples can be found even when specific antigen is not present (Kupfer et al., 1987a; Sanders et al., 1986) and we find them difficult to distinguish from specific couples by light microscopy. Therefore, we can use the talin redistribution in an individual cell couple we are examining as an indication that the T cell has recognized the antigen/ class II on the B cell and that a true "interaction" is taking place. Thus, we can identify collaborating T cell-B cell couples and then examine these to identify other events associated with interaction.

We stained mixtures of T and B cells with antibodies directed to T cell surface proteins thought to be involved in T cell recognition of antigen/class II. D10.G4.1 uses a T cell receptor (TCR) employing $V_{\beta 8}$ so we were able to visualize the distribution of the TCR with KJ16 (Haskins et al., 1984). In interacting T-B cell couples (i.e., ones in which talin was concentrated in the T cell) the TCR was seen to be markedly concentrated on the T cell membrane to the area of interaction between T and B cells. This aggregation/capping was specific and occurred under the same sets of conditions found for the intracellular T cell event (Kupfer et al., 1987b).

Next, we examined the fate of CD4/L3T4 molecules during T-B interaction. CD4 molecules were found to be concentrated to the interaction area of specific couples just like molecules of the TCR (Kupfer et al., 1987b). Class I MHC molecules and surface Ig on the B cell showed no redistribution, and like CD4 and TCR in nonspecific interactions, remained evenly distributed around the membrane of appropriate cells.

Recently, we have examined LFA-1, a non antigen/MHC specific adhesion molecule. LFA-1 also became redistributed like the TCR and CD4. Again, the redistribution occurs only during specific recognition and only in the T cell partner (Kupfer et al., unpublished).

Thus we have observed a number of impressive events which occur in the T cell as a consequence of specific recognition of antigen/class II on the B cell. These include the polarization of the MTOC/golgi complex, cytoskeletal rearrangements which result in the concentration of talin under the area of T-B contact, and the congregation into the area of T-B membrane contact of several T cell molecules thought to be involved in recognition or binding to the B cell including the TCR, CD4 and LFA-1. These events are illustrated in Figure 1.

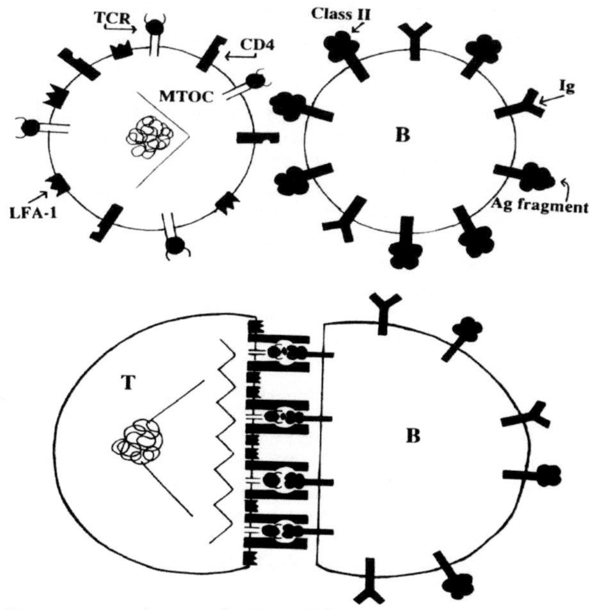

Fig. 1. Congregation of T cell receptor and accessory molecules during T-B collaboration.

DISCUSSION

Several novel facets of T-B interaction are indicated by these observations, though we still know very little about the mechanism of the events we have observed.

First, it is possible to visualize specific T-B interactions by fluorescence microscopy. This visualization is possible because of the use of clonal T and B cell populations and a variety of antibodies which stain T and B cell structures. We have established that when an antigen-specific T cell is spun together with a B cell presenting antigen and appropriate class II, that considerable numbers of T-B cell couples are formed and the T cell rapidly undergoes major changes associated with specific recognition. This occurs in the majority of T cells seen to be in contact with B cells under optimal conditions. Sanders et al. (1986) have also observed T-B cell conjugates and have studied some of the factors affecting them. In these studies, nonspecific interactions also occur but their data suggests that there are more conjugates under conditions of specific recognition. In that system, one has the potential to study what variables effect the frequencies of conjugates, though the existence of both specific and nonspecific conjugates makes the detailed analysis of the results somewhat problematic.

In our system where we examine individual couples, we can determine the frequency of interacting T-B cells, identify those couples which are interacting and then study what other events occur. Of course, we can also study what things effect these events. For instance, all the T cell responses require specific recognition of processed antigen when soluble antigen is used, and specific presentation by appropriate class II. This implies that engagement of the TCR is a prerequisite for all the other events.

What can we say about the significance of the intracellular T cell events? Polarization of the golgi apparatus has been associated with directed motility (Kupfer et al., 1984) as well as other directional events involving granular secretion. Thus, reorientation may be a part of a process whose final purpose is the deposition of new membrane or membrane components into a particular area of the membrane or the release of secretory granules or products in a particular direction. It is tempting to consider the possibility that soluble lymphokines produced by the helper T cell and designed to regulate B cell activity may be secreted in a polar fashion. Another possibility is that some lymphokines are actually not generally found as soluble products but function in a membrane associated form as has been suggested for IL1 (Kurt-Jones et al., 1985) and recently for GMCSF (Gordon et al., 1987). It should be noted, however, that even in these partially activated T cell lines and hybridomas, induction of lymphokine synthesis appears to require at least 8-12 hours so if polar lymphokine secretion is to be envisaged as the purpose for the golgi reorientation, the T and B cell would need to interact for a prolonged period.

Another polar event within the T cell is the redistribution of the cytoskeleton which is inferred from talin concentration to the area of T cell membrane interaction with the B cell. This is a specialized event involving some but not all cytoskeletal elements and there really is very little evidence as to what is its purpose, except that it also occurs in T cell effector target interactions. One can speculate that there are some causal relationships among the different redistributions, but at the moment there is little data to indicate which events are first. Two facts are known. The MTOC orientation but not the talin redistribution is Ca^{++}-dependent (Kupfer et al., 1986). Suggesting at the least, that the talin concentration does not depend on reorientation of the MTOC. Secondly, antibody induced capping of L3T4 (without TCR engagement) does not lead to capping of TCR or LFA-1 (Kupfer et al., 1987b) nor does it lead to talin concentration (Kupfer, Swain, Janeway and Singer, unpublished).

It is easier to speculate about the significance of redistribution of putative membrane receptors. One is quite sure that TCR binds to antigen/class II and we and others have suggested that CD4 also binds to class II (Swain, 1983; Swain et al., 1983; and reviewed Swain and Dutton, 1987). LFA-1 is involved in nonspecific as well as specific cell-cell adhesion and appears to bind to ICAM-1 (reviewed in Springer et al., 1987). Thus the congregation and concentration of many putative receptors along the membrane-membrane contact area is likely to lead to an avid and perhaps long-lived interaction between the T cell and B cell. Another expected consequence is the concommitant redistribution of the ligands of the receptors. Such a postulated aggregation on the B cell surface is a good candidate for an event required for B cell triggering. Indeed, several recent reports suggest that class II molecules can be signal transducers for B cells (Palacios et al., 1983; Bishop and Haughton, 1986; Cambier et al., 1986). Thus we imagine that the redistribution are important for both B and T cell triggering. Again the mechanism and the identification of the particular signal transducers remain to be elucidated. Several bits of data are germane. The massive T cell redistributions appear to depend on some form of T cell triggering since they occur only in specific interaction even thought the putative ligands for the CD4 and LFA-1 are present in nonspecific interactions. Furthermore, T cell activation can be mediated by fixed APCs as long as antigen is "preprocessed" (Shimonevitz et al., 1983), and we have confirmed that D10 lymphokine production occurs with the same efficiency with fixed LK cells preincubated with antigen. This suggests that T cell triggering perse does not depend on the cocapping of T and B cell molecules.

FUTURE DIRECTIONS

These studies and the other direct studies of T-B interaction raise many questions that will need to be resolved in future studies. One general area that needs examining is the sequence of events and how they are causally related. Also, we know little at this time about the concommitant events in the B cell (redistribution of specific class II?) It will be important to determine the consequence of the direct interaction with the T cells for the B cell. What signals are given? What is/are their role in the B cell response?

Also important, are kinetic considerations: When in the response does the T cell-B cell interaction occur? How long does it last?

Some answers to these questions and many others should be facilitated by the possibility of doing direct studies of T-B cell interaction such as those discussed here.

REFERENCES

Berke, C., 1983, Cytotoxic T lymphocytes. How do they function?, Nature, 162:107.

Bishop, G.A., and Haughton, G., 1986, Induced differentiation of a transformed clone of Ly1 positive B cells by clonal T cells and antigen, Proc. Natl. Acad. Sci (USA) 83:7410.

Cambier, J.C., Ransom, J.T., Harris, L.K., Coggeshall, K.M., Chen, Z.Z., Newell, and Justement, L.B., 1986, Coupling of B-cell surface Ig, Ia and BSF1 receptors to intracellar "second messengers.", in: "Proceedings of the Conference on Lymphocyte Activation and Immune Reaction," S. Gupta, W.E. Paul, and A.S. Fauci ed., Plenum Press, New York, in press.

Haskins, K., Hannum, C., White, J., Roehm, N., Kubo, R., Kappler, J., and Marrack, P., 1984, The major histocompatibility complex-restricted antigen receptor on T cells. VI. An antibody to a receptor allotype, J. Exp. Med. 160:452.

Gordon, M.Y., Riley, G.P., Watt, S.M., and Greaves, M.F., 1987, Compartmentalization of a haematopoietic growth factor (GM-CSF) by glycosaminoglycans in the bone marrow microenvironment, Nature 326:403.

Kappler, J.W., White, J., Wegmann, R., Mustain, E., and Marrack, P., 1982, Antigen presentation by Ia^{+} B cell hybridomas, Proc. Natl. Acad. Sci (USA) 79:3604.

Kaye, J., Procelli, S., Tite, J., Jones, B. & Janeway, C.A., 1983, Both a monoclonal antibody and antisera specific for determinants unique to individual cloned helper T cells can substitute for antigen and antigen-presenting cells in the activation of T cells. J. Exp. Med. 158:836.

Kupfer, A., Louvard, D., and Singer, S.J., 1984, Polarization of the elements of the golgi apparatus with microtubules. Golgi apparatus and the microtubule-organizing center in cultured fibroblasts at the edge of an experimental wound, Proc. Natl. Acad. Sci. (USA) 79:2603.

Kupfer, A., Dennert, G., and Singer, S.J., 1985, The reorientation of the golgi apparatus and the microtubule organizing center in the cytotoxic effector cells is a prerequisite in the lysis of bound targets, J. Mol. Cell. Immunol. 2:37.

Kupfer, A., Singer, S.J., and Dennert, G., 1986a, On the mechanism of unidirectional killing in mixtures of two cytotoxic T lymphocytyes. Unidirectional polarization of cytoplasmic organelles and the membane-associated cytoskeleton in the effector cell, J. Exp. Med. 163:489.

Kupfer, A., Swain, S., Janeway, C.A., and Singer, S., 1986b, The specific direct interaction of helper T cells and antigen-presenting B cells, Proc. Natl. Acad. Sci. (USA) 83:6080.

Kupfer, A., Swain, S., and Singer, S.J., 1987a, The specific direct interaction of helper T cells and antigen-presenting B cells. II. Reorientation of the microtubule organizing center and reorganization of the membrane associated cytoskeleton inside the bound helper cell, J. Exp.Med. 165:1565.

Kupfer, A., Janeway, C.A., Singer, S.J., and Swain, S., 1987a, Co-clustering of CD4 (L3T4) with the T cell receptor is induced by specific direct interaction of helper T cells and antigen-presenting cells, Proc. Natl. Acad. Sci. (USA), in press.

Kupfer, A., and Singer, S.J., 1987, Membrane dynamics in cell-cell interactions, with application to immunology, in: The T Cell Receptor, UCLA Symposium on Molecular and Cellular Biology, New Series, Vol. 73, eds, J. Kappler and M. Davis, Alan R. Liss, Inc., New York, in press.

Kurt-Jones, E.A., Beller, D.I., Mizel, S.B., and Unanue, E.R., 1985, Identification of a membrane-associated interleukin 1 in macrophages, Proc. Natl. Acad. Sci. (USA) 82:1204.

Mitchison, N.A., 1971, The carrier effect in the secondary response to hapten-protein conjugates. II. Cellular cooperation, Eur. J. Immunol. 1:18.

Noelle, R.J., Krammer, P.H., O'Hara, T., Uhr, J.W., and Vitetta, E.S., 1984, Increased expression of Ia antigens on resting B cells: An additional role for B cell growth factor, Proc. Natl. Acad. Sci (USA) 81:6149.

Podack, E.R., and Konigsberg, P.J., 1984, Cytolytic T cell granules. Isolation, structural, biochemical and functional characterization, J. Exp. Med. 160:695.

Sanders, V.M. Synder, J.M., Uhr, J.W., and Vitetta, E.S., 1986, Characterization of the physical interaction

between antigen-specific B and T cells. J. Immunol. 137:2395.
Shimonkevitz, R., Kappler, J., Marrack, P., and Grey, H., 1983, Antigen recognition by H-2 restricted T cells. I. Cell-free antigen processing. J. Exp. Med. 158:303.
Springer, T.A., Dustin, M.L., Kishimoto, T.K., and Martin, S.D., 1987, The lymphocyte function-associated LFA-1, CD-2 and LFA-3 molecules: Cell adhesion receptors of the immune system, Ann. Rev. Immunol. 5:223.
Swain, S.L., 1983, T cell subsets and the recognition of MHC class, Immunol. Rev. 74:129.
Swain, S.L., Dutton, R.W., Schwab, R., and Yamamoto, J., 1983 Xenogeneic human anti-mouse T cell responses are due to the same functional T cell subsets responsible for allospecific and major histocompatibility complex-restricted responses, J. Exp. Med. 157:720.
Swain, S.L., and Dutton, R.W., 1987, Consequences of the direct interaction of helper T cell with B cells presenting antigen, Immunol. Rev. 99 in press.
Swain, S.L., Kubota, E., and Dutton, R.W., 1987, Receptor redistribution and other signals in T and B cell triggering, in: The T Cell Receptor, UCLA Symposium on Molecular and Cellular Biology, New Series, Vol. 73, eds. J. Kappler and M. Davis, Alan R. Liss, Inc., New York, in press.
Vitetta, E., Bessie, A., Fernandez-Botran, R., Myers, C.D., Oliver, K.G., Sanders, V.M., and Stevens, T.L., 1987, Interaction and activation of antigen-specific T and B cells. Immunol. Rev. 99, in press.

A ROLE FOR Ia ANTIGENS IN B CELL ACTIVATION: STUDIES WITH NORMAL B CELLS AND A B CELL LYMPHOMA[+]

Arthur R. Baluyut, V. Udhyakumar, J. Morris, and Bondada Subbarao

Department of Microbiology and Immunology
Sanders-Brown Center on Aging, University of Kentucky
Lexington, KY 40536, USA

ABSTRACT

Monoclonal anti-Ia antibodies enhanced anti-μ induced proliferation of murine B lymphocytes. Anti-Ia induced augmentation of B cell proliferation was allele specific and did not require participation by T cells and adherent cells. The effects of anti-Ia antibodies on B cell activation are neither due to induction of interleukin-1 secretion in the cultures nor due to interaction with the Fc receptors and can be demonstrated under serum-free culture conditions. Monoclonal antibodies against both IA and IE region encoded Ia molecules were able to synergize with anti-μ in inducing B cell proliferation. Antibodies to both IA and IE coded antigens induced IgM secretion from the B lymphoma cell lines BKS3 and BKL. The anti-Ia antibodies did not affect the proliferation of the B lymphoma cells. These results suggest that the interaction of B cell surface Ia with the anti-Ia antibodies results in an activation signal and that the B cell surface Ia antigens may function as signal transducer molecules.

INTRODUCTION

A variety of external stimuli can stimulate small resting B cells to enter cell cycle and differentiate into immunoglobulin (Ig) secreting cells (Subbarao and Mosier, 1982; Howard et al., 1984; and Melchers and Corbel, 1984). One of the signals for initiation of B cell growth can be generated by the interaction of antigen or anti-Ig antibodies with the cell surface Ig. The perturbation of B cell surface Ig initiates a number of the early events such as phosphatidylinositol (PI) turnover, Ca^{++} mobilization, membrane depolarization and activation of protein kinase C (Cambier and Ransom, 1982). These early events have been shown to be on the pathway of inducing cell growth or differentiation in a number of mammalian cell systems. In B cells, all these early events are required for anti-Ig antibody induced hyper Ia expression at the B cell surface (Mond et al, 1981; Cambier and Ransom, 1987). However, it is becoming clear that additional signals are necessary to initiate B cell growth or differentiation. Recent studies have shown that lymphokines

[+]This work is supported by the grants AI-21490 and AG-05731, small research project award and PSP funds from the University of Kentucky. V.U. is supported by a PSP postdoctoral fellowship.

like interleukins 4 and 5 (formerly BSF-1, BCGF II) can synergise with other stimuli in inducing B cell proliferation (Howard et al, 1984; Melchers and Corbel, 1984; Klaus, 1986). One of these lymphokines, IL-4 has also been shown to induce hyper-expression of B cell surface Ia but does not initiate any of the other events such as PI turnover, Ca^{++} mobilization, etc (Noelle et al, 1984; Cambier and Ransom, 1987). Even though, it is well established that Ia antigens are critical recognition structures in T-B interactions (Julius, 1987), currently it is not known if B cell surface Ia has any direct role in induction of B cell growth. However, several studies have suggested that Ia antigens may be important for B cell maturation. Thus, T cells specific for B cell surface Ia can induce Ig secretion in normal B cells or a B cell lymphoma (Locasio et al, 1984; Pobor et al, 1984; and Nagarkatti, et al., 1985). In addition, monoclonal anti-Ia antibodies have been shown to inhibit mitogen (LPS) induced B cell activation (Niederhuber et al, 1975; Forsgren et al, 1984).

In this report we propose a direct role for the Ia molecules in induction of B cell growth. Utilizing monoclonal anti-Ia antibodies directed against Ia antigens under serum free conditions, we have demonstrated an enhancement of anti- induced B cell proliferation by anti-Ia antibody. The synergistic action of anti-Ia and anti-μ antibodies did not require the presence of T cells, was allele specific, and could be observed with IA as well as IE region specific monoclonal antibodies. Also we have demonstrated that macrophages did not play a major role in this synergy. In addition, we have shown that antibodies to both IA and IE region specified antigens induced IgM secretion in two surface IgM^+ B cell lymphomas BKS3 and BKL, isolated in our laboratory recently.

MATERIALS AND METHODS

Mice. Six to eight week old mice of the strains DBA-2/J ($H-2^d$); Balb/c ($H-2^d$); C57BL/6 ($H-2^b$); B10.BR ($H-2^k$); and C3H/HeJ were obtained from Jackson Laboratories, Bar Harbor, MA.

Preparation of T depleted spleen cells. T cell depletion was accomplished through treatment of spleen cells with monoclonal anti-Thy 1.2 ascities (clone 13-4), anti-Lyt 1 (clone 53-7), and anti-Lyt 2 (clone 53-6) antibodies for 45 minutes on ice (Ledbetter and Herzenberg, 1979; Marshak-Rothstein et al, 1979) and with monoclonal mouse anti-rat kappa antibody (Kung et al, 1981) and rabbit complement at 37° for 30 minutes. Success of treatment was shown through a 95% decrease in the proliferative response to concanavalin A (Con A) in treated versus untreated groups.

To obtain highly purified B cells, spleen cells were incubated on plastic dishes at 37° to remove adherent cells and the nonadherent cells were stained with fluoresceinated anti-Thy 1.2 antibodies. Fluorescence negative cells were obtained by cell sorting using a fluorescence activated cell sorter (FACS 420, Becton Dickinson Laboratories, Mountain View, CA).

Reagents used: Affinity pure anti-μ was prepared by us as described before (Subbarao and Mosier, 1983). 10.3.6.2, MKD6, 11.4.1 and 14.4.4 are monoclonal antibodies of IgG 2a subclass and react with antigens specified by IA^k, IA^d, $H2K^k$ and $IE^{d,k}$ subregions respectively (Oi et al, 1978; Marrack et al, 1981; Ozato et al, 1980). These hybridomas were obtained from ATCC, Rockville, MD. and the antibodies were purified on a protein A Sepharose column. These anti-Ia antibodies were shown to contain < 0.015 ng endotoxin as determined by the Limulus Amebocyte Lysate assay. Antibodies from the clones H-39-49.5, H7.8-26.2, H39-352-4 and H40-164-3 were obtained from Drs. M. Pierres and C.S. David and were employed as supernatants from the hybridoma cultures (Pierres et al, 1980, 1981). Monoclonal anti-Lyb2 was derived from the clone 10.1.D2 and was prepared as described previously (Subbarao and Mosier, 1983). Before plating each time, the anti-Ia antibodies were airfuged at 100,000 x g to remove any macromolecular aggregates.

Purified interleukin-1 (IL-1) was obtained from Genzyme at 100 units/ml concentration and was quantitated by the thymocyte costimulation assay (Mizel et al, 1978). Supernatant from a turkey gamma globulin specific long term T cell line (TGG sup) was used as a source of IL-4 and other T cell factors and was provided by D. Casatt and D. Cohen of our university.

Culture conditions and Cell Proliferation Assay. 2.5 x 10^5 cells were cultured in each well of a 96 well culture plate in a final volume of 200ul of serum free Iscove/F12 medium (Mosier, 1981). The final concentration of each reagent per ml was as follows: Lipopolysaccharide (LPS):50μg; anti-μ 50μg; anti-Ia:50μg (unless specified otherwise); control Ig:50μg;, Con A:0.2 μg. Cultures were incubated for 48 hours in 5% CO_2 at 37°C and then pulsed with tritiated thymidine (6.0 mCi/mM, New England Nuclear) for 4 hours and were harvested onto glass fibre filters. They were counted in a Packard liquid scintillation counter. Results were expressed as geometric mean (and S.E.) of triplicate cultures.

Induction of IgM secretion in the B lymphoma cell lines: We have isolated several B cell lymphomas that originated spontaneously in 22 month old CBA/Ca mice. Two of these lymphoid tumors, BKS3 and BKL were adapted to in vitro culture and have been maintained in the culture continuously for the last 5 months. Both the cell lines are surface IgM^+, IgD^+, $Ly1^+$, IA^+, IE^+ and Thy 1.2^- (Udhyakumar and Subbarao manuscript in preparation). These B lymphoma cells were cultured in IF 12 + 5% fetal calf serum at 10^5cells/well in presence or absence of various stimulants. After culture for 3-4 days supernatants were harvested. The amount of secreted IgM was quantitated by an enzyme linked immunospecific assay (ELISA). Briefly, the assay consisted of coating wells of a 96 well plate with affinity pure goat anti-u, blocking with a buffer containing 1% egg albumin and titering the culture supernatants or standard IgM protein. The level of IgM was determined by adding alkaline phosphatase coupled goat anti-mouse IgM (Sigma Chemical Co., St. Louis, MO) and measuring the bound enzyme activity by the hydrolysis of p-nitrophenyl phosphate.

RESULTS

Anti-Ia antibodies synergise with anti- antibodies in inducing B cell proliferation: In order to determine the role of Ia molecules in B cell growth we studied the effect of purified monoclonal anti-Ia antibodies on anti-μ induced B cell proliferation. In serum free cultures anti-u antibodies elicited a small amount of B cell proliferation when T-depleted spleen cells were cultured at a density of 2.5 x 10^5 cells per microwell. MKD6 and several other monoclonal anti-Ia antibodies alone did not have much effect on thymidine incorporation by B cells. However, when MKD6 antibodies were added along with anti-μ antibodies, the B cell proliferative response was much more than with either antibody alone. These results are summarized in figure 1. There appeared to be a synergistic effect, since proliferation in the presence of both anti-μ and anti-Ia antibodies was more than the sum of the effect with each antibody alone. The synergy between anti-μ and MKD6 was observed at all the doses of anti-Ia antibody tested. The expected additive responses in the absence of any synergy are indicated by an arrow in fig. 1 and all the other figures. In these experiments there was no inhibition or enhancement of the proliferative response to LPS by the MKD6 antibody.

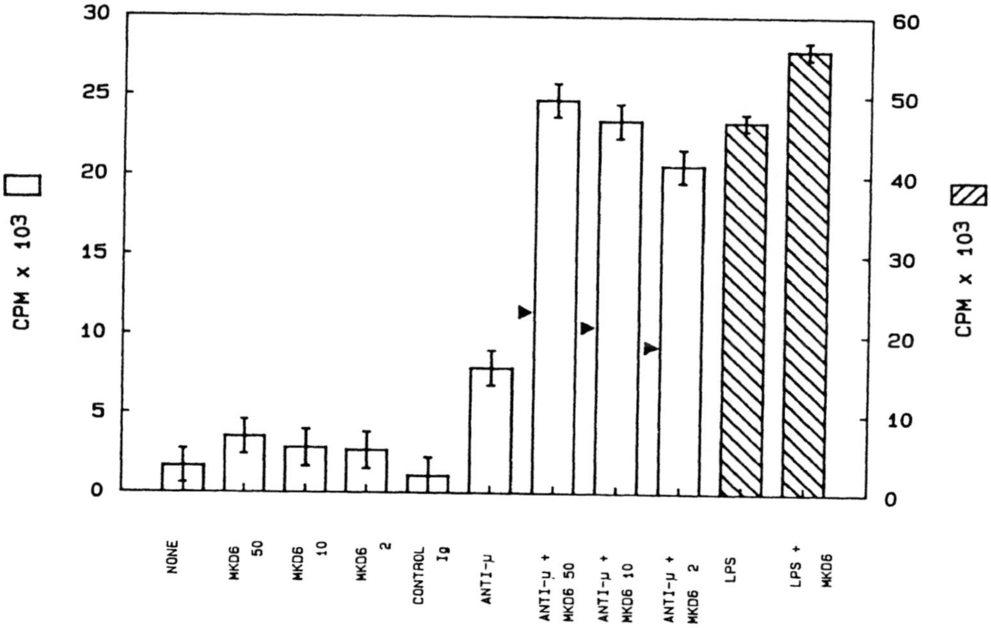

Fig. 1 Synergistic activation of T-depleted spleen cells with anti-IgM and anti-Ia antibodies. DBA-2/J spleen cells were T-cell depleted and cultured in serum free IF-12 medium as outlined in Materials and Methods. The arrows depict the predicted additive effect of the two stimuli. ConA responses of untreated cells and the T-depleted cells were respectively 56,500 and 4,670 CPM.

The ability of anti-Ia antibody to enhance anti-μ induced proliferative response was not unique to MKD6 or IA region specific antibodies, since 14.4.4, a monoclonal antibody that reacts with IE region specified Ia antigens was also able to synergise with anti-μ in inducing B cell growth. However two other monoclonal anti-IA^k antibodies (10.3.6.2 and H39.49.5) did not enhance anti-μ induced B cell proliferation. The action of anti-Ia antibody required interaction with the appropriate allelic determinant since synergistic response was seen when MKD6 (anti-Ia^d) antibodies were added to DBA/2 but not to B10.BR (Ia^k) spleen cells cultured in presence of anti-u (figure 2). Even though the low density, serum free culture conditions appeared better to demonstrate the synergy, anti-Ia antibodies 14.4.4 and MKD6 increased anti-u induced B cell proliferation at all cell densities studied and even in the presence of fetal calf serum. Similar results were obtained with a monoclonal rat-anti-u (Bet 2) antibody instead of the affinity purified goat anti-μ antibodies (data not shown).

Since these positive effects of anti-Ia antibodies on anti-μ induced B cell proliferation are in contrast to their inhibitory effects on mitogen induced B cell activation in both murine (Forsgren et al, 1984) and human systems (Clement et al, 1986) we repeated these experiments several times. We find that in 24 different experiments the average synergy index, as defined by the ratio of response obtained in presence of both anti-Ia and anti-μ antibodies to the theoretically expected (if there was no synergy) sum of the responses in presence of each individual antibody, was 2.61 $\pm$ 0.22. Finally the stimulatory effects were not due to endotoxin contamination of the antibodies, since the endotoxin levels in

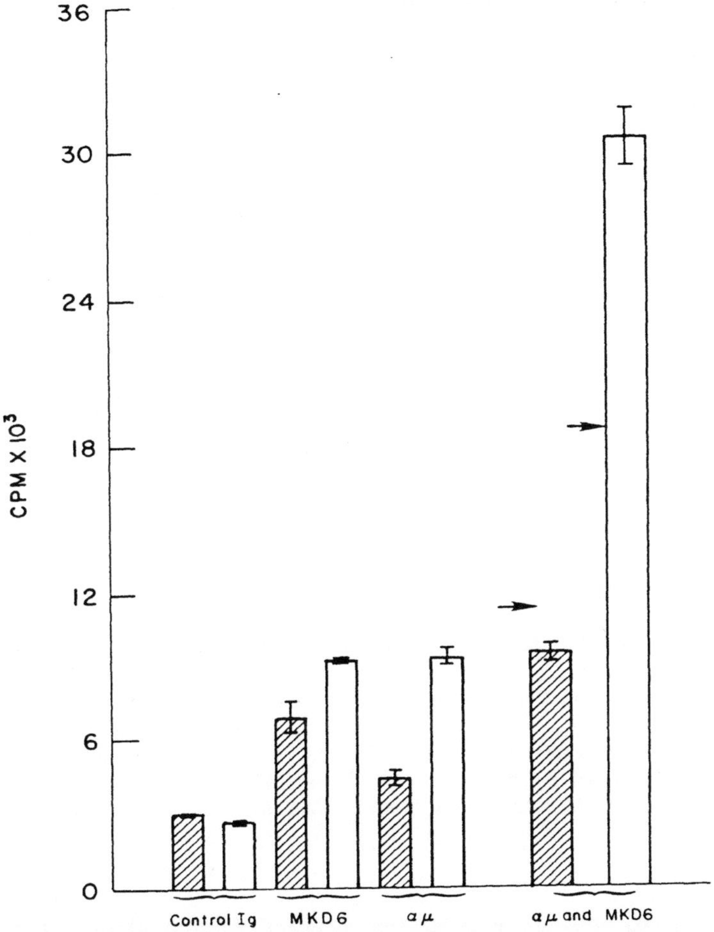

Fig. 2. Activation of B cells with anti-Ia (MKD6) and anti-IgM is allele specific. B10.BR (H-2^k) spleen cells and DBA-2/J (H-2^d) spleen cells were both T-cell depleted and cultured under the same conditions as in Fig. 1. Hashed bars depict the responses of B10.BR (H-2^k) while those of DBA-2/J (H-2^d) are shown by clear bars. Once again arrows show the expected additive effect of the two stimuli if there was no synergy.

MKD6 and 14.4.4 antibodies were less than the amounts that can be detected by the Limulus amebocyte lysate assay.

Role of adherent cells and interleukin-1 in the synergistic action of anti-Ia and anti-μ in inducing B cell proliferation. Since Ia antigens are expressed by both B cells and adherent-cells, the activating effects of anti-Ia antibodies may be due to stimulation of accessory cells, which inturn may help B cells. Therefore macrophage like cells were depleted by plastic adherence and then the purified small B cells were obtained by cell sorting for Thy 1.2⁻ small lymphocytes after staining with a fluoresceinated anti-Thy 1.2 antibody. Responses of these highly purified

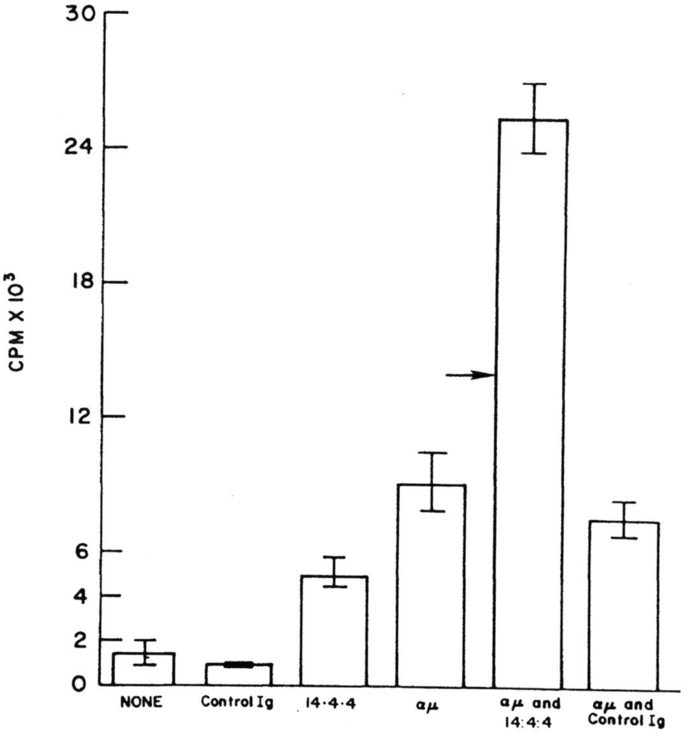

Fig. 3. Anti-IgM and anti-Ia synergism is also present in small B lymphocytes purified by adherent cell depletion and cell sorting to remove Thy 1.2$^+$ cells. Other culture conditions are as described previously.

small B cells to anti-Ia and anti-μ antibodies are shown in figure 3. The proliferative response induced in these enriched B cells by anti-Ia (14.4.4) plus anti-μ was significantly more than by either antibody alone or the sum of the responses with each individual antibody.

Several studies have demonstrated that interleukin-1 (IL-1) can increase B lymphocyte responses to various stimuli (Howard et al, 1983; Nossal and Pike, 1985). Further, a recent report suggests that anti-Ia may stimulate monocytes to secrete IL-1 (Palacios, 1985). Since the cell depletion experiments cannot completely rule out efffects due to lymphokine secretion by small numbers of contaminating cells, we determined the contribution of IL-1 in our assay system by two methods. First, we added purified IL-1 to cultures of B cells plus anti-μ and determined if IL-1 would replace anti-Ia antibodies and enhance the response to anti-μ. As shown in figure 4, the addition of purified IL-1 did not substitute for anti-Ia antibodies. Moreover the enhancement of B cell response by anti-Ia antibodies could be seen even in the presence of purified IL-1. These preparations of IL-1 have been assayed in our laboratory and were shown to

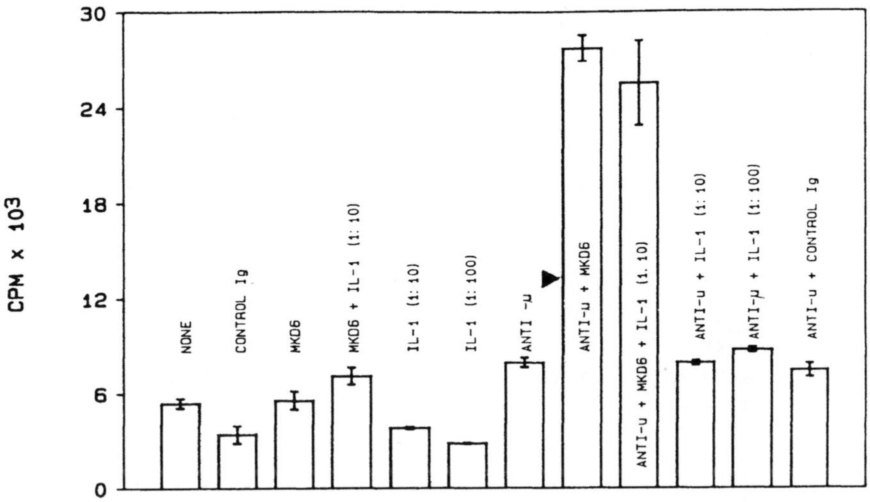

Fig. 4. Interleukin-1 does not substitute for anti-Ia antibodies in augmenting anti-IgM induced B cell proliferation. Conditions in culture are the same as in Figs. 1 and 2. Purified human IL-1 was used at 10 units/ml and 1 unit/ml concentration in the well. Arrow again depicts expected additive effects of anti-Ia and anti-IgM antibodies, if they do not act synergistically.

be potent in the thymocyte co-stimulation assay. Secondly, we measured the amounts of IL-1 secreted in the B cell cultures with various stimulating antigens. We were able to detect small amounts of IL-1 (0.2 to 0.3 units) in the cultures of T depleted spleen cells. However, the amount of IL-1 secreted was not higher in cultures stimulated with anti-Ia plus anti-μ than that in the cultures stimulated with control Ig plus anti-μ (data not shown).

The effect of anti-Ia plus anti-μ antibodies are neither due to nonspecific membrane perturbation nor due to interaction with Fc receptors: Since addition of antibodies to two cell surface antigens may simply perturb the membrane more and may cause nonspecific activation, we determined the effect of adding antibodies to cell surface antigens other than Ia on the anti-μ induced B cell activation. Addition of anti-class I (data not shown) or anti-Lyb2 antibodies (Table 1) did not augment B cell proliferation induced by anti-μ. Further, antibodies to Lyb2, which are similar to anti-μ in their ability to induce B cell proliferation, also did not synergize with anti-Ia antibodies. The activating effects of anti-Ia did not appear to be due to interaction with Fc receptors since anti-Fc receptor antibodies (2.4G2) (Unkless, 1978) did not inhibit the synergistic response with anti-μ (Table 1). These results suggest that the increase in B cell proliferation induced by Ia specific antibodies is due to a specific positive signal induced by interaction of the antibody with the Ia antigens.

Table 1

Specificity of the synergistic B cell activation induced by Ia and μ specific antibodies

Expt	Reagents	Poliferative response
1	anti-μ	51.5 (1.10)
	anti-Lyb2	20.6 (1.05)
	anti-μ + anti-Lyb2	78.4 (1.10)*
2	anti-Lyb2	3.62 (1.05)
	MKD6	3.51 (1.10)
	anti-Lyb2 + MKD6	7.44 (1.06)*
	anti-μ	7.88 (1.11)
	anti-μ + MKD6	24.7 (1.07)+
3	anti-μ	11.7 (1.11)
	MKD6	11.5 (1.09)
	2.4G2	3.5 (1.10)
	MKD6 + 2.4G2	12.4 (1.14)
	anti-μ + MKD6	33.4 (1.03)+
	anti-μ + MKD6 + 2.4G2	40.4 (1.01)

*In these groups the observed response with two stimulants is very close to the sum of the responses obtained with the individual antibodies and therefore no synergistic response is obtained.

+In these groups the observed response is greater than the sum of the responses obtained with the individual antibodies indicating a synergistic effect.

Anti-Ia antibodies induce IgM secretion in B cell lymphomas: Since the studies with normal B cells are always subject to contamination with small numbers of macrophages and T cells we decided to evaluate the effects of anti-Ia antibodies on homogeneous populations of B lymphocytes. Recently we have isolated several B cell lymphomas from old mice and have adapted two of these cell lines to *in vitro* culture. The cell lines, BKS3 and BKL, express IgM, IgD and Ia antigens on the cell surface but secrete very little IgM. We have observed that both these B lymphoma cell lines secreted IgM if they were stimulated with monoclonal antibodies to Ia antigens (Table 2).

As shown in Table 2, supernatant from a long term T cell line as well as LPS were also able to induce IgM secretion from these B cell lines. Moreover, anti-Ia antibody was able to induce better Ig secretion in presence of the lymphokine. Ia antigens appear to be uniquely important in delivering a positive signal, since antibodies to class I antigens were without any effect (Table 3).

Antibodies to both IA and IE subregion coded Ia antigens were effective in inducing increased IgM secretion from the BKS3 cells (Table 3). Of the eight different anti-Ia monoclonals tested only two each of IA and IE specific antibodies were able to significantly augment IgM secretion. Currently studies are in progress to determine if certain epitopes on Ia molecules are more important than others in providing a signal to these B lymphoma cells. The anti-Ia antibodies were at least as effective as LPS or a mixture of T cell derived lymphokines (Tables 2 and 3).

Table 2

Effect of anti-Ia antibody on secretion of IgM by B lymphoma cell lines+

Stimulant	BKL	BKS3.1	BKS3
	IgM secreted ($x10^{-2}$ ng/ml)@		
None	1.58	1.6	0.92
Control Ig	1.96	N.D.	0.53
LPS	4.7 (3.0)	5.8 (3.6)	2.9 (3.2)
14.4.4	1.1 (0.7)	6.2 (3.9)	0.69 (0.7)
10.3.6.2	8.2 (5.2)	5.25 (3.3)	4.73 (5.15)
TGG Sup	24.6 (15.6)	3.84 (2.4)	5.62 (6.11)
10.3.6.2 + TGG Sup	27.8 (17.6)	17.5 (10.9)	6.94 (7.5)

+B lymphoma cells (10^5/well) were cultured with various stimulants for four days. The supernatants were harvested from quadriplicate cultures, pooled and assayed for IgM.

*BKS3 is a subline derived from BKS3.1 by growing in presence of TGG Sup, which is a supernatant from TGG specific long term T cell line.

@Values in the parenthesis indicate stimulation index which is the ratio of IgM secreted in the stimulated culture to the IgM level in the unstimulated group. Responses with a stimulation index greater than 3 are underlined.

It has been observed that some B cell lymphomas (e.g.: CH12 B cell lymphoma) can be induced to secrete IgM with agents like hydroxyurea that inhibit DNA synthesis (Haughton et al, 1986). In our system the inductive effects of anti-Ia antibodies were not due to growth inhibition since the cell proliferation was virtually unaffected by the presence of anti-Ia antibodies (Table 3). Both LPS and TGG sup, however, augmented cell proliferation as well as IgM secretion.

DISCUSSION

B lymphocytes constitute a major portion of the Ia$^+$ cells of the lymphoid system. The significance of Ia expression by B cells is however not well understood. There is good evidence for a functional role for B cell surface Ia in the interaction of B cells with T cells. Antigen presentation by B cells to T cells involves recognition of antigen plus Ia at the B cell surface by T cells (Chestnut and Gray, 1985; Julius, 1987). H-2 restricted activation of B cells by T cells also appears to involve T cell recognition of B cell surface Ia molecules (Sprent, 1978; Andersson et al, 1980; Julius, 1987). A specific role for surface Ia in B lymphocyte activation has been proposed by several studies but has not been demonstrated directly. Thus, T cells specific for syngeneic or allogeneic Ia antigens alone have been shown to be able to directly activate B cells or B lymphoma cells to Ig secretion (Locassio et al 1984; Pobor et al, 1984; Finnegan et al, 1984; Nagarkatti et al, 1985; Bishop and Haughton, 1986). However, in these systems it was not clear if the interaction of T cells and B cells through Ia molecules resulted in an activation signal for B cells directly. Thus it is conceivable that the T cells are activated after interaction with B cell Ia and release soluble factors that

Table 3

Effect of different monoclonal antibodies to H-2^k and Ia^k antigens on IgM secretion by the BKS3 lymphoma cells*

Clone Designation*	Clone Specificity	IgM secreted by 10^5 cells@ (μg/ml)	Proliferation CPM/10^4 cells
Medium		1.15 ± 0.3	5,417
LPS		2.13 ± 0.3	53,243
TGG Sup		7.0 ± 0.16	59,110
11.4.1	H-2K	2.2 ± 0.51	ND
H39 - 49.5	IA	4.02 ± 0.5	ND
10.2.16	IA	1.86 ± 0.2	ND
10.3.6.2	IA	4.6 ± 0.95	9,052
14.4.4	IE	1.17 ± 0.15	4,280
H7.8-26.2	IE	4.0 ± 0.5	ND
H39-352-4	IE	4.05 ± 0.6	ND
H40-164-3	IA & IE	2.8 ± 0.24	ND
M5/114	IA & IE	1.72 ± 0.15	ND

*BKS3 lymphoma cells (10^5) were stimulated for four days with various agents and were assayed for IgM by the ELISA assay. For proliferation 10^4 cells were cultured and were pulsed with ^{3}H thymidine on days 2 and 3. Day 2 responses are provided in the table and the pattern of response was identical on day 3.

+Antibodies 14.4.4, 10.3.6.2 and 11.4.1 and were used at 50 ug/ml. The remaining antibodies were used as culture supernatants and were diluted 1:4 in the assay cultures.

@Arithmetic mean ± S.E. of quadriplicate determinations of IgM secreted is provided. Responses which are greater than three fold over unstimulated groups are underlined. Proliferative responses are reported as geometric mean of triplicate cultures.

mediate B cell activation. Our present studies were concerned with the possibility that B cells may receive direct activation signals through the surface Ia molecules. Thus we have shown that monoclonal anti-Ia antibodies could augment B cell proliferation induced by anti-μ antibodies in serum free cultures. It appeared that the augmentation of B cell growth by anti-Ia occurred via interaction of the anti-Ia antibodies with the Ia antigens since the effects were allele specific. Importantly, the synergy between anti-μ and anti-Ia could be achieved in the apparent absence of T cells. We have been able to show that the antibodies to Ia molecules specified by IA as well as IE loci were effective in this system. However, all anti-Ia antibodies cannot synergize with anti-u antibodies in causing increased B cell proliferation. For example, the augmentation of B cell growth by 10.3.6.2 and H39-49.5 two Ia^k specific monoclonal antibodies was very small and irreproducible. This, however, is not surprising since only some but not all monoclonal anti-μ antibodies are able to induce B cell proliferation (Julius, et al, 1984).

Since the contribution of non-B cells to the enhanced B cell growth is potentially crucial, we made special efforts to determine if the observed effects of anti-Ia antibodies are being exerted on B cells directly. Especially the role of accessory cells in our system was important because the Ia^+ accessory cells may be affected by anti-Ia antibodies. Recently Palacios et al (1985) have shown that anti-DR antibodies activate human monocytes to secrete IL-1. Interleukin-1 augments anti-μ plus IL-4 induced B cell proliferation (Howard et al, 1983) and increases the cloning efficiency of FITC specific B cells (Pike and Nossal, 1985). In the present study, we have three observations which suggest that interaction of accesesory cells with anti-Ia may not play a major role in the observed synergy between anti-μ and anti-Ia. First, the anti-Ia antibodies MKD6 or 14.4.4 and anti-μ exhibit same synergism when added to adherent cell depleted, cell sorter purified small B lymphocytes. Second, addition of purified IL-1 did not remove the requirement for anti-Ia antibodies for the observed synergy. Thirdly, during the tested time period (24-48 hours) IL-1 secretion in T depleted spleen cell cultures with anti-μ plus anti-Ia was not more than in the cultures with anti-μ plus a control antibody. Our inability to demonstrate large amounts of IL-1 secretion in these cultures with anti-Ia (for 2 days only) may not be in contradiction to the results of Palacios et al (1985) since they were able to detect large amounts of IL-1 only in cultures of purified monocytes stimulated with anti-DR antibodies.

The augmentation of B cell growth by anti-Ia may be due to non specific effects such as increased perturbation of B cell membranes induced by antibodies to two different B cell surface antigens or due to nonspecific interaction of the antibodies with Fc receptors. The former possibility appears unlikely since no synergy is obtained when antibodies to Ia are added along with Lyb2 specific antibody. Also, there was no synergy between u and class I or Lyb2 antigen specific antibodies. The likelihood of interactions with the Fc receptor being important is lessened since the anti-Ia antibodies exhibited the expected allele specificity. Further, addition of 2.4G2, an anti-Fc receptor specific antibody did not diminish the synergy beween anti-Ia and anti-μ. Instead, the proliferative response was slightly better in presence of all the three antibodies (anti-Ia, anti-μ and the antibody to the Fc receptor). One explanation for the 2.4G2 induced enhancement is that our affinity purified goat anti-μ antibody may have caused some Fc mediated inhibition similar to that reported for rabbit anti-μ antibodies by Parker et al (1980).

Anti-Ia and DR antibodies have been shown respectively to inhibit B cell responses to LPS (Niederhuber et al, 1975; Forsgren et al, 1984 and 1987) and mitogen induced human B cell proliferation (Clement et al, 1987). In the experiments presented here, there was no inhibition of LPS induced B cell growth. In the recent studies of Forsgren et al. (1987) the inhibitory effects of anti-Ia antibodies appear to be dependent on using a mixture of numerous anti-Ia monoclonal antibodies in the same culture. Thus, the number of different anti-Ia antibodies in the culture varied from 5 to 21 in these studies. We do not know if such inhibition was due to direct effects of the anti-Ia antibodies on B cells or a combination of Ia and Fc receptor mediated effects or due to inhibiton of the accessory cell function.

Recently Cambier et al (1987) have demonstrated that anti-Ia antibodies increased intracellular cyclic AMP levels in B cells. Since enhanced cyclic AMP is known to be anti-proliferative, we investigated the possibility that anti-Ia antibodies may promote B cell differentiation. A B cell lymphoma model was employed, since it permitted the evaluation of the functional role of B cell Ia in the complete absence of other accessory cells. In both the B cell lymphoma lines studies, anti-Ia antibodies significantly increased secretion of IgM. However, only four out of eight different monoclonal anti-Ia antibodies tested were effective in augmenting Ig secretion. Three different anti-IA antibodies were evaluated so far and had differential effects on the differentiative response. These three antibodies were shown to recognize three different Ia epitope regions (Pierres et al, 1981) suggesting that certain epitopes may be more important functionally than others. Our results are in agreement with the reported ability of anti-DR antibodies to increase Ig secretion from mitogen activated human B cells (Palacios et al, 1983). The only other example of induction of IgM secretion from a B cell tumor line with anti-Ia antibody consists in induction of the CH12 B cell lymphoma (Bishop and Haughton, 1986). In this system IE-subregion but not the IA-subregion coded molecules were important in induction. Together with the data presented here, both IA and IE region specified Ia molecules appear to serve as functional receptors on B cells. However, different B cells may use Ia molecules defined by IA or IE subregions or both.

It appears highly likely that the synergistic effects of the Ia and μ specific antibodies are due to generation of a positive signal generated as a result of the direct interaction of B cell Ia with anti-Ia antibodies. The mechanism by which the anti-Ia antibody increases anti-induced B cell growth is however not clear. Also, we do not know if one of the two signals (those mediated through Ia and surface IgM) is required earlier than the other. It is conceivable that anti-u enhances B cell Ia as reported by others and the hyper Ia expression at the B cell surface facilitates the action of anti-Ia antibodies. Cell surface Ia measurements suggest that the effect of anti-Ia was not due to alterations in the total amount of Ia expressed at the B cell surface (data not shown). Culturing B cells with anti-Ia may have resulted in continued modulation and reexpression of Ia on B cells resulting in a signal for B cell growth. This signal is not likely to affect the phosphatidylinositol metabolism, since we have found that in B cells phosphatidylinositol turnover was not significantly affected by anti-Ia antibodies (Grupp, S., J. Harmony, Baluyut, A.R., and Subbarao, B., unpublished observations). We and others (Cambier et al, 1987) have also shown that anti-Ia antibodies neither induce calcium mobilization nor affect the anti-μ induced calcium response. Therefore, the effects of anti-Ia antibodies may be at a later stage of B cell activation. Recent observations of Chen et al (1987) on the ability of anti-Ia antibodies to induce relocalization of protein kinase C into the nuclear fraction, and to increase intracellular cyclic AMP (Cambier et al, 1987) is consistent with such a notion.

In conclusion, we have shown that anti-Ia antibodies enhance the proliferative response of B cells to anti-μ antibodies and this enhancement can be observed in the absence of measurable numbers of T cells and macrophages. Murine B cell lymphoma cell lines can be directly activated by anti-Ia antibodies to secrete IgM. Our data strongly suggest that B cell surface Ia molecules can mediate some activation signals necessary for B cell growth and differentiation.

ACKNOWLEDGEMENTS

We thank N.H. Hansberger for expert technical assistance and A. Neilsen for her excellent secretarial assistance in preparation of this manuscript. Our thanks are also due to C. Brandt and R.J. Cross for their help with the flow cytometric analysis.

REFERENCES

Andersson, J., Schreier, M.H. and Melchers, F. T-cell dependent B-cell stimulation is H-2 restricted and antigen dependent only at the resting B-cell level. Proc. Natl. Acad. Sci. USA. 77:1612-1616, 1980.

Andersson, J. and Melchers, F. T cell-dependent activation of resting B cells: Requirements for both nonspecific unrestricted and antigen-specific Ia-restricted soluble factors. Proc. Natl. Acad. Sci. USA. 78:2497, 1981.

Bishop, G.A. and Haughton, G. Induced differentiation of a transformed clone of Ly-1$^+$ B cells by clonal T cells and antigen. Proc. Natl. Acad. Sci. USA 83:7410-7414, 1986.

Cambier, J.C. and Ransom, J.T. Molecular mechanisms of transmembrane signalling in B lymphocytes. Ann. Rev. Immunol. 5:175-199, 1987.

Cambier, J.C., Justement, L.B., Newell, M.K., Chen, Z.Z., Harris, L.K., Sandoval, V.M., Klemsz, M.F., and Ransom, J.T. Transmembrane signals and intracellular "second messengers" in the regulation of quiescent B lymphocyte activation. Immunol. Rev. 95:37-85, 1987.

Chen. Z.Z., McGuire, J.C., Leach, K.L. and Cambier, J.C. Transmembrane signaling through B cell MHC class II molecules: Anti-Ia antibodies induce protein kinase C translocation to the nuclear fraction. J. Immunol. 138:2345-2352, 1987.

Chestnut, R.W. and Grey, H.M. Studies on the capacity of B cells to serve as antigen-presenting cells. J. Immunol. 126:1075-1079, 1981.

Clement, L.T., Tedder, T.F. and Gartland, G.L. Antibodies reactive with class II antigens encoded for by the major histocompatibility complex inhibit human B cell activation. J. Immunol. 136:2375-2381, 1986.

Corbel, C., and Melchers, F. The synergism of accessory cells and of soluble -factors derived from them in the activation of B cells to proliferation. Immunol. Rev. 78:51-75, 1984.

Finnegan, A., Needleman, B. and Hodes, R.J. Activation of B cells by autoreactive T cells: Cloned autoreactive T cells activate B cells by two distinct pathways. J. Immunol. 133:78-85, 1984.

Forsgren,, S., Martinez, C. and Coutinho, A. The role of I-A/E molecules in B lymphocyte activation II. Mechanism of inhibition of the responses to lipopolysaccharide by anti-I-A/E antibodies. Scand. J. Immunol. 25:225-234, 1987.

Forsgren, S., Pobor, G., Coutinho, A., and Pierres, M. The role of I-A/E molecules in B lymphocyte activation: Inhibition of lipopolysaccharide-induced responses by monoclonal antibodies. J. Immunol. 133:2104-2110, 1984.

Haughton, G., Arnold, L.W., Bishop, G.A., and Mercolino, T.J. The CH series of murine B cell lymphomas: Neoplastic analogues of Ly-1$^+$ normal B cells. Immunol. Rev. 93:35-52, 1986.

Howard, M., Mizel, S.B., Lachman, L., Assel,J., Johnson, B. and Paul, W.E. Role of interleukin-1 in anti-immunoglobulin induced B cell proliferation. J. Exp. Med. 157:1529-1543, 1983.

Howard, M., Nakanishi, K. and Paul, W.E. B cell growth and differentiation factors. Immunol. Rev. 78:185-210, 1984.

Julius, M.H. Reciprocity in lymphocyte interactions. Immunol. Rev. 95:177-194, 1987.

Julius, M.H., Heusser, C.H. and Hartmann, K.U. Induction of resting B cells to DNA synthesis by soluble monoclonal anti-immunoglobulin. Eur. J. Immunol. 14:753-757, 1984.

Klaus, G.G.B. Unravelling the control of B cells. Nature 324:16-17, 1986.

Kung, J.T., Sharrow, S.O, Sieckmann, D.G., Lieberman, R., and Paul, W.E.. A mouse IgM allotypic determinant (Igh 6.5) recognized by a monoclonal rat antibody. J. Immunol. 127:873-876, 1981.

Ledbetter, J.A. and Herzenberg, LA. Xenogeneic monoclonal antibodies to mouse lymphoid differentiation antigens. Immunol. Rev. 47:63-90, 1979.

Locascio, N.J., Haughton, G., Arnold, L.W., and Corley, R.G. Role of cell surface immunoglobulin in B-lymphocyte activation. Proc. Natl. Acad. Sci. USA. 81:2466-2469, 1984.

Marrack, P., Kappler, J.W., Skidmore, B., and White, J. Antigen-induced, H-2 restricted, interleukin-2 producing T cell hybridomas. J. Exp. Med. 153:1198-1214, 1981.

Marshak-Rothstein, A., Fink, P., Gridley, T., Raulet, D.G., Bevan, M.J., and Gefter, M.L. Properties and application of monoclonal antibodies directed against determinants of the Thy-1 locus. J. Immunol. 122:2491-2497, 1979.

Melchers, F. and Lernhardt, W. Three restriction points in the cell cycle of activated murine B lymphocytes. Proc. Natl. Acad. Sci. USA 82:7681-7685, 1985.

Mi[illegible], S.B., Oppenheim, J.J., and Rosenstreich, P.L. Characterization of lymphocyte activating factor (LAF) produced by the macrophage cell line, P388D1. J. Immunol. 120:1497-1503, 1978.

Mond, J.J., Seghal, E., Kung, J., and Finkelman, F.D. Increased expression of I-region associated antigens (IA) on B cells after cross-linking of surface Ig. J. Immunol. 127:881-888, 1981.

Mosier, D.E. Primary in vitro antibody responses by purified murine B lymphocytes in serum-free defined medium. J. Immunol. 127:1490-1493, 1981.

Nagarkatti, P.S., Snow, E.C., and Kaplan, A.M. Characterization and function of autoreactive T lymphocyte clones isolated from normal unprimed mice. Cell Immunol. 94:32-48, 1985.

Niederhuber, J.E., Frelinger, J.A., Dugan, E., Coutinho, A., and Shreffler, D.C. Effects of anti-Ia serum on mitogenic responses: Inhibiton of the proliferative response to B cell mitogen. J. Immunol. 115:1672-1676, 1975.

Noelle, R., Krammer, P.H., O'Hara, J., Uhr, J.W., and Vitteta.E.S. Increased expression of Ia antigens on resting B cells: An additional role for B-cell growth factor. Proc. Natl. Acad. Sci. USA. 81:6149-6153, 1984.

Oi, V.T., Jones, P.P., Goding, J.W., Herzenberg, L.A., and Herzenberg, L.A. Properties of monoclonal antibodies to mouse Ig allotypes and Ia antigens. Current Topics in Microbiol. and Immunol. 81:115-129, 1978.

Ozato, K., Mayer, N., and Sachs, D.H. Hybridoma cell lines secreting monoclonal antibodies to mouse H-2 and Ia antigens. J. Immunol. 124:533-540, 1980.

Palacios, R. Monoclonal antibodies against human Ia antigens stimulate monocytes to secrete interleukin-1. Proc. Natl. Acad. Sci. USA. 82:6652-6656, 1985.

Palacios, R., Martinez-Maza, D. and Guy, K. Monoclonal antibodies against HLA-DR antigens replace T helper cells in activation of B lymphocytes. Proc. Natl. Acad. Sci. USA 80:3456-3460, 1983.

Phyllips, N.E. and Parker, D.C. Crosslinking of B lymphocyte Fc-γ receptors and membrane immunoglobulin inhibits anti-immunoglobulin-induced blastogenesis. J. Immunol. 132:627-632, 1982.

Pierres, M., Devaux, C., Dosseto, M., and Marchetto, S. Clonal analysis of B- and T-cell responses to Ia antigents. 1. Topology of epitope regions on I-A^k and I-E^k molecules analyzied with 35 monoclonal antibodies. Immunogenetics 14:481-495, 1981.

Pierres, M., Kourilsky, F.M., Rebouah, J.P., Dosseto, M., and Carillol, D. Distinct epitopes on I^k gene products identified by monoclonal antibodies. Eur. J. Immunol. 10:950-957, 1980.

Pike, B.L. and Nossal, G.J.V. Interleukin-1 can act as a B cell growth and differentiation factor. Proc. Natl. Acad. Sci. USA. 82:8153-8157, 1985.

Pobor, G., Pettersson, S., Bundeira, A., Martinez, A.C., and Coutinho, A. B lymphocyte activation upon exclusive recognition of major histocompatibility antigens by T helper cells. Eur. J. Immunol. 14:222-227, 1984.

Sprent, J. Role of H-2 gene products in the function of T-helper cells from normal and chimeric mice in vivo. Immunol. Rev. 42:108-137, 1978.

Subbarao, B. and Mosier, D.E. Role of B cell differentation antigens in the activation of B lymphocytes. Immunol. Rev. 69:81-97, 1982.

Subbarao, B. and Mosier, D.E. Induction of B lymphocyte proliferation by monoclonal anti-Lyb2 antibody. J. Immunol. 130:2033-2037, 1983.

Unkeless, J. Characterization of a monoclonal antibody directed against mouse macrophage and lymphocyte Fc receptors. J. Exp. Med. 150:580-596, 1979.

THE CLASS II MOLECULE AS A SIGNAL TRANSDUCER TO THE B CELL: CELLULAR AND MOLECULAR APPROACHES

Gail A. Bishop and Jeffrey A. Frelinger
Department of Microbiology and Immunology and
The Lineberger Cancer Research Center
The University of North Carolina
Chapel Hill, NC 27514

INTRODUCTION

The ultimate function of B lymphocytes is the production and secretion of specific immunoglobulin (Ig). This process is regulated by interactions between cells, cell products, and antigen. Particularly significant are antigen-specific interactions between B and T helper (Th) lymphocytes. Activation of the Th cell in such interactions requires that an antigen-presenting cell, such as a macrophage, dendritic cell, or B cell, present antigen to the Th cell in association with molecules encoded by genes of the class II region of the major histocompatibility complex (MHC). The function of class II antigens in T cell activation has been the subject of intense investigation in recent years (Schwartz, 1985; Germain and Malissen, 1986; Guillet et. al., 1987). There is little understanding, however, of the role of the B cell class II molecule in transmitting a differentiative signal to the B cell itself. This question has been technically difficult to approach, since all antigen-presenting cells express class II antigens. Thus, the unavoidable contamination of uncloned B cells with at least a small percentage of macrophages makes the use of such cells to define the signaling function of B cell Ia problematic. Although long-term culture of untransformed B cells has met with some success (Braun et. al., 1986; Pike and Nossal, 1986), such cell lines are not yet widely available. An alternative approach employs transformed, immortal B cell lines to study the process of B cell differentiation (Arnold et. al., 1986). A major limitation in the study of many B cell tumors is that the specificity of the Ig which they produce is unknown. Therefore, it is difficult to use them to study antigen-specific interactions. However, several clones of transformed murine B cells have been characterized which bear Ig of defined antigenic specificity and are responsive to immunoregulatory signals (Bishop et. al., 1986a). The CH series of murine B cell lymphomas has proven useful in studying B cell differentiation (Haughton et. al., 1986; Bishop and Haughton, 1987).

THE MODEL SYSTEM

CH12.LX is a surface IgM^+, IgD^-, $Ly\text{-}1^+$ B cell clone derived by single-cell cloning from the murine B cell lymphoma CH12, with which it shares phenotypic and functional characteristics (Arnold et. al., 1983). The surface and secreted Ig of CH12.LX binds specifically to the phosphatidyl choline moeity of sheep and bromelainated mouse erythrocytes (SRBC, BrMRBC; Mercolino et. al., 1986). CH12.LX cells bear the I-A^k and I-E^k-encoded antigens of their H-2^a haplotype, in abundant and approximately equal amounts (G. Bishop, unpublished).

Under normal culture conditions, about 0.1-1.0% of CH12.LX cells spontaneously secrete IgM which is hemolytic for SRBC and BrMRBC. This fraction is unaffected by the addition of antigen (SRBC) to the cultures. However, a 5-20-fold increase in plaque-forming cells (pfc) is induced when CH12.LX cells are cultured for 48 hours in the presence of both SRBC and E^k-restricted or E^k-reactive Th cell hybrids (Bishop and Haughton, 1986). Although both A^k and E^k-specific Th cells can recognize Ia antigens on CH12.LX cells, as demonstrated by the production of interleukin-2 (IL-2), A^k-specific Th cells do not induce CH12.LX cells to differentiate (ibid). The secretion of Th cell-derived lymphokines is not essential to induce differentiation of CH12.LX cells, since fixed Th cells, in the presence of SRBC, can induce differentiation (ibid). In a further simplification of this system, it was found that monoclonal antibodies (Mabs) specific for E^k could substitute for Th cells in inducing CH12.LX to secrete IgM. As with results using Th cells, differentiation occurs only if SRBC are also present, and A^k-specific Mabs are ineffective (ibid).

The two A^k-specific Mabs used in the previous studies are specific for determinants present on the ß chain of the A^k molecule. The location of the determinants recognized by the A^k-restricted or alloreactive Th hybridomas is unknown. It was therefore possible that the observed preference of CH12.LX for receiving differentiative signals by way of its E^k molecules was actually a preference for signals generated by binding the α chain rather than the ß chain of the Ia molecule. We have recently examined the ability of ten additional Ia^k-specific Mabs to induce differentiation of CH12.LX cells, in the presence of SRBC. The results, which will be presented in detail elsewhere[1] , are summarized in Table 1. These composite results of both studies clearly demonstrate that only $E_\alpha{}^k$ or $E_\beta{}^k$-specific Mabs, in the presence of SRBC, can induce CH12.LX cells to differentiate. Mabs specific for either $A_\alpha{}^k$ or $A_\beta{}^k$ are ineffective, either in the presence or absence of SRBC. To determine whether the inability of the A^k molecules of CH12.LX to transmit a differentiative signal is due to an alteration in the A^k molecule, two-dimensional (2-D) gel electrophoresis was performed upon the A^k and E^k molecules of CH12.LX cells and normal mouse splenocytes. We found that the electrophoretic pattern of the E^k molecules of CH12.LX was indistinguishable from that of normal splenocytes (G. Bishop and M. McMillan, unpublished. CH12.LX A^k molecules, however, show electrophoretic differences in size and isoelectric point from their normal spleen cell counterparts.[1]

The 2-D gel differences which we observed can be explained by either post-translational modification or protein sequence differences in the CH12.LX A^k molecule. To distinguish between these possibilities,

---

1 Bishop, G.A., McMillan, M.S., Haughton, G., and Frelinger, J.A. Induced differentiation of a B cell clone by anti-Ia is locus-specific. in preparation.

we prepared a cDNA library from CH12.LX cells, and isolated clones corresponding to the α and β chains of A^k. We have recently completed the DNA sequence of the α chain clones, with the result that no differences were found between the $I\text{-}A_\alpha^k$ cDNA of CH12.LX (G. Bishop and J. Frelinger, unpublished) and the reported wild-type $I\text{-}A_\alpha^k$ sequence (Benoist et. al., 1983). We are now in the process of obtaining the $I\text{-}A_\beta^k$ CH12.LX cDNA sequence, which we expect will be completed shortly.

Whatever the underlying reason for the failure of the A^k molecule of CH12.LX to transmit differentiative signals to the B cell, this failure demonstrates that activation of Th cells is not necessarily the only requirement for induction of B cell differentiation. Thus, while the class II molecule is being examined by others to determine which portions are important in antigen presentation to the Th cell (Brown et. al., 1986; Lechler et. al., 1986), these portions will not necessarily be those which are crucial to transmission of differentiative signals to the B cell. It is this question which we wish to examine, using CH12.LX cells as a model system.

Table 1. Specificity of Monoclonal Antibodies and Ability to Induce Differentiation of CH12.LX Cells.

Antibody	Ia Specificity	Chain Specificity	PFC Induction
14-4-4S	E^k	alpha	+
17-3-3S	E^k	beta	+
9A	E^k	beta	+
Y-17	E^k	beta	+
39G	E^k	beta	+
40K	E^k	beta	+
40B	$E^k + A^k$	beta	+
10-2.16	A^k	beta	-
10-3.6.2	A^k	beta	-
11-5.2.1.9	A^k	alpha	-
H116-3.2	A^k	alpha	-
H118-4.9	A^k	alpha	-
39C	A^k	alpha	-
39F	A^k	alpha	-

THE APPROACH

The availability of genomic clones corresponding to the genes for murine class II molecules has opened the possibility of transfection experiments as a direct probe of class II function. A variety of permanent T and B cell lines have been transfected with genes encoding class II molecules (Malissen et. al., 1984; Germain and Malissen, 1986). The class II genes appear to function normally in these new environments, including mutant (Brown et. al., 1986) or exon-shuffled (Germain and Malissen, 1986) class II genes. Previous studies have focused upon the ability of class II molecules produced by introduced genes to be recognized by antibodies and T cells. These experiments thus examined the important structural features of class II molecules as viewed by the T cell.

In contrast, we plan to utilize CH12.LX cells, coupled with DNA-mediated gene transfer, to explore the role of class II molecules as receptors of differentiative signals on B cells, a function which is also supported by the results of Palacios et. al. (1983) and the recent experiments of Chen et. al. (1987). The first aspect of this goal will be to transfect class II genes of other haplotypes into CH12.LX cells, using an electroporation method which has proven highly successful in our laboratory, combined with the mycophenolic acid selection (Mulligan and Berg, 1981) for transfectants. Expression of class II molecules by genes introduced into CH12.LX cells will be detected by Mab binding and antigen presentation to Th cells, as previously described (Macchi et. al., 1984; Bishop and Haughton, 1986). The final test of normal function of transfected class II genes will be whether they can transduce a differentiative signal to CH12.LX cells, as described above.

The successful transmission of differentiative signals to CH12.LX cells by introduced class II molecules will allow us to use genetic manipulations to pinpoint the portions of the class II molecule important to this function. The first constructions which we shall make will replace the transmembrane and cytoplasmic portion (exon 4) of (e.g.) the I-E^d gene with exon 4 of (e.g.) the I-A^b gene. This type of construction was chosen because we believe that the transmembrane and cytoplasmic regions of the class II molecule will prove important in signal transduction to the B cell. The exon replacement constructions will be performed upon both the class II α and β chain genes. These constructions will be mixed and transfected together; they should produce a hybrid molecule which is E^d outside the cell and A^b inside. If anti-E Mabs or Th cells plus antigen (SRBC) do not induce the transfected cells to differentiate, reciprocal constructions will be made and tested. These experiments will determine which class II domains are crucial in signal transduction.

Results obtained from the exon-shuffling experiments will determine the portion(s) of the class II molecule to focus upon next, using a mutagenesis approach. We shall use a method recently developed by our colleagues Hutchison et. al. (1986), for producing and identifying every possible single base substitution mutation within a region. This method has been used successfully in our laboratory to produce a complete library of point mutations in the DP α_1 gene segment (R. Murray and J. Frelinger, in preparation). The method is based upon the automated synthesis of two complementary DNA strands with cohesive terminii, corresponding to the region of interest in a given gene. During oligonucleotide synthesis, random mutations are produced in the DNA sequence by "spiking" each of the four nucleotide phosphoramidites (A, C, G, T) with a low level of the other three nucleotides. This yields a preparation of oligonucleotides with a controllable, calculated frequency of random point mutations. The oligonucleotides are annealed to construct an entire exon, and cloned into an M13 phage vector, providing a library of point mutations. These mutant exons can then be used in exon-replacement constructions, and transfected into CH12.LX cells as described above. The transfectants in which a previously effective class II molecule has lost the ability to transduce a differentiative signal will be identified by functional assay (Bishop and Haughton, 1986). The clones containing these mutations can then be selected from the M13 library and rapidly sequenced in the M13 vector. The work of Hutchison et. al. (1986) has shown that such a library can contain all of the possible point substitution mutations for a given sequence. It should thus be possible, using this method, to identify the residues within the class II genes necessary for transmitting a differentiative signal to the B cell by way of its class II molecules.

CONCLUSIONS

Both our work and that of others has demonstrated that the class II MHC molecule, in addition to its more well-known function as an integral component in antigen presentation to Th cells, can also function in the direct transmission of differentiative signals to the B cell. The cellular system provided by the CH12.LX clone has made possible a biological assay for this class II function. Use of the molecular techniques outlined here should allow definition of the structural features of the class II molecule which determine this function.

ACKNOWLEDGEMENT

Supported by NIH grant CA42771.

REFERENCES

Arnold, L.W., LoCascio, N.J., Lutz. P.M., Pennell, C.A., Klapper, D., and Haughton, G. Antigen-induced lymphomagenesis: Identification of a murine B cell lymphoma with known antigen specificity. J. Immunol. 131: 2064-2068, 1983.

Arnold, L.W., Lutz, P.M., Pennell, C.A., Bishop, G.A., Corley, R.B., Haughton, G., and LoCascio, N.J. B cell tumors as models of B lymphocyte differentiation. in Cambier, J., Ed. B Lymphocyte Differentiation CRC Press, Boca Raton, pp. 109-135, 1986.

Benoist, C.O., Mathis, D.J., Kanter, M.R., Williams, V.E.II, and McDevitt, H.O. The murine IA alpha chains E-alpha and A-alpha show a surprising degree of sequence homology. Proc. Natl. Acad. Sci. (USA) 80: 534-538, 1983.

Bishop, G.A., and Haughton, G. Induced differentiation of a transformed clone of Ly-1+ B cells by clonal T cells and antigen. Proc. Natl. Acad. Sci. (USA) 83: 7410-7414, 1986.

Bishop, G.A., Arnold, L.W., and Haughton, G. Antigen-specific B cell tumors of mice. CRC Crit. Rev. Immunol. 6: 105-122, 1986.

Bishop, G.A., and Haughton, G. Use of the CH lymphomas as models of murine B cell differentiation. Immunol. Res. 5: 263-270, 1987.

Braun, J., Citri, Y., Baltimore, D., Forouzanpour, F., King, L., Theranizadeh, K., Bray, M., and Kliever, S. B-Ly1 cells: Immortal Ly-1+ B lymphocyte cell lines spontaneously arising in murine splenic cultures. Immunol. Rev. 93: 5-22, 1986.

Brown, M.A., Glimcher, L.A., Nielsen, E.A., Paul, W.E., and Germain, R.N. T-cell recognition of Ia molecules selectively altered by a single amino acid substitution. Science 231: 255-258, 1986.

Chen, Z.Z., McGuire, J.C., Leach, K.L., and Cambier, J.C. Transmembrane signaling through B cell MHC class II molecules: Anti-Ia antibodies induce protein kinase C translocation to the nuclear fraction. J. Immunol. 138: 2345-2352, 1987.

Germain, R.N. and Malissen, B. Analysis of the expression and function of class II MHC-encoded molecules by DNA-mediated gene transfer. Ann. Rev. Immunol. 4: 281-316, 1986.

Guillet, J.G., Lai, M.-Z., Briner, T.J., Buus, S., Sette, A., Grey, H.M., Smith J.A., and Gefter, M.L. Immunological self, nonself discrimination. Science 235: 865-870, 1987.

Haughton, G., Arnold, L.W., Bishop, G.A., and Mercolino, T.J. The CH series of murine B cell lymphomas: Neoplastic analogues of Ly-1+ normal B cells. Immunol. Rev. 93: 35-52, 1986.

Hutchison, C.A.III, Nordeen, S.K., Vogt, K., and Edgell, M.H. A complete library of point substitution mutations in the glucocorticoid element of mouse mammary tumor virus. Proc. Natl. Acad. Sci. (USA) 83: 710-714, 1986.

Lechler, R.I., Ronchese, F., Braunstein, N.S., and Germain, R.N. I-A restricted T cell antigen recognition. Analysis of the roles of A_α and A_β using DNA-mediated gene transfer. J. Exp. Med. 163: 678-696, 1986.

Macchi, M., Woodward, J., McLaughlin-Taylor, E., Griffin, J., Hood, L., and Frelinger, J.A. Cloning and identification of the H-2D^p gene. Immunogenetics 19: 195-204, 1984.

Malissen, B., Price, M.P., Goverman, J.M., McMillan, M., White, J., Kappler, J., Marrack, P., Pierres, A., Pierres, M., and Hood, L. Gene transfer of H-2 class II genes: Antigen presentation by mouse fibroblast and hamster B-cell lines. Cell 36: 319-327, 1984.

Mercolino, T.J., Arnold, L.W., and Haughton, G. Phosphatidyl choline is recognized by a series of Ly-1+ murine B cell lymphomas specific for erythrocyte membranes. J. Exp. Med. 163: 155-165, 1986.

Mulligan, R.C., and Berg, P. Selection for animal cells that express the E. coli. gene coding for xanthine-guanine phospohribosyltransferase. Proc. Natl. Acad. Sci. (USA) 78: 2072-2076, 1981.

Palacios, R., Martinez-Maza, O., and Guy, K. Monoclonal antibodies against HLA-DR antigens replace T helper cells in activation of B lymphocytes. Proc. Natl. Acad. Sci. (USA) 80: 3456-3460, 1983.

Pike, B.L., and Nossal, G.J.V. Growth and differentiation of B cell clones in vitro. in Cambier, J., ED. B Lymphocyte Differentiation, CRC Press, Boca Raton, pp. 79-108, 1986.

Schwartz, R.H. T lymphocyte recognition of antigen in association with gene products of the MHC. Ann. Rev. Immunol. 3: 237-261, 1985.

THE ORIGIN OF Lyt-2$^+$ CLASS II SPECIFIC ALLOGENEIC CTL

Nobukata Shinohara

Transplantation Biology Section,
Immunology Branch, NCI, NIH, Bethesda, Maryland

INTRODUCTION

T lymphocytes recognize antigens in the context of MHC molecules and can be divided into two major subpopulations according to the expression of the two types of murine accessory molecules, Lyt-2 and L3T4 antigens. A general correlation has been noted between the class of MHC antigens recognized by T cells and the type of accessory molecules they express, with Lyt-2$^+$ lymphocytes recognizing antigens in the context of class I molecules and L3T4$^+$ lymphocytes in the context of class II molecules (1,2). However, CTLs specific for class II alloantigens do not follow this rule. In fact, allogeneic CTLs induced against disparities at class II loci were found to consist of comparable numbers of Lyt-2$^+$ and L3T4$^+$ cells (3,4). A part of such Lyt-2$^+$ exceptions could be explained by the existence of clones recognizing allogeneic class II antigens in the context of class I antigens as exemplified by several isolated CTL clones (5). Nevertheless, there still remains a major population of Lyt-2$^+$ cells with genuine class II specificity, as judged from four lines of evidence; genetic mapping, sensitivity to the blocking effect of monoclonal antibodies, failure to recognize I-A mutant cells, and ability to lyse cells transfected with alpha and beta genes of the I-A antigen (6). This population of CTL turned out to be extremely insensitive to the blocking effect of antibodies to the Lyt-2 antigen (3,4,6). Thus, such cells with "wrong phenotype" may have been triggered by class II antigens because of their independence from function of the accessory molecule.

Since there is no obvious specialization among V gene sets of the T cell receptor for a particular class of MHC antigens, the general correlation between the class of the restricting MHC antigen and the phenotype of T cells implies the existence of a selective process involving actual testing of T cell receptors for reactivity with MHC antigens during ontogeny of T cells or during induction of immune responses to maintain the concordance. If the former is the case, the abundance of Lyt-2$^+$ cells among class II specific CTL suggests the existence of another pathway in which T precursor cells are allowed to mature without such selection. Recent works from several laboratories indicate existence of a subpopulation of cells differentiating into mature T cells without entering the thymus (7). A lymphocyte surface protein, Ly6.c has been reported to subdivide Lyt-2$^+$ populations of peripheral mature T cells and not to be expressed on detectable numbers of thymic lymphoctyes (8,9). This gene product is thought to be a possible candidate for a marker of extrathymic T cells. If Lyt-2$^+$ class II specific CTL truly represent the putative extrathymic maturation pathway, it was expected that such cells would be absent in the thymus and express Ly6.c on the surface. Based on these speculations, the origin of Lyt-2$^+$ class II specific CTLs was studied with special references to thymic and extrathymic populations and expression of the Lyt-6 antigen. The results indicate that such Lyt-2$^+$ class II specific CTL are not confined to any particular subpopulations of Lyt-2$^+$ T cells as distinguished by the expression of Ly6.c surface antigen or by organ distribution.

RESULTS AND DISCUSSION

<u>Lyt-2$^\pm$ class II specific CTL precursors are found in thymocyte populations.</u> Class I and class II MHC antigen specific allogeneic CTL were induced in primary MLC from thymocytes and spleen cells of A.TH mice using irradiated A.TL (for class II specific CTL) or A.AL (for class I specific CTL) splenic lymphocytes as stimulators (see legend for Fig. 1). Phenotypes of CTL were studied by treating with the relevant antibody and complement (Fig. 1). Splenic responder cells generated a mixture of Lyt-2$^+$L3T4$^-$ and Lyt-2$^-$L3T4$^+$ class II specific CTL as indicated by partial depletion of the killing activity by either antibody alone and complete depletion by the combined treatment with the two antibodies (panel B). Likewise, thymic responder cells

<u>Legend for Fig. 1.</u> Spleen and thymus cells of A.TH mice were stimulated in the primary MLC using irradiated A.TL (class II specific CTL) or A.AL (class I specific CTL) cells as stimulators in the presence of 10% rat ConA culture supernatant. Treatment of cells at the effector phase was carried out on cells plated in microtiter wells. After treating effector cells, labeled targets were added to the wells to carry out CML. Thus, cell numbers were adjusted for starting cell numbers rather than for number of cells recovered. Class II specific CTL were tested on B10.A LPS blasts to avoid contamination by CTL specific for Qa-1-like antigens (3), and class I specific CTL on B10.A ConA blasts depleted for Ia$^+$ cells. Monoclonal antibodies used were GK1.5 (anti-L3T4), 83-12-5 (anti-Lyt-2.2), 15-1-5 (anti-K^k), and 10-2-16 (anti-I-A^k). CTL shown in panels C and F were induced from responders depleted for Lyt-2$^+$ (-2) cells prior to MLC.

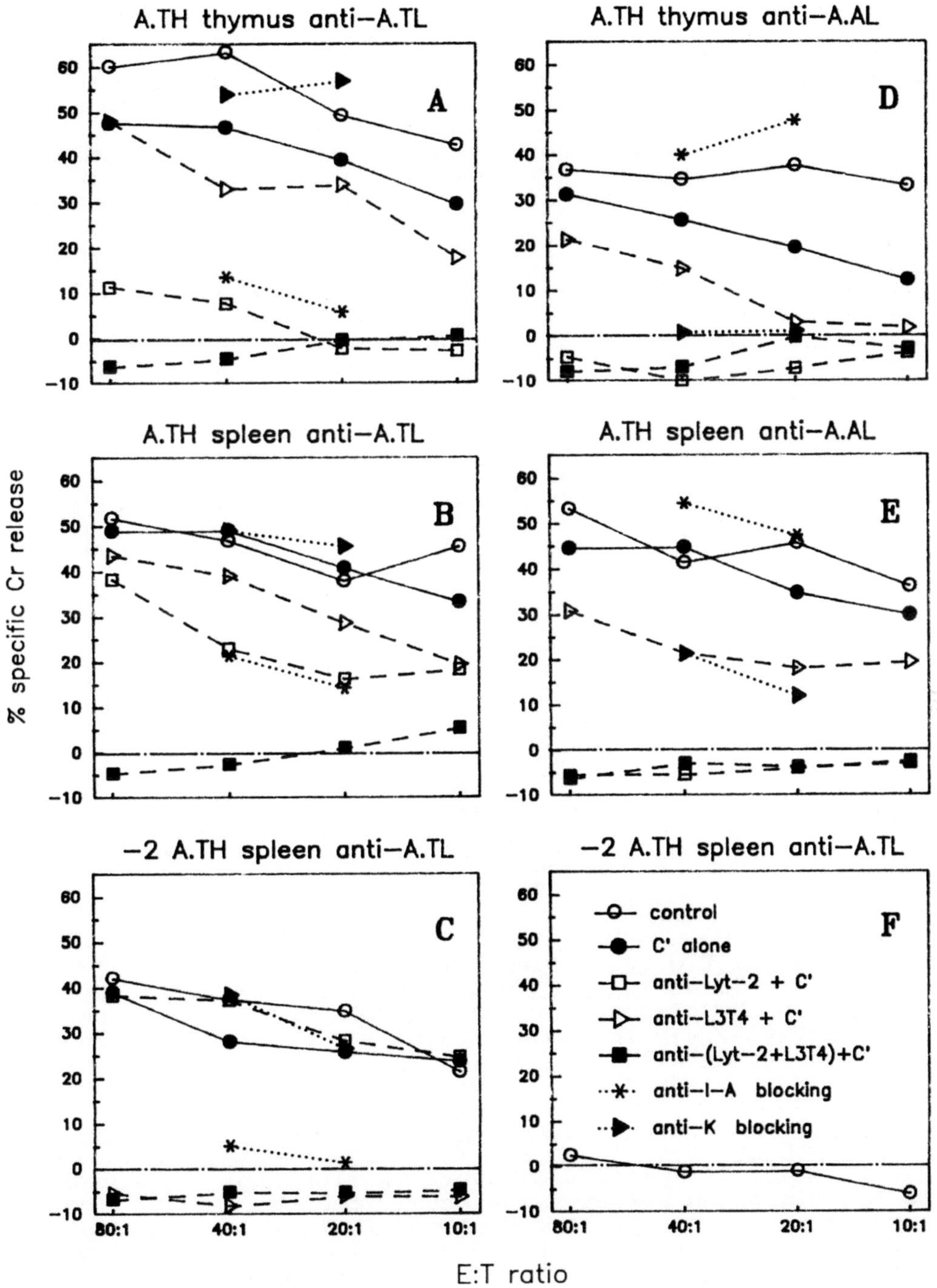

Fig. 1 Lyt-2+ and L3T4+ class II specific CTL

generated both types of class II specific CTL, although the activity of L3T4$^+$ cells was much lower compared to that of splenic responders in this experiment (panel A). This result clearly indicates that the thymic CTL precursor pool includes Lyt-2$^+$ class II specific cells as well as L3T4$^+$ cells and is not different from the splenic precursor pool. Class I specific CTL consisted exclusively of Lyt-2$^+$ cells (panels D,E), and could not be induced from Lyt-2-depleted population of cells whereas class II specific CTL were (panels C, F).

Further studies were carried out in another combination, bm12 anti B6, in which the genetic difference is confined to I-A gene product alone. As primary CTL were not induced from thymocytes, bm12 responders were stimulated three times in the presence of TCGF *in vitro* to generate reasonable level of CTL activity. This population of CTL also consisted of Lyt-2$^+$ cells L3T4$^+$ cells, the former being the major population (Fig. 2). Thus the results obtained on two different strain combinations indicate that the thymic T cell population is not devoid of Lyt-2$^+$ class II specific CTL precursors.

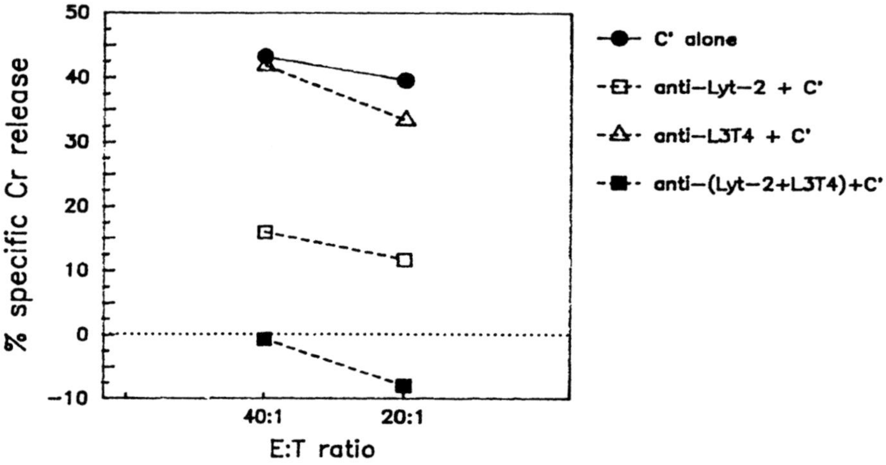

Fig. 2 bm12 thymus anti−B6 CTL

Legend for Fig. 2. Splenic lymphocytes of B6.CH-2^{bm12} were stimulated *in vitro* with B6 stimulator cells three times in the presence of 10% rat ConA culture supernatant. CTL activity was tested on LPS blasts of B6. See legend for Fig. 1 for details

Precursors of Lyt-2$^{\pm}$ class II specific CTL are found among both Ly6.c-positive and -negative populations

Lyt-2$^+$ class II specific CTL were examined for expression of Ly6.c antigen marker which subdivides the Lyt-2$^+$ T cell population. Lyt-2- or L3T4-depleted (A.THxB10.QBR)F_1 spleen cells were stimulated with B10.MBR cells and examined for expression of the Ly6.c at the effector phase (Fig. 3). Class II specific CTL generated from thymocytes consisted of Lyt-2$^+$ and L3T4$^+$ cells and were not sensitive to treatment with anti-Ly6.c antibody and complement (difference between the open and solid bars). On the other hand, a large portion of class II specific CTL induced from spleen cells were sensitive to the anti-Ly6 treatment. CTL induced from Lyt-2-depleted spleen cells were entirely $L3T4^+$ and were $Ly6.c^-$. The $Lyt\text{-}2^+$ CTL population obtained by stimulating L3T4-depleted spleen cells was a mixture of $Ly6.c^+$ and $Ly6.c^-$ cells indicating that $Lyt\text{-}2^+$ class II specific CTL are distributed in both populations.

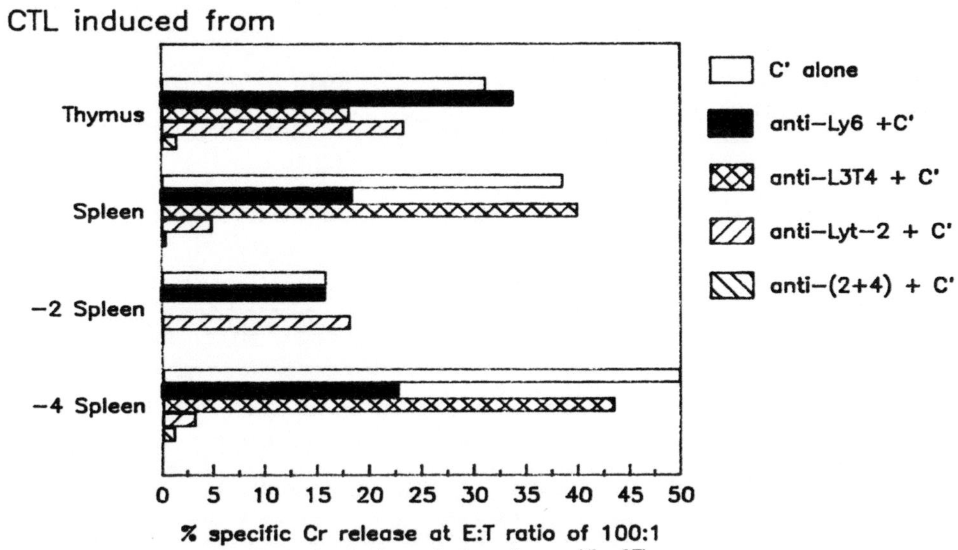

Fig. 3 Ly6.c typing of class II specific CTL

<u>Legend for Fig. 3.</u> Primary $(A.THxB10.QBR)F_1$ anti-B10.MBR CTL were tested on B.10.A(4R) LPS blasts. In this combination, killing specificity is confined to the <u>I-A</u> subregion. Anti-Ly6.c antibody was 34-2-11. See legend for Fig. 1 for treatment of effectors.

Finally class II specific CTL were generated from Ly6-depleted spleen cells of $(A.THxB10.QBR)F_1$ to confirm the existence of $Lyt\text{-}2^+Ly6^-$ class II specific CTL (Fig. 4). This population of CTL was not sensitive to anti-Ly6 treatment confirming the absence of $Ly6^+$ cells. The major portion of the class II specific killing activity of this population of cells was $Lyt\text{-}2^+$ as indicated by the sensitivity to anti-Lyt-2 + complement treatment. Similar observations were made on <u>in vitro</u> tertiary class II specific CTL induced in the combination bm12 anti-B6 (data not shown). This result, together with the data shown in Fig. 3 indicates that $Lyt\text{-}2^+$ class II specific CTL are present in the Ly6.c negative as well as the positive population.

The $Lyt\text{-}2^+$ cells constitute a major population among class II specific CTL rather than rare exceptions(3-6). This

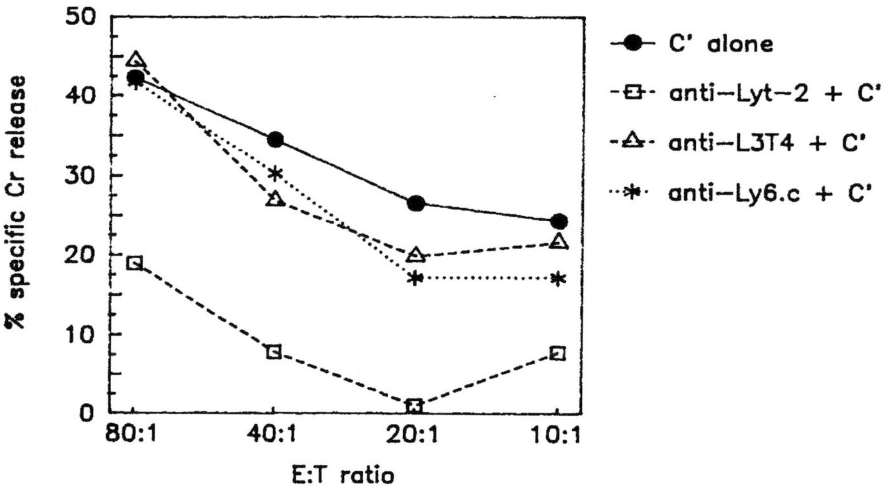

Fig. 4 Ly6.c-depleted class II specific CTL

Legend for Fig. 4. (A.THxB10.QBR)F_1 responders were depleted for Ly6.c positive cells before MLC. See legend for Fig. 1 for detail.

population of CTL is a conspicuous exception to the general correlation between the accessory molecule expressed, i.e., Lyt-2 or L3T4, and the class of MHC antigens recognized by T cells. The results of this series of experiments clearly indicated that precursors of Lyt-2^+ class II specific CTL are distributed among thymocytes as well as spleen cells, and among the Ly6.c negative as well as the Ly6.c positive populations in the spleen. Thus the speculation that such T cells with exceptional combination of the accessory molecule and the receptor specificity might represent a particular subset of Lyt-2^+ T cell population.

Thus far, no major exception have been found among L3T4^+ helper cell population in terms of the MHC class specificity. This population of T cells has been shown to be under strict selection with respoect to the allelic specificity of class II antigens as restricting element such that mature cells of this population recognize antigens exclusively in the context of thymic type class II antigens (10). On the contrary, the repertoir of precursors of Lyt-2^+ CTL have been found not to be strongly skewed toward self MHC restriction (10). Thus it appears possible that the entire Lyt-2^+ CTL precursor population is not subject to strict cognate type positive selection during ontogeny. If this is the case, the precursor pool of Lyt-2^+ CTL should contain a large number of cells expressing receptors compatible with class II + X antigens. Nevertheless, such cells with "wrong combination" of receptor and accessoty molecule are predicted to have a disadvantage in recognizing the antigens in the context of class II molecules because of the lack of the L3T4 molecule. Thus the skewing of Lyt-2^+ cells toward class I antigen may be the result of selection imposed upon antigenic triggering. Only those cells whose receptors happened to show high affinity to the stimulating antigen class II complex are expected to respond to the antigenic stimulation in the absence of the L3T4 molecule. Consistent with this explanation is that Lyt-2^{+} class II specific CTL do not show any dependence on the function of the Lyt-2 molecule. An alternative possibility is that the entire Lyt-2^{+} population is subject to positive selection by class I antigens and that the observed class II reactivity of Lyt-2^{+} cells is due to cross-reactive recognition of certain class II antigens by such cells, as reported on an alloreactive CTL clone (11). However, the absence of such cross-reaction in the other direction, i.e., L3T4^{+} cells cross-reacting with allogeneic class I antigens, makes this possibility less likely (12).

REFERECES

1. S.L. Swain, Significance of Lyt phenotypes: Lyt2 antibodies block activities of T cells that recognize class I major histocompatibility complex antigens regardless of their function. Proc. Natl. Acad. Sci. USA 78:7101 (1981).

2. D.P. Dialynas, D.B. Wilde, P. Marrack, A. Pierres, K.A. Wall, W. Havran, G. Otten, M.R. Loken, M. Pierres, J. Kappler, and F.W. Fitch. Characterization of the murine antigenic determinant, designated L3T4a recognized by monoclonal antibody GK1.5: Expression of L3T4a by functional T cell clones appears to correlate primarily with class II MHC antigen reactivity. Immunol. Rev. 74:29 (1983).

3. N. Shinohara, and M. Kojima. Mouse alloantibodies capable of blocking cytotoxic T cell function. V. The majority of I region-specific CTL are Lyt-2^{+}but are relatively resistant to anti-Lyt-2 blocking. J. Immunol. 132:578 (1984).

4. N. Shinohara. Class II antigen-specific murine cytolytic T lymphocytes (CTL). I. analysis of bulk populations and establishment of Lyt-2^{+}L3T4^{-} and Lyt-2^{-}L3T4^{+} bulk CTL lines. Cell. Immunol. in press (1987).

5. N. Shinohara, J.A. Bluestone, and D.H. Sachs. Cloned CTL which recognize and I-A region product in the context of a class I antigen. J. Exp. Med. 163:972 (1986).

6. N. Shinohara, N. Hozumi, M. Watanabe, J.A. Bluestone, R. Johnson-Leva, and D.H. Sachs. Class II antigen specific murine cytolytic T lymphocytes (CTL). II. Genuine class II specificity of Lyt-2^{+} CTL clones. submitted (1987).

7. A.M. Kruisbeek, S.O. Sharrow, B.J. Mathieson and A. Singer The H-2 phenotype of the thymus dictates the self-specificity expressed thy thymic but not splenic cytotoxic T lymphocyte presursors in thymus-engrafted nude mice. J. Immunol. 127:2168 (1981).

8. H. Auchincloss, Jr., K. Ozato and D.H. Sachs. Two distinct murine differentiation antigens determined by genes linked to the Ly-6 locus. J. Immunol. 127:1839 (1981).

9. F.J. Dumont, L.Z. Coker, R.C. Habbersett and J.A. Treffinger. Xenogeneic monoclonal antibody to an Ly-6-linked murine cell surface antigen: Differential reactivity with T cell subpopulations and bone marrow cells. J. Immunol. 134:2357 (1985).

10. S.M. Bradley, A.M. Kruisbeek and A. Singer. Cytotoxic T lymphocyte responses in allogeneic radiation bone marrow chimeras: The chimeric host strictly dictates the self-repertoire of Ia-restricted T cells but not H-2K/D-restriced T cells. J. Exp. Med. 156:1650 (1982).

11. M.W. Schilham, R. Lang, R. Benner, R.M. Zinkernagel. Characterization of an Lyt-2^+ alloreactive cytotoxic T cell clone specific for H-$2D^b$ that cross-reacts with I-E^k. J. Immunol. 137:2748 (1986).

12. T. Mizuochi, S. Ono, T.R. Malek and A. Singer. Characterization of two distinct primary T cell populations that secrete inter leukin-2 upon recognition of class I or class II major histocompatibility antigens. J. Exp. Med. 163:603 (1986).

DO CLASS II MAJOR HISTOCOMPATIBILITY MOLECULES FUNCTION AS SIGNAL TRANSDUCERS DURING B LYMPHOCYTE ACTIVATION?

M.K. Newell,[1,2] L.B. Justement,[1] K. Lehman,[1] K. Caldwell,[2] D.M.F. Cooper,[2] J.H. Freed,[1,2] and J.C. Cambier[1,2]

[1]National Jewish Center for Immunology and Respiratory Medicine
[2]University of Colorado Health Sciences Center
Denver, CO

INTRODUCTION

The studies described here address the hypothesis that class II molecules (Ia) serve not only as restriction elements for cognate T cell:B cell interaction, but also as signal transducers involved in B cell activation. We have tested this hypothesis by studying modulation of B cell physiology by anti-Ia antibodies. Specifically, we have assessed the ability of these antibodies to induce "second" messenger generation and to modulate cell proliferative and differentiative responses to LPS and anti IgM antibodies.

A large and growing body of evidence attests to the complexity of regulation of B lymphocyte activation by antigens, cytokines, and cell-cell contact. In the mouse, 80-90% of peripheral B cells are quiescent, non-cycling cells. The state of activation of these cells can be modulated by a variety of agents ranging from antigen, surrogate antigen in the form of anti-immunoglobulin antibodies (anti-Ig), IL-4 (Noelle et al. 1984), gamma interferon,(Mond et al. 1981), B cell activating factor BCAF (Leclerq et al. 1984), lipopolysaccharide (LPS) (Andersson et al. 1980), and ligands which bind to major histocompatibility class II (Ia) molecules (Chen et al. 1987). B cells in proliferative cycles are regulated by these species and by additional interleukins, including IL-5 (BCGF-2), IL-2, IL-1 and less well defined B cell differentiation factors. The fact that each of these regulators affects the biology of B cells differently suggests that each has a distinct receptor on the B cell surface. In addition these findings suggest that the respective receptors must be coupled to distinct intracellular second messenger generating systems.

Ligation of the B cell antigen receptor (membrane immunoglobulin, mIg) induces proto-oncogene expression (M.J. Klemz, E. Palmer and J.C. Cambier, submitted for publication), increased Ia expression (Monroe and Cambier 1984), in some cases, G_0 to G_1 transition and B cell proliferation (for review see Finkelman). The receptor mediates these effects through the hydrolysis of phosphatidylinositol-4,5-bisphosphate ($PtdInsP_2$). The consequence of this hydrolysis is the generation of the second messengers diacylglycerol (DAG) and inositol trisphosphate ($InsP_3$) (Bijsterbosch et al. 1985.

The hypothesis that Ia molecules also function as signal transducers is supported by a number of experimental observations. Recent studies have documented effects of anti-Ia antibodies, presumably acting as surrogates of T cells, on B cell proliferation and differentiation (Forsgren et al. 1984, Niederhuber et al. 1975, Palacios et al. 1983). Anti-Ia antibodies inhibit LPS and anti-Ig-induced B cell mitogenesis (Niederhuber et al. 1975). Anti-Ia antibodies reportedly augment *in vitro* plaque forming cell responses (Palacios et al. 1983). Finally, Bishop and Haughton have reported that anti-Ia induces differentiation of the B cell lymphoma CH12 into antibody secreting cells (Bishop and Haughton 1986). Considered in view of recent studies which indicate that cognate T-B (Ia involving) interactions are essential for generating plaque forming cells, but not for proliferative responses (DeFranco and Paul 1984, Julius and Cambier, submitted for publication) these findings suggest that T cell-B cell contact via T cell receptor and Ia may mediate signals which promote B cell differentiation. Here we report experiments designed to address the possibility that Ia mediates signaling by cAMP generation leading to B cell differentiation.

Several published reports (Forsgren et al. 1984, Niederhuber et al. 1975) indicate that pretreatment of non-separated (by density) B cells can be inhibited by pretreating the cells with anti-Ia antibodies or analogues of cAMP. Based on these observations, we investigated the effects of anti-Ia antibodies on Ia expression, proliferation and differentiation. In addition, we directly measured cAMP levels in these cells following Ia perturbation.

RESULTS

Anti-Ia Antibodies and Analogues of cAMP can Inhibit LPS-Induced B Cell Proliferative Responses

Small (>1.075 g/ml) B cells were cultured with or without anti-Ia or anti-H-2K antibodies for 6 hr, followed by the addition of LPS. In the presence of the anti-Ia antibody, but not the anti-H-2K antibody, the proliferative response generated by LPS was inhibited by approximately 50% (Fig. 1A).

In parallel experiments, analogues of cAMP were examined to see whether they could mimic the inhibition of the proliferative response produced by anti-Ia antibodies. A significant inhibition of LPS and rabbit anti-mouse immunoglobulin (Ramig) induced proliferation following pretreatment with cAMP was observed. This effect was dose dependent. When the cAMP concentration was lower than 10^{-6}M, the proliferative response was slightly enhanced overbackground (Fig. 1B).

Anti-Ia and cAMP Analogues Inhibit Mitogen-Induced Increases in Ia Expression

We next determined whether binding of anti-Ia leads to inhibition of earlier events in B cell activation, specifically induction of Ia expression. In Fig. 2A are shown data demonstrating that pretreatment of quiescent B cells (ρ>1.075 g/ml) with monoclonal anti-I-A antibodies for 6 hr, could completely inhibit the LPS-induced I-E hyper-expression measured 30 hr after stimulation. Anti-class I antibodies of the same isotype did not inhibit LPS-induced Ia expression (data not shown). This effect could be mimicked by the pretreatment of these cells with analogues of cAMP, either 8-bromo-cAMP (Fig. 2B) or dibutyryl cAMP (data not shown).

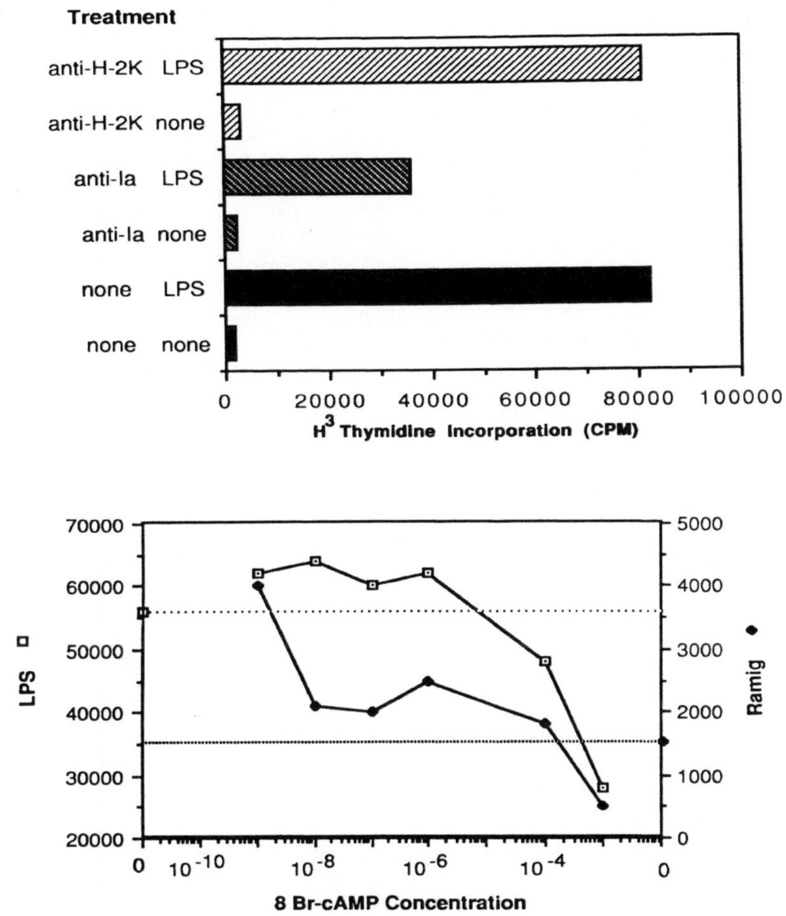

Fig. 1. Inhibition of LPS-induced proliferative responses. A. Small (ρ>1.075 g/ml) normal AKR B cells (5×10^5/well) were cultured in the presence or absence of 20 µg/ml of anti-class II (10-3.6) or anti-class I (11-4.1) for 6 hr prior to the addition of 20 µg/ml LPS. The cells were incubated for 30 hr at 37° in 5% CO_2. At this time 1 µCi of ^{3}H-thymidine was added per culture. After 4 hr the cells were harvested and counted. Results are recorded as uptake of ^{3}H-thymidine in counts per minute. B. The anti-proliferative effects of anti-class II antibodies can be mimicked by analogues of cAMP. Small B cells were cultured in the presence or absence of titered doses of 8 Br-cAMP, followed by the addition of LPS at 20 µg/ml on the left Y axis, or rabbit anti-mouse immunoglobulin (Ramig) at 50 µg/ml, on the right Y axis. Note that at doses below 10^{-6}M the inhibitory effect of the 8-Br-cAMP appears to be reversed and apparent stimulation of proliferation is observed. A box on the left axis and the associated dotted line mark the result of LPS alone in the cell cultures. A diamond on the right axis and the associated dotted line indicate Ramig stimulation alone.

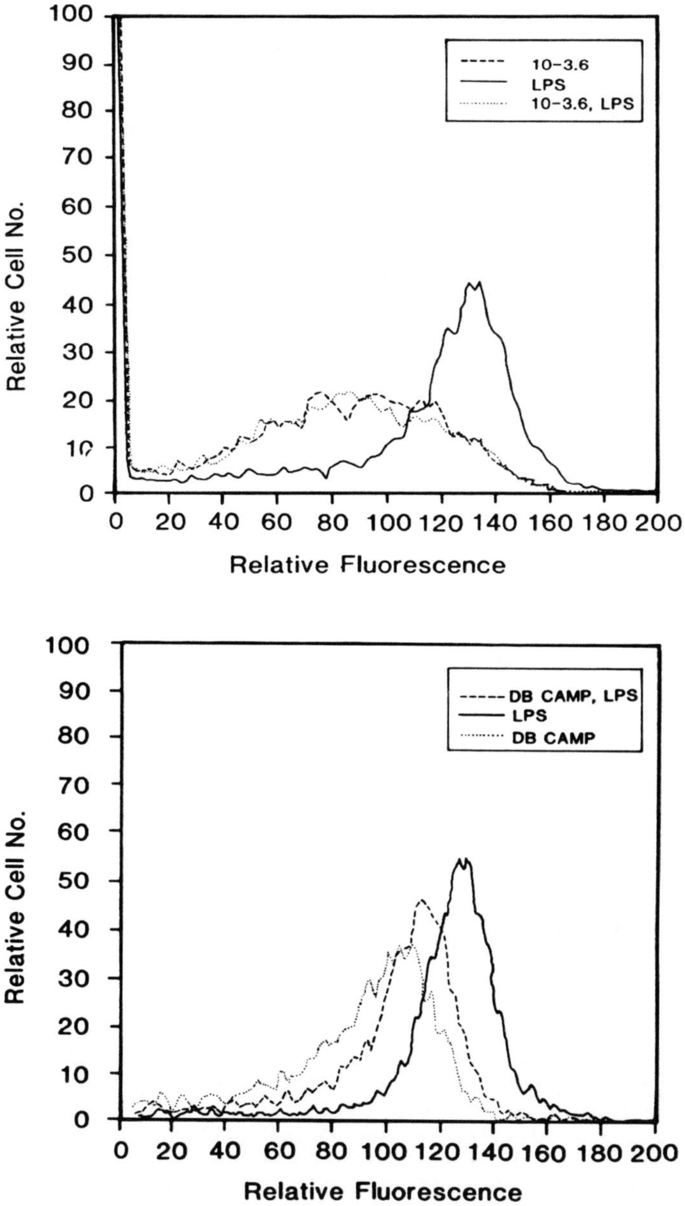

Fig. 2. Inhibition of Ia hyper-expression. A. Duplicate cultures of small normal AKR B cells, as described in Fig. 1, were cultured with and without the anti-class II antibody, 10-3.6 at 50 µg/ml, for 6 hr. Cells were then stimulated with LPS for 18 hr. Expression of the I-E antigen was measured with the 14-4-4S monoclonal antibody. Results are recorded as relative fluorescence intensity on the X axis and cell number on the Y. B. cAMP inhibits subsequent LPS-induced Ia hyper-expression. Cells were cultured in the presence or absence of 8 Br-cAMP at 10^{-5}M for 6 hr. The cells were then stimulated with LPS for 18 hr and analyzed for I-E expression by flow cytometric analysis.

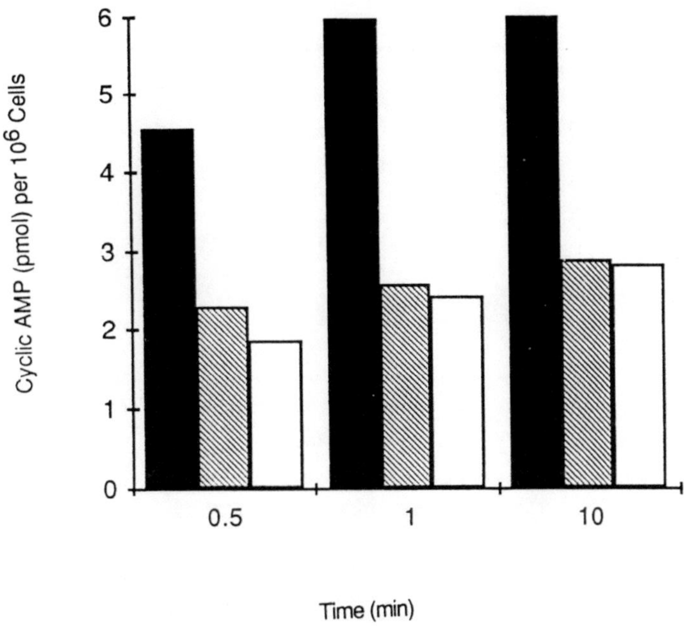

Fig. 3. Radioimmunoassay measuring cAMP levels in small (ρ>1.075 g/ml) AKR B cells as a result of anti-Ia treatment. Cells, at 10^6/ml, were cultured in the presence of 10% BSF1 (stippled bars); or 10-3.6, anti-I-A^k at 50 μg/ml (solid bars) or in the absence of both (open bars), for the indicated times. Results are depicted as levels of total intracellular cAMP (pmol) at the indicated time points.

Anti-Ia Induces an Increase in cAMP Levels

The results of the preceding experiments indicate that anti-Ia antibodies and cAMP affect B cell physiology similarly suggesting that Ia may mediate signals via induction of cAMP generation. To address this possibility, we assessed the affects of anti-Ia antibodies on cellular cAMP levels. As shown in Fig. 3, anti-Ia antibodies induced a rapid (within 1 min) 2 to 3-fold increase in cellular levels of cAMP. Control antibody binding, i.e., to class I and to mIg molecules, produced no such increase (data not shown). Nitta et al. (1982), have demonstrated that binding of IgG_{2a} and IgG_{2b} Fc to membrane immunoglobulin receptors causes increased intracellular cAMP levels. Because most of the antibodies employed were of the IgG_{2a} subclass, we addressed the possibility that the increases in cAMP observed were a result of Fc mediated cAMP generation. $F(ab')_2$ fragments of the Ia binding antibodies were also found to increase cAMP levels.

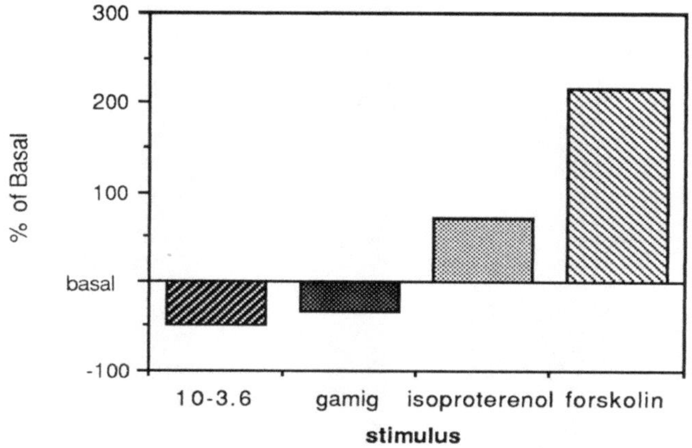

Fig. 4. Adenylate cyclase activity in lymphocyte membranes after anti-Ia treatment. Plasma membranes from AKR B cells were isolated by sucrose density centrifugation following osmotic lysis and homogenization of small lymphocytes. Membranes, 25 µg protein/point, were treated with 25 µg of anti-I-A^k, or goat anti-mouse immunoglobulin for 10 min. Isoproterenol (10^{-5} M) and forskolin (10^{-5} M) were used a positive controls. Cyclase activity was recorded as pmol/mg/min and subsequently were converted to % basal activity as shown.

Effects of Anti-Ia Antibodies on Adenylate Cyclase

An increase in cellular cAMP can occur as a result of altered activities of several metabolic pathways including the activation of adenylate cyclase. Adenylate cyclase converts ATP to cyclic-3',5'-AMP, which has been established to be a most powerful "second messenger" in receptor mediated signaling. This enzymatic activation can be the direct result of receptor ligation, or alternatively a secondary metabolite may feedback to activate the enzyme. The results summarized in Fig. 4 illustrate that these antibodies do not activate the cyclase in these membranes preparations. In fact, the anti-Ia appears to inhibit adenylate cyclase enzyme in GTP independently (data not shown). The implications of these results will be discussed below.

Anti-Ia Antibodies Enhance LPS Induced Staphylococcal Protein A Plaques and Ig Secretion

We next assessed the effects of anti-Ia antibodies on differentiation of B cells to antibody secreting cells. Polystyrene plates were precoated with antibodies, including D3, 10-2.16 or 11-4.1 or with fetal calf serum overnight and then washed three times. Small B cells, from either (C57BL/6 x DBA/2)F_1 (BDF1) or AKR, were separated as described and treated with several mitogenic stimuli, including IL-4 and LPS. At the end of six days the wells were harvested and analyzed by two parameters, either immunoglobulin secretion or plaque formation. Fig. 5 demonstrates that the presence of anti-Ia (only of the appropriate haplotype specificity) increases both plaque formation and immunoglobulin secretion.

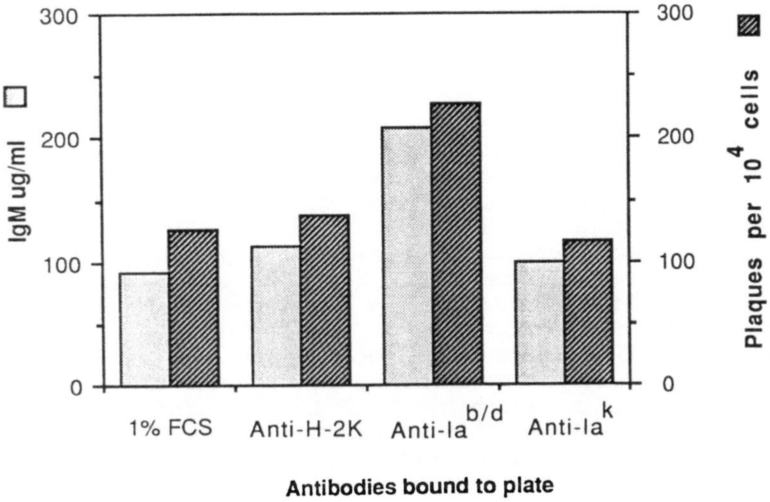

Fig. 5. Anti-Ia-induced increases in plaque formation and immunoglobulin secretion. Small B cells were isolated from BDF1 mice. Microtitier plates were coated with 1% FCS, anti-H-2K^{b} (M1.42), D-3 (anti-I-A$^{b/d}$), or anti-I-A^{k} (10-2.16) overnight at 4°C. Small B cells (5 x 10^{5}) were added to the microtiter plates in the presence of 25% D9 supernatant (IL-4) and 0.1 µg/ml LPS. Protein A plaque analysis was performed on day 4. Supernatants from duplicate cultures were harvested after 6 days and assayed for immunoglobulin secretion by ELISA.

Interestingly, when anti-Ia antibodies were added in soluble form, the enhancing effects were demonstrable only when the antibodies were added at concentrations ≥50 µg/ul). These doses of antibody lead to cell agglutination presumably mediated by cell-cell bridging by antibody.

DISCUSSION

To gain an understanding of the molecular basis for signal transduction by Ia, physiologic changes in cells stimulated by anti-Ia antibodies have been examined. Ligands specific for I-A and I-E molecules do not induce detectable increases in phospholipid metabolism or Ca^{++} mobilization (data not shown). However, they induce a rapid loss of >80% of cytoplasmic protein kinase C (Chen et al. 1987) and promote differentiation to antibody secretion. The results reported here demonstrate the anti-proliferative effects of anti-Ia antibodies as well as anti-Ia mediated inhibition of mitogen induced Ia hyper-expression.

Initially, the molecular basis of anti-Ia mediated effects on B cell physiology were obscure. Noting however, that the anti-proliferative and differentiative effects of the anti-Ia antibodies were similar to effects mediated by cAMP in other tissues, the possibility that increased cAMP levels result from mIa ligation was explored. As shown in Fig. 2, cAMP analogues mimicked the effects of anti-Ia antibodies in inhibiting LPS-induced proifertive responses. LPS-induced increases in expression of I-E could be inhibited by 0.1 mM dibutyryl cAMP, again analogously to anti-Ia antibodies. Finally, as shown in Fig. 2, anti-Ia antibodies induce a significant increase in intracellular levels of cAMP.

Based on these observations, it is hypothesized that ligation of Ia by T cells leads to activation of membrane associated adenylate cyclase, rising cellular levels of cAMP. However, while anti-Ia induced an increase in cAMP in the cell, the same antibodies inhibit the activity of adenylate cyclase in purified membranes, Fig. 4. The interpretation of this result remains obscure. A possible explanation is that a key component ofo the signal generating complex may be coupled to the cytoskeleton. When membranes are isolated and the structural constraints provided by an intact cytoskeleton are removed, the appropriate second messenger can no longer be generated. This hypothesis supported by the observation that α_s, the GTP-binding α chain of the G protein complex, which regulates the effector β and γ subunits, copurifies with filamentous actin (Kawahara et al. 1980). Only when the receptor is coupled in the appropriate macromolecular context to the correct components is the appropriate signal delivered. This may be particularly relevant to signaling which results from cell to cell contact, i.e., T cell:B cell conjugate formation. Furthermore, in parallel studies, we have demonstrated that class II molecules are clearly associated with actin and perhaps with components of the adenyl cyclase and/or PKA systems (M.K. Newell and J.H. Freed, manuscript in preparation).

The inhibitory effects of soluble anti-Ia antibodies are well documented (Niederhuber et al. 1975, Forsgren et al. 1984). The fact that anti-Ia-induced inhibition of Ia hyper-expression and proliferation can be mimicked by analogues of cAMP suggest that cAMP mediates inhibition.

In a number of systems, including B cells, elevation of cAMP is associated with cell differentiation. Consistent with these findings are results reported here which indicate that anti-Ia antibodies enhance differentiation. From these data, the following model for thymus dependent B cell activation has been proposed. Binding of thymus-dependent antigen to quiescent B cells evokes inositol lipid hydrolysis, Ca^{++} mobilization and increased expression of Ia molecules. The antigen is internalized, processed and reexpressed in the context of Ia antigens. These events confer on the B cell competence to present antigens to helper T cells. T cells bind to B cell antigen-Ia complexes stimulating an elevation in intracellular cAMP, interpreted by the B cell as a differentiative signal. Lymphokines released by T cells following T-B interaction stimulate proliferation. This hypothesis differs from generally accepted paradigm in suggesting that cognate T cell-B cell contact mediated signals exert their affect on B cell differentiation rather than proliferation.

This work was supported in part by PHS grants AI 20519 and AI 21768 and USPHS grant CA 36700.

REFERENCES

Andersson, J., Schrier, M. H., and Melchers, F.: T cell dependent B cell stimulation is H-2 restricted and antigen dependent only at the resting B cell level. Proc. Natl. Acad. Sci. U.S.A. 77:1612-1616, 1980.

Arad, H., Rasenbusch, J. P., and Lenitzki, A.: Stimulatory GTP regulatory unit Ns and the catalytic unit of adenylate cyclase are tightly associated: Mechanistic consequences. Proc. Natl. Acad. Sci. U.S.A. 81:6579-6583, 1984.

Benovic, J. R., Schorr, G. L., Caron, M. G., and Lefkowitz, R. J.: The mammalian β-adrenergic receptor: Purification and characterization. Biochem. 23:4510-4518, 1984.

Bijsterbosch, M. K., Meade, J. C., Turner, G. A., and Klaus, G. G. B.: B lymphocyte receptors and polyphosphoinositide degradation. Cell 41:999-1006, 1985.

Bishop, G. A., and Haughton, G.: Induction of differentiation of a transformed clone of Ly1+ B cells by clonal T cells and antibodies, Proc. Natl. Acad. Sci. U.S.A. 83:7410-7418, 1986.

Bourn, H. R.: "Wrong subunit" regulates cardiac potassium channels. Nature 325:296-297, 1987.

Cambier, J. C., and Ransom, J. T.: Molecular mechanism of transmembrane signaling in B lymphocytes. Immunol. Rev. 5:175, 1987.

Chen, Z. Z., McGuire, J. C., Leach, K. L., and Cambier, J. C.: Transmembrane signaling through B cell MHC class II molecules: Anti-Ia antibodies induce protein kinase C translocation to the nuclear fraction. J. Immunol. 138:2345-2352, 1987.

DeFranco, A. L., Ashwell, J. D., Schwartz, R. H., and Paul, W. E.: Polyclonal stimulation of resting B lymphocytes by antigen specific T lymphocytes. J. Exp. Med. 159:861-880, 1984.

Forsgren, S., Pobor, G., Coutinho, A., and Pierres, M.: The role of I-A/E molecules in B lymphocyte activation. I. Inhibition of LPS induced responses by monoclonal antibodies. J. Immunol. 133:2104-2110, 1984.

Kahn, R.: The molecular mechanism of insulin action. Ann. Rev. Med. 36:429-451, 1985.

Kawahara, Y., Takai, Y., Minakuchi, R., Sno, K., and Nishizuka, Y.: Phospholipid turnover as a possible transmembrane signal for protein phosphorylation during human platelet activation by thrombin, Biochem. Biophys. Res. Commun. 97:309-317, 1980.

Leclerq, L., Bismuth, G., and Theze, J.: Antigen specific helper T cell clone supernatant is sufficient to induce both polyclonal proliferation and differentiation of small resting B lymphocytes. Proc. Natl. Acad. Sci. U.S.A. 81:6491-6495, 1984.

Mond, J. J., Seghal, E., Kung, J., and Finkelman, F. D.: Increased expression of I-region-associated antigen (Ia) on B cells after crosslinking of surface immunoglobulin. J. Immunol. 127:881-888, 1981.

Monroe, J. G., and Cambier, J. C.: B cell activation. III. B cell plasma membrane depolarization and hyper I-A antigen expression induced by receptor immunoglobulin crosslinking are coupled. J. Exp. Med. 158:1589-1599, 1983.

Niederhuber, J. E., Frelinger, J. A., Dugan, E., Coutinho, A., and Shrefler, D.: Effects of anti-Ia serum on mitogenic responses. I. Inhibition of proliferative response to B cell mitogen, LPS, by specific anti-Ia sera. J. Immunol. 115:1672-1676, 1975.

Nishizuka, Y.: The role of protein kinase C in cell surface signal transduction and tumor promotion. Nature 308:693-698, 1984.

Nitta, Y., and Suzuki, T.: Biochemical signals transmitted by FcY receptors: Triggering mechanisms of the increased synthesis of adenosine-3',5'-cyclic monophosphate mediated by FcY_{2a} and FcY_{2b} receptors of a murine macrophage-like cell line ($P388D_1$). J. Immunol. 129:2708-2714, 1982.

Noelle, R. H., Krammer, P. H., Ohara, T., Uhr, J. W., and Vitetta, E. S.: Increased expression of Ia antigens on resting B cells: an additional role for B cell growth factor. Proc. Natl. Acad. Sci. U.S.A. 81:6149-6153, 1984.

Palacios, R., Martinez-Maza, O., and Guy, K.: Monoclonal antibodies against HLA-DR antigens replace T helper cells in activation of B lymphocytes. Proc. Natl. Acad. Sci. U.S.A. 80:3456-3460, 1983.
Sahyoun, N. E., Levine, III, H. E., Davis, J., Hebdon, G. M., and Cuatrecasas, P.: Molecular complexes involved in the regulation of adenylate cyclase. Proc. Natl. Acad. Sci. U.S.A. 78:6158-6162, 1981.
Snow, E. C., Fetherston, J. D., and Zimmes, S.: Induction of c-myc after antigen binding to hapten-specific B cells. J. Exp. Med. 164:944-950, 1986.

ANALYSIS OF ANTIGEN-SPECIFIC T CELL-MEDIATED SUPPRESSION AT THE CLONAL LEVEL[1]

Barbara A. Araneo and Tad Dowell
University of Utah Medical Center
Salt Lake City, Utah 84132

ABSTRACT

For the purpose of investigating inhibition of T cell activation at a molecular level, we have assembled a panel of T cell hybridomas whose members respond to antigen and Class II molecules by production of the cytokine, IL-2, and have established bulk cultured Ts cells which inactivate certain T hybridomas. Several important observations concerning the interaction between T hybridomas and Ts cells have contributed to our understanding of inhibitory cellular interactions. These findings are 1) antigen-induced cytokine production by HEL/I-A^b specific T hybridomas is specifically and completely inhibited by HEL-induced Ts cells, 2) T cell hybridomas of other specificities (e.g. HEL/I-A^d) are not inhibited by HEL-Ts cells, 3) bulk cultured Ts cells are functionally superior to primary Ts cells following their short term culture in lymphokine supplemented media. This experimental system now provides an excellent opportunity to learn how helper T cells become inactivated by Ts and to describe the mechanism of inactivation in molecular terms.

INTRODUCTION

The anti-HEL response developed by H-2^b haplotype mice (referred to as low responders) is remarkably compartmentalized, since antibody against HEL may or may not be observed depending upon the route of immunization. Within 7-10 days of intraperitoneal immunization, HEL-specific suppressor T cells (Ts) are established in the spleens of low responder mice. This is to the exclusion of helper T cells. Within 7-10 days of footpad immunization high levels of HEL-specific helper T cells are found in the draining popliteal lymph nodes (1). The relative level of helper activity developed by low responder (LR) or high responder (HR) T cells is nearly equivalent at this early 7-10 day time point.

A unique feature of low responder Th cells, defined by their invariant specificity for HEL/I-A^b, is an extreme sensitivity to HEL-activated Ts cells(1). Ts, like LR Th, are derived from H-2^b haplotype mice, e.g. B10 and BDF1 strains. We believe the

[1]This work supported by PHS research grant CA-38349

relationship between HEL Th and HEL Ts cells is established early in T cell development, during intrathymic selection of the Th cell repertoire in the absence of antigen. This hypothesis derives from the observation that in mice, selection of T cells lacking I-Ab restricted Th cells, (F1-->D2 bone marrow chimaeras), also selects against development of suppressor T cells capable of inhibiting HEL/I-A^b Th cells (2). This feature is even more exceptional in light of the fact that F1 bone marrowcan donate precursors of T cells that are able to mature into Ts in a B10 irradiated mouse (2).

Suppression of in vitro Th cells requires a minimun of three interacting T cell subsets; Ts cells which function as inhibitors, T cells auxiliary to Ts acting as inducers or transducers, and Th cells which appear to be the targets of inhibition. Research in this laboratory has recently begun to focus on detailing the mechanism of inhibitory cellular interactions, especially those affecting Th cells. To achieve this goal we needed to develop a simple and direct assay for Th cell inhibition by Ts. It was decided to use their T hybridoma equivalents. This report describes the analysis of a panel of T cell hybridomas which respond to a ligand, antigen/Class II MHC molecular complexes, by production of IL-2. We also describe how inhibition of IL-2 production is mediated by HEL-activated, bulk-cultured Ts cells. The important feature of this report is that inhibition of T hybridomas is antigen/MHC specific. On the basis of present and former observations we believe that Ts cells and LR-Th cells are linked by the antigen and MHC, perhaps through Ts recognition of an idiotypic determinant on the Th cell's receptors for antigen. We have no solid information concerning the nature of the recognition structure on Ts cells.

METHODS

Mice. Six to eight week old male or female C57B1/10 (B10), B10.D2/oSnJ (B10.D2), and (B10 x B10.D2) F1 (BDF1) hybrid mice have been purchased from the Jackson Laboratories (Bar Harbor, ME) or bred within the Medical Center animal facility. All mice are maintained in the animal facility until 12 to 16 weeks of age.

Antigens. HEL (chicken egg-white lysozyme) and huTrf (human apotransferrin) are purchased from Sigma Chemical Co. (St. Louis, MO), and used without further purification.

Preparation of T cell hybridomas. The method of Kappler et. al. (3) has been successsful in constructing antigen-specific T cell hybridomas. Mice are injected subcutaneously in the hindfootpads with a total of 100ug of antigen in CFA. After 7 days, popliteal and inguinal lymph nodes are excised and the cells cultured with 100ug antigen/ml/culture in Eagles High Amino Acid medium. After 3-4 days, the cultured cells are harvested, counted and re-cultured for 4 days in MEM containing 1000 Units/ml of Con A-induced cell free supernatant. The resulting blast T cells were fused with BW5147 according to the procedure of Marrack (4). Following fusion, primary wells with dividing cells were split and the duplicate well screened for antigen/MHC reactive T hybridomas. Selected primary wells were then cloned and the clones retested for antigen/MHC-specific induction of IL-2 production. We have constructed a variety of hybridomas using this procedure (5). T hybridomas described in this report are assayed under optimal conditions; and inhibition by Ts also utilize these conditions (see Table legends). Each of these studies have been conducted numerous times to confirm the observations. However, only single represenative examples have been compiled.

Ts cell enrichment. Either B10 or (B10 x B10.D2)F1 mice are immunized by ip. injection of 100ug HEL in CFA. Ten days later spleens of LR mice are excised and a single cell suspension is prepared. First we select for the T cell fraction of spleen cells using

Rabbit anti-mouse Ig plates, then deplete T cells bearing the I-J, Lyt-1 and CD4 cell surface markers by lysis with specific monoclonal antibodies and complement. This Lyt-2 selected T cell population which is now functionally enriched for 1° Ts cells specifically inhibits HEL/I-A^b specific helper T cell function. Primary Ts are cultured for at least four days in flasks at a concentration of 5 x 10^5/ml in Mishell-Dutton media supplemented with 1000 U/ml of IL-2; from then on they are referred to as bulk cultured Ts lines. The source of IL-2 is culture supernatant of 24-hour, Con-A activated mouse spleen cells. On the fourth day, some of the Ts cells are harvested from flasks, washed free of lymphokines and then prepared for an experiment by resuspending in complete media at a concentration of 2 x 10^6/ml.

Assay for T cell induction by antigen/Class II and inhibition of T cell function by specific suppressor T cells. Routinely, 1 x 10^5 T cell hybridomas are co-cultured with 5 x 10^5 irradiated spleen cells(or 1 x 10^5 I-$A^{b,d}$ expressing B lymphoma cells) as accessory cells plus a predetermined optimal concentration of soluble antigen, which is 200ug/ml for high responder and 4mg/ml for low responder T cell hybridomas. Following an 18-24 hr incubation, culture supernatants are assayed for the titer of IL-2 using viability of the IL-2 dependent cell line, HT-2. Suppressor T cell activity in this system, is assayed by inhibition of IL-2 production by LR T hybridomas compared to HR hybridomas (Ts insensitive). Thus, bulk cultured Ts cells, 1-2 x 10^5, are added to parallel cultures of T cell hybridomas, accessory cells and soluble antigen.

RESULTS AND DISCUSSION

HEL-specific T cell hybridomas used in the following experiments were derived from a single fusion of HEL-primed, and propagated, lymph node T cell blasts using the method of Kappler (3). T cell hybridomas specific for human transferrin were derived from a single fusion using a similar protocol. The notation "Hbd" identifies HEL-induced (B10 x D2) F1 T cell clones and "Tb" signifies Transferrin-specific B10 T cell clones. While the Hbd clones are genetically identical they are phenotypically distinct in their specificity for HEL. Hbd 30.4 is one of many HEL-reactive clones selected from this fusion that exhibits a low responder phenotype, specificity for HEL/I-A^b-specificity and inhibition by HEL-Ts cells. The clone Hbd 31.1, and many other clones, is a high responder to HEL displaying an MHC-specificity for the d haplotype and resistance to suppression.

HEL-specific, LR phenotype T cell hybridomas express a traditional T cell receptor for antigen (TCR) complex. In the past, we have assessed the behavior of LR T cells in both helper (1) and proliferation assays (6). We had observed that by comparison to HR T cells, LR T cells develop a nearly equivalent level of responsiveness to HEL. With the objective of studying T cell induction at the clonal level, we constructed T hybridomas that respond to several stimuli with production of the cytokine, IL-2. This approach would allows us to compare, for each stimulus, response achieved by both LR and HR HEL-specific T hybridomas and thus detect any unusual characteristics associated with the LR-phenotype T cells. The hybridomas listed in Table 1 are two of many such HEL-helper T cell equivalents. First, we determined whether the TCR complex of LR-hybridomas functions as efficiently as TCR of a genetically identical HR T hybridoma, using anti-CD3 and several other monoclonal antibodies to inhibit hybridoma induction by antigen/Class II molecules. For example in Table II, when anti-CD3 (1452C-11.4.5) antibodies were added to cultures containing hybridoma T cells, antigen and the antigen-presenting lymphoma (LB15.13), Table I, we observed strong inhibition of both LR and HR T hybridomas. This was also true for anti-CD4 and the appropriate monoclonal anti-I-A antibodies, even though HR T hybridomas are more resistant to

Table I. T cell hybridomas blocked by anti-CD3 and anti-I-A antibodies.

	hybridoma* + ab+	antigen	U IL-2/ml#
1.	(LR) Hbd 30.4	HEL	1280
	Hbd 30.4 + anti-I-A^d	HEL	1280
	Hbd 30.4 + anti-I-A^b	HEL	40
	Hbd 30.4 + anti-CD4	HEL	80
	Hbd 30.4 + anti-CD3	HEL	40
2.	(HR) Hbd 31.1	HEL	2560
	Hbd 31.1 + anti-I- A^d	HEL	80
	Hbd 31.1 + anti-I-A^b	HEL	2560
	Hbd 31.1 + anti-CD4	HEL	320
	Hbd 31.1 + anti-CD3	HEL	20

*Hybridomas were cultured at 1 x 10^5/well of a 96-well culture plate with 2 x 10^5 accessory cells plus soluble HEL for 24 hours. Hbd 31.1 gives an optimal IL-2 response with 200ug/ml HEL in culture, while Hbd 30.4 responds to 4mg/ml HEL. The lymphoma, LB 15.13, is an I-$A^{b,d}$ expressing accessory cell which is added at 2 x 10^5/culture.

+Monoclonal antibodies were prepared in this laboratory by purification of Ig from culture supernatants using caprylic acid. Antibodies purified in this manner are dialyzed against PBS, concentrated to 4mg/ml and stored as a sterile 50% glycerol solution at -20°C. For functional studies, a final concentration of 1-2 ug/ml of the final culture volume achieved optimal, and specific blocking of antigen induced activation.

#The amount of IL-2 produced in any given culture was determined by pooling supernatants of triplicate wells followed by serial two-fold dilution. 4,000 HT-2 cells were added to each culture. The viability of HT-2 was assessed at the end of a 24-hour incubation to determine the relative titer of IL-2 in each sample.

inhibition by anti-CD4. The data in Table I indicate that activation of HEL/I-A^b-specific (LR) hybridomas by HEL is easily and completely blocked by the monoclonal antibody 25-9-3S (anti-I-A^b) but not by MKD6 (anti-I-A^d). Conversely, HEL/I-A^d-specific (HR) T hybridomas, Hbd 31.1, are inhibited by anti-I-A^d but not anti-I-A^b monoclonal antibodies. The results of these inhibition studies suggest that the LR T cell hybridomas are induced by their appropriate ligand via a functionally traditional TCR complex.

Induction of T cell hybridomas via Ti/CD3 receptor complex. The demonstration that non-aggregated anti-CD3 antibodies block T hybridoma induction, indicates that TCR (*excluding* the idiotype, Ti) of LR and HR T hybridomas function similarly. Nevertheless LR T hybridomas have very different requirements for activation. For example, HEL-LR T cell hybridomas require a minimum of 4mg/ml of antigen (compared to 200 ug/ml for some HR clones) and produce a maximum IL-2 titer that is 2-4 fold less than HR clones. We are currently investigating whether the weaker response by LR T hybridomas to HEL may be a reflection of lower affinity between LR-TCR and ligand, and/or less ligand (inefficient antigen/Ia-complex formation). To begin to address this question, we assumed that the only difference between F1-derived LR and

Table II. Induction of T cell hybridomas by antigen and anti-receptor antibodies

	T cells (origin)	induction	U IL-2/ml
1.	Hbd 30.4 hybridoma	HEL/I-A^b	640-1280
		anti-CD4	20
		anti-CD3	2560
2.	Hbd 31.1hybridoma	HEL/I-Ad	1280-2560
		anti-CD4	<10
		anti-CD3	2560
3.	Tb 8.3 hybridoma	huTf/I-A^b	640-1280
		anti-CD4	10
		anti-CD3	2560

*Hybridomas were cultured at 5 x 10^4/well of a 96-well culture plate in the presence of 2 x 10^5 lymphoma cells, LB15.13. Concentrations of antigen were 4 mg/ml HEL for Hbd 30.4, 200 ug/ml HEL for Hbd 31.1, and 4 mg/ml transferrin for Tb 8.3.

+Monoclonal antibodies were prepared in this laboratory and used at a concentration of 20 ug/ml of the final culture volume, *in the absence of soluble antigen*

#The amount of IL-2 produced in any given cultured was determined by pooling supernatants of triplicate wells followed by serial two-fold dilution into the base culture media. 4,000 HT-2 cells were added to each culture. The viability of HT-2 was assessed at the end of a 24 hour incubation to determine the relative titer of IL-2 in each sample.

HR T hybridomas is their TCR, each with specificity for a unique ligand. Therefore, we felt any non-TCR associated deficiencies in T cell activation could be ruled out by induction with anti-CD3 antibodies. To do this, anti-CD3 would have to become aggregated into a polymeric form in culture by accessory cells in the absence of soluble antigen. We predicted that induction with anti-CD3 would stimulate strong responses by both LR and HR T hybridomas. The results of this experiment are detailed in Table II. We observed that anti-CD3, but not anti-CD4, could elicit equivalent and vigorous responses by both LR and HR T hybridomas and at an equivalent optimal dose, 10 ug/ml. In LR hybridomas, the intensity of the response to anti-CD3 clearly contrasts the intensity of responses induced by antigen. While induction with anti-CD3indicates that a normal cellular response can be developed by LR hybridomas, it is important to emphasize that the weak response to antigen is the feature which mimicks the response potential of LR Th cells in vivo. Because LR Th are known to be regulated by HEL-activated Ts, it is possible that one factor contributing to effective Th-Ts interaction is lesion in TCR binding to antigen.

Inhibition of cytokine production by T cell hybridomas is linked to the antigen/class II specifictiy of the T cell hybridoma. In a prior report, we demonstrated that low responsiveness to HEL by H-2^b haplotype mice is due to active inhibition by suppressor T cells; where HEL-induced helper and proliferating T cells are primarily affected (1,7).With the technology available for cloning T cells, it becomes appropriate to ask questions aimed at understanding the biochemical basis of T cell regulatory actions. In an effort to improve our own methodology for evaluating the cellular physiology of suppression, a protocol was designed to test the ability of HEL-induced suppressor T cells to specifically inhibit cytokine production by LR T

Table III. IL-2 production by HEL/I-A^b specific T cell hybridomas are inhibited by Ts cells in an antigen/MHC-specific manner.

T cell hybridomas *+ Ts cells	antigen	U IL-2/ml#
1. Hbd 30.4	HEL	1280
Hbd 30.4 + SPL TS cells	HEL	20
Hbd 30.4 + SPL Ts membranes	HEL	40
2. Hbd 31.1	HEL	2560
Hbd 31.1 + SPL Ts cells	HEL	2560
Hbd 31.1 + SPL Ts membranes	HEL	2560
3. Tb 8.3	hu Tf	1280
Tb 8.3	HEL	<10
Tb 8.3	hu Tf + HEL	1280
Tb 8.3 + SPL Ts membranes	hu Tf + HEL	1280
Tb 8.3 + SPL Ts membranes	hu Tf + HEL	1280

*T cell hybridomas are assayed as described in Table I, with the addition of bulk cultured Ts cells in some experimental groups. Ts cells do not respond to antigen either directly or association with MHC macromolecules. We routinely culture T hybridomas and Ts cells in a 1:1 ratio but have measured complete inhibition at ratios of 10:1 Vesicles are prepared by incubation of cells in 1 mM phenylarsine oxide at 0°C, followed by centrifugation and resuspension in a balanced salt solution at 37°C. We culture the vesicles at concentrations equivalent to the original cell concentrations.

#The relative titer of IL-2 was determined by pooling supernatants of triplicate wells followed by serial two-fold dilution. The viability of the added HT-2 cells was assessed at the end of a 24-hour incubation period to assign an endpoint and Units of IL-2/ml.

hybridomas. We discovered that suppression mediated by primary splenic Ts cells, those obtained from spleens on the day of the experiment, is somewhat dependent upon the presence of inducer T cells. (Suppression of HEL-helper T cells is absolutely dependent upon inducer T cells (1).) We, therefore, devised a pre-culture system for Ts cells that would allow us to eliminate the inducer population in the hybridoma suppression assay. We found that Lyt-2-enriched, splenic T cells from HEL-primed LR mice could be pre-cultured in lymphokine supplemented media, such that over a four-day period, Ts became potent inhibitors of LR Th as well as independent of inducer T cells. In Table III we illustrate 1) suppression mediated by intact cells or their membrane vesicles, and 2) Ts specificity for LR, HEL-reactive T hybridomas. We observed that Ts cells and their membrane vesicles inhibit T hybridoma activation not only with strict antigen specificity but definite MHC-linkage, resulting in exclusive inhibition of HEL/I-A^b specific T cells. Transferrin-specific hybridomas are not inhibited even though they possess the I-A^b-specificity of Hbd 30.4. The Hbd 31.1 clone (HR) is not inhibited even though it expresses an HEL-specificity. The data suggest linked-recognition between the LR T hybridoma and Ts cells, such that Transferrin-specific hybridomas are not able to be inhibited by Ts cells even if HEL is added to the culture system. This result suggests two plausible modes of recognition between helper and suppressor T cells; an antigen-bridge or direct receptor-anti-receptor contact.

Summary

To date, a variety of different T cell hybridomas which display both antigen-specificity and MHC-restriction have been derived by us. Some of this work has already been published (5). As is the case with T cell hybridomas produced in other laboratories, we can assess induction of our T hybridomas by measuring production of the cytokine, IL-2. Both LR and HR HEL-specific hybridomas are capable of producing significant quantities of IL-2 over a 24-hour period when induced by either antigen/class II or anti-CD3 antibodies. The data in Table III demonstrate the ability of Ts cells to specifically inhibit T hybridoma production of IL-2. The specificity of inhibition rules out the possibility that Ts cells simply utilize IL-2 as a growth hormone during the 24-hour culture period, because HR T hybridoma IL-2 production is not decreased significantly.

We believe that the experimental approach described in this study is superior to our former helper T cell studies, because Th cell assays are limited to measuring the indirect affect of Ts on LR-Th that stimulate antibody producing cells. With the present clonal assay we believe we can begin to appreciate how Ts affect Th cell activation at a molecular level. It is our hypothesis that Ts cells and T hybridoma target cells are linked by the Ti of the hybridoma. Two possible modes of recognition between Ts and Th are 1) the antigen-bridge and 2) direct receptor (Ti) contact by an anti-receptor (anti-Ti) structure on Ts.

Part of being able to resolve these two mechanisms is to establish clones of Ts and characterize their antigen receptor system. So far, we have been able to establish suppressor cell bulk lines which can be grown for a short time in T cell growth factors. These cells actively divide, transform into blast cells and then become very potent inhibitors of our HEL/I-A^b-specific T hybridomas. Unlike the requirement for non-Th, non-Ts auxilliary T cells in helper assays, Ts and their membrane vesicles act independently to inhiibt T hybridoma induction by antigen. Kinetic studies suggest that inactivation occurs during the first hour following T cell co-culture with antigen-pulsed accessory cells. Finally, we have also conducted a flow cytometric analysis of Ts bulk lines to determine the heterogeneity of phenotypes. Once clones of Ts have been established, these will be incorporated into the hybridoma assay system so that we might detail the important regulatory cellular interactions that so drastically affect the development of antibody-mediated immunity.

REFERENCES

1. B.A. Araneo, R.L. Yowell, and E.E. Sercarz. (1979). *J. Immunol.* 123:961
2. B.A. Araneo. 1986. *J. Molec. Cell. Immunol.* 2:219
3. J.W. Kappler, B. Skidmore, J. White, P. Marrack. (1981). *J. Exp. Med.* 153:1198.
4. P. Marrack, et. al. (1982). in "Isolation, characterization and utilization of T lymphocyte clones," C.G. Fathman and F.W. Fitch, eds., Academic Press, p.508.
5. B.C. Cole, B.A. Araneo, G.J. Sullivan. (1986). J. Immunol. 136:3572.
6. R.L. Yowell, B.A. Araneo and e.E, Sercarz. (1980). J. Immunol 124:2160.
7. R.L. Yowell, B.A. Araneo, A. Miller and E.E. Sercarz. (1979) Nature 279:70

AUTOLOGOUS MIXED LYMPHOCYTE REACTION INDUCED IN MICE BY XENOGENEIC IMMUNIZATION WITH SOLUBLE HLA-DR ANTIGENS

Patrice Debre and Mireille Viguier

Laboratoire d'Immunogenetique
Departement d'Hematologie
Hopital Pitie Salpetriere
91, Bd de L'Hopital, 75013, Paris, France

Abstract

In order to study the effects of in vivo immunization of mice with xenogeneic human MHC class II antigens, mice were injected with cellular or purified HLA-DR antigens and their T cell proliferative response tested in secondary in vitro cultures. Our data indicated that small amounts of soluble HLA-DR antigens were able to prime the animals and that the xenogeneic MLR depends on the expression of HLA class II antigens on the stimulating cells. No proliferative response was obtained with cells expressing only HLA class I molecules. Using a pannel of human cells with various haplotypes our results showed that non polymorphic determinants of HLA class II antigens trigger dominantly the murine T cells and that the xenogeneic response was inhibited by anti I-E but not anti I-A or anti-HLA class II MAb. In addition, our data demonstrated that such immunization proceedure could also stimulate a murine auto-MLR since HLA class II primed murine lymph node cells reacted against autologous spleen cells or dendritic cells. These results suggested that HLA class II antigens acting as nominal antigens can induce murine T cells to recognize cross-reactive determinants at the surface of autologous cells.

Introduction

The crucial role of MHC class II molecules in activation of T lymphocytes is widely documented. Studies on mixed lymphocyte reactions (MLR) showed that differences in MHC class II polymorphic determinants are sufficient to induce an allogeneic proliferative response in mice (Schwartz et al,1976) and in human (Albrechtsen et al,1977). Moreover in the xenogeneic MLR, MHC class II molecules appeared to be the most potent xenogeneic molecules responsible for induction of T cell proliferative responses (Widmer and Bach,1972). In human anti-mouse xenogeneic system it was clearly demonstrated that polymorphic determinants of MHC antigens induce a xenogeneic response of T lymphocytes (Lindahl and Bach,1976). The opposite mouse anti-human xenogeneic MLR has been studied in a lesser extend and appeared to be induced by others than polymorphic determinants on HLA class II antigens (Engelhard et al,1980, Yoshizawa and Yano,1984). More striking results were reported in the last decade on the syngeneic or autologous MLR. First described in mice (Howe,1973, Von Boehmer and Adams,1973) and further explored in human (Opelz et al,1975, Kuntz et al,1976, Weksler and Kosak,1977) the syngeneic MLR was reported in different experimental conditions and appeared to involve responding T helper cells and MHC class II positive cells as syngeneic stimulating cells.

In our study we compared the ability of human HLA class II molecules in soluble and cellular forms to induce a murine xenogeneic T cell proliferative response. Lymph node cells from mice previously immunized with human HLA class II antigens (Ag) were tested in MLR either with xenogeneic HLA class II positive cells or with murine syngeneic Ia positive cells. Our results showed that immunization of mice with soluble or cellular HLA-DR Ag induced similar proliferative responses. Murine T cells primed in vivo with a panel of human peripheral blood lymphocytes (PBL) did not distinguish the polymorphism of the various haplotypes. Ia molecules played a critical role since both syngeneic and xenogeneic proliferative responses were inhibited by anti-I-E but not anti-I-A monoclonal antibodies (MAb). In such a xenogeneic mouse anti-human reactivity HLA-DR Ag seemed to act as nominal antigens inducing a proliferative response against cross-reactive epitopes shared by human cells of various haplotypes and murine Ia positive cells.

Materials and methods

Animals : BALB/c, DBA/2 (H-2d) and C3H/He (H-2k) female mice, 2-3 months of age were purchased at the IFFA Credo bredder institute (Saint Germain sur l'Arbresle, France).

Human cells : human cell lines or peripheral blood leukocyte (PBL) used in these experiments were previously described (Viguier et al,1987). All human cell lines were maintained in RPMI 1640 supplemented with 10% heat inactivated fetal calf serum (FCS), 2mM L-Glutamine, 1mM Sodium pyruvate.

Syngeneic murine stimulating cells : Dendritic enriched spleen cells were prepared as described by Knight et al. (1985). Spleen cells were collected from normal untreated mice, washed and suspensed in RPMI 1640 medium supplemented with 2.10^{-5} mercaptoethanol and 5% heat inactivated FCS. Approximatively 5 to 8 ml of suspension at 5.10^{6} cells/ml were layered on to 3 ml metrizamide (Nyegaard analyticalgrade 14,5 g/100 ml RPMI-1640), centrifuged at 600 x g for 15 minutes. Mononuclear cells were collected at the interface, washed once and suspensed in culture medium.

Monoclonal antibodies : anti-Ia monoclonal used as purified MAb at a concentration of 1 µg/ml were previously described (Pierres et al,1982) - Anti L3T4 MAb was a culture supernatant of GK1.5 hybridoma and was used at 1:150 dilution in blocking assays of proliferative response.

Purification of HLA-DR proteins by affinity chromatography : 1,2 g of CNBr activated CL4 B (Pharmacia Fine Chemicals) were coupled with 20 mg of D1.12 MAb previously purified over a Protein-A-Sepharose CL4B coupled column (Pharmacia Fine Chemicals). The anti-HLA-DR column was charged with 0,5% NP40 whole cell extract (14 ml per 10^9 cells) washed with lysate buffer (0,5 % NP40, 0,015M Tris, 0,140 M NaCl, pH 7,4) supplemented with protease inhibitors (dithiotreithol 1mM and PMSF 2.10^5M).Elution of non specific bound material was done by Tris 1M buffer pH:7,8. The colum was then equilibrated with elution buffer without KSCN. The specific elution was obtained using elution buffer containing 50mM Tris, 0,1M NaCl, 30mM N-octylglucosid, 2M KSCN, pH:7,8. Protein dosage of each sample was carried out by the method of Lowry et al. (1951) on 12,5% TCA precipated sample. HLA-DR content of each fraction was evaluated by dot-immunobinding assay on nitro-cellulose filters using D1.12 MAb as previously described (Teyton et al, 1986). The purity was assessed by analysis on 2-D gel electrophoresiss gel of ^{125}I iodinated sample.

Immunization of mice : mice were injected subcutaneously in the base of the tail with purified HLA-DR antigens or with human cells emulsified (v/v) with complete Freund adjuvant (CFA). A negative control was done by immunization with CFA alone.

T cell proliferation assays : paraortic and inguinal lymph node from immunized mice were collected and suspensed in click's medium (Click et al, 1972) supplementend with 1% normal mouse serum and 2.10^5M 2-mercaptoethanol-0,2 ml of culture (3.10^5cells) were set up in 96T.microculture plates (Falcon) with or without irradiated (5000 rads) stimulating cells. The cultures were allowed to proliferate in 5% CO_2 at 37°C over a period of 5 days. 1µCi of [^{3}H]TdR (1Ci:mMole, CEA, France) and [^{3}H] TdR uptake was measured 8-18H later. Data were expressed as the mean count per minute (mean cpm) ± standard error of the mean (SEM) for triplicate determinations.

Effects of various MAb on xenogeneic and syngeneic MLR : to analyse the subpopulations of cells required to elicit a T cell proliferative response, anti Ia and anti-L3T4 MAb were added at various dilutions to the xenogeneic and syngeneic MLR. Effects of these MAb were measured by incorporation of [^{3}H] TdR of specific proliferative cells.

Results and Discussion

To detect a cellular immune response against human MHC class II Ag, BALB/c mice were immunized with various amounts of purified HLA-DR 4/4 proteins or with EBV-transformed BM cells (HLA-DR 4/4) from which the solubilized MHC Ag were extracted. Results of table 1 clearly showed that 5.10^6BM cells were able to prime mice for a secondary in vitro MLR. No proliferative response was observed with the class II negative, class I positive Molt4 T cell line. Moreover they demonstrated that various amounts of solubilized HLA-DR Ag were immunogeneic in mice in dose dependant manner.

To further investigate the specificity of the xenogeneic murine response, we then tested the reactivity of the HLA class II primed T cells in different strains of mice against various syngeneic or xenogeneic stimulating cells. Target cells were whole spleen cells, dendritic enriched spleen cells or human PBL. Results of table 2 showed that murine lymphoïd cells in vivo primed with human cells, were able to proliferate in secondary MLR with xenogeneic or syngeneic stimulating cells. Similar results were obtained with DBA/2 (H-2d), BALB/c(H-2d) or C3H/He(H-2k) mice. Dendritic cells were more effective than whole spleen cells when used in MLR assays.

Together results of table 1 and 2 demonstrated that solubilized and cellular HLA-DR Ag induced both a xenogeneic and syngeneic proliferative response in mice. Our data strongly suggested that histocompatibiliy antigens could act as nominal antigens in triggering xenoreactive T cells. They also showed that immunogeneic determinants are shared by solubilized and native HLA class II molecules on the lymphoïd cell surface. In proliferative responses our results and others showed that the xenogeneic murine T cells were primarily specific for human MHC class II Ag (Yoshizawa and Yano,1984; Viguier et al,1987). In contrast, there was no proliferative response induced by class I positive class II negative stimulating cells, indicating that human MHC molecules have different effects in T cell activation (Viguier et al,1987, Greensteinetal,1986).

Our data showed that the syngeneic and xenogeneic secondary MLR have a comparable proliferative index. In previous reports the syngeneic MLR was first described in new-born and neonatal

table 1 : xenogeneic mouse anti-human MLR after in vivo priming with solubilized or cellular HLA class II antigens.

Primary in vivo immunization with[a]	[3H] TdR incorporation (mean+SEM)[c]			
	Secondary in vitro immunization with[b]			
	Medium	BM cells	Molt4 cells	Con A
CFA	703±501	1384±451	722±152	7378± 841
0,24µgHLA.DR4/4	256± 48	3628±328	1350±326	6198±2115
0,80µgHLA.DR4/4	156± 52	7277±1825	1689±300	13149±2027
2,40µgHLA.DR4/4	923±329	16588±3307	2156±202	18958±6751
5.10^6BM cells	640±329	29284±2555	411±300	8981±1393

[a]. BALB/c mice were subcutaneously injected in the base of the tail with various doses of HLA-DR proteins or with BM cells emulsified in complete Freund Adjuvant (CFA). The soluble material was extracted from BM cells (HLA DR4/4) and purified over an anti-HLA DR MAb-coupled affinity column (as described in Materials and Methods). 5 days later 3.10^5 cells from inguinal and para-aortic lymph node were tested in a proliferation assay.[b]. Responding cells were incubated with or without 3.10^4 irradiated (5000 rads) human stimulating cells : the class II positive BM cells (an Epstein Barr Virus transformed B cell line), the class I$^+$, class II$^-$ Molt 4 cells (a lymphoblastoïd T cell line). Controls were done with medium alone and with 2,5 ug/ml concanavaline A (Con A).[c]. MLR response was evaluated by [3H] TdR uptake at day 5 of culture. Results were expressed as mean of count per minutes incorporated ± standard error of the mean (cpm + SEM) for triplicate determinations.

table 2 : Immunization of various strains of mice with xenogeneic HLA class II positive cells induced a syngeneic MLR.

Primary (a) in vivo immunization		[3H] TdR incorporation (mean cpm)				
		Secondary in vitro immunization with (b)				
in	with	Medium	ConA	Spleen cells	Dendritic cells	human PBLDR3/6
DBA/2						
	CFA	461	26738	471	613	722
	WT46(DR6/6)	287	13790	17304	53332	55164
BALB/c						
	CFA	1433	15469	1410	3744	3658
	WT46(DR6/6)	681	8981	14830	47433	49592
C3H/He						
	CFA	120	7552	62	69	46
	PBL(DR3/6)	895	7356	16168	26911	49088

(a). DBA/2 and BALB/c ($H-2^d$) and C3H/He ($H-2^k$) strain mice were immunized as described in table 1 with HLA class II positive cells emulsified in CFA. 5.10^6 lymph node cells were assaied for in vitro proliferation at day 5. A negative control was done by injection of mice with CFA alone.(b). 3.10^4 irradiated whole spleen cells or dendritic enriched spleen cells (prepared as previously described (Knight et al,1985) were added to stimulating cells. Controls were done with medium alone ; 2,5 µg/ml of Concanavaline A or with 3.10^4 human stimulating cells. Results were expressed as described in table 1.

table 3. Human immunizing cells with various HLA-DR haplotypes gave similar xenogeneic and syngeneic MLR.

Primary in vivo(a) immunization by human PBL cells of HLA-DR haplotypes	[3H] TdR incorporation (mean of cpm+SEM)		
	Secondary in vitro immunization with (b)		
	Medium	Syngeneic dendritic cells	Xenogeneic human cells
DR3/6	1766±1249	106286±28532	69263±47666
DR7/1	1540±1171	11138± 2480	97239±23929
DR4/5	1256± 410	141400±29918	42816± 9972
DR5/2	1180± 405	148389±17228	149512±14782

(a). BALB/c mice were immunized as described in table 1. Human PBL (5.10^6/mice) from various HLA-DR haplotypes were used. Murine immune lymph node cells (3.10^5) were assaied for in vitro MLR 5 days later.(b).3.10^4irradiated (5000 rads) syngeneic murine dendritic enriched spleen cells or xenogeneic human PBL identical to in vivo priming or medium alone were added to the responding cells. Results were expressed as described in table 1.

mice (Howe,1973, Von Boehmer and Adams,1973) but because of the weakness of the response, results were reported sporadically in adult mice. The syngeneic MLR has been reported in various experimental conditions such as Ag specific T cells lines or clones or induced differenciated T cell line (Howe,1973, Von Boehmer and Adams,1973, Opelz et al,1975, Kuntz et al,1976, Weksler and Kosak,1977, Rock and Benacerraf,1983, Clayberger et al,1984, Faherty et al,1985, Tilkin et al,1986, De Talance et al,1986). We clearly evidenced the potent stimulatory role of Ia+ dendritic cells when compared to whole spleen cells. Similarly our previous studies have shown that the amount of class II Ag in human lymphoïd cells was critical for triggering murine T cells (Viguier et al,1987). The fact that HLA-DR primed murine T cells responded to both syngeneic or xenogeneic MHC class II positive target cells strongly suggested that cross-reactive epitopes shared by Ia and HLA-DR Ag were responsible for the cellular immune xenogeneic response in mice. Similarly in testing antibody responses of mice against human class II Ag, previous studies showed that several murine monoclonal anti I-Ak and anti I-Ek antibodies cross-react with HLA-DR supertypic and subtypic determinants (Pierres et al,1982).

In order to further characterize the immunogeneic role of polymorphic or non polymorphic determinants of HLA-DR Ag, we then investigated if murine responses were influenced by the various haplotypes of the human immunizing cells. Table 3 showed similar results in xenogeneic and syngeneic MLR of cells from mice primed with human PBL of various donors. These results corroborated our previous studies (Viguier et al,1987) and others

table 4 : Comparative inhibitory effect of anti-Ia MAb in xenogeneic and syngeneic MLR.

Culture conditions (a)	3H TdR incorporation (mean cpm)	
	Xenogeneic MLR	Syngeneic MLR
Medium	1896	1303
Stimulating cells (SC)	264194	126080
SC+anti-I.E.$^{(d)}$(H10-81-10)	66758	47086
SC+anti-I.E.$^{(d)}$(H39-91-1)	61645	48486
C+anti-I.E$^{(d)}$(H10-199-9)	101832	111373
C+anti-I.E$^{(d)}$(H40-242-3)	201229	32733
SC+anti-I.A.$^{(d)}$(H8-15-9)	193209	145692
SC+anti-I.A$^{(d)}$(H39-58-11)	182237	96068
SC+anti H-2D$^{(d)}$(H97-76-7)	213094	98560

a). Lymph node cells (3.10^5) from BALB/c mice, injected 5 days before with 5.10^6human PBL were assaied either for xenogeneic or syngeneic MLR. Irradiated (5000 rads) stimulating cells were respectively human PBL (3.10^4/well) for xenogeneic MLR and normal untreated BALB/c spleen cells (8.10^4well) for syngeneic MLR. Various anti-Ia MAb which biochemical and functional characterization were previously reported (Pierres et al,1982) were added in MLR culture at a concentration of 1 µg/ml.$^{(b)}$ The proliferative response in those various culture conditions was evaluated at 5 days of culture by [3H] TdR incorporation. Results were expressed as mean of cpm in triplicate determinations.

(Yoshizawa and Yano,1984) indicating that xenoreactive murine T cells recognize primarily non polymorphic determinants of HLA class II Ag. In contrast, Lindahl and Bach(1972) demonstrated that human lymphocytes recognized polymorphic determinants of Ia antigens in human anti-mouse MLR. These authors and others also showed that the human cytolytic T lymphocytes could recognize polymorphic determinants of murine class I Ag (Achour et al,1986, Maryanski et al,1987). Those differences between xenogeneic proliferative and cytolytic responses to MHC Ag might be due to the fact that HLA class II molecules could act as nominal antigens in which non polymorphic determinants are immunodominant in mice.

In order, to dissect the influence of H-2 molecules in xenogeneic and syngeneic MLR, various anti-H-2 MAb were used to tentatively inhibit the secondary in vitro proliferative response. Table 4 showed results of MLR incubated with anti-Ia MAb whose biochemical and functional properties have been previously reported (Pierres et al,1982). Several anti I-E but not anti-I-A MAb were able to significantly block both syngeneic and xenogeneic responses. Among the anti-I-E MAb tested, H10-199-9 MAb inhibited the xenogeneic proliferative response but not the syngeneic MLR, conversely H40-242-3 MAb inhibited the syngeneic but not the xenogeneic proliferative response.

Yoshizawa et al.(1984) reported that I-A on APC had a dominant role in triggering murine xenoreactive T cells whereas I-E molecules were not involved in such responses. In our experiments only I-E molecules appeared to be involved. Two anti-I-E MAb evidenced differences in Ia epitopes involved in xenogeneic and syngeneic MLR. These data emphasize the role of Ia molecules in recognition process of HLA-DR antigens. In addition to the fact that HLA-DR and Ia Ag share cross-reactive epitopes, our results suggest that human HLA-DR molecules are recognized in mice in the context of murine MHC class II molecules. Similar results were reported for CTL responses demonstrating that cellular immune responses to HLA class I Ag were restricted by murine H-2 K or H-2D Ag (Achour et al,1986, Maryanski et al,1987).

Together these findings support the generality of a model for CTL and proliferative T cell responses against HLA antigens in which human nominal antigens are presented in the context of the corresponding murine class I or II restricting molecules. The human critical association (self Ia + xenogeneic HLA-DR) on the APC cell surface is in addition responsible for a cellular anti-self (Ia) response, a result which could help to better understand the mecanism of auto-immunity.

References

Achour, A., Begue,B., Gomard, E., Paul, P., Sayagh, B., Van Pel, A. and Levy, J.P : Specific lysis of murine cells expressing HLA molecules by allospecific human and H-2 restricted murine anti-HLA T killer lymphocytes. Eur.J.Immunol.16:597,1986

Albrechtsen, D., Solheim, B.G. and Thorsby, E. : Antiserum inhibition of the mixed lymphocyte culture (MLC) interaction. Inhibitory effect of antibodies reactive with

HLA-D associated determinants. Cell Immunol.28:258,1977
Clayberger, C., Dekruyff, R.H. and Cantor, H. : Immunoregulatory activities of autoreactives T cells:an I-A specific T cell clone mediates both help and suppression of antibody responses. J. Immunol.132:2237,1984
Click, R.E., Benck, L. and Alter, B.J. : Immune responses in vitro. I. Culture conditions for antibody synthesis. Cell. Immunol.3:264,1972
Engelhard, V.H., Kaufman, J.F., Strominger, J.L. and Burakoff, S.J. : Specificity of mouse cytotoxic T lymphocytes stimulated with either HLA-A and B or HLA DR antigens reconstituted into phospholipid vesicles. J.Exp.Med.152:54s,1980
Faherty, D., Jonhson, A. and Zunderer, M. : Origin and specificty of autoreactive T cells in antigen induced populations. J.Exp.Med.161:1293,1985
Greenstein, J.L., Foran, J.A., Gorga, J.C. and Burakoff, S.J. : The role of T cell accessory molecules in the generation of class II specific xenogeneic cytolytic T cells. J. Immunol.136:2358,1986
Howe, M.L : Isogenic lymphocyte interaction : responsiveness of murine thymocytes to self antigens. J. Immunol.100:1090,1973
Knight, S.C., Krejci, J., Malkovsky, M., Coli, V., Gautran, A. and Asherson, G.L. : The role of dendritic cells in the initiation of immune responses to contact sensitisers. In vivo exposure to antigens. Cell. Immunol.94:427,1985
Kuntz, M.M., Innes, J.B. and Weksler, M.E. : Lymphocyte transformation induced by autologous cells : IV. Human T-lymphocyte proliferation induced by autologous or allogeneic non-T lymphocytes. J.Exp.Med.143:1042,1976
Lindahl, K.F. and Bach, F.H. : Genetic and cellular aspects of xenogeneic mixed leukocyte culture reaction. J.Exp.Med.144:305,1976
Lowry, O.H., Rosebrough, N.J., Farr, A.L. and Randall, R.J. : Protein measurement with the folin phenol reagent. J.Biol.Chem.193:265,1951
Maryanski, J.L., Accola, R.S. and Jordan, B. : H-2 restricted recognition of cloned HLA class I gene products expressed in mouse cells. J.Immunol, in press,1987
Opelz, G., Kiuchi, M., Takasugi, M. and Terasaki, P.J. : Autologous stimulation of human lymphocyte subpopulations. J.Exp.Med.142:1327,1975
Pierres, M., Mercier, P., Madsen, M., Mawas, C. and Kristensen, T. : Monoclonal mouse anti-I-A^K and anti-I-E^K antibodies cross reacting with HLA-DR supertypic and subtypic determinants rather than classical DR allelic specificities. Tissue antigens.40:289,1982
Rock, K.L. and Benacerraf, B. : The role of Ia molecules in the activation of T lymphocytes : III Antigen specific Ia restricted interleukin-2 producing T cell hybridomas with detectable affinity for the restricting IA molecules. J.Exp.Med.157:359,1983
Schwartz, R.H., Fathman, C.G. and Sachs, D.H. : Inhibition of stimulation of murine mixed lymphocyte cultures with an allo-antiserum directed against a shared Ia determinant. J.Immunol.116:929,1976
Teyton, L., Lotteau, V., Boyer, B. and Charon, D.J. : A quantitative dot immunobinding assay for human HLA class II antigens using nitro-cellulose membrane filters. J. of Immunol.Meth. 89:73,1986
Tilkin, A.F., Michon, J., Juy, D., Kayibanda, M., Henin, Y.,

Sterckers, G., Betuel, H. and Levy, J.P. : Autoreactive T cell clones of MHC class II specificities are produced during responses against foreign antigens in man. J. Immunol. 138:674,1986

Viguier, M., Lotteau, V., Charron, D.J. and Debré, P. : Xenogeneic recognition of soluble and cell surface HLA class II antigens by proliferative murine T cells. Eur.J.Immunol, in press,1987

Von Boehmer, H. and Adams, P.B. : Syngeneic mixed lymphocyte reaction between thymocytes and peripheral lymphoïd cells in mice : stain specificity and nature of the target cell. J. Immunol. 110:376,1973

Weskler, M.E. and Kosak, R. : Lymphocyte transformation induced by autologous cells. V. Generation of immunologic memory and specificity during the autologous mixed lymphocyte reaction. J.Exp.Med. 146:1833,1977

Widmer, M.B. and Bach, F.H. : Allogeneic and xenogeneic response in mixed leukocyte cultures. J.Exp.Med. 135:1204,1972

Yoshizawa, K. and Yano, A. : Mouse T lymphocytes proliferative responses specific for human MHC products in mouse anti-human xenogeneic MLR. J. Immunol. 132:2320,1984

Ia GENE EXPRESSION IN NON-BONE MARROW DERIVED CELLS DURING GRAFT VS HOST DISEASE IN THE MOUSE

P. Michael Stuart and Jerold G. Woodward

Department of Microbiology and Immunology
University of Kentucky Medical Center
Lexington, KY 40536-0084 USA

ABSTRACT

We have examined the capacity of non-bone marrow-derived (NBMD) cells to express endogenous Ia genes by evaluating E alpha mRNA expression in various tissues derived from long term bone marrow chimeras. These chimeras were produced in the combination B10.A(4R) into B10.A and allowed to rest for greater than 100 days before use. Since B10.A(4R) is incapable of transcribing the E gene, E mRNA expression would most likely represent Ia expression by the host B10.A NBMD tissues in these long term chimeras. Our results demonstrate that host E alpha mRNA expression was readily detectable in kidney, lung and thymus, but not in the spleen of chimeric animals. During graft-vs-host disease (GVHD) E alpha expression was enhanced up to 4-fold in kidney and was also detectable in heart extracts as well. These experiments demonstrate that resident host cells, most likely NBMD, in a variety of organs are capable of Ia gene expression. This expression appears to be both constituitive and inducible. Furthermore, different tissues show a marked quantitative difference in the magnitude of NBMD Ia expression with kidney showing the highest level.

INTRODUCTION

The I region of the mouse major histocompatibility complex (MHC) contains four class II genes which encode the classical Ia antigens I-A and I-E. These dimeric cell surface proteins play a pivotal role in the initiation of most T cell dependent immune responses and have been equated with the immune response (Ir) genes mapping to the same region (Schwartz et al. 1978). The basis of this control lies in the fact that the T cell receptor specifically recognizes the Ia molecule either alone or in association with foreign antigen on the surface of an antigen presenting cell. Although antigen presenting cells or stimulator cells were once thought to be restricted to macrophages or related cells, it is now apparent that many different cell types can effectively interact with T cells as long as they express Ia antigens (Shevach and Rosenthal 1973, Kappler et al. 1982, Malissen et al. 1984, Fierz et al 1985, Ben-Nun et al 1985).

Because of the importance of the Ia antigens in Ia restricted T cell responses, a considerable effort has gone into defining which cell types are capable of Ia expression. Although it was originally thought that Ia expressing cells were primarily hematopoietic in derivation, a number ofcell types of non-bone marrow derived (NBMD) origin have since been described that express Ia antigens to varying degrees. These include epidermal cells (Lampert et al. 1981, Daynes et al 1983), vascular endothelium (de Waal et al. 1983, Pober et al. 1983), renal tuble cells (Halloran et al. 1980, Wadgymar et al. 1984), thymic epithelium (Jenkinson et al. 1981), astrocytes (Fierz et al. 1985) and gut epithelium (Mason et al. 1983). With the exception of thymic epithelium and renal tubule cells, Ia expression is only observed after <u>in vivo</u> induction such as graft vs. host disease (GVHD) or allografting. While both mouse and human NBMD cells have been shown to express Ia antigens, one striking difference between mouse and human class II expression is in their <u>in vitro</u> inducibility with interferon gamma. While human NBMD cells are readily inducible <u>in vitro</u> with IFN (Pober et al. 1983, Basham et al. 1984), we know of no mouse NBMD cell lines that are inducible for Ia <u>in vitro</u> with IFN (Wong et al. 1984).

One of the difficulties in the serological detection of Ia on NBMD cells is that there is always the possibility of passive attachment of Ia shed from infiltrating or resident monocytes. This is a particular problem in situations where <u>in vivo</u> induction is utilized since there is usually a concurrent infiltration of large numbers of monocytes. Although some of the serological studies mentioned above have ruled out passive attachment by using bone marrow chimeras (Halloran et al. 1980), or cytoplasmic localization of class II antigen (Lampert et al. 1981, Mason et al. 1983), others have not. In addition, actual gene expression or biosynthesis of class II antigens in NBMD cells has not yet been examined. It would also be of value to compare the amount of NBMD Ia expression from one tissue to the next and to measure the magnitude of induction that is seen. Thus, do all tissues have the same capacity for NBMD class II expression or are there clearly some organs with higher overall NBMD class II expression than others?

Here, we describe a mouse chimera system that allows the direct visualization of NBMD Ia gene expression within individual organs and tissues. Using northern blot analysis of total RNA extracted from various organs, we show that class II mRNA can readily be detected from NBMD tissues in kidney, heart, lung and thymus. In addition, induction of class II RNA expression was observed in mice undergoing GVHD.

MATERIALS AND METHODS

Mice. Female B10.A/SgSN, B10.A(4R) and SJL/J mice were purchased from the Jackson Labs, Bar Harbor, ME). Mice were housed in the University of Kentucky Medical Center Animal Care Facility.

Chimeras. Chimeras were produced as previously described (Woodward et al. 1982) with some modifications. Briefly, recipient B10.A mice were irradiated with 1100 rads from a ^{137}Cs source irradiator. These mice were reconstituted by injection of $2x10^7$ anti-Thy 1.2+C' treated B10.A(4R) bone marrow cells. Chimeras were not used until 100+ days had elapsed to allow for complete turnover of tissue resident, host Ia positive cells (Woodward et al. 1982, Frelinger et al. 1979).

Cell line: A20/2J, a BALB/c derived B cell lymphoma was used as an Ia positive control.

RNA Extraction. Total RNA was extracted from heart, kidney, lung, skin, spleen and thymus by the guanidine-HCl procedure (Chirgwin et al. 1979). Organs from individual mice were first homogenized in 2ml of guanidine thiocyanate using a Tissumizer (Tek-Mar) tissue homogenizer. RNA was then purified by centrifugation through cesium chloride. Skin RNA represents RNA derived from the tail skin of a single mouse. For the B10. A experiments organs from two mice were pooled before RNA extraction.

Hybridization analysis of RNA. For Northern blot analysis, 20ug of total organ RNA was electrophoresed on a 1% agarose gel containing 2.2M formaldehyde (Maniatis et al. 1982). RNA was transferred to nitrocellulose filters and hybridized to ^{32}P-labeled cDNA probes. Hybridization was carried out at 42°C in 50% formamide, 5x denhardt's solution, 100ug/ml denatured salmon sperm DNA and 100ug/ml yeast tRNA. Probes used for hybridization were gel purified inserts derived from pEAC11 (E alpha) (Mathis et al. 1983a), pAAC6 (A alpha) (Benoist et al. 1983), and pHF5 (human actin) (Gunning et al. 1983). Blots were washed in 2xSSC (0.3M NaCl, 0.03M Na Citrate), 0.1% SDS at 25°C and then in 0.1xSSC (0.015M NaCl, 0.0015M Na Citrate), 0.1% SDS at 55°C. They were then dried and subjected to autoradiography. The autoradiographs were quantitated by densitometric scanning using actin hybridization as the correction for the amount of input RNA. For each figure, the hybridization with the three different probes represents sequential hybridization of the same blot. Between each hybridization, the previous probe was removed by washing in 0.1x SSC, 0.1% SDS at 100°C for 5 min. Removal of the old probe was confirmed by autoradiography.

Induction of GVHD. Chimeras of greater than 100 days were subjected to whole-body irradiation (450 rads) 24 hours prior to tail vein injection of $4x10^7$ SJL/J (H-2^s, E alpha negative) spleen cells. Animals were sacrificed 8, 9, 10, 12 and 15 days following induction of GVHD and appropriate organs were removed for RNA extraction as described above. At the time of sacrifice characteristic GVHD enlargement of the spleen was noted in all animals.

RESULTS

The purpose of this study was to define a system in which we could compare the relative contribution of NBMD tissues to class II expression among different organs. In order to differentiate between host (NBMD) and donor (BMD) tissues by RNA hybridization, we made use of the fact that mice of the _b_ haplotype are incapable of transcribing the E alpha gene due to a deletion in the 5' region of the gene (Mathis et al. 1983). Since the E alpha probe used does not cross hybridize with A alpha mRNA, it is possible to distinguish between _H-2_^{b} haplotype Ia expression and _H-2_^{a} haplotype Ia expression in chimeric mice. Chimeras were produced in the combination B10.A(4R) (E alpha negative) into B10.A (E alpha positive) and were not utilized until at least 100 days had elapsed. This period of time has previously been shown to be sufficient for complete turnover of tissue resident, host Ia positive cells (17-18). In addition, the mice received 1100 rads irradiation before bone marrow reconstitution to insure complete elimination of radioresistant, tissue specific monocytes from the host.

To confirm that BIO.A(4R) mice lack E alpha expression as well as to verify probe specificity, we performed Northern blot analysis on a variety of organs from B10.A(4R) mice. As shown in Fig. 1, there was detectable hybridization to RNA from all organs tested with the A alpha probe. In contrast, the E alpha probe showed no detectable hybridization to RNA derived from B10.A(4R) mice, but good hybridization to RNA from the E alpha positive B cell line, A20/2J. The results in figure 2 show that both the E alpha and A alpha probes hybridize well with RNA derived from BIO.A organs. Surprisingly, very little Ia expression was detected in skin from both BIO.A and BIO.A(4R) mice.

Athough in this experiment, Ia expression in BIO.A skin was practically nonexistent, similar gels from other BIO.A mice revealed low but detectable levels of Ia mRNA. When these gels were re-probed with a class I probe, very low class I expression was also observed in tail skin (data not shown).

As the above results demonstrate, Ia expression is clearly detectable in a variety of organs. In order to determine the relative contribution of BMD and NBMD cells to the expression observed, we performed Northern blots using RNA derived from B10.A(4R) into B10.A long term chimeras. As shown in Figure 3, the E alpha probe did not hybridize to spleen RNA whereas the A alpha probe hybridized very well. These results demonstrate that this mouse was a true chimera and most, if not all, host lymphoid cells had been replaced by E alpha negative donor cells (we estimate that our level of detection is between 1 and 5% contaminating E alpha positive cells). Interestingly, E alpha expression was clearly detectable in kidney, lung and thymus, apparently representing consitutive Ia expression by the NBMD cells in these tissues. When probed with the A alpha probe, Ia expression was detectable in all tissues as was observed for the normal BIO.A(4R) and B10.A mice.

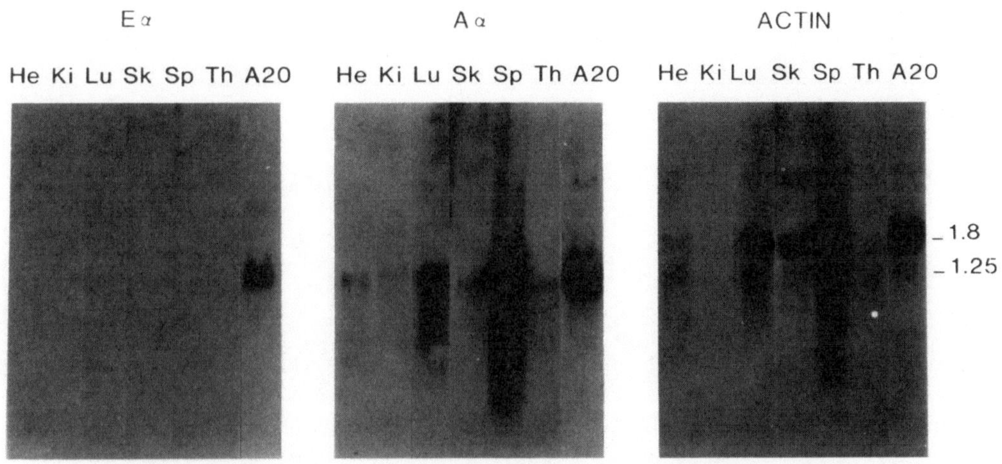

Figure 1. Northern blot analysis of E alpha, A alpha and Actin RNA expression in tissues derived from a normal B10.A 4R) mouse. Total RNA was isolated from Heart (He), Kidney (Ki), Lung (Lu), Skin (Sk), Spleen (Sp), Thymus(Th), and the BALB/c plasmacytoma A20/2J (A20) and analysed with pEAC11 (Ealpha), pAAC6(A alpha), and pHF5 (actin) cDNA probes. The three panels represent successive re-probing of the same blot.

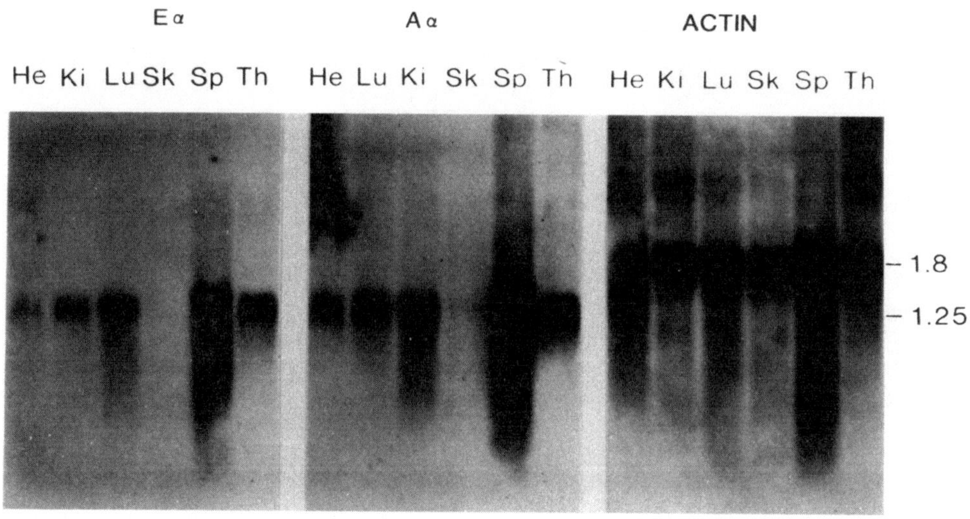

Figure 2. Northern Blot analysis of E alpha, A alpha and actin RNA expression in tissues derived from a B10.A mouse. See figure 1 legend for details.

We next sought to determine the inducibility of Ia on NBMD tissues following induction of graft vs host disease. Long term B10.A(4R) into B10.A chimeras were irradiated with 450 rads and injected intravenously with 4 x 10^7 SJL ($\underline{H-2^s}$, E alpha negative) spleen cells. Figure 4 presents data concerning the Ia expression in chimeras 9 days after the initiation of GVHD. GVHD was apparent in these mice since they exhibited classical splenomegally as well as severe blanching of most of the internal organs. In contrast to the normal chimeras, E alpha mRNA was detectable not only in kidney and lung, but in heart as well. The lack of E alpha hybridization to spleen RNA again verifies the chimeric nature of these mice as well as the lack of E alpha expression by the SJL spleen cells used to induce the GVHD. Thymus was not included due to the difficulty of harvesting enough tissue to sufficiently isolate RNA. When normalized to hybridization by an actin probe, the E alpha mRNA was found to be increased for both heart and kidney but not lung as compared to the non-GVH induced chimera. We were unable to detect E alpha expression in the heart of normal chimeras but clearly detected expression during GVHD. Although kidney E alpha expression was demonstrable in normal chimeras, it was markedly increased during GVHD. Using a scanning densitometer and normalizing the E alpha band to actin, we estimate that kidney E alpha expression increased approximately 4 fold following GVHD. The same pattern was observed in chimeras 8 and 10 days following induction of GVHD (data not shown).

DISCUSSION

In this study, we describe a system whereby class II gene expression within non-bone marrow derived tissues can be evaluated and compared without the complication of resident or infiltrating lymphoid or macrophage-like cells. Our results demonstrate that the host component in long term bone marrow chimeras is capable of Ia gene expression and that this expression is induced during graft vs. host disease. Furthermore, we see an interesting variation of the level of NBMD Ia expression between different organs. In the uninduced chimera, kidney, lung, and thymus show roughly equivalent levels of NBMD Ia expression when normalized to expression of the actin gene. We did not detect any NBMD Ia expression in heart, skin or spleen. Following induction of GVHD, NBMD Ia expression was induced roughly four fold in the kidney, and was detectable in heart. Lung Ia remained about the same and expression was still negative in skin and spleen. These experiments demonstrate that there is a considerable variation in the level of Ia expression in NBMD tissues and that GVHD induces NBMD Ia gene expression most notably in kidney and heart.

The term "non-bone marrow derived" is used operationally in this system to indicate cells of recipient origin that remain in long term bone marrow chimeras. We cannot completely rule out that a radioresistant (1100 rad) bone marrow derived cell is persisting in long term chimeras and contributing to the Ia expression observed. Although studies on epidermal Langerhans cells indicate that the bulk of these cells are completely eliminated from the recipient and repopulated from donor bone marrow in long term radiation chimeras (Woodward et al. 1982, Frelinger et al. 1979), there is no data on the half life of comparable cells in kidney, lung and heart. We are currently addressing this question using in situ hybridization analysis.

Regardless, it is clear that a variety of NBMD cells are capable of Ia expression. Using antisera absorption, Halloran et al. (1980) demonstrated Ia expression on both marrow derived and non-marrow derived cells in kidneys of long term chimeras. In addition, NBMD Ia expression was found to be increased 10 fold in kidneys of mice undergoing GVHD (Wadgymer et al. 1984). While the NBMD Ia positive cells in normal

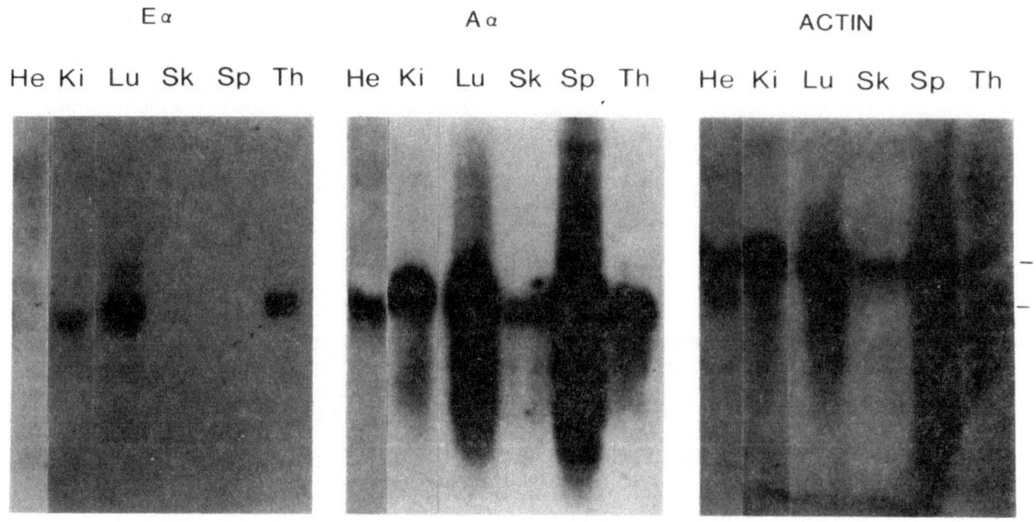

Figure 3. Northern blot analysis of E alpha, A alpha and Actin RNA expression in tissues derived from a B10.A(4R) into B10.A chimeric mouse. Chimeras were produced by irradiating B10.A recipients with 1100 rads followed by intravenous injection of 2 X 10^7 anti-Thy 1.2 + C' treated bone marrow cells from B10.A(4R) mice. Chimeras were not used until 100 + days had elapsed. See figure 1 legend for details.

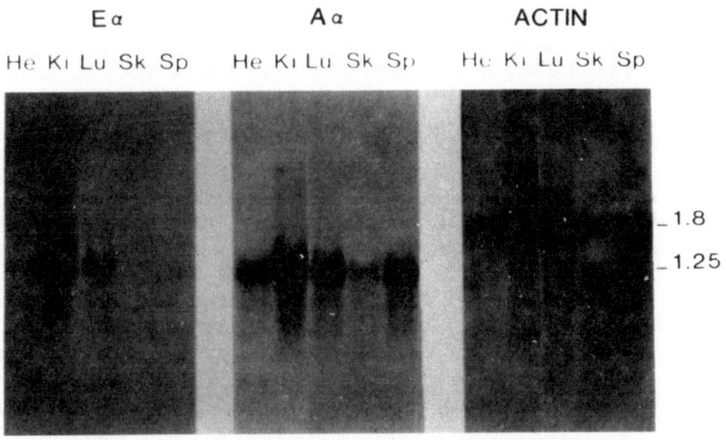

Figure 4. Northern blot analysis of E alpha, A alpha, and actin RNA expression in tissues from a B10.A(4R) into B10.A chimeric mouse undergoing graft versus host disease. Chimeras were produced as described in the legend for Fig. 3. Graft versus host disease was initiated by irradiating mice with 450 rads and injecting 4 X 10^7 spleen cells from an SJL/J mouse intravenously. Tissue was removed from the chimera 9 days following induction of graft versus host disease. See figure 1 legend for details.

kidneys were believed to be endothelial cells of the peritubular capillaries, the majority of Ia positive cells in GVHD induced kidneys were renal tubule epithelial cells. Our results are in close agreement with these studies and indicate that at least part of the induction is at the messenger RNA level and therefore, most likely transcriptional.

Our results demonstrate that NBMD Ia expression in the lung is as high as in the kidney. Although we are not aware of any reports specifically addressing the identity of Ia positive, NBMD cells in the lung, the high degree of vascularization in the lung would suggest that a major portion of the NBMD Ia expression is due to vascular endothelial cells which have been previously shown to express Ia (de Waal et al. 1983, Pober et al. 1983). Interestingly, we do not see any appreciable induction of lung NBMD Ia expression during GVHD. This could be due to the relative differences in intensity of immune reactions in the kidney versus lung or that lung NBMD cells are unresponsive to the inductive signals. In order to distinguish between these two mechanisms it is necessary to ensure that both organs receive equal induction stimuli.

In contrast to the lung, induction of Ia expression in heart was observed during GVHD. In fact, we could not detect heart NBMD Ia expression in normal chimeras. As in the lung, vascular endothelial cells in the heart could account for the expression we observed. Whether the differences in levels reflect different endothelial cell densities between organs or different levels of cellular expression is not known.

At first glance, our inability to detect NBMD Ia expression in skin may seem somewhat surprising. Lampert et al. (1981) has reported expression of Ia on epidermal keratinocytes during GVHD in the rat. Their detection of Ia intracellularly suggests de novo synthesis by these cells. Daynes et al. (1983) also reported the induction of Ia expression on epidermal cells following skin grafting of normal skin onto nude mice. However, our results with normal B10.A and B10.A(4R) mice indicate that tail skin is inherently low in expression of class II and class I (data not shown) genes. Recent experiments with ear skin indicate that Ia expression in this tissue is similar to that of other organs. Thus our inability to detect Ia expression in NBMD skin seems to reflect a peculiarity of tail skin. We are currently evaluating NBMD Ia expression in skin derived from other sites.

We have presented a method that allows the semi-quantitative analysis of Ia expression in NBMD tissues under various experimental situations. In order to gain a better understanding of the tissue levels and distribution of NBMD Ia expression we are currently evaluating the effects of graft rejection and autoimmune responses on NBMD Ia expression in various organs.

Acknowledgements. We would like to thank Diane Mathis and Christophe Benoist for providing plasmids pEAC11 and pAAC6, and Larry Kedes for providing pHF5. We also thank Eileen Vernon and Kathy Omer for technical assistance and Charles Snow for critical reading of this manuscript. This work was supported in part by NIH grant CA-39070. JGW is a recipient of a National Arthritis Foundation Investigator Award. PMS is supported by NIH Training Grant T32CA09509.

REFERENCES

Basham, T.Y., B.J. Nickoloff, T.C. Merigan and V.B. Morhenn. Recombinant gamma interferon induces HLA-DR expression on cultured human keratinocytes. J. Invest. Derm. 83:88-90, 1984.

Ben-Nun, A., W. Strauss, S.A. Leeman, L.E. Cohn, C. Murre, A. Duby, J.G. eidman and L.H. Glimcher. An Ia-positive mouse T-cell clone is functional in presenting antigen to other T cells. Immunogenetics. 22:123-130, 1985.

Benoist, C.O., D.J. Mathis, M.R. Kanter, V.E. Williams II and H.O. McDevitt. The murine Ia alpha chains, E alpha and A alpha, show a surprising degree of sequence homology. Proc. Natl. Acad. Sci. USA 80:534-538, 1983.

Chirgwin. J.M., A.E. Przbyla, R.J. MacDonald and W.J. Rutter. Isolation of biologically active ribonucleic acid from sources enriched in ribonuclease. Biochemistry 18:5294-5299, 1979.

Daynes, R.A., M. Emam, G.G. Krueger, and L.K. Roberts. Expression of Ia antigens on epidermal keratinocytes after the grafting of normal skin to nude mice. J. Immunol. 130:1536-1539, 1983.

de Waal, R.M.W., M.J.J. Bogman, C.N. Maass, L.M.H. Cornelissen, W.J.M. Tax, and R.A.P. Koene. Variable expression of Ia antigens on the vascular endothelium of mouse skin allografts. Nature 303:426-429, 1983.

Fierz, W., B. Endler, K. Reske, H. Wekerle and A. Fontana. Astrocytes as antigen presenting cells. I. Induction of Ia antigen expression on astrocytes by T cells via immune interferon and its effect on antigen presentation. J. Immunol. 134:3785-3793, 1985.

Frelinger, J.G., L. Hood, S. Hill, and J.A. Frelinger. Mouse epidermal Ia molecules have a bone marrow origin. Nature 232:321-323, 1979.

Gunning, P., P. Ponte, H. Okayama, J. Engel, H. Blau and L. Kedes. Isolation and characterization of full-length cDNA clones for human alpha, beta and gamma actin mRNA's: Skeletal but not cytoplasmic actins have an amino terminal cysteine that is subsequently removed. Mol. and Cell. Biol. 3:787-795, 1983.
Halloran, P.F., S.K. Stylianos, M. Stubbs, and D. Dutton. Expression of Ia in mouse kidney. II. Evidence for expression on marrow-derived and nonmarrow-derived cells. Transplantation 30:264-288, 1980.
Jenkinson, E.J., W. Van Ewijk and J.J.T. Owen. Major Histocompatibility complex antigen expression on the epithelium of the developing thymus in normal and nude mice. J. Exp. Med. 153:280-292, 1981.
Kappler, J., J. White, D. Wegmann, E. Mustain, and P. Marrack. Antigen presentation by Ia^+ B cell hybridomas to H-2 restricted T cell hybridomas. Proc. Natl. Acad. Sci. USA: 79:3604-3607, 1982.Lampert, I.A., A.J. Suitters and P.M. Chisholm. Expression of Ia antigen on epidermal keratinocytes in graft-versus-host disease. Nature 293:149-150, 1981.
Malissen, B., M. Peele Price, J.M. Goverman, M. McMillan, J. White, J. Kappler, P. Marrack, A. Pierres and L. Hood. Gene transfer of H-2 class II genes: Antigen presentation by mouse fibroblast and Hamster B-cell lines. Cell 36:319-327, 1984.
Maniatis, T., E. Fritsch and J. Sambrook. Molecular Cloning: A laboratory manual. Cold Spring Harbor Laboratory, New York, 1982.
Mason, D.W., M. Dallman, and A.N. Barclay. Graft-versus-host disease induces expression of Ia antigen in rat epidermal cells and gut epithelium. Nature. 293:150-151, 1983.
Mathis, D.J., C.O. Benoist, V.E. Williams II, M.R. Kanter and H.O. McDevitt. The murine E-alpha immune response gene. Cell 32:745-754, 1983a.
Mathis, D., C. Benoist, V. Williams II, M. Kanter, and H. McDevitt. Several mechanisms can account for defective E alpha gene expression in different mouse haplotypes. Proc. Natl. Acad. Sci. USA. 80:273-277, 1983b.
Pober, J.S., T. Collins, M.A. Gimbrone, Jr., R.S. Cotran, J.D. Gittin, W. Fiers, C. Clayberger, A.M. Krensky, S.J. Burakoff and C. Reiss. Lymphocytes recognize human vascular endothelial and dermal fibroblast Ia antigens induced by recombinant immune interferon. Nature 305:726-729, 1983.
Schwartz, R.H., A. Yano, and W.E. Paul. Interaction between antigen presenting cells and primed T lymphocytes. Immunol. Rev. 40:153-180, 1978.
Shevach, E.M. and A. Rosenthal. Function of macrophages in antigen recognition by guinea pig T lymphocytes. II. Role of the macrophage in the regulation of genetic control of the immune response. J. Exp. Med. 138:1213-1229, 1978.
Wadgymar, A., J. Urmson, R. Baumal, and P.F. Halloran. Changes in Ia expression in mouse kidney during acute graft vs. host disease. J. Immunol. 132:1826-1832, 1984.
Wong, G.H.W., I. Clark-Lewis, A.W. Harris and J.W. Schrader. Effect of cloned interferon-gamma on expression of H-2 and Ia antigens on cell lines of hematopoietic, lymphoid, epithelial, fibroblastic and neuronal origin. Eur. J. Immunol. 14:52-56, 1984.
Woodward, J.G., B.L. Shigekawa, and J.A. Frelinger. Bone marrow-derived cells are responsible for stimulating I region-incompatible skin graft rejection. Transplantation 33:254-259, 1982.

GENETIC CONTROL OF T-CELL AND NK-CELL PROTECTION AGAINST LETHAL SENDAI VIRUS INFECTION

W. Martin Kast, Arie C. Voordouw and Cornelis J.M. Melief

The Netherlands Cancer Institute
Antoni van Leeuwenhoek Huis
Amsterdam, The Netherlands

SUMMARY

The in vivo importance of class I MHC regulation of the cytotoxic T cell (Tc) response to a natural pathogenic agent of high virulence was studied on the basis of our demonstration of a major difference in the capacity to generate a Sendai virus-specific Tc response between C57BL/6 (B6, H-2^b) mice and H-$2K^b$ mutant B6.C-H-2^{bm1} (bm1) mice. These two mouse strains differ from each other only in three amino acids in the crucial H-$2K^b$ restriction element for this response. Bm1 mice, in contrast to B6 mice, are Tc nonresponders against this virus, but show Sendai-specific T cell proliferation, antibody production, and delayed type hypersensitivity (DTH) reactions, as well as natural killer (NK) cell activity, equal to those of B6 mice. Another H-2^b mouse strain, the 129/J, also shows equal Sendai virus-specific Tc, T helper cell (Th), B cell and DTH responses compared to B6, but is virtually deficient in generating an NK cell response. B6, Sendai Tc-deficient bm1, T cell-deficient B6 nu/nu and NK low-responder 129/J mice differ from each other in susceptibility to lethal pneumonia induced by intranasal (i.n.) inoculation of virulent Sendai virus. The lethal dose (LD_{50}) in B6 mice averages 152 $TCID_{50}$, in bm1 mice 14 $TCID_{50}$, in B6 nu/nu mice 0.5 $TCID_{50}$ and in 129/J mice 0.2 $TCID_{50}$. The importance of Tc is shown by the difference in susceptibility between B6 and bm1 mice and also by the complete protection of B6 nu/nu mice against infection with a lethal virus dose by i.v. injection of a Sendai virus-specific, IL-2 dependent and H-$2K^b$ restricted B6 Tc clone. In vivo protection by this Tc clone is H-$2K^b$ restricted. Apart from Tc, an important role for virus-specific Th cells is evident from the difference in susceptibility between bm1 and B6 nu/nu mice. This conclusion is supported by the demonstration that the mean survival time of B6 nu/nu and bm1 nu/nu mice can be significantly prolonged, in an I-A^b restricted manner, by the injection of in vitro-propagated, Sendai-specific B6 or bm1 Th clones after a lethal dose of Sendai virus, and by the demonstration that inoculation of these Th clones provides help to virus-specific Tc by means of IL-2 production. Strikingly, Th and Tc cooperate in anti-Sendai virus immunity, since permanent survival of lethally infected nu/nu mice is only achieved by inoculation of a mixture of Tc and Th clones or a mixture of a Tc clone and rIL-2. Furthermore, the difference in susceptibility to Sendai virus infection between B6 and bm1 mice provides a unique model for the study of MHC-disease associations. The importance of NK cells is revealed by the high susceptibility of 129/J mice to Sendai virus infection, although all other immune parameters measured appear to be normal.

INTRODUCTION

Immune regulation by MHC molecules might be an important mechanism to explain MHC-disease associations, although solid evidence for this is missing.

The opportunity to study the in vivo importance of class I MHC regulation of the Tc response to a natural pathogenic agent of high virulence came with our previous demonstration (1) of a major difference in the capacity to generate a Sendai virus-specific Tc response between C57BL/6 (B6, H-2^b) mice and H-$2K^b$ mutant B6.C-H-2^{bm1} (bm1) mice. These mice differ from each other only in three amino acids in the H-$2K^b$ molecule (2,3). B6 mice are responders to Sendai virus measured by the generation of virus-specific Tc, virus-specific Th proliferation, and natural killer (NK) cell activity in vitro and by anti-viral antibody production and virus-specific delayed type hypersensitivity (DTH) in vivo (1,4,5, and this study). In contrast, bm1 mice are Tc nonresponders against this virus, but do not differ in any of the other immune parameters (1,4,5, and this study). These immune parameters were also studied in thymus deficient nu/nu mice. These mice show not only deficient Tc responses, but also deficient Th responses and thus deficient DTH and antibody responses, although their baseline NK activity is increased in comparison with normal mice (1,4,5, and this study). Another H-2^b mouse strain, 129/J, also shows equal Sendai virus-specific Tc, Th, B cell and DTH responses compared to B6, but is almost completely defective in generating an NK response.

We now report that B6, bm1, B6 nu/nu, and 129/J mice differ from each other in susceptibility to lethal pneumonia induced by intranasal (i.n.) inoculation of virulent Sendai virus. NK cell deficient 129/J mice and T-cell deficient B6 nu/nu animals were most susceptible to the lethal effects of the virus, whereas B6 mice were most resistant. Bm1 mice showed intermediate susceptibility. The difference in susceptibility between B6 and bm1 mice is ascribed to the defective Sendai-specific Tc response in bm1 mice. The importance of Tc was further demonstrated by the complete protection of B6 nu/nu mice (in an H-$2K^b$ restricted manner) against a lethal virus dose by i.v. injection of an IL-2 dependent Sendai-specific and H-$2K^b$ restricted B6 Tc clone. Thus, in this case, an association between MHC and susceptibility to a natural pathogenic agent of high virulence is linked to Tc nonresponsiveness on the basis of class I MHC regulation. Apart from Tc, an important role for virus-specific Th cells in the protection against the virus is evident from the difference in susceptibility between bm1 and B6 nu/nu mice. This conclusion was supported by the demonstration that inoculation of I-A^b-restricted Sendai-specific Th clones clearly prolonged the lifespan of B6 nu/nu mice and bm1 nu/nu mice in an I-A^b-restricted manner, after challenge with a lethal dose of virus, and by the demonstration that inoculation of these Th clones provided help to virus-specific Tc. Finally the importance of NK cells is revealed by the high susceptibility of 129/J mice to Sendai virus infection, although all other immune parameters measured appear to be normal. This study provides a unique model for the further investigation of MHC-disease associations, it shows that antigen-specific Tc and Th cells cooperate in in vivo protection against virus infection and indicates the importance of NK cells in anti-viral function.

Table 1. H-2 haplotypes of mouse strains used in this study

mouse strain	abbreviation	H-2 K	H-2 I-A	H-2 D	structural alteration
C57BL/6	B6	b	b	b	-
C57BL/6 nu/nu	B6 nu/nu	b	b	b	-
129/J	129/J	b	b	b	-
B10.A(4R)	4R	k	k	b	-
B10.A (5R)	5R	b	b	d	-
B10.MBR	MBR	b	k	q	-
B6.C-H-2bm1[a]	bm1	bm1	b	b	Glu → Ala at position 152[b] Arg → Tyr at position 155[c] Leu → Tyr at position 156[c]
B6.C-H-2bm1 nu/nu	bm1 nu/nu	bm1	b	b	Same as bm1
B6.C-H-2bm12[a]	bm12	b	bm12	b	Ile → Phe at position 67[d] Arg → Glu at position 70[d] Thr → Lys at position 71[d]
B6.C-H-2bm12 nu/nu	bm12 nu/nu	b	bm12	b	Same as bm12

[a]Congenic or coisogenic with C57BL/6 (B6, H-2b)
[b]According to Pease et al. (2)
[c]According to Nairn et al. (2)
[d]According to McIntyre et al. (7)

MATERIALS AND METHODS

Animals

C57BL/6, 129/J, B10.A(4R), B10.A(5R) and B10.MBR mice, H-2 mutant (B6.C-H-2bm1 (bm1) and B6.C-H-2bm12 (bm12) mice and C57BL/6 nu/nu mice were bred in our laboratory under specific pathogen-free conditions. Bm1 nu/nu mice were bred as described previously (4). Bm12 nu/nu mice were bred by mating normal bm12 with C57BL/6 nu/nu mice. The F_1 mice were mated and the F_2 nu/nu mice were H-2 typed by cytofluorographic analysis on lipopolysaccharide (LPS) induced (30 μg/ml), 4-days cultured lymphoblasts obtained from lymph node cells. For typing, we used monoclonal antibody (mAb) 34-5-3S, a gift from Dr. D.H. Sachs (Bethesda, MD), which reacts strongly with the lymphocytes of I-Ab but not of I-Abm12 mice (6). The mouse strains used in this study, their H-2 haplotypes and the structural alterations in the H-2 molecules of the mutant mouse strains are listed in Table 1. All mice were used at 6-12 weeks of age.

Viruses

Nonvirulent Sendai virus, lot 40340087, was obtained from Flow Laboratories (McLean, VA). This virus had been propagated in pathogen-free eggs. The titer was 10^4 hemagglutinating units (HAU)/ml. Virulent Sendai virus, strain P3193, was a gift of Dr. J.C. Parker (Microbiological Associates, Bethesda, MD). This virus was propagated in the lungs of 129/J mice. Homogenates of infected lungs (10% suspension (wt/vol) in basal (Eagle's) medium with antibiotics clarified at 2,300 x g for 20 min at 4°C) were inoculated by i.n. instillation of 0.02 ml of 10% suspension of infected mouse lung cells. Lungs of mice were harvested 6 days after inoculation. P3193 virus was tested by the mouse antibody-production test (8) and found not to contain other murine virus contaminants. The titer was 3.2 x 10^6 50% tissue culture infective dose ($TCID_{50}$)/ml. Both viruses were stored at -70°C.

Virus titration and quantitation

Virus titration and quantitation were performed essentially as described (9) with slight modifications. For virus titration in tissue culture, clarified 10% suspensions of infected lung cells were diluted 10-fold and 0.1 ml was inoculated into each of four 2-ml wells of a 24-wells plate (Nunc, Roskilde, Denmark) containing a monolayer of primary rhesus-monkey kidney cells (a gift from Dr. M. Jonker, T.N.O., Rijswijk, The Netherlands). Cells were observed for cytopathic effects daily for 14 days, and end-point titers were calculated by the methods of Kārber (10). Virus titration and quantitation in vivo was done using four mice from each of the strains B6, bm1 or B6 nu/nu at each titration point. They were inoculated i.n., each with 0.02 ml of a 3.33-fold virus dilution. The same person (W.M. Kast) made all inoculations throughout the titration experiments. Infected mice were observed for disease and death up to day 28 or longer. During these experiments, mice were housed in an isolator in which the airflow was directed from cages with mice infected with low doses of virus to cages with mice infected with high doses of virus to avoid contamination. Virus titers are expressed as the number of $TCID_{50}$/0.02 ml required to cause a lethal infection (LD_{50}).

Immunizations and elicitation of DTH

Sendai virus-specific DTH responses were elicited in the ear. Mice were primed with 10^2 HAU noninfectious Sendai virus 6 days before challenge by i.n. instillation of 20 µl of Sendai virus suspension diluted in PBS. The challenge was given by injecting into the dorsal surface of the ear a total volume of 25 µl of either PBS (right ear) or 10^2 HAU Sendai virus diluted in PBS (left ear) using a 50 µl Hamilton syringe fitted with a 30-gauge needle. The same procedure was performed in nonimmunized (naive) control mice. Ear swelling was measured with a Mitutoyo model 102-217 micrometer (Steenkist-Rooymans, Eindhoven, The Netherlands). The percentage increase in ear swelling was calculated as:

$$\frac{\text{thickness of left ear - thickness of right ear}}{\text{thickness of right ear}}$$

T-cell clones

Culture conditions for generation of T-cell clones were essentially the same as described before (1). In brief, C57BL/6 and bm1 mice were injected intraperitoneally (i.p.) with 10^2 HAU Sendai virus. Three weeks later, spleen cells of these mice were restimulated in vitro with syngeneic Sendai virus-infected irradiated (25 Gy) spleen cells (stimulator cells) for 5 days. Culture medium consisted of Iscove's modified Dulbecco's medium (IMDM) (Gibco, Grand Island, NY), supplemented with 10% pooled human serum, penicillin (100 IU/ml), streptomycin (100 µg/ml) and 2-mercaptoethanol (2.10^{-5} M). Effector cells were run on a density gradient (Lympholyte M, Cedarlane, Hornby, Ontario, Canada) and cultured again in the same way. This procedure was repeated three times after which a precursor frequency was established in a limiting-dilution assay, using 96 U-shaped well plates (Titertek, Flow Laboratories, McLean, VA) with 1.5 x 10^5 Sendai-coated syngeneic stimulator cells and 12.5% rat cell supernatant (RF) as lymphokine source (4) in a total volume of 200 µl culture medium. Wells that showed cell growth at a dilution below 10% of the precursor frequency were transferred into 24-mm Costar wells (Costar, Cambridge, MA). Cells were routinely subcultured once a week. Th clone 6C3 (Th-6C3) derived from a B6 mouse has the marker profile Thy-1+, L3T4+, Lyt 2^- and produces IL-2 and gamma-IFN after concanavalin A (Con

A) stimulation (not shown). Tc clone 5 (Tc-5) derived from a B6 mouse, has the marker profile Thy-1+, L3T4$^-$, Lyt 2+. This clone produces gamma-IFN but did not produce IL-2 after Con A stimulation (not shown). They were tested in in vivo and in vitro assays approximately two months after establishment. Th clone EA-7, specific for egg albumin and derived from a B6 mouse, was originally described by Dr. M.H. Schreier (11) and obtained through the kind courtesy of Dr. R. Benner (Erasmus University, Rotterdam, The Netherlands).

To explore the protective capabilities of these clones, naive mice were inoculated i.n. with 10 LD_{50} Sendai virus and 1 hour later were given one i.v. injection of cloned T cells in PBS or PBS alone. The results of these tests are given in mean survival time ± SD. For statistical analysis of these results the Mann-Whitney U test was used.

Recombinant IL-2

Recombinant IL-2 (batch RNB 85738/09Y) was obtained from Biogen (Geneva, Switzerland). In protection experiments it was administered as a single subcutaneous injection of 1.25 x 10^4 U/mouse in complete Freund adjuvant, with 0.5% bovine serum albumin.

NK cell assay

Varying numbers of spleen cells of different mouse strains were used as effector cells at different time points after i.p. inoculation with 3 x 10^2 HAU Sendai virus against 5 x 10^3 Na ^{51}Cr-labelled YAC-1 target cells in 0.2 ml culture medium in wells of roundbottomed microtiter plates. After six hours incubation at 37°C in humidified air with 5% CO_2 the percent specific ^{51}Cr release was determined as described (1). Background release was always <15%. The standard error of triplicate cultures was always <3% specific ^{51}Cr release.

Proliferation response in MLC

Responder spleen cells (4 x 10^5) of mice primed against Sendai virus were cultured with 6 x 10^5 Sendai virus infected irradiated (20 Gy) spleen cells in flatbottomed tissue culture plates (Costar, Cambridge, MA) in a total volume of 0.2 ml culture medium. Cultures were incubated at 37°C and 5% CO_2 for 4 days, the last 4 hours in the presence of 0.4 μ Ci (^{3}H)-thymidine added in 20 μl. The cells were harvested with an automated cell harvester and radioactivity was measured in a liquid scintillation counter. Data are presented as the mean value ± SE of five replicate wells in cpm.

Determination of Sendai-specific antibody titers

The titer of Sendai-specific antibodies in mouse sera was determined with a hemagglutination inhibition test and an enzyme-linked immunosorbent assay (ELISA). The ELISA was performed by coating microtiter plates with 0.2 ml/well Sendai virus (0.005 mg protein/ml) by overnight incubation at 4°C. After washing in PBS with 0.1% Tween 20, 0.05 ml diluted test serum was added. The sera were diluted in PBS/Tween containing 10% FCS. Subsequently, the plates were incubated for 1 hour at 37°C and were then washed three times in PBS/Tween. Finally, 50 μl of peroxidase-labeled rabbit anti-mouse IgG (Miles Laboratories, Elkhart, IN), at a 1 : 1000 dilution in PBS/Tween/FCS, was added. After 1 hour at 37°C, the plates were washed three times with PBS/Tween, and the diluted substrate (orthophenylenediamine/H_2O_2) was added. After 30 min, the reaction was stopped by adding 0.1 ml 3 N H_2SO_4. The optical density of the reaction, as a measure of the amount of specific IgG, was determined by spectrophotometry (Titertek Mullisham; Flow Laboratories).

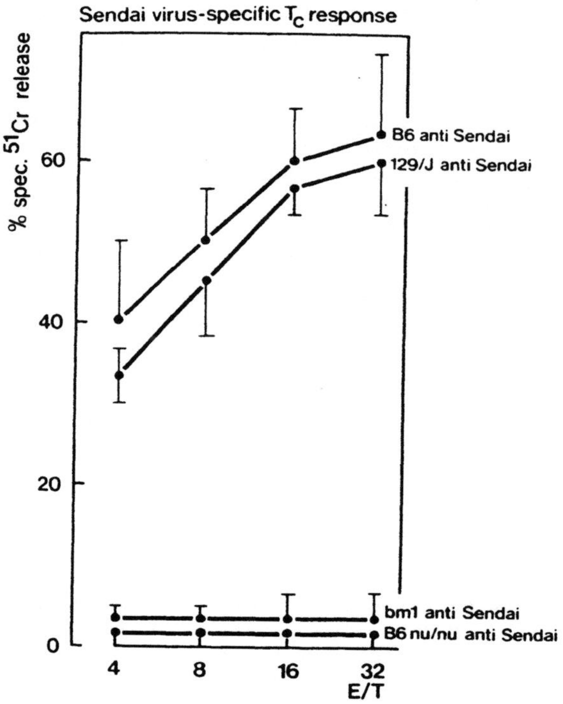

Fig. 1. Sendai virus-specific Tc response. Mice were primed with 10^2 HAU Flow Sendai virus and 3 weeks later their spleen cells were restimulated with irradiated syngeneic Sendai virus-infected stimulator spleen cells. Five days later the effector cells were tested on syngeneic Sendai virus-infected Con A stimulated target cells. Data are expressed as the mean percentage specific ^{51}Cr release ± S.E. of six mice. ^{51}Cr release on uninfected target cells was always <5%.

Measurement of Tc effector activity

Sendai virus-specific Tc effector activity of bulk cultures was essentially measured as described (1). As targets we used ^{51}Cr labelled Con A induced (2.5 μg/ml) lymphoblasts (3-days cultures). Percent specific ^{51}Cr release was determined as described (1). Background release was always <25%. The standard error of triplicate cultures was always <5% specific ^{51}Cr release.

RESULTS

Sendai virus-specific Tc response

Primed B6, bm1, B6 nu/nu and 129/J mice were tested for their ability to generate a Sendai virus-specific Tc response. As shown in Fig. 1, B6

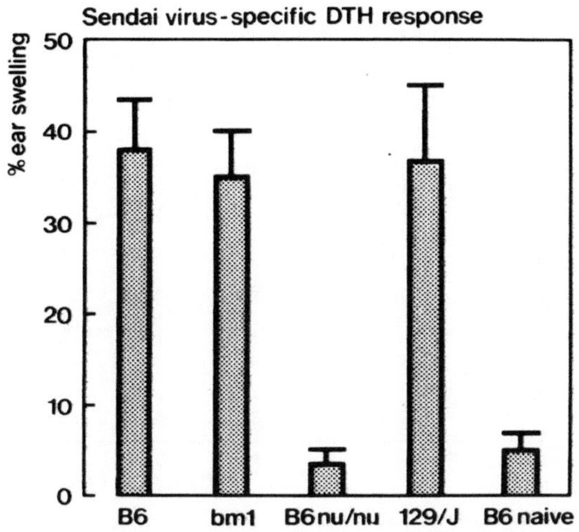

Fig. 2. Sendai virus-specific DTH response. Mice were naive (not primed) or were primed with 10^2 HAU Flow Sendai virus 6 days before challenge by i.n. instillation of a total volume of 25 µl of either PBS (right ear) or 10^2 HAU Flow Sendai virus diluted in PBS (left ear). The same procedure was performed in nonimmunized (naive) control mice. Ear swelling was measured at 48 hours. Data are expressed as the mean percentage ± S.E. of 100 x {(left ear thickness) - (right ear thickness)} / (right ear thickness) for groups of 35 B6, 12 bm1, 17 B6 nu/nu, 6 129/J, and 6 B6 naive mice.

and 129/J mice showed equally strong Tc activity against syngeneic Sendai infected target cells. In contrast, bm1 and B6 nu/nu mice did not generate a Sendai virus-specific Tc response, illustrating a Sendai virus-specific Tc response defect.

Sendai virus-specific DTH response

Primed B6, bm1, and B6 nu/nu and 129/J mice as well as unprimed (naive) B6 mice were tested for their ability to generate a Sendai virus-specific DTH response. As shown in Fig. 2, unprimed B6 mice did not generate a Sendai virus-specific DTH response. Primed B6, bm1 and 129/J mice showed equal percentages of ear swelling after challenge with Sendai virus. Thus, these three mouse strains did not differ in the DTH response to Sendai virus. In contrast, B6 nu/nu mice did not generate a Sendai-specific DTH response, illustrating the T-cell dependency of the DTH response.

NK cell activity

The time course of NK cell activity was studied in naive B6, bm1, B6 nu/nu and 129/J mice following 3.10^2 HAU Sendai virus inoculation per mouse (Fig. 3). NK cell activity in control mice was 31 ± 2% specific ^{51}Cr

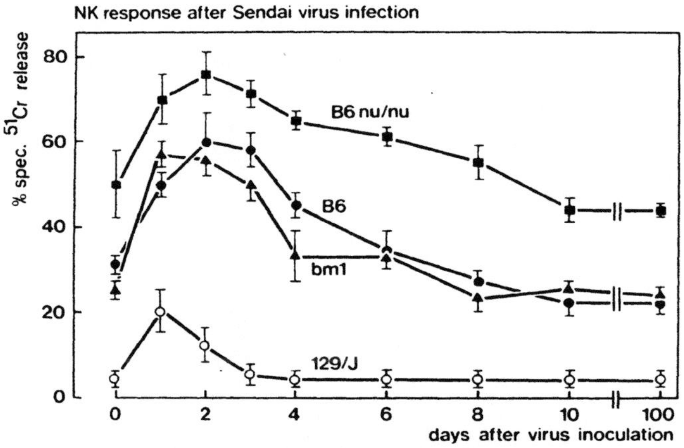

Fig. 3. Time course of NK activity in spleen cells of different mouse strains after i.p. inoculation with 3 x 10^2 HAU Sendai virus per mouse. Symbols represent NK activity of: ▲ , bm1 mice; ● , B6 mice; ■ , B6 nu/nu mice; ○ , 129/J mice. Cytotoxic activity was measured by ^{51}Cr release assay using ^{51}Cr-labelled YAC-1 cells as targets. E/T ratio was 100 : 1. Each data point represents the mean ± SEM of six mice.

release at an effector/target (E/T) ratio of 100 : 1 for B6 mice, 26 ± 2% for bm1 mice, 50 ± 8% for B6 nu/nu mice and 3 ± 1% for 129/J mice (mean ± SEM of six mice). The initial elevation in NK cell cytotoxic activity was observed 1 day after infection. Peak levels of NK activity occurred on the second day and by the 8th day it had declined to normal levels. B6 and bm1 mice showed equal kinetics of NK cell activity before and after priming with Sendai virus. B6 nu/nu mice, though displaying the same time course of NK cell activity showed a higher basic level of NK activity with a return to similar values after infection. In contrast, 129/J mice showed a very low basic level of NK activity, which only slightly increased 1 day after infection and which declined rapidly to the baseline level 3 days after infection. Thus B6 and bm1 mice did not differ in NK cell activity and NK cell activity kinetics after challenge with Sendai virus whereas B6 nu/nu mice had high baseline, and 129/J mice very low baseline NK cell activity before and after challenge with Sendai virus.

Sendai virus-specific T-cell proliferative response

Primed B6, bm1, B6 nu/nu and 129/J mice were tested for their ability to generate a Sendai virus-specific proliferative response in MLC. As shown in Table 2, spleen cells of B6, bm1 and 129/J mice showed equal amounts of Sendai virus-specific proliferation. But spleen cells of B6 nu/nu mice did not proliferate at all indicating a normal Th cell pathway in the first three mouse strains and a Th defect in the B6 nu/nu mouse strain.

Table 2. Sendai virus-specific T-cell proliferative response

responder cells	stimulator cells	cpm	stimulation index
B6	B6 Sendai	8477	5.3
	B6	1611	
bm1	bm1 Sendai	9181	5.6
	bm1	1628	
B6 nu/nu	B6 Sendai	1023	1.0
	B6	1002	
129/J	129/J Sendai	9856	4.9
	129/J	1989	

Responder cells were derived from animals primed with 10^2 HAU Flow Sendai virus i.p. Stimulator cells were treated with NH_4Cl, irradiated (20 Gy) and infected with Sendai virus or were left untreated.

Sendai virus-specific antibody response

B6, bm1, B6 nu/nu and 129/J mice were tested for their capacity to form Sendai virus-specific antibodies. As shown in Table 3, B6, bm1 and 129/J mice formed equal amounts of Sendai virus-specific antibody titers after immunization with 10^2 HAU Flow Sendai virus. In contrast, B6 nu/nu mice did not form these antibodies, again indicating a normal Th pathway (B cells are Th dependent) in the first three strains and a defective Th cell pathway in the B6 nu/nu mice.

Susceptibility to virulent Sendai virus infection

B6, bm1 and B6 nu/nu and 129/J mice were challenged i.n. with virulent Sendai virus to investigate their susceptibility (Table 4). We found that the LD_{50} for the Sendai Tc deficient bm1 strain was

Table 3. Sendai virus-specific antibody response

serum source	Sendai virus immunization	Sendai virus-specific antibody titer
B6	+	1/200[a]
B6	-	0
bm1	+	1/200
bm1	-	0
B6 nu/nu	+	0
B6 nu/nu	-	0
129/J	+	1/400
129/J	-	0

[a]Hemagglutination inhibition.

Table 4. Susceptibility to virulent Sendai virus infection

mouse strain	LD_{50}[a] (expressed in $TCID_{50}$[b])
B6	150.0 ± 74.9
bm1	14.7 ± 4.8
B6 nu/nu	0.5 ± 0.6
129/J	0.2 ± 0.2

[a]LD_{50} lethal dose for 50% of animals.
[b]$TCID_{50}$ tissue culture infectious dose for 50% of animals.

approximately 10 times lower than for the B6 strain, compatible with an important role of virus-specific Tc. The LD_{50} for the T-cell deficient B6 nu/nu strain, in turn, was 30 times lower than for the bm1 strain, indicating an important role of T cells other than Tc, notably Th cells, in anti-viral immunity. The LD_{50} for the NK lowresponder 129/J mice was the lowest of all strains tested, indicating the importance of NK cells in antiviral immunity. To further confirm the notion that both Th and Tc cells are important in anti-viral immunity nude mouse protection experiments with Th and Tc clones were carried out.

Protection against lethal Sendai virus infection in nu/nu mice by T cell clones

In the experiments described in Table 5 we determined whether the Th and Tc clones could protect against a lethal Sendai virus infection. Therefore, B6 nu/nu, bm1 nu/nu and bm12 nu/nu mice were given a Sendai virus dose of 10 LD_{50} i.n., and simultaneously, T cell clones or PBS i.v. Table 5 shows that B6 nu/nu mice die around day 18. Injection of B6 Th clone 6C3 extended the survival time of B6 nu/nu mice by a factor of two but no permanent survivors were observed. The H-2 I-A^b restriction of Th 6C3 was apparent in vivo, because bm12 nu/nu mice could not be protected

Table 5. Protection against lethal Sendai virus infection in different mouse strains by Th and Tc clones

mouse strain	n	injected with: (no. of cells)	mean survival time (days ± S.D.)	range
B6 nu/nu	38	-	18.6 ± 5.4	(11-28)
	13	Th 6C3 (3.10^6)	38.5 ± 10.2	(21-62)
	7	Tc 5 (3.10^6)	24.1 ± 2.7	(22-26)
	7	Th 6C3 (3.10^6) + Tc 5 (3.10^6)	>100.0	
	3	Tc 5 (3.10^6) + rec. IL-2	>100.0	
	4	rec. IL-2	16.7 ± 2.4	(15-20)
	3	Th EA-7 (3.10^6)	21.2 ± 3.8	(16-25)
bm12 nu/nu	7	Th 6C3 (3.10^6)	19.5 ± 4.3	(13-25)
bm1 nu/nu	4	Tc 5 (3.10^6) + rec. IL-2	13.7 ± 2.9	(12-18)

from death by this clone. Injection, however, of an H-2 I-A^b restricted B6 Th clone specific for egg albumin had no protective effect, illustrating that the life prolongation by the Sendai-specific Th clone was specific. The Sendai virus-specific B6 Tc-5 clone by itself only marginally extended the survival time of B6 nu/nu mice. However, upon injection of a combination of 3 x 10^6 Tc-5 and 3 x 10^6 Th-6C3 cloned T cells all mice survived and remained healthy indicating cooperation between Th and Tc in antiviral immunity. Probably, Th cells mediate their activity in this cell-cell cooperation at least partially by IL-2 release, because permanent survival was also achieved by injection of a mixture of 3 x 10^6 Tc-5 and rIL-2. rIL-2 by itself had no protective effect. The in vitro H-$2K^b$ restriction specificity of Tc-5 was also apparent in vivo because bm1 nu/nu mice could not be protected from death by this clone under conditions where B6 nu/nu mice could be protected.

DISCUSSION

This study establishes a clear association between MHC type and susceptibility to Sendai virus-induced lethal pneumonia. Mutation of three amino acids in the H-2 K^b class I molecule in bm1 mice causes a higher susceptibility to the lethal effect of the virus, compared with B6, the strain of origin. The only measurable difference in Sendai-specific immune responses between bm1 and B6 mice is the inability of the mutant to generate Sendai-specific Tc (Fig. 1; Table 6). This difference is also the only expected difference because class I MHC molecules, of all immune responses studied, only restrict and regulate Tc responses and because no other genetic differences between B6 and bm1 mice are known to exist. Indeed, all other immune responses measured against the virus such as DTH (Fig. 2), T-cell proliferation (Table 2), and antibody production (Table 3), as well as NK activity (Fig. 3) of these two mouse strains were identical. The likelihood that the increased virus susceptibility and the Tc nonresponsiveness of the bm1 mouse are causally related is further enhanced by the fact that the H-$2K^b$ molecule is the only functional class I MHC restricting element for Sendai virus specific Tc in B6 mice (1).

The importance of virus-specific Tc in anti-viral immunity was further revealed by the fact that B6 nu/nu mice could be protected from death by transfer of a B6 Sendai virus-specific Tc clone. A positive control for

Table 6. Summary of immune responses against Sendai virus

assay of immune response	mouse strain			
	B6	bm1	B6 nu/nu	129/J
In vitro				
Tc	+	-	-	+
T-cell proliferation	+	+	-	+
NK	+	+	++	-
In vitro				
antibody production	+	+	-	+
DTH	+	+	-	+
resistance against infection	+	±	-	-

the importance of Tc against Sendai virus in bm1 mice would be a transfer of bm1 Sendai specific Tc clones into lethally infected bm1 mice. However, bm1 mice are Tc nonresponders against Sendai virus, therefore such bm1 Sendai specific Tc clones are non-existent, even after prolonged cell culture in vitro with IL-2 (W.M. Kast, unpublished observations). Moreover, transfer of B6 Tc clones specific for Sendai virus into lethally infected bm1 mice is unlikely to have any protective effect because of the MHC restriction of these Tc clones.

One of the most striking features of anti-viral T cell immunity in the current study is the cooperation between Th and Tc cells in anti-viral immunity. Permanent survival of lethally infected nu/nu mice was achieved only with a mixture of virus specific Th and Tc or a mixture of Tc and rIL-2 (Table 5). The cooperative effect of Th cells can at least partially be explained by the release of IL-2, because 1) Th-6C3 produces IL-2, whereas the Tc-5 does not (data not shown), and 2) the Th cell in this cell-cell cooperation can be replaced by rIL-2 (Table 5). IL-2 release does not explain the fact, however, that Th clones by themselves, without Tc, also display a marked protective effect, because rIL-2 by itself has no protective effect. (Table 5).

The importance of Th cells was further revealed by the difference in susceptibility (to Sendai virus infection) between T-cell deficient B6 nu/nu mice and Tc-deficient bm1 mice for Sendai virus infection (Tables 4 and 6). It seems likely that this difference is due (directly or indirectly) to the generation of Sendai-specific Th cells in bm1 mice. The importance of NK cells is revealed by the high susceptibility of NK low-responder 129/J mice to Sendai virus infection, although all other immune parameters measured seem to be normal. Transfer of NK cell clones, as done in a murine cytomegalo virus model (12), would be the ultimate experiment and is currently undertaken by us.

Transfer of immune T cells was shown (13-15) to protect against several viruses such as influenza virus, Herpes Simplex virus type 1 (16) and lymphocytic choriomeningitis virus (LCMV) (17,18). Usually, Tc clones were transferred in the same, or even higher amounts than in this study. When Th cells were used, they sometimes worsen (10) or ameliorate (20) virus-induced disease. Our Th clone 6C3 could not protect I-A^b-disparate bm12 nu/nu mice from death (Table 5). Furthermore the Tc clone could not protect H-$2K^b$-disparate bm1 nu/nu mice from death (Table 5). In vivo protection with immune T cells against virus infection only functions in syngeneic situations (16,17). In these studies, completely different allogeneic strains were used so that the exact genetic restriction element was not identified. We now show that the in vivo protection by cloned Th cells shows the same I-A^b restriction as previously found in vitro (5).

The exact mechanism(s) by which both Th and Tc clones exert their protection remain(s) to be solved. One possible protective mechanism of Th and Tc is production of gamma-IFN which is released by both our Th and Tc clones (data not shown). In experiments with influenza virus (14) and with Herpes virus (16), only those Tc clones which produced gamma-IFN could clear the virus in vivo. However, recent experiments (15) also in the influenza-system, showed that the protective effect of cloned Tc was highly specific and probably not correlated with gamma-IFN production. Therefore the straightforward possibility that Tc protect by killing virus infected cells, remains a distinct one.

A direct link between MHC type and susceptibility to acute viral illness has not been established before. On the other hand, the association between MHC type and susceptibility to chronic disease induction by RNA tumor viruses, where immune mechanisms are probably responsible for protection, is well established (21-27). In this case, again, the ability to generate a strong MHC-regulated immune response is associated with resistance to the induction of disease. In lethal LCMV-induced choriomeningitis however, the generation of a strong MHC-regulated immune response (notably class I-restricted Tc) is associated with susceptibility to the induction of disease. In this model (e.g. intracerebral inoculation of LCM virus), the autoaggressive potential of the antiviral immune response outweighs the beneficial effects of the T-cell response (28-31). Indeed, recently (32) it was demonstrated that mice producing Tc against LCMV because they have an appropriate H-2D-restricting element, die after infection, whereas mice that do not generate Tc because they lack a proper H-2D-restricting element, survive (32). Thus, generation of a strong class-I MHC-regulated anti-viral Tc response can have two final results: increased resistance to the induction of disease, as demonstrated in this study, or increased susceptibility to the induction of disease (e.g. LCMV) (32). The outcome depends on a series of factors, including cytopathogenicity and virulence of the virus and the beneficial versus harmful effects of T cell activity (33).

This work was supported in part by the Foundation for Medical and Health research (MEDIGON), which is subsidized by the Netherlands Organization for the Advancement of Pure Research (ZWO).

REFERENCES

1. L.P. de Waal, W.M. Kast, R.W. Melvold, and C.J.M. Melief, Regulation of the cytotoxic T-lymphocyte response against Sendai virus analyzed with H-2 mutants. J. Immunol. 130:1090 (1980).
2. R. Nairn, K. Yamaga, and S.G. Nathenson, Biochemistry of the gene product from murine MHC mutants. Ann. Rev. Genet. 14:241 (1980).
3. L.R. Pease, D.H. Schulze, G.M. Pfaffenbach, and S.G. Nathenson, Spontaneous H-2 mutants provide evidence that a copy mechanism analogous to gene conversion generates polymorphism in the major histocompatibility complex. Proc. Natl. Acad. Sci. USA 80:242 (1983).
4. W.M. Kast, L.P. de Waal, and C.J.M. Melief, Thymus dictates major histocompatibility comples (MHC) specificity and immune-response gene phenotype of class-II MHC-restricted T cells but not of class-I MHC-restricted T cells. J. Exp. Med. 160:1752 (1984).
5. W.M. Kast, A.M. Bronkhorst, L.P. de Waal, and C.J.M. Melief, Cooperation between cytotoxic and helper T lymphocytes in protection against lethal Sendai virus infection. Protection by T cells is MHC-restricted and MHC-regulated; a model for MHC-disease associations. J. Exp. Med. 164:723 (1986).
6. M.R. Melino, S.L. Epstein, D.H. Sachs, and T.H. Hansen, Idiotypic and fluorometric analysis of the antibodies that distinguish the lesion of the I-A mutant B6.C-H-2^{bm12}. J. Immunol. 131:359 (1983).
7. K.R. McIntyre and J.G. Seidman, Nucleotide sequence of mutant I-A-$beta^{bm12}$ gene is evidence for genetic exchange between mouse immune-response genes. Nature (Lond.) 308:551 (1984).
8. M.J. Collins Jr. and J.C. Parker, Murine virus contaminants of leukemia viruses and transplantable tumors. J. Natl. Cancer Inst. 49:1139 (1972).
9. J.C. Parker, M.D. Whiteman, and C.B. Richter, Susceptibility of inbred and outbred mouse strains to Sendai virus and prevalence of infection in laboratory rodents. Infect. Immun. 19:123 (1978).
10. E.H. Lenette, General principles underlying laboratory diagnosis of virus and rickettsial infections, in: Diagnostic Procedures for Viral and Rickettsial Infections, 4th ed., American Public Health Association, Inc., New York (1969).

11. M.H. Schreier, R. Tees, A.A. Nordin, R. Benner, A.T.J. Bianchi, and M.J. van Zwieten, Functional aspects of helper T cell clones. Immunobiology 161:107 (1982).
12. J.F. Bukowski, J.F. Warner, G. Dennert, and R.M. Welsh, Adoptive transfer studies demonstrating the antiviral effect of natural killer cells in vivo. J. Exp. Med. 161:40 (1985).
13. Y.L.Lin and B.A. Askonas, Biological properties of an influenza- A virus-specific killer T-cell clone. Inhibition of virus replication in vivo and induction of delayed-type hypersensitivity reactions. J. Exp. Med. 154:225 (1981).
14. P.M. Taylor and B.A. Askonas, Diversity in the biological properties of anti-influenza cytotoxic T-cell clones. Eur. J. Immunol. 13:707 (1983).
15. A.E. Lukacher, V.L. Braciale, and T.J. Braciale, In-vivo effector function of influenza virus-specific cytotoxic T-lymphocyte clones is highly specific. J. Exp. Med. 160:814 (1984).
16. K.K. Sethi, Y. Omata, and K.E. Schneweis, Protection of mice from fatal herpes-simplex virus type-1 infection by adoptive transfer of cloned virus-specific and H-2 restricted cytotoxic T lymphocytes. J. Gen. Virol. 64:443 (1983).
17. J.A. Byrne and M.B.A. Oldstone, Biology of cloned cytotoxic T lymphocytes specific for lymphocytic choriomeningitis virus: clearance of virus in vivo. J. Virol. 51:682 (1984).
18. F. Lehmann-Grube, U. Assmann, C. Loliger, D. Moskophidis, and J. Lohler, Mechanism of recovery from acute virus infection. I. Role of T lymphocytes in the clearance of lymphocytic choriomeningitis virus from spleens of mice. J. Immunol. 134:608 (1985).
19. G.L. Ada, K.-N. Leung, and H.C.J. Ertl, An analysis of effector T-cell generation and function in mice exposed to influenza A or Sendai virus. Immunol. Rev. 58:6 (1981).
20. E.L. Howes, W. Taylor, N.A. Mitchison, and E. Simpson, MHC matching shows that at least two T-cell subsets determine resistance to HSV. Nature (Lond.). 277:67 (1979).
21. D. Meruelo, H-2D control of leukemia susceptibility: mechanism and implications. J. Immunogenet. 7:81 (1980).
22. P. Debre, B. Boyer, S. Gisselbrecht, A. Bismuth, and J.P. Levy, Genetic control of sensitivity to Moloney virus in mice. III. The three H-2-linked Rmv genes are immune response genes controlling the antiviral antibody response. Eur. J. Immunol. 10:914 (1980).
23. W.J. Britt and B. Chesebro, H-2D control of recovery from Friend virus leukemia: H-2D region influences the kinetics of the T-lymphocyte response to Friend virus. J. Exp. Med. 157:1736 (1983).
24. A. Vlug, H.J. Schoenmakers, and C.J.M. Melief, Genes of the H-2 complex regulate the antibody response to murine leukemia virus. J. Immunol. 126:2355 (1981).
25. A. Vlug, M. Zijlstra, R.E.Y. de Goede, W.G. Hesselink, H.J. Schoenmakers, and C.J.M. Melief, H-2 control of the cytotoxic antibody response against a newly defined MuLV-related cell-surface antigen: g(B10.A). Int. J. Cancer 31:617 (1983).
26. M. Zijlstra, R.E.Y. de Goede, H. Schoenmakers, T. Radaszkiewics, and C.J.M. Melief, Ecotropic and dualtropic mink-cell focus-inducing murine leukemia viruses can induce a wide spectrum of H-2 controlled lymphoma types. Virology 138:198 (1984).
27. F. Lilly and T. Pincus, Genetic control of murine viral leukemogenesis. Adv. Cancer Res. 17:231 (1983).
28. P.C. Doherty and R.M. Zinkernagel, Capacity of sensitized thymus-derived lymphocytes to induce fatal lymphocytic choriomeningitis is restricted by the H-2 gene complex. J. Immunol. 114:30 (1975).
29. P.C. Doherty, M.B.C. Dunlop, C.R. Parish, and R.M. Zinkernagel, Inflammatory process in murine lymphocytic choriomeningitis is

maximal in H-2K- or H-2D-compatibele interactions. J. Immunol. 117:187 (1976).
30. J.E. Allan and P.C. Doherty, Immune T cells can protect or induce fatal neurological disease in murine lymphocytic choriomeningitis. Cell. Immunol. 90:401 (1985).
31. M.B.A. Oldstone, R. Ahmed, J. Byrne, M.J Buchmeier, Y. Riviere, and P. Southern, Virus and immune responses: lymphocytic choriomeningitis virus as a prototype model of viral pathogenesis. Brit. Med. Bull. 41:70 (1985).
32. R.M. Zinkernagel, C.J. Pfau, H. Hengartner, and A. Althage, Susceptibility to murine lymphocytic choriomeningitis maps to class-I MHC genes - A model for MHC/disease associations. Nature (Lond.) 316:814 (1985).
33. R.M. Zinkernagel, H. Hengartner, and L. Stitz, On the role of viruses in the evaluation of immune responses. Brit. Med. Bull. 41:92 (1985).

SECTION V

EXPRESSION OF H-2 GENES ON NEOPLASTIC CELLS

MHC ANTIGEN EXPRESSION IN MALIGNANT TUMOURS AND THEIR EFFECTS ON HOST-TUMOUR INTERACTION

Hilliard Festenstein and Mario Labeta

Department of Immunology
The London Hospital Medical College
London, UK.

The development of malignant tumours and their immune regulation depends on a variety of factors including the presence or absence of tumour cell associated antigens (TAA) and the quantitative and qualitative representation of major histocompatibility complex (MHC) determinants in the tumour cells. Investigations of the latter and their importance in relation to host tumour interaction has been the main thrust of our research in this area over the last ten years. Increased or decreased expression of syngeneic Class I and Class II molecules as well as the expression of aberrant "allospecificities" may in different ways affect the immunosurveillance of tumours, their growth rate, as well as their metastatic potential. Our original experimental findings included the observations that certain tumour cells (a) selectively fail or express very weakly the specificities of one of the syngeneic H-2 Class I loci and/or (b) express novel H-2 "allospecificities" as determined by antibody testing.

The experiments were done with the following tumours: Meth.A (a methylcholanthrene induced tumour in BALB/c mice), Gardner tumour (an oestrogen induced tumour of C3H mice) and SL2 (a spontaneous Thy 1 positive mouse lymphoma of DBA/2 origin). In our experiments we used a variety of serological techniques and assays of cell-mediated immunity including mixed lymphocyte culture tests, tests of cell-mediated cytotoxicity and cytostasis (Festenstein et al, 1977). For the serological testing we included a specifically devised post labelling radioassay depending on the capacity of tumour cells to incorporate radiolabelled ^{14}C-uridine/thymidine before and after treatment with specific antibody and complement. After treating the tumour cells with specific antibody and complement there is a substantial reduction in the uptake of the radiolabel. The reduction of isotope incorporated in the test culture was compared with the controls which were treated with normal serum and complement and expressed as percent reduction. The results of testing the Gardner and SL2 tumours are summarised in Table 1 & 2.

The H-2D^k specificity of the Gardner tumour was easily identified while the H-2K^k specificity was virtually undetectable. In contrast, while the SL2 tumour expresses its syngeneic H-2K^d and H-2D^d specificities it also expresses a novel H-2D^k-like specificity apparently sharing epitope/s with H-2.32. When the anti H-2.32 alloantiserum

Table 1. No Serologically Detectable H-2K^k on Gardner (of C3H - H-2^k origin) and Extra "Alloreactive" H-2D^k-like specificity on SL2 Lymphoma (of DBA/2-H-2^d origin).

H-2 Allo Antisera Employed	Tumour Target Cells	
	SL2 Lymphoma (H-2K^d,H-2D^d)	Gardner Tumour ("H-2K^k",H-2D^k)
NIL	$6x10^{-3}$cpm	$8x10^{-3}$cpm
NIL (normal mouse serum plus C')	$6x10^{-3}$cpm	$6x10^{-3}$cpm
H-2.23(αH-2K^k)	NEG	**NEG**
H-2.32(αH-2D^k)	**POS(++)**	POS(+++)
H-2.31(αH-2K^d)	POS(+++)	NEG
H-2.4 (αH-2D^d)	POS(+++)	NEG

POS(+++) = 80-100%, POS(++) = 75%, NEG = 0% reduction of cpm of ^{14}C-thymidine uptake by SL2 and Gardner tumours after pretreatment with H-2 alloantisera and complement.

Adapted from Garrido, Festenstein & Schirrmacher Nature: 261: 705 (1976).

was absorbed with an H-2D^k negative cell (B10.A) its reactivity against the SL2 tumour was relatively unchanged but when absorbed with B10.BR (H-2D^k positive) its reactivity was removed indicating that the novel H-2D^k molecule shares relevant epitope/s with the H-2D^k specificities (H-2.32), (Garrido et al, 1976a) (Table 2).

Similar results were obtained with Class II alloantisera specific for antigens of the H-2^b and H-2^k haplotypes. Not only were inappropriate H-2 "allospecificities" found on in vivo propagated tumour cell lines but such changes in the H-2 profiles were also brought about by passaging the Meth.A tumour in BALB/c mice together with vaccinia virus (Garrido et al, 1976b; Garrido et al, 1977). In these experiments the Meth.A tumour typed, as expected for H-2^d specificities but the Meth.A 'vaccinia' tumour typed in addition with a whole variety of alloantisera normally reacting only with specifities of non H-2^d haplotypes. These included both the H-2K and H-2D private specificities of the H-2^k haplotype. Again H-2D^k and H-2K^k positive cells removed the reactivity from the sera so that they no longer reacted with the tumour while absorbtion with H-2K^k and H-2D^k negative cells had no such effect. The changes in the profiles of vaccinia treated cells were however transient and after about a week the "allospecificities" were no longer detectable.

At about the same time the groups of Parmiani (Invernizzi & Parmiani, 1975) and Martin (1975) showed that the growth of syngeneic tumours could be dramatically inhibited by preimmunising mice with allogeneic tissues before challenging them with the syngeneic tumours. At first, it was suggested that these findings could be explained by the expression of allogeneic minor histocompatibility antigens which

Table 2. Specific Removal of Anti H-2D^k Reactivity Against SL2 and Gardner Tumours by Absorbing the H-2.32 Alloantibody with B10.BR cells.

H-2 Allo-Antisera Employed	°Absorbtion/Non Absorbtion of H-2 Alloantisera	Tumour Target Cells	
		SL2 Lymphoma (H-2K^d,H-2D^d)	Gardner Tumour ("H-2K^k",H-2D^k)
NIL		18x10^{-3}*	13x10^{-3}cpm
NIL (normal mouse serum plus C')		15x10^{-3}cpm	15x10^{-3}cpm
H-2.32(αH-2D^k)	**(a) not absorbed**	**POS(++)**	**POS(++)**
	(b) absorbed with spleen cells from:		
	(i) B10.A (H-2.32 NEG)	**POS(+++)**	**POS(++)**
	(ii) B10.BR(H-2.32 POS)	**NEG**	**NEG**
H-2.31(αH-2K^d) (control)	(a) not absorbed	POS(+++)	NEG
	(b) absorbed with spleen cells from:		
	(i) B10.D2(H-2.31 POS)	NEG	NEG
	(ii) B10.BR(H-2.31 NEG)	POS(+++)	NEG

° Absorbed with 5x10^7 spleen cells.

* cpm of ^{14}C-Uridine uptake by SL2 and Gardner Tumours: reduction of cpm after pretreatment of these tumour target cells with specific absorbed/non absorbed H-2 alloantisera and complement: POS(+++) = 80-100%, POS(++) = 70-79% and NEG = 0% reduction of cpm.

Adapted from Garrido, Festenstein & Schirrmacher, Nature 261: 705 (1976)

are normally not expressed in the tumour bearing strains of mice but are derepressed in the tumours. Later data was presented supporting the hypothesis that the relevant antigens in these systems may also be H-2-like "allospecificities" (Parmiani, 1977; Martin et al, 1976).

Inappropriate MHC Class I and I-E like specificities were also found by Bonavida's group (Bonavida, 1986) on reticulum cell sarcomas of the H-2^s strain which does not normally express I-E antigens. In Martin's experiments several transplacentally induced malignant alveologenic lung adenocarcinomas induced by 1-ethyl-1-nitroso-urea in C3Hf mice apparently expressed an H-2K associated antigen designated 'K unique' not normally present in C3Hf mice.

Soon after our original findings of changing antigenic MHC profiles on tumour cells outlined above, we began to study a series of AKR leukaemic cell lines, one of which, K36 was obtained from J.P. Levy in Paris. This spontaneous leukaemia was made into a cell line in Lloyd Old's laboratory at The Sloan Kettering Institute in New York (Old et al, 1965). Several others were obtained from Peter Krammer in Heidelberg. We had originally planned to study the H-2 Class I-like "allospecificities" following in vivo passage together with vaccinia virus - experiments which were originally prompted by an outbreak of ectromelia in our colony and because vaccinia was used to immunise the mice. But as the vaccinia virus caused only transient changes in the MHC antigenic profiles we selected initially for more detailed study the spontaneous leukaemic cell line, K36 in which the presence

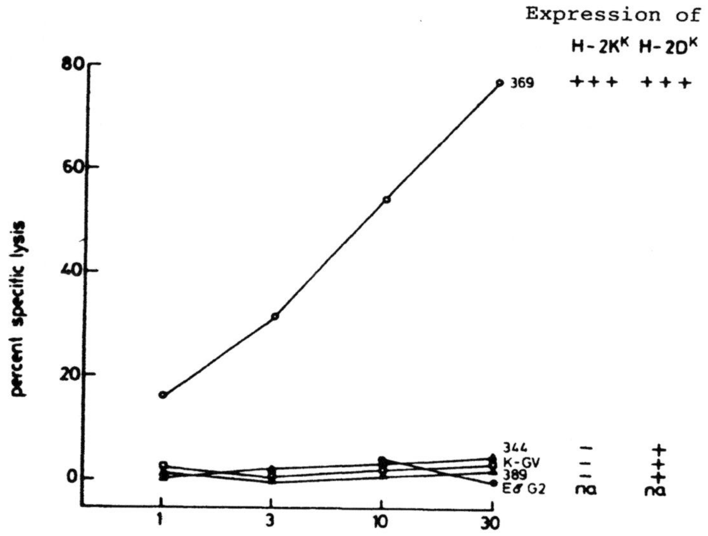

Fig. 1. H-2K^k restricted cytolysis of spontaneous AKR leukaemias. Effectors: AKR sensitised by AKR tumour 369.

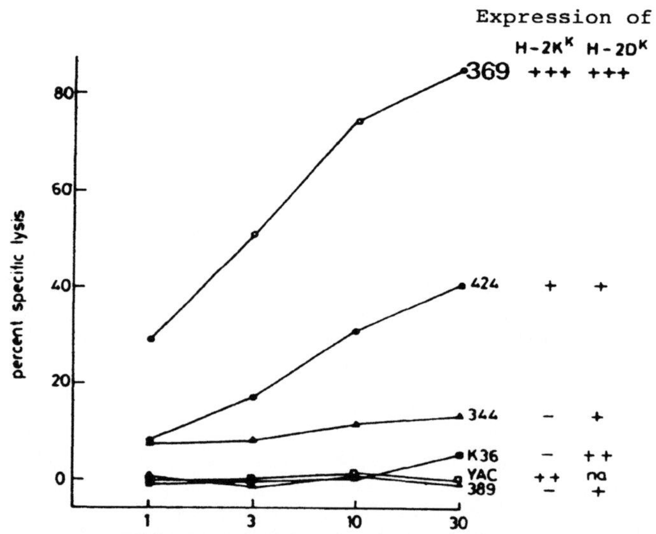

Fig. 2. H-2K^k restricted cytolysis of spontaneous AKR leukaemias. Effectors: AKR sensitised by AKR tumour 369.

of an aberrant extra $H-2D^d$-like "allospecificity" as well as the selective absence of the syngeneic $H-2K^k$ Class I specificity (and not $H-2D^k$) were found.

IMBALANCE OF H-2K/H-2D EXPRESSION ON AKR LEUKAEMIAS

The K36 tumour was cloned and the 16th clone designated K36.16 was studied in detail. The absence of the $H-2K^k$ specificity of this tumour was established as follows: (1) The $H-2K^k$ antigenic specificities were undetectable serologically on its cell surface. Similar results were obtained with the K-GV tumour derived from BALB.K. (2) No antibody responses against H-2.23, 11, 25 and 45 $H-2K^k$ specificities could be elicited by immunising H-2 allogeneic mice with K36. (3) Cytotoxic T cells sensitised against the $H-2K^k$ antigen using H-2 congenic combinations were not, or were only weakly cytotoxic for the tumours. (4) Anti-$H-2K^k$ CTL could not be stimulated in allogeneic mice after immunisation with the tumours. (5) No $H-2K^k$ antigens could be detected by indirect immunoprecipitation in radiolabelled detergent lysed tumour extract, i.e. neither in the glycoprotein nor in the protein fraction. In contrast, the $H-2D^k$ antigen was found both by serological and cellular techniques. It is structurally unaltered and identical to $H-2D^k$ from normal lymphocytes as determined by peptide mapping (Festenstein & Schmidt, 1981). (6) Specific $H-2K^k$ messenger RNA was also not readily detectable by an SI nuclease protection assay (Hui et al, 1984). This tumour grows very easily in the mouse with inoculations of less than 10^3 cells and is able to kill the mouse within approximately 2-3 weeks after injection. Other AKR tumours which express H-2K, grow less well and can be killed by T cells. These results suggested that the $H-2K^k$ epitopes may be the restriction element for T cell cytotoxicity against AKR leukaemic cells and may be biologically important in the immune surveillance of the leukaemias.

Frank Lilly (1966) was the first to observe that the K end of the H-2 haplotype is important in Gross virus leukaemogenesis. In accordance with this observation we designed experiments to test the hypothesis that the decrease or absence of expression of the H-2K antigen is not only important in in vitro MHC restriction but also in in vivo surveillance. To test the in vitro hypothesis AKR mice were sensitised by intraperitoneal injection with the AKR tumour 369 which expresses large amounts of H-2K. After 10-14 days the spleen cells were restimulated in culture with irradiated tumour cells - the same as those used for the original immunisation. After 5 days, the potential effectors were tested in cell mediated cytotoxicity against chromium labelled AKR leukaemic and other target cell lines. The H-2K/H-2D antigen expression on these target cells varied. The effectors were tested against tumour targets having normal or increased amounts of $H-2K^k$. There was a proportional amount of killing of target cells relative to the amount of $H-2K^k$ expressed. The cytotoxic effectors were T cells, as indicated by their sensitivity to anti-Thy-1 and complement. However, when the targets lacked the $H-2K^k$ antigens there was low or no killing (see AKR effectors against 344, 389, K36, K-GV) (Figures 1, 2). The H-2 and virus controls were E♂G2 ($H-2^b$) and YAC ($H-2^a$). E♂G2 has Gross virus but no $H-2K^k$ antigens, while YAC is $H-2K^k$ positive but is a Moloney virus tumour and is the classical NK target. Neither are killed in these experiments. These results indicate that $H-2K^k$ antigen expression is necessary for $H-2K^k$ restricted cytotoxicity of AKR Gross virus leukaemias (Schmidt & Festenstein, 1982; Festenstein & Schmidt, 1981; Schmidt et al, 1981) (Figures 1, 2 and 3).

Specific blocking of anti 369 CTL by anti H-2K^k MoAb

Specific blocking of anti 369 CTL by anti H-2K^k MoAb

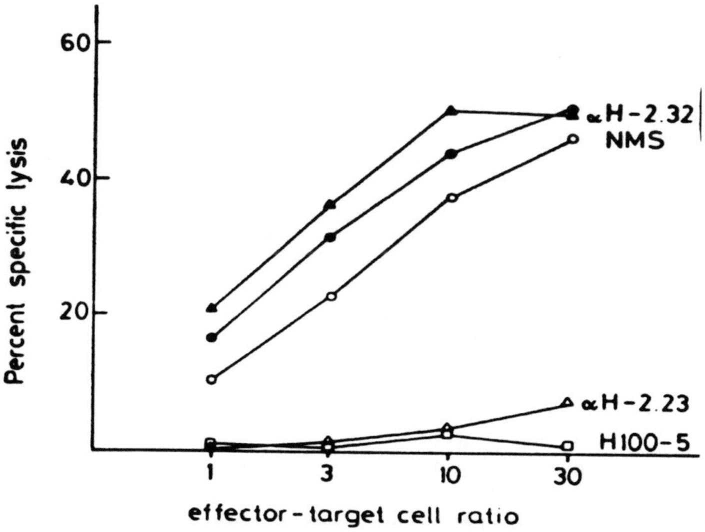

Fig. 3. Inhibition of Gross/AKR-MuLV specific cytotoxic T lymphocytes by alloantisera and monoclonal antibodies. Cytotoxic effectors were AKR/J splenic lymphocytes immunised and restimulated in vitro with 369 tumour cells. ^{51}Cr-labelled 369 tumour target cells were preincubated for 30 min with normal mouse serum (NMS,O), anti H-2.23 (△) and anti H-2.32 (▲) serum at a final dilution of 1/10 and with MoAbs H100-5 (with specificity for H-2K^k antigens) (□) at a final dilution of 1/100. Untreated target cells were also included as a control (●). (Schmidt & Festenstein 1982).

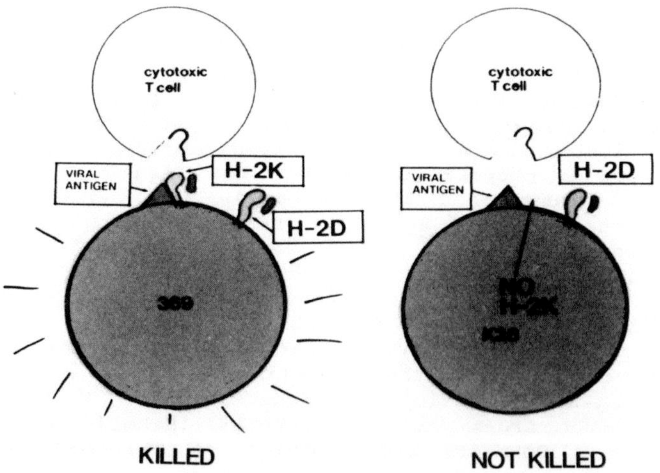

Fig. 4. H-2K^k restricted killing of Gross-virus leukaemias.

To find out if $H-2K^k$ antigens alone are sufficient or whether $H-2D^k$ antigens can also function as restriction elements in this system, we tried to inhibit the cytotoxicity with monoclonal antibodies and alloantisera against the $H-2K^k$ and $H-2D^k$ antigens. The results of these experiments are shown in Figure 3. When anti-H-2.32 ($H-2D^k$) antibody was used, there was no inhibition, but when anti-H-2.23 alloantibody and anti-$H-2K^k$ monoclonal antibodies were used there was no cytotoxicity of the 369 tumour target ($H-2K^kD^k$ positive). These experiments confirm the specific role of $H-2K^k$ in anti-Gross virus induced tumour cytotoxicity (Schmidt & Festenstein, 1982).

Recent experiments by Schäfer & Schmidt (1986) have confirmed that the $H-2K^k$ negative AKR leukaemic lines can not be lysed by AKR Gross MuLV-specific CTL and are unable to induce a cellular immune response. However some of these lines become susceptible to lysis after stimulation with interferon presumably due to the expression of the relevant $H-2K^k$ restriction epitopes. Although all the $H-2K^k$ positive lines tested were able to induce cytotoxic T cells capable of killing 369, some were not able to kill the syngeneic AKR leukaemic lines used for the induction of T cell cytotoxicity. These leukaemias were also resistant to lysis by anti 369 CTL suggesting either that the specific effector restriction epitope/s of $H-2K^k$ are obscured e.g. by excessive sialylation (see below) or that the $H-2K^k$ antigens on these tumours are defective.

We then investigated the balance between the expression of H-2K and H-2D in the various AKR leukaemic cell lines kindly provided by Peter Krammer and the K-GV BALB.K Gross virus leukaemic line kindly provided by Frank Lilly. Quantitative absorbtion experiments were done using specific H-2 alloantisera and an imbalance in the expression of the H-2K and H-2D antigens was found in several lines e.g. K36, 344 and 389 where $H-2K^k$ is virtually absent but $H-2D^k$ is normally expressed. However in other lines like K-GV and 422 both H-2K and H-2D are greatly reduced and in the 369 line both H-2K and H-2D are greatly increased. In the 424 cell line both H-2K and H-2D are normally expressed. These differences in expression are clearly important in the way the immune system reacts to these cells (Figures 1, 2 & 4) (Festenstein & Schmidt, 1981).

If the expression of H-2K is important in the prevention of Gross virus leukaemias one might wonder how leukaemic cell lines like the 369 cell line which expresses a large amount of the $H-2K^k$ antigen escaped immune surveillance. The initial observation that AKR mice inoculated with this tumour produce an "autoantibody" which reacts with the 369 tumour has now been extended. The findings clearly indicate that an "autoantibody" in the serum is directed against H-2K antigens which could be precipitated from lysates of leukaemic cells. The experiments reported by Schmidt (1987) included inhibition experiments with H-2 negative leukaemic cells and certain allogeneic lymphocytes which excluded the possibility that the precipitation was due to antiviral antibodies. However the antibody reacted not only with the tumour cells but also with mitogen activated AKR cells. These antibodies may thus have a direct effect on immune surveillance in vivo by covering up the relevant potential restriction elements (all the CTL experiments in vitro do not contain this antibody). In addition this antibody reacts with certain allogeneic cells especially of the $H-2^b$ and $H-2^d$ haplotypes but not normal AKR cells. This finding is especially intriguing since the 369 cell also expresses an $H-2D^d$-like antigen which reacts with the 34-5-8 anti $H-2D^d$ monoclonal antibody which we have previously demonstrated in the K36, 424 and other leukaemic lines (Figure 9). This antibody may be reacting with a gene converted

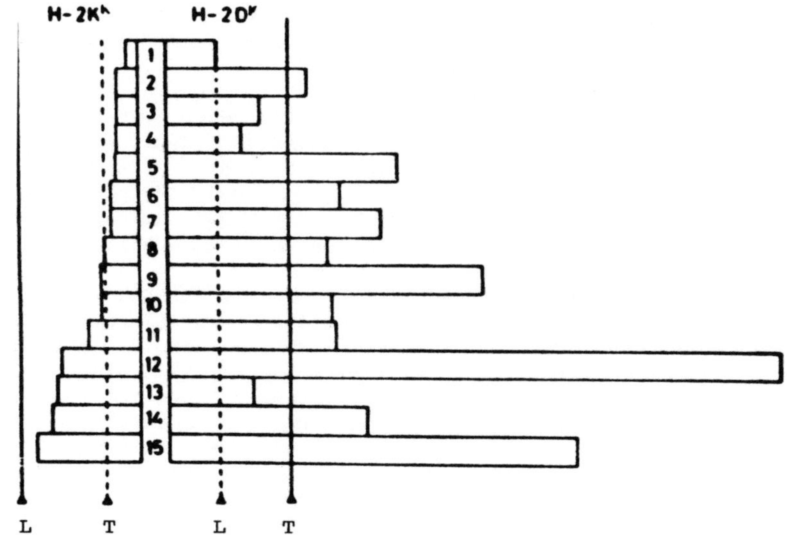

L = Lymphocytes.   T = Thymocytes.

Fig. 5. H-2K and H-2D antigen expression on primary AKR leukaemias (Festenstein & Schmidt, 1981).

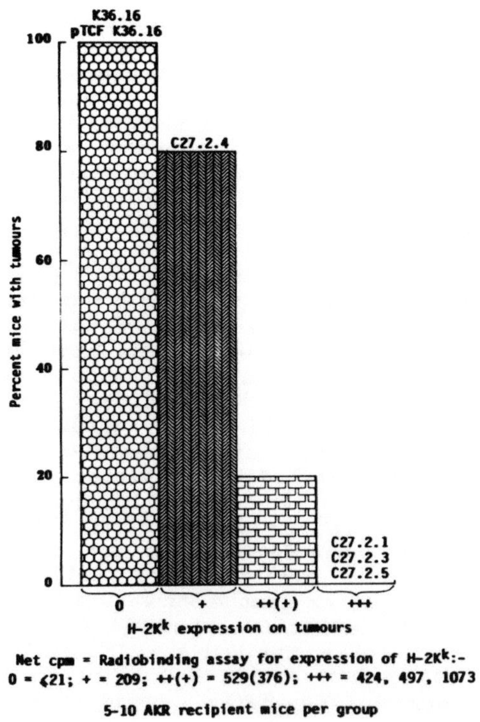

Fig. 6. Tumour incidence varies according to H-2K expression

Qa/TL-like specificity which could cross react with this antibody (see section on Aberrant Extra "Allospecificities") and may be involved in tumour promotion. These concepts are supported by the observations of Schmidt in that the development of spontaneous leukaemias are greatly facilitated and speeded up by immunising AKR mice with the leukaemic line 369 (Schmidt, 1987).

We also made a special study of the amount of H-2K and H-2D expressed on spontaneous primary tumours derived from AKR mice. They were typed not only for the representation of their H-2 antigens but also for Thy-1 and viral antigens using monoclonal antibodies and alloantisera in complement dependent cytotoxicity and absorbtion assays. We confirmed that the H-$2K^k$ antigen/s are either completely lost or greatly reduced in many of the spontaneous AKR leukaemias. The results of testing are shown in Figure 5 (Festenstein & Schmidt, 1981). In approximately half these leukaemias H-$2K^k$ antigen expression was reduced to less than one finds on normal thymic cells. The remainder had H-$2K^k$ expression either equivalent to or slightly more than the amount present on normal AKR thymic cells but less than one finds on normal AKR lymph node cells. In contrast the H-$2D^k$ antigens were uniformly increased by 2 to 12x in 14/15 of the leukaemic cells. All these leukaemias expressed more H-$2D^k$ than are normally expressed on thymocytes and 11/14 had more H-$2D^k$ than are normally present on lymph node cells. However the overall balance between H-2K and H-2D expression in the AKR leukaemias is generally in favour of H-2D, suggesting that the latter may be relevant for tumour promotion, results consistent with those of Meruello (1980), Segal, Feldman (Katzav et al, 1983), and Rigby (Brickell et al, 1985).

H-2 CLASS I TRANSFECTION EXPERIMENTS

As the degree of H-2K expression is generally correlated with the extent of anti AKR leukaemia T cell cytotoxicity, high levels of H-2K expression may also be indicative of potential resistance to Gross virus leukaemogenesis.

We then designed experiments in collaboration with Dr Grosveld at the NIMR to test this hypothesis and to ascertain whether the H-$2K^k$ molecule was essential for effective host anti tumour interaction to occur. The experiments were devised to cause the H-$2K^k$ antigen to become expressed in the H-$2K^k$-deficient cell line K36.16 and, if so to find whether they would grow less easily that the original tumour which is H-$2K^k$-deficient. Accordingly, we introduced into K36.16 by DNA-mediated gene transfer, a normal AKR H-$2K^k$ cloned gene, c27.2 together with the G418-resistant plasmid pTCF. Different amounts of the H-$2K^k$ molecules were found in the various transformant clones. The presence of H-$2K^k$ specific mRNA was shown to be present by SI nuclease protection mapping. The H-$2K^k$ gene products are immunoprecipitable from the transformants which express the largest amount of the H-$2K^k$ molecule The results of these experiments showed that the ability of the H-$2K^k$ deficient leukaemia K36.16 to grow in vivo was impaired when the normal H-$2K^k$ gene became expressed after DNA-mediated gene transfer (Hui, Grosveld & Festenstein, 1984).

These findings suggest that the relative absence of the H-$2K^k$ specificity gave the tumour cells a selection advantage in vivo. Because high H-$2K^k$ antigen-expressing transformants were rejected more efficiently than low expressors, it implies that a certain minimum of H-$2K^k$ antigen is needed to elicit the rejection response. These responses may include the early generation of cytostasis effectors that appear to be important in the prevention of the development of the tumour (Hui et al 1985), (Figure 6).

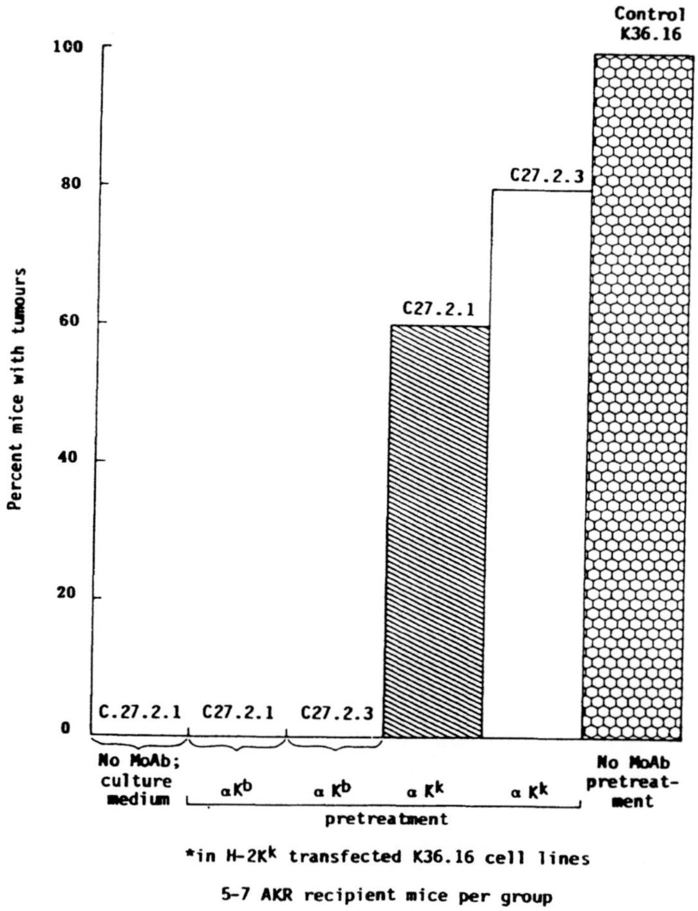

Fig. 7. Reversal of $H\text{-}2K^k$ protection by anti $H\text{-}2K^k$ MoAb pretreatment

(Adapted from Hui, Grosveld & Festenstein, Nature, 311: 750-752, 1984).

Table 3. Mice Immunised with the Transfected Clones Reject a Second Challenge of the Original K36.16 Tumour Cells

AKR mice primed with clone	No. of mice with tumours 30 days after challenge with K36.16
C27.2.3	0/5
C27.2.3 *(mitomycin C treated)	4/5
C27.2.2	0/5
C27.2.4	0/2
K36.16 *(mitomycin C treated)	5/5

AKR mice were injected s.c. with 10^5 C27.2 transfected tumour cells. The mice rejected the tumours. After 3-4 weeks, the mice were challenged with 10^5 K36.16 tumour cells.

*Mitomycin C treatment consisted of 50 $\mu g/ml^{-1}$ 10^6 cells for 30 min at 37°C, followed by 4 washings with PBS. These control cells were also injected s.c. as indicated above.

Adapted from Hui et al. Nature 311: 750, 1984.

We were also able to reverse the protection by "covering up" the transfected gene product by exposing the tumours to anti K^k MoAbs prior to inoculation and then injecting the mice with the anti H-$2K^k$ monoclonal antibodies (Figure 7). Similar results of transfection experiments were also obtained by the groups of Shraga Segal, Gunter Hammerling and Michael Feldman (Wallich et al, 1985; Hammerling et al, 1986) working with several other tumour systems where H-2K gene expression was decreased and in which metastasis appeared to be dependent upon low H-2K and high H-2D expression. Transfection of the H-2K gene was also effective in preventing growth of the tumours and/or metastatic spread. An interesting additional observation with respect to the AKR leukaemias but not with the other tumours is that after rejecting the transfected K36 tumour they were protected when challenged with the original K36 tumour. The transfected tumour thus appeared to behave like a "vaccine" (Table 3).

The MHC antigenic profile of tumour cells may be modified by a variety of factors and mechanisms and it is clear from the work reviewed here that the consequences of decreased expression or loss of determinants affect T cell surveillance of the tumour and hence its ability to grow. In contrast the unexpected gain of novel histocompatibility "allospecificities" on syngeneic tumours may provide the means in some instances by which the immune system can bring them under control. However, these novel "allospecificities" may, instead of initiating rejection of the tumours, be tumour promoting e.g. through the stimulation of suppressor cells. Although there are many possible mechanisms which cause variations in the MHC antigenic profiles of tumour cells, definitive evidence for specific mechanisms have not yet been established in many instances. Disturbances in genetic regulatory mechanisms are obviously important in the selective decrease in expression of the H-$2K^k$ gene product. Southern blot experiments with the K36.16 tumour have ruled out the possibility that there is structural gene deletion of the H-$2K^k$ gene (Hui et al, 1986). Cell

H-2D^d expression on K36.16

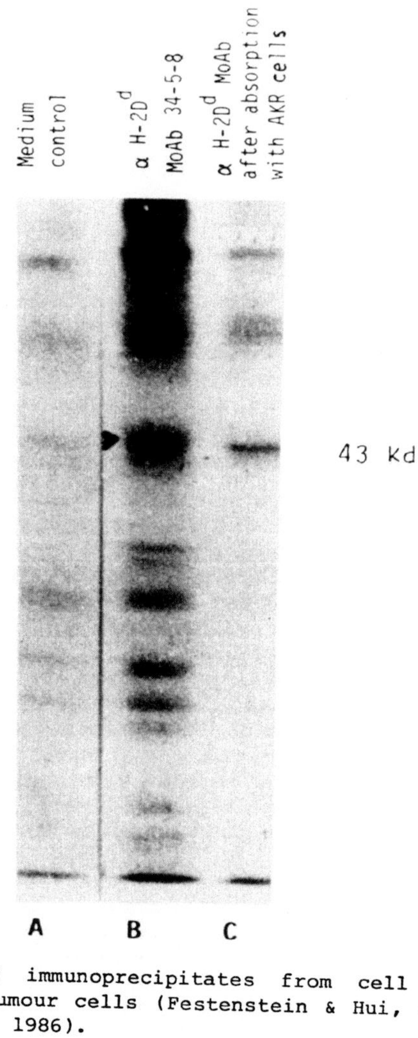

Fig. 8. SDS-PAGE of immunoprecipitates from cell membrane extract of K36.16 tumour cells (Festenstein & Hui, J. Immunogenetics, 13: 113-116, 1986).

fusion experiments performed by Bishop et al, (1982) in this laboratory indicate that a specific dominant gene is probably involved in the down regulation of the representation of $H-2K^k$ in the K36 leukaemia. Fusion with $H-2K^k$ normal lymphocytes resulted in hybrids expressing the $H-2D^k$ specificity in normal amounts but having a substantially reduced level of the $H-2K^k$ gene product. Furthermore, fusion with $H-2^b$ cells failed to induce reexpression of this gene product, while the $H-2K^b$ levels were not suppressed. The mechanism is not yet established. Gene methylation may be involved, associated with reduced $H-2K^k$ mRNA and excessive selective sialylation of $H-2K^k$. Attempts to clone the $H-2K^k$ gene from K36 have so far been unsuccessful.

The role of viruses in MHC gene regulation and/or rearrangements was also investigated by Schrier et al, (1985) who showed that adenovirus 12 in transformed rat cells switches off the expression of Class I MHC antigens and as a result such cells are highly oncogenic. In contrast, non-oncogenic adenovirus strain A5, which does express MHC antigens, albeit at a lower level, is resistant to oncogenesis. H-2 Class I transfection experiments by Tanaka et al, (1986) potentiated immune recognition of murine tumour cells induced by adenovirus 12.

ABERRANT EXTRA "ALLOSPECIFICITIES" ON AKR LEUKAEMIAS

The finding of aberrant MHC-like "allospecificities" on malignant cells has been the subject of intensive research during the past decade. Initially, many difficulties were encountered in establishing the true nature of these aberrant molecules because of the transient expression of some of these specificities (Garrido et al, 1976), the low level of representation on the tumour cell surface in other instances (Festenstein & Schmidt, 1981) and the presence of anti-viral antibodies in many of the alloantisera employed. But recent technological advances, particularly the development of monoclonal antibodies (MoAbs) and molecular biological techniques, have led to rapid progress in this field of research. As indicated above, the K36.16 spontaneous thymoma, expresses an aberrant $H-2D^d$-like "allospecificity" (Schmidt & Festenstein, 1980). In addition it is Thy-1.1 and $H-2D^k$ positive. It is also TL negative but expresses a variety of Gross virus surface antigens (gp70, p30, p15, and G_{IX}). The extra $H-2D^d$ "allospecificity" proved to be a M_r 45kD glycoprotein which was precipitated from radiolabelled K36.16 cell membrane lysates using anti-H-2 alloantisera. (The total amount of the $H-2D^d$ was 50-100 times less than the normal $H-2D^d$ on BALB/c lymphoid cells). Peptide maps were then done. The tryptic peptides of ^3H-arginine labelled K36.16 precipitated by $H-2D^d$ alloantiserum were compared with a ^{14}C-arginine labelled $H-2D^d$ positive control. Although all the specific $H-2D^d$ peaks were apparently included in the K36.16 pattern, there were also a number of extra peaks which did not correspond with the $H-2D^d$ and we were unable to account for and which we attributed to viral products (Schmidt & Festenstein, 1980; Festenstein & Schmidt 1981). The results of direct and cold target inhibition functional assays were also consistent with the conclusion that the aberrant "allospecificity" is $H-2D^d$-like. So, when anti $H-2D^d$ MoAbs became available (Ozato et al, 1982) we used them to investigate further these findings using radiobinding and immunoprecipitation studies (Festenstein & Hui, 1986).

The results of immunoprecipitation are shown in Figure 8. Three lanes are shown: (A) medium control, (B) immunoprecipitate with MoAb 34-5-8 (anti-$H-2D^d$) and (C) with anti-D^d 34-5-8 after absorbtion with AKR spleen cells. An M_r 43 kD band was evident and became much clearer when precipitated with the pre-absorbed 34-5-8 antibody (Figure 8).

Radiobinding Assays of AKR leukaemia using H-2K^k, H-2D^k and H-2D^d MoAbs

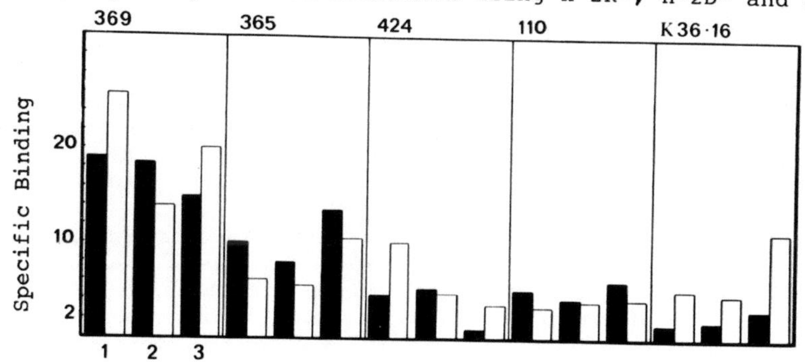

Fig. 9: Cell-binding radioimmunoassays before (solid bars) and after (open bars) neuraminidase treatment of the AKR derived leukaemias. The affinity purified MoAbs used were (1) 15-1-5, anti H-2K^k, H-2D^k; (2) H100-5 anti H-2K^k and (3) 34-5-8, anti H-2D^d. 2x10^5 tumour cells were incubated overnight at 4°C with the specific MoAb. ^{125}I-F(ab')$_2$ sheep anti-mouse immunoglobulin was used as a second antibody. Each bar represents an average of three independent sets of experiments done in triplicate (S.D. less than 5%). The specific binding is expressed as times the background values (250 cpm).

Immunoprecipitations from affinity purified 424 glycoproteins (gps)

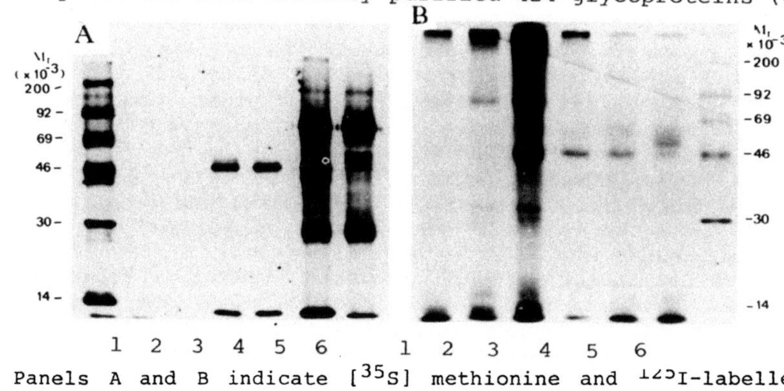

Fig. 10: Panels A and B indicate [^{35}S] methionine and ^{125}I-labelled gps. Panel A, lane 1: tissue culture medium (RPMI 1640). Lane 2: 34-5-8. Lane 3: 15-1-5. Lane 4: supernatant from the previous immunoprecipitation (lane 3) incubated with 34-5-8 MoAb. Lane 6: C3H/He with 34-5-8. Panel B, lanes 1-4: the same distribution as Panel A. Lane 5: BALB/c with 34-5-8. Lane 6: BALB/c with 34-1-2 (HB 79, anti-H-2K^d, H-2D^d) MoAb. MoAb supernatants were used.

It is interesting to note that the 34-5-8 antibody, which does not give a positive radiobinding result, nevertheless gives a positive immunoprecipitation result. Since not all the anti-H-2D^d MoAbs react with the K36.16 tumour line it implies that there is heterogeneity of reactivity of these different antibodies. It could be that the positive reactions are due to the presence of specific epitopes which are common to the H-2D^d specificity but that the specificity with which the antibody reacts is not a classical H-2D^d molecule. The genetic basis of the expression of this H-2D^d-like "allospecificity" is not yet understood. However, there is sufficient homology with the H-2D^d-like antigen as judged not only by the above techniques but by cellular assays as previously described (Festenstein et al, 1983).

We are currently investigating other AKR leukaemias to see if they also express this H-2D^d-like antigen. Preliminary results indicate that this aberrant H-2D^d-like "allospecificity" is indeed present on other AKR leukaemic lines.

Five of Peter Krammer's AKR leukaemic lines were studied. The results of radiobinding experiments using H-2 monoclonal antibodies are shown in Figure 9. All these leukaemic lines were tested before and after treatment with neuraminidase and all are positive although the levels of binding varied somewhat. The results confirmed the low-level of expression of the H-2D^d-like antigen on K36 and 424 without pretreatment with neuraminidase. After treatment with neuraminidase the levels increased to 10 and 3.5 times background respectively. Both cell lines 365 and 369 express high levels of the H-2D^d-like "allospecificity" both before and after neuraminidase treatment. Significantly positive but lower levels of expression were found on cell line 110. Direct immunoprecipitations of ^{35}S-metabolically labelled glycoproteins from 369 were also done with 34-5-8 MoAb. They showed the classical H-2 Class I 46 kD and 12 kD patterns.

These results clearly indicate that the expression of the H-2D^d-like "allospecificity" is likely to be general for all AKR leukaemias and that in those instances where the specificities could not readily be detected by binding without neuraminidase treatment, e.g. in 424, a heavy 46kD immunoprecipitate was obtained with the H-2D^d specific alloantibody 34-5-8 but only after preclearance of the syngeneic H-2K^k and H-2D^k specificities (Figures 10 and 11). Two-dimensional gel electrophoresis of the H-2D^d reactive molecule shows a unique pattern differnt from those of the normal H-2D^d,H-2K^k and H-2D^k. Structural analysis of the likely homology of this molecule with that of the classical H-2D^d from BALB/c strain is in progress.

As the putative novel H-2D^d-reactive molecule escapes detection by direct cell-binding radioimmunoassay and immunoprecipitation and could only be detected after preclearing of the syngeneic specificities from the 424 glycoprotein pool or after enzymatic treatment of the tumour cells it suggests that epigenetic phenomena may account for these anomalies: (a) the specificities may be obscured by excessive sialylation and/or (b) the relevant epitopes may be hidden by macromolecular associations with syngeneic H-2 Class I antigens. Sialic acid is found in the terminal or inside positions of the oligosaccharide chain on MHC Class I glycoproteins. Thus, it is feasible that the bulky, negatively charged sialic acid residue, together with the large and often branched oligosaccharide chain, covers the polypeptide part of a neighbouring molecule in the cell membrane or influences its conformation so that it is not recognised by the immune system (unpublished data).

Sequential immunoprecipitation of the H-2D^d-like antigen

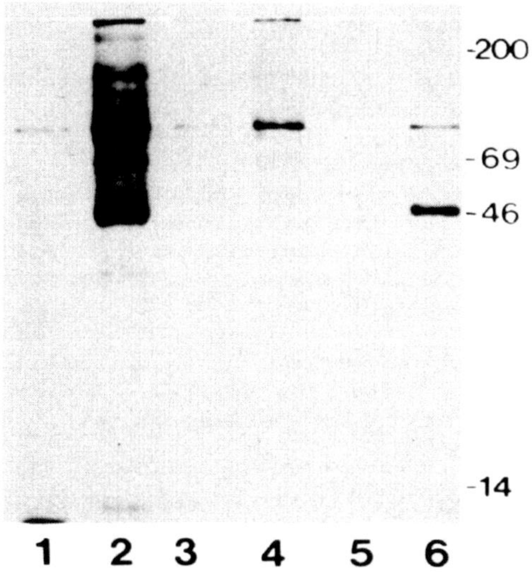

Fig. 11: Sequential immunodepletion of the [^{35}S] labelled 424 tumour glycoproteins. Lane 1: PBS. Lane 2: 15-1-5 (anti-H-2K^k, H-2D^k) MoAb. Lane 3: Supernatant from previous immunoprecipitation (Lane 2) with 15-1-5. Lane 4: Supernatant from Lane 3 with 15-1-5. Lane 5: Supernatant from Lane 4 with excess of protein A. Lane 6: Supernatant from Lane 5, with 34-5-8 (anti-H-2D^d) MoAb.

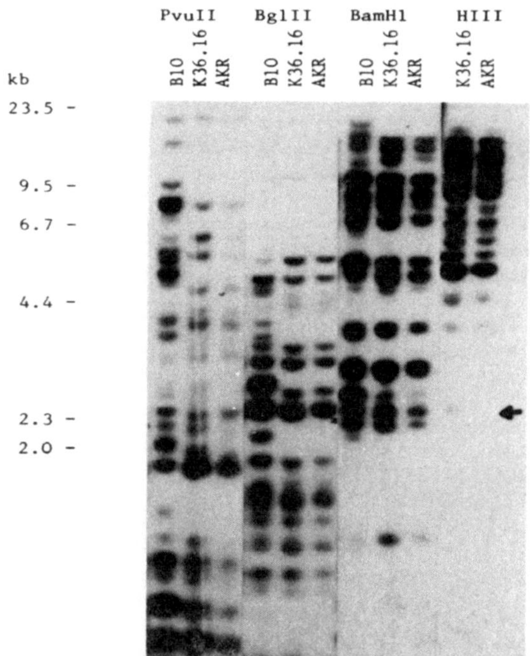

Fig. 12: Southern blots of normal AKR thymus and K36.16. Probe: pH-2IIa, c' cDNA gene (Hui et al 1986).

The use of nonionic detergents (NP-40,Triton X-100) to solubilise the 424 glycoproteins may lead to the formation of soluble protein complexes in which the novel antigen is selectively associated with at least one of the Class I specificities. This association may render the H-2D^d reactive epitopes inaccessible to the specific monoclonal antibody. The anti H-2K^k and H-2D^k MoAb (15-1-5) may disrupt such complexes. Thus after "preclearing" the syngeneic antigens, the H-2D^d reactive epitopes become reactive with the 34-5-8 specific MoAb.

To test this hypothesis, a zwitterionic detergent (CHAPS) was used to solubilise the 424 glycoproteins. It is known that this type of detergent is highly efficient at breaking protein-protein interactions. Immunoprecipitations done with the 34-5-8 MoAb are consistent with this hypothesis: 46kD and 12kD bands compared with the classical H-2 Class I pattern were obtained by SDS-PAGE after **direct precipitation** with the anti-H-2D^d MoAb using the CHAPS solubilized glycoprotein pool (Labeta et al, 1987).

To investigate the genetic basis of the altered MHC profiles, DNA from normal AKR thymus, K36.16 thymoma and normal C57BL/10 thymus was digested with endonucleases and hybridized with the probes mentioned above. No differences were seen between the K36.16 tumour DNA and the DNA of the strain of origin (AKR) using either the 5' flanking probe or the pH-2III probe. But as expected, differences were seen with the C57BL/10 (H-2^b) thymus DNA. However, hybridisation of the Hind III digested DNA with the pH-2IIa probe (Steinmetz et al, 1981) revealed a fragment of about 2.8 kb which is present in the K36.16 genomic DNA but absent from that of the AKR thymus DNA (Figure 12). Although these results rule out gross rearrangements and deletions in the H-2 region of the K36.16 cells, the assay is not sensitive enough to detect point mutations or minor changes resulting from gene conversion or small deletions. Nevertheless, we can detect differences between the AKR thymoma and the normal AKR DNA but are, as yet, unable to assign the 2.8 kb band to any particular MHC gene. As a consequence we do not know whether this particular change has any relation to the K36.16 oncogenic phenotype, the lack of expression of the H-2K^k molecule or the aberrant H-2D^d-like "allospecificities". These changes in the Southern blots nevertheless, indicate that some variations in the MHC genome must have taken place in the tumours and may be responsible for some of the altered biological properties. This should become clear once we have cloned and sequenced the H-2K gene from K36.16. These experiments are currently in progress (Hui et al, 1986).

MECHANISMS

Disturbances in the genetic regulation could result in the expression of genes with failure of expression of normal syngeneic antigens and the derepression of silent Qa/Tla structural genes homologous to H-2D^d.

Such mechanisms involving regulatory genes have already been invoked to explain the "anomalous" expression of TL antigens in some leukaemias. For example, in Gross virus leukaemia TL antigens not only of the relevant syngeneic strain but also those of allogeneic strains may be expressed as a result of derepression of the Tla genes.

The TL antigens are antigens of differentiation as well as antigens which occur anomalously on leukaemias. Tla^b strains like AKR do not express TL antigens on their normal thymocytes. But when spontaneous AKR leukaemias develop, approximately 11% become TL positive and express TL 1,2 and 4. Other strains like BALB/c and DBA/2 of the Tla^c haplotype express the TL2 differentiation antigen only on normal thymocytes but TL1 or TL1 and TL4 in addition to TL2 on TL positive leukaemias. TL4 is not a differentiation antigen. It is expressed only on leukaemic cells (Old & Stockert, 1977). If the TL antigens cross react with H-2D^{d} this could explain our results. However, all our AKR leukaemic cell lines have been tested for the TL4 antigen by radiobinding with MoAb before and after neuraminidase treatment as well as by immunoprecipitation and none have so far been positive.

Another possible explanation for the presence of an H-D^{d} epitope on the AKR leukaemias is that certain Qa DNA sequences that are not normally expressed may be transferred to another Qa or H-2K^{k} gene by gene conversion. The 424 tumour expresses H-2K^{k} as well as reacting with the H-2D^{d} monoclonal antibody 34-5-8. The reactivity of the H-2D^{d} monoclonal antibody is extremely strong especially after preclearance of the syngeneic H-2K^{k} and H-2D^{k} specificities. This result indicates that the H-2D^{d} reactivity cannot be due to gene conversion of the H-2K^{k} gene. Neither can it be due to viral alteration of the H-2K^{k} gene product. It is therefore clear that the structural gene for the H-2D^{d} epitope must be present in all the AKR leukaemias so far studied. It is structurally distinct from the syngeneic H-2K^{k} specificity but could be part of a macromolecular complex involving the syngeneic Class I specificities. Activation of the oncogenic Gross virus has apparently enabled the relevant gene sequence to become expressed. Such a product may be central to the leukaemogenic process. Expression of this normally silent gene (it is absent from normal resting AKR cells) could come about through several possible mechanisms: (1) the Gross retrovirus may integrate close to the regulatory control of this DNA sequence and cause it to become expressed. (2) The Gross virus may initiate a recombinational event thus removing putative codon stops or other inhibitory DNA sequences and causing a Qa gene with close homology to H-2D^{d} to become expressed. (3) Through gene conversion to another Class I gene other than H-2K. The donor sequence could be derived from a Qa or Tla gene homologous to the H-2D^{d} gene.

Genetic recombination is also a likely mechanism for the production of aberrant "allospecificities" on syngeneic tumours. It is similar to the one proposed by Nathenson and colleagues (1986) for the generation of H-2K^{b} mutants. The mechanism implies the transfer of DNA sequences from one Class I gene to another, by reciprocal crossing over, by unequal crossing over or by gene conversion and postmeiotic or mitotic segregation. It has been clearly established by Nathenson that the various H-2K^{b} mutants have their origin in the transfer of a minimum of 5 nucleotides e.g. from Q4 to H-2K^{b} to produce the mutants bm6 and bm9 and from Q10 to produce the mutants bm1 and bm23. The donor DNA sequences for the mutants bm10 and bm11 are probably derived from K1 and H-2D^{d} respectively.

ABERRANT MHC "ALLOSPECIFICITIES" IN OTHER TUMOURS

A system that has been studied by Marelli and colleagues (1982) for the expression of allodeterminants is the L1210 Cr (DBA/2-H-2^{d}, - a methyl cholanthrene induced lymphoma). Previous reports showed that the L1210 Cr, treated in vivo with DTIC (Dacarbazine) became immunogenic and was rejected by the syngeneic host. CTL's raised against the H-2^{d} xenogenised line reacted with H-2K^{k} blast cells indicating the presence of an H-2^{k}like Class I "allospecificity" on the tumour cells.

The original L1210 Cr was cloned by limiting dilution in vitro and subcloned in vivo. One of these subclones expresses an "allospecificity" resembling $H-2K^k$ by monoclonal antibody testing, before and after treatment with neuraminidase. In addition when the same subclone was treated with DTIC there was a dramatic increase of the "allospecifcity" $H-2K^k$ and also of the syngeneic $H-2D^d$ and $H-2K^d$ specificities. The reaction with the public specificity monoclonal antibody (anti $H-2K^k$, $H-2D^k$), was not increased by neuraminidase treatment although there is twice the amount of this specificity on the DTIC tumour compared with the untreated L1210 Cr tumour. After neuraminidase treatment and testing the DTIC tumour with anti $H-2K^k$ monoclonal antibody there was a substantial increase in expression, comparable to the level of the syngeneic $H-2K^d$ specificity. Molecular studies are in progress.

More recent reports of aberrant specificities have been made by the groups of Schreiber, Goodenow and McMillan working with UV-induced mouse tumours Philipps et al, (1986), Stauss et al, (1986) and by Schmidt working with Rous sarcoma-induced tumours in mice. These tumours are additional examples in which H-2-like "allospecificities" are expressed on syngeneic tumours. The mechanism involved could be similar to the ones described above for the AKR leukaemias.

In another model Karre studied YAC-I tumour cells induced by Moloney virus. Increased amounts of H-2 antigen expression is directly related to increased metastatic potential. The host response in this case is dependent on natural killer cell activity, which operates best when H-2 antigens are absent from the target cells (Ljunggren and Karre, 1986).

Expression of MHC antigens on human tumour cells also vary. Extra HLA Class I-like specificities of the HLA-Aw19 cross-reactive group on HTLV-1 infected cells have been described by Mann et al, (1983) and HLA Class I and II specificity gains and losses in adult T cell leukaemia-lymphoma patients and family members by Sonoda et al, (1986). They have been attributed by Mann to the high degree of cross-reactivity between virally-induced, tumour associated antigens and these HLA specificities.

CONCLUSION

The understanding of the genetic and molecular biological mechanisms responsible for the expression of aberrant (extra) MHC-like "allospecificities" on tumour cells is of critical importance also for the understanding of the genetic organisation and control of expression of the MHC genes themselves.

DNA rearrangement and gene conversion events involving the multiple silent Qa and Tla-like genes and MHC pseudogenes which have a considerable degree of homology with other MHC genes could provide the genetic basis of aberrant MHC antigenic expression. Toxic chemicals, radiation effects and viruses may all play a part in initiating the process. Such aberrant MHC molecules may function either as tumour associated transplantation antigens in one context or may even be intrinsically suppressor and tumour promoting in another genetic context.

ACKNOWLEDGEMENT

We are grateful for the generous financial support provided by the Cancer Research Campaign and The Medical Research Council of Great Britain. We are also greatly indebted to Valerie Verbi and Denny Williams for preparing this manuscript for publication.

REFERENCES

Bishop, C.E., Lewis, C.M. & Festenstein, H.: Dominant allele-specific regulation of expression of H-2K^k gene products revealed by somatic cell hybridisation. Somatic Cell Genetics, 8: 623-634, 1982.

Bonavida, B.: The SLJ/J spontaneous reticulum cell sarcoma: new insights in the fields of neoantigens, host-tumour interactions, and the regulation of tumour growth. Adv. Cancer Res., 38: 1-22, 1983.

Brickell, P., Latchman, D., Murphy D., Willison, K. & Rigby, P.W.J.: The Class I major histocompatibility antigen gene activated in a line of SV-40-transformed mouse cells is H-2D^d, not Qa/Tla. Nature 316: 162-163, 1985.

Festenstein, H., Garrido, F., Matossian-Rogers, A., Schirrmacher, V., Schmidt, W., DeGiorgi, L., Biasi, G. & Jaraquemada, D.: The major histocompatibility system, tumours and viruses, in: HLA System, New Aspects (ed. G.B. Ferrara), Elsevier/North Holland Biomedical Press, p.53-67, 1977.

Festenstein, H. & Schmidt, W.: Variation in MHC antigenic profiles of tumour cells and its biological effects. Immunological Rev., 60: 85-127, 1981.

Festenstein, H., Alonzo, A., Ferluga, J., Ma, B.L., Santamaria, O., Marelli, O., Schmidt, W. & Flavell, R.A.: Further molecular and functional evidence for the expression of H-2 allodeterminants on the AKR leukaemia, K36. Transpl. Proc., 15: 2107-2110, 1983.

Festenstein, H. & Hui, K.M.: Aberrant H-2-like allospecificities on K36.16 thymoma. Studies of radiobinding and immunoprecipitation with anti-H-2 monoclonal antibodies. J. Immunogenetics, 13: 113-116, 1986.

Garrido, F., Festenstein, H. & Schirrmacher, V.: Further evidence for derepression of H-2 and Ia-like specificities of foreign haplotypes in mouse tumour cell lines. Nature, 261: 705-707, 1976a.

Garrido, F., Schirrmacher, V. & Festenstein, H.: H-2-like specificities of foreign haplotypes appearing on a mouse sarcoma after vaccinia virus infection. Nature, 259: 228-230, 1976b.

Garrido, F., Schirrmacher, V. & Festenstein, H.: Studies on H-2 specificities on mouse tumour cells by a new microradioassay. J. Immunogenetics, 4: 15-27.

Garrido, F., Schmidt, W. & Festenstein, H.: Immunogenetic studies on Meth.A vaccinia tumour cells in vivo and in vitro. J. Immunogenetics, 4: 115-125, 1977.

Hammerling, G.J., Klar, D., Katzav, S., Segal, S., Feldman, M., Wallich, R. & Hammerling, A.: Manipulation of metastasis and tumour growth by transfection with histocompatibility Class I genes. J. Immunogenetics, 13: 153-157, 1986.

Hui, K.M., Grosveld, F. & Festenstein, H.: Rejection of transplantable AKR leukaemia following MHC DNA-mediated cell transformation. Nature, 311: 750-752, 1984.

Hui, K.M., Matossian-Rogers, A., Festenstein, H. & Grosveld, F.: Demonstration of cytostasis and H-2K^k antigen expression in an H-2K^k-deficient AKR leukaemia following DNA-mediated gene transfer. Transpl. Proc., 17: 955-956, 1985.

Hui, K.M., Minamide, L., Prandoni, N., Festenstein, H. & Grosveld, F.G.: Structural variations in the H-2 genes of AKR lymphomas. J. Immunogenetics, 13: 117-121, 1986.

Invernizzi, G. & Parmiani, G.: Tumour associated transplantation antigens of chemically induced sarcoma cross-reacting with allogeneic histocompatibility antigens. Nature, 254: 713, 1975.

Katzav, S., Tartokovsky, B., de Baetselier, P., Isakov, N., Feldman, M. & Segal, S.: H-2 and other major histocompatibility complexes; Biologic function. Transpl. Proc., 15: 162-170, 1983.

Labeta, M.O., Fernandez, N. & Festenstein, H.: Solubilisation effect of Nonidet P-40, Triton X-100 and CHAPS in the detection of MHC-like glycoproteins. (Submitted).

Lilly, F.: The inheritance of susceptibility to the Gross leukaemia virus in mice. Genetics, 53: 529, 1966.

Ljunggren, H-G. & Karre, K.: Variations in MHC antigen expression on tumours and its significance. Experimental strategies and interpretations in the analysis of changes in MHC gene expression during tumour progression: opposing influences of T cell and natural killer mediated resistance. J. Immunogenetics, 13: 141-151, 1986.

Mann, D., Popovic, M., Sarin, P., Murray, C., Reitz, M.S., Strong, D.M., Haynes, B.F., Gallo, R.C. & Blattner, W.A.: Cell lines producing human T-cell lymphoma virus show altered HLA expression. Nature, 305: 58-59, 1983.

Marelli, O., Testorelli, C., Canti, G., Festenstein, H. & Nicolin, A.: Immunological cross-reactivity between H-2D^K product and DTIC-treated H-2^d lymphoma. J. Immunogenetics, 9: 407-412, 1982.

Martin, W.J.: Immune surveillance directed against derepressed cellular and viral antigens. Cell. Immunol., 15: 1, 1975.

Martin, W.J., Gibson, T.G., Martin, S.W. & Rice, J.M.: Derepressed alloantigen on lung tumour cells transplacentally induced, coded by H-2 liked gene. Science, 194: 532, 1976.

Meruello, D.: H-2D control of leukaemia susceptibility: mechanisms and implications. J. Immunogenetics, 7: 81-90, 1980.

Old, E., Boyse, E.A. & Stockert, E.: The G (Gross) leukaemia antigen. Cancer Res., 25: 813, 1965.

Old, L.J. & Stockert, E.: Immunogenetics of cell surface antigens of mouse leukaemia. Ann. Rev. Genet., 17: 127-160, 1977.

Parmiani, G.: Foreign histocompatibility determinants as tumour associated transplantation antigens of chemically induced murine fibrosarcoma. In: HLA System - New Aspects (ed. G.B. Ferrara), Elsevier/North Holland Biomedical Press, p.45, 1977.

Philipps, G., Stauss, H.J., Wortzel, R.D. & Schreiber, H.: Unusual or aberrant MHC antigen expression on tumours. A novel MHC Class I molecule as a tumour-specific antigen. Correlation between the antibody-defined and the CTL-defined target structure. J. of Immunogenetics, 13: 93-99, 1986.

Schäfer, A. & Schmidt, W.: Resistance to cellular immune response in AKR leukaemias. Eur. J. Immunol., 16: 753, 1986.

Schmidt, W., Leben, L., Atfield, G. & Festenstein, H.: Variation of expression of histocompatibility antigens on tumour cells: absence of H-2K^k gene products from a Gross virus induced leukaemia in BALB.K. Immunogenetics, 14: 323-339, 1981.

Schmidt, W., Alonzo, A., Leben, L. & Festenstein, H.: Differential regulation of H-2 antigen expression in tumours and its biological consequences. Transpl. Proc., 13: 1814-1818, 1981.

Schmidt, W. & Festenstein, H.: Resistance to cell-mediated cytotoxicity is correlated with reduction of H-2K gene products in AKR leukaemia. Immunogenetics, 16: 257-264, 1982.

Schmidt, W.: H-2 specific antibodies induced by injection of syngeneic leukaemia cells. Immunogenetics, 25: 215-221, 1987.

Schrier, P.I., Bernards, R., Vaessen, R.T.M.J., Houweling, A. & van der Eb, A.J.: Expression of Class I major histocompatibility antigens switched off by highly oncogenic adenovirus 12 in transformed rat cells. Nature, 309: 771, 1983.

Sonoda, S., Yashiki, S., Takahashi, K., Matsumoto, T., Matsumoto, M., Yunoki, K., Sato, K., Inoko, H. & Tsuji, K.: Altered expression of MHC Class I and II antigens in T and B lymphocytes of adult T cell leukaemia-lymphoma patients. Proceedings from the Third Asia-Oceania Histocompatibility Workshop Conference (ed. M. Aizawa), Hokkaido University Press, Sapporo, Japan, p.628-631.

Stauss, H.J., Linsk, R., Fischer, A., Watts, S., Banasiak, D., Haberman, A., Clark, I., Forman, J., McMillan, M., Schreiber, H. & Goodenow, R.S.: The MHC genes encoding the tumour specific Class I antigens expressed on a murine fibrosarcoma. J. Immunogenetics, 13: 101-112, 1986.

Steinmetz, M., Frelinger, J.S., Fisher, D., Hunkapiller, T., Pereira, D., Weissman, S.M., Uehara, H., Nathenson, S. & Hood, L.: Three cDNA clones encoding mouse transplantation antigens: Homology to Immunoglobulin genes. Cell, 24: 125-134, 1981.

Tanaka, K., Hayashi, H., Hamada, C., Khoury, G. & Gilbert, J.: Expression of major histocompatibility complex Class I antigens as a strategy for the potentiation of immune recognition of tumour cells. Proc. Natl. Acad. Sci. (USA), 83: 8723-8727, 1986.

Wallich, R., Bulbuc, N., Hammerling, G., Katzav, S., Segal, S. & Feldman, M.: Abrogation of metastatic properties of tumour cells by de novo expression of H-2K antigens following H-2 gene transfection. Nature, 315: 301, 1985.

CLASS I ANTIGEN EXPRESSION IN LINE 1 CELLS: MOLECULAR BIOLOGY AND IMMUNOLOGICAL EFFECTS

John G. Frelinger, Karen M. Cerosaletti, David W. Bahler, Lee W. Harwell and Edith M. Lord

Department of Microbiology and Immunology, University of Rochester Cancer Center, Rochester, N.Y.

ABSTRACT

Cultured line 1 murine lung carcinoma cells normally express very low levels of class I H-2 antigens. We have continued our investigations of line 1 lung carcinoma cells to understand the molecular basis of decreased expression of class I H-2 antigens and class I antigen induction with dimethyl sulfoxide (DMSO). We show that line 1, a murine lung carcinoma cell line, has low levels of class I antigens (H-2K, D, and L) because it is deficient in both class I and beta$_2$-microglobulin (B2M) RNAs, and that the mRNAs can be coordinately induced with dimethyl sulfoxide (DMSO). Our experiments suggest that interferon can induce surface expression of class I antigens but may act through a different mechanism than DMSO in inducing class I antigens. To further evaluate the regulation of class I expression, H-2D^p genes were transfected into line 1 cells. The transfected H-2 genes appear to be constitutively expressed at much higher levels than are the endogenous class I genes and are associated with endogenous B2M protein. Surface expression of the D^p antigens on the transfectants is induced similar to the endogenous H-2^d haplotype class I antigens following treatment with DMSO. All the D^p transfectants had increased levels of B2M mRNA as well as higher levels of class I RNA when compared to control or untransfected line 1 cells. These results suggest that the regulation of class I and B2M genes is linked and that expression of class I genes can affect expression of B2M genes.

In order to investigate how the expression of class I antigens affects the *in vivo* growth of this spontaneous tumor, we transplanted the H-2D^p expressing transfectants into mice. Marked differences in tumorigenicity (defined as tumor growth in immunologically competent hosts) were observed between the D^p transfected cells and untransfected or control transfected line 1 cells in syngeneic mice only if the animals had previously received injections of irradiated D^p transfectants. Our *in vivo* results show that increased expression of class I antigens can reduce the growth of tumors like line 1 which lack all class I antigens.

INTRODUCTION

Class I major histocompatibility complex (MHC) antigens are the major transplantation antigens in graft rejection and serve as restriction elements for cytotoxic T lymphocytes during the recognition of foreign antigens such as viruses (Zinkernagel and Doherty, 1979). Recognition of non-MHC encoded molecules by cytotoxic T lymphocytes depends on the expression of both the appropriate target antigen and MHC antigens. Limiting quantities of either type of antigen can prevent cell lysis. It has also been suggested that class I molecules may play an important role in the killing of neoplastic cells (reviewed by Goodenow et al., 1985). This has been suggested initially by studies in which the aggressiveness of tumors correlated inversely with the expression of class I antigens. Using recombinant DNA transfection techniques, we and others have shown that class I antigen expression can have an effect on tumor growth in several spontaneous, chemically or virally induced tumors (Bahler et al., 1987, Wallich et al., 1985, Tanaka et al., 1985, and Hui et al., 1984).

The class I antigens have some interesting regulatory aspects. While most somatic cells in the adult express class I antigens, the antigens do not appear to be expressed in very early stages of embryonic life but are activated later in development. The level of class I antigen expression in adult mice also varies enormously between different cell types. For example, spleen cells express 100 times as much class I antigen per cell as heart, brain, or skeletal muscle cells (reviewed in Klein et al., 1975). Further, the levels of these antigens can be modulated in some cells by gamma interferon. All class I antigens are composed of two non-covalently associated subunits. The larger subunit or heavy chain is a 45,000 molecular weight component encoded in the MHC on chromosome 17 of the mouse. The smaller subunit is called beta$_2$-microglobulin (B2M) and is encoded on chromosome 2. The expression of a class I molecule on the cell surface requires both these subunits and thus the expression of these unlinked genes requires coordinate regulation (reviewed in Hood et al., 1983). The class I molecule can therefore serve as a relatively simple system to study this common problem of coordinately regulated unlinked genes. These regulatory aspects of class I expression and their importance in cellular interactions has led us to examine class I expression in detail.

In this paper, we will summarize and review our work with line 1 cells, a lung carcinoma cell line derived from a BALB/c mouse (Yuhas et al., 1974), to study both the regulation of class I genes and the biological effects of their expression. We have focussed on line 1 cells for a variety of reasons. First, the expression of class I proteins in line 1 cells is normally low but is both inducible and reversible over approximately a 50 fold range. Second, these cells are easily transfected making them amenable to various genetic studies. Finally, the line 1 cells are similar in many respects to small lung cell carcinoma (Bahler et al., 1987, and Doyle et al., 1985), and thus may serve as a good model system for this type of human tumor.

MATERIALS AND METHODS

Antigen Expression Assays

Radioimmunoassays were performed by incubating cells with first step antibody at saturating conditions at 4°C overnight. The cells were washed 3 times, incubated with ^{125}I-protein A at 4°C overnight. Cells were washed 3 times and radioactivity determined using a gamma counter.

Flow cytometry and density calculations were performed as described previously (Bahler and Lord, 1985a). Cells were induced using DMSO by culturing them for 3 days in media containing 3% DMSO.

Northern and Dot Blot Analysis

RNA was isolated using either the protocol of Cheley and Andersen, 1984 or Chirgwin et al., 1979 as noted in the Figures. Blots were performed as described by Thomas, 1980. The probes pH2III (Steinmetz et al., 1981) actin DmA2 (Fryberg et al., 1980) tubulin pBr 44-11, (Cleveland et al., 1980) or B2 pBRcB-3 (Parnes et al., 1981) were nick translated as described by Maniatis (Maniatis, et al., 1982).

Transfection Studies

Cells were cotransfected with pko-neo (Van Doren et al., 1984) and the DP plasmid F12 (Darsley et al., 1987) using calcium phosphate as described (Bahler et al., 1987). The B2M genomic clone psv227 (Parnes and Seidman, 1982) from a C57BL/6 mouse cloned into the psv2-gpt plasmid and was generously provided by Dr. Jane Parnes, Stanford University. The monoclonal antibody mc-B2M-B-clone 23 which detects the products of this allele of B2M was generously provided by Dr. Fung-Win Shen, Sloan Kettering Cancer Center (Chorney et al., 1982). The monoclonal antibody 7-16.10 which recognizes the D^p molecule was described previously (Harmon et al., 1983). The rabbit anti-B2M antibody was made against purified rat B2M and has been used previously on mouse cells (Frelinger et al., 1984).

Tumor Growth

Line 1 cells transfected with the pko-neo alone or a clone C13.10, derived from cells transfected with pko-neo and the D^p plasmid F12, were injected intramuscularly in the hind leg and tumor size followed over time as described. Mice were measured individually using calipers and the average diameter determined from two measurements.

RESULTS

DMSO and Gamma Interferon Induce the Expression of Class I Antigens

Line 1 cells express a very low level of class I antigens which are barely detectable using indirect immunofluorescence and flow cytometry. However, these cells can be induced to express approximately 50 fold more class I antigen upon exposure to either dimethyl sulfoxide (DMSO) or gamma interferon (Bahler and Lord, 1985a). This induction increases the density of class I antigens on line 1 cells to levels comparable to those found on other tumor cells or spleen cells (Figure 1). This expression depends upon the continued presence of the inducing agent. If the inducing agent is removed the class I antigen expression returns to the levels found in the untreated line 1 cells in approximately 72 hours (Bahler and Lord, 1985a). This expression is functionally significant in that the uninduced cells are not susceptible to lysis by treatment with anti-H-2^d reactive antibody and complement or by class I H-2^d reactive cytotoxic T lymphocytes (CTL) whereas the induced cells are effectively lysed (Bahler and Lord, 1985b).

DMSO Induces B2M and Class I mRNA

Our initial results showed that mRNA levels for both subunits of a class I molecule closely paralleled antigen expression in the induced and uninduced state. Thus, in the uninduced state, there was very little if any B2M or heavy chain class I mRNA, while exposure to DMSO dramatically induced the steady state levels of both these mRNAs (Figure 2). Southern blot analysis using a class I gene probe suggested that there were no dramatic changes in the class I genes (data not shown)

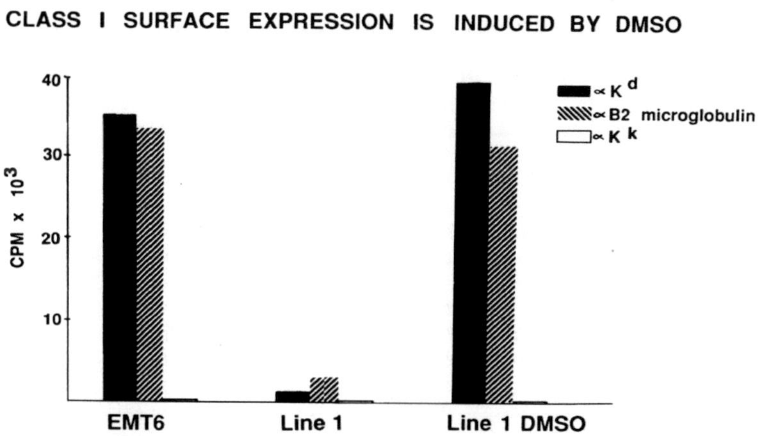

Figure 1. Expression of class I and B2M on line 1 and DMSO treated line 1 cells. Surface expression was quantitated using a radioimmunoassay as described in materials and methods. Cells used were EMT6, an $H\text{-}2^d$ expressing mammary tumor line (Rockwell et al., 1972), untreated line 1 cells, and line 1 cells cultured for 5 days in media containing 3% DMSO. Antibodies used were SF1-1.1 (anti-K^d) (Lorber et al., 1982), a polyclonal anti-rat B2M which crossreacts with all mouse B2M (anti-B2M) (Frelinger et al., 1981), and AF3-12.1 (anti-K^k) (Lorber et al., 1982).

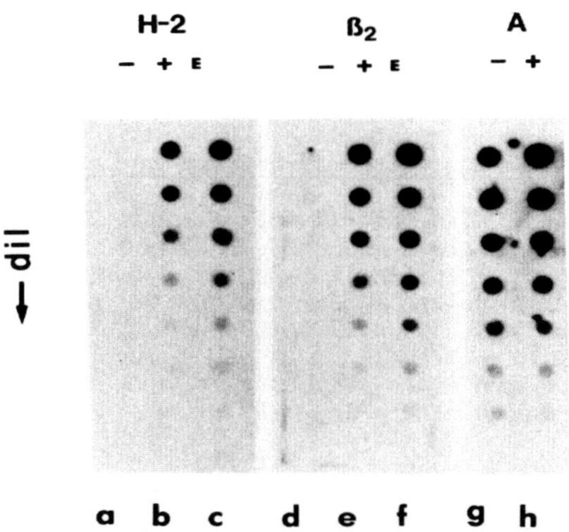

Figure 2. RNA dot blot analysis of line 1 cells, line 1 cells treated with DMSO, and EMT6. Each line shows 2 fold dilutions (arrow) of RNA extracted from 10^7 cells. The probes used were nick translated cDNA clones pH-2III (class I), pBRcB-3 (B2M), or DmA2 (actin). The line 1 cells were either untreated (-) or treated with 3% DMSO for 5 days prior to RNA isolation (+). EMT6 (E) serves as a positive control since it expresses high levels of both class I and B2M.

that could account for this lower expression unlike the gene alterations which occur with radiation leukemia viruses (Meruelo et al., 1986).

Cycloheximide Induces Class I mRNA

In light of the possibility that an active repressor molecule was present in line 1 cells which prevented the expression of class I antigens, we treated line 1 cells with cycloheximide to see if this drug induced expression of class I antigens. The rationale for this experiment, as suggested previously in other systems (Ringold et al., 1984), is that a repressor might be short lived and depend on continued protein synthesis. Thus, in the absence of protein synthesis, class I mRNA might be increased due to decreased levels of the putative repressor. We do see about a 2-4 fold increase in class I mRNA following treatment of line 1 cells with cycloheximide as measured by dot blot analysis (Figure 3). Since this effect is not dramatic a repressor mechanism may not account for all the regulation of the class I genes in line 1 cells.

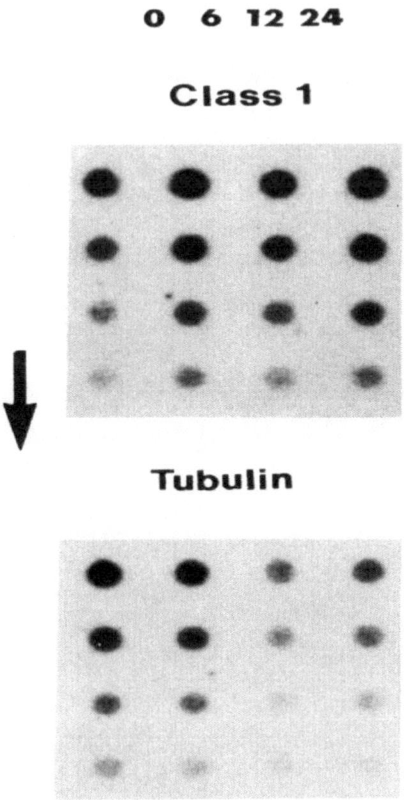

Figure 3. Dot blot analysis of class I expression of line 1 cells. Line 1 cells were incubated with 1 microgram/ml cycloheximide for 0, 6, 12, or 24 hours and RNA isolated from 10^7 cells using the Cheley and Anderson procedure. Each lane shows serial 2 fold dilutions. Duplicate blots were probed with pH-2III or tubulin which served as a control for the amount of RNA loaded on the gel.

Line 1 Cells Can Constitutively Express Transfected Class I Genes with Endogenous B2M

Line 1 transfection experiments were done in an attempt to understand the regulation of class I genes in these cells and to generate line 1 cell lines which expressed class I antigens constitutively. We initially performed these transfection experiments by introducing an allogeneic or foreign class I gene, in this case the D^p class I gene from the P/J strain of mice, into line 1 cells. We could distinguish the transfected D^p gene product from the recipient line 1 class I genes by its reaction with a specific anti-D^p monoclonal antibody 7-16.10, which does not react with the endogenous $H\text{-}2^d$ gene products. We found that we could generate class I expressing line 1 cells by introducing only the heavy chain of the class I molecule into line 1 cells despite the observation that line 1 cells are deficient in B2M. This is demonstrated by the flow cytometry data shown in Table 1. This result was surprising since earlier genetic data in other systems showed that B2M was obligatory to obtain class I antigen expression (Arce-Gomez et al., 1978, Hyman and Stallings, 1977, Parnes and Seidman, 1982, Severinsson and Peterson, 1984). The putative transfectants were screened both in the presence and absence of DMSO to ensure that the level of B2M was not limiting our ability to detect D^p expressing line 1 cells. No transfectants were found which expressed D^p only when induced, which suggests that the constitutive D^p expressing cells are not the result of transfecting a rare B2M expressing subpopulation of line 1 cells. Further analysis showed that the transfectants had increased levels of the endogenous B2M protein (Figure 4) and mRNA (data not shown). Our results suggested that the increased expression of a class I gene seemed to induce or coregulate the expression of the B2M mRNA and protein.

B2M Transfection Does not Seem to Induce Class I Antigen Expression

In order to see the effect of B2M expression in line 1 cells we transfected these cells with a genomic clone of B2M ($B2M^b$) cloned

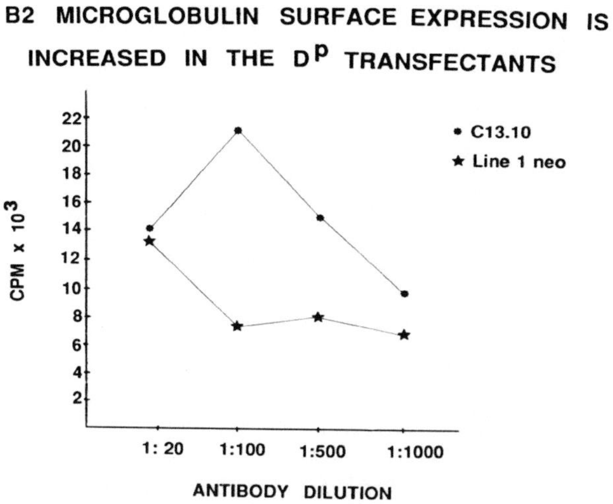

Figure 4. Expression of B2M on line 1 transfected with the neomycin gene only and on C13.10 a D^p expressing transfectant. Antibody dilution represents the final concentration of rabbit anti-rat B2M polyclonal antisera. Radioimmunoassay was performed as described in the Materials and Methods.

TABLE 1. Class I Antigen Expression of Transfected Line 1 Clones

Cell line	Surface Density*	
	D^p	D^d**
C1.2	20	2
C1.6	21	4
C13.10	7	7
Line 1-neo	0	1
Line 1	0	1
Spleen	100	100

* Percentage relative to BALB/c x P/J spleen cells determined by flow cytometry.

** D^d and D^p expression were evaluated using monoclonal antibodies AF3 62.4 (anti-D^d) (Lorber et al., 1982) and 7-16.10 (anti-D^p) (Harmon et al., 1983)

into psv2-gpt vector. The gene product of the B2M and allele in this construct is recognized by the monoclonal antibody mc-B2M-B-clone 23 which does not react with the product of the endogenous B2M allele present on induced line 1 cells. Thus we have a monoclonal antibody which is specific for the transfected gene product. Our preliminary experiments with a limited number of these B2M transfectants do not show constitutive expression of $B2M^b$ or a significant increase in the levels of class I antigens. The transfected B2M gene is capable of functioning in these cells since the transfectants express substantial amounts of B2M b allele when treated with DMSO (Table 2). We are currently investigating the apparent lack of expression of B2 microglobulin and whether this indicates that coregulation of B2 microglobulin is unidirectional or alternatively is due to this particular construct, repression of the transfected gene, or is a reflection of the small number of transfectants analyzed.

The Expression of a Class I Antigen Can Result in Decreased Tumor Growth In Vivo

We have utilized the D^p transfectants to examine the role of class I antigen expression on the growth of a spontaneous tumor *in vivo*. Because we introduced a p haplotype gene into an $H\text{-}2^d$ tumor, we tested the ability of these cells to grow in (BALB/c x P/J) F1 ($H\text{-}2^{d/p}$) animals which are H-2 compatible with the transfected cells. In initial experiments with unprimed mice, both the normal and transfected line 1 cells grew, though the D^p expressing transfectants grew somewhat more slowly. As one can see from Fig. 5, in mice previously primed with a D^p expressing transfectant the C13.10 transfectants were efficiently rejected whereas line 1 cells transfected with neo alone grew. Thus, in certain circumstances, the expression of a class I antigen can have a dramatic effect on the growth of tumors.

DISCUSSION

There are several possible mechanisms for the origin of class I negative cells. It is clear that oncogenic viruses can directly interfere with the expression of class I antigens (Bernards et al., 1983,

TABLE 2. Analysis of B2 Microglobulin and Class I Expression on Transfectant Clones

Cell Line	^{125}I-Protein A Binding (cpm)[1]			
	Uninduced		DMSO Induced[2]	
	$B2M^b$	K^d	$B2M^b$	K^d
L1B2A4	0	2,224	25,761	44,095
L1B2B7	22	1,633	21,760	30,060
L1B2A7	10	6,352	6,414	25,801

[1] The cells were incubated in microtubes with anti-$B2M^b$ (mc-B2M-B-clone 23) or anti-K^d (SF1-1.1) monoclonal antibodies, washed, ^{125}I- protein A added. The cells were washed again and then counted in a gamma counter.
[2] The cells were cultured in the presence of 3% DMSO for 7 days prior to analysis.

Hayashi et al., 1984). Cells which have lost the expression of a class I antigen, which serves as a restriction element for a particular virus or

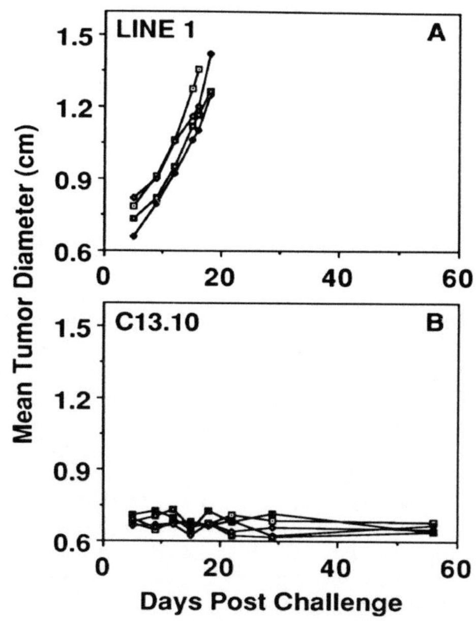

Figure 5. <u>In vivo</u> growth of line 1 and a D^p line 1 expressing transfectant, C13.10. (BALB/c x P/J)F1 mice were injected intramuscularly with 50,000 cells and the size of the tumor measured over time. These mice had been previously immunized with 5 x 10^6 cells of a D^p expressing line 1 transfectant. Each line represents the measurements of the tumor in a single mouse.

tumor antigen might be selected _in vivo_ by cytotoxic T cells. The methylcholanthrene induced tumor, T10 (Katzav et al., 1981), and the SV40 transformed cell lines described in detail by Gooding, 1982, might be examples of such a mechanism since they have lost the expression of one or more but not all the class I antigens. Line 1 cells, like embryonal carcinoma cells (Morello et al., 1982, Croce et al., 1981) and small lung cell carcinoma cells (Doyle et al., 1985) may represent a third class of tumors which normally express very low levels of class I antigens. Histological staining of tissues suggest that there is normally a population of cells in a variety of tissues which express low levels of class I antigens (Fleming et al., 1981, Klein, 1975). It is interesting that line 1 tumors expressing a class I antigen can be recognized as foreign. One interesting speculation is that an organism might not be truly tolerant of such class I negative cells but rather fails to respond to such cells because of their lack of MHC molecules and their inability to serve as good targets for cytotoxic cells.

There appear to be several ways in which the levels of class I antigen can be regulated. The transfected gene appears to be inducible with DMSO since we can show that the level of D^p mRNA increases when the cells are treated with DMSO (data not shown). Whether this is at the level of transcription or mRNA stability is yet unknown since we have only examined steady state levels of D^p mRNA. In addition, there appears to be a level of regulation previously unrecognized in the expression of class I antigen expression in that the level of either class I protein or mRNA seems to influence the amount of B2M expressed. Taking these observations into account we have formulated a working model presented in Fig. 6. We are currently defining the putative regulatory regions of class I and B2M to see if the inducing agents DMSO and gamma interferon work at the same or different sites. To address the question of coregulation directly, we are using class I genes under the control of the inducible metallothionein promoter. This will allow us to vary the levels of class I in a given cell to determine if the levels of class I and B2M vary coordinately. It is interesting that there is precedent for this phenomenon of one gene inducing another in the immune system. The transfection of a functional beta chain gene of the T cell receptor into a Jurkat cell line with a mutant beta chain resulted in the increased expression of the alpha chain mRNA (Ohashi et al., 1985). This raises the possibility that the phenomenon of coregulation of genetically unlinked but physically associated proteins such as the class I heavy chain and B2M may be a specific example of a more common mechanism of gene regulation.

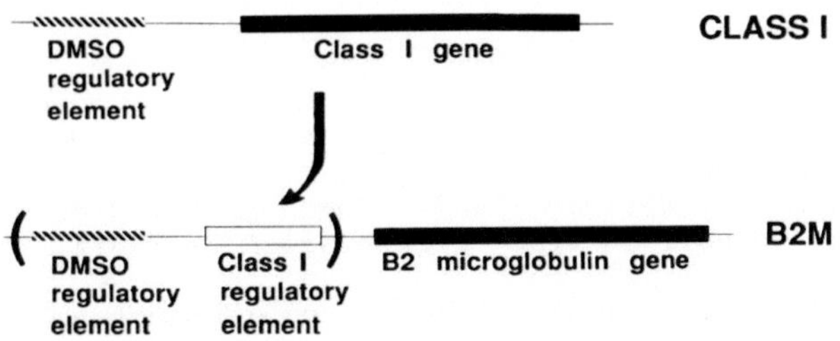

Figure 6. A hypothetical model for the control of class I and B2 microblobulin expression indicating the possibility of multiple controlling regions and a possible regulatory effect of class I on B2 microglobulin.

The expression of a class I antigen can clearly have dramatic effects on the growth of line 1 cells in vivo in primed syngeneic mice. However, it must be remembered that these cells have the ability to be induced to express higher levels of class I antigens by exogenous agents. We believe it is significant that the transfected cell lines, though expressing different levels of class I antigen, can still be rejected in vivo. It is possible that the main role of the D^p class I antigen is to help initiate an immune response which in turn causes various lymphokines such as gamma interferon to be produced. Gamma interferon and other lymphokines released in the context of the immune response might then induce both the transfected gene and the endogenous gene products in these transfectants resulting in a further amplification of the response. Consistent with this theory, we have been able to isolate T cells restricted to the d haplotype gene products from tumors grown in vivo from line 1 transfected cells. Thus, the role of the inducibility of these cells and its effect on tumor growth needs to be examined more closely in this system.

ACKNOWLEDGEMENTS

This work was supported by research grants CA 28332 and CA 41448 from the National Institutes of Health and a grant from the United Cancer Council and is publication number 30 from the Immunology unit of the University of Rochester Cancer Center. John G. Frelinger is supported by Junior Faculty Research Award JFRA 142 from the American Cancer Society. Karen M. Cerosaletti is supported by HSS training grant 1 T32 AI 07285 from the National Institutes of Health. David W. Bahler is supported by MSTP training grant 5 T32 GM 07356 from the National Institutes of Health.

The authors thank Lynne Palmiere and Mary LeRoy-Jacobs for typing the manuscript.

REFERENCES

Arce-Gomez, B., E.A. Jones, C.J. Barnstable, E. Solomon, and W.F. Bodmer. 1978. The genetic control of HLA-A and B antigens in somatic cell hybrids: requirement for B2 microglobulin. Tissue Antigens. 11: 96.

Bahler, D.W. and E.M. Lord. 1985a. Dimethyl sulfoxide induces expression of H-2 antigens on mouse lung carcinoma cells. J. Immunol. 134: 2790.

Bahler, D.W. and E.M. Lord 1985b. Enhanced immune recognition of H-2 antigen deficient murine lung carcinoma cells following treatment with dimethyl sulfoxide. Cancer Res. 45: 5362.

Bahler, D.W., J.G. Frelinger, L.W. Harwell, and E.M. Lord. 1987. Reduced tumorigenicity of a spontaneous mouse lung carcinoma following H-2 gene transfection. Proc. Natl. Acad. Sci., in press.

Bernards, R., P.I. Schrier, A. Houweling, J. Bos, A.J. van der Eb, M. Zijlstra, and C.J.M. Melief. 1983. Tumorigenicity of cells transformed by adenovirus type 12 by evasion of T-cell immunity. Nature 305: 776.

Cheley, S. and R. Anderson. 1984. A reproducible microanalytical method for the detection of specific RNA sequences by dot-blot hybridization. Analyt. Biochem. 137: 15.

Chirgwin, J.M., A.E. Przybyla, R.J. MacDonald, and W.J. Rutter. 1979. Isolation of biologically active ribonucleic acid from sources enriched in ribonuclease. Biochem. 18: 5294.

Chorney, M., F-W Shen, J. Michaelson, and E.A. Boyse. 1982. Monoclonal antibody to an alloantigenic determinant on B2 microglobulin (B2M) of the mouse. Immunogenetics 16: 91.

Cleveland, D.W., M.A. Lopata, R.J. MacDonald, N.J. Cowan, W.J. Rutter, and M.W. Kirschner. 1980. Number and evolutionary conservation of -and tubulin and cytoplasmic - and -actin genes using specific cloned cDNA probes. Cell 20:95.

Croce, C.M., A. Linnenbach, K. Huebner, J.R. Parnes, D.H. Marguilles, E. Apella, and J.G. Seidman. 1981. Control of expression of histocompatibility antigens (H-2) and B2-microglobulin in F9 teratocarcinoma stem cells. Proc. Natl. Acad. Sci. USA. 78: 5754.

Darsley, M.J., H. Takahahi, M.J. Macchi, J.A. Frelinger, K. Ozata, and E. Apella. 1987. New family of exon shuffled recombinant genes reveals extensive interdomain interactions in class I histocompatibility antigens and identifies residues involved. J. Exp. Med. 165: 211.

Doyle, A., W.J. Martin, K. Funa, A. Gazday, D. Carney, S.E. Martin, I. Linoila, F. Cuttitta, J. Mulshine, P. Bunn, and J. Minna. 1985. Markedly decreased expression of class I histocompatibility antigens, proteins, and mRNA in human small-cell lung carcinoma. J. Exp. Med. 161: 1135.

Fleming, K.A., A. McMichael, J.A. Morton, J. Woods, and J.O.D. McGee. 1981. Distribution of HLA class I antigens in normal human tissue and in mammary cancer. J. Clin. Pathol. 34: 779.

Frelinger, J.G., L. Hood, and P. Wettstein. 1981. Analysis of RT1 products using two-dimensional polyacrylamide gels. Transplant. Proc. 18: 1360.

Frelinger, J.G., A. Sing, A. Infante, and C.G. Fathman. 1984. Clonotypic antibodies which stimulate T cell clone proliferation. Ann. Rev. Immunol. 81: 21.

Fryberg, E.A., K.L. Kindel, N. Davidson, and A. Sodja. 1980. The actin genes of Drosophila: a dispersed multigene family. Cell. 19: 356.

Goodenow, R.S., J.M. Vogel, and R.L. Linsk. 1985. Histocompatibility antigens on murine tumors. Science 230: 777.

Gooding, L.R. 1982. Characterization of a progressive tumor from C3H fibroblasts transformed in vitro with SV40 virus. Immunoresistance in vivo correlates with phenotypic loss of $H\text{-}2K^k$. J. Immunol. 129: 1306.

Harmon, R., N. Stein, and J.A. Frelinger. 1983. Monoclonal antibodies reactive with H-2 determinants. Immunogenetics. 18: 541.

Hayashi, H., K. Tanaka, F. Jay, G. Khoury, and G. Jay. 1985. Modulation of the tumorigenicity of human adenovirus-12-transformed cells by interferon. Cell 43: 263.

Hood, L., M. Steinmetz, and B. Malissen. 1983. Genes of the major histocompatibility complex of the mouse. Ann. Rev. Immunol. 1: 529.

Hui, K., F. Growveld, and H. Festenstein. 1984. Rejection of transplantable AKR leukemia cells following MHC DNA-mediated cell transformation. Nature 311: 750.

Hyman, R. and V. Stallings. 1977. Analysis of hybrids between an $H\text{-}2^+$, TL^- lymphoma and an $H\text{-}2^+$, TL^+ lymphoma and its $H\text{-}2^-$, TL^- variant subline. Immunogenetics. 4: 171.

Katzav, S., P. De Baetseiler, E. Gorelik, M. Feldman, and S. Segal. Immunogenetic control of metastasis formation by a methylcholantrene-induced tumor (T10) in mice: Differential expression of H-2 gene products. Transpl. Proc. 13: 742.

Klein, J. 1975. Biology of the Mouse Histocompatibility -2 Complex. Springer-Verlag, New York.

Lorber, M.I., M. Loken, A. Stall, and F. Fitch. 1982. I-A antigens on cloned alloreactive murine T lymphocytes are acquired passively. J. Immunol. 128: 2798.

Maniatis, T., E. Fritsch, and J. Sambrook. 1982. Molecular Cloning: A Laboratory Manual. Cold Spring Harbor Laboratories, Cold Spring Harbor, New York.

Meruelo, D., R. Kornreich, A. Rossamando, C. Pampeno, A. Boral, J. Silver, J. Buxbaum, E. Weiss, J. Devlin, A. Mellor, R.A. Flavell, and A. Pellicer. 1986. Lack of class I H-2 antigens in cells transformed by radiation leukemia virus is associated with methylation and rearrangement of H-2 DNA. Proc. Natl. Acad. Sci. USA. 83: 4504.

Morello, D., F. Daniel, P. Baldacci, Y. Cayre, G. Gachelin, and P. Kourilsky. 1982. Absence of significant H-2 and B_2-microglobulin mRNA expression by mouse embryonal carcinoma cells. Nature 296: 260.

Ohashi, P.S., T. Mak, P. Van den Elsen, Y. Yanagai, Y. Yoshikai, A. Claman, C. Terhorstay, J. Stobo, A. Weiss. 1985. Reconstitution of an active surface T3/T cell antigen receptor by DNA transfer. Nature 316:606.

Parnes, J.R. and J.G. Seidman. 1982. Structure of wild type and mutant mouse B_2 microglobulin. Cell 29: 661.

Parnes, J.R., B. Velan, A. Felsenfeld, L. Ramanathan, U. Ferini, E. Appella, and J.G. Seidman. 1981. Mouse B_2-microglobulin cDNA clones: a screening procedure for cDNA clones corresponding to rare mRNA's. Proc. Natl. Acad. Sci. USA. 78: 2253.

Ringold, G.M., B. Dieckmann, J.L. Vannice, M. Trahey, and F. McCormick. 1984. Inhibition of protein synthesis stimulates the transcription of human B interferon genes in Chinese hamster ovary cells. Proc. Nat. Acad. Sci. USA, 81: 3964.

Rockwell, S.C., R.F. Kallman, and L.F. Fajardo. 1972. Characteristics of a serially transplanted mouse mammary tumor and its tissue-culture-adapted derivative. J. Natl. Cancer Inst. 49: 735.

Severinsson, L. and P.A. Peterson. 1984. B_2-microglobulin induces intracellular transport of human class I transplantation antigen heavy chains in Xenopus laevis oocytes. J. Cell Biol. 99: 226.

Steinmetz, M., J.G. Frelinger, D. Fisher, T. Hunkapiller, D. Pereira, S.M. Weissman, H. Uehara, S. Nathenson, and L. Hood. 1981. Three cDNA clones encoding mouse transplantation antigens: homology to immunoglobulin genes. Cell. 24: 125.

Tanaka, K., K.J. Isselbacher, G. Khoury, and G. Jay. 1985. Reversal of oncogenesis by the expression of a major histocompatibility complex class I gene. Science 228: 26.

Thomas, P.S. 1980. Hybridization of denatured RNA and small DNA fragments transferred to nitrocellulose. Proc. Natl. Acad. Sci. USA. 77: 5201.

Van Doren, K., D. Hanahan, and Y. Gluzman. 1984. Infection of eucaryotic cells by helper-independent recombinant adenoviruses: Early region 1 is not obligatory for integration of viral DNA. J. Virol. 50: 606.

Wallich, R., N. Bulbuc, G.J. Hammerling, S. Katzav, S. Segal, and M. Feldman. 1985. Abrogation of metastatic properties of tumor cells by de-novo expression of H-2K antigens following H-2 gene transfection. Nature 315: 301.

Yuhas, J.M., N.H. Pazmino, J.O. Proctor, and R.E. Toya. 1974. A direct relationship between immune competence and the subcutaneous growth rate of a malignant murine lung tumor. Cancer Res. 34: 722.

Zinkernagel, R.M. and P.C. Doherty. 1979. MHC-restricted cytotoxic T cells: studies on the biologic role of polymorphic major transplantation antigens determining T cell restriction-specificity, function and responsiveness. Adv. Immunol. 27: 51.

THE BIOLOGICAL IMPLICATIONS OF THE ABNORMAL EXPRESSION OF HISTOCOMPATIBILITY ANTIGENS ON MURINE AND HUMAN TUMORS

Federico Garrido

Servicio Análisis Clínicos

Hospital Virgen de las Nieves, 18014 Granada-Spain

There is increasing evidence indicating that the expression of histocompatibility antigens is altered in experimental tumors induced in mice as well as in human tumors (1,2,). Two different types of alterations have been described:

a) Total or selective loss of class I molecules (K,D,L or HLA, A,B,C) whose reexpression can in most cases be induced after γIFN treatment. Examples of this are absence of the K^k molecule of Gardner lymphoma (3) or the disappearence of four $H\text{-}2^d$ antigenic specificities on an $H\text{-}2^d$ sarcoma (4).

These losses may represent an escape route from T cell immunosurveillance or a mechanism to induce NK sensitive tumor targets, (19).

b) The appearance of aberrant class I like molecules which may behave like alloantigens and are capable of triggering an immune response like that seen in allograft rejection (5,6). The aberrant molecules on these clones may be tumor associated transplantation antigen (TATA).

Rearrangements of class I genes exist in 5 to 10% of ultraviolet light induced tumors (7) and have also been described in Gross virus induced AKR leukemias (9) and Rous virus induced sarcomas (10). Such genetic rearrangements may well represent the mechanism of appearence of aberrant class I molecules on tumors (8).

The alteration of the expression of MHC molecules may also have important implications in the growth and development of primary tumors (11). It is also becoming evident that the immune response and tumor growth are not only the consequence of the presence or absence of tumor associated antigens (TAA) but also depend to a considerable extent on the nature and expression of MHC antigens (1).

Our laboratory is interested in this type of problem and we have been involved in developing a research program on murine as well as on human tumors for several years. On murine tumors we are using different inducing agents (chemicals, viruses and radiation) in the BALB/c ($H\text{-}2^d$) mouse strain.

THE MURINE TUMOR SYSTEM GR9

Heterogeneity of expression of H-2 molecules on GR9 clones.

This tumor system was induced with methylcholantrene and adapted to in vitro growth without any passage in vivo in syngeneic BALB/c mice (11). After cloning, the tumor was typed for H-2. We used alloantisera of restricted specificity, monoclonal antibodies against class I and II antigens, absortion of sera with normal lymphoid cells and tumor cells and alloreactive cytotoxic T lymphocytes against K^d and D^d molecules. A summary of the results obtained is presented in Table I. Different clones were obtained with different class I antigen expression (K,D,L). For example clones G2, A7 and D8 present a high class I expression; B7 or B3 express moderate amounts and clones like B10 and B9 have a very low expression of H-2 specificities, similar to that observed in the negative controls (13). This heterogeneity among the different clones in class I expression was also observed for other tumors induced with metylcholantrene, such as the tumor GRB7.1 (Table I). This heterogeneity is in marked contrast with the homogeneous composition of other long term established tumors.

We further investigated two GR9 clones A7 and B9, with high and low H-2 (K,D) antigen expression respectively. Using Southern Blot techniques we could not detect differences in the RFLP's between these clones using different probes and different restriction enzymes (14). Hence we have no evidences for class I gene rearrangement. However differences in the methylation pattern of A7 and B9 class I genes were detected. The incubation of B9 cells with 5 azacitidine was furthermore suficient to reexpress moderate amounts of H-2 molecules (K^d, D^d) (14). Interestingly, by using Northern Blot techniques we detected clear differences in class I gene transcription that correlated with the previously observed high and low levels of class I expression (15).

In vivo growth of GR9 clones

GR9 tumor clones were subcutaneously injected in syngeneic BALB/c mice and local tumor growth measured. We observed that the growth was at times inversely correlated with the expression of class I antigens (Fig. IA). Clones with higher class I expression grew slowly i.e. were more immunogeneic. In contrast, those clones with low class I antigens were more locally malignant. In irradiated BALB/c mice these differences were clearly reduced, indicating that a radiosensitive mechanism is responsible for the differences observed in local tumor growth of the different clones (Fig. 1B). We also transfected the D^d gene to the B9 GR9 clone (low class I) and measured syngeneic growth of the D^d-B9 transfected clones (K^d negative D^d positive). Interestingly, no differences were observed in comparison to the B9 control growth pattern (K^d negative D^d negative) (18).

TABLE I.- CLASS I AND II ANTIGEN EXPRESSION ON MURINE TUMORS

GR9 TUMOR CLONES

CLONES	$H\text{-}2K^d$	$H\text{-}2D^d$	$H\text{-}2L^d$	Ia
G2	+++	+++	++	−
D8	+++	+++	+++	−
A7	+++	+++	+	−
D6	++	++	−	−
B11	++	++	−	−
B7	+	++	−	−
B3	+	+++	−	−
C11	−	−	−	−
B10	−	−	−	−

GR B7.1 TUMOR CLONES

CLONES				
38	+++	+++	+++	−
1	+++	+++	+++	−
3	+++	+++	+++	−
4	+	+	+	−
41	−	−	−	−

We used a binding assay with MoAbs against K^d, D^d, $H\text{-}2^d$ and Ia antigens and a sheep antimouse ^{125}I (Fab) Ig.
+++ (high binding); ++ (moderate binding); − (low binding). As positive and negative controls we used BALB/c and CBA/H normal lymphoid cells.

Effects of γ IFN on the class I antigen expression

B10 and B9, GR9 clones that expressed low amounts of class I antigens were incubated with 100 I.U. of murine recombinant γ IFN. After a few hours of incubation class I antigens were reexpressed on both clones in high amounts, higher in fact than the positive controls. (Fig. 2). This effect was maintained for 6 days, returning subsequently to the original figures for class I expression on B10 and B9 clones (15).

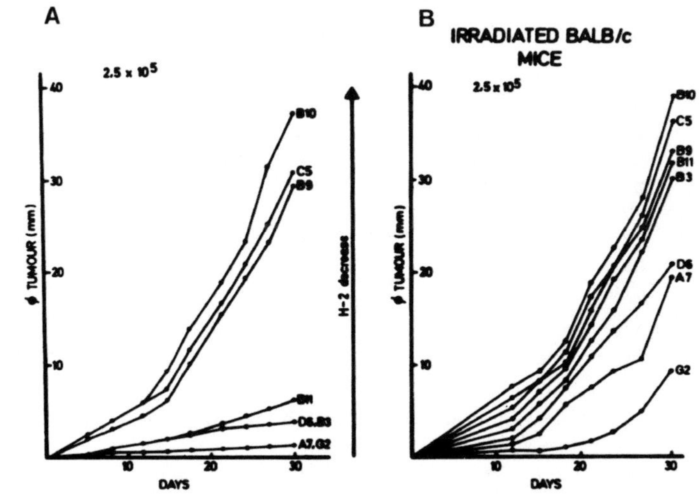

Fig. 1A.- 2.5 x 10^5 GR9 tumor clones were subcutaneously injected in BALB/c mice and tumor growth measured every 3 days.
Fig. 1B.- The same number of GR9 tumor cell clones were injected in sublethally irradiated BALB/c mice.

CLASS I EXPRESSION

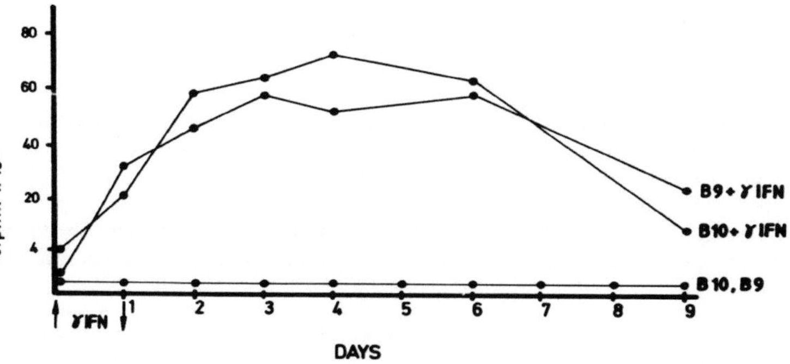

Fig. 2.- B10 and B9 GR9 clones were incubated with 100 I.U. of murine recombinant γ IFN. Class I antigens were expressed as asessed by a binding assay using an anti H-2^d MoAb.

Control of the BALB/c origin of metylcholantrene induced tumors

In order to confirm the BALB/c origin of the different GR9 tumor clones we compared the electrophoretic mobility of different isoenzymes obtained from normal tissues of our BALB/c colony and from different GR9 clones. The isoenzymes studied were: malic enzyme (MOD) Glucosa GP Isomerase (GPi) and Isocitrate Dehydrogenase. The results obtained in our experiments indicated that GR9 clone isoenzymes had the same electrophoretic mobility as BALB/c isoenzymes, while differing from other mouse strains (C57 Bl/6, CBA, DBA.....) (Fig. 3).

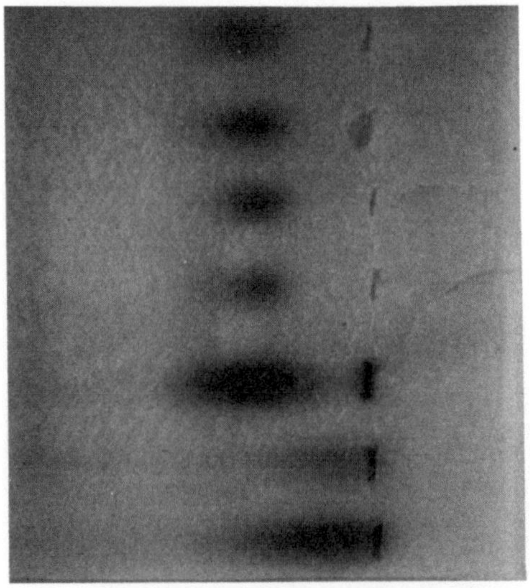

Fig. 3.- Isoenzyme pattern of four GR9 clones, showing identical mobility in GR9 clones and BALB/c tissues. Malic Enzyme (MOD).

Immune response against the GR9 tumor

One of the most important aims of the study of the GR9 tumor system was to determine the mechanism of immune response that may be responsible for tumor rejection. We had previously demonstrated that A7 GR9 clone (K^d D^d positive) did have tumor associated transplantation antigens (TATA) and was capable of protecting against the syngeneic growth of other GR9 clones (13).

We first turned our attention to the humoral immune response. BALB/c mice were immunized with increasing numbers of A7 cells, (a K^d D^d positive GR9 clone) and a series of monoclonal antibodies were obtained (16). Two of them, named A7.2 and A7.6, recognized a 70 KD peptide that was identified by immunoprecipitation and electrophoresis in SDS polyacrilamide gel assays (Fig. 4).

The tissue and cellular distribution of this antigen showed restricted expression to the majority of GR9 clones with the exception of B3 and B7 (Fig. 5). However, it was not present in normal cells or in tumors induced with different agents (viruses, radiation, chemicals) in various strains of mice (Figs. 6A, 6B, 6C) (15). We have also observed that conventional anti GP 70 monoclonal antibodies precipitated other molecules from GR9 clones than those recognized by A7.2 and A7.6 syngeneic monoclonal antibodies. In addition, A7.2 and A7.6 MoAbs were negative in tumor cells that expressed the GP70 conventional antigen induced with MuLv (17).

An interesting observation was that A7.2 and A7.6 MoAbs did bind to other methylcholantrene induced tumors of BALB/c origin obtained in our laboratory, including MCG11, GRIR5, GRA51 and GRB7.1 (Fig. 6).

To sum up, this 70 KD peptide could represent a tumor associated antigen (TAA) present on GR9 clones (with the exception of three) and also found in other M.C. induced BALB/c tumors. It is absent in normal cells and a large number of tumor cells produced in different laboratories.

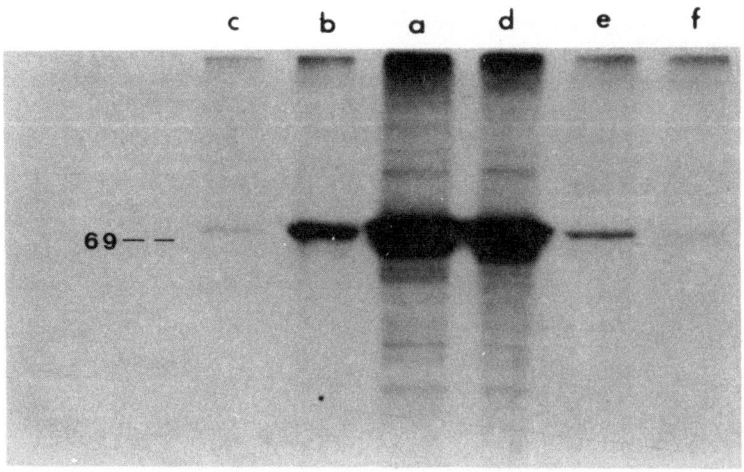

Fig. 4.- Immunoprecipitation of the peptide recognized by MoAbs A7.2 and A7.6. Two sequential immunoprecipitations were performed on iodine labelled B9 cells with A7.2 and A7.6 MoAbs (lane a, b and d, e respectively). Later, a third precipitation with the irrelevant MoAb (A7.6 and A7.2 lanes c and f)demonstrated that both MoAbs recognize the same peptide present on most GR9 clones as a candidate for tumor associated antigen (TAA).

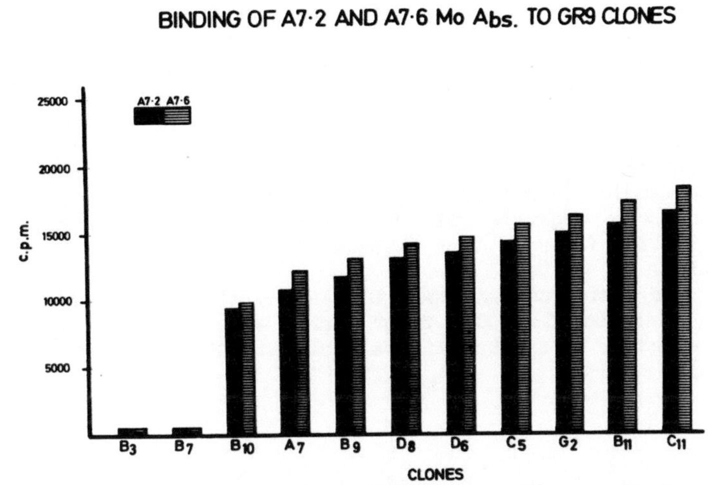

Fig. 5.- Binding of A7.2 and A7.6 to GR9 clones. The syngeneic antitumor MoAbs A7.2 and A7.6 recognized antigen present on most of GR9 clones with the exception of B3 and B7.

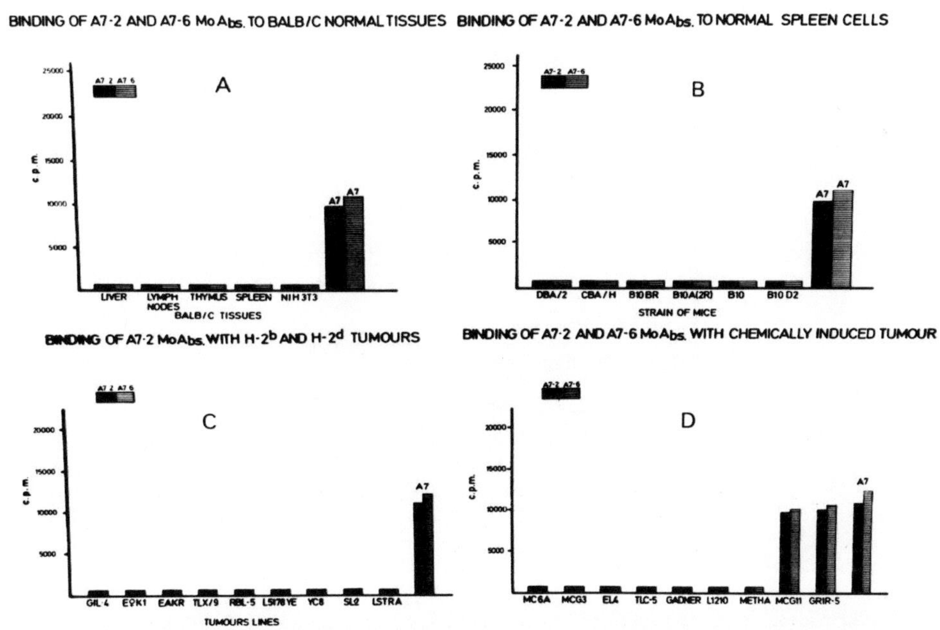

Fig. 6A.B.C.D. Pattern of reaction of A7.2 and A7.6 anti tumor MoAbs with normal and tumor cells.- A7.2 and A7.6 MoAbs did not react with normal cells from different strains of mice (6A,6B), nor with tumors of different H-2 haplotypes and origin including several methylcholantrene induced tumors (6C,6D). However, these MoAbs reacted with other M.C. induced BALB/c tumors produced in our laboratory.6D

Generation of antitumor cytotoxic T lymphocytes

It was also possible to induce antitumor CTL's by immunizing syngeneic BALB/c mice with A7 tumor cells (K^d D^d positive) and restimulating in vitro the spleen cells for five days with Mitomicin treated A7 cells (15). These secondary CTL's lysed the GR9 clones with the exception of B10, B7, and B3 (Fig. 7). Lysis was inhibited after treatment with anti Thy 1.2. plus complement. Different target cells were assayed including ConA blasts from various strains of mice with different recombinant haplotypes; different tumor cells such as MethA ($H\text{-}2^d$ MC induced); YC8 and LSTRA ($H\text{-}2^d$ Moloney virus induced). Our anti GR9 CTL's were negative with all target cells (15). We are currently investigating the role that these anti tumor CTL's may play in tumor rejection.

We also have evidence that NK cytotoxicity is involved in GR9 tumor rejection. Some GR9 tumor clones were sensitive to NK lysis (I. Algarra and K. Karré, Karolinska Institute Stockolm, personal communication).

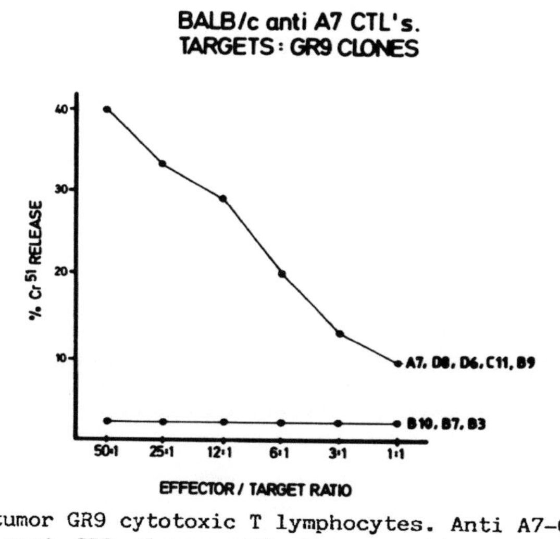

Fig. 7.- Antitumor GR9 cytotoxic T lymphocytes. Anti A7-GR9 CTL's were able to lyse most GR9 clones with the exception of B10, B7 and B3. Other $H\text{-}2^d$ tumor cells such as MethA, LSTRA or YC8 were also spared.

Tumor associated transplantation antigens (TATA) on GR9 clones

We have data indicating that GR9 clones share TATA. A7-GR9 cells can protect against the challenge of other GR9 clones, independently of its H-2 class I expression (13) or the presence of the 70 KD peptide (TAA). For instance, A7 (K^d D^d positive) protect B9 and B10 (K^d D^d low) and also B3 and B7 (TAA negative).

THE EXPRESSION OF MHC ANTIGENS ON HUMAN TUMORS

Data obtained from different laboratories are indicating that MHC class I and II antigenic expression is also altered on human tumors (1, 22, 21, 25, 33, 26).

Our interest in MHC antigen expression, has led us to investigate a total of 284 neoplasias comprising 193 primitive and 91 metastasis with immunohistological techniques including peroxidase, alkaline phosphatase and immunofluorescence (21, 22, 26). The following monoclonal antibodies were used: W6/32 against HLA class I antigen heavy chains, GRH1 against B2 microglobulin (27), two HLA B locus specific monoclonal antibodies kindly provide by Doctors Milstein and Vives, and a group of allospecific monoclonal antibodies obtained at the X International Workshop on HLA Antigens. Class II antigens were studied with GRB1, which recognizes monomorphic DR (28) Tu22, against DQ (29) and B7/21 to detect DP (30). Other MoAbs including GRT2 were also used to detect leukocytic common antigen (LCA) and thus served as a useful measure of leukocytic infiltration in tumors.

Histocompatibility antigen expression on colon tumors

No class I antigen expression was seen in 5 of the 34 primary colon tumors studied (Table 1, Fig. 8). In all other tumors expression was intense, approaching 100% of all cells examined.
Class II antigen expression however was heterogeneous in 18 of 34 cases studied, with significant differences in levels of expression: DR > DP > DQ molecules. All metastases studied expressed class I antigens, with fewer cells positive in 8 of 13 metastatic lesions in comparison to primary tumors. Very low levels of class II antigen expression were found, with 5 of 8 cases positive and frequently showing a focal distribution.

Parallel studies were carried out on normal colon mucosa from all patients, in which class I antigens only were detected. Exceptions to this finding were those cases in which mucosa adjacent to the tumor were also examined and found to express the DR molecule.

A total of 25 polyps were also studied for antigen expression, with similar results to those found in normal mucosa. All polyps were HLA class I positive while class II antigen expression paralleled the degree of cellular dysplasia. A further finding, analogous to results in tumor studies, showed the DR antigen to be most frequently expressed, followed in decreasing order by DQ and DP molecules.

Histocompatibility antigen expression on melanomas

Class I antigen expression in melanomas varied depending on whether the tumor was primary or metastatic. HLA-ABC antigens were observed on 17 of the 19 primary melanomas studies, although in 5 cases staining was heterogeneous, affecting less than 50% of the cells (Table 1). The percentage of positive cells could be correlated with the Clark level of invasion. High levels of expression were obtained on all primary tumors at Clark levels I and II of invasion, while both HLA class I negative tumors had invaded the reticular dermis (Clark level IV).

In contrast, class I antigen expression was not seen on 11 of 23 metastatic tumors representing 6 of 15 ganglion metastases and 5 of 8 cutaneous metastases. In three cases differential expression was found between the primitive tumor and autologous metastases (Table 3). These findings concur with those of other authors (31,32) and suggest that class I antigens are less expressed by tumors with a greater potential for invasion and metastasis.

Fewer primary melanoma cells were positive for class II antigen expression, and only 6 of 19 such cases showed positive staining. On the other hand between 25 and 75% of all cells were stained positive in 7 of the 23 metastatic lesions examined. Significant differences were furthermore noted when lymphatic (7 of 15 cases positive) and cutaneous (1 of 8 cases positive) were compared for HLA DR reactivity.

TABLE II. CLASS I AND II ANTIGEN EXPRESSION IN PRIMARY AND METASTATIC TUMORS

PRIMARY TUMORS

	Class I (+/total)		Class II (+/total)		
Tumors	B-2m	H chain	DR	DP	DQ
Colon	29/34	29/34	18/34	5/34	3/34
Stomach	18/21	18/21	3/21	3/21	3/21
Breast	33/39	33/39	15/39	N.T.	N.T.
Larynx	24/29	24/29	2/24	0/24	0/24
Melanoma	17/19	17/19	6/19	N.T.	N.T.
Renal	12/13	12/13	7/13	2/7	3/7
Sarcoma	0/4	0/4	1/4	1/4	1/4
Epidermoid	7/8	7/8	5/8	N.T.	N.T.
Basal.cell	17/26	17/26	2/6	N.T.	N.T.

METASTATIC TUMORS

	Class I (+/total)		Class II (+/total)		
Tumors	B-2m	H chain	DR	DP	DQ
Colon	13/13	13/13	5/13	1/13	0/13
Stomach	27/30	27/30	3/30	2/30	2/30
Breast	0/1	0/1	0/1	0/1	0/1
Larynx	18/21	18/21	2/21	0/21	0/21
Melanoma	12/23	12/23	7/23	N.T.	N.T.
Renal	1/1	1/1	1/1	1/1	1/1
Rhabdomyo-sarcoma	0/1	0/1	0/1	0/1	0/1
Epidermoidal	1/1	1/1	1/1	1/1	1/1

A total of 193 cases of primary tumor were studied. The figures show numbers of positive cases in comparison to total cases.

91 metastasis were studied located at different anatomic sites but predominating lymph node metastasis.

Histocompatibility antigen expression in breast cancer

HLA class I antigens were observed in 33 of 39 cases diagnosed as ductal infiltrating carcinoma. In many instances, expression was rather heterogeneous and could not be correlated to the degree of differentiation in these tumors (19). HLA-DR antigen was detected in 15 of 39 cases although expression in most tumors was weak and heterogeneous.

Histocompatibility antigen expression in stomach cancer

A total of 21 cases of stomach cancer and 31 metastatic tumors were examined. Generally speaking, HLA-ABC antigen expression was quite strong, with only 3 cases negative and 4 showing heterogeneous expression. More than 75% of all cells were positive in all remaining cases. A noteworthy finding in all undifferentiated tumors was the high rate of class I antigen expression, in contrast with moderately or well differentiated lesions, 3 of which were negative and 4 of which showed heterogeneous expression. These findings seem to parallel antigen expression on normal gastric mucosa, which was scarce overall and absent in many cases.

In 30 ganglionar metastases located in the vicinity of the tumor, HLA class I antigen expression was similar to that seen on primiti· ˋ tumors. In only one case a contrast between the primary lesion and the autologous metastasis was observed.

Class II antigen expression was very weak and noticiable in only 3 of the 21 primary tumors. The greatest number of positive cells expressed the DR antigen, while the lowest number of reactive cells were positive for DP. This observation contrasts with findings in normal mucosa, which in a large portion of cases were class II antigen positive, even though staining tended to be focal and associated with the presence of lymphocytic infiltrate.

Histocompatibility antigen expression in larynx cancer

A total of 29 cases of primitive tumors and 21 metastases of larynx cancer were tested. Positive reactions for HLA class I antigens were noted in 18 of 29 cases, while expression was heterogeneous in 6 of 29 and null in 5 cases. The majority of positive tumors were well differentiated. All undifferentiated tumors, on the other hand, presented heterogeneous or null staining for class I HLA antigens.

Most larynx cancer tumors failed to express class II antigens, with only 2 well differentiated tumors showing positive HLA-DR expression.

TABLE III. EXPRESSION OF CLASS I AND II ANTIGENS IN PRIMARY TUMORS AND AUTOLOGOUS METASTASES

		Class I Antigens		Class II Antigen	
Case	Site	Primary	Metastasis	Primary	Metastasis
Stomach	l.node	+	–	–	–
Larynx	"	–	+	–	–
Larynx	"	–	+	–	–
Larynx	"	+	–	–	–
Larynx	"	+	–	–	–
Melanoma	"	+	–	–	–
Melanoma	"	–	+	+	+
Melanoma	"	–	+	+	–

Of 60 primary tumors with autologous metastases we found divergences of expression in the eight cases shown above.

TABLE IV. SELECTIVE LOSS OF HLA CLASS I ANTIGENS IN HUMAN TUMORS

	Lymphocytic typing	Tumor typing
Colon	A2,-/B5,B21	A2,-/,-
Larynx	A2,-/B5,B44	A2,-/,-
Stomach	A11,-/B14,B44	-,-/-,-

Lymphocytic typing was performed with conventional serological techniques. Tumors were typed in cryostatic sections using the following monoclonal antibodies: anti-heavy chain, anti-B2 microglobulin, anti B locus, anti BW4, anti-BW6 and allospecific MoAbs.

Histocompatibility antigen expression in other human tumors

Other kinds of tumors investigated in the present study were: 11 renal cancers, 4 sarcomas, 8 squamous cell epitheliomas and 26 basal cell epitheliomas. These tumors revealed notable differences in class I antigen expression inasmuch as most kidney cancers and squamous cell epitheliomas showed marked positivity(12 of 13 and 7 of 8 cases respectively), whereas 9 of 26 cases of basal cell epithelioma were negative, along with all 4 cases of rhabdomyosarcoma. These findings highlight the heterogeneous nature of HLA class I antigen expression among the various histologic types studied. We consider this a key observation, bearing as it does on the significance which may have the altered levels of expression of such antigens. A case in point is melanoma, a tumor in which there is apparently a particular relationship between a low class I antigen expression and increasing invasiveness. However, no close correlation seems to exist between the lack of expression of these antigens and greater tumor aggressiveness, as exemplified by basal cell epithelioma of the skin, a nonmetastatic tumor presenting a high rate of loss of expression. Some alternative mechanisms to CTL immunosurveillance may operate in some tumors (10).

Selective loss of HLA class I antigens

We believe that the use of monomorphic monoclonal antibodies against class I antigens allows us to present a more precise picture of their actual expression. There is a possibility that an imbalance in expression between the three HLA-ABC molecules may go unnoticed with conventional immunohistologic procedures used up to now. This finding has been described in murine tumoral clones (35)as a factor having substantial relevance upon the metastatic behavior of these clones(12)We have also employed B locus specific monoclonal antibodies. Allospecific monoclonal antibodies have been used in those cases where discrepancies arose between the results obtained with B locus specific and conventional anti-heavy chain or anti-B2 microglobulin MoAbs. With this procedure we have detected alterations in these molecules in three tumors previously classified as HLA class I positive (Table 4). In the first case, lymphocyte typing in a patient with colon cancer was A2,-/B5, B21, but tumor cells failed to reveal the presence of antigens B5 or B21. A case of larynx cancer in an individual whose normal typing was A2,-/B5, B44 was negative for antigens B5 and B44. The final instance was a stomach cancer in a patient typed as A11,-/B12, B14, in which no A or B antigens could be detected on the tumor, hence in this case there is a possibility that other molecules of the human Qa-Tl like system (TCA) may be expressed as was observed in human teratocarcinomas (34).

Study of HLA class I genes in human tumors

We were interested in investigating whether any changes could be discerned at the gene level of HLA class I antigens which would explain the drops or alterations in expression by the tumors discussed in the present study. To this end, Southern blotting techniques were used to compare these genes in tumoral and normal (i. e. lymphocytes or normal mucosa) tissue.

In most cases studied (15 tumors) we could detect no difference between tumoral and normal tissue DNAs (Fig. 9). Although point mutations or small deletions cannot be ruled out, no significant rearrangements appear to take place, a finding which supports induction study results obtained in our laboratory with tumors adapted to short term culture, upon which HLA class I and class II antigen expression could be readily induced (melanoma, colon cancer and stomach cancer). This would in principle suggest the participation of normal regulatory mechanisms in the down regulation of class I genes.

Preliminary data suggest that a rearrangement of class I genes may take place in some tumors (5 to 10%) and may be detectable on comparing RFLP's of normal mucosa and tumor DNA. Our findings to date suggest that gene rearrangements in a small group of tumors may explain the phenotypic variations shown by these malignant cells. It should moreover be kept in mind that such rearrangements might also

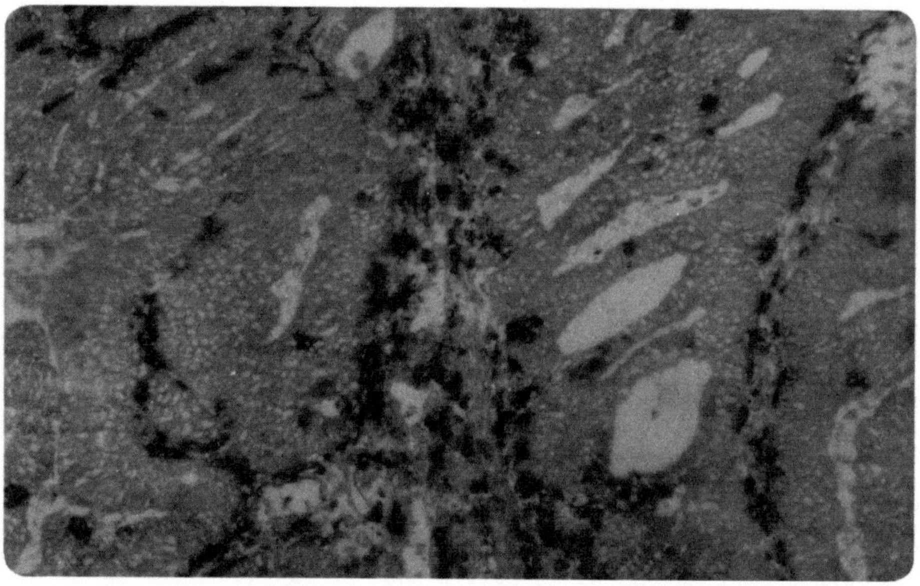

Fig. 8. Cryostatic section of a colon carcinoma stained with the MoAb W6/32 (anti heavy chain) and the immunephosphatase alkaline technique. It is a class I negative tumor. The stroma surrounding the tumor is class I positive.

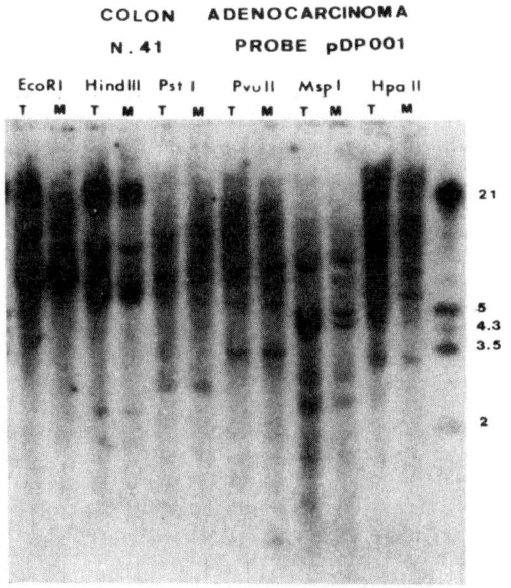

Fig. 9. Southern blot analysis of class I genes of the colon tumor nº 41 (class I positive), using DNA from the tumor tissue (T) and normal mucosa (M) of the same patient. No rearrengements of class I gene were detected.

be involved in the appearance of aberrant class I molecules. In other words, we may be dealing with true alloantigens, which behave like tumor antigens in some cases and supressor antigens in others, as has previously been described in murine models (1) . Tumors may therefore exist which failto express HLA-ABC self antigens (allodeterminants) while at the same time showing positive reactivity with monoclonal antibodies against B2 microglobulin or heavy chain monomorphic determinants.

There is undoubtably much that remains to be learned about the role of histocompatibility antigens in the appearance and development of human tumors and host immune responses. But there is no doubt also that MHC antigen manipulation could be a way to induce rejection of tumors in some cases or loss of immunogenicity in others (transplants). If this can be done, we may approach an understanding of the preoccupation of the immune system with histocompatibility antigens and the surveillance of transplants and tumors.(36).

Acknowledgments

The authors would like to acknowledge funding receive from the "Fondo de Investigaciones Sanitarias de la Seguridad Social" and the CAICYT, SPAIN. Thanks are also due to Dr. Biro, Dr. L. Eisenbach, Dr. Milstein, Dr. M. Steinmetz, Dr. T. Strachan, Dr. J. Vives and Dr. Wernet for providing with MoAbs and class I probes and to Dr. A. Ferrón, F. Esteban, J. Gutierrez, C. Huelin, R. Oliva, C. Romero, F. Ruiz-Cabello, T. Cabrera, B. de la Higuera, A. Caballero, M. Pérez, A. Garrido, E. Pareja, Mª.J. Mialdea, for their cooperation in this paper, and Ms Rosa Fernández for typing the manuscript. We thank Dr.M.A. Lopez Nevot for providing with impublished results and Dr. S. David for H-2 recombinant mice.

1. H. Festenstein, F. Garrido. MHC antigens and malignancy. Nature 322 502-503. (1986).
2. H. Festenstein. The biological consequences of altered MHC expression on tumours. British Medical Bulletin 43,1, 217-227. (1987).
3. F. Garrido, H. Festenstein, V. Schirrmacher. Further evidence for derepression of H-2 and Ia-like specificities of foreign haplotypes in mouse tumour cell lines. Nature 261-705. (1976).
4. F. Garrido, M. Pérez, M.D. Torres. Absence of four $H-2^d$ antigenic specificities in an $H-2^d$ sarcoma. J. of. Immunogenetics 6, 83-86. (1979).
5. V. Schirrmacher, D. Hübsch, F. Garrido. Syngeneic tumor cells can induce alloreactive T killer cells: A biological role for transplantation antigens. Proc. Natl. Acad. Sci. 77, 9, 5409-5413.(1980)
6. F. Garrido, M. Pérez, M.D. Torres, E. Garcia-Olivares, P. Ivanyi, V. Schirrmacher. A syngeneic anti tumor serum recognizing a complex H-2 alloantigen. Immunobiol. 156, 110-120. (1979).
7. H.J. Stauss, R. Linsk, A. Fischer, S. Watts, D. Banasiak, A. Haberman, I. Clark, J. Forman, M. McMillan, H. Schreiber, R.S. Goodenow. Isolation of the MHC genes encoding the tumour-specific class I antigens expressed on a murine fibrosarcoma. J. of Immunogenetics. 13, 101-111. (1986).
8. R.S.Goodenow, J.M. Vogel, R.L. Linsk. Histocompatibility antigens on murine tumors. Science 230, 777. (1985).
9. K. Hui, L. Minamide, N. Padroni, H. Festenstein, F.G. Grosveld. Structural variations in the H-2 genes AKR lymphomas. J. of Immunogenetics 13, 117-121. (1986).

10. W. Schmidt, G. Noll, D. Bevec, U. Henseling. Aberrant MHC antigens in a sarcoma virus-induced mouse tumour. J. of Immunogenetics. 13, 123-132. (1986).
11. A. Garrido, M. Pérez, C. Delgado, M.L. Garrido, J. Rojano, I. Algarra, F. Garrido. Influence of class I H-2 gene expression on local tumor growth. Exp. and Clinical Immunogenetics. 3, 98-110 (1986).
12. L. Eisenbach, S. Segal, M. Feldman. MHC imbalance and metastatic spread in Lewis lung carcinoma clones. International J. of Cancer 32, 113. (1983).
13. M.L. Garrido, M. Pérez, C. Delgado, J. Rojano, I. Algarra, A. Garrido, F. Garrido. Immunogenicity of H-2 positive and H-2 negative clones of a mouse tumour GR9. J. of Immunogenetics. 13, 159-167. (1986).
14. F.J. Bonal, E. Pareja, J. Martín, C. Romero, F. Garrido. Repression of class I H-2K, H-2D antigens on GR9 methylcholanthrene-induced tumour cell clones is related to the level of DNA methylation. 13, 179-186. (1986).
15. A. Caballero, MD. Collado, I. Algarra, A. Garrido, M. Pérez, F. Garrido. H-2 antigen expression, tumor associated transplantation antigens any anti tumor CTL's in clones derived from a chemically induced tumours. (in press) (1987).
16. C. Delgado, A. Garrido, M. Pérez, M.L. Garrido, I. Algarra, F. Garrido. Characterization of the syngeneic anti-tumour response against the GR9 tumour with the production of isoantisera and monoclonal antibodies. J. of Immunogenetics. 13, 169-177. (1986).
17. A. Watson, F.H. Bach. The role of gp70 in the target antigen recognized by murine leukemia virus immune cytotoxic T-lymphocytes. Int. J. Cancer. 26, 483. (1980).
18. E. Pareja, E. Cañadas, C. Romero, J. Martín M.J. Mialdea, F. Garrido. MHC-DNA class I gene transfection and expression in a murine class I negative tumour cell clone. Inmunologia (in press). (1987).
19. M. Pérez, T. Cabrera, M.A. López Nevot, M. Gomez, F. Peran, F. Garrido. Heterogeneity of the expression of class I and II HLA antigens in human breast carcinoma. J.of Immunogenetics.13,247-253
20. H.G. Ljunggren, K. Kärre. Experimental strategies and interpretations in the analysis of changes in MHC gene expression during tumour progression: opposing influences of T cell natural killer cell mediated resistance. J. of Immunogenetics. 13, 141-151.(1986)
21. M.A. López Nevot, E. Garcia, E. Pareja, F.J. Bonal, J. Martín, F. Differential expression of HLA class I and II antigens in primary and metastatic melanomas. J. of Immunogenetics. 13, 219-227. (1986).
22. J. Gutierrez, M.A. López Nevot, T. Cabrera, R. Oliva, J. Esquivias F. Ruiz-Cabello, F. Garrido. Class I and II HLA antigen distribution in normal mucosa, adenoma and colon carcinoma: Relation with malignancy and invasiveness. Clin. and Exp. Immunogenetics (in press. (1987).
23. M. Pérez, A. Garrido, I. Algarra, F. Garrido. Different H-2 phenotypes in clones derived from a new BALB/c solid tumor. Its relevance for local tumor growth. Inmunología. 4,2, 60-69. (1985).
24. P.I. Schrier, R. Bernards, R.T.M.J. Vaessen, A. Houweling, A.J. Van Der Eb. Expression of class I major histocompatibility antigens swiched off by highly oncogenic adenovirus 12 in transformed rat cells. Nature. 305, 771. (1983).

25. F. Momburg, P. Möller, G. Moldenhauer, G.J. Hämmerling. Loss of HLA-A,B,C, in colorectal carcinoma is related to the degree of de-differentiation. J. of Immunogenetics. 13, 195-199. (1986).
26. F. Ruiz-Cabello, M.A. López Nevot, J. Gutierrez, A. Ferrón, F. Esteban, C. Rivas, M.A. Piris, F. Garrido. Phenotypic expression of histocompatibility antigens in human primary tumors and metastases. Cancer Research. (in press). (1987).
27. M.A. López Nevot, T. Cabrera, B. de la Higuera, F. Ruiz-Cabello F. Garrido. Production and characterization of monoclonal antibodies against human leukaemia cells. Inmunologia. 5, 2. 51-59. (1986).
28. T. Cabrera, F. Ruiz-Cabello, M.A. López Nevot, B. de la Higuera, M. Sanchez, F. Garrido. Characterization of monoclonal antibodies directed against HLA class II molecules. Hybridoma. 5,3, 191-197. (1986).
29. A. Ziegler, B. Uchanska-Ziegler, G. Rosenfelder, D.G. Braun, P. Wernet. Heterogeneity of established human hematopoietic cell lines: Surface antigens detected by monoclonal antibodies and glycosphilipid patterns. In: Leukaemia markers. Proceedings of the leukaemia marker conference held in Vienna. Academic Press. 137. (1981).
30. A.J. Watson, R. Demars, I.S. Trowbridge, F.H. Bach. Detection of a novel human HLA antigen. Nature. 304, 358-361. (1983).
31. D.J. Ruiter, W. Bergman, K. Welvaart, E. Scheffer, W.A. van Vloten C. Russo, S. Ferrone. Immunohistological analysis of malignant melanomas and nevocellular nevi with monoclonal antibodies to distinct monomorphic determinants of HLA antigens. Cancer Res. 44, 3930. (1984).
32. E.B. Bröcker, L. Suter, J. Brüggen, D.J. Ruiter, E. Macher, C. Sorg. Phenotypic dynamics of tumor progression in human malignant melanoma. Int. J. of Cancer. 36, 29. (1985).
33. F. Ruiz-Cabello, M.A. López Nevot, F. Garrido. MHC class I and II gene expression on human tumors. Cancer Metastasis, Bolonia, Italy Plenum Publishing Corporation. (In press). May 13-15 (1987).
34. P.L. Stern, N. Beresford, S.M. Bell, S. Thompson, K. Jones, A. Mellor. Murine embryonal carcinoma cells express class I MHC like antigens. J. of Immunogenet. 13, 133. (1986).
35. G.J. Hämmeling, D. Klar, S. Katzav, S. Segal, M. Feldman, R. Wallich, A. Hämmerling. Manipulation of metastasis and tumor growth by transfection with histocompatibility class I genes. J. of Immunogenet. 13, 153. (1986).
36. F. Garrido, V. Schirrmacher, H. Festenstein. H-2 like specificities of foreign haplotypes appearing on a mouse sarcoma after vaccinia virus infection. Nature. 259, 5540, 228-230. (1976).

ALTERED MHC CLASS I GENES CAN ENCODE IMMUNOGENIC ANTIGENS THAT CAUSE TUMOR REJECTION

Hans J. Stauss, Mary Ann Fink, Barbara Starr and Hans Schreiber

The University of Chicago
Department of Pathology
5841 S. Maryland - Box 414
Chicago, IL 60637

ABSTRACT

The C3H UV-induced skin tumor 1591 is highly immunogenic and is rejected when transplanted into immunocompetent syngeneic C3H mice. We have isolated three MHC class I genes from a genomic tumor library and we show that these genes encode novel class I antigens expressed in 1591 tumor cells but not in normal C3H cells. All three genes account for a restriction fragment length polymorphism in the tumor DNA relative to normal C3H DNA, indicating that the genes were not preexistant in the C3H genome but arose by mutation or recombination. We show that one of the tumor class I genes encodes a highly immunogenic class I antigen which is a target antigen for tumor rejection in immunocompetent hosts.

INTRODUCTION

Tumor-specific transplantation antigens are antigens that can lead to immune destruction of a transplanted cancer by syngeneic hosts. Such antigens, which are often found on cancers induced by chemical or physical carcinogens, are usually unique, i.e., antigenically different for each independently induced tumor (Prehn and Main, 1957; Klein et al., 1960). Although the molecular nature of these unique, tumor-specific antigens has not yet been determined, evidence has been accumulated suggesting that tumors can express novel MHC class I antigens (Parmiani et al., 1979; Doherty et al., 1984). The apparent expression of anomalous class I antigens in tumor cells is intriguing, because these molecules of the MHC are known to play an essential role in immune regulation. Self-class I antigens function as restriction elements, directing the attack of cytotoxic T lymphocytes (CTL) against virally-infected and transformed target cells (Doherty and Zinkernagel, 1975). Non-self class I antigens are extremely immunogenic and efficiently mediate rejection of histoincompatible transplanted tissue (Alter et al., 1973). It is, therefore, essential to establish the molecular nature of novel class I antigens on tumor cells and to elucidate the function of these antigens during tumor rejection and tumor progression.

In order to address these questions, we studied the C3H-derived UV-induced skin tumor, 1591 (Fisher and Kripke, 1977). This tumor is highly immunogenic when transplanted into normal syngeneic mice. Analysis of tumor variants with cloned CTL lines suggested that the 1591 tumor expresses several independent antigens which account for its immunogenicity (Wortzel et al., 1984). Two syngeneic monoclonal antibodies (mAbs) which recognize tumor-specific antigens on 1591 have recently been generated (Philipps et al., 1985). Mapping studies with H-2 congenic mouse strains and biochemical analyses revealed that these antibodies recognize unique class I products expressed on tumor cells but not on normal C3H cells (Philipps et al., 1985; McMillan et al., 1985). The genetic origin of these novel class I molecules remained obscure, however, and it was possible that they were derived by alternative processing or by de novo activation of endogenous class I genes. Furthermore, the relationship between the antibody-recognized novel class I antigens and the T cell-recognized rejection antigens (Wortzel et al., 1983) remained unclear. Since the antibodies did not block the activity of tumor-specific CTL clones (Philipps et al., 1986) it was possible that the two probes recognized distinct molecules.

We now show that the 1591 tumor contains three novel class I genes which encode the antibody-recognized tumor-specific class I antigens. All three genes appear to be the result of mutation or recombination because they are not preexistant in the C3H genome. One of the novel class I genes encodes an antigen that is recognized by a tumor-specific CTL clone. We used gene transfection to show that the expression of this antigen in tumor cells is sufficient to cause complete tumor rejection in immunocompetent animals.

MATERIALS AND METHODS

Tumor Lines

The 1591 tumor originated from a C3H/HeN (MTV-) mouse and was induced by UV-irradiation (Fisher and Kripke, 1977). The C3H origin of the tumor has been confirmed by the electrophoretic analysis of seven polymorphic isoenzymes and by staining with nine mAbs specific for H-2^k haplotype class I antigens (Philipps et al., 1985). 1591-VAR8 is a progressor variant isolated from a normal C3H mouse that failed to reject a 1591 tumor challenge (Urban et al., 1982).

Serological Analyses

The following mAbs were used in this study: CP28 and CP3F4 are two C3H-derived antibodies which recognize unique tumor-specific class I determinants expressed by the 1591 tumor (Philipps et al., 1985); the antibodies 30-5-7 and 28-14-8 were generated against the H-$2L^d$ antigen (Ozato et al., 1980) and cross-react with the 1591 tumor (Philipps et al., 1985). The fluorescence-activated cell sorter, FACS IVB (Becton and Dickinson), was used to quantify the degree of MHC class I antigen expression of tumor cells and of class I gene transfectants. Cells were incubated with the MHC class I-specific antibodies first and then with fluorescein-coupled goat anti-mouse immunoglobulin antibodies. The binding ratio was determined as the amount of fluorescence after staining with both antibodies divided by the amount of fluorescence after staining with the second antibody alone.

Construction and Screening of Genomic Library

Genomic DNA from 1591 tumor cells was isolated and partially digested with the restriction enzyme Mbo I. The genomic DNA fragments were inserted into the Bam HI site of the lambda vector EMBL 3 (Frischauf et al., 1983). The average size of inserts was approximately 20 kb. Phage containing class I inserts were identified by filter hybridization using the class I-specific probe, pH-2IIa (Steinmetz et al., 1981).

Transfection of Cloned Class I Genes

Lambda clones containing complete class I genes were introduced into thymidine kinase-negative C3H L cells (Ltk-) by calcium phosphate co-precipitation with the HSV tk gene (Parker and Stark, 1979). Approximately 5 x 10^6 L cells were transfected with 50 ng ptk5 DNA, 2 μg cloned class I DNA, and 10 μg carrier DNA. The transformants were selected in media which contained hypoxanthine, aminopterin, and

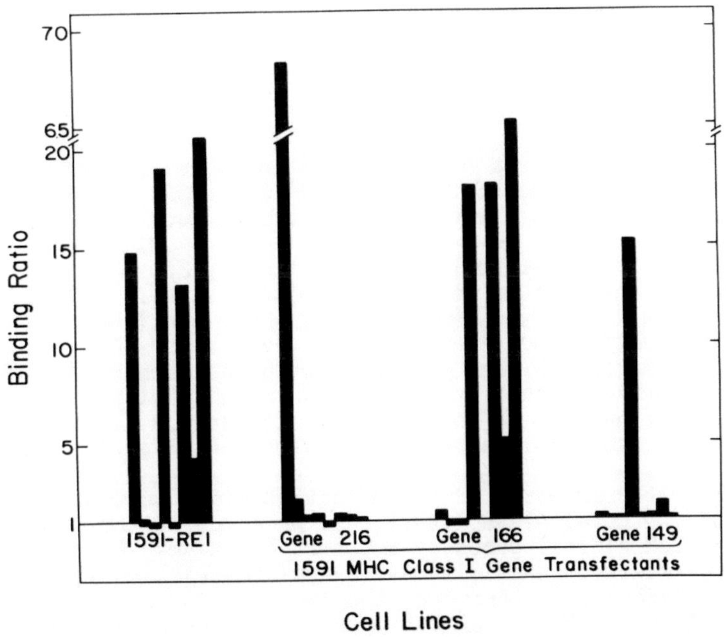

Fig. 1. The 1591 class I genes 216, 166 and 149 account for all the novel MHC class I antigens that have previously been detected on 1591-RE using MHC class I-specific antibodies. The novel class I gene 216 selectively encodes for the antigen reactive with the syngeneic tumor-specific monoclonal antibody CP28. The fluorescence-activated cell sorter, FACS IVB, was used to determine the indirect fluorescence listed as binding ratio, i.e. fluorescence of the tumor cells stained with the first and second antibody over the fluorescence of the tumor cells stained with the second antibody alone for background (for details see Materials and Methods). The bars (left to right) indicate the binding of CP28, 34-2-12 (D^d), 34-5-8 (D^d), 28-14-8 ($L^dD^{b,q}$), 34-4-20 (L^dD^d), 30-5-7 ($L^dD^qL^qL^b$), 23-5-21 ($D^bD^dD^{s,q,p}$), and CP3F4 to the parental 1591 regressor tumor or the gene transfected L cells (Reprinted with permission from Stauss et al., 1986b).

thymidine. The progressor variant 1591-VAR8 was co-transfected with the cloned 1591 class I genes and with the plasmid pZipNeo (Cepko et al., 1984), which contains the gene encoding the aminoglycoside phosphotransferase. The cells that acquired aminoglycoside phosphotransferase activity were selected by their ability to grow in the presence of 500 μg/ml of the antibiotic G418 (untransfected cells consistently died after 1 wk under those conditions). Gene transfected cells were cloned by limiting dilution and the individual clones were analyzed with the FACS IVB for class I antigen expression.

Southern Blotting

DNA was extracted from tumor cell lines grown in vitro or from spleen cells of inbred mouse strains and was digested to completion using an excess of restriction enzyme (New England BioLabs, Beverly, MA). The digested DNA was separated on 0.9 percent agarose gels and blotted onto zetabind membrane (AMF-Cuno, Meriden, CT) by capillary flow using 20 x SSC as transfer buffer. The conditions of the hybridization and the origin of the MHC class I-specific probe 149.6-6 have been described (Stauss et al., 1986a).

RESULTS

The 1591 tumor expresses novel class I antigens that are recognized by the syngeneic monoclonal antibodies CP28 and CP3F4 (Philipps et al., 1985). These novel class I antigens also cross-react with the antibodies 28-14-8 (anti-L^d, D^b) and 30-5-7 (anti-L^d, D^b, D^q, L^q). From a genomic 1591 library, we isolated approximately 250 MHC class I genes and transfected them into mouse L cells (Stauss et al., 1986a). The transfected L cells were screened with the above mentioned monoclonal antibodies to identify the genes encoding novel tumor-specific class I antigens. Figure 1 shows that the genes with the number 149, 166 and 216 encode class I antigens that are expressed in the 1591 tumor. Furthermore, together the three genes can account for all the novel class I determinants present on the parental 1591 tumor (Fig. 1).

To test whether mutation or recombination might account for the expression of the novel class I antigens, we compared the tumor class I genes and the C3H class I genes by Southern blotting. Figure 2 shows that the tumor class I genes display several restriction fragment length polymorphisms (RFLP). Furthermore, the 166 and 216 genes account for two RFLP's present in the tumor DNA but absent from normal C3H DNA (Fig. 2). The 149 gene contains a polymorphic restriction fragment identical in size to the polymorphic fragment of the 166 gene (Stauss et al., 1986a). Together, this indicates that the 149, 166 and 216 genes were not preexistent in the C3H genome and it is possible that they were generated by mutation or recombination.

In a previous study, we have shown that progressor variants of the 1591 regressor tumor always lost the 149, 166 and 216 genes simultaneously (Stauss et al., 1986b). It remained therefore unclear whether all three genes were required to cause tumor rejection or whether the expression of only one of these genes would be sufficient to cause tumor regression. To test this, we introduced by transfection the 216 gene into a progressively growing 1591 variant, designated 1591-VAR8, which had lost all 3 novel class I genes. This progressor tumor was co-transfected with the 216 gene and the gene encoding the enzyme aminoglycoside phosphotransferase, which confers resistance to the drug G418. The G418-resistant cell population was cloned and two 216 gene expressing clones, designated $TR216^+.1$ and $TR216^+.2$, and two negative

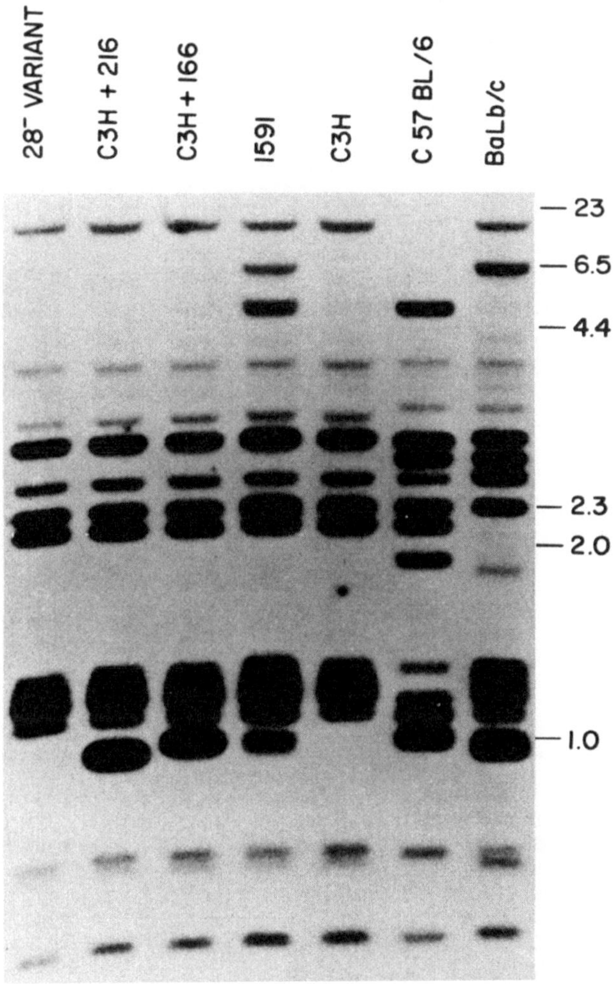

Fig. 2. Southern blot analysis of tumor DNA compared to normal C3H DNA. C3H spleen DNA (lane 5) was compared to 1591 tumor DNA (lane 4). Lanes 2 and 3 contain C3H DNA plus approximately 3 ng of gene 216 and 166 DNA, respectively. Lane 1 contains DNA from a tumor variant that lost expression of the novel class I antigens. DNA of the inbred strains C57BL/6 (lane 6) and BALB/c (lane 7) is shown for comparison. All DNAs were digested with the restriction enzyme Pst 1 and the blots were probed with the 3' class I probe 149.6-6 generated from the 1 kb polymorphic Pst 1 fragment of the 149 gene. The position of the size markers is indicated (Reprinted with permission from Stauss et al., 1986a).

clones, designated TR216⁻.3 and TR216⁻.4, which were G418 resistant but did not express the 216 gene-encoded antigen, were analyzed further. Cells of these four clones were injected into nude mice and fragments of the growing tumors were used to challenge normal animals. The 216 gene expressing $TR216^+.1$ clone grew out in only 1 of 5 animals and that the 216 gene expressing $TR216^+.2$ clone was rejected in all animals. In contrast, the clones $TR216^-.3$ and $TR216^-.4$, which do not express the 216 gene-encoded antigen, grew in 5 of 5 and 4 of 5 mice, respectively.

Table 1. Reversal of Malignant Growth in Normal Mice by Transfection of the Novel Class I Gene 216

Cell line[a]	Expression of the 216 gene product[b]	Tumor incidence (%)[c] Normal mice	Nude mice
1591-VAR8 $TR216^+.1$	+	[d]1/5	2/2
1591-VAR8 $TR216^+.2$	+	0/5	2/2
		Total 1/10 (10)	
1591-VAR8 $TR216^-.3$	–	5/5	2/2
1591-VAR8 $TR216^-.4$	–	4/5	2/2
		Total 9/10 (90)	
1591-VAR8 TR216.1 Reisolated[d]	–	5/5 (100)	ND
1591-VAR8	–	8/10 (80)	ND
1591-RE	+	0/10 (0)	2/2

[a]A clone of the 1591-VAR8 tumor (clone VAR8.7) was transfected with the 216 gene and the neomycin resistance gene. The G418 drug-resistant cell population was cloned and two clones which expressed the 216 gene-encoded antigen and two clones which did not express the 216 gene-encoded antigen were used to challenge 5 normal mice with tumor fragments (each animal was injected with a total of 10 tumor fragments of approximately 1 mm^3 in size) or 2 nude mice (with five 1 mm^3 tumor fragments each).

[b]Expression of the 216 gene product was determined by FACS IVB analysis using the monoclonal antibody CP 28 that specifically recognizes this gene product and a fluoresceinated second antibody. Cell lines designated positive for expression of the 216 gene product stained at least 2 times above background (binding ratio >2) while all cell lines designated negative for 216 gene expression stained less that 1.5-fold above background (binding ratio <1.5).

[c]Number of mice with progressively growing tumors/number of mice challenged. Mice receiving the 216^- clones died within approximately 6 wk due to the large tumor burden. The mice that were challenged with the 216^+ transfectants did not develop tumors even after 4 months except for one mouse that grew out an antigen loss variant approximately 2.5 wk after injection. All cell lines used in this experiment readily formed tumors in nude mice.

[d]One of the mice injected with the transfected 1591-VAR8 $TR216^+.1$ cell line developed a progressively growing tumor that was reisolated (designated 1591-VAR8 TR216.1 Reisolate) and reanalyzed for expression of the 216 gene by FACS IVB and for tumor incidence in normal mice (Modified from Stauss et al., 1986b).

The single tumor which grew out in one of the animals that were challenged with the TR216^{+}.1 clone was readapted to culture and analyzed for the expression of the 216 gene-encoded antigen. FACS analysis showed that all cells of the reisolated tumor were negative for the 216 antigen (Fig. 3), indicating that the cells either lost the transfected 216 gene or that its expression was prevented by some other mechanism. Together, these data indicate that the stable expression of the 216 gene-encoded antigen is sufficient to change the phenotype of a

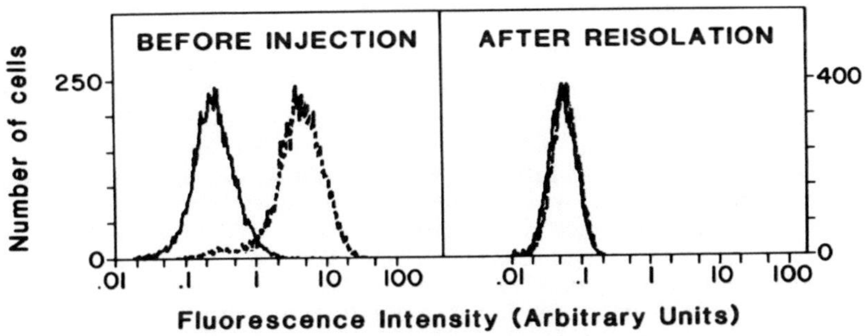

Fig. 3. Loss of expression of the transfected 216 gene in a reisolated 1591-VAR8 tumor that grew progressively despite transfection with the 216 gene. The 216 gene-transfected tumors analyzed are the same as those used for the experiments described in Table 1. The first panel show the histogram of the 1591-VAR8 TR 216^{+}. 1 cell line and the second panel shows the histogram of the 1591-VAR8 TR216.1 reisolate. Cells were incubated with the monoclonal antibody CP28 followed by incubation with fluorescein-coupled goat anti-mouse immunoglobulin antibodies (---) or incubated with only the goat anti-mouse immunoglobulin (__). Ten thousand cells were analyzed with the FACS IVB (Reprinted with permission from Stauss et al., 1986b).

progressor tumor and to cause tumor rejection in normal animals. Furthermore, the loss of the expression of the 216 antigen in transfected tumor cells allows these cells to escape immune destruction and to display the phenotype of the untransfected parental progressor tumor.

DISCUSSION

We have identified three functional class I genes from a 1591 genomic library and demonstrated that these genes encode molecules recognized by several monoclonal antibodies reactive with the tumor. Southern blot analysis suggests that the three genes were generated by mutational events since they contain polymorphic restriction enzyme fragments which are only found in the tumor but not in the normal C3H genome. The C3H origin of the tumor is indicated by the well documented history of 1591 and by immunological and biochemical analyses (see Materials and Methods). To establish that the novel antigens expressed on the 1591 tumor were generated by mutational events involving C3H class I genes, it will be important to identify the endogenous C3H loci from which the tumor genes were derived.

Southern blot analysis of three tumors that were isolated together with 1591 in the same experiment from the same batch of mice showed that all three tumors displayed a restriction fragment pattern characteristic for the class I genes of the C3H strain and none contained the RFLP's present in 1591 (data not shown). This excludes the possiblity that genetic drift of the present day C3H strain (Bailey, 1982) accounts for the detection of the polymorphic class I sequences in 1591.

The fact that the novel class I antigens were found on the tumor immediately after *in vitro* adaptation (Philipps et al., 1985) indicates that the genes encoding the antigens did not arise during long-term passage *in vitro* or *in vivo*. Normal cells from the animal in which the 1591 tumor arose are not available, and therefore, we cannot determine whether the mutant C3H genes were generated by germ line mutations or by somatic mutations during tumor induction. Since UV-induced tumors frequently express immunogenic antigens and are rejected in immunocompetent syngeneic hosts (Kripke, 1981), it seems unlikely that germ line mutations can account for the high frequency at which these immunogenic antigens are observed. It appears more likely that somatic mutations, possibly due to the extensive UV exposure during tumor induction, lead to the expression of tumor-specific antigens.

We have shown that the novel MHC class I gene 216 encodes an antigen that causes tumor-rejection in immunocompetent mice. Transfection of the 216 gene into a progressively growing 1591 tumor variant leads to the rejection of the cells expressing the 216 gene-encoded antigen. We found that the 216 antigen must be lost before the tumor can grow progressively in a normal mouse. Therefore, the presented data have shown that an altered MHC class I gene can encode a unique tumor-specific rejection antigen. Work in progress will determine whether the novel class I genes 149 and 166 also encode tumor-specific rejection antigens and whether the expression of these antigens will prevent tumor progression in normal mice.

Unique tumor-specific transplantation antigens are antigenically distinct for independently induced tumors. These different antigens may be the result of mutational changes of different unrelated genes. Alternatively, these antigens might be encoded by the members of a gene family such as the immunoglobulin genes, the T cell receptor genes, the MHC class I and class II genes or the genes of the multiple retroviral proviruses which are present in the murine genome. It has been shown that even a single malignant cell can express multiple unique tumor-specific antigens (Uyttenhove et al., 1983; Wortzel et al., 1983). To resolve multiple unanswered questions concerning the origin of these antigens and to determine if they are encoded by a family of related genes, it will be necessary to identify molecularly and genetically the unique tumor-specific transplantation antigens of other tumors.

We have generated a new bank of UV-induced tumors in which normal control cells are concurrently isolated from each tumor-bearing mouse. These new tumors will be useful to determine to what extent tumor-specific rejection antigens of other highly immunogenic regressor tumors are encoded by novel MHC class I genes and whether these genes represent germ line mutations or somatic mutations caused by the carcinogen treatment.

REFERENCES

Alter, B. J., Schendel, D. J., Bach, M. L., Bach, F. H., and Stimpfling, J. H., 1973, Cell-mediated lympholysis. Importance of serologically defined H-2 regions., J. Exp. Med., 137:1303.

Baily, D. W., 1982, How pure are inbred strains of mice., Immunol. Today, 3:210.

Cepko, C. L., Roberts, B. E., and Mulligan, R. C., 1984, Construction and applications of a highly transmissible retrovirus shuttle vector., Cell, 37:1053.

Doherty, P. C., and Zinkernagel, R. M., 1975, H-2 compatibility is required for T cell-mediated lysis of target cells infected with lymphocytic choriomeningitis virus., J. Exp. Med., 141:502.

Doherty, P. C., Knowles, B. B., and Wettstein, P. J., 1984, Immunological surveillance of tumors in the context of major histocompatibility complex restriction of T cell function., Adv. Cancer Res., 42:1.

Fisher, M. S., and Kripke, M. L., 1978, Systemic alteration induced in mice by ultraviolet light irradiation and its relationship to ultraviolet carcinogenesis., Proc. Natl. Acad. Sci. USA, 74:1688.

Frischauf, A., Lehrach, H., Poustka, A., and Murray, N., 1983, Lambda replacement vectors carrying polylinker sequences., J. Mole. Bio., 170:827.

Klein, G., Sjogren, H. O., Klein, E., and Hellstrom, K. E., 1960, Demonstration of resistance against methylcholanthrene-induced sarcomas in the primary autochthonous host., Cancer Res., 20:1561.

Kripke, M. L., 1981, Immunologic mechanisms in UV radiation carcinogenesis., Adv. Cancer Res., 34:69.

McMillan, M., Lewis, K. D., and Rovner, D. M., 1985, Molecular characterization of novel H-2 class I molecules expressed by a C3H UV-induced fibrosarcoma., Proc. Natl. Acad. Sci. USA, 82:5485.

Ozato, K., Hansen, T. H., and Sachs, D., 1980, Monoclonal antibodies to mouse MHC antigens., J. Immunol., 125:2473.

Parmiani, G., Carbone, G., Invernizzi, G., Pierotti, M. A., Sensi, M. L., Rogers, M. J., and Appela, E., 1979, Alien histocompatibility antigens on tumor cells., Immunogenetics, 9:1.

Philipps, C., McMillan, M., Flood, P. M., Murphy, D. B., Forman, J., Lancki, D., Womack, J. E., Goodenow, R. S., and Schreiber, H., 1985, Identification of a unique tumor-specific antigen as a novel class I major histocompatibility molecule., Proc. Natl. Acad. Sci. USA, 82:5140.

Philipps, C., Stauss, H. J., Wortzel, R. D., and Schreiber, H., 1986, A novel MHC class I molecule as tumor-specific antigen: correlation between the antibody-defined and the CTL-defined target structure., J. Immunogenet., (Oxf.), in press.

Prehn, R. T., and Main, J. M., 1957, Immunity to methlcholanthrene-induced sarcomas., J. Natl. Cancer Inst., 18:769.

Stauss, H. J., Linsk, R., Fischer, A., Watts, S., Banasiak, D.,

Haberman, A., Clark, I., Forman, J., McMillan, M., Schreiber, H., and Goodenow, R., 1986a, Isolation of the MHC genes encoding the tumor-specific class I antigens expressed on a murine fibrosarcoma., J. Immunogenet., 13:101.

Stauss, H. J., Van Waes, C., Fink, M. A., Starr, B., and Schreiber, H., 1986b, Identification of a unique tumor antigen as rejection antigen by molecular cloning and gene transfer., J. Exp. Med., 164:1516.

Steinmetz, M., Frelinger, J. G., Fisher, D., Hunkapiller, T., Pereira, D., Weissman, S. W., Uehara, H., Nathenson, S. and Hood, L., 1981, Three cDNA clones encoding mouse transplantation antigens: homology to immunoglobulin genes., Cell, 24:125.

Urban, J. L., Burton, R. C., Holland, J. M., Kripke, M., and Schreiber, H., 1982, Mechanisms of syngeneic tumor rejection. Susceptibility of host-selected progressor variants to various immunological effector cells., J. Exp. Med., 155:557.

Uyttenhove, C., Maryanski, J., and Boon, T., 1983, Escape of mouse mastocytoma P815 after nearly complete rejection is due to antigen-loss variants rather than immunosuppression., J. Exp. Med., 157:1040.

Wortzel, R. D., Philipps, C., and Schreiber, H., 1983, Multiple tumor-specific antigens expressed on a single tumor cell., Nature, 304:165.

Wortzel, R. D., Urban, J. L., and Schreiber, H., 1984, Malignant growth in the normal host after variant selection in vitro with cytolytic T cell lines., Proc. Natl. Acad. Sci. USA, 81:2186.

REGULATION OF H-2 CLASS I GENE EXPRESSION IN VIRUS TRANSFORMED AND/OR INFECTED CELLS

Daniel Meruelo

Department of Pathology and Kaplan Cancer Center

New York University Medical Center

New York, New York 10016

Virally-induced Tumors: Early studies from our laboratory

Our group first documented that viral infections and virus-induced transformations can significantly affect class I gene expression. These virally-induced alterations in H-2 (class I) antigen expression were shown to play a striking role in resistance to neoplasia[18]. Similar observations which have recently been made by numerous investigators in a variety of other systems [6, 8, 12, 24, 26].

Our early studies showed that resistance to RadLV induced leukemia is mediated by gene(s) in the H-2D region of the major murine histocompatibility complex (MHC)[17]. These experiments correlated disease resistance with changes in H-2 expression occurring immediately after virus inoculation and after tumorigenesis[13,18]. For example, H-2D antigen expression is elevated immediately after virus inoculation on thymocytes of resistant but not of susceptible mice[18]. An inverse relationship was shown to exist between expression of H-2 and viral antigens[18]. After RadLV infection, viral antigen expression is greater in susceptible animals which show little if any changes in H-2 antigen expression. In virus-infected resistant mice, having maximal H-2 antigen expression, rapid elimination of viral antigen expressing cells occurs[18]. Finally, H-2 antigens usually disappear from the surface of RadLV transformed cells when overt leukemia develops[18]. Thus, resistance to RadLV-induced neoplasia is associated with increased H-2 antigenic expression, whereas the onset of leukemia is associated with disappearance of these antigens.

Further experiments demonstrated that elevated H-2 antigen expression enhances the effectiveness of the host's immune response to virus-infected cells and functions in resistance to leukemogenesis[13]. Cell-mediated immunity against RadLV transformed or infected cells could be easily detected in resistant mice when H-2 positive, RadLV positive target cells were substituted in the cell-mediated lympholysis (CML) assay for the normally H-2 nonexpressing, RadLV transformed cells[13]. (The still unexplained observation was made in these studies that H-2 nonexpressing,

RadLV transformed cells, could be induced to reexpress H-2 antigens by *in vivo* passage[13]. Also, resistant mice were shown to have many more effector cells when infected with RadLV than did susceptible mice. Injection of normal (uninfected) thymocytes into syngeneic recipients of resistant or susceptible H-2 type does not stimulate a CML response[13]. However, injection of RadLV infected thymocytes from resistant mice elicits the most vigorous CML response at a time when both H-2 and viral antigens are found on their cell surface at high levels[13]. By contrast, injection of infected thymocytes from susceptible mice, which express viral antigens but low levels of H-2 antigens, does not stimulate a CML reaction[13]. Furthermore, target recognition appears to be specificfor certain H-2 antigens since cytolytic T lymphocytes (CTL) from F1 mice challenged with infected, resistant thymocytes can lyse resistant target cells but not susceptible targets despite adequate amounts of H-2 antigens in bothtarget cell types[13].

Other experiments indicated that transfer of thymocytes infected with RadLV for a short time (e.g. 3 wk), from resistant or susceptible mice, into irradiated, adult, syngeneic F1 mice leads to death from tumorigenesis in a relatively short time[13]. It is unlikely that such death results from the induction of leukemia by virus present in transformed cells because the progress of disease is too rapid and RadLV is not known to induce leukemia when injected into adult mice. Rather, preleukemic cells are probably generated quickly in the thymus by RadLV infection of both resistant or susceptible mice, and transfer of these cells to the irradiated host environment permits theirescape from the immunological control that normally prevents their growth. These observations clearly indicated the importance of immunosurveillance in controlling tumorigenesis by RadLV, and the impact that altered H-2 antigen expression has in the effectiveness of the host's immune response to deal with virus-infected cells.

(A) RadLV transformation is associated with increased methylation of Class I genes

A finding which is consistent with the lack of Class I gene transcription and expression observed in RadLV transformed cells is the drastic alterations in the degree of methylation of Class I DNA observed in the tumor cells[14]. Every RadLV induced tumor examined (over 40) shows altered methylation patterns for Class DNA when compared to normal cells[14]. Furthermore, alterations in methylation induced by RadLV appear to be specific for Class I genes, since none of the multiple other genes examined display similar alterations[14].

Others[20, 21, 25] have also shown that changes in the levels of DNAmethylation associated with Class I genes might be relevant to the issue of Class I gene expression. For example, both metastatic and non-metastatic phenotypes could be imparted to subclones of the Lewis lung carcinoma by treatment with 5-azacytidine, which is thought to specifically inhibit the enzymes involved in the maintenance of DNA methylation patterns[21]. The changes in metastatic potential of the cells thus achieved were accompanied by altered expression of specific Class I genes[21]. This observation suggests that changes in Class I gene expression induced by certain agents is reversible, and is consistent with our observations in the RadLV system. I have previously stated that H-2 antigen nonexpressing tumor cells can be converted into H-2 antigen expressing cells by passaging them *in vivo* through normal, syngeneic, healthy mice[13].

(B) Novel Class I RFLPs are observed in 10-20% of RadLV induced tumors

Rearrangements in MHC DNA also appear to accompany RadLV transformation as detected by digestion with various restriction enzymes[14]. Again, there seems to be specificity in this phenomena[14]. In RadLV transformed cells. novel RFLPs are only associated with Class I genes[14]. However, tumors with novel Class I RFLPs are seen less frequently than tumors with changed methylation patterns[14].

While studies to determine more precisely which Class I genes are methylated and rearranged in DNA from RadLV transformed cells are still preliminary, it is possible to conclude that alterations in methylation appear to affect numerous Class I genes[14]. However, novel RFLPs involve a more limited number of H-2 genes[14]. Thus while rearrangements can play a role in loss of expression of a specific Class I gene, it is difficult to envision amechanism by which limited rearrangements would affect expression of all Class I genes. Nonetheless, the study of such rearrangements, as by cloning some of the novel RFLPs and determining the Class I genes involved and the orientation of any viral sequences with respect to the former, should be most informative in understanding the interactions between viruses and MHC genes, and remains an important goal of our research. We have recently cloned some of these rearranged RFLPs and will now begin to characterize them.

(C) Interactions of viruses with promoter and enhancer-like sequences of Class I genes

Several promoter elements are crucial to the accuracy and efficiency of transcription by RNA polymerase II[4, 9]. The cap site identifies the point at which transcription starts. The Goldberg-Hogness or TATA box is usually located some 30 bp upstream (+1 refers to the cap site), a sequence of the CAAT type[5,9] or a GC-rich region[9, 10] also important for transcription has been found in the -50 to -90 region. Finally sequences located even further upstream, or sometimes within the genes (or downstream), known as enhancer elements, have been shown to stimulate transcription from homologous or heterologous promoters in a manner relatively independent of their distance and orientation with regard to the promoters[7, 9]. Enhancers found in cellular genes have also been implicated in the regulation of the tissue specific transcription of the latter[1, 9].

Naturally, given the above described effects of viruses on Class I gene transcription, it is of general interest to determine the interactions of viruses with these regulatory sequences. Kimura et al.[9]. have recently demonstrated that enhancer sequences associated with the $H\text{-}2K^b$ gene are notthe target of the inhibition of expression observed in Ad12 transformed cells. These investigators also found that the $H\text{-}2K^b$ promoter is repressed about eight to ten times more efficiently by Ad12 than by Ad5. These experiments reproduce in a transient assay, and with the $H\text{-}2K^b$ promoter alone, what is observed in vivo with the $H\text{-}2K^b$ gene. Furthermore, these workers point to the E1a region of the virus as the important viral element in this interaction. However, because as was pointed earlier, during acute infection by Ad5 and Ad12, $H\text{-}2K^b$ transcription is stimulated rather than repressed, the relationship between H-2 promoters, enhancers and viral elements is likely to be quite complex. It will not be explained solely by a direct inhibitory effect of E1a protein as has been found by Borelli et al.[3] on several viral enhancers.

In collaboration with the laboratories of Drs. George Scangos and Gilbert Jay we have examined the RadLV-induced deregulation of MHC antigen expression in transgenic mice and etablished that trans-activation is involved in RadLV-induced deregulation of MHC antigen expression and that cis-regulatory elements exist and can be found within a 2 kb span of DNA flanking the 5'-end and/or 3 kb piece of DNA flanking the 3'-end of Class I genes. Various CAT constructs have been generated to study this issue further in vitro. Studies using these will be next in our efforts to dissect the effects of RadLV on MHC antigen expression. By examining cloned RadLV variants we have begun the analysis required to determine precisely the viral elements involved in RadLV-induced deregulation of MHC antigen expression.

Given these observation and reports by others that tissue specific regulatory signals for Class I gene transcription are also found within the gene and in the 3' flanking region, we shall construct appropriate CAT vectors for transient expression assays with various segments of 5', 3' flanking andcoding sequences of Class I genes and determine the effect RadLV has on the expression of these vectors.

(D) Evidence for Insertion of Viral Sequences in the MHC

One mechanism by which viruses can impact on Class I expression is by their integration in the MHC. A number of studies from my laboratory have now conclusively demonstrated that exogenous virus can integrate in the MHC, and that in wild or laboratory mice, endogenous viruses can be found flanking many Class I genes.

Our studies with C57BL/10 (B10) mice provided the first example of a mouse strain which carries endogenous viruses in the MHC. Examination of a battery of 38 Class I gene containing cosmids, isolated from two large genomic libraries constructed from B10 spleen DNA, led to localization of viral sequences within the murine MHC[15]. Extensive analysis, including cloning and sequencing of these viral sequences showed that two viral genomes, TLev-1 and TLev-2, were located in a region of 90 kb of DNA in the TL region[22]. At least one of these, TLev-1 is complete, it contains the typical LTR-gag-pol-env-LTR configuration of retroviruses. So far, TLev-2 has been shown to encode gag and pol sequences[22]. Detailed restriction analyses have shown that there is a minimum distance of between 600-1000 bp between viral and H-2 sequences[22]. Similar viral sequences are present in many wild and inbred strains of mice.

In collaboration with Dr. L. Hood and colleagues, we have now conducted and extensive analysis to determine whether viral sequences are associated with other Class I genes[11]. These studies indicate that viral sequences flank a substantial number of Class I genes[11].

The above studies are complemented by other studies from our laboratory[16,19,23] and at least two other groups[2, 27, 28]. These studies demonstrate that viral sequences are often found adjacent to minor histocompatibility genes (MIH) and genes encoding several lymphocyte differentiation antigens (Ly). For example, RFLPs hybridizing with viral probes are associated with Ly-17 on chromosome 1; Ly-21 on chromosome 7, Ly-6 on chromosome 2, Thy-1 on chromosome 9, etc. and at least fifteen MIH genes[19,23].

From our previous studies[15, 19, 23], it was evident that the question of RadLV insertions within the MHC was best approached by preparing a cosmid library of genomic DNA from cells transformed by this virus. Preliminary analysis of this library suggests that at least three RadLV-like sequences are present in the MHC. On a preliminiary basis one of the viral insertions in this cell line appears to be in the K region, and another two in the TL region. The effect of these insertions, as well as their mode of insertion in the MHC remains to be determined, and is clearly one of our main goals.

These observations may have evolutionary and functional connotations and raise several important questions. First, are the associations between viral and Class I sequences significant? Second, could the simplest explanation to these findings be that MIH are viral genomes? Third, are there such large numbers of both MIH and endogenous retroviruses that, on a purely random basis, one should expect to find these two type of sequences linked as frequently as we have? Finally, if as we believe to be the case, specificity and functional significance exists, what then is the mechanism(s) by which theactual integration site is determined?

3. Experiments to study the function of retroviral sequences in the human MHC

The HLA gene complex of man represents the strongest transplantation barrier. Already, its study has proven of great importance from the clinical point of view. Progress in understanding the functioning and biology of this gene complex has greatly improved transplantation of organs and tissue. Furthermore, a second major aspect of this gene complex which has been widely studied is its association with susceptibility to many diseases, including leukemias and lymphomas. While an understanding of disease associations has not yet been achieved, it is likely that the presence of immune response genes in the HLA complex, and the extensive polymorphisms uniquely observed for genes of this complex, play significant roles.

An additional component of these disease associations, whose potential is as yet unknown, is the role that endogenous or exogenous retroviruses integrated next to HLA genes may play. My laboratory has postulated that endogenous retroviruses are located in the HLA complex. These viruses have the potential to (1) alter the transcription and expression of HLA gene products and thereby change the capacity of the host to defend itself against disease, and (2) greatly increase the polymorphism of HLA genes. We are currently devoting substantial effort to determining whether these possibilities are correct.

This work was supported by NIH grants CA22247, CA31346, and CA41420. D.M. in an Established Investigator of the American Heart Association.

REFERENCES

1. Banerji, J., Olsson, L., and Shaffner, W., A lymphocyte specific cellular enhancer is located downstream of the joining region in immunoglobulin heavy chains, Cell, 33, 729, 1983.
2. Blatt, C., Milham, K., Haas, M., Nesbitt, M. N., Harper, M. E., and Simon, M. I., Chromosomal mapping of the mink cell focus-inducing and xenotropic env gene family in the mouse, Proc. Natl. Acad. Sci. USA, 80, 6298, 1983.

3. Borelli, E., Hen, R., and Chambon, P., Adenovirus-2 E1A products repress enhancer-induced stimulation of transcription, Nature (London), 312, 608, 1984.
4. Burgert, H. G. and Kvist, S., An adenovirus type 2 glycoprotein blocks cell 41. Dierks, P., Ooyen, A. V. A. N., Cochran, M. D., Dobkin, C., Reiser, J., and Weissman, C., Three regions upstream from the cat site are required for effective and accurate transcription of the rabbit globin gene in mouse 3T6 cells, Cell, 32, 695, 1983.
5. Dierks, P., Ooyen, A. V. A. N., Cochran, M. D., Dobkin, C., Reiser, J., and Weissman, C., Three regions upstream from the cat site are required for effective and accurate transcription of the rabbit globin gene in mouse 3T6 cells, Cell, 32, 695, 1983.
6. Eager, K. B., Williams, J., Breiding, D., Pan, S., Knowles, B., Apella, E., and Ricciardi, R. P., Expression of histocompatibility antigens H-2K, D, and K is reduced in adenovirus-12-transformed mouse oells and is restored by interferon gamma, Proc. Natl. Acad. Sci. USA, 82, 5525, 1985.
7. Gluzman, Y. and Shenk, T., Eds., Enhancers and eukaryotic gene expression, Cold Spring Harbor Laboratory, Cold Spring Harbor, 1983.
8. Hui, K., Grosveld, F., and Festenstein, H., Rejection of transplantable AKR leukaemia cells following MHC DNA-mediated cell transformation, Nature (London), 311, 750, 1984.
9. Kimura, A., Israel, A., LeBail, O., and Kourilsky, P., Detailed analysis of the mouse H-$2K^b$ promoter: enhancer-like sequences and the role in the regulation of class I gene expression, Cell, 44, 261, 1986.
10. McKnight, S. L. and Kingsbury, R., Transcriptional control signals of a eukaryotic protein-coding gene, Science, 217, 316, 1982.
11. Meruelo, D.: Retroviral sequences flanking histocompatibility genes alter their expression, function and evolution. A Hypothesis. In "Genetic Control of Host Resistance to Infection and Immunity," Skamene, E. (ed) Alan R. Liss, Inc. New York, pp 655-669, 1985.
12. Mellow, G. H., Fohring, B., Doughert, J., Gallimore, P. H., and Raska, K., Tumorigenicity of adenovirus-transformed rat cells and expression of Class I histocompatibility antigen, Virology, 134, 460, 1984.
13. Meruelo, D., A role for elevated H-2 antigen expression in resistance to RadLV-induced leukemogenesis: Enhancement of effective tumor surveillance by killer lymphocytes, J. Exp. Med., 149, 898, 1979.
14. Meruelo, D., Kornreich, R., Rossomando, A., Pampeno, C., Boral, A., Silver, J. L., Buxbaum, J., and Weiss, E. H., Devlin, J. J., Mellor, A. L., Flavell, R. A. and Pellicer, A., Lack of class I H-2 antigens in cells transformed by radiation leukemia virus is associated with methylation and rearrangement of H-2 DNA, Proc. Natl. Acad. Sci. USA, 83, 4504, 1986.
15. Meruelo, D., Kornreich, R., Rossomando, A., Pampeno, C., Mellor, A. L., Weiss, E. H., Flavell, R. A., and Pellicer, A., Murine leukemia virus sequences are encoded in the murine major histocompatibility complex, Proc.Natl. Acad. Sci. USA, 81, 1804, 1984.
16. Meruelo, D. and Kramer, J., H2-D control of radiation leukemia virus induced neoplasia: Evidence for interaction of viral and H-2 genomic information, Transplant. Proc., 13, 1858, 1981.
17. Meruelo, D., Lieberman, M., Ginzten, M., Deak, B., and McDevitt, H. O., Genetic control of Radiation Leukemia virus-induced tumorigenesis. I. Role of the murine major histocompatibility

complex H-2, J. Exp. Med., 146, 1079, 1977.
18. Meruelo, D., Nimelstein, S. H., Jones, P. P., Lieberman, M., and McDevitt, H. O., Increased synthesis and expression of H-2 antigens on lymphocytes as a result of radiation leukemia virus infection: A possible mechanism for H-2 linked control of virus-induced neoplasia, J. Exp. Med., 147, 470, 1978.
19. Meruelo, D., Rossomando, A., Offer, M., Buxbaum, J., and Pellicer, A., Association of endogenous viral loci with genes encoding murine histocompatibility and lymphocyte differentiation antigens, Proc. Natl. Acad. Sci. USA, 80, 5032, 1983.
20. Olsson, L., Identification of a gene and its product associated with metastatic activity, Fed. Proc. Fed. Am. Soc. Exp. Biol., 44, 1336, 1985.
21. Olsson, L. and Forchhamer, J., Induction of the metastatic phenotype in a mouse tumor by 5-azacytine and characterization of an antigen associated with metastatic activity, Proc. Natl. Acad. Sci. USA, 81, 3389, 1984.
22. Pampeno, C. L. and Meruelo, D., Isolation of a retroviruslike sequence from the TL locus of the C57BL/10 murine major histocompatibility complex, J. Virol., 58, 296, 1986.
23. Rossomando, A. and Meruelo, D., Viral sequences are associated with many histocompatibility genes, Immunogenetics, 23, 233, 1986.
24. Schrier, P. I., Bernards, R., Vaessen, R. T. M. J., Houweling, A., and van der Eb, A. J., Expression of class I major histocompatibility antigens switched off by highly oncogenic adenovirus 12 in transformed rat cell, Nature (London), 305, 771, 1983.
25. Tanaka, K., Isselbacher, K. J., Khoury, G., and Jay, G., Reversal of oncogenesis by the expression of a MHC class I gene, Science, 228, 26, 1985.
26. Wallick, R., Bulbuc, N., Hammerling, G. J., Katzav, S., Segal, S., and Feldman, M., Abrogation of metastatic properties of tumor cells by de novo expression of H-2K antigens following H-2 gene transfection, Nature (London), 315, 301, 1985.
27. Wejman, J. C., Taylor, B. A., Jenkins, N. A., and Copeland, N. G., Endogenous xenotropic murine leukemia virus-related sequences map to chromosomal regions encoding mouse lymphocyte antigens, J. Virol., 50, 237, 1984.
28. Wettstein, P. J. and Melvold, R. W., Xenotropic virus related restriction patterns of non-H2 histocompatibility mutant mice strains, Immunogenetics, 23, 156, 1986.

MONOCLONAL H-2 CLASS I SPECIFIC ANTIBODIES ISOLATED AFTER IMMUNIZATION OF C57Bl/6 MICE WITH SYNGENEIC SENDAI VIRUS--COATED CELLS

F. Kievits[1], A. Opolski[2], W.J. Boerenkamp[1], M. Pla[2] and P. Ivanyi[1]

[1]Central Laboratory of the Netherlands Red Cross Blood Transfusion Service, and Laboratory of Experimental and Clinical Immunology of the University of Amsterdam, Amsterdam, The Netherlands and [2]U93, INSERM, Hopital St. Louis, Paris, France[2]

ABSTRACT. Two alloreactive H-2 (class I) specific cytotoxic IgM monoclonal antibodies (McAbs), B6-1 and B6-2, were isolated from C57Bl/6 (B6) mice after injections of syngeneic Sendai virus-coated (SV+) spleen cells. McAb B6-1 recognizes the public H-2 class I specificity H-2.25, shared by the $H-2^k(K^k)$ and $H-2^r$ haplotypes and cross-reacts with $H-2^z$ antigens on SV-infected (SVi) lymphoblasts. McAb B6-2 recognizes the private $H-2K^f$ determinant H-2.26 on normal Sendai virus-negative (SV-) spleen cells but cross--reacts with $H-2K^k$ and $H-2D^d$ antigens on SVi blast cells. A polymorphic reaction pattern, that was dependent on the presence of Sendai virus, as tested on a panel of B10 target cells, was also observed with the cytotoxic immune sera from the mice whose cells were used in fusion experiments. Given the fact that each immune serum is an extensive mixture of anti-H-2 antibodies with different specificities, the isolated McAbs can be seen as illustrative examples which explain the reaction pattern of the immune sera. The recognition of polymorphic determinants on SV-infected, positive cells, is presumably due to a modified exposure of cross-reacting public H-2 class I determinants. Taken together, the lymphocytotoxic McAbs induced by injections of syngeneic SV+ cells recognize neither viral antigen nor self--MHC+X composite determinants, but allogeneic H-2 determinants as presented on normal, SV-coated or SV-infected cells.

INTRODUCTION

The T-cell repertoire is dedicated to the recognition of membrane expressed foreign antigens in the context of self-MHC molecules (Zinkernagel and Doherty 1979). In contrast, the B-cell repertoire is developed to recognize foreign antigen per se (Singer et al. 1979, Sprent and Bruce 1979). However, MHC-restricted recognition of antigens has also been reported as a component of the humoral immune response (Katz et al. 1978, Gorczynski et al. 1980, Nisbet-Brown et al. 1981, Hodes and Singer 1984). A limited number of studies have shown that some antibodies, produced in response to membrane-expressed antigens, recognized those antigens only in the context of self-MHC (van Leeuwen et al. 1979, Wylie et al. 1981, Froscher et al. 1986, Schmidt 1987).

In a previous work we have examined whether injection of Sendai virus--'modified' syngeneic cells could trigger the production of MHC-restriced anti-viral antibodies (Kievits et al. 1987). Almost all injected B6 mice produced auto and alloreactive H-2-specific lymphocytotoxic antibodies. Although these cytotoxic antibodies exhibited an enhanced binding for SV-coated (SV+) target cells, detailed study showed that they were directed against H-2 class I molecules (Kievits et al. 1987). In the present report we describe the isolation and the specificity of two McAbs obtained from two B6 mice injected with syngeneic SV+ lymphocytes. The sera of these mice contained cytotoxic antibodies reactive with a broad panel of H-2 haplotypes. Two IgM-producing hybridomas B6-1 and B6-2, were isolated. The antibodies they produced both had affinity for normal (SV-) allogeneic target cells; B6-1 for $H\text{-}2^k(K^k)$ and $H\text{-}2^r$, B6-2 for $H\text{-}2^f(K^f)$. Moreover, McAb B6-1 was also weakly reactive with $H\text{-}2^z$ and McAb B6-2 with $H\text{-}2K^k$ and $H\text{-}2D^d$ molecules on SV-infected (SVi) lymphoblasts. No cytotoxicity for syngeneic ($H\text{-}2^b$) SV-, SV+ or SVi target cells was observed. The binding of McAbs B6-1 and B6-2 to certain SV-infected lymphoblasts is interpreted as being due to a distant signal of SV which can modify the exposure of cross-reacting public H-2 class I determinants.

MATERIAL AND METHODS

Mice. All mice, except the B10.W ($H\text{-}2^{wild}$) strains, were bred in the

Animal house of our Institute and used at 8 to 16 weeks of age. The B10.W strains, i.e. B10-congenic strains with an H-2 haplotype derived from wild mice, were kindly provided by Prof. J. Klein and Dr. F. Figueroa (Max-Planck Institute for Biology, Tübingen, FRG).

Immunization. C57Bl/6 (B6, H-2^b) mice were injected i.p. weekly with 10^7 syngeneic Sendai virus-coated (SV+) spleen cells as described in detail (Kievits et al. 1987). SV, the nonpathogenic Cantell strain, obtained from Flow Laboratories (Ayshire, United Kingdom; lot no. 40340089), was used. Coating with SV was performed by a technique routinely used for the preparation of stimulator and target cells in SV-specific cytotoxic T lymphocytes (CTL) assays (Kast et al. 1984).

Serology. The microlymphocytotoxicity test (MLCT) on normal (SV-), SV-coated (SV+) and SV-infected (SVi) lymphocytes and lymphoblasts was performed as described (Ivanyi et al. 1978, Kievits et al. 1987). SVi cells were obtained by coculturing lymphocytes with 600 hemagglutination units (HAU) of SV in 50 ml culture medium per 10^7 cells for 18 h at 37°C. Lymphoblast were prepared by stimulation of lymphocytes with 2.5 μg Concanavalin A (Con A) per ml for two days.

Cell fusion. From a serie of immunized mice McAbs were obtained from two mice by different techniques. Spleen cells (1.25 x10^6) from mouse no.3 were mixed with the same concentration of syngeneic irradiated (2500 rad) SV+ lymphocytes and adoptively transferred intravenously into immunized (B6) mice 7 days after the last injection with syngeneic SV+ cells. The recipient mice received 350 rad whole body irradiation 24 h before cell transfer. Seven days after cell transfer, recipient spleens were used for fusion. From mouse no.88 lymph node cells were used for fusion. Fusion experiments were performed by hybridizing lymphocytes with SP2/OAg14 myeloma cells at the given ratio.

Hypoxanthine/aminopterin/thimidine (HAT) selection was done as described (van Mourik et al. 1984). After 12 to 21 days, supernatants from growing hybridomas were screened in MLCT on panel of SVi Con A lymphoblasts from eight H-2 congenic mouse strains on the B10 background. Hybridomas weer cloned by 1 ml cultures, followed by limiting dilution. Hybridoma cells producing McAbs were injected in pristan-treated (B6xBALB/c)F_1 hybrid mice to produce ascites, and various batches of ascites were tested.

Table 1. Reaction pattern of two immune sera (no. 3 and 88) from B6 ($H-2^b$) mice immunized with syngeneic SV-coated cells[1].

Serum	H-2 haplotypes of target cells							
	b	k	r	s	d	q	f	p
No.3								
SV+ cells	32[2]	2	32	0	4	16	0	64
SV- cells	0	0	0	0	0	0	0	2
No.88								
SV+ cells	16	32	32	4	8	8	32	64
SV- cells	2	0	0	0	0	4	0	2

1) Cells from these two mice were used in fusion experiments.

2) Reciprocal of the highest serum dilution with positive (≧ 60%) cell lysis. Immune sera were tested against a panel of normal (SV-) and SV--coated (SV+) lymphocytes from H-2 congenic mouse strains on the B10 background, namely B10 ($H-2^b$), B10.BR ($H-2^k$), B10.RIII ($H-2^r$), B10.S ($H-2^s$), B10.D2/n ($H-2^d$), B10.Q ($H-2^q$), B10.M ($H-2^f$) and B10.Y ($H-2^p$).

RESULTS

Serum antibodies in B6 mice. Syngeneic SV+ spleen cells were used to immunize B6 mice (Kievits et al. 1987). Thirty one of the 71 injected B6 mice (44%) produced antibodies cytotoxic for SV- lymphocytes. When the sera were tested on SV+ cells, 89% (63/71) of the sera were cytotoxic. The reaction pattern of the lymphocytotoxic sera from individual mice, as tested on a panel of various syngeneic and allogeneic inbred mouse strains, was shown to be not only dependent on the H-2 haplotype but also on the presence of SV, and ranged from almost anti-private to widely cross-reacting serotypes (Kievits et al, 1987). We intended to obtain, by fusion experiments, McAbs with the H-2 specificities detected in the sera of B6 mice injected with syngeneic SV+ spleen cells. Two mice, one (no.3) from the described (Kievits et al. 1987) immunization groups and another (no.88) from a later immunization experiment, both with a representative serum reaction pattern (Table 1), were selected for fusion experiments.

Fusion experiments. Spleen cells from mouse no.3 were adoptively transferred to irradiated B6 mice previously primed with syngeneic SV+ cells. After 7 days spleen cells were isolated and fused with mouse myeloma cells. From mouse no.88 lymph node cells were directly used for fusion. Culture supernatants from wells with good cell growth were assayed for the presence of lymphocytotoxic antibodies on a panel of SV-infected Con A lymphoblasts from H-2 congenic strains on the B10 background. Of 288 supernatants which originated from cells of mouse no.88, one contained cytotoxic antibodies (Table 2). This supernatant reacted strongly with $H\text{-}2^f$. Cells from this positive wells were further cloned in 1 ml cultures and McAb B6-2 was established. Among the primary supernatants which originated from mouse no.3, good hybridoma cell growth was observed in 110 wells (Table 2). Hence, the fusion efficiency was low (29%). One out of 110 supernatants was lymphocytotoxic and reacted strongly with $H\text{-}2^k$ and $H\text{-}2^r$ target cells.

Table 2. Summary of fusion experiments with lymphocytes from B6 mice no.3 and no.88 after syngeneic immunization with SV-coated spleen cells.

Mouse	Fusion[1)] ratio	No. of seeded wells	No. of growing clones	Fusion efficiency %	Postive[2)] primary supernatants n	%	McAb
no.3	1:1	384	110	29	1	1	B6-1
no.88	1:4	288	178	62	1	2	B6-2

1) Ratio of SP2 myeloma cells /lymphocytes

2) Supernatants were tested on Sendai virus-infected Con A lymphoblasts of eight H-2 congeneic B10 mouse strains. Supernatants were scored as positive when ≧20% cells of at least one haplotype were lysed.

A stable hybridoma (B6-1) was obtained which produced cytotoxic antibodies reactive with $H\text{-}2^k$ and $H\text{-}2^r$ target cells, a specificity that was already found in the primary supernatant. Immunodiffusion with specific anti-mouse IgG and IgM antibodies showed that McAbs B6-1 and B6-2 were both of the IgM class (data not shown).

Specificity of McAb B6 -1 and B6-2. An extensive panel of spleen cells from inbred mouse strains and from recently introduced B10.W strains with H-2 haplotypes from wild mice was used for detailed analysis of the H-2 specificity of McAb B6-1 and B6-2 (Table 3). McAb B6-1 lysed only target cells expressing the $H\text{-}2K^k$ and $H\text{-}2^r$ antigens, indicating the recognition of the public K determinant, H-2.25. McAb B6-2, recognized only a private determinant on $H\text{-}2K^f$-positive target cells, a specificity recorded as H-2.26. Neither McAb B6-1 nor McAb B6-2 were reactive with syngeneic $H\text{-}2^b$ lymphocytes. Moreover, no reactivity of McAbs B6-1 and B6-2 was observed with any of the tested B10.W strains with the following H-2 haplotypes: w4, w5, w6, w13, w15, w16, w17, w23, w27 (data not shown).

Reactivity of McAb B6-1 and B6-2 on normal (SV-), SV-coated (SV+) and SV-infected (SVi) lymphocytes and lymphoblasts. McAbs B6-1 and B6-2 were obtained from B6 mice with a high titer of lymphocytotoxic serum antibodies after syngeneic immunization with SV+ spleen cells. These serum antibodies reacted preferentially with SV+ spleen cells (Table 1). Both McAbs B6-1 and B6-2 also distinguished between SV+ and SV- cells, although the differences in cytotoxic titers were small (Table 4). Moreover, reactivity on SV- lymphoblasts was stronger than on SV+ lymphocytes, indicating the role of H-2 class I antigen expression for McAb binding. Strongly increased lysis was found for SVi lymphoblasts, which remarkably, was still specific for the determinants H-2.25 and H-2.26 which were already detectable on SV- cells. Thus, there is the possibility of misinterpretation of the results, if only cells of certain haplotypes are tested and the antibodies are examined only in certain dilutions. Furthermore, some "extra" reactions were detectable on SVi lymphoblasts. McAb B6-1 reacts, albeit weakly but reproducibly, with $H\text{-}2^z$ SVi lymphoblasts, and McAb B6-2 was found to be reactive with $H\text{-}2^d$, and $H\text{-}2^k$ on SVi lymphoblasts. The latter reactions were specified as anti-K^k and anti-D^d by testings on H-2 recombinant SVi lymphoblasts (data not shown).

In conclusion, two McAbs B6-1 and B6-2 were isolated. McAb B6-1 reacts preferentially with $H\text{-}2K^k$ and $H\text{-}2^r$ and cross-reacts with determinants on $H\text{-}2^z$. McAb B6-2 reacts preferentially with $H\text{-}2K^f$ and crossreacts with

H-2K^k and H-2D^d determinants. The cross-reactions of both McAbs were shown to be dependent on SV infection of the target cells, suggesting a modification of exposed H-2 molecules by Sendai viral infection.

Table 3. Reaction pattern of McAbs B6-1 and B6-2 on a panel of normal (SV-) lymphocytes from H-2 congenic mouse strains with various H-2 haplotypes and genetic backgrounds.

Target cell	H-genotype		Cytotoxic titer[1)] of McAb	
	K	D	B6-1	B6-2
B10	b	b	0	0
B10.D2/n	d	d	0	0
B10.HTG	d	b	0	0
B10.A(5R)	b	d	0	0
B10.Y	p	p	0	0
B10.Q	q	q	0	0
B10.S	s	s	0	0
B10.SM	v	v	0	0
B10.M	f	f	0	128
B10.M(17R)	k	f	512	0
A.TFR2	f	d	0	128
A.CA	f	f	0	128
B10.RIII	r	r	64	0
BALB.K	k	k	128	0
BALB.B	b	b	0	0
BALB/c	d	d	0	0
C3H/He	k	k	128	0
C3H.OH	d	k	0	0
B10.BR	k	k	64	0
B10.A	k	d	128	0
B10.AKM	k	q	64	0
B10.A (2R)	k	b	256	0

1) Reciprocal of the highest ascites dilution with positive (≧60%) cell lysis

Table 4. The reaction patterns of McAbs B6-1 and B6-2 on normal (SV-), SV--coated (SV+) and SV-infected (SVi) lymphocytes and Con-A lymphoblasts.

	cytotoxic titer)[1] on					
H-2 haplotype[2]	Lymphocytes			Con-A lymphoblasts		
McAb B6-1	SV-	SV+	SVi	SV-	SV+	SVi
k	64	256	64 000	64 000	64 000	256 000
r	64	256	64 000	64 000	64 000	128 000
z	0	0	0	0	0	32
f	0	0	0	0	0	0
b	0	0	0	0	0	0
d	0	0	0	0	0	0
s	0	0	0	0	0	0
p	0	0	0	0	0	0
q	0	0	0	0	0	0
v	0	0	0	0	0	0
McAb B6-2						
f	128	512	1024	1024	2048	8192
k	0	0	0	0	0	32
d	0	0	0	0	0	16
b	0	0	0	0	0	0
r	0	0	0	0	0	0
s	0	0	0	0	0	0
p	0	0	0	0	0	0
q	0	0	0	0	0	0
z	0	0	0	0	0	0
v	0	0	0	0	0	0

1) Reciprocal of the highest ascites dilution with positive (≧60%) cell lysis.
2) $H\text{-}2^z$ haplotype was of the NZW strain, all other haplotypes of H-2 congeneic B10 strains (see Table 3).

DISCUSSION

In a previous paper (Kievits et al. 1987) it was shown that the immune response to injections of syngeneic SV+ spleen cells resulted in the regular induction of lymphocytotoxic H-2 (class I) specific serum antibodies. In contrast, injections of normal spleen cells or SV alone did not trigger the production of this type of antibody. These results indicated that virus-"modified" syngeneic cells are a prerequisite for the selective stimulation of the B-cell response to syngeneic SV+ cells.

However, the role of SV in the induction of H-2-specific antibodies remains unclear. One possible explanation for triggering H-2-specific antibodies by viral antigens or virus-infected syngeneic cells is based upon the interaction between MHC and foreign antigen (Wylie et al. 1982, Cerny--Provaznik et al. 1985, Schmidt 1987). New conformational determinants may be formed by physical and functional association of foreign antigen (X) and H-2 (composite determinants) (Matzinger 1981, Babbit et al. 1985, Ashwell and Schwartz, 1986) or arise on H-2 molecules by interaction with foreign antigen (interaction determinants) (Sherman 1982, Allen et al. 1984). We have recently proposed that Sendai viral antigens might act as a "distant signal" to induce the above mentioned interaction determinants (Kievits et al. 1987). Syngeneic antibodies directed against composite or interaction determinants will be specific for self-MHC+X, i.e. they are MHC restricted. Such antibodies have been described for Influenza virus (Wylie et al. 1982), Simian virus 40 (Froscher et al. 1986), murine leukemia virus (Schmidt 1987) and human H-Y antigens (van Leeuwen et al. 1979). However, in our model of syngeneic immunization with SV+ cells, we could not find antibodies which we would designate as anti-viral MHC restricted (Kievits et al. 1987). Although the induced cytotoxic antibodies imitated MHC-restricted antibodies by an enhanced binding to syngeneic SV+ cells, a detailed study of the reaction pattern allowed us to conclude that the induced cytotoxic serum antibodies were a mixture of various alloreactive H-2 (class I) specific antibodies (Kievits et al. 1987). That study included absorption experiments with SV- and SV+ syngeneic, allogeneic and xenogeneic cells or with SV alone, capping experiments, immunoprecipitation, analysis of the specificity of individual mouse sera (Kievits et al. 1987) and the isolation and analysis of a first McAb (Q-1) obtained from an analogous immunization experiment in B10.Q mice (Opolski et al. 1986). Most serum antibodies were anti-H-2 public, and in some instances recognized also syngeneic H-2 determinants. However autoreactivity was never exclusive.

In this report we describe two McAbs, B6-1 and B6-2, which can be seen as illustrative examples that explain the reaction pattern of the syngeneic immune sera. McAb B6-1 recognizes a public determinant, probably H-2.25 on H-$2K^k$ and H-2^r molecules, whereas McAb B6-2 recognizes a private determinant (H-2.26) on H-$2K^f$ molecules. Both McAb B6-1 and B6-2 discriminate between SV-, SV+ and SVi lymphocytes, and thus behave as cytotoxic serum antibodies present in mice injected with syngeneic SV+ cells (Kievits et al. 1987). McAb binding to SVi cells is the strongest, but the difference between SV- and SV+ cells is minimal (Table 4). However, binding to SV- ConA lymphoblasts was more intense than binding to SV+ lymphocytes and similar as binding to SVi lymphocytes. This effective McAb binding to virus negative lymphoblasts suggests, that it is the mode of H-2 exposure which enhance antibody binding rather than the specific presence of SV. Most intense was antibody binding to SVi ConA lymphoblasts (Table 4). These findings also indicate possibilities of misinterpretation. If the antibodies had not been titrated and tested only in a certain dilution against normal cells and SVi cells of some haplotypes, the role of SV might appear as more specific. However, the antibodies are not antiviral but anti-H-2 and SV only modify H-2 exposure (Kievits et al. 1987). We proposed that SV might act on the cell membrane as a "distant signal" to H-2 class I molecules and causes a modified exposure of public class I determinants. Accordingly, weak but distinct reactions with cells of other haplotypes were detected, but only on SVi ConA lymphoblasts (H-2^z for B6-1 and H-2^d, H-2^k for B6-2; see Table 4). Possibly, some modifications of H-2 molecules induced by SV can be detected by antibodies only on cells with an increased density of class I molecules (i.e. on ConA blast cells).

In variance to the reaction pattern of serum antibodies induced by multiple injections of syngeneic SV+ cells (Kievits et al. 1987) and some other H-2 McAb isolated from mice without prior alloimmunization (Cerny--Provaznik et al. 1985), McAb's B6-1 and B6-2 did not recognize normal or virus infected syngeneic cells, i.e. they are not autoreactive. This might be due to the relatively lower affinity of B6-1 and B6-2 as compared with McAb Q-1 (Opolski et al. 1986) which was also isolated after injections of syngeneic SV+ cells.

It remains unclear whether the suggested modified exposure of public class I determinants is also able to trigger the induction of cytotoxic H-2-specific serum antibodies after injections of syngeneic SV+ cells.

ACKNOWLEDGEMENTS. This investigation was in part supported by the Foundation for Medical Research FUNGO, which is subsidized by the Netherlands Organization for the Advancement of Pure Research (ZWO) (grant no. 509-087) and in part by the Deutsche Forschungsgemeinschaft (grant no.5/1-2).

References

Allen, H., Wraith, d., Pala, P., Askonas B., and Flavell, R.A.: Domain interactions of H-2 class I antigens after cytotoxic T-cell recognition sites. *Nature 309:*279-281, 1984

Ashwell, J.D., and Schwartz, R.H.: T-cell recognition of antigen and Ia molecules as ternary complex. *Nature 320:*176-179, 1986 Babbit, B.P., Allen, P.M., Matsueda, G., Haber, E., and Unanue, E.R.: Binding of immunogenic peptides to Ia histocompatibility molecules. *Nature 317:*357-316, 1985.

Cerny-Provaznik, R., van Mourik, P., Limpens, J., Leupers, T., and Ivanyi, P.: Anti-MHC immunity detected prior intentional alloimmunization. III. Natural autoreactive H-2 specific antibodies. *Immunogenetics 21:* 461--504, 1985

Froscher, B.G., and Klinman, N.R.: Immunization with SV40-transformed cells yields mainly MHC-restricted monoclonale antibodies. *J. Exp. Med. 164:* 196-210, 1986.

Gorczynski, R.M., Kennedy, M.J., MacRae, S., Steele, E.J., and Cunningham, A.J.: Restriction of antigen recognition in mouse B lymphocytes by genes mapping within the major histocompatibility complex. *J. Immunol. 124:* 590-596, 1980

Hodes, R.J., and Singer, A.: MHC restricted recognition by antigen-specific B cells: fact or artefact? *Immunology Today 5:*50-54, 1984

Ivanyi, P., van den Berg-Loonen, E., and de Greeve, P.: Individual mice of one inbred strain produce anti-H-2 and anti-HLA antibodies of different specificities. *Tissue Antigens 12:*32-38, 1978

Kast, W.M., de Waal, L.P., and Melief, C.J.M.: Thymus dictates major histocompatibility complex (MHC) specificity and immune response gene phenotype of class II MHC-restricted T cells but not class I MHC-restricted T cells. *J. Exp. Med. 160:*1752-1766, 1984

Katz, D.H. Skidmore B.J., Katz, L.R., and Bogowitz C.A.: Adaptive differentation of murine lymphocytes. I. Both T and B lymphocytes differentiating in $F_1 \rightarrow$ parental chimeras manifest preferential cooperative activity for partner lymphocytes derived from the same parental type corresponding to the chimeric host. *J. Exp. Med. 148:*727-745, 1978

Kievits, F., Rocca, A., Opolski, A., Limpens, J., Leupers, T., Kloosterman, T., Boerenkamp, W.P., Pla, M., and Ivanyi, P.: Induction of H-2 specific antibodies by injections of syngeneic Sendai virus-coated cells. *Eur. J. Immunol. 17:*27-35, 1987

Van Leeuwen, A.E., Goulmy, A., and van Rood, J.J.: Major histocompatibility complex restricted antibody reactivity mainly, but not exclusively, directed against cells from male donors. *J. Exp. Med. 150:*1075-1083, 1979

Matzinger, P.: A one-receptor view of T-cell behaviour. *Nature 292:*497-501, 1981

Van Mourik, P., Rivero, R.A., van der Kwast, T.H., Lansdorp, P.M., and Zeijlemaker, W.P.: Density separation of spleen cells increases fusion sequency and yiels of Ig-producing hybridomas. *J. Immunol. Methods 68:* 45-55, 1984

Nisbet-Brown, E., Singh, B., and Diener, E.: Antigen recognition. V. Requirement for histocompatibility between antigen-presenting cell and B-cell in the response to a thymus-dependent antigen, and lack of allogeneic restriction between T and B cells. *J. Exp. Med. 154:*676-687, 1981

Opolski, A., Kievits, F., and Ivanyi, P.: Polymorphic and autoreactive H-2 specific monoclonal antibodies isolated after injections of syngeneic Sendai virus-coated lymphocytes. *Immunogenetics 24:*402-408, 1986

Sherman, L.A.: Recognition of conformational determinants on H-2 by cytotoxic T lymphocytes. *Nature 297:*511-513, 1982

Singer, A., Hathcock, K.S., and Hodes, R.J.: Cellular and genetic control of antibody responses. V. Helper T-cell recognition of H-2 determinants on accessory cells but not B cells. *J. Exp. Med. 149:*1208-1229, 1979

Sprent, J., and Bruce, J.: Lymphoid function in $F_1 \rightarrow$ parent chimeras. Lack of evidence for adaptive differentation of B cells or antigen-presenting cells. *J. Exp. Med. 150:*715-720, 1979

Wylie, D.E., Sherman, L.A., and Klinman, N.R.: Participation of the major histocompatibility complex in antibody recognition of viral antigens expressed on infected cells. *J. Exp. Med. 155:*403-414, 1982

Zinkernagel, R.M., and Doherty, P.C.: MHC-restricted cytotoxic T cells: Studies on the biological role of polymorphic major transplantation antigens determing T cell restriction-specificity. *Adv. Immunol. 27:*51-77, 1979

ANALYSIS OF ANTI-REOVIRUS CYTOTOXIC T LYMPHOCYTES (CTL) USING THE $H\text{-}2^{dm1}$ MUTANT

Duane W. Sears, Suezanne E. Parker and Donna Zeger

Department of Biological Sciences, University of California, Santa Barbara, CA 93106

Abstract

The murine cytotoxic T lymphocyte response to reovirus -- a double-stranded, segmented RNA virus -- has been analyzed using the *dml* mutant and its *d* parent strain. Reovirus stimulates a strong CTL response in mice of both haplotypes. The $H\text{-}2D/L^{dm1}$, $H\text{-}2D^d$ and $H\text{-}2L^d$ antigens all serve as anti-reovirus CTL restricting elements. These CTL most likely recognize nonmembrane structures of reovirus because this "naked" virus is nonenveloped and nonbudding with no known membrane maturation stage in its replication cycle. The fine-specificity of the H-2 restriction imposed by the individual class I molecules of these haplotypes has been examined by analyzing the crossreactivity patterns of parent and mutant CTL tested with L cells transformed with various cloned *H-2* genes. Preliminary data indicates that *d* anti-reovirus CTL generally do not crossreact with infected targets expressing the mutant $H\text{-}2D/L^{dm1}$ antigen whereas *dml* anti-reovirus CTL frequently cross-lyse reovirus infected targets expressing either the $H\text{-}D^d$ or $H\text{-}L^d$ antigens. The nonreciprocity of the *d* and *dml* CTL response suggests that fundamentally different immunodominant determinants are selected for CTL recognition in *d* as compared to *dml* mice although substantial sequence homology exists between the $H\text{-}2D/L^{dm1}$ hybrid antigen and the two parent antigens from which the mutant class I molecule arose. Based on the unique hybrid nature of the $H\text{-}2D/L^{dm1}$ antigen, additional hybrid class I molecules have been constructed in collaboration with Drs. Iwona Stroynowski and Lee Hood, using the mutant and parent genes for exon-shuffled gene constructs. Preliminary data is presented showing that *dml* CTL can recognize reovirus infected L cell transformants expressing the class I variant, $[D^d]\text{-}[D/L^{dm1}]\text{-}[D^d]$, with the brackets denoting the boundaries between the $[\alpha 1]\text{-}[\alpha 2]\text{-}[\alpha 3]$ extracellular domains. Eventually additional variants of this type will be constructed and expressed in L cells. In conjunction with the recently-isolated cloned reovirus genes, these novel class I genes will provide further insight into the structural elements of these molecules which govern anti-viral CTL recognition.

Introduction

The complex nature of antigen recognition by CTL has intrigued and puzzled immunologists for some time now. In particular, the way in which virus specific CTL simultaneously recognize viral antigens and "restricting" class I MHC molecules remains elusive. One approach to this complex phenomenon of CTL recognition is to identify and study the structural features of class I molecules which impose the restrictions on antigen detection by CTL. The availability of cloned class I genes and MHC genetic mutant strains provide a useful starting point for such studies.

One mutation which has been valuable in the study of the anti-viral CTL response and the structure/function relationships of class I antigens is the *dml* mutant (Egorov, 1967; Shumova *et al.*, 1972; Vederinikov and Egorov, 1973). This mutant is unique from other *H-2* mutants in that it appears to have arisen from the fusion of portions of two class I antigen genes, the *H-2D*^{d} and *H-2L*^{d} genes of the parent *d* haplotype (Wilson *et al*, 1982; Burnside *et al*, 1984; Hunt *et al.*, 1985, Sun *et al.*, 1985). In general, class I genes are split into eight exons with intervening sequences (Hood *et al.*, 1983). The *dml* mutant gene is found to encompass the 5' end of the *H-2D*^{d} gene -- including the first exon, (leader sequence) the second exon, ($\alpha1$ domain), and the first half of the third exon ($\alpha2$ domain) -- and the 3' end of the *H-2L*^{d} gene -- beginning at the third exon ($\alpha2$ domain) and including the remaining 3' portion of the *H-2L*^{d} gene (exons 5-8 which encode the $\alpha3$, transmembrane, and cytoplasmic domains of the H-2L^d antigen). The *H-2D/L*^{dml} gene is of normal size. The mutant protein expressed from this gene is identical to H-2D^d in the $\alpha1$ domain and two-thirds of the $\alpha2$ domain, and it is identical to the H-2L^d antigen in the latter third of the $\alpha2$ domain, the whole $\alpha3$ domain, and the remaining C-terminal regions. The extracellular domains of the H-2D/L^{dml} antigen are designated as follows: [D^d]-[D^d/L^d]-[L^d].

Using the genes encoding the H-2D^d, H-2L^d, and H-2D/L^{dml} class I antigens (Evans *et al*, 1982a; Moore *et al.*, 1982; Goodenow *et al.*, 1982a, 1982b; Margulies *et al.*, 1983; Sun *et al.*, 1985), it has been possible to create "novel" class I genes by exchanging homologous exons between different class I DNA sequences through the applications of recombinant DNA technology. For example, the technique of exon shuffling *between H-2* class I genes has been used to construct recombinant H-2D^d and H-2L^d genes (Evans *et al.*, 1982b; Ozato *et al.*, 1983; Reiss *et al.*, 1984a, 1984b; Murre *et al.*, 1984; Stroynowski *et al.*, 1984, 1985). The introduction of these recombinant genes into mouse L cells by DNA mediated gene transfer has resulted in the expression by these transformed cells of hybrid or "mosaic" class I antigens that have been tested for their capacity to function in restricting antigen recognition by CTL. Functional CTL analysis with transformants bearing exon shuffled H-2D^d and H-2L^d antigens has revealed that the $\alpha1$ and/or $\alpha2$ domains of a class I molecule may be the most important components of H-2 antigens for the recognition by most CTL of alloantigens or certain viral antigens (Ozato *et al.*, 1983; Reiss *et al.*, 1984a, 1984b; Murre *et al.*, 1984; Stroynowski *et al.*, 1984, 1985).

In the present study we have extended this type of analysis of the recognition properties of CTL and the H-2 restricting properties of class I molecules using H-2D/L^{dml} antigen as the prototypic exon-shuffled molecule and reovirus as the model virus. The crossreactive patterns of *d* parent and *dml* mutant reovirus immune CTL were tested on a variety of transformed L cells expressing either natural or variant *H-2* genes. Specifically, CTL generated in *dml* mice were examined for specific lysis of reovirus infected targets expressing the H-2D/L^{dml}, H-2D^d or H-2L^d antigen. Conversely, CTL generated in mice of the parental *d* haplotype were examined for the lysis of targets expressing the *d* parent antigens and or the mutant H-2D/L^{dml} antigen. Preliminary lytic data with a novel exon shuffled molecule is also described. A surprising nonreciprocity in the crossreactivity patterns was observed. An understanding of this phenomenon could provide important insights into the ways in which CTL recognize viral antigens and the ways in which certain regions on class I molecules act to restrict antigen recognition.

Materials and Methods

Mice: Mice from 6-8 weeks of age of both sexes were used from colonies bred in this laboratory.

Murine cell lines: The following murine cells (*H-2* haplotype in parenthesis) were used as targets: L ($H\text{-}2^k$) fibroblasts derived from C3H mice; T1.1.1 ($H\text{-}2K^k, D^k, L^d$), $H\text{-}2L^d$ transformed L fibroblasts (Evans *et al.*, 1982a); T4.8.3 ($H\text{-}2K^k, D^k, D^d$), $H\text{-}2D^d$ transformed L fibroblasts (Marguiles *et al.*, 1983); and K31.25.19($H\text{-}2K^k, D^k, D/L^{dm1}$), $H\text{-}2D/L^{dm1}$ transformed L fibroblasts (Sun *et al.*, 1985). The T1.1.1 and T4.8.3 cell lines were generously provided by Dr. J. G. Seidman, Harvard University (Boston, MA). The K31.25.19 cell line was developed by Y. H. Sun at the California Institute of Technology (Pasadena, CA). The cells were maintained in standard complete culture medium (CM) defined here as RPMI 1640 supplemented with 10 *mM* Hepes; 23 *mM* $NaHCO_3$; 0.14% reduced glutathione; 2 mM glutamine; 50 *U*/ml penicillin; 50 μg/ml streptomycin and 10% heat inactivated FCS.

Virus: Reovirus T3 (Dearing strain) was grown and isolated according to standard procedures as described elsewhere (S. E. Parker, Ph.D. Thesis, UCSB).

Anti-reovirus CTL immunizations: Mice were immunized by i.p. inoculation with 1 x 10^7 plaque forming units (PFU) of reovirus T3 or T1 in Puck's saline. Seven days post primary immunization with reovirus, the mice were sacrificed, and their spleens were removed and teased apart in PBS. The splenocytes (responder cells) were washed 2X, and placed in Costar 24 well tissue culture plates at 7 x 10^6 cells in a final volume of 2 ml CM supplemented with 50 μM β-mercaptoethanol (CM-βme). For secondary in vitro stimulation, 1 x 10^7 PFU reovirus were added to each well and the cultures were incubated at 37°C in CO_2/air for 5 days as previously described (Kauffman *et al.*, 1983).

Target cell preparation: Prior to being infected with reovirus, fibroblasts were trypsinized and grown in suspension for 24 hrs in CM. The fibroblasts were then washed 2X in Puck's saline + 1% FCS (Puck's-FCS), resuspended at 5 x 10^6/ml in Puck's-FCS, and incubated with virus at an MOI of 5 for 1 hr at 37°C in CO_2/air with occasional shaking. After 1 hr, the reovirus infected cells were washed 1X in Puck's-FCS, resuspended in CM-βME and cultured at 37° in CO_2/air for an additional 18 hrs. One hr prior to a CTL assay, infected fibroblasts were harvested, washed 1X in Puck's-FCS, resuspended in CM-βME and incubated for 1 hr in 50-100 μC $Na^{51}CrO_4$ (New England Nuclear, Boston MA) at 37°C in CO_2/air with occasional shaking. The radiolabeled and infected cells were then harvested, washed 3X in PBS and resuspended in CM-βME and used as targets for CTL assay. Radiolabeled, uninfected targets were prepared in the same fashion omitting the virus infection steps above.

^{51}Cr Release CTL assay: 10^4 labeled target cells were incubated for 4-5 hr at 37°C in CO_2/air with varying numbers of effector cells in 200 μl CM-βME in 96 well round bottom microtiter plates (initially centrifuged for 1 min at 500 x *g*). At the end of the assay, 100 μl supernatant aliquots were withdrawn, mixed with a scintillation fluor (Ecoscint) and cpm values were determined in a liquid scintillation counter. The data presented are average values of triplicate samples within a single experiment. The specific ^{51}Cr release is equivalent to the following: 100 x [(ER) - (SRC)]/[(FRC) - (SRC)] where ER is the average cpm release value for the experimental sample point, SRC is the average "spontaneous release control" for targets without effectors and FRC is the average "full release control" determined as 75% of the cpm in 100 μl of supernatant from

targets lysed with NP40. (This method of determining the FRC closely approximates FRC values determined from supernatants of labeled targets frozen and thawed 3X.)

Results

In order to characterize the CTL response in mutant *dml* mice, it was first necessary to establish that the novel H-2D/L^{dml} antigen could serve as a restricting element for *dml* reovirus-specific CTL. The results of this analysis are shown in Fig. 1 on the next page. By ^{51}Cr-release assay, the *dml* effectors primed against reovirus *in vivo* and restimulated *in vitro* were tested for cytotoxicity against T3 infected, *H-2D/L*^{dml} transformed L cells (K31.25.19) or infected, nontransformed L cells. The data shown in this figure demonstrate that the H-2D/L^{dml} antigen serves as a restricting element for reovirus specific CTL generated in *dml* mice as these CTL effectively lyse infected transformants but failed to lyse infected L targets of the allogeneic *k* haplotype. The failure of the *dml* anti-viral CTL to lyse infected L targets was not due to the inability of these cells to serve as suitable targets for viral specific effectors because they were effectively lysed by the syngeneic B10.BR (H-2K^k, H-2D^k) anti-viral CTL (data not shown) indicating that the H-2K^k and H-2D^k antigens expressed on L cells cannot substitute for the H-2D/L^{dml} antigen for target cell recognition by *dml* anti-viral CTL.

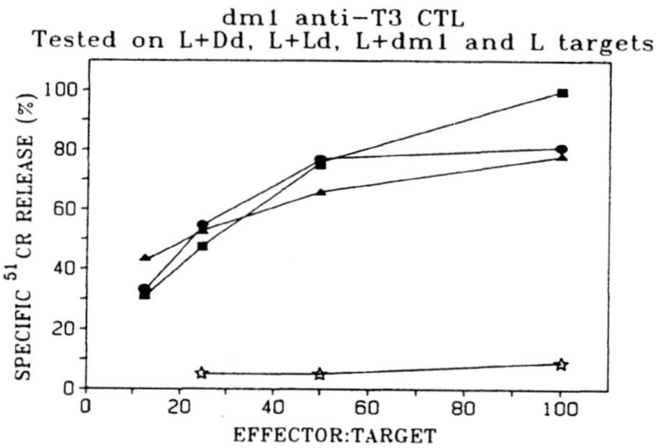

Fig. 1. Crossreactive lysis of reovirus infected L^d and D^d expressing target cells by dml specific anti-reovirus CTL. L^d expressing L cell transformant, T1.1.1 (▲); D^d expressing L cell transformant, T4.8.3 (●); D/L^{dml} expressing L cell transformant, K31.25.19 (■); untransformed L cells (☆). The reovirus specific CTL failed to lyse uninfected targets (data not shown).

Having established in Fig. 1 that the H-2D/L^{dml} antigen can serve as a restricting element for CTL generated in *dml* mice, we proceeded to characterize the potential crossreactive lysis of *dml* anti-reovirus CTL tested against infected cells expressing either the H-2D^d or H-2L^d class I antigens. The results of the crossreactivity analysis of *dml* effectors are also shown in Fig. 1. In this experiment *dml* anti-reovirus CTL effectively lysed infected targets expressing the H-2D^d (T4.8.3) or the H-2L^d (T1.1.1) antigen. The same degree of crossreactivity was not observed in all experiments but crossreactivity on cells expressing parent antigens was generally detected with *dml* CTL in most experiments.

The lack of reciprocal cross-lysis of *H-2D/L*^{dm1}-transformants by *d* anti-reovirus CTL cells is shown in Fig. 2. Whereas parent-derived CTL readily

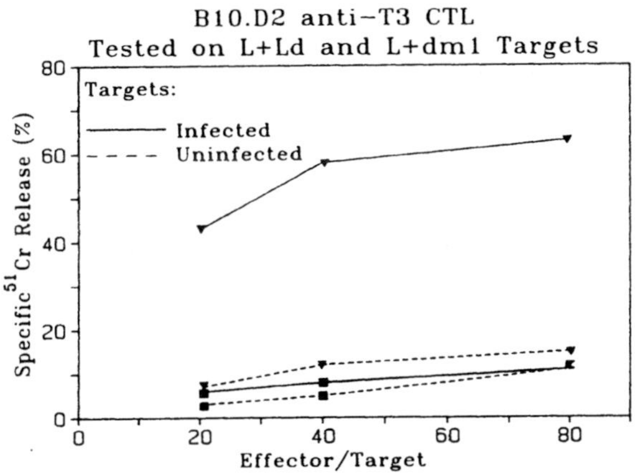

Fig. 2. The mutant *dml* class I antigen did not serve as a restricting element for anti-reovirus CTL generated in mice of the parental H-2^d haplotype. Anti-reovirus CTL generated in B10.D2 mice (H-2^d) efficiently lyse virus-infected syngeneic targets (▼), an H-2L^d expressing L cell transformant, T1.1.1) yet fail to lyse virus-infected K31.25.19 targets that express the *dml* mutant antigen (■).

lysed virus infected *H-2L*^{d} transformants (and *H-2D*^{d} tranformants, data not shown), they typically did not lyse the *H-2D/L*^{dm1}-transformants.

In order to define further the H-2-restricting structures on these class I molecules which account for the nonreciprocal crossreactivity, we have initiated a project to construct a series of class I variants of the *H-2D/L*^{dm1} gene in collaboration with Drs. Stroynowski and Hood at Caltech. Novel *H-2* gene variants have been created by replacing exons encoding the extracellular domains of the *H-2D/L*^{dm1} gene with the corresponding exons of the *H-2D*^{d} or *H-2L*^{d} genes. These variants have been used to make stable L cell transformants. The organization of the extracellular domains of the parent molecules and variants are shown in Table 1 on the next page where the origins of the [α1]-[α2]-[α3] domains are indicated in brackets.

A stable transformant (K70.25) has been created using variant 1 in

Table 1. The ability of this variant class I H-2 antigen to serve as a restricting element for *dml* anti-reovirus CTL effectors is shown in Fig. 3 on the next page. Consistent with previous data assigning the α1 and α2 domains, but not the α3 domain, as the most important for CTL recognition (Ozato *et al.*, 1983; Reiss *et al.*, 1984a, 1984b; Murre *et al.*, 1984; Stroynowski *et al.*, 1984, 1985), it was not unexpected that the replacement of the α3 domain of the H-D/L^{dm1} antigen by the α3 domain of the H-$2D^d$

Table 1

Extracellular Domain Organization of Parent, Mutant, and Variant Class I Molecules

Class I Antigen	[α1]	-	[α2]	-	[α3]
D^d	[D^d]	-	[D^d]	-	[D^d]
L^d	[L^d]	-	[L^d]	-	[L^d]
D^{dm1}	[D^d]	-	[D^d/L^d]	-	[L^d]
Variant 1	[D^d]	-	[D^d/L^d]	-	[D^d]
Variant 2	[L^d]	-	[D^d/L^d]	-	[L^d]

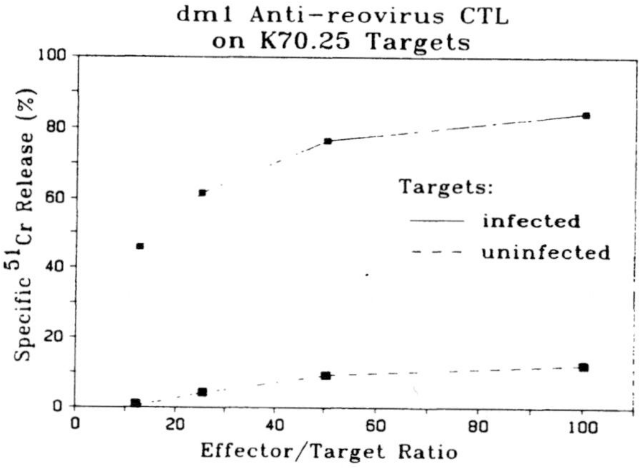

Fig. 3. Lysis of reovirus infected K70.25 targets by *dml* anti-reovirus CTL. The novel class I antigen (variant 1, Table 1) expressed on K70.25 targets shares only the α1 and α2 domains in common with the D/L^{dm1} antigen and yet these targets are lysed by the *dml* effectors. This demonstrates that the first two extracellular domains of the H-2D/L^{dm1} antigen are sufficient to achieve lysis by the *dml* anti-reovirus CTL.

antigen had no effect on the ability of *dm1* CTL to recognize these transformed targets.

Discussion

We have sought to establish a preliminary characterization of the bulk population CTL response to reovirus in mice of the parent *d* and mutant *dm1* haplotypes. Both *d* and *dm1* mice give vigorous anti-reovirus responses, thus establishing that the mutation has not impaired the CTL response to this virus. It was found that *dm1* specific anti-reovirus CTL usually crosslyse virally infected H-$2D^d$- or H-$2L^d$-expressing L cell transformants whereas *d* specific anti-reovirus CTL generally failed to crosslyse H-$2D/L^{dm1}$-expressing transformants. The lack of reciprocity between the *dm1* and *d* effectors in recognizing the H-2D^d and H-2D/L^{dm1} antigens was surprising given that the amino acid sequences in the $\alpha1$ and the $\alpha2$ domains are nearly identical (98% homology). The crosslysis of *dm1* CTL with the H-2L^d transformants was also surprising given the number of amino acid sequence difference in the first two extracellular domains, there being 19 differences (85% homology). However, if one includes the $\alpha3$ domain in this homology comparison, then the H-2L^d and H-2D/L^{dm1} antigens are 91% homologous for the first three extracellular domains. The crossreactivity in this case suggests that the $\alpha3$ domain may be directly involved in the *H-2*-restricted recognition of *dm1* anti-reovirus CTL even though this domain is generally found to be nonessential in determining *H-2* restriction (see Introduction).

While the lack of crossreactivity of parent *d* CTL with mutant H-$2D/L^{dm1}$ transformants is a finding generally consistent with findings for other viruses and *H-2* mutants, the crossreactive lysis of infected H-$2D^d$- or H-$2L^d$-transformants by *dm1* CTL is atypical. However, this result is generally consistent with the observation that anti-ectromelia virus CTL of the *b* haplotype do cross-lyse ectromelia virus infected targets expressing *bm8* mutant antigens while *bm8* anti-ectromelia CTL do not cross-lyse infected targets expressing parental K^b antigens (Blanden *et al.*, 1976).

Given these findings, we propose a model which may explain our data. This model is based on the concept of "agretope" developed to explain MHC restriction by class II antigens (Schwartz, 1985). According to the agretope concept, foreign antigens associate with specific sequences on class II molecules and are recognized as such by T cells thereby accounting for the *H-2* restriction. Likewise, it is assumed that reovirus proteins (or fragments thereof) associate with the H-2D^d, H-2L^d or H-2D/L^{dm1} antigens. In the most simple case, the D/L^{dm1} antigen would be viewed as having a minimum of three *H-2* restricting sequences or structures: one structure unique to D/L^{dm1} and not found on either D^d or L^d; and two other structures which are homologous to corresponding structures on D^d and L^d, respectively. Conversely, the D^d and L^d antigens, in the most simple case would be viewed as having a minimum of two *H-2* restricting structures: one unique structure not found on the other two antigens; and one structure common to H-2D/L^{dm1} in each case. By this model the nonreciprocity of the *dm1* and *d* CTL response to reovirus would be explained by arguing that different *dm1* CTL clones in the bulk CTL population detect virus in the context of different restricting structures on the H-2D/L^{dm1} antigen. One set of these *dm1* clones detects the common restricting structure on the H-2D^d antigen; another detects the common restricting structure on the H-2L^d antigen; and the third set detects the unique structure of the H-2D/L^{dm1} antigen. The restricting structures present on the H-2D/L^{dm1} antigen would also be present on the novel class I variant antigen expressed by the K70.25 transformant (see Fig. 3) since *dm1* CTL readily cross-lysed these cells when infected with reovirus. In contrast to the crossreactivity of *dm1* CTL, *d* CTL preferentially detect viral antigens only in the context of the restricting structures which are unique to either the H-2D^d or H-2L^d antigens and which are not common to the restricting structures of the H-2D/L^{dm1} antigen.

In conclusion, the immunodominant forms of reovirus antigens are different in the parent and mutant mice even though the parent class I molecules can present reovirus antigens in a class I context which is suitable for *dm1* CTL recognition. The observations made in these studies invite a more detailed analysis of the class I restricting structures recognized by anti-viral CTL. With additional variants (like variant 2 in Table 1) and using the recently cloned genes for reovirus proteins, it should be possible to clone anti-reovirus CTL and analyze their specificities in much greater molecular detail.

References

Blanden, R. V., Dunlop, M. B. C., Doherty, P. C., and Kohn, H. I.: Effects of four *H-2K* mutations on virus-induced antigens recognized by cytotoxic T cells. *Immunogenetics 3:* 541-548, 1976

Burnside, S. S., P. Hunt, K. Ozato, and D. W. Sears. A molecular hybrid of the *H-2D*^{d} and *H-2L*^{d} genes expressed in the *dm1* mutant. *Proc. Natl. Acad. Sci. USA 81:* 5204-5208, 1984.

Clark, S. S., and J. Forman. Allogeneic and associative recognition determinants of H-2 molecules. *Transplant. Proc. 15:* 20290-20292,1983.

Egorov, I. K. A mutation of the histocompatibility-2 locus in the mouse. *Genetika (Moscow) 3:* 136-144, 1967.

Egorov, I. K., and Z. K. Blandova. The genetic homogenicity of the inbred mice bred at the Stolbovya farm. II. Skin grafting tests. *Geneteka 12:*, 1968.

Evans, G. A., D. H. Margulies, R. D. Camerini-Otero, K. Ozato, and J. G. Seidman. Structure and expression of a mouse major histocompatibility antigen gene, *H-2L*^{d}. *Proc. Natl. Acad. Sci. USA 79:* 1994-1998, 1982a.

Evans, G. A., D. H. Margulies, B. Shykind, J. G. Seidman, and K. Ozato. Exon shuffling: mapping polymorphic determinants on hybrid mouse transplantation antigens. *Nature 300:* 755-757, 1982b.

Goodenow, R. S., M. McMillan, M. Nicolson, B. T. Sher, K. Eakle, N. Davidson, and L. Hood. Identification of the class I genes of the mouse major histocompatibility complex by DNA-mediated gene transfer. *Nature 300:* 231-237, 1982a.

Goodenow, R. S., M. McMillan, A. Orn, M. Nicolson, N. Davidson, J. A. Frelinger, and L. Hood. Identification of a BALB/c H-2L^d gene by DNA-mediated gene transfer. *Science 215:* 677-679, 1982b.

Hood, L., M. Steinmetz, and B. Malissen. Genes of the major histocompatibility complex of the mouse. *Ann. Rev. Immunol. 1:* 529-568, 1983.

Hunt, P., S. S. Burnside, and D. W. Sears. Evidence of only one H-2D/L-related glycoprotein in *H- 2*^{dm1} mutant cells. *J. Immunogenet. 12:* 33-44, 1985.

Kauffman, R. S., Lee, S., and Finberg, R.: Cytolytic T-cell mediated lysis of reovirus-infected cells: Requirements for infectious virus, viral particles and viral proteins in infected target cells. *Virology 131:* 265-273, 1983

Margulies, D. H., G. A. Evans, K. Ozato, R. D. Camerini-Otero, K. Tanaka, E. Appella, and J. G. Seidman. Expression of H-2D^d and H-2L^d mouse major histocompatibility antigen genes in L cells after DNA-mediated gene transfer. *J. Immunol. 130:* 463-470, 1983.

Moore, K. W., B. T. Sher, Y. H. Sun, K. A. Eakle, and L. Hood. DNA sequence of a gene encoding a BALB/c mouse L^d transplantation antigen. *Science 215:* 679-682, 1982.

Murre, C., E. Choi, J. Weis, J. G. Seidman, K. Ozato, L. Liu, S. J. Burakoff, and C. S. Reiss. Dissection of serological and cytolytic T lymphocyte epitopes on murine major histocompatibility antigens by a recombinant H-2 gene separating the first two external domains. *J. Exp. Med. 160:* 167-178, 1984.

Ozato, K., G. A. Evans, B. Shykind, D. H. Margulies, and J. G. Seidman. Hybrid *H-2* histocompatibility gene products assign domains recognized by alloreactive T cells. *Proc. Natl. Acad. Sci. USA 80:* 2040-2043, 1983.

Parker, S. E. Characterization of the murine CTL Response to Reovirus. Ph.D. Thesis, UCSB, 1987.

Reiss, C. S., G. A. Evans, D. H. Margulies, J. G. Seidman, and S. J. Burakoff. Allospecific and virus-specific cytolytic T lymphocytes are restricted to the N or C1 domain of H-2 antigens expressed on L cells after DNA-mediated gene transfer. *Proc. Natl. Acad. Sci. USA 80:* 2709-2712, 1983.

Reiss, C. S., G. A. Evans, C. Murre, D. H. Margulies, J. G. Seidman, and S. J. Burakoff. Cytotoxic T lymphocyte recognition of class I H-2 antigens after DNA-mediated gene transfer. *Fed. Proc. 43:* 271-275, 1984

Schwartz, R. H. T-lymphocyte recognition of antigen in association with gene products of the major histocompatibility complex. *Ann. Rev. Immunol. 3:* 237-261, 1985.

Shumova, T. E., V. P. Kryshkina, and I. K. Egorov. Study of *H-2* mutations in mice. I. Analysis of the mutation 504 by the F_1 hybrid test. *Genetika (Moscow) 8:* 171-173, 1972.

Stroynowski, I., S. Clark, L. A. Henderson, L. Hood, M. McMillan, and J. Forman. Interaction of α1 with α2 region in class I MHC proteins contributes determinants recognized by antibodies and cytotoxic T cells. *J. Immunol. 135:* 2160-2166, 1985.

Stroynowski, I., A. Orn, R. S. Goodenow, M. McMillan, J. Forman, P. R. Brayton, J. Frelinger, and L. Hood. Cytotoxic T lymphocytes recognize determinants on the BALB/c-H- $2L^d$ molecule controlled by α1 and α2 but not α3 external domains. *Immunogenetics 20:* 141-154, 1984.

Sun, Y. H., R. S. Goodenow, and L. Hood. Molecular basis of the dml mutation in the major histocompatibility complex of the mouse: a D/L hybrid gene. *J. Exp. Med. 162:* 1588-1602, 1985.

Vedernikov, A. A., and I. K. Egorov. Study of H-2 mutations in mice. II. Recombination analysis of the mutation 504. *Genetika (Moscow) 9:* 60-66, 1973.

Wilson, P. H., R. Nairn, S. G. Nathenson, and D. W. Sears. Unexpected complexity of the *dml* mutation revealed in the structure of three H-2D/L-related antigens. *Immunogenetics 15:* 225-237, 1982.

THE H-2 COMPLEX AND THE HORMONAL FACTORS IN MAMMARY TUMORIGENESIS IN MICE

G. Röpcke, M. Sluyser and P. Demant

Departments of Molecular Genetics and Tumor Biology
The Netherlands Cancer Institute, Plesmanlaan 121
1066 CX Amsterdam, The Netherlands

Abstract Induction of mammary tumors by hormonal stimulation from heterotopic hypophyseal isografts has been studied in H-2 congenic mouse strains free of infectious mammary tumor virus. Significant differences in tumor incidence have been observed, indicating that H-2-linked genes influence the tumorigenesis in hormonally stimulated mammary glands. In addition, significant differences between the H-2 congenic strains were found in estrogen receptor levels measured in the hypophyseal isografts. These differences do not appear to correlate in any obvious way with the induction of mammary tumors. Our data indicate that the MHC or MHC-linked genes influence one or more steps related to hormonal regulation of the mammary gland.

Introduction

Extensive studies have demonstrated an influence of the H-2 gene complex on the resistance of mice to a variety of MuLV (Murine leukemia virus) induced tumors of haemopoietic cells. In the instances where the mechanism of this resistance has been studied, it was found to be based on the well-known functions of the class I and class II antigens in antigen presentation to cytotoxic and helper T lymphocytes, respectively (Zijlstra et al., 1986). Extensive studies with mammary tumors induced by the mammary tumor virus (MTV) showed H-2 haplotype effects on resistance. These effects are specific for individual MTV strains, suggesting an immunological mechanism (reviewed by Mühlbock and Dux, 1981). This is indirectly supported by the finding of Dux and Demant (1987) that H-2-linked resistance against C3H-MTV-induced mammary tumors is systemic rather than local. However, non-immunological functions of the H-2 gene complex may also have influence on tumor development in the mammary gland, because the development and function of this organ are hormonally regulated. Mühlbock and Dux (1971; 1981) demonstrated that H-2 haplotypes influence the incidence of mammary tumors induced by the method of hormonal stimulation in mice free of infectious MTV (Boot et al., 1981).

Here we provide further evidence for H-2-dependent differences in hormonal induction of mammary tumors, using heterotopic pituitary isografts in MTV-free mice. We also show that the H-2 genotype influences the levels of estrogen receptors in these isografts.

Materials and Methods

Mice. H-2 congenic strains were obtained from dr. G.D. Snell and are maintained as SPF-colonies in this Institute. Their haplotypes are given in Table 1a. For composition of recombinant haplotypes see Klein et al. (1983). All strains are free of infectious MTV.

Hormonal stimulation. Isogenic pituitary glands, transplanted under the kidney capsule, are not under hypothalamic control any more. They are not reached by the pituitary inhibiting factor from the hypothalamus and therefore produce prolactin continuously, which stimulates the growth of the mammary gland (Boot et al., 1981). Female mice, 50 days old, were grafted with two hypophyses, which were placed under the capsule of the left kidney. The donors were adult male mice of the same strain. All mice were kept in groups of two or three in plastic cages. They were palpated for the presence of mammary tumors once a week. Mammary tumors were recorded when first palpable. The mice were killed and all tumors were examined histologically. The hypophyseal isografts were removed, weighed, and stored at -70°C for estrogen and progesterone receptor measurements. The mice without tumors were killed when moribund and their hypophyseal isografts were analyzed in the same way. The strain differences in tumor appearance were evaluated by the test of Mantel (1966).

Hormone receptor assay has been carried out as described earlier (Sluyser et al., 1978). Receptor levels were expressed as fmol/mg cytosol protein. Briefly, cytosols of hypophyseal isografts were incubated for 16 hours in the cold with 2nM ^{3}H-estradiol. Excess nafoxidine was added in controls. Unbound ligand was removed by incubation with dextran-coated charcoal.

Prolactin assay. Radioimmunoassay for plasma prolactin was performed according to Kwa et al.(1972).

Results

The data on mammary tumors in hormonally stimulated females in six H-2 congenic strains is summarized in Table 1a. Most mice without mammary tumors reached a very high age (more than 2 years). Earlier deaths were due to a variety of causes: tumorous growth of the hypophyseal implant, skin defects, leukemias (mostly in the strain B10.AKM), lung and liver tumors, and sporadic technical accidents. The mammary tumors were classified according to Dunn (1959). Most of the tumors (83%) were adenoacanthomas. This type of tumor is typical for strains of mice free of infectious MTV. The proportion of other tumors (adenocarcinomas type B, carcino-sarcomas, mixed tumors) was approximately the same in all strains. The mammary tumor incidence ranges from the low 21% [B10.A(4R)] and 24% (B10.A) to the high 63% [B10.A(2R)]. The mean age of tumor appearance varies from 561 days [B10.A(2R)] to 659 days [B10.A(4R)].

We used the statistical evaluation based on the actuarial survival curves (Mantel, 1966). This method takes into account both the proportion of mice with tumors and the time at which the tumors appear. The results are given in Table 1b. Highly significant differences were seen between the susceptible strain B10.A(2R) and the strains B10.A, B10.A(4R), B10, and B10.A(5R). The other susceptible strain, B10.AKM, differs significantly only from the most resistant strains, B10.A and B10.A(4R). B10.AKM has intermediate tumor incidence, but the mean age of tumor appearance is similar to that of B10.A(2R).

Table 1a. INCIDENCE OF MAMMARY TUMORS IN FEMALE MICE WITH TWO PITUITARY ISOGRAFTS IN THE LEFT KIDNEY

STRAIN	H-2	% Ma tumors	Ma tumor age (days)	Age without tumor (days)	Number of mice	Mean Prolactin level (ng/ml) at 12 months
C57BL/10	b	41	653	706	22	3000 ± 980
B10.A	a	24	627	648	42	3400 ± 420
B10.A(2R)	h2	63	561	537	30	6400 ± 1200
B10.A(4R)	h4	21	659	630	42	2500 ± 420
B10.A(5R)	i5	33	620	613	36	1700 ± 490
B10.AKM	m	44	572	578	36	2700 ± 260

Plasma levels of prolactin were determined in six females from each strain at the age of 12 months. The mean values show no obvious correlation with the tumor susceptibility of the strain (Table 1a), nor do the prolactin values observed in individual mice correlate with the subsequent appearance of tumors (data not shown).

The level of estrogen receptors in hypophyseal isografts was measured at the time of sacrifice of the individual mice and is given in Table 2. The values found in strain B10 are lower than in the strain

Table 1b. STATISTICAL SIGNIFICANCE (P VALUES)

	B10.A	4R	B10	5R	AKM	2R
B10.A	--	.88	.86	.19	.009	<.0001
B10.A(4R)		--	.76	.07	.004	<.0001
B10			--	.39	.07	.0001
B10.A(5R)				--	.16	.0002
B10.AKM					--	.035
B10.A(2R)						--

B10.A. Although in some mice of the latter strain low values similar to B10 were found, in most B10.A mice much higher values were present.

The mean of the estrogen receptor levels in the 'high' strain B10.A is 2.5 times higher than in the 'low' strain B10 (114.3 ± 16.6 vs. 46.0 ± 8.8 fmol/mg protein). The difference between the two strains is highly significant (Wilcoxon test, $P < 0.005$). The estrogen receptor levels in hypophyseal isografts did not correlate with the age of the mice and the time of tumor appearance (Table 2).

Table 2. ESTROGEN RECEPTOR LEVELS IN HYPOPHYSEAL ISOGRAFTS IN H-2 CONGENIC STRAINS (fmol/mg CYTOSOL PROTEIN)

B10 ER	Age (days)	B10.A ER	Age (days)
11.6	680	32.7	688
27.3	680	35.1	609
28.8	729	66.1	723
33.8	902	67.0	673
51.5	699	76.6	625
62.2	736	82.0	723
66.6	709	100.1	607
86.5	730	104.2	718
		114.3	761
		115.0	715
		134.5	688
		174.2	666
		222.8	743
		235.4	726

Discussion

The incidence and time of appearance of mammary tumors in females bearing hypophyseal grafts from males of the same strain under the kidney capsule were significantly different in some H-2 congenic strains on C57BL/10ScSn (B10) genetic background. The strain B10.A and B10.A(4R) are resistant. The strain B10.A(2R) is the most susceptible, the strain B10.AKM is also susceptible but less than B10.A(2R). The strains B10 and B10.A(5R) are less resistant than the strains B10.A and B10.A(4R). The observed pattern of strain differences indicates that more than one gene is involved. The strains B10.A (resistant) and B10.A(2R) (susceptible) differ at the segment to the right of <u>S</u>, including the <u>D</u> and <u>Qa-Tla</u> regions. Both the <u>D</u> region and the <u>Qa-Tla</u> region have been implicated in resistance against MTV-induced mammary tumors (Mühlbock and Dux, 1981, Dux, 1983). However, the resistant strains B10.A(4R) and B10 share the <u>D-Qa-Tla</u> segment with the susceptible B10.A(2R). They both differ from

B10.A(2R) at the central E-S regions of the H-2 complex. Possibly the interaction of E-S and D-Qa-Tla segments alters the resistance pattern. The validity of these interpretations is only conditional, they have to be confirmed by testing other recombinant haplotypes. More than one MHC region have been shown to affect the resistance to MTV-induced mammary tumors in mice (Dux, 1983, Mühlbock and Dux, 1981).

The mechanism of the observed influence of the H-2 gene complex on the development of mammary tumors is not known. An effect based on the well-known function of class I and II antigens during antigen presentation of viral antigens (Zijlstra et al., 1986) is known to be the basis of the role of the H-2 complex in resistance against viral leukemias. It is not likely that this type of effect is responsible for the phenomenon described here. The immune responses in mice with leukemias are directed against viral (MuLV-related) antigens. However, the mammary tumors induced in infectious MTV-free mice by hormonal stimulation, in contrast to MTV-induced tumors, express no immunohistologically detectable MTV antigens (Hageman, personal communication) and contain no or only minimal amounts of MTV mRNA (Ashley et al., 1980) In addition Long et al. (1980) found no differences in the number and structure of endogenous MTV proviruses nor in their expression in H-2 congenic strains. However, H-2 regulation of an immune response against a hypothetical non-viral tumor antigen cannot be excluded.

The second possibility is the effect of the MHC on the stimulation by the hypophyseal isografts. However, there was no correlation between plasma prolactin levels and appearance of tumors. Conceivably, the levels reached in our experiments exceed the threshold value necessary for induction of tumors and the actual appearance of tumors and their growth are regulated by other factors as well. The transplanted hypophyseal glands were from male donors, because transplants from males are more effective than from females in induction of mammary tumors (Röpcke, 1975). Although the H-2 complex regulates the rejection of H-Y incompatible grafts (Bailey and Hoste, 1971), the size of the hypophyseal transplants is not correlated with the appearance of tumors (Röpcke, in preparation).

Finally, the H-2 gene complex might affect the susceptibility of the mammary gland to hormonal stimulation. Nagasawa et al. (1976) compared the proliferative and differentiative response of the mammary glands to hormonal stimulation by hypophyseal isografts between two strains which differ in susceptibility to the induction of mammary tumors by hormonal stimulation. The mammary glands of the susceptible strain were more responsive than those of the resistant strain. Experiments are currently being carried out to ascertain whether any differences in susceptibility of mammary glands to hormonal stimulation exist between H-2 congenic strains.

The estrogen receptor levels in hypophyseal isografts were measured because they may be relevant for the stimulatory effect of the hypophyseal isograft. In female mice the estrogens cause indirectly stimulation of the mammary gland by prolactine, because they stimulate the secretion of this hormone by hypophysis, while progesterone acts directly on the mammary gland (for references see Sluyser et al., 1978). No correlation between the estrogen receptor levels and the time of tumor appearance has been observed (Table 2). This result is in accordance with the lack of correlation between plasma prolactin levels and tumor susceptibility (see above).

The significant difference between the estrogen receptor levels in hypophyseal isografts in the strains B10.A and B10 is an intriguing observation which cannot be explained by the presently known functions of the MHC. The observed difference may be due to two or more genes which may be involved in non-additive interactions, since we did not yet succeed in mapping the relevant gene. In order to further elucidate the influence of the H-2 gene complex on the estrogen receptor levels, more information is needed about the nature of the interstrain differences. They may be caused by different saturation grade of the existing receptor molecules, or by differences in the numbers of receptor molecules present. These may in turn be caused by intrinsic differences in the production of the receptor molecules in the hypophysis, or by the differences in the regulatory network which includes also gonads and adrenal gland. In that case, the primary cause of the observed H-2 influence can lie outside the hypophysis.

Palumbo and Vladutiu (1979) observed differences in estrogen receptor levels in uteri of mice of different strains. Some of these differences were caused by genes not linked with H-2. However, comparison of H-2 congenic strains of different haplotypes revealed that H-2 also influences the estrogen receptor levels. The haplotype used in both this study and in their study has been $\underline{H\text{-}2}^{b}$. Both in our study with hypophyseal isografts and in that of Palumbo and Vladutiu with uteri, this haplotype is associated with low levels of estrogen receptors.

The mammary gland is an organ under complex control of steroid and pituitary hormones. The study of the effects of the H-2 gene complex on mammary tumorigenesis in such organs may be useful in providing insight into the presently unknown effects of the H-2 gene complex on certain steps of hormonal regulation. Lung is another organ under multihormonal control. The differentiation and specific functions of lung fibroblasts and alveolar cells are known to be under cell-specific multihormonal control by glucocorticoids, insulin, and thyroxin which have stimulatory effects and by testosterone, which has inhibitory effects (Hitchcock, 1980; Ballard, 1983; Smith and Sabry, 1983; Carlsson et al., 1984). The H-2 gene complex influences the numbers and growth rate of lung tumors induced by prenatal treatment of mice with the carcinogen ethylnitrosourea (Oomen et al., 1983). Recently, evidence has been obtained in our laboratory that the H-2 effect on lung tumorigenesis involves hormonal factors (Oomen et al., in preparation). When the carcinogen is administered to congenic mice together with the glucocorticoid hormone triamcinolone, the tumorigenesis is enhanced in some H-2 haplotypes and inhibited in others (Oomen et al., in preparation). This effect is in some strains sex-dependent and indicates direct or indirect functional interactions between the H-2 complex and adrenal and sex steroids activity in the lung. The effects of the H-2 complex on sensitivity of mouse embryos to glucocorticoid-induced teratogenesis were amply demonstrated (for references see Demant, 1985). The cellular basis for these effects of H-2 must be understood before their molecular-biological analysis is possible.

The data presented in this paper suggest that the H-2 complex has two apparently independent effects during hormonal induction of mammary tumors. It may modulate the function of hypophyseal isografts through influence on the estrogen receptor levels. It affects the tumor susceptibility, possibly through regulation of susceptibility of the target tissue to hormonal stimulation.

Acknowledgement

We thank Dr. A. Dux and Dr. R. van Nie for numerous discussions during this work and the preparation of the manuscript, Dr. M. Oudshoorn-Snoek for careful reading of the manuscript, Dr. A. van der Gugten for measurements of prolactin levels, Mrs. A. de Moes and Mr. C. de Goey for skilful technical assistance, and Mrs. M. Sonne and Mrs. T. van Diepen for excellent secretarial work.

References

Ashley, R.L., Cardiff, R.D., and Fanning, T.G.: Reevaluation of the effect of mouse mammary tumor virus infection on the BALB/c mouse hyperplastic outgrowth. J. Natl. Cancer Inst. 65: 977-986, 1980

Bailey, D.W., and Hoste, J.: A gene governing the female immune response to the male antigen in mice. Transplantation 11: 404-407, 1971

Ballard, P.L.: Hormones and receptors in developing lung. Progr. Clin. Biol. Res. 140: 103-117, 1983

Boot, L.M., Kwa, H.G., and Röpcke, G.: Hormonal induction of the mouse mammary tumors. In J. Hilgers and M. Sluyser (eds.): Mammary tumors in the mouse, pp. 117-200, Elsevier/North-Holland Biomedical Press, Amsterdam, 1981

Carlsson, K.S., Smith, B.T., and Post, M.: Insulin acts on the fibroblast to inhibit glucocorticoid stimulation of lung maturation. J. Appl. Physiol. 57: 1577-1579, 1984

Demant, P.: Corticosteroid-induced cleft palate: Cis interaction of MHC genes and hybrid resistance. Immunogenetics 22: 183-188, 1985

Dunn, T.B.: Morphology of mammary tumors in mice. In F. Homburger (ed.): Physiopathology of Cancer, 2nd ed., pp. 38-84, Hoeber, New York, 1959

Dux, A.: Multiple genetic factors in the MHC and predominant role of D-end in the resistance against C3H-MTV-induced mammary tumors. Transpl. Proc. 15: 2101-2103, 1983

Dux, A., and Demant, P.: The influence of the MHC on resistance against C3H-MTV induced mammary tumors is predominantly systemic rather than local. Int. J. Cancer: in press

Hitchcock, K.R.: Lung development and the pulmonary surfactant system: hormonal influences. Anat. Rec. 198: 13-34, 1980

Klein, J., Figueroa, R., and David, C.S.: H-2 haplotypes, genes and antigens: Second listing. II. The H-2 complex. Immunogenetics 17: 553-596, 1983

Kwa, H.G., Verstraeten, A.A., and Scheijde-Bakker, M.G.M.: Isolation of prolactin from the 'granular fraction' of pituitary tumour transplants: Improved method for the isolation of mouse and rat prolactin for radioimmunoassay. Eur. J. Cancer 8: 33-38, 1972

Long, C.A., Vaidya, A.B., and Dumaswala, U.J.: Influence of the major histocompatibility complex on susceptibility to MuMTV. Abstract, 12th meeting on mammary cancer in experimental animals and man, Maastricht, 1980

Mantel, N.: Evaluation of survival data and two new rank order statistics arising and its consideration. Cancer Chemother. Rep. 50: 163-170, 1966

Mühlbock, O., and Dux, A.: Histocompatibility genes and susceptibility to mammary tumor virus (MTV) in mice. Transpl. Proc. 3: 1247-1250, 1971

Mühlbock, O., and Dux, A.: Histocompatibility genes and mammary cancer. In J. Hilgers and M. Sluyser (eds.): Mammary tumors in the mouse, pp. 545-572, Elsevier/North-Holland Biomedical Press, Amsterdam, 1981

Nagasawa, H., Yanai, R., Taniguchi, H., Tokuzen, R., and Nakahara, W.: Two way selection of a stock of Swiss albino mice for mammary tumorigenesis: Establishment of two new strains (SHN and SLN). J. Natl. Cancer Inst. 57: 425-429, 1976

Oomen, L.C.J.M., Demant, P., Hart, A.A.M., and Emmelot, P.: Multiple genes in the H-2 complex affect differently the number and growth rate of transplacentally induced lung tumors in mice. Int. J. Cancer 31: 447-454, 1983

Palumbo, D.A., and Vladutiu, A.O.: Estrogen receptor in uteri of mice of different H-2 genotypes. Experientia 35: 1103-1104, 1979

Röpcke, G.: Interaction of hypophyseal isografts and ovarian hormones in mammary tumour development in mice. Thesis, University of Amsterdam, 1975

Sluyser, M., Boot, L.M., and Röpcke, G.: High estrogen and low progestin receptor levels in outgrowths of hypophyseal isografts. Cancer Res. 38: 2859-2860, 1978

Smith, B.T., and Sabry, K.: Glucocorticoid-thyroid synergism in lung maturation: A mechanism involving epithelial-mesenchyneal interaction. Proc. Natl. Acad. Sci. USA 80: 1951-1954, 1983

Zijlstra, M., Vasmel, W.L.E., Radaskiewicz, T., Matthews, E., and Melief, C.J.M.: The H-2 complex regulates both the susceptibility to murine viral lymphomagenesis and the phenotype of the virus-induced lymphomas. J. of Immunogenetics 13: 69-76, 1986

IN VIVO ANTITUMOR EFFECTS OF ANTI-I-A ANTIBODIES

Sandra H. Bridges[1] and Dan L. Longo[2]

[1]Medicine Branch, National Cancer Institute, National Institutes of Health, Bethesda, MD, and Centro di Endocrinologia ed Oncologia del CNR, Naples, Italy;
[2]Biological Response Modifiers Program, Division of Cancer Treatment, National Cancer Institute, Bethesda, MD

In addition to their expression on various normal cells of the immune system, Ia molecules are present on a variety of neoplastic cells, most importantly for the work described here on the surface of virtually all B-cell lymphomas and leukemias[1]. As an extension of our previous studies[2-4] on the in vivo effects of I-A-specific monoclonal antibodies (Mab), we have investigated their effects on an I-A-bearing B cell lymphoma. Differential effects on normal and neoplastic cells were observed, suggesting that Ia molecules on neoplastic cells are excellent targets for antibody attack in vivo.

The components of our experimental system are: 1) a B cell lymphoma (L10A) characterized as strongly $\underline{I\text{-}A}^d$ positive and more weakly IgM and FcR positive and 2) a purified Mab reactive with $\underline{I\text{-}A}^d$ (MK-D6), which was given intraperitoneally according to various schedules initiated soon after tumor inoculation: 1 or 2 mg of MK-D6 given at 2 hrs after tumor inoculation and again on days 2, 4, 6, and 8 (schedule nos. 1 and 5, respectively), or 2 mg at 2 hrs after L10A cells and again at 48 hrs (no. 2), or the same as no. 2 with additional 2 mg doses on days 11 and 13 (no. 3) or days 11, 13, 23, 25, 34, and 36 (no. 4). L10A cells, 2.5 X 10^4 per mouse, were given intravenously to BALB/c mice and effects on tumor growth were judged in two ways: a) by a short term assay, which depends on the formation of tumor nodules in the spleen, and b) by survival.

In previous studies, it had been shown that anti-I-A treatment of adult mice results in a short term abrogation of antigen presenting cell (APC) function which correlates with the modulation of Ia molecules from the surface of thymus and spleen cells[4]. Our current studies, comparing spleen cells from normal mice and mice bearing large splenic L10A burdens, are partially illustrated in fig. 1. Briefly, we found that I-A was diminished on normal and tumor cell populations at 16 hrs after a single injection of 3 mg of MK-D6 (panel C, L10A-bearing mice). Normal cells, however, had modulated the antibody-antigen complexes, as demonstrated by the absence of cell bound MK-D6, while splenic L10A cells were clearly positive for IgG2a (panel B), the isotype of MK-D6. These results suggested that the Ia molecules on L10A do not modulate or internalize in the same manner as Ia molecules on normal cells. Thus, a differential effect of anti-I-A on normal and neoplastic cells was established.

Next we monitored APC activity in the spleens of mice inoculated with L10A and treated with MK-D6 according to schedule 1 (above). At 24 hrs after the last injection of Mab, the spleens of treated, tumor-inoculated mice displayed APC activity comparable to that of normal, untreated mice, and by 72 hrs the two were indistinguishable, suggesting the clearance or growth inhibition of the majority of tumor cells and the recovery of I-A expression on normal cells. Spleen cells from untreated, tumor-bearing mice had higher than normal activity at both time points, reflecting the well-known ability of I-A bearing lymphomas to present antigen[5,6], and spleen cells from normal, treated animals had greatly diminished activity at the first time point but had recovered by the second time point, as previously reported[4]. We had again confirmed the feasibility of our approach since we showed that tumor cell expansion had been inhibited by Mab, as demonstrated by the presence of normal levels of APC activity in the spleen, a primary site of tumor colonization.

Dramatic effects of anti-I-A on tumor growth were seen using spleen colony formation as a quantitative measure of efficacy[7]. Groups of BALB/c mice were given L10A cells i.v., treated with Mab according to one of our protocols, and 12 days later sacrificed for the enumeration of splenic tumor colonies. Antibody-treated mice had a mean number of colonies of less than 1 per spleen, whereas untreated mice or mice treated with an isotype matched myeloma Ig had from 52 to 61 colonies per spleen (3 experiments). When CB6 mice ($\underline{I\text{-}A}^d$ X $\underline{I\text{-}A}^b$) were used as hosts and liver colonies enumerated (2 additional experiments), comparable inhibitory effects were obtained with MK-D6 but no effect was seen with Y-3P, a Mab reactive with the irrelevant $\underline{I\text{-}A}^b$ molecule, that is, an I-A molecule present on normal host cells but not on the tumor cells ($\underline{I\text{-}A}^d$).

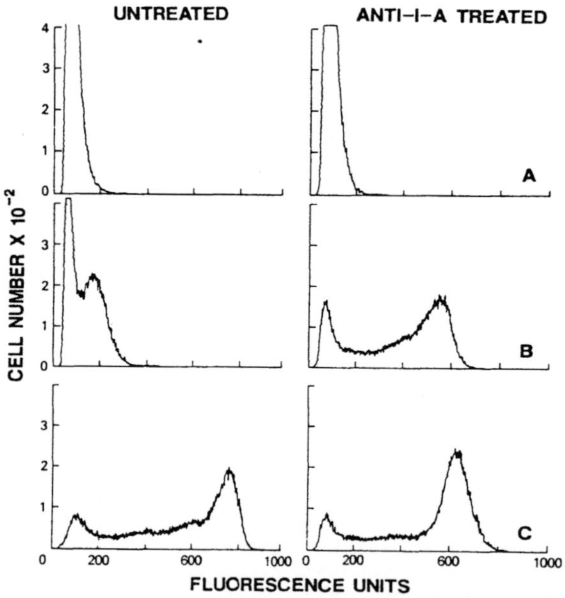

Figure 1. Spleen cells from untreated (left) and anti-I-A treated (right) tumor-bearing mice: unstained (A), stained with FITC-anti-IgG (B) or with FITC-anti-I-A (C). Treated mice received 3 mg of MK-D6 16 hrs prior to analysis.

To determine whether the treatment was inhibitory or caused the actual elimination of tumor cells, we followed several groups of treated mice for extended periods of time. Depending on the protocol used, we had long term survival of 30 to 50% of the mice and an extended survival time in those that were not cured. On several occasions we looked at I-A expression on tumors from treated mice which developed well after those in the respective control groups and found that resistance to Mab treatment was not due to loss of the target antigen or the epitope recognized by the Mab used, as has been reported with idiotype[8,9] or Thy 1.1 antigen targets[10].

As for direct effects of anti-I-A on L10A in vitro, none were seen as judged by effects on proliferation. We examined a range of concentrations, from 1 to 100 ug/ml, and various means of cross-linking I-A molecules, including the use of irradiated spleen cells (FcR-mediated cross linking that is also theoretically possible through the FcR on L10A itself) and insolubilized anti-I-A (covalently linked to beads).

Another direct effect of antibody could be mediated by complement, especially since L10A cells can be lysed in vitro by MK-D6 and complement. To examine this possibility, we used nude BALB/c mice depleted of C3 with cobra venom factor as tumor recipients. There was no effect on splenic tumor colony formation despite a 94% depletion of C3, when anti-I-A was given in vivo (schedule no. 2). When L10A cells were precoated with anti-I-A, to reduce the amount of circulating MK-D6 during the 12 day in vivo growth of the tumor, a modest increase in the number of colonies with respect to the non-depleted, Mab-treated mice was noted, indicating that some tumor cells may indeed be removed by complement mediated lysis or other mechanisms involving complement. However, if this were the primary mechanism a much greater effect would have been expected to result from a C3 depletion of 94%.

Two lines of evidence suggested that T lymphocytes were not involved in the observed tumor cell elimination: 1) Mab treatment was as effective in nude mice as in normal mice as judged by the spleen colony forming assay, and 2) survivors of tumor inoculation and Mab treatment showed no increased resistance to a second tumor challenge.

An often suggested mechanism for Mab-mediated effects on tumor growth is antibody dependent cellular cytotoxicity (ADCC). We directly examined this possibility by depleting nude mice of asialo GM1-bearing cells before giving tumor cells and anti-I-A. NK cell activity was shown to be minimal or absent at the time of tumor inoculation by an in vitro ^{51}Cr assay and results obtained in vivo were consistent with this, that is, mice given anti-asialo GM1 alone had a greatly increased tumor burden at the time of sacrifice, as has been described for a variety of experimental tumors grown in NK-depleted mice[11,12]. Mice given both anti-asialo GM1 and anti-I-A were uncompromised with regard to their ability to deal with the injected tumor cells, thus demonstrating that NK cells are not involved in the mechanism of the antitumor effect of anti-I-A antibodies.

A primary objection to the use of a widely distributed, physiologically important molecule such as Ia as a tumor target for Mab is the potential for widespread disturbances in normal functions. Thus, we looked for acute and long-term deficiencies in Ia-related immune activities. We investigated the effects of multiple doses of anti-I-A on normal spleen cells and found that surface expression of I-A and APC activity rebounded within 72 hrs of the cessation of treatment, as we had reported for a single dose[4]. With regard to possible long-term effects, we examined the immune reactivity of spleen cells from a group of long term survivors (>3 mos) that had been treated extensively with anti-I-A (on days 0,2,11,13,23,25,34, and 36 after tumor inoculation), and thus should have shown immune defects if any had been induced by the treatment. Briefly, our experiments showed that spleen cells from these mice were quite active, both in antigen presentation and in the recognition of alloantigens (fig. 2). In addition, as an indication of the status of the humoral immune system, we measured serum Ig levels in another group of long term survivors. The results of these experiments showed that IgG levels were as much as two-fold increased and suggested that multiple administrations of anti-I-A antibodies in vivo can cause polyclonal B cell activation.

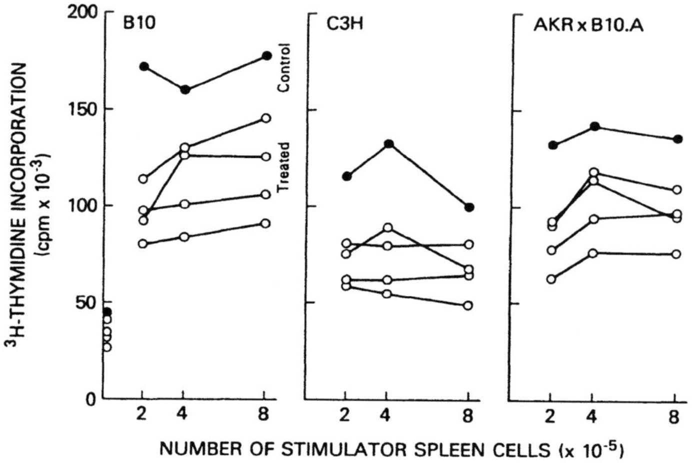

Figure 2. Recognition of alloantigens by spleen cells of mice cured of L10A following extensive treatment with anti-I-A. Responder spleen cells (4 X 10^5) from normal (•) or anti-I-A treated (o) mice were cultured with the indicated number of irradiated spleen cells from B10, C3H, or AKR X B10A mice. Proliferation was determined on day 4, as judged by ^{3}H-thymidine incorporation.

In summary, we have studied the biological consequences of using Ia-specific Mab for the in vivo elimination of a B cell lymphoma. We found that, despite the presence of I-A on a variety of cell types and its propensity to modulate in response to in vivo treatment with anti-I-A, a dramatic effect on lymphoma growth could be obtained without acute or long-term detrimental effects on the immune system. Tumor I-A did not modulate in vivo, thus providing an excellent target for antibody attack.

With regard to the mechanism of the observed effects on tumor growth in vivo, we ruled out the participation of T lymphocytes, complement, and antibody dependent cellular cytotoxicity by NK cells. We favor the idea that MK-D6 functions directly to inhibit tumor cell growth. This seems reasonable in light of the effects of Ia-specific Mab on activation and differentiation of normal[13-15] and neoplastic[16] B cells reported by others. These effects, seen in vitro, required the use of mitogens or specific antigen in addition to anti-Ia. We have been unable to demonstrate direct inhibition of proliferation of L10A by MK-D6 in vitro; thus, it would appear that anti-Ia alone is not capable of eliciting such effects in vitro and suggests that in vivo additional factors may be involved. A direct manifestation of the ability of anti-Ia to transduce regulatory signals, the translocation of protein kinase C from the cytoplasm to the nucleus, was recently reported[17]. Further studies on signal transduction through the Ia molecule on normal and neoplastic B cells are underway.

With our colleague, Jonathan Ashwell, we recently reported that in vivo activation of antigen-specific T cell hybridomas via the T cell receptor results in tumor elimination due to 1) direct cytotoxic effects related to antigen activation and 2) the induction of host immunity[18]. In vitro certain mitogenic Mab elicit many, if not all, the signs of activation elicited by antigen by binding to particular epitopes of signal transducing molecules of the T-hybridoma cell surface[18,19]. With regard to the B cell lineage, surface immunoglobulin (Ig) has long been recognized as a signal transducing molecule[20], and inhibitory effects of anti-Ig reagents on neoplastic murine B cells have been described[8,21-23]. Our observation that multiple administrations of anti-I-A appear to induce polyclonal B cell activation in addition to tumor cell elimination would suggest that activation can be equated with tumor cell killing in our system, an idea we are actively pursuing.

ACKNOWLEDGMENT

S. Bridges was partially supported by the National Research Council (Italy) finalized project "Oncology."

REFERENCES

1. A. S. Freedman and L. M. Nadler, Cell surface markers in hematologic malignancies, Sem. Oncol. 14:193 (1987).

2. A. M. Kruisbeek, J. J. Mond, B. J. Fowlkes, J. A. Carmen, S. Bridges, and D. L. Longo, Absence of the $Lyt2^{-}$,$L3T4^{+}$ lineage of T cells in mice treated neonatally with anti-I-A correlates with absence of intrathymic I-A-bearing antigen-presenting cell function, J. Exp. Med. 161:1029 (1985).

3. A. M. Kruisbeek, S. Bridges, J. Carmen, D. L. Longo, and J. J. Mond, In vivo treatment of neonatal mice with anti-I-A antibodies interferes with the development of the class I, class II, and Mls-reactive proliferating T cell subset, J. Immunol. 134:3597 (1985).

4. A. M. Kruisbeek, J. A. Titus, D. A. Stephany, B. L. Gause, and D. L. Longo, In vivo treatment with monoclonal anti-I-A antibodies: disappearance of splenic antigen-presenting cell function concomitant with modulation of splenic cell surface I-A and I-E antigens, J. Immunol. 134:3605 (1985).

5. E. Walker, N. L. Warner, R. Chesnut, J. Kappler, and P. Marrack, Antigen-specific, I region-restricted interactions in vitro between tumor cell lines and T-cell hybridomas, J. Immunol. 128:2164 (1982).

6. L. H. Glimcher, K. J. Kim, I. Green, and W. E. Paul, Ia antigen-bearing B cell tumor lines can present protein antigen and alloantigen in a major histocompatibility complex-restricted fashion to antigen-reactive T-cells, J. Exp. Med. 155:445 (1982).

7. M. Daley, S. H. Bridges, and R. G. Lynch, Plasmacytoma spleen colonization: a sensitive in vivo assay for idiotype-specific immune suppression, J. Immunol. Methods 24:47 (1978).

8. S. H. Bridges, C. Le Guern, and C. Gurgo, Inhibition of in vivo growth of murine plasmacytoma MOPC-460 by monoclonal anti-idiotypic antibodies directed at distinct idiotypes of the immunoglobulin on the surface of MOPC-460, Cancer Res. 44:5051 (1984).

9. T. Meeker, J. Lowder, M. L. Cleary, S. Stewart, R. Warnke, J. Sklar, and R. Levy, Emergence of idiotype variants during treatment of B-cell lymphoma with anti-idiotype antibodies, N. Engl. J. Med. 312: 1658 (1985).

10. C. C. Badger and I. D. Bernstein, Therapy of murine leukemia with monoclonal antibody against a normal differentiation antigen, J. Exp. Med. 157:828 (1983).

11. S. Habu, J. Fukui, K. Shimamura, M. Kasai, Y. Nagai, K. Okumura, and N. Tamaoki, In vivo effects of anti-asialo GM1. 1. Reduction of NK activity and enhancement of transplanted tumor growth in nude mice, J. Immunol. 127:34 (1981).

12. M. Kasai, T. Yoneda, S. Habu, U. Maruyama, K. Okumura, and T. Tokunaga, In vivo effect of anti-asialo GM1 antibody on natural killer activity, Nature 291:334 (1981).

13. S. Forsgren, G. Pobor, A. Coutinho, and M. Pierres, The role of I-A/E molecules in B lymphocyte activation. I. Inhibition of lipopolysaccharide induced responses by monoclonal antibodies, J. Immunol. 133:2104 (1984).

14. L. Clement, T. F. Tedder, and G. L. Gartland, Antibodies reactive with class II antigens encoded for by the major histocompatibility complex inhibit human B cell activation, J. Immunol. 136:2375 (1986).

15. R. Palacios, O. Martinez-Maza, and K. Guy, Monoclonal antibodies against HLA-DR antigens replace T helper cells in activation of B lymphocytes, Proc. Natl. Acad. Sci. USA 80:3456 (1983).

16. G. B. Bishop and G. Haughton, Induced differentiation of a transformed clone of $Ly\text{-}1^+$ B cells by clonal T cells and antigen, Proc. Natl. Acad. Sci. USA 83:7410 (1986).

17. Z. Z. Chen, J. C. McGuire, K. L. Leach, and J. C. Cambier, Transmembrane signaling through B cell MHC class II molecules: anti-Ia antibodies induce protein kinase C translocation to the nuclear fraction, J. Immunol. 138:2345 (1987).

18. J. D. Ashwell, D. L. Longo, and S. H. Bridges, T-cell tumor elimination as a result of T-cell receptor-mediated activation, Science 237:61 (1987).

19. M. Mercep, J. J. Sussman, and J. D. Ashwell, Stimulation of murine T cell hybridomas with anti-Thy-1 monoclonal antibodies results in IL-2 production and inhibition of growth, Fed. Proc. 46:1051 (1987).

20. E. S. Vitetta, K. Brooks, P. Isakson, J. Layton, E. Puré, and D. Yuan, B lymphocyte receptors, In: "Fundamental Immunology," W. Paul, ed., Raven Press, New York (1984).

21. P. C. Isakson, K. A. Krolick, J. W. Uhr, and E. S. Vitetta, The effect of anti-immunoglobulin antibodies on the in vitro proliferation and differentiation of normal and neoplastic murine B cells, J. Immunol. 125:886 (1980).

22. A. W. Boyd and J. W. Schrader, The regulation of growth and differentiation of a murine B cell lymphoma, J. Immunol. 126:2466 (1981).

23. D. W. Scott, D. Livnat, C. A. Pennell, and P. Keng, Lymphoma models for B cell activation and tolerance, J. Exp. Med. 164:156 (1986).

HOST-RCS TUMOR INTERACTIONS IN SJL/J MICE

Benjamin Bonavida[1] and Kazunori Ohnishi

Department of Microbiology and Immunology
and the Jonsson Comprehensive Cancer Center
UCLA School of Medicine, University of California
Los Angeles, California 90024

INTRODUCTION

Spontaneous reticulum cell sarcoma (RCS) tumors arise spontaneously in SJL/J mice between the ages of 8-12 months. Since its original description by Murphy (1963) several studies have been undertaken to investigate this unusual tumor that expresses several unique properties. A general description of this tumor system has been recently reviewed (Bonavida, 1983, 1985). The most prominent features of this tumor are characteristics not shared by other studied tumor systems i.e. the RCS tumor expresses inappropriate Ia antigens on the surface, it stimulates syngeneic T cells to proliferate both *in vivo* and *in vitro*, and its growth is dependent on host T cells and on both the MHC and non-MHC genetic background of the host mouse. The tumor is difficult to establish in culture and only a few spontaneous tumors can be transplanted in syngeneic hosts and become transplantable lines.

Interest in this experimental RCS tumor system has arisen initially because of its resemblance to Hodgkin's lymphoma but this premise does not appear to hold at present. Nevertheless, because SJL/J RCS is a spontaneous tumor, it is useful to study it experimentally and apply various experimental manipulations the results of which may be benefical clinically as well as in fundamental tumor immunobiology. There are several pertinent questions pertinent to the RCS tumor system that have been partially addressed but require further investigation. For instance, these issues include the mechanism of tumor induction and latency, the cellular origin of RCS and clonality, the role of MHC and non-MHC genes and genetic background of the permissive host, the biochemical and molecular nature of tumor associated antigens, the delineation of the underlying mechanism of intimate tumor-host interactions, and the biochemical nature of host or tumor factors needed for RCS growth and maintenance *in vivo*. The following sections will describe briefly our studies addressing these various topics with reference to related investigations.

---

[1]Acknowledgement: This work was supported in part by grant CA19753 from the National Cancer Institute, DHHS and in part by a gift from Chugai Pharmaceuticals, Japan.

TUMOR INDUCTION AND LATENCY

The RCS tumor arises spontaneously in SJL/J mice at the ages 8-12 months. The majority of the mice will succumb to the tumor but a small percentage survives (Murphy 1963;1969). It is not clear whether the survivals rejected the tumor or that the tumor never arose. The long latency for tumor development has not been accounted for. Earlier studies have indicated that immunoregulatory mechanisms do not operate properly in SJL/J mice as tolerance induction to soluble antigens in mice >3 months could not be established (Owens and Bonavida, 1976). It is possible that immune functions directed against the tumor may be operable and which may dictate the onset of the tumor. Attempts to shorten the latency period have not been examined.

Recent evidence from our laboratory has demonstrated the presence of activated protooncogenes in RCS (Pulciani et al., 1987). DNA from RCS transform both murine NIH-3T3 and rat F2408 fibroblast cell lines. The observed high frequency of transformation of the RCS tumor DNA suggests that a common mechanism of oncogene activation is occuring in tumor tissues and this is concordant with the high incidence of RCS in SJL/J mice. Germ line transmission of the oncogene is unlikely because DNA from normal tissue did not transform mouse fibroblasts. Based on these studies we postulate that the induction of RCS tumors arise from alterations in individual somatic cells and that factors at present unknown of predisposing malignancy are genetically transmitted in this strain of mice.

ORIGIN AND CLONALITY OF RCS

The cellular origin and nature of the RCS tumor is controversial (Carswell et al., 1976; Ford et al., 1981; Pattengale and Taylor, 1983). Some studies suggest that it is a non T non B cell and the tumor does not share properties characteristic of mature macrophages. It expresses IA on the surface and stimulates syngeneic T cells to proliferate. Other studies suggest that the tumor is in the B cell lineage. Thus, mice pretreated neonatally with anti-IgM antibody showed reduction in tumor induction. The precise indentification of the cellular origin of this tumor must await further studies at the molecular level.

ROLE OF MHC AND NON-MHC GENETIC BACKGROUND IN TUMOR GROWTH

RCS tumors arise spontaneously in SJL/J mice (H-2^s) and can only be transplanted in SJL/J but not in other MHC identical strains such as A.SW or B10.S. However, a genetic influence has been demonstrated in the ability of F1 to support RCS growth. Studies using F1, F2, and backcrosses of A.SW (H-2^s) have indentified a single, non-H-2 gene capable of suppressing spontaneous RCS development (Katz et al., 1980). More recently, we examined the growth of RCS in several congenic and recombinant inbred strains between Balb/cKe (H-2^d) and SJL/J (H-2^s) mice (Sakano et al., 1985). SJA 20 mice congenic with SJL/J except at the Igh locus supported RCS growth. Recombinant mice of the H-2^d haplotype did not support RCS growth. However, recombinant inbred mice of the H-2^s haplotype varied in their susceptibility to permit RCS growth *in vivo*, supporting a role of non-H-2 gene(s) controlling growth of RCS. The various recombinant strains used in these studies exhibited different immunological properties and it may be postulated that non-H-2 genes controlling the T cell repertoire are involved such as strains in which the presence of T cells that respond to RCS will be permissive for RCS growth.

NATURE OF RCS TAA

RCS tumor expresses IA antigens on the cell surface that have been shown to be involved in the syngeneic stimulation of T cells. The addition of antibody to IA^s block the proliferative response *in vitro* (Ponzio et al., 1977). Furthermore, passive administration of mAb to IA^s inhibits RCS growth *in vivo* (Sakano and Bonavida, 1986). These results suggest that tumor associated Ia antigens play an important role in regulating RCS tumor growth. In additon to IA^s, the tumor also expresses IE-like specificities, even though the host strain does not express on the surface hybrid IE molecules (Wilbur and Bonavida, 1981; Wilbur et al., 1981). Strains of $H\text{-}2^{b,s}$ haplotypes do not synthesize the $E\alpha$ polypeptide but have a cytoplasmic $E\beta$ chain and lack messenger RNA for the $E\alpha$ polypeptide in the cytoplasm (Jones et al., 1981). The nature of the IE aberrant specificities in RCS has been examined in a variety of experimental systems briefly reviewed below. Initially, we noticed that RCS cells stimulation of syngeneic T cells can be partially inhibited by IE directed mAb and the tumor binds such antibodies by absorption experiments (Wilbur and Bonavida, 1981; Wilbur et al., 1981). Direct demonstration of IE antigens by biochemical means has met with little convincing evidence.

Another approach was undertaken to characterize RCS TAA at the clonal level by generating T cell hybridomas with specificity for RCS tumors. Several T cell hybridomas were generated and selected for a specific response to RCS by their ability to secrete IL-2 following activation. Four such hybridomas were chosen for further study two of which responded to RCS and IE^k and IE^d bearing allogeneic cells respectively, and the other two hybridomas were RCS tumor specific. None of these hybridomas responded to normal or LPS induced B cells blasts from the host SJL/J mouse. Antibodies directed against the $IA\beta^s$ polypeptide of the IA hybrid molecule blocked the antitumor response by all four hybridomas. However, the response to allogeneic IE^+ cells was not blocked by anti-IA^s but was blocked by antibodies directed against either the $IA^{k,d}$ or $IE^{k,d}$ hybrid molecules or the corresponding α or β chains. The four hybridomas were $L3T4^+$ and their response can be blocked by L3T4 mAb. These results therefore demonstrated that among the repertoire of T cells responding to RCS there exists cells that show cross-reactivity between RCS and allogeneic cells (Ohnishi and Bonavida, 1986 (a)).

Further confirmation of T cell cross-reactivity was demonstrated in T lymphocyte-target conjugate formation at the single cell level. The frequency of conjugate formation ranged from 20-40% above background. Conjugate formation was antigen specific and correlated well with the hybridomas specificity determined by IL-2 response following antigenic stimulation. The cross-reactive hybridomas formed conjugates with RCS and LPS blasts from $H\text{-}2^k$ or $H\text{-}2^d$ origin but not with cells of syngeneic or other allogeneic haplotypes (Ohnishi and Bonavida, 1986 (b)).

The expression of allogeneic Ia specificities on RCS tumors suggests that the RCS IA antigens must have undergone structural changes. Several plausible mechanisms may be invoked such as (a) the RCS tumor might have undergone genetic changes and expresses on the surface IE hybrid molecules through gene expression of the $E\alpha$ gene, normally defective because of deletion of the promoter region (b) the tumor might express the $E\beta^s$ chain on the surface by hybridization with the $A\alpha^s$ molecule, (c) the tumor might express multiple forms of $IA\alpha$ and $IA\beta$ chains (d) gene conversion between the $A\alpha$ and $E\beta$ chains might have taken place and (e) antigenic modulation of Ia antigens may have resulted from oncogenic transformation. These and other possibilities can be verified experimentally and are underway in our laboratory.

RCS TUMOR-HOST INTERACTIONS

RCS tumor cells stimulate syngeneic Thyl$^+$ L3 T4$^+$ cells both *in vitro* and *in vivo*. Indirect studies have revealed that RCS growth *in vivo* is dependent on host T cells. Direct evidence for the role of L3T4$^+$ T cells *in vivo* in regulating tumor growth was obtained in studies of passive adminstration of L3T4 mAb in SJL/J mice. Mice that received L3T4 mAb and inoculated with a lethal dose of RCS tumor survived with no apparent sign of RCS growth. The adminstration of a single dose of L3T4 mAb 4 days before tumor inoculation resulted in complete depletion of L3T4$^+$ cells and complete inhibition of tumor growth. These results demonstrated that the initiation of tumor growth is dependent on host L3T4$^+$ cells. Administration of mAb as late as 7 days after tumor inoculation resulted in inhibition of tumor growth demonstrating that continued tumor growth *in vivo* is dependent or the presence of L3T4$^+$ cells. Thus, the presence of L3T4$^+$ T cells is important for initiation and continued progression of tumor growth (Ohinishi and Bonavida, 1987 (a)).

An observation made in these studies suggested that tumor growth or proliferation and tumor maintenance may be under different regulatory mechanisms. Tumor bearing mice that were treated with L3T4 mAb resulted in tumor arrest as the tumor was maintained at the stage of arrest for several days therafter. We postulated that while RCS proliferation is dependent on L3T4$^+$ T cells, its maintenance is not and therefore tumor bearers treated with L3T4 mAb establish a state of tumor dormancy. We examined dormancy by passive administration of cells derived from treated mice into naive mice and observed signs of tumor growth. The results of such studies demonstrated that recipient mice develop tumor with the same growth kinetics as tumors derived from untreated mice. Furthermore, the IA^{+s} cell concentration, denoting primarily RCS tumor, coincided with controls. The state of dormancy could be demonstrated for as late as 11 weeks post antibody treatment but subsided thereafter (Ohnishi and Bonavida, 1987 (b)). The mechanism of tumor dormancy was not due to the induction of suppressor cells inhibiting the syngeneic anti-RCS response. Thus, even in the presence of recovered L3T4$^+$ cells, the tumor remained dormant. Thus, other factors may be involved that establish dormancy and these may not be derived from L3T4$^+$ cells. Further studies of this state of dormancy are required to determine underlying mechanisms.

CONCLUDING REMARKS

The spontaneous RCS tumor in SJL/J mice exhibits several unusual characteristics that are important to decipher. This tumor provides an opportunity to explore tumor related properties that are pertinent to its growth and maintenance in the host. Likewise, the intimate host interaction with the tumor that dictates the tumor outcome raises important issues that may be pertinent to human tumors and metastases.

REFERENCES

Bonavida, B. 1983. The SJL/J spontaneous reticulum cell sarcoma: new insights in the field of neoantigen, host-tumor interaction, and regulation of tumor growth. *Adv. Cancer Res.* 38:1.

Bonavida, B. 1985. "Intimate host-tumor interaction in the spontaneous reticulum cell sarcoma of SJL/J mice: Is it an exceptional case? *Surveys Imm. Res.* 4:271.

Carswell, E.A., Lerman, S.P., and Thorbecke, G.J. 1976. Properties of reticulum cell sarcomas in SJL/J mice. II. Fate of labeled tumor cells in normal and irradiated syngeneic mice. Cell. Imm. 23:39.

Ford, R.J., Ruppert, B., and Maizel, M. 1981. The SJL/J tumor: a neoplasm involving macrophages. Clin Invest 45:111.

Jones, P.P., Murphy, D.B., and McDevitt, H.O. 1981. Variable synthesis and expression of $E\alpha$ and $Ae\beta(E\alpha)$ Ia polypeptide chains in mice of different H-2 haplotypes. Immunogenetics 12:321.

Katz, I.R., Lerman, S.P., Ponzio, N.M., Schreffler, D.C., and Thorbecke, G.J. 1980. Growth in SJL/J derived transplantable reticulum cell sarcoma as related to its ability to induce T-cell proliferation in the host I. Dominant negative genetic influence of other parent haplotypes in F1 hybrids of SJL/J mice. J. Exp. Med. 151:247.

Lerman, S.P., Chapman, J.M., Carswell, E.A., and Thorbecke, G.J. 1974. Properties of reticulum cell sarcomas in SJL/J mice I. Proliferative response to tumor cells of T-derived lymphoid cells from normal mice. Int. J. Cancer 14:808.

Murphy, E.D. 1963. SJL/J, a new inbred strain of mouse with a high, early incidence of reticulum cell sarcoma. Proc. Am. Assoc. Cancer Res. 4:46.

Murphy, E.D. 1969. Transplantation behavior of Hodgkin's-like reticulum cell neoplasms of strain SJL/J mice and results of tumor inoculation. J. Natl. Cancer Inst. 42:797.

Ohnishi, K., and Bonavida, B. 1986(a). Mapping of SJL/J reticulum cell sarcoma tumor associated Ia antigens by T cell hybridomas: characterization of tumor specific and shared epitopes detected on IE^+ allogeneic cells. J. Immunol. 137:733.

Ohnishi, K., and Bonavida, B. 1986(b). Specific lymphocyte-target cell conjugate formation between tumor specific helper T-cell hybridomas and IA bearing allogeneic cells. I. Role of Ia and both L3T4 and LFA-1 antigens in recognition/binding. J. Immunol. 137:3681.

Ohnishi, K., and Bonavida, B. 1987. Regulation of Ia^+ reticulum cell sarcoma (RCS) growth in syngeneic SJL/J mice I. Inhibition of tumor growth by passive administration of L3T4 monoclonal antibody before or after tumor inoculation. J. Immunology. 138:4524, 1987.

Ohnishi, K., and Bonavida, B. Regulation of Ia^+ reticulum cell sarcoma (RCS) growth in syngeneic SJL/J mice II. Establishment of tumor dormancy in tumor bearers by passive administration of L3T4 monoclonal antibody (Submitted).

Owens, M.H., and Bonavida, B. 1976. Immune functions characteristic of SJL/J mice and their association with age and spontaneous reticulum cell sarcoma. Cancer Research 36:1007.

Pattengale, P.K., and Taylor C.R. 1983. Experimental models of lymphoproliferative disease. The mouse as a model for human non-Hodgkin's lymphomas and related leukemia. Am. J. Path. 113:237.

Ponzio, N.H., David, C.S., Schreffler, D.C., and Thorbecke, G.J. 1977. Properties of reticulum cell sarcomas in SJL/J mice IV. Nature of reticulum cell sarcoma surface antigen which induces proliferation of normal SJL/J T cells. J. Exp. Med. 146:132, 1977.

Pulciani, S., Sakano, T., Ohnishi, K., Anastasi, A.M., Pecorelli, A., Fiorucci, G., Oppi, C., Rossi, G.B., and Bonavida, B. 1987. Detection of a transforming gene in spontaneous reticulum cell sarcoma of SJL/J mice: A genetically linked and host-dependent neoplasia. Cancer Research. 47:523, 1987.

Sakano, T., and Bonavida, B. 1986. Inhibition of IA positive RCS tumor cell growth in syngeneic SJL/J mice by monoclonal anti-IA antibody. Cancer Research 46:3245.

Sakano, T., Wilbur, S.M., Bonavida, B., and Cohn, M. 1985. Non-H_2 linked control of in vivo growth of SJL/J derived reticulum cell sarcoma in recombinant inbred strains between BALB/c ke and SJL/K mice. J. Natl. Cancer Inst. 75:669.

Wilbur, S.M., and Bonavida, B. 1981. Expression of hybrid Ia molecules on the cell surface of reticulum cell sarcomas that are undetectable on host SJL/J lymphocytes. J. Exp. Med. 153:510.

Wilbur, S.M., Marelli, O., and Bonavida, B. 1983. Serological demonstration of an allogeneic Ia.7 antigen on the cellular surface of SJL/J-derived reticulum cell sarcomas. Cancer Res. 43:4266.

THE ROLE OF DEFECTIVE MHC CLASS I EXPRESSION FOR TUMOR GROWTH AND METASTASIS

Günter J. Hämmerling, Daniela Klar, Uwe Maschek,
Wolfgang Pülm, and Knut Sturmhöfel

Institute for Immunology and Genetics
German Cancer Research Center
Heidelberg, W.-Germany

INTRODUCTION

The very early work on transplantation of murine tumors and "tumor rejection antigens" by pioneers such as Tyzzer, Little and Snell lead 50 years ago to the discovery of the major histocompatibility antigens. In the present overview it is discussed that MHC class I antigens induce not only the rejection of tumors in allogeneic hosts but that they are also fundamental for the rejection of tumors and metastasis in syngeneic hosts. The studies demonstrate that for induction of a specific T cell response the tumor cells have to express not only a novel tumor associated antigen but also MHC class I antigens. Numerous reports have demonstrated strong variations in the expression of class I antigens on mouse and rat tumors, e.g. on thymomas (Schmidt et al., 1979), on spontaneous lung carcinomas (Eisenbach et al., 1983), on methyl-cholantrene A induced fibrosarcomas (De Baetselier et al., 1980; Hämmerling et al., 1987), cells transformed with human adenovirus strain 12 (Bernards et al., 1983), etc.. On many human tumors variable expression of HLA antigens was also observed (see Table 4). Because cytotoxic T cells can recognize foreign antigens only in conjunction with MHC class I structures the decreased class I expression on tumors was interpreted to facilitate the escape from immune surveillance. However, all these assumptions were based on indirect evidence, namely on a correlation between the absence of class I antigens and the tumorigenic properties of the tumor cells.

In this report direct experimental evidence is summarized demonstrating that class I expression influences indeed immunogenicity and thereby the tumorigenic and metastatic potential of tumor cells. High expression of H-2 class I antigens obtained after H-2 gene transfection of tumor cells rendered these cells immunogenic and lead to induction of an H-2 restricted T cell response and rejection of the tumor cells and metastasis in vivo. However, we will also discuss new findings suggesting that sometimes high expression of H-2 class I antigens can have the opposite effect. It seems that in these cases High H-2 expression is paralelled by increased resistance to NK cell mediated lysis which can facilitate more vigorous outgrowth of tumors and metastasis in vivo.

RESULTS AND DISCUSSION

Studies on the molecular defect of H-2 deficient tumor cells

Before the biological effect of deficient H-2 and HLA expression is discussed, studies on the molecular nature of the defect will be summarized.

Analysis of a large number of H-2 deficient tumor lines showed that there exist two broad categories depending on their responsiveness to interferon-Y. In the vast majority of tumor lines investigated by us H-2 expression could be induced by in vitro treatment with IFN-Y. In few other tumor lines IFN treatment had no effect on H-2 expression.

One of the latter tumors was investigated in more detail. The Meth.A induced fibrosarcoma IC9 (see below) is heterozygous but expresses only the D^b molecule whereas the D^k, K^k and K^b genes are completely silent. Treatment with IFN-Y or with the demethylating reagent 5′-azacytidine did not result in H-2 expression. In order to see if the silent genes were defective the K^b gene was cloned from IC9 cells. No modifications were observed in this K^b gene or in its 5′ flanking region.

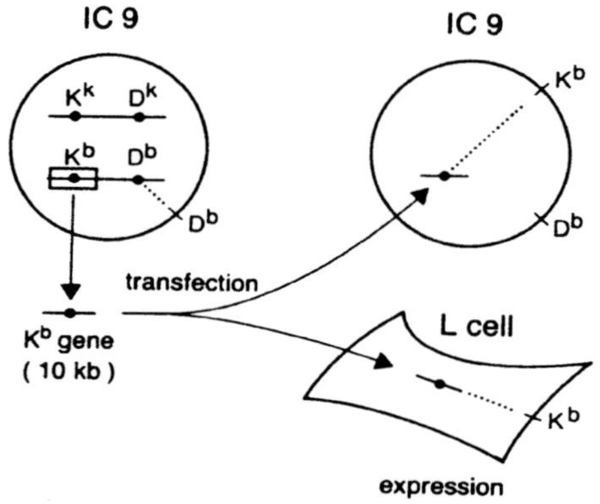

Fig. 1 The silent K^b gene of IC9 cells is functional after cloning. The silent K^b gene from IC9 tumor cells was cloned and identified with the help of K^b specific oligonucleotides. Expression was obtained after transfection into L cells or IC9 cells.

Transfection into L-cells (see Fig. 1) showed that the gene could be expressed and therefore, was fully functional. Moreover, when this K^b gene was transfected back into the IC9 tumor cell (from which it was originally isolated) expression was observed (U. Maschek, W. Pülm, unpublished). Since transfected genes will integrate randomly into the genome, these findings show that the location of the gene in the genome is important for expression. It is not yet clear why the endogeneous K^b gene is not expressed. Possibly alterations in the chromatine structure around the MHC region on chromosome 17 prevents its expression. Studies on the IFN inducible tumor cells showed that treatment with IFN-Y induced transcription of the silent H-2 genes. During the course of these investigations we observed that these cells displayed simultaneously an additional defect which provided new information about the assembly of H-2 heavy chains and β2m. A spontaneous lung carcinoma (CMT), a Meth. A fibrosarcoma (Bc20) and a spontaneous melanoma (B16) were analysed. In all these H-2 negative cell lines H-2 expression could be induced by IFN-γ. When these tumor cells were transfected with H-2 genes cell surface expression of the transfected H-2 was only observed after IFN-γ treatment.

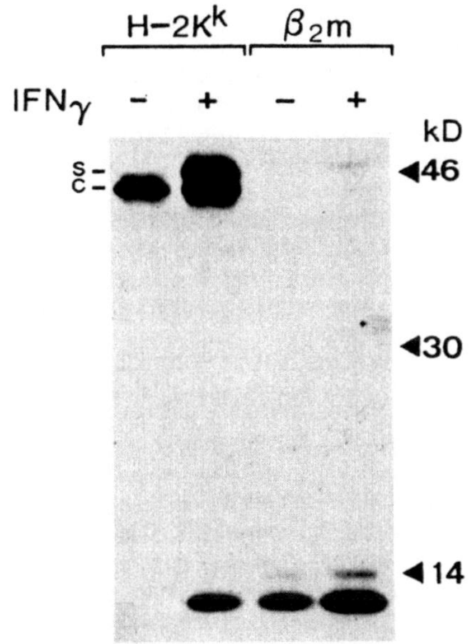

Fig. 2 Assembly of H-2 heavy chain and β2m is a regulated process and can can be induced by IFN-γ. The IFN inducible fibrosarcoma Bc20 of C57Bl/6 origin was transfected with the allogeneic K^k gene. After 2 hrs labeling with ^{35}S methionine the K^k antigen was immunoprecipitated with mAb H100-27 and separated on a 10% SDS gel. β2m was precipitated with a rabbit anti-mouse β2m serum. Coprecipitation of the K^k antigen and β2m with the anti-K^k antibody was observed only after treatment with IFN-γ (48 hrs). c indicates the cytoplasmic form of the K^k heavy chain and s indicates the cell surface form.

In order to differentiate between the endogenous and the transfected H-2 gene for this experiment products allogeneic H-2 genes (e.g. K^k) were transfected into H-2^b cells. Although no surface expression was obtained large amounts of transfected K^k specific mRNA and K^k protein were observed in the cytoplasm without IFN-γ.

Immunoprecipitation studies with anti-K^k and anti-β2m antibodies showed that these cells contained not only K^k antigens but also considerable amounts of β2m (see Fig. 2).

However, it is evident that the K^k protein and β2m are not associated in the absence of IFN-γ: the anti-K^k antibody precipitates only the free K^k heavy chain but no β2m is coprecipitated. The free K^k chain obtained in the absence of IFN-γ is the cytoplasmic form (c) with incompletely processed carbohydrates. In contrast, after treatment with IFN-γ the processed surface form(s) of the K^k heavy chain was observed which was coprecipitated and therefore assembled with β2m.

These studies demonstrate for the first time that assembly of the H-2 heavy chain and β2m, and possibly the transport, is a regulated process. It is of interest to note that all three cell lines randomly investigated by us display simultaneously these two types of defect, namely blockade of the transcription of the endogeneous H-2 genes and association of H-2 and β2m. Therefore it can be assumed that blockade of heavy and light chain assembly occurs frequently in IFN inducible cells. Since in other systems proteins such as the immunoglobulin binding protein appear to be involved in the assembly of secreted and membrane bound proteins (Munro and Pelham, 1986), it remains to be seen if similar mechanisms apply to the assembly of class I antigens.

De novo expression of H-2 antigens obtained by H-2 gene transfection abrogates of tumor growth and metastasis in vivo

In the following section the biological effects of deficient class I expression on tumors are discussed.

The tumor line 3LL is a spontaneous lung carcinoma derived from C57Bl/6 mice. It was found to express only the H-2 D^b antigens but not K^b. This tumor grows rapidly in C57Bl/6 mice and forms many metastases in the lung. In order to investigate if restoration of the expression of the missing K^b antigen would change the tumorigenic and metastatic properties the 3LL cells were transfected with a cloned K^b gene (Table 1). The transfectants were found to express the K^b molecules on the cell surface. In contrast to the K^b deficient parental 3LL cells the K^b positive transfectants grew much slower in syngeneic C57Bl/6 mice. More strikingly, their metastatic potential in immunocompetent hosts was completely abrogated (Table 1, own unpublished observations). These data suggest that expression of the syngeneic K^b molecule is important for rejection of the 3LL tumor cells.

Table 1 Growth and metastasis of K^b transfected 3LL tumor in syngeneic C57Bl/6 mice

Cell line	transfected gene	H-2 phenotype	growth in C57Bl/6: primary tumor	growth in C57Bl/6: metastasis nodules/lung
3LL	-	-, D^b	fast	>100
3LL.K^b-1	K^b	K^b, D^b	slow	0

The C57Bl/6 derived spontaneous lung carcinoma 3LL, which is deficient for K^b expression, was transfected with the K^b gene. The tumorigenic and metastatic potential of the transfectants was tested in syngeneic C57Bl/6 mice after inoculation of 5×10^5 cells into the hind foot pads.

In another study performed in collaboration with Drs. S. Segal and M. Feldman the Meth. A induced fibrosarcoma IC9 from $(C3H \times C57Bl/6)F_1$ mice was chosen (de Baetselier et al., 1980). This tumor expresses only the D^b molecule but not the K^b, K^k and D^k antigens which are found on normal F_1 cells. Restoration of cell surface expression of the "missing" H-2 antigens was achieved by transfection with the K^b, K^k or D^k genes. After inoculation into syngeneic F_1 mice it was found that only expression of the K^b molecule abrogated the tumor growth in vivo (but not in vitro), whereas expression of K^k or D^k did not influence the tumor growth (Table 2) (Wallich et al., 1985). Testing of a large number of independently derived transfectants verified that the observed effect was indeed due to the de novo expressed H-2 antigen and not caused by the transfection procedure. Tumor growth of the K^b transfectants was observed in immunodeficient (irradiated) mice indicating that the immune system mediates the rejection in normal mice. In fact, in further studies tumor specific, H-2 restricted CTL were only found when syngeneic F_1 mice were immunized with an H-2K transfected IC9 cell. No CTL response against the parental IC9 cells was observed (Wallich et al., 1985). These data suggest that there is a hierarchy among the various H-2 alleles to function as H-2 restriction elements, and that T lymphocytes recognize the putative tumor associated antigen of IC9 cells only efficiently when it is associated with the K^b antigen.

Table 2 Growth and metastasis of H-2 gene transfected IC9 and IE7tumor in syngeneic F_1 mice

cell line	transfected gene	H-2 phenotype	tumor growth	metastasis nodules/lung
IC9	-	-, D^b	fast	0
IC9.D^k-1	D^k	D^k, D^b	fast	0
IC9.K^k-1	K^k	K^k, D^b	fast	0
IC9.K^b-1	K^b	K^b, D^b	none/slow	0
IE7	-	-, D^b, D^k	fast	>100
IE7.K^k-1	K^k	K^k, D^b, D^k	fast	0

IC9 is a (C3HxC57Bl/6)F_1 derived sarcoma which expresses only the D^b molecule. Restoration of H-2 K^k, D^k or K^b expression was achieved by transfection with H-2 genes. Tumor growth of the transfectants was determined after inoculation into the hind foot pad of syngeneic F_1 mice as described by Wallich et al., 1985.

When a metastatic variant (IE7) of the IC9 tumor was transfected with a K^k gene formation of metastasis was no longer observed in F_1 mice, although the presence of the K^k molecule did not affect the growth of the primary tumor (Table 2,Wallich et al., 1985). Probably in this case the resulting K^k restricted T cell response is not strong enough to eliminate the subcutaneously growing tumor, but it appears to be strong enough for elimination of the few metastasizing cells in the periphery which are more easily accessible to the attacking immunocytes.

Similar transfection studies have also been performed by other investigators. They are summarized in Table 3. Hui et al. (1985) have found that restoration of K^k expression of the K^k deficient thymoma K36 blocked the in vivo growth. Tanaka et al. (1986) have also observed that transfection of a class I gene into adenovirus 12 transformed cells decreased their tumorigenicity. In conclusion, our studies and those of the other investigators demonstrate clearly that the de novo expression of MHC class I antigens obtained after H-2 gene transfection can render the tumor cells highly immunogenic and thus prevent tumor growth and metastatic spread in immunocompetent hosts.

Table 3 Studies on abrogation of tumorigenicity by H-2 gene transfection

Tumor	origin	parental H-2 phenotype K	D	transf. gene	foot note
K36	AKR Thymoma	-	D^k	K^k	(1)
C57ATl	Adenovirus 12	-	-	L^d	(2)
IC9	$(C3HxB6)F_1$ Meth.A sarc.	--	$-,D^d$	K^b,K^k,D^k	(3)
IE7	$(C3HxB6)F_1$ Meth.A sarc.	--	D^k,D^b	K^b,K^k	(4)
3LL	C57Bl/6 lung carc.	-	D^b	K^b	(5)

Foot note
(1) Hui et al., 1984 - K^k decreased tumor growth in AKR mice
(2) Tanaka et al., 1985 - L^d decreased tumor growth in (B6xBALB/c) mice
(3) Wallich et al., 1985 - K^b, but not K^k or D^k abrogated tumor growth in $(C3HxB6)F_1$ mice
(4) Wallich et al., 1985 - K^k abrogated metastasis but not the primary tumor
(5) Hämmerling, unpublished - K^b decreased growth of primary tumor and metastasis in C57Bl/6 mice

HLA-A,B,C expression on human tumors

A considerable percentage of human tumors of various origins have been found to be deficient for HLA-A,B,C expression (in general 10-15%). The crucial question is if the observed lack of HLA antigens on the tumors leads to a decrease of their immunogenicity as was described above for the mouse tumors. Therefore several investigators have tried to correlate the lack of HLA antigens with pathological criteria.

Some of these reports are summarized in Table 4. In most cases the authors have compared HLA expression on benign forms of the tumors with the malignant tumors. For some tumors, such as the mammary carcinoma, the equine porocarcinoma, etc. loss of class I antigens was more frequently observed on the malignant form. In studies where the case numbers were large enough a statistical evaluation of the relationship of loss of class I with the malignant phenotype was performed. In the cases of colorectal carcinoma (Momburg et al., 1986) and B cell malignancies (Möller et al., 1987) a highly significant statistical correlation between loss of class I and the malignant phenotype was found. These studies suggest that also in the human the loss of MHC class I antigens can contribute to their malignancy.

Table 4 Correlation between deficient HLA-A,B,C expression on tumors with the malignant phenotype

Correlation observed	
Cutaneous sqamous cell carcinoma[1]	Turbitt & Mackie, 1981
Mammary carcinoma[1]	Bhan et al., 1983
Eccrine procarcinoma[1]	Holden et al., 1983
Colorectal carcinoma[2]	Momburg et al., 1986
B cell lymphoma[2]	Möller et al., 1987
No correlation observed	
Malignant melanoma	Ruiter et. al, 1982
Cervical carcinoma	Ferguson et al., 1985
Endometrical carcinoma	Ferguson et al., 1985
Small cell lung carcinoma	Doyle et al., 1985
Neuroblastoma	Whelan et al., 1985

HLA-A,B,C and/or β2m expression was determined by immunohistochemical staining. Correlation with the malignant phenotype was done by
(1) comparison of malignant with benign tumors
(2) statistical evaluation of a large number of cases in relationship to the pathological grading.

However, it is also evident from the lower part of Table 4 that for many tumors no relationship between HLA expression and the malignant phenotype was observed. But here one has to bear in mind that in many studies the case number was not high enough to yield significant statistical information. Moreover, all authors used monomorphic HLA reagents which did not differentiate between the individual HLA alleles. In analogy to the work with mouse tumors where only certain H-2 alleles were found to be important for syngeneic tumor rejection (see Table 3) it is conceivable that analysis of the human tumors with HLA allele specific antibodies would yield more information. In fact, our preliminary studies show that there also exist fresh human tumors which have lost expression of only one of their HLA alleles (Momburg et al., unpublished). Certainly more work is required in this field.

Relationship between H-2 class I expression, NK cell mediated lysis and tumor growth in vivo

Several investigators have observed that treatment of IFN-inducible cell lines not only enhances H-2 class I expression but simultaneously can decrease their sensitivity for NK cell mediated lysis. Since NK cells have been implicated to control in vivo tumor growth and the metastatic spread, IFN treated tumor cells were injected i.v. into syngeneic mice. Three to four weeks later the number of metastatic nodules was determined. Table 5 shows the results of a typical experiment which was obtained with the spontaneous lung carcinoma CMT 64.5 of C57Bl/6 origin. It can be seen that induction of H-2 expression by IFN-γ strongly decreased the NK sensitivity and that these cells formed more metastasis in vivo.

Table 5 Increase of H-2 expression and experimental metastasis after IFN treatment of CMT tumor cells

IFN-γ	H-2 expression (CPM) D^b	K^b	Nk lysis (%)	Metastasis No. nodules in lung (range)
-	214	106	49.8	28 (2 - 50)
+	23.161	4.438	27.2	80 (60 - 100)

The spontaneous lung carcinoma CMT 64.5 of C57Bl/6 origin was treated in vitro for 48 hrs with IFN-γ (10 μ/ml). H-2 expression was monitored in a cellular radioimmunoassay with monoclonal antibodies. NK susceptibility was measured with poly I:C induced spleen cells from young CBA mice. Experimental metastasis (number of nodules in the lung) was determined 2 weeks after injection of 10^5 cells i.v. into C57Bl/6 mice.

Another example is shown in Table 6 where the H-2 positive thymoma EL4 was compared with its H-2 negative variants obtained after cell sorting. Our preliminary results suggest that the H-2 negative variants did not grow as primary tumors in vivo in syngeneic C57Bl/6 mice whereas the parental H-2 positive cells grew readily. Again, the H-2 positive cells were more resistant to NK mediated lysis than the H-2 negative variants (unpublished).

Table 6 Increase of H-2 expression on the EL4 tumor correlates with NK resistance and tumor growth in vivo

cell line	H-2 expression (CPM) Kb	Db	Nk lysis (%)	tumor growth in C57Bl/6
EL4	11.356	20.752	20.7	yes
EL4.null	438	690	45.7	no

An H-2 negative EL4 variant was selected by cell sorter. H-2 expression and NK lysis was determined as indicated in Table 5. Tumor growth in C57Bl/6 mice was determined after i.p. injection.

Hence, it appears that the NK cells can control not only the metastatic spread but also the growth of primary tumors, and that H-2 class I antigen expression may contribute to resistance to NK mediated lysis. Similar findings have been reported by various other investigators, e.g. Kawano et al. (1986), Harel-Bellan et al., (1986) and Kärre et al. (1986). The latter author has proposed that the function of NK cells is to discriminate between cells expressing a self-signal (MHC antigens) and none self (MHC negative) and that the absence of class I antigens will provide a signal for killing of the "foreign" cell ("foreign" for the NK cells because MHC class I is missing). According to this hypothesis the immune system has two ways for elimination of tumor cells in both of which class I antigens are involved. In a first line of defense NK cells, which do not need to be immunized, are able to eliminate tumor cells with low class I expression. A second line of defense is provided by the induction of an H-2 restricted specific T cell response which requires class I expression on the tumor cells.

The idea that the class I molecules themselves are directly responsible for NK resistance is intriguing but so far there is no direct experimental evidence. There exist also several studies where no correlation between NK sensitivity and class I expression was observed (e.g. Dalianis et al., 1981). The studies outlined above are reminiscent of the hybrid resistant phenomenon where F_1 mice reject parental hemapoietic grafts. This rejection seems to be mediated by NK cells, and the antigens encoded by the H-2D loci have been implicated as target antigens. However, a recent study has clearly shown that H-2D antigens are not required for graft rejection and that the hybrid resistant locus Hh-1 can be separated from the H-2D locus by recombination (Daley et al., 1987).

Therefore the frequently observed association between NK resistance and class I expression could be a coincidence. The possibility has to be considered that the unknown NK target structures and class I antigens can sometimes influence each other in their expression, conformation, etc.. In this context recent findings are of interest demonstrating that there exists an inverse relationship between expression of class I genes and certain oncogenes.

Oncogenes and class I expression

Bernards et al. (1987) have reported that high levels of N-myc achieved by transfection of the N-myc gene into human neuroblastoma cells will drastically decrease HLA-A,B,C expression. Similarly Schriers et al. have found an inverse relationship between c-myc and HLA expression on human melanoma cells (personal communication). Alon et al. (1987) have shown that transfection of the IC9 fibrosarcoma with the H-2D^k gene will strongly decrease Ki-ras expression. All these studies suggest that class I gene transcription can be influenced by other cellular genes and vice versa, which may lead to important changes of the immunological properties of the cells.

In fact, very recently increased Ha-ras expression in fibroblasts was found to be accompanied by enhanced NK susceptibility (Johnson et al., 1987). Future studies have to show if increased oncogene expression, decreased class I expression, or other events are responsible for augmented NK susceptibility, and if these events are causatively linked.

SUMMARY

The immune system has two principle pathways for elimination of neoplastic cells, namely antigen specific T lymphocytes and nonspecific NK cells. MHC class I antigens play an important role in both pathways although with opposite effects. High expression of class I antigens on tumors is necessary for induction of an H-2 restricted immune response, whereas in the case of NK cells high class I expression on tumors appears to prevent their lysis by NK cells.

For these studies H-2 negative tumors were used. Restoration of H-2 expression by H-2 gene transfection abrogated tumor growth and metastasis in vivo. Studies on the mechanism showed that H-2 class I expression renders the tumor cells highly immunogenic and that in vivo CTL could be induced which recognized the putative tumor antigen in conjunction with the transfected H-2 antigens. However, the data also showed that only certain H-2 alleles function efficiently as H-2 restriction elements. These results demonstrate convincingly that class I antigens are required for induction of a specific T cell response. Similar mechanisms may also apply for rejection of human tumors because for several types of tumors a correlation between loss of HLA-A,B,C antigens and the malignant phenotype was observed.

With a different set of murine tumor cells it was observed that high expression of class I antigens can have an opposite effect. In these tumors class I expression enhanced the resistance for NK mediated lysis and therefore these tumors metastasized more readily in vivo. In contrast variants of these tumors with low class I expression were more NK susceptible and therefore were less tumorigenic or metastatic in immunocompetent hosts. However, it is not yet clear if H-2 antigens directly or indirectly prevent lysis by NK cells. The recently observed inverse relationships between oncogene and class I expression and also between oncogene expression and NK resistance indicate that secondary events are involved and suggest the intriguing possibility that class I antigens, oncogenes, and NK target structures influence each other by yet unknown mechanisms.

REFERENCES

Alon, Y., Hämmerling, G.J., Segal, S. & Bar-Eli, M. (1987) Cancer Res., **47**, 2553.

Bernards, R., Schrier, P.I., Houweling, A., Bos, J.L. & van der Eb, A.J. (1983). Nature, **305**, 776

Bernards, R., Dessain, S.K., Weinberg, R.A. (1986) Cell, **47**, 667.

Bhan, A.K. & DesMarais, C.L. (1983). J. Nat. Canc. Inst., **71**, 507.

Daley, J.P., Wroblewski, J.M., Kaminsky, S.G. & Nakamura, I. (1987). Immunogenetics, **26**, 21.

Dalianis, T., Ahrlund-Richter, L., Merino, F., Klein, E. & Klein, G. (1981). Immunogenetics, **12**, 371.

De Baetselier, P., Katzav, S., Gorelik, E., Feldman, M. & Segal, S. (1980). Nature, **288**, 179.

Doyle, A., Martin, W.J. & Funa, K. (1985). J. Exp. Med., **161**, 1135.

Eisenbach, L., Segal, S. & Feldman, M. (1983). Int. J. Canc., **32**, 113.

Ferguson, A., Moore, M. & Fox, H. (1985). Brit. J. Canc., **52**, 551.

Harel-Bellan, A., Quillet, A., Marchiol, C., DeMars, R., Tursz, T. & Fradelizi, D. (1986). Proc. Nat. Acad. Sci., USA, **83**, 5688.

Hämmerling, G.J., Klar, D., Moldenhauer, G., Momburg, F. & Pülm, W. (1986). Progress in Immunology VI, Eds. B. Cinader & R.A. Miller, Academic Press, p. 684.

Hämmerling, G.J., Klar, D., Pülm, W., Momburg, F. & Moldenhauer, G. (1987). Biochimica et Biophysica Acta, Elsevier Science Publishers, Biomedical Division - Amsterdam, in press.

Holden, C.A., Shaw, M., McKee, P.H., Sanderson, A.R. & MacDonald, D.M. (1984). Arch. Dermatol., **120**, 732.

Hui, K., Grosveld, F. and Festenstein, H. (1984). Nature, **311**, 750-752.

Johnson, p. W., Trumble, W. S., Hozumi, N. and Roder, J. C., (1987). J. Immunol., **138**, 3996-4003.

Kawano, Y.-I., Taniguchi, K., Toshitani, A. and Nomoto, K., (1986). J. Immunol., **136**, 4729-4732.

Kärre, K., Ljunggren, H. G., Piontek, G. and Kiessling, R., (1986). Nature, **119**, 675.

Momburg, F., Degner, T., Bacchus, E., Moldenhauer, G., Hämmerling, G. J. & Möller, P., (1986a). Int. J. Canc., **37**, 179.

Möller, P., Herrmann, B., Moldenhauer, G. & Momburg, F., (1987). Int. J. Cancer, **40**, 32.

Munro, S. & Pelham, H. R. B., (1986). Cell, **46**, 291.

Ruiter, D. J., Bhan, A. K., Harrist, T. J., Sober, A. J. & Mihm, M. C., (1982). J. Immunol., **129**, 2808.

Schmidt, W., Altfield, G. & Festenstein, H., (1979). Immungenetics, **8**, 311.

Tanaka, K., Isselbacher, K. J., Khoury, G. & Jay, G., (1985). Science, **228**, 26.

Turbitt, M.L. & Mackie, R.M. (1981). Brit. J. Dermatol., **107**, 507.

Wallich, R., Bulbuc, N., Hämmerling, G.J., Katzav, S., Segal, S. & Feldman, M. (1985). Nature, **315**, 301.

Whelan, J.P., Chatten, J. & Lampson, L.A. (1985). Canc. Res., **45**, 5976.

SECTION VI

ROLE OF H-2 GENES IN DISEASE

H-2-LINKED CONTROL OF THE SUSCEPTIBILITY OF MICE TO CLEFT PALATE INDUCED BY CORTISONE AND TESTOSTERONE

David L. Gasser, Chhanda Gupta and Allen S. Goldman*

Department of Human Genetics
University of Pennsylvania School of Medicine, and
Children's Hospital of Philadelphia, Philadelphia, PA
19104

Abstract. In the course of mapping H-2-linked genes which control susceptibility to cortisone-induced cleft palate, we have observed that certain pairs of congenic strains which have been considered to have the same H-2-recombinant chromosomes differ in their susceptibility. The B10.A(1R) and B10.A(2R) congenic strains have been believed to possess the same a/b crossover in the S/D interval, but B10.A(2R) is significantly more susceptible than B10.A(1R). Likewise, the B10.A(18R) and B10.BAR5 strains have been considered to have the same b/a crossover in the S/D interval, but B10.BAR5 is significantly more susceptible than B10.A(18R). In order to assess the possible effects of these genes on susceptibility to other steroids, we have injected pregnant mice on days 11 through 14 with testosterone. We have observed significant differences among H-2 congenic strains in the frequency of testosterone-induced fetal resorption. Among surviving fetuses, there were significant differences in the frequency of testosterone-induced cleft palate.

INTRODUCTION

It is well established that genes in the H-2 region affect the susceptibility of mice to cortisone-induced cleft palate (Bonner and Slavkin, 1975; Biddle and Fraser, 1977; Tyan and Miller, 1978; Gasser et al., 1981; Gasser and Goldman, 1983; Bonner and Tyan, 1984, Demant, 1985). Investigators in several of these laboratories have tested congenic strains with recombinant H-2 haplotypes, and have obtained evidence that more than one H-2-linked gene is involved in determining susceptibility. We now report that certain pairs of congenic strains which have been believed to have the same recombinant haplotypes differ in their susceptibility to cortisone-induced cleft palate. All of the genes known to be shared by these strains can therefore be ruled out as determinants of susceptibility.

In order to determine whether the genes that we have been studying may be related to H-2-linked genes that are known to affect testosterone metabo-

* Current address: Center for Craniofacial Anomalies and Department of Pediatrics, The University of Illinois College of Medicine at Chicago, IL 60680

lism (Ivanyi et al., 1972a) and the target organs of testosterone (Ivanyi et al., 1972b; Gregorova et al., 1973), we have injected pregnant females with testosterone and have studied abnormalities in the progeny. Our results indicate that the rate of testosterone-induced fetal resorption is influenced by an H-2-linked gene. We have also observed cleft palates in the progeny of treated females, and have found that the frequency of testosterone-induced cleft palate is associated with the H-2 haplotype.

MATERIALS AND METHODS

Mice B10, B10.A, B10.A(2R) and B10.D2 mice were obtained from The Jackson Laboratory, Bar Harbor, Maine. Dr. Jack Stimpfling (McLaughlin Research Institute, Columbus Hospital, Great Falls, Montana) kindly provided the B10.A(1R), B10.A(18R), B10.S and B10.Q strains, and Dr. Donald C. Shreffler (Department of Genetics, Washington University, St. Louis, Missouri) generously supplied the B10.BAR8 and B10.BAR12 animals.

Treatment Female mice were mated overnight with syngeneic males, and checked for plugs and weighed the following morning. Those judged to be pregnant were injected on days 11, 12, 13, and 14, with the plug day being considered day 0. The steroids were dissolved in dimethyl sulfoxide (DMSO), and the indicated dosages were injected subcutaneously. Mice were dissected and examined on day 18 or 19.

Statistical Analysis The litter rather than the fetus has been used as the unit of analysis (Haseman and Hogan, 1975), and we have done this by comparing percentages of affected fetuses using the Mann-Whitney U Test. In order to avoid errors arising from small litters, we have excluded from statistical analysis all litters with fewer than three fetuses. However all litters, including those with one or two fetuses, have been included in the tables.

RESULTS

The results of testing several strains with the vehicle alone are shown in Table 1. Out of 20 litters consisting of 169 fetuses, only one cleft palate was observed and there were only four fetal resorptions. The results of injecting pregnant females with cortisone are shown in Table 2. Although B10.A(1R) and B10.A(2R) have been considered to have the same genes in the H-2 region (Klein et al., 1978), the frequency of cleft palate was significantly greater in B10.A(2R) than in B10.A(1R) ($p < 0.002$). B10.A(18R) was significantly less susceptible than both B10.BAR5 ($p < 0.05$) and B10.BAR12 ($p < 0.05$), despite the fact that these three strains are also believed to share the same H-2 haplotype.

When pregnant mice of various congenic strains were injected with testosterone, the results shown in Table 3 were obtained. Although not enough litters in all of these strains have yet been tested for valid comparisons, there are several conclusions which can already be made. The first point is that the congenic strains differ in their overall sensitivity to the toxic effects of testosterone. At 20 mg of testosterone per kg of body weight, there were significantly fewer fetal resorptions among the B10.A(1R) mice than in either B10.BAR8 ($p < 0.02$) or B10.Q ($p = 0.02$). The frequency of resorptions at 20 mg/kg in B10.BAR8 was significantly greater than in B10.BAR12 ($p < 0.002$), which is interesting because H-2-linked differences have not yet been detected in these strains. There is considerable variation among the other strains at both doses of testosterone, but not enough litters have been done yet to properly test the significance of these differences.

Among the surviving fetuses, there were significant differences in the frequencies of testosterone-induced cleft palate. B10.A(1R) was significantly less susceptible than B10.Q at 20 mg/kg ($p < 0.05$). B10.A(1R) was also significantly less susceptible than B10.A(2R) at 10 mg/kg ($p = 0.012.$), but many more litters are needed in these groups before one can be confident of the result.

DISCUSSION

The interpretation of the data presented in this report is very much dependent upon the degree to which we can accept the assumption that H-2 congenic strains differ from their parental strain only with respect to H-2-linked loci. If this assumption is valid for the congenic strains utilized in these experiments, then we have demonstrated that susceptibility to cortisone-induced cleft palate is affected by at least one H-2-linked gene which is not the same as any of the antigen-coding loci which have been defined so far. This follows from our demonstration that B10.A(1R) and B10.A(2R), which have been believed to have the same a/b recombinant haplotype, differ significantly in their susceptibility (Table 2). B10.A(18R) and B10.BAR5 are believed to have the same b/a crossover in the S/D interval (Klein et al., 1978), and they also differ significantly from each other in their susceptibility (Table 2). B10.BAR12 appears to have the same H-2 haplotype (D. C. Shreffler, personal communication), and it also differs significantly from B10.A(18R).

It has been reported that the effect of H-2 on adenosine cyclic 3', 5'-monophosphate (cAMP) may be due to an effect of glucagon binding to receptors (Lafuse and Edidin, 1980), and that this effect can be inhibited by anti-H-2 antisera (Meruelo and Edidin, 1980). A similar mechanism with regard to cortisone-induced cleft palate would seem to be ruled out insofar as the K, I-A, I-E, D and Tla antigens are concerned. The fact that both groups of "H-2-compatible" congenic strains which differ in their susceptibility involve S/D crossovers provides evidence for the assignment of a susceptibility gene in the S/D interval (Bonner and Tyan, 1984).

There have been previous reports of H-2-linked genes which affect testosterone metabolism and the target tissues of testosterone (Ivanyi et al., 1972a; 1972b; Gregorova and Ivanyi, 1973). In Table 3, we present data which demonstrate H-2-linked effects on both testosterone-induced fetal resorption and cleft palate. The data are insufficient to establish whether these genes are the same as those reported earlier, and whether they might be the same as those which affect cortisone-induced cleft palate. It does appear however, that there is a distinction between testosterone-induced fetal resorption and cleft palate, since these traits are dissociated in B10.Q. The fact that B10.BAR8 and B10.BAR12 differ significantly in testosterone-induced fetal resorption seems to place a gene for this trait in the S/D interval.

These genes could cause these effects by any one of several mechanisms. Steroid hormones are known to interact with receptors which then interact with specific DNA sequences associated with target genes. One possibility would involve receptor differences, but the glucocorticoid receptor is known to map on chromosome 18 (Francke and Gehring, 1980) and the testosterone receptor is on the X-chromosome (Bullock et al., 19871). A variant form of the glucocorticoid receptor, designated IB, was discovered in rats and is known to bind several additional hormones including testosterone (Litwack and Rosenfield, 1975). A similar receptor has been observed in the mouse, and it appears to be controlled by an H-2-linked gene (Goldman and Katsumata, 1986). However, there are other possibilities involving the hormone-receptor complex. It is known that hormone responsive elements which bind the receptors for glucocorticoids, androgens and progestins are

Table 1. Results of injecting pregnant congenic mice with DMSO.

Strain	Total No. of Litters	Resorptions		Fetuses with Cleft Palate	
		No./Total	%	No./Total	%
B10.A(1R)	9	3/79	4	1/76	1
B10.S	6	0/55	0	0/55	0
B10.Q	5	1/39	3	0/38	0

Table 2. Incidence of cortisone-induced cleft palate and fetal resorption in various congenic strains.*

STRAIN	H-2 Region								No. of litters	Fetuses with Cleft palate		Resorptions	
	K	A_β	A_α	E_β	E_α	S	D	Tla		No./ Total	%	No./ Total	%
B10	b	b	b	b	b	b	b	d	15	23/105	22	21/126	17
B10.A	k	k	k	k	k	d	d	a	21	127/147	86	47/194	24
B10.A(1R)	k	k	k	k	k	d	b	b	23	53/163	33	42/205	20
B10.A(2R)	k	k	k	k	k	d	b	b	16	79/113	70	47/160	29
B10.D2	d	d	d	d	d	d	d	c	12	3/78	4	9/87	10
B10.A(18R)	b	b	b	b	b	b	d		23	54/164	33	28/192	15
B10.BAR5	b	b	b	b	b	b	d		24	105/175	60	65/240	27
B10.BAR8	b	b	b	b	b	b	d		23	65/133	49	28/161	17
B10.BAR12	b	b	b	b	b	b	d		22	100/172	58	21/191	11

*All pregnant mothers were injected with 100 mg of cortisone per kg of body weight on days 11, 12, 13 and 14 of gestation.

Table 3. Results of injecting pregnant congenic mice with testosterone.

Strain	Dose of testosterone	Total No. of Litters	Resorptions		Fetuses with cleft palate		Litters with any fetuses with cleft palate	
			No./Total	%	No./Total	%	No./Total*	%
B10	10 mg/kg	3	0/18	0	0/18	0	0/3	0
	20 "	5	3/24	13	0/21	0	0/4	0
B10.A	10 mg/kg	5	1/34	3	0/33	0	0/5	0
	20 "	14	49/130	38	3/81	4	3/12	25
B10.A(1R)	10 mg/kg	7	10/61	16	0/51	0	0/6	0
	20 "	28	94/229	41	3/135	2	3/21	14
B10.A(2R)	10 mg/kg	3	1/10	10	3/13	23	3/3	100
"	20 "	2	9/15	60	0/6	0	0/2	0
B10.BAR8	10 mg/kg	8	22/72	31	0/50	0	0/8	0
"	20 "	18	99/143	69	3/42	7	3/11	27
B10.BAR12	10 mg/kg	3	2/27	7	0/25	0	0/2	0
	20 "	7	16/68	24	0/44	0	0/6	0
B10.S	10 mg/kg	4	1/32	3	1/31	3	1/4	25
	20 "	27	105/219	48	7/112	6	6/19	32
B10.G	10 mg/kg	5	6/42	14	0/36	0	0/5	0
	20 "	8	5/69	7	7/64	11	5/8	63

* The litters in this column include only those in which there were at least three intact fetuses.

closely associated upstream of the mouse mammary tumor virus (Darbre et al., 1986; Cato et al., 1987). Thus there could be one or more target genes in the S/D interval which are associated with glucocorticoid- and androgen-responsive elements, and these elements may have been separated by some of the crossovers in our series.

We must also consider the possibility that steroid-binding proteins similar to those which map on chromosome 7 (Dlouhy et al., 1987) may be encoded by H-2-linked genes. One final possibility is that genes similar to the Preimplantation-Embryo-Development (Ped) gene may play a role. The strain distribution of Ped alleles does not correspond to our susceptibility data, but the possibility exists that similar genes map in the S/D interval. In any case, there seems to be a very interesting series of genes in the H-2 region which are involved with embryonic development, teratogenic susceptibility and steroid-responsive tissues.

ACKNOWLEDGEMENTS. We wish to thank Drs. Stimpfling and Shreffler for providing valuable strains of mice and Eva Peak, Marianne Webster and Karen Yadvish for excellent technical assistance. This work was supported by Public Health Service grant #DE07466 and a grant from the University of Pennsylvania Research Foundation.

REFERENCES

Biddle, F.G. And Fraser, F.C.: Cortisone-induced cleft palate in the mouse. A search for the genetic control of the embryonic response trait. Genetics 85: 289-302, 1977

Bonner, J.J. and Slavkin, H.C.: Cleft palate susceptibility linked to histocompatibility-2 (H-2) in the mouse. Immunogenetics 2: 213-218, 1975

Bonner, J.J. and Tyan, M.L.: Glucocorticoid-induced cleft palate genes in chromosome 17: Genetic linkage and mapping analyses. Immunogentics 20: 169-183, 1984

Cato, A.C.B., Henderson, D. and Ponta, H.: The hormone response element of the mouse mammary tumor virus DNA mediates the progestin and androgen induction of transcription in the proviral long terminal repeat region. EMBO Journal 6: 363-368, 1987

Darbre, P., Page, M. and King, R.J.B.: Androgen regulation by the long terminal repeat of mouse mammary tumor virus. Mol. Cell Biol. 6: 2847-2854, 1986

Demant, P.: Corticosteroid-induced cleft palate: Cis interaction of MHC genes and hybrid resistance. Immunogenetics 22: 183-188, 1985

Dlouhy, S.R., Taylor, B.A. and Karn, R.C.: The genes for mouse salivary androgen-binding protein (ABP) subunits alpha and gamma are located on chromsome 7. Genetics 115: 535-543, 1987

Francke, V. and Gehring, U.: Chromosome assignment of a murine glucocorticoid receptor gene (Grl-1) using intraspecies somatic cell hybrids. Cell 22: 657-664, 1980

Gasser, D.L. and Goldman, A.S.: Genetic and biochemical studies on glucocorticoid-induced cleft palate. Biochemical Actions of Hormones 10: 357-382, 1983

Gasser, D.L., Mele, L., Lees, D.D. and Goldman, A.S.: Genes in mice that affect susceptibility to cortisone-induced cleft palate are closely linked to Ir genes on chromsomes 2 and 17. Proc. Natl. Acad. Sci. USA 78: 3147-3150, 1981

Goldman, A.S. and Katsumata, M.: Murine glucocorticoid receptors: New evidence for a discrete receptor influenced by H-2. Arch. Biochem. Biophys. 249: 316-325, 1986

Gregorova, S. and Ivanyi, P.: H-2-Associated genetic differences in androgen-dependent traits. The effect of testosterone injections. Foila biologica 19: 337-345, 1973

Haseman, J.K. and Hogan, M.D.: Selection of the experimental unit in teratology studies. Teratology 12: 165-172, 1975

Ivanyi, P., Gregorova, S. and Mickova, M.: Genetic differences in thymus, lymph node, testes and vesicular gland weight among inbred mouse strains. Association with the major histocompatibility (H-2) system. Foila biologica 18: 81-97, 1972a

Ivanyi, P., Hampl, R., Starka, L. and Mickova, M.: Genetic association between H-2 gene and testosterone metabolism in mice. Nature New Biology 238: 280-281, 1972b

Klein, J., Flaherty, L., VandeBerg, J.L. and Shreffler, D.C.: H-2 haplotypes, genes, regions and antigens: First listing. Immunogenetics 6: 489-512, 1978

Lafuse, W. and Edidin, M.: Influence of the major histocompatibility complex, H-2, on liver adenylate cyclase activity and on glucagon binding to liver cell membranes. Biochemistry 19: 49-54, 1980

Litwack, G. and Rosenfield, S.A.: Liver cytosol corticosteroid binder IB, a new binding protein. J Biol. Chem. 250: 6799-6805, 1975

Meruelo, D. and Edidin, M.: The biological function of the major histocompatibility complex: Hypotheses. Contemp. Topics Immunobiol. 9: 231-253, 1980

Tyan, M.L. and Miller, K.K.: Genetic and environmental factors in cortisone-induced cleft palate. Proc. Soc. Exp. Biol. Med. 158: 618-621, 1978

Warner, C.M., Gollnick, S.O. and Goldbard, S.B.: Linkage of the Preimplantation-Embryo-Development (Ped) gene to the mouse major histocompatibility complex (MHC). Biol. Reprod. 36: 606-610, 1987

THE ROLE OF IMMUNE RESPONSE GENE AND I-A MOLECULE IN MURINE MYASTHENIA GRAVIS PATHOGENESIS

Premkumar Christadoss

Department of Pathology
University of Vermont
College of Medicine
Burlington, Vermont 05405 USA

ABSTRACT

Myasthenia gravis (MG[1]) is an autoimmune neuromuscular disease characterized by muscle weakness. Antibody mediated destruction of muscle membrane acetylcholine receptors (AChR) is the primary pathology in MG. Because of the association of HLA-DR3 gene in MG, we studied the role of class II genes and their product in the murine model of MG, experimental autoimmune MG (EAMG), which mimics human MG in all respects. Initial studies on B10 congenic and recombinants suggested the involvement of IA subregion gene on EAMG pathogenesis. Later, evaluation of IA beta chain mutant bml2 revealed that IA molecule is one of the determinants which mediates EAMG. Recent studies pointed out that L3T4+ helper T cells, which participate in T cell response to class II antigens is required for EAMG pathogenesis. Therefore, specific therapy of MG is possible by modulating the functions of DQ/CD4 determinants, which are analogous to IA/L3T4 determinants in the mouse.

INTRODUCTION

Myasthenia gravis (MG) is a neuromuscular disease in which there is a defect in the neuromuscular transmission causing weakness and fatigue of the voluntary muscles. Much evidence suggests that the defect is due to the destructive effect of antibodies to nicotinic acetylcholine receptors (AChR) leading to a diminution in the amount of muscle AChR at the post synaptic membrane (Drachman 1981, Engel 1979, Lennon 1979, Lindstrom *et al*. 1976). Although there may be definite genetic predisposition to the development of MG, the mechanism by which an autoimmune response to AChR is triggered is still not understood.

Studies in humans and mice have demonstrated a relationship between histocompatibility antigens, immune responsiveness and certain autoimmune diseases (McDevitt and Bodmar 1972). Thus, an increase in HLA-B8 antigen frequency was found among young Caucasian MG patients (Safwen-

[1]Abbreviations used in this paper

MG, myasthenia gravis; AChR, acetylcholine receptors; EAMG, experimental autoimmune myasthenia gravis; MHC, major histocompatibility complex; Mepp, miniature end plate potentials; APC, antigen presenting cells.

berg *et al*. 1978). Yoshida *et al*. reported HLA-A10 and HLA-B12 as the most frequent haplotypes found in Japanese patients with MG (Yoshida *et al*. 1977). When MG phenotypic frequencies were examined, severe symptoms of MG were less frequent in the HLA-B8$^+$, GM1$^-$ group as compared to the HLA-B8$^+$ GM1$^+$ group (Smith *et al*. 1983). In the Seventh Histocompatibility Workshop, it was shown that MG was associated with A1, B8 and DRW3 in Caucasoides. In contrast, there appeared to be a slight increase of AW19, B5, B40, and CW3 interalia among the Japanese. Thus, HLA antigen association with MG differs between various ethnic groups. A suggestion was made that there may be an association between the presence of anti-AChR antibodies and A1, B8, DRW3, and BW38. Recently, HLA-DR3 restricted AChR specific T cell lines were generated from a patient with MG (Hohlfeld *et al*. 1984). More interestingly, with a cDNA probe for a DQ beta gene (human equivalent of mouse I-A beta gene) a 15 kb Hinc II restriction fragment has been demonstrated in genomic DNA from seven of sixteen HLA-DR3 patients with MG and one of nineteen healthy DR3 controls. Thus, HLA-DQ beta-chain polymorphism was linked to MG (Bell *et al*. 1986). These findings suggest the crucial role of HLA and GM antigen in MG susceptibility. Although certain HLA antigens are associated with MG susceptibility, the immunological mechanism by which Ir genes within the HLA complex control the induction and development of MG is not known. The murine model of experimental autoimmune myasthenia gravis (EAMG) produced by AChR autoimmunity provides an opportunity to study the mechanism by which Ir genes and their product operate in the induction and maintenance of an autoimmune response to AChR. Since the Ir genes and their product, the Ia antigen in the mouse is analogous to the human Ir genes, and their product HLA-DR/DQ, studies on the role of Ir genes and Ia antigens in the induction of EAMG may serve as a model for similar studies in human MG. What follows is a review of our work in exploring the role of Ir genes and Ia antigens on the induction and development of EAMG. The possible immunotherapeutic strategies to modulate the Ir gene effect, to down regulate the autoimmune response to AChR in murine EAMG and its potential application in human MG immunotherapy is also discussed. This work was done in collaboration with Drs. C.S. David, V. Lennon, E. Lambert, C. Krco (Mayo Clinic), Jon Lindstrom (Salk Institute), R. Melvold (Chicago), N. Talal, and M. Dauphinee (San Antonio).

Influence of H-2 Linked Gene(s) in EAMG Susceptibility

In 1976, Fuchs *et al*. reported strain differences in EAMG susceptibility. However, in that study, H-2 congenic animals were not used, and the H-2 influence on EAMG pathogenesis was neither suggested nor discussed. To evaluate the role of major histocompatibility complex (MHC) gene(s) in EAMG susceptibility, we initiated studies in H-2 congenic mice. B10 congenic mice were immunized with *Torpedo* AChR in complete Freund's adjuvant and screened for: (1) *In vitro* T cell proliferative response to *Torpedo* AChR, (2) autoantibodies to mouse muscle AChR, (3) degree to which muscle AChR complexed with antibodies, (4) amplitude of miniature end plate potentials, (Mepp; an electrophysiological measurement to detect defects in neuromuscular transmission) and (5) clinical signs of EAMG.

In 1979, we (Christadoss, Lennon, Lambert, and David) reported for the first time an H-2 linkage of EAMG susceptibility (Christadoss *et al*. 1979). Following inoculation with AChR, strains bearing the H-2^b haplotype (B6, B10), demonstrated the highest AChR specific lymphocyte proliferation and serum autoantibody titer, and their muscle ACHR complexed with antibodies roughly in proportion to the amount of antibodies in their serum. Most of the mice had an electrophysiological defect and approximately 30% developed clinical muscle weakness (Table I). B10 congenic mice bearing the H-2^p haplotype (B10.P) demonstrated a lower

Table I. Features of EAMG in B6 and B10 Congenic Mice

Strain	H-2 Haplo-type	Cellular Response	Serum Auto-Ab	Muscle AChR Complexed with Ig	Muscle AChR Loss (%)	Electro-Physiological Defect	Clinical MG
B6	b	H*	H	H	>50	Yes	Yes
B6.H-2^k	k	L*	L	L	NT+	No	No
B10	b	H	H	H	>50	Yes	Yes
B10.S	s	I	I	I	NT	Yes	No
B10.P	p	L	L	L	NT	No	No
B10.BR	k	L	L	L	<20	No	No

* H - high; L - low; I - intermediate; + NT - not tested

cellular and humoral immune response to AChR, and low concentration of muscle AChR were complexed with antibody. None of the B10.P animals developed clinical muscle weakness and electrophysiological defect. The B10.S strain (H-2^s) had intermediate cellular and humoral immune response to AChR; muscle AChR were complexed with antibodies roughly in proportion to the amount of antibodies in the serum. None of the animals developed clinical muscle weakness, they showed minimal electrophysiological defect. Therefore, the difference in EAMG among B10 congenic mice expressing various H-2 haplotypes indicated that gene(s) within the H-2 complex influenced susceptibility to EAMG (Christadoss et al. 1979). Later, several other B10 and B6 congenic strains were screened for EAMG (Christadoss et al. 1981, Christadoss et al. 1985). In these studies, we also evaluated the loss of muscle AChR (an index for EAMG pathology). EAMG susceptible B6 and B10 mice lost >50%, while resistant B10.BR lost <20% total muscle AChR.

Influence of I-A Gene in EAMG Susceptibility

To map the gene within the H-2 complex which influence EAMG susceptibility, we screened several B10 recombinant strains bearing susceptible and resistant alleles within the H-2. B10.A(5R) mice bearing $K^bA^bJ^kE^kS^dD^d$ alleles demonstrated an optimal cellular and moderate humoral immune response to AChR, and good amount of muscle AChR were complexed with antibody. The mice also demonstrated a reduction in Mepp amplitude and developed clinical muscle weakness (Table II). B10.A(4R) ($K^kA^kJ^bE^bS^bD^b$) and B10.MBR ($K^bA^kJ^kE^kS^kD^q$) mice demonstrated lower cellular and humoral immune response to AChR, less than 1% muscle AChR were complexed with antibody, and had a normal Mepp amplitude. These data suggest that an immune response gene at the I-A subregion influences EAMG susceptibility (Christadoss et al. 1981a).

The Role of I-A Molecule in EAMG Pathogenesis

To determine the importance of the Ir gene product, the Ia antigens, in EAMG pathogenesis, the degree of EAMG susceptibility an I-A mutant, the B6 C-H-2^{bm12} (bm12), and its parent B6/Kh were evaluated.

Table II. Features of EAMG In B10 Recombinant Strain

Strain	I-A Allele	Cellular Response	Serum Auto-Ab	Muscle AChR Complexed With Ig	Muscle AChR Loss (%)	Electro-Physiological Defect	Clinical MG
B10.A (5R)	b	H*	I*	I	NT++	Yes	Yes
B10.A (4R)	k	L*	L	L	<20	No	No
B10.MBR	k	L	L	L	NT	No	No

* + same as Table I

In one of the experiments, three of eleven B6 mice developed clinical muscle weakness after two immunizations with AChR. None of the bm12 mice developed clinical muscle weakness. AChR specific lymphocyte proliferation of bm12 was significantly lower than that of B6. Likewise, the autoantibody titer of bm12 was significantly lower than that of B6. B6 mice lost significantly higher amount of muscle AChR (42.3%) as compared with bm12 mice (19.7%). The finding suggested that I-A beta chain mutation converted an EAMG susceptible strain into a relatively resistant strain. To confirm the above results, we performed another experiment on B6 and bm12 animals. In this experiment, we also quantitated the fraction of available muscle AChR complexed with antibody. The bm12 lymphocyte response, serum autoantibody titer, fraction of muscle AChR complexed with antibody, and percent muscle AChR loss were significantly lower than that of B6 mice. Two of nine B6 animals developed clinical muscle weakness, while none of the ten bm12 did. Although only two of the nine B6 animals developed muscle weakness, all seven animals tested lost a significant amount of muscle AChR (35-90%). This data confirmed that a mutation at the I-A beta chain prevented the development of EAMG (Christadoss et al. 1985).

The relative resistance to EAMG induction in bm12 may be due to lack of Ia8 and/or quantitative expression of Ia antigens and/or the alteration of three amino acids in the $I\text{-}A_B$ chain believed to have occurred due to a gene conversion event. This study clearly suggests that the I-A molecule is one of the crucial determinants which mediate EAMG pathogenesis.

From our studies in mice, we speculate that the HLA-DQ antigens may be one of the determinants which mediate cellular and humoral autoimmunity to AChR in human MG. Following our publication, Bell et al. (1986) with a cDNA probe for a DQ beta gene demonstrated a 15 Kb Hinc II restriction fragment in genomic DNA from seven of sixteen HLA-DR3 patients with MG and one of nineteen healthy DR3 controls. Thus, HLA-DQ beta chain polymorphism was linked to MG. These studies demonstrate the crucial role of IA/DQ beta-chain gene in EAMG/MG susceptibility. Therefore, one might hope to suppress the development of MG by modulating the function of HLA-DQ determinants.

The Effect of *In Vivo* Anti-I-A Antibody Administration in EAMG

Waldor and co-workers could suppress the cellular and humoral immune response to *Torpedo* AChR by *in vivo* administration of monoclonal anti-I-A antibodies in SJL/J and B6/J (22). But their study failed to demonstrate suppression of an autoimmune response to mouse muscle AChR or prevention of EAMG, since the data lacked the critical parameters (muscle AChR loss or EAMG decrement) to evaluate the degree of EAMG pathogenesis. Therefore, we studied the *in vivo* effect of polyclonal as well as monoclonal anti-I-A antibodies not only before the induction of EAMG, but also after established disease.

Monoclonal anti-I-A antibodies 25-9-3, directed against $I-A^b$ private specificity Ia 20, 28-16-8, directed against $I-A^b$ public specificity Ia8, 25-9-17, directed against an unidentified Ia^b specificity; and 26-8-16, directed against Ia^k determinant (specificity control) were administered intraperitoneally (i.p.) into B6 mice a day before primary and secondary immunization with AChR. Thereafter the antibody was given once a week. The experiment was terminated a month after the second immunization. The above treatment did not suppress the cellular and serum autoantibody response to AChR. Neither did they prevent the development of clinical muscle weakness or muscle AChR loss.

I-A Gene Dose Effect in EAMG Pathogenesis

Recently, we screened the F_1 hybrids between susceptible B6 and resistant B10.A(4R) strain to study the mode of EAMG inheritance. The F_1 mice demonstrated an intermediate autoantibody response, without developing clinical EAMG. The intermediate autoantibody response to AChR in the F_1 suggests that a co-dominant gene controls this response. The relative resistance to induction of EAMG in F_1 bearing the $I-A^{b/k}$ genotype suggests that for full expression of EAMG, $I-A^{b/b}$ homozygosity is required. Thus, an I-A gene dose influences the development of EAMG. (Christadoss *et al.*, submitted).

Role of L3T4 Antigen in EAMG Pathogenesis

The L3T4 antigen in the mouse, which is analogous to the human CD4 antigen expressed on helper T lymphocytes participate in T cell response to class II antigens. Because I-A gene and its product influence EAMG pathogenesis, we evaluated the role of L3T4 antigen (Christadoss and Dauphinee 1986).

Initially, we evaluated the effect of monoclonal antibody mAb GK1.5 which recognizes the L3T4 antigen on the *in vitro* AChR-specific lymphocyte proliferation response, which is under class II MHC gene control. It was found that mAb GK1.5 inhibited approximately 83-97% of B6 AChR-specific lymphocyte proliferation. The data emphasized the crucial role played by L3T4+ helper T lymphocytes on AChR-specific lymphocyte response.

Next we (Christadoss and Dauphinee 1986) tested the *in vivo* effect of mAb GK1.5 on established autoimmunity to AChR on B6 mice. The mAb GK1.5 treated mice demonstrated significantly lower mean ($9-10.5 \times 10^{-10}$ M) autoantibody responses to AChR at any given point of time when compared with saline treated controls ($26-35 \times 10^{-10}$ M). Four of eleven saline treated mice developed muscle weakness compared to none of 10 mAb GK1.5 treated mice. Moreover, the saline treated group lost muscle ACHR to a greater extent (45.5%) than the mAb GK1.5 treated group (13.9%). Thus, *in vivo* mAb GK1.5 not only suppressed the autoimmune response to AChR but also helped in preventing and delaying the development of muscle weakness characteristic of EAMG.

Eventually, the effect of *in vivo* mAb GK1.5 on established clinical EAMG was studied. Five mice bearing I-A^b genotype exhibiting muscle weakness were administered with 160 ug of mAb GK1.5 after they started to show clinical remission in all five mice. The seven control mice from the same strains, which had established clinical disease treated with saline, died within 15 days of the treatment.

The following may be the potential mechanisms by which GK1.5 induces immunological and clinical remissions of EAMG. GK1.5 can suppress anti-AChR antibody production by partial elimination of L3T4+ lymphocytes in the lymph nodes and circulation and/or preventing interaction of AChR-I-A complex with L3T4+ lymphocytes, thus blocking AChR-specific helper cell proliferation and/or generating AChR specific suppressor cells and/or factors. This finding implies that functional L3T4+ helper T cells are required to mediate EAMG pathogenesis.

Role of Non-H-2 Gene(s) in EAMG Susceptibility

Except for AKR/J (H-2^k), strains bearing H-2^k haplotype are relatively resistant to EAMG development (Christadoss *et al*. 1981). The EAMG susceptibility of AKR/J, a non-B6 or B10 background strain which expresses H-2^k, is evidence for the additional influence of non-H-2 linked background gene(s) in EAMG susceptibility. Lack of demonstrable AChR specific lymphocyte proliferation of AKR/J suggests the possibility of an alternative pathway of EAMG induction in the absence of the appropriate Ia molecule.

The data of Berman and Patrick (1980) suggests that the H-2 complex and Igl locus influence the frequency of muscular weakness after immunization with AChR in CFA. But according to our data, the B6.H-2^k strain which bears H-2^k haplotype and Ig-1^b allotype is resistant to the development of EAMG. If Igl locus influences EAMG development as suggested by Berman and Patrick (1980), then B6.H-2^k should have shown high or moderate susceptibility. Thus, our finding conflicts with the data of Berman and Patrick. Although non-H-2 genes play a role, it is still not clear where these non-H-2 gene(s) are situated. My recent study (Christadoss, submitted) suggests that C5 gene can influence EAMG pathogenesis at the efferent limb of an autoimmune response to AChR. From our studies, it is clear that the I-A gene is one of the primary gene which controls EAMG susceptibility, while non-H-2 genes (ex: T cell receptor and complement genes) and other factors may also modulate EAMG susceptibility.

Mechanism of Cellular Autoimmunity to AChR

The *in vitro* cellular immune response to AChR, which is controlled by a Mendelian dominant I-A gene (Christadoss *et al*. 1982), is dependent on Lyt1+ helper T lymphocytes, and adherent accessory cells (Christadoss *et al*. 1982, 1981b). Also, AChR specific lymphocyte proliferation is mediated by the I-A molecule since (1) monoclonal anti-I-A antibodies inhibited lymphocyte proliferation in response to AChR (Christadoss *et al*. 1983a) and (2) the I-A mutant bm12 strain gave a low response (Christadoss *et al*. 1982).

The cellular unresponsiveness to AChR in EAMG resistant strain bearing Ia^k gene product (B6.H-2^k, B10.BR) may be due to failure of AChR to associate with the Ia^k molecule, which would prevent appropriate presentation of AChR to the helper T cells or failure of helper T cells to recognize AChR in association with Ia^k. More recent studies suggest that antigen presenting cells (APC) from EAMG resistant strain B10.A(4R) are inefficient in processing and/or presenting ACHR to AChR immune F_1 T cells to provoke AChR-specific proliferation (Christadoss *et al*., submitted). Thus, the low responder APC play a crucial role in determining unresponsiveness to AChR at the cellular level. EAMG resistance of 4R may be partly due to inefficient processing and/or presentation of AChR by low responder APC to T helper cells. Since HLA-DQ antigen is analogous to murine I-A molecule, it is tempting to speculate that HLA-DQ antigen on the APC as one of the determinants which conditions responsiveness, or lack or it, to AChR in humans. The linkage of HLA-DQ polymorphism to MG further supports this notion (Bell et al. 1986).

A Hypothetical Pathway of MG Immunopathogenesis

The initial molecular event triggering autoimmunity to AChR in MG is not known. From our data in murine EAMG, we suggest that AChR is taken up by the high responder (EX: B6) APC and is processed and presented in the context of appropriate Ia antigen to T helper cells (CD4+). T helper cells recognize AChR plus Ia antigen through its receptor for AChR plus Ia. Helper T cells undergo proliferation and collaborate with AChR specific B cells that differentiate into plasma cells and generate pathogenic antibodies to AChR.

Immunotherapy for MG through Modulating the Function of Ir Gene Products and/or T Helper Cells which Participate in Response to I-A/DQ Antigens

(a) Anti-I-A Therapy Logically, one could prevent the development of EAMG by modulating the function of class II antigens, since these antigens control the induction and development of EAMG. In this regard, Waldor et al. (1983) suppressed the antibody response to Torpedo AChR by in vivo administration of anti-I-A monoclonal antibody. However, this study only demonstrated a suppression of a xenogeneic response (antibody to Torpedo AChR) but not an autoimmune response (antibody to mouse muscle AChR). Moreover, they failed to measure EAMG pathology (muscle AChR loss) or an electrophysiological defect in AChR immunized mice. Further, the effect of monoclonal anti-I-A antibody after established autoimmunity to AChR was not studied. Thus, further studies are required to conclude that in vivo therapy with monoclonal anti-I-A antibodies can prevent EAMG development. Thus, therapy of human MG with antibody to HLA-DR/DQ should not be attempted until data in the mouse is available.

(b) Anti-L3T4 Therapy More recent studies have shown that in vivo therapy with GK1.5, a monoclonal antibody that recognized a glycoprotein antigen designated L3T4 on murine helper T lymphocytes, suppressed the development of murine lupus (Wofsy et al. 1985) and experimental autoimmune encephelomyelitis (Waldor et al. 1985). The L3T4 antigen expressed on mouse T cells is analogous to CD4 antigen expressed on human helper T lymphocytes, since they both participate in the T cell response to class II MHC antigens (Dialynas et al. 1983a, Wilde et al. 1983). Our studies have established the crucial role of class II MHC gene and its product, on EAMG pathogenesis (Christadoss et al. 1981, 1985). Also, immune response to Torpedo AChR can be suppressed by either in vitro or in vivo anti-I-A mAb treatment (Christadoss et al. 1983a, Waldor et al. 1983). Moreover, the AChR specific lymphocyte response is dependent on Lyt1+ helper T lymphocytes (Christadoss et al. 1981b). Thus, the mouse EAMG model is an ideal system to study the immunotherapeutic efficacy of mAb GK1.5.

Recent studies in my laboratory has demonstrated suppression of the AChR specific lymphocyte response in vitro with mAb GK1.5. Also, mAb GK1.5, administration in vivo, suppressed the autoantibody production and muscle AChR loss and reduced the amount of muscle AChR complexed with Ig. Moreover, mAb GK1.5 therapy induced permanent clinical remission, if given after established disease (Christadoss et al. 1986).

By eliminating or suppressing the function of AChR specific helper T cells (CD4 cells which presumably trigger B cells to produce anti-AChR antibody), one could induce permanent immunological and clinical remission of MG. Thus, antibody to CD4 antigen may be utilized for MG therapy, although, the long term side effects of in vivo anti CD4 antibody have not been evaluated. Thus, therapy for MG is feasible by modulating the function of AChR responder Ia antigens and/or AChR responsive T helper cells.

REFERENCES

Bell, J., Rassenti, L., Smoot, S., Smith, K., Newby, C., Hohlfeld, R., Toyka, K., McDevitt, H., and Steinman, L.: HLA-DQ Beta-chain polymorphism linked by myasthenia gravis. Lancet. May 10:1058-1060, 1986.

Berman, P.W. and Patrick, J.: Linkage between the frequency of muscle weakness and loci that regulate immune responsiveness in murine experimental myasthenia gravis. J. Exp. Med. 152:507-520, 1980.

CHristadoss, P., Lennon, V.A., Lambert, E.H., and David, C.S.: Genetic control of experimental autoimmune myasthenia gravis in mice. In T and E Lymphocytes: Recognition and Function. F.H. Bach, B. Bonavida, E.S. Vitetta, and C.F. Fox, Eds.:249-256. Academic Press, New York, NY, 1979.

Christadoss, P., Lennon, V.A., Krco, C.J., Lambert, E.H., and David, C.S.: Genetic control of autoimmunity to acetylcholine receptors - Role of Ia molecules. Ann. NY Acad. Sci. 377:258-276, 1981a.

Christadoss, P., Lindstrom, J.M., Melvold, R.W., and Talal, N.: Mutation at I-A beta chain prevents experimental autoimmune myasthenia gravis. Immunogenetics 21:33-38, 1985a.

Christadoss, P., Lennon, V.A., and David, C.S.: Genetic control of experimental autoimmune myasthenia gravis in mice. I. Lymphocyte proliferative response to acetylcholine receptor is under H-2 linked Ir gene control. J. Immunol. 123:2540-2543, 1979.

Christadoss, P., Lennon, V.A., Krco, C.J., and David, C.S.: Genetic control of experimental autoimmune myasthenia gravis in mice. III. Ia molecules mediate cellular immune responsiveness to acetylcholine receptors. J. Immunol. 128:1141-1144, 1982.

Christadoss, P., Krco, C.J., Lennon, V.A., and David, C.S.: Genetic control of experimental autoimmune myasthenia gravis in mice. II. Lymphocyte proliferative response to acetylcholine receptor is dependent on Lyt-1 23 cells. J. Immunol. 126:1646-1647, 1981b.

Christadoss, P., Lindstrom, J., and Talal, N.: Cellular immune response to acetylcholine receptors in murine experimental autoimmune myasthenia gravis: Inhibition with monoclonal anti-I-A antibodies. Cell Immunol. 81:1-8, 1983a.

Christadoss, P. and Dauphinee, M.J.: Immunotherapy for myasthenia gravis: A murine model. J. Immunol. 136:2437-2440, 1986.

Drachman, D.: The biology of myasthenia gravis. Ann. Rev. Neurosci. 4: 195-225, 1981.

Dialynas, D.P., Quan, Z.S., Wall, K.A., Pierres, A., Quintans, J., Loken, M.R., Pierres, M., and Fitch, F.W.: Characterization of murine T cells surface molecule designated L3T4 to human Leu3/T4 molecule. J. Immunol. 131:2445-2451, 1983.

Dialynas, D.P., Wilde, D.B., Marrack, P., Pierres, A., Wall, K.A., Havram, W., Otten, G., Loken, M.R., Pierres, M., Kappler, J., and Fitch, F.W.: Characterization of the murine antigenic determinant L3T4a, recognized by monoclonal antibody GK1.5 expression of L3T4a by functional T cell clones appears to correlate primarily with class II MHC antigen reactivity. Immunol. Rev. 74:29-56, 1983.

Fuchs, S., Neiro, D., Tarrab-Hazdai, and Yarr, G.: Strain differences in the autoimmune response of mice to acetylcholine receptors. Nature 263:329-330, 1976.

Hohlfeld, R., Toyka, K.V., Heininger, K., Grosse-Wilde, H., and Kalies, I.: Autoimmune human T-lymphocytes specific for acetylcholine receptor. Nature 310:244-246, 1984.

Lennon, V.A.: Immunologic mechanisms in myasthenia gravis - a model of a receptor disease. In Clinical Immunology Update - Reviews for Physicians. E.C. Franklin, Ed. Elsevier, New York, NY, 1979.

Lindstrom, J.: Autoimmune response to acetylcholine receptors in maysthenia gravis and its animal model. Adv. Immunol. 27:1-50, 1979.

McDevitt, H.O. and Bodmer, W.F.: Histocompatibility antigen, immune responsiveness, and susceptibility to disease. Am. J. Med. 52, 1-8, 1972.

Safwenberg, J., Hammarstrom, L., Lindblom, J.B., Matell, G., Moller, E., Osterman, P.O., and Smith, S.I.E.: HLA-A, -B, -C, and -D antigens in male patients with myasthenia gravis. Tissue Antigens 12:136-142, 1978.

Smith, C.I.E., Grubb, R., and Hammarstrom, L.: GM allotypes in Swedish myasthenia gravis patients. J. Immunogenetics 10:1-9.

Waldor, M.K., Hardy, R.R., Hayakawa, K., Steinman, L., Herzenberg, L.A., and Herzenberg, L.A.: Proc. Natl. Acad. Sci. 81:2855-2858, 1984.

Waldor, M.K., Sriram, S., McDevitt, H.D., and Steinman, L.: In vivo therapy with monoclonal anti-Ia antibody suppress immune response to acetylcholine receptors. Proc. Natl. Acad. Sci. 80:2713-2717, 1983.

Waldor, M.K., Sriram, S., Hardy, R., Herzenberg, L.A., Lanier, L., Linn, M., and Steinman, L.: Reversal of experimental allergic encephalomyelitis with monoclonal antibody to a T-cell subset marker. Science 227:415-417, 1985.

Wilde, D.B., Marrack, P., Kappler, J., Dialynas, D.P., and Fitch, F.W.: Evidence implicating L3T4 in class II MHC antigen reactivity: Monoclonal antibody GK1.5 (anti-L3T4a) blocks class II MHC antigen-specific proliferation, release of lymphokines and binding by cloned murine helper T lymphocyte lines. J. Immunol. 131: 2178-2183, 1983.

Wofsy, D. and Seaman, W.E.: Successful treatment of autoimmunity in NZB/NZW F_1 mice with monoclonal antibody to L3T4. J. Exp. Med. 161:378-391, 1985.

Yoshida, I., Isuchtya, M., Ono, A., Yoshimatus, H., Satoyoski, E., and Tsuji, K.: HLA antigens and myasthenia gravis in Japan. J. Neurol. Sci. 32:195-201, 1977.

H-2 GENES IN TMEV-INDUCED DEMYELINATION, A MODEL FOR MULTIPLE SCLEROSIS

Roger W. Melvold [1], Diane M. Jokinen [1], Stephen D. Miller [1], Mauro C. Dal Canto [2,3] and Howard L. Lipton [3]

[1] Department of Microbiology-Immunology and the Cancer Center, [2] Department of Pathology and [3] Department of Neurology, Northwestern University Medical and Dental Schools, 303 East Chicago Avenue, Chicago IL 60611.

ABSTRACT

Theiler's murine encephalomyelitis virus (TMEV) is a natural enteric pathogen of mice which, upon entry into the CNS, sets up a persistent infection that, in some strains of mice, results in an immunologically-mediated, progressive chronic demyelinating disease with histopathological and clinical similarities to human multiple sclerosis. Although the CNS virus infection persists in all strains, only some go on to develop the demyelinating disease. This susceptibility has a strong genetic basis which involves both H-2 and non-H-2 loci. Comparisons involving different combinations of susceptible and resistant strains indicate the involvement of numerous loci, not all of which are apparent in any given comparison. The differences between the susceptible DBA/2J and resistant C57BL/6 and C57BL/10 strains are primarily dependent upon H-2 genotype and at least one non-H-2 gene, with resistance being dominant to susceptibility. The D region of H-2 has a strong influence ($\underline{H\text{-}2^b}$ associated with resistance and $\underline{H\text{-}2^d}$ with susceptibility) and substitution, in appropriate hybrids, of single gene mutations of the $\underline{H\text{-}2D^b}$ gene abrogates resistance. This may mean that resistance is, in fact, an active process mediated, for example, by specific suppression.

In DBA/2, the $\underline{H\text{-}2^d}$ haplotype is associated with susceptibility, unlike the H-2 identical, but resistant, BALB/c strain. The resistance associated with $\underline{H\text{-}2^b}$ is not absolute and can, in segregating populations be overcome by the non-H-2 genome. It is likely that critical combinations of genes, e.g. those encoding H-2 and the T cell receptor chains, are the determining factors in disease susceptibility or resistance.

INTRODUCTION

Theiler's murine encephalomyelitis virus (TMEV), a member of the picornavirus group, is a natural enteric pathogen of wild and laboratory mice which, when it gains access to the central nervous system (CNS), causes a biphasic disease in mice (Theiler 1937, Daniels et al. 1940, Theiler and Gard 1940, Lipton 1975, Lehrich et al. 1976). An early, polio-like phase, caused by the lytic activity virus infecting neurons, results in flaccid paralysis similar to human poliomyelitis (Theiler 1937, Lipton 1975). Mice which survive the early disease phase later develop a chronic, progressive CNS demyelinating disease, similar to human multiple sclerosis (MS), which is characterized clinically by the development of motor difficulty leading to an abnormal waddling gait, limb spasms and incontinence (Lipton 1975, Lehrich et al. 1976, Lipton and Dal Canto 1976, Dal Canto & Lipton 1976).

In the late stage disease, the virus persists permanently in the CNS, particularly the spinal cord, and the demyelination is believed to result from damage inflicted by the immune system acting against the virus (Lipton and Dal Canto 1979, Roos et al. 1982, Clatch et al. 1985, 1986). Such studies have been aided by the development of a tissue culture adapted strain of TMEV, BeAn 8386, which does not cause the early polio-like disease, but efficiently causes the late MS-like disease. Histopathology of the affected CNS tissues shows demyelination and substantial mononuclear cell infiltration. The immune responses causing the damage are believed to be cellular in nature, with some investigators having evidence of DTH involvement, while others propose CTL activity as the destructive agent (Clatch et al. 1985, 1986, Lipton et al. 1986, Rodriguez et al. 1986b, Clatch et al. 1987). Other immune parameters, such as titer of anti-viral antibody and virus-specific T cell proliferative response, appear to have no correlation with disease incidence.

The susceptibility or resistance to development of the late phase demyelinating disease clearly has a genetic component (Lipton and Dal Canto 1979, Lipton and Melvold 1984). Some inbred strains (such as SJL, SWR, DBA/1, DBA/2 and PL) are highly susceptible while others (such as C57BL/6, C57BL/10, C57L, C57BR and BALB/c) are resistant. In analyses of hybrids between susceptible and resistant strains, susceptibility is sometimes dominant (e.g., hybrids between DBA/2 and C57BL/6) and sometimes recessive (e.g., hybrids between SWR and C57L). The H-2 complex often contributes to this genetic predisposition (Lipton and Melvold 1984, Clatch et al. 1985, Rodriguez and David 1985, Lipton et al. 1986, Rodriguez et al. 1986a & b, Clatch et al. 1986, 1987), but not always as in the cases of resistant BALB/c ($\underline{H\text{-}2^d}$) vs. susceptible SJL ($\underline{H\text{-}2^s}$) (Melvold et al. 1987) and resistant BALB/c vs. susceptible DBA/2 (both of which are $H\text{-}2^d$). Non-H-2 genes, however, also are important as demonstrated by studies utilizing both congenic and segregating populations derived from crosses between susceptible and resistant strains (Lipton and Melvold 1984, Melvold et al. 1987). The only involved non-H-2 locus which has thus far been mapped appears to be on chromosome 6, near the constant region gene of the T cell receptor beta chain (Melvold et al. 1987).

Comparisons between different combinations of resistant and susceptible strains implicate different sets of loci as having primary roles in the differential susceptibility, and numerous strain comparisons will be required for a good understanding of the genetic factors involved. In this report, we analyze the relevant genetic differences between the susceptible DBA/2 strains and the resistant C57BL/6 and C57BL/10 strains.

MATERIALS AND METHODS

Animals and inoculations

All of the mice used were bred in our facility at Northwestern University. The strains used and their genotypes are presented in Table 1. The mice were caged and maintained in accordance with AALAS standards and received standard mouse chow and acidified water ad libidum. Mice, at 4-6 weeks of age, were anesthetized with methoxyfluorane and inoculated in the right cerebral hemisphere with 1.3×10^6 PFU of BeAn 8386 virus. All animals were examined daily for the first three weeks, and weekly thereafter, for 105-120 days for development of clinical neurologic symptoms, particularly the chronic gait abnormality caused by demyelination.

Virus and cells

BeAn 8386 was isolated from a feral mouse in Belem, Brazil in 1957 and was later classified as a TMEV by complement fixation serology. After plaque purification and amplification of the titer by several passages in BHK-21 cells, two sequential working stocks were prepared, A20 and 173J which had titers of 1.3×10^6 and 2.6×10^6 PFU/ml, respectively.

Histology

Mice were anesthetized and sacrificed by perfusion through the left ventricle with 10 ml of PBS (pH 7.3), followed by 100 ml of chilled 3% glutaraldehyde in phosphate buffer (pH 7.3). Spinal cords were dissected from the vertebral canal, sectioned at approximately 1 mm intervals, post-fixed in 1% osmic acid for 1 hr and processed for Epon embedding. Fifteen 1 um thick sections from each spinal cord were stained with toluidine blue and examined by light microscopy.

H-2 typing

H-2 genotypes of backcross and F2 progeny were determined by standard complement-mediated microcytoxicity tests using vital dye exclusion as described previously (Lipton and Melvold 1984). Antisera used for typing of the H-2 haplotypes in segregating crosses were F-33 (K^b), Anti-Ia 11.16 (K^d), B22-249R1 (D^b) and 3-25.2 (D^d). F-33 and Anti-Ia 11.16 were obtained from the NIH Antisera Bank, B22-249R1 and 3.25.2 were gifts from Drs. Stanley Nathenson and Jeffrey Frelinger, respectively.

Determination of T cell proliferative responses and antiviral antibody titers

T cell proliferation was determined as previously described (Clatch et al. 1985). Total serum antibodies against the BeAn 8386 strain of TMEV were quantified through an indirect ELISA assay as described by Clatch et al. (1985).

Measurement of delayed type hypersensitivity (DTH)

At appropriate times (90-120 days) after intracerebral inoculation of TMEV, the ears of infected and control uninfected (negative control) mice were measured with a Mitutoya Model 7326 micrometer. Immediately thereafter, the dorsal side of each ear received a dermal injection of purified BeAn 8386 virus (5 ug of virus in 10 ul of PBS, pH 7.2) to elicit TMEV-specific DTH responses. Twenty-four hours after challenge, each ear was again measured to determine the increase in thickness (swelling) due to mononuclear cell infiltration. The increases in thickness were expressed in units of 10^{-4} inches.

Statistics

Statistical comparisons between disease incidences in segregating populations (backcross and F2) were made using the standard 2 x 2 test for independence. Statistical analysis of viral titers, viral antibody titers, and DTH responses employed the Student t-test and one-way analysis of variance.

RESULTS

Genetics of susceptibility

The susceptibility of the DBA/2 strain is dependent upon both H-2 and non-H-2 genes (Table 1). A single copy of the "susceptible" H-2 and non-H-2 genomes is insufficient, in that (B6 x D2)F1 hybrids are fully resistant. Thus, resistance is dominant to susceptibility in this comparison. However, homozygosity for $H\text{-}2^{d}$ in the presence of at least one copy of the "susceptible" non-H-2 genome does lead to disease, as seen in the (B10.D2 x D2)F1 hybrids. The reverse combination, heterozygosity for H-2 and homozygosity for the DBA/2 background, was not possible with the available strains. This data could be interpreted either to mean that (a) more than half of the genome (H-2 and non-H-2) must derive from the susceptible strain in order to permit disease development, or that (b) some particular combination(s) of H-2 and non-H-2 genes from the resistant B6 genome will prevent disease.

Previous reports on the role of H-2 genes in susceptibility to TMEV-induced demyelinating disease, where an effect of H-2 is evident, have implicated the D region (Rodriguez et al. 1986, Clatch et al. 1986). In preliminary evaluations of the role of specific H-2 loci in the DBA/2 - C57BL/6 combination, we utilized H-2 mutants. Two mutations of the $H\text{-}2D^{b}$ gene ($H\text{-}2^{bm13}$ and $H\text{-}2^{bm14}$) and one involving the I region ($H\text{-}2^{bm12}$), all on the C57BL/6 background, were used (no such mutations are available on the DBA/2 strain

Table 1. Involvement of both H-2 and non-H-2 genes in differential susceptibilities of C57BL/10, C57BL/6 AND DBA/2 mice to TMEV-induced demyelinating disease.

STRAIN	GENOME H-2	GENOME NON-H-2	% AFFECTED	N
C57BL/6 (B6)	b	B6	0	20
C57BL/10 (B10)	b	B10	0	20
DBA/2J (D2)	d	D2	90	20
B10.D2	d	B10	0	5
(B6 x D2)F1	b/d	B6/D2	0	22
(B10 x D2)F1	b/d	B10/D2	0	5
(B10.D2 x D2)F1	d	B10/D2	75	12
B6.C-$\underline{H-2}^{bm13}$ (bm13)[a]	bm13	B6	0	5
(bm13 x D2)F1	bm13/d	B6/D2	100	8
B6.C-$\underline{H-2}^{bm14}$ (bm14)[a]	bm14	B6	0	5
(bm14 x D2)F1	bm14/d	B6/D2	63	11

[a] These strains carry single gene mutations of H-D^{b}.

background). While the I region mutation (bm12) had no effect (data not shown), the D locus mutations (bm13 and bm14), when substituted for the parental B6 gene in hybrids with DBA/2, resulted in susceptible rather than resistant animals (Table 1). Thus, minor changes in a gene ($\underline{H-2D^{b}}$) associated with resistance (as opposed to substitution with a comparable allele from a susceptible strain) were sufficient to produce susceptibility. This suggests, that resistance may be an active component, rather than merely the absence of sufficient "susceptibility" genes. Other H-2 recombinant and mutant analyses are in progress.

Susceptibility in segregating populations. Data from the congenic and mutant studies suggested that, whatever non-H-2 genes are present, the presence of the $\underline{H-2^{b}}$ haplotype conferred resistance to TMEV-induced demyelinating disease. To try to confirm this, as well as to estimate the number of relevant non-H-2 genes, we examined disease susceptibility in backcrosses of B6D2 hybrids to the susceptible (recessive phenotype) D2 parent and in F2 hybrids (Table 2). The backcross segregation data (33/39 $\underline{H-2^{d}}$ homozygotes and 10/25 $\underline{H-2^{b}}/\underline{H-2^{d}}$ heterozygotes) is compatible with a small number (one or a few) of non-H-2 loci being involved. It is of

Table 2. Susceptibility (affected/total) to TMEV-induced Demyelinating Disease in Populations Segregating at H-2

GENOTYPE	H-2 GENOTYPE $H\text{-}2^b/H\text{-}2^b$	$H\text{-}2^b/H\text{-}2^d$	$H\text{-}2^d/H\text{-}2^d$	N
B6	0%	--	--	20
D2	--	--	90%	20
B6D2F1	--	0%	--	22
B6D2F1 x D2	--	29%	85%	74
B6D2F2	0%	16%	54%	47

Table 3. DTH Responsiveness Against TMEV in Comparisons of B6 and D2 Using Congenic and Mutant Strains

STRAIN	INFECTED	NAIVE	DTH	P
<u>D2</u>[a]	21.0 ± 0.9	4.2 ± 0.9	16.8	< 0.001
B6	6.5 ± 1.6	2.4 ± 0.1	4.1	n.s.
B10	9.1 ± 1.2	4.9 ± 4.5	4.2	n.s.
(B6 x D2)F1	9.1 ± 1.2	4.8 ± 1.0	4.3	n.s.
(B10 x D2)F1	8.0 ± 2.5	8.7 ± 2.3	-0.7	n.s.
B10.D2	5.2 ± 1.3	5.0 ± 2.8	0.2	n.s.
<u>(B10.D2 x D2)F1</u>	17.9 ± 2.2	3.3 ± 1.1	14.6	< 0.01
bm13	10.1 ± 1.1	9.5 ± 5.0	0.6	n.s.
<u>(bm13 x D2)F1</u>	20.8 ± 1.4	3.2 ± 3.5	17.6	< 0.01
bm14	9.2 ± 2.5	8.7 ± 7.1	0.5	n.s.
<u>(bm14 x D2)F1</u>	27.7 ± 1.9	6.5 ± 2.1	21.2	< 0.01

[a] Susceptible genotypes are underlined.

interest that some H-2^b/H-2^d heterozygotes clearly developed the disease. Thus a single copy of the H-2^b haplotype, by itself, cannot confer absolute resistance and can be "overridden", presumably by the presence of sufficient other relevant genes from the susceptible genome.

Correlation of particular immune responses with disease

In the inbred and congenic animals, the ability to mount significant TMEV-specific DTH responses correlated perfectly (Table 3) with susceptibility. Other parameters, such as specific anti-TMEV antibodies and TMEV-specific splenic T cell proliferative responses, showed no correlation with development of disease (data not shown).

CNS viral titer

The titer of TMEV recovered appeared to be generally higher among diseased animals than normal animals, but the correlation was not perfect (Table 4). For example, titers were not significantly different between resistant B6.C-$H\text{-}2^{bm14}$ and susceptible (bm14 x D2)F1 animals.

Table 4. CNS viral titer (log_{10}) in susceptible and resistant genotypes

SUSCEPTIBLE GENOTYPE	MEAN	SEM [a]	RESISTANT GENOTYPE	MEAN	SEM
D2	3.24	0.10	B6	2.14	0.73
(B10.D2 X D2)F1	2.95	0.23	B10	2.24	0.44
(bm13 x D2)F1	2.76	0.37	(B6 x D2)F1	1.5	0.20
(bm14 x D2)F1	2.41	0.31	(B10 x D2)F1	1.97	0.30
			B10.D2	1.85	0.45
			bm13	2.33	0.44
			bm14	2.17	0.46
B6D2F1 x D2			B6D2F1 x D2		
$H\text{-}2^b/H\text{-}2^d$	3.36	0.21	$H\text{-}2^b/H\text{-}2^d$	1.68	0.30
$H\text{-}2^d/H\text{-}2^d$	3.48	0.11	$H\text{-}2^d/H\text{-}2^d$	1.97	0.60

[a] Standard error of the mean

Histopathology

Examination of 1 um think sections from infected DBA/2

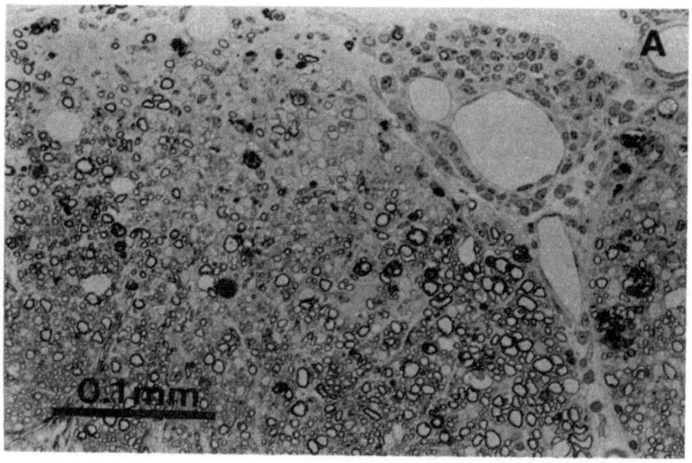

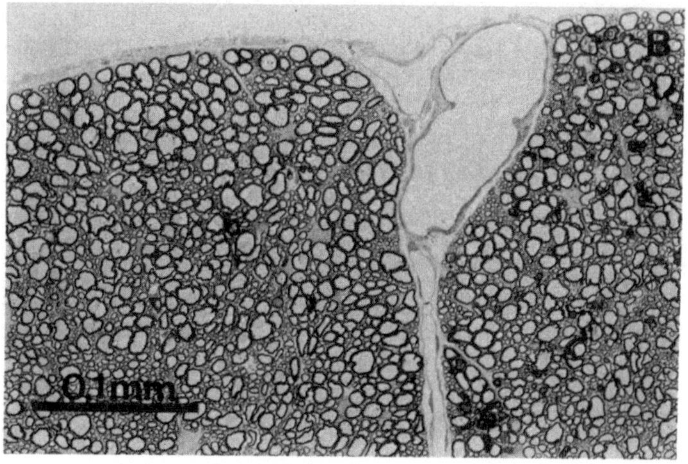

Figure 1. CNS histopathology of demyelinating disease after inoculation with BeAn 8386 strain of TMEV

A. Typical section from spinal cord of susceptible strain showing meningeal inflammatory mononuclear cell infiltration and primary demyelination in the adjacent CNS parenchyma at 120 days post-inoculation. One um thick Epon embedded section stained with toluidine blue.

B. Typical section from spinal cord of resistant strain showing no pathological changes at 120 days post-inoculation. One um thick Epon embedded section stained with toluidine blue.

animals showed numerous foci of meningeal and parenchymal inflammation (Figure 1A). Inflammatory cells consisted of lymphocytes, plasma cells and macrophages and were particularly numerous around venules. In adjacent areas of the spinal cord, particularly in the anterior and lateral columns, there was extensive destruction of myelin sheaths around axons which showed otherwise normal morphology. Demyelinated areas were rather well demarcated from the surrounding unaffected white matter. The macrophages and large numbers of mononuclear cells in the lesions were consistent with persistent activity of demyelinating disease approximately 4 months after infection. The lesions were similar in number and severity with those observed in the "classical" susceptible strain, SJL. Figure 1B shows a comparably treated section from an infected resistant strain.

DISCUSSION

Development of TMEV-induced demyelinating disease in mice has many characteristics which make it an excellent model for human multiple sclerosis (Lipton et al. 1986, Rodriguez et al. 1986b). Multiple sclerosis is one of many diseases which show associations with particular HLA genes and a genetic component in risk of MS is also apparent from family and twin studies (Nathanson and Miller 1978, Spielman and Nathanson 1982, Waksman and Reynolds 1984, Lipton et al. 1986). It is hoped that identification and study of relevant genes in the mouse model may provide clues as to the roles of comparable human genes.

In the comparisons of susceptible DBA/2 and resistant C57BL/6, C57BL/10 mice, the major histocompatibility complex is clearly important. As in other reports, the $\underline{H\text{-}2^{b}}$ haplotype is associated with resistance, but the $\underline{H\text{-}2^{d}}$ haplotype here, unlike previous reports (Lipton an Melvold 1984, Rodriguez and David 1985, Clatch et al. 1985, Rodriguez et al. 1986a & b, Melvold et al. 1987), is associated with susceptibility when carried in the context of the DBA/2 genome.

As in other analyses, the class I gene(s) of the D region of the H-2 complex appears to be important. Introduction of single gene mutations, differing from the parental molecule by only one or a few amino acids, into appropriate hybrids was sufficient for conversion from resistance to susceptibility. Rodriguez et al. (1986a) also found that the $H\text{-}2^{dm1}$ mutation, involving a deletion of a portion of the D molecule, also altered resistance. In that case, however, the mutation involved the $\underline{H\text{-}2^{d}}$ haplotype in a resistant strain (B10.D2). The $\underline{H\text{-}2^{d}}$ haplotype is variable, associated with resistance in some strains (BALB/c) and susceptibility in others (DBA/2). The $\underline{H\text{-}2^{b}}$ haplotype is consistently associated with resistant strains (B6, B10, C57L, etc.). The abrogation of resistance to TMEV-induced demyelinating disease by substitution of one or a few amino acids in the D molecule, rather than the substitution of alleles from susceptible strains, suggests that resistance may be due to an active process, such as immune suppression, rather than merely resulting from the lack of enough "susceptibility" genes. Similar conclusions were drawn from the results involving the $H\text{-}2^{dm1}$ deletion mutant (Rodriguez et al. 1986a).

It is also clear that the H-2 genotype, while important, is not sufficient in and of itself, to determine susceptibility. The characterization of the non-H-2 genes, and the ways in which they interact with H-2, will also be important to defining the genetic components of disease susceptibility. We previously have reported that, in the comparison of susceptible SJL/J and resistant BALB/c mice, the H-2 complex has little or no effect on disease incidence, but that a gene(s) mapped to chromosome 6, very near the constant region gene of the T cell receptor beta chain, played a major role. It may be that particular combinations of T cell receptor genotypes and MHC genotypes are critical, and this possibility is currently being tested. In addition, relevant non-MHC genes are currently being studied in a variety of other susceptible-resistant strain combinations, utilizing recombinant inbred strains.

LITERATURE CITED

Clatch, R.J., Melvold, R.W., Miller, S.D. and Lipton, H.L., 1985, Theiler's murine encephalomyelitis virus (TMEV)-induced demyelinating disease in mice is influenced by the H-2D region: correlation with TMEV-specific delayed-type hypersensitivity, J. Immunol. 135:1408.

Clatch, R.L., Lipton, H.L. and Miller, S.D., 1986, Characterization of Theiler's murine encephalomyelitis virus (TMEV)-specific delayed type hypersensitivity responses in TMEV-induced demyelinating disease: correlation with clinical signs, J. Immunol. 136:920.

Clatch, R.J., Melvold, R.W., Dal Canto, M.C., Miller, S.D. and Lipton, H.L., 1987, The Theiler's murine encephalomyelitis virus (TMEV) model for multiple sclerosis shows a strong influence of the murine equivalents of HLA-A, -B and -C, J. Neuroimmunol.: (in press).

Dal Canto, M.C. and Lipton, H.L., 1976, Primary demyelination in Theiler's virus infection, Lab. Invest. 33:626.

Daniels, J.B., Pappenheimer, A.M. and Richardson, S., 1952, Observations on encephalomyelitis of mice (DA strain), J. Exp. Med. 96:517.

Lehrich, J.R., Arnason, B.G. and Hochberg, F.,1976, Demyelinative myelopathy in mice induced by the DA virus, J. Neurol. Sci. 29:149.

Lipton, H.L., 1975, Theiler's virus infection in mice: an unusual biphasic disease process leading to demyelination, Infect. Immun. 11:1147.

Lipton, H.L. and Dal Canto, M.C., 1976, Chronic neurologic disease in Theiler's virus infection of SJL/J mice, J. Neurol. Sci. 30:201.

Lipton, H.L. and Dal Canto, M.C., 1976, Theiler's virus-induced demyelination: prevention by immunosuppression, Science 192:62.

Lipton, H.L. and Dal Canto, M. C., 1979, Susceptibility of inbred mice to chronic central nervous system infection by Theiler's murine encephalomyelitis virus, Infect. Immun. 26:369.

Lipton, H.L. and Melvold, R.W., 1984, Genetic analysis of susceptibility to Theiler's virus induced demyelinating disease in mice, J. Immunol. 132:1821.

Lipton, H.L., Miller, S., Melvold, R., and Fujinami, R.S.,1986, Theiler's murine encephalomyelitis virus (TMEV) infection in mice as a model for multiple sclerosis, in: "Concepts in Viral Pathogenesis II", A.L. Notkins and M.B.A. Oldstone, eds., Springer-Verlag, New York.

Melvold, R.W. Jokinen, D.M., Knobler, R.L. and Lipton, H.L., 1987, Variations in genetic control of susceptibility to Theiler's murine encephalomyelitis virus (TMEV)-induced demyelinating disease. I. Differences between susceptible SJL/J and resistant BALB/c strains map near the T cell B-chain constant gene on chromosome 6, J. Immunol. 138:1429.

Nathanson, N. and Miller, A., 1978, Epidemiology of multiple sclerosis: critique of evidence for a viral etiology, Am. J. Epidem. 107:451.

Rodriguez, M., Pease, L.R. and David, C.S., 1986, Immune mediated injury of virus-infected oligodendrocytes, Immunol. Today 7:359.

Rodriguez, M. and David, C.S., 1985, Demyelination induced by Theiler's virus: influence of the H-2 complex, J. Immunol. 135:2145.

Rodriguez, M., Leibowitz, J. and David, C.S., 1986, Susceptibility to Theiler's virus-induced demyelination. Mapping of the gene within the H-2 region, J. Exp. Med. 163:620.

Roos, R.P., Fireston, S., Wollman, R., Variakojis, D. and Arnason, B.G.W., 1982, The effect of short-term and chronic immunosuppression on Theiler's virus demyelination, J. Neuroimmunol. 2:223.

Spielman, R.S. and Nathanson, N., 1982, The genetics of susceptibility to multiple sclerosis, Epidemiol. Rev. 4:45.

Theiler, M., 1937, Spontaneous encephalomyelitis of mice, a new virus disease, J. Exp. Med. 65:705.

Theiler, M. and Gard, S., 1940, Encephalomyelitis of mice. III. Epidemiology, J. Exp. Med. 72:79.

Waksman, B.H. and Reynolds, W.E., 1984, Multiple sclerosis as a disease of immune regulation, Proc. Soc. Exp. Biol. Med. 175:282.

THE CONTRIBUTION OF MHC GENE PRODUCTS TO DEMYELINATION BY THEILER'S VIRUS

Moses Rodriguez[*,+], Chella S. David[+] and Larry R. Pease[+]

Department of Neurology[*] and the Department of Immunology[+]

Mayo Clinic and Mayo Foundation, Rochester, MN 55905

INTRODUCTION

Infection with Theiler's murine encephalomyelitis virus (TMEV) provides an opportunity to study viral persistence and neuropathologic abnormalities in the central nervous system. This picornavirus was first recovered by Max Theiler in 1934 from a mouse suffering from spontaneous flaccid paralysis of the hind legs (Theiler, 1934). The virus is similar in size, virulence, buoyant density and viral structural proteins to poliovirus (Lorch et al., 1981). Early studies showed that intracerebral or intranasal inoculation of the virus into neonatal or weanling mice resulted in spinal cord lesions characterized by neuronal necrosis, especially of anterior horn cells, which is very similar to human poliomyelitis. This virus received little attention until Daniels et al. (1952) described an isolate of TMEV, subsequently designated DA strain, which had the propensity to induce in young adult mice primary demyelination in the central nervous system. The pathology in the spinal cord was characterized by an intense inflammatory infiltrate associated with primary destruction of myelin sheaths with relative preservation of axons (Dal Canto and Lipton, 1975; Lehrich et al., 1976).

The model has been particularly attractive because the viral induced demyelination in young adult mice has many similarities to the pathology in multiple sclerosis (Dal Canto and Lipton, 1975; Rodriguez et al., 1983). Since epidemiolgic, virologic, and immunologic data suggest that multiple sclerosis results from an immune-mediated response triggered by virus, TMEV has received wide attention as the single best model of the human disease (Dal Canto and Rabinowitz, 1982). The model exhibits the following advantages: 1) pathologic abnormalities (demyelination) limited to the CNS, 2) naturally occurring viral persistence, 3) infection in the mouse (a species in which there is vast immunologic, virologic, and genetic information), 4) infection by a family of viruses (picornaviridae) in which there is detailed information on molecular biology, and 5) immune system playing a role in myelin destruction.

PATHOLOGY AND BIOLOGY OF TMEV INFECTION

Intracerebral inoculation of TMEV into neonatal mice produces flaccid paralysis or death in the majority of animals within 7-10 days after infection (Rodriguez et al., 1983a). There is severe encephalitis characterized by neuronal necrosis, inflammatory infiltrates including lymphocytes and polymorphonuclear cells, and a diffuse spongy state of the white matter. Electron microscopy of infected neurons reveals intra-cytoplasmic inclusions containing numerous 25-29 nm in diameter virion particles at times clustered in paracrystalline arrays (Fig. 1a). Viral replication occurs primarily in neurons but in addition astrocytes and oligodendrocytes are infected. In the neonate, virus antigen is found throughout the cerebral cortex, basal ganglia, thalamus, hypothalamus and anterior horn cells of the spinal cord.

In contrast, infection of young adult mice (4 to 6 weeks of age) results in an unusual biphasic disease (Lehrich et al., 1976; Lipton, 1975). Depending on the strain of TMEV, there is an acute disease characterized by viral replication in neurons of the brain and spinal cord which may be associated with paralysis within the first two weeks of infection. This is then followed by a late demyelinating phase. Two relatively distinct groups of TMEV viruses have been identified (Lorch et al., 1981). The more virulent GDVII and FA brain-adapted Theiler's strains result in flaccid paralysis of the hind limbs followed by death in many animals (Lorch et al., 1981). In contrast, intracerebral injection of tissue culture adapted strains (DA, WW, YALE and BeAN) results in minimal early neuronal disease but more prominent chronic demyelinating disease (Lipton and Dal Canto, 1979). Electron microscopy reveals infiltrates of mononuclear cells in intimate contact with demyelinated axons (Fig. 1b,c). Active ongoing demyelination is present for as long as one year after infection which roughly parallels the persistence of virus in the CNS. Ultrastructural immunoperoxidase studies (Dal Canto and Lipton, 1982; Rodriguez et al., 1983) as well as _in situ_ hybridization (Cash et al., 1985; Chamorro et al., 1986) using cDNA from viral RNA have demonstrated chronic infection of macrophages, astrocytes and oligodendrocytes (the myelin-producing cell) during the demyelinating phase. Attempts to visualize the virus by electron microscopy during the late phase have been unsuccessful because single picorna-virions resemble host ribosomes in size and structure.

CRITICAL ROLE OF CLASS I MHC GENE PRODUCTS

One of the most interesting aspects of the pathogenesis of demyelination induced by TMEV has been the demonstration of genetic control to resistance/susceptibility that maps to the major histocompatibility complex (MHC). Initial studies of Lipton and Dal Canto (1979a) demonstrated a wide range of susceptibility of inbred strains to chronic disease which was most severe in SJL, intermediate in CBA and C3H, and least in C57BL/6 mice. These early investigations were performed with a brain-derived strain of DA that produced both acute poliomyelitis followed by chronic demyelinating disease. Subsequent investigations by Lipton and Melvold (1984) using a tissue culture adapted strain (BeAN 8386) examined various crosses between susceptible SJL(H-2^s) and resistant C57BL6(H-2^b). Six of 39 F_1 hybrid progeny developed clinical disease. Seventy-three percent of (B6 x SJL)F_1 x SJL developed clinical signs while only 2 percent of (B6 x SJL)F_1 x B6 developed disease. The presence of clinical signs correlated with high titers of virus from the CNS.

To further explore the role of H-2 on demyelination, we performed a series of ultrastructural morphologic studies in nonrecombinant H-2 congeneic strains of mice on common background genes expressing independent haplotypes (Rodriguez and David, 1985). Mice with _s_, _f_, _p_, _r_, _v_ or _q_ haplotypes on B10 background showed demyelination and perivascular inflammation while mice with _b_, _k_, or _d_ haplotypes showed no pathologic abnormalities. A follow-up study of TMEV infection of mouse strains with

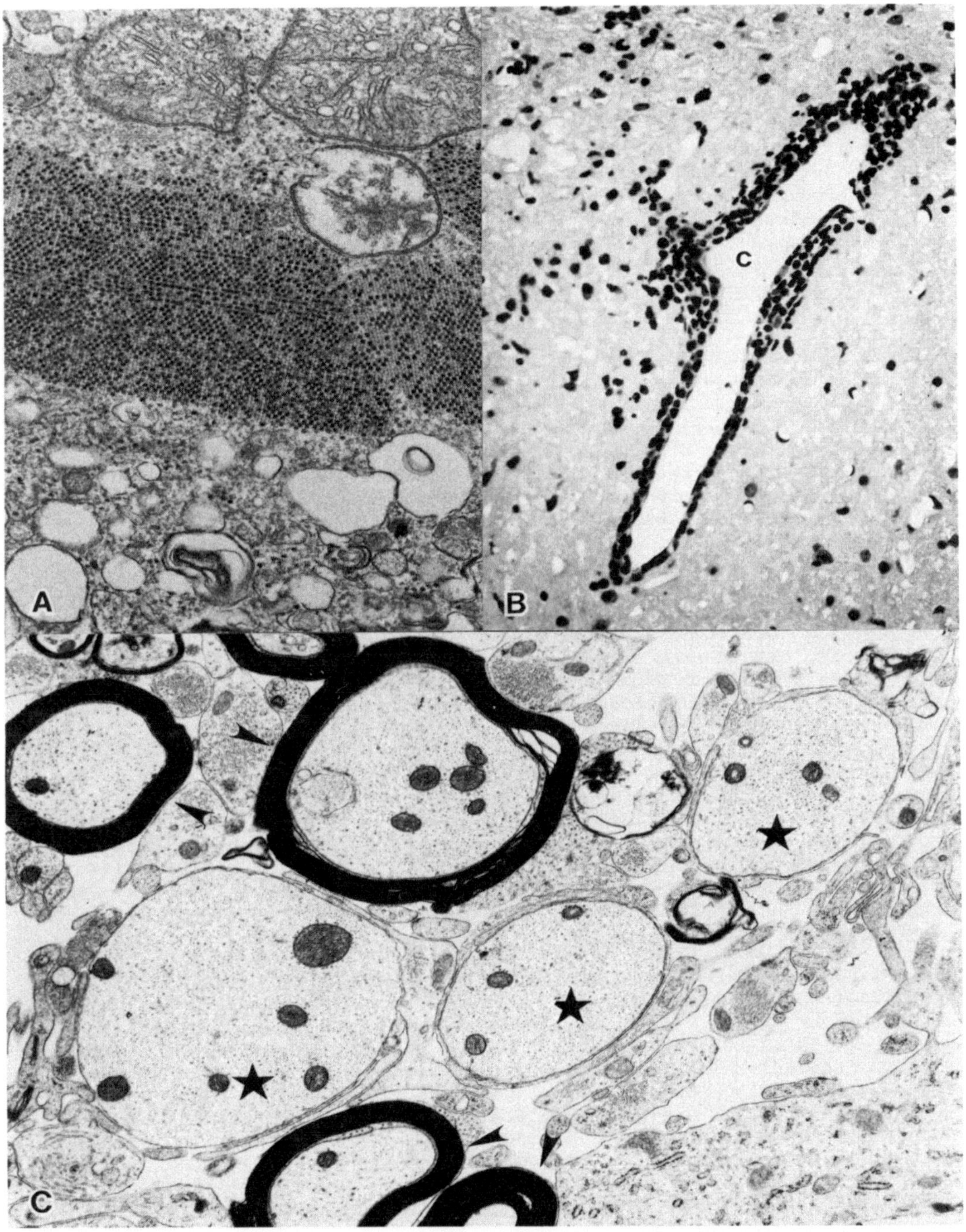

Fig. 1. Pathologic abnormalities in the central nervous system produced by Theiler's virus. A) Viral particles in the cytoplasm of an infected neuron from the spinal cord of a 6-day-old SJL mouse infected at birth with the DA strain of TMEV. Note that the virions tend to form a paracrystalline array. Empty capsomeres are seen intermingled with fully formed virus particles. The bottom of the electron micrograph shows vacuolar degeneration in the cytoplasm of this neuron which is a frequent finding during neonatal

(continued)

infection with TMEV (ultra-thin section stained with uranyl acetate and lead citrate). B) Mononuclear inflammatory cells surrounding a capillary (c) in the spinal cord white matter of an SJL/J mouse infected with virus at 4 weeks of age and examined 45 days following infection. Note that inflammatory cells are also invading the substance of white matter and are associated with areas of myelin damage, (glycol methacrylate section stained with modified hematoxylin and eosin). C) Electron micrograph showing multiple demyelinated axons (stars) within the substance of the white matter of an SJL mouse 63 days following infection. Mice showing these pathologic changes are frequently paralyzed and spastic. Note the adjacent normally myelinated axons (arrows). The myelin destruction is very specific since the axons are well-preserved (i.e. primary demyelination rather than secondary demyelination due to destruction of axons).

congeneic recombinant haplotypes demononstrated that the D region of H-2 determines susceptibility/resistance to infection (Rodriguez et al., 1986a). Mice which expressed the D^s gene were susceptible to demyelination even if resistant alleles were present on other regions of MHC. In contrast, mice that expressed D^d or D^b were resistant even if they had susceptible alleles on K, I or S. To further map the susceptibility gene within the D region, we examined mouse strain $B10.D2^{dml}$ and Balb/C dm2 for infection. As expected, B10.D2 or Balb/C parental mice showed no or minimal pathologic abnormalities. However, all dml mice showed extensive demyelination and inflammation where almost every spinal cord section showed prominent pathologic abnormalities. The finding was confirmed in B10.D2 (R106) mice (K^bD^{dml}) which express the same mutation. However, dm2 mice showed no demonstrable pathologic abnormalities. Since the dml mutation is a deletion encompassing the 3' exon of D^d and the 5' exons of L^d, while the dm2 mutation is a deletion of the complete L gene between the D gene and the gene of the Qa region, deductive reasoning suggests that D^d is one of the genes that controls resistance and/or susceptibility to TMEV.

Virologic studies at 45 days post-infection demonstrated that 3 to 4 logs of virus (plaque-forming units per gram of CNS tissue) could be recovered from mice exhibiting demyelination (i.e., B10.S, SJL, $B10.D2^{dml}$). In contrast, no virus could be isolated from the CNS of mice failing to show clinical signs of demyelination (i.e., B10.D2, B10, Balb/C ^{dm2}). This suggested that the D region genes were either important in clearing virus from the CNS in resistant mice or helping to maintain persistent infection in susceptible mice.

Similar results have been obtained independently by Clatch et al. (1985, 1986) using crosses between SJL and several congeneic H-2 recombinant mouse strains bearing different combinations of MHC genes. Animals homozygous for $H\text{-}2^s$ allele in the D region showed evidence of late paralytic disease indicative indirectly of demyelination in contrast to $H\text{-}2^s$ homozygotes in K or I. The data correlated with TMEV-specific delayed-type hypersensitivity but did not correlate with level of TMEV-specific humoral immunity (Clatch et al., 1985; Clatch et al., 1986).

POSSIBLE ADDITIONAL ROLE OF CLASS II GENE PRODUCTS IN DETERMINING THE SEVERITY OF DEMYELINATION

In an effort to define additional contributions of immune response gene products on virus-induced demyelination, we performed a quantitative analysis of the pathology in the spinal cord of mice with differences only within the class II genes (Table I). Our strategy was to choose strains with susceptible haplotypes on the D region (i.e., q, s, f) and keep the haplotypes on the D and K regions constant while varying immune response

Table 1. Effect of Immune Response (Ir) Genes on the Severity of Demyelination

Strain	K	A	A	E	E	D	Pathologic Score Inflammation	Pathologic Score Demyelination
B10.MBR	b	k	k	k	k	q	38.0 ± 20	38.6 ± 22
B10.RBQ1	b	b	b	b	b	q	3.2 ± 6.3	2.4 ± 5.3
B10.RSF3	s	k	k	k	k	f	19.2 ± 8.2	24.1 ± 7.9
B10.RSF5	s	s	s	s	p	f	4.7 ± 4.9	4.7 ± 4.6
B10.S(8R)	k	k	k	k	s	s	6.1 ± 4.5	7.4 ± 3.9
B10.ASR2	k	k	k	k	k	s	7.8 ± 3.2	10.9 ± 5.7
B10.RKF1	k	k	k	k	k	f	4.82 ± 10.7	5.5 ± 12.2
B10.RKF2	k	k	k	b	b	f	7.6 ± 6.2	9.9 ± 6.0
B10.RSF2	s	k	k	k	b	f	8.4 ± 8.1	8.5 ± 8.1
B10.RSF4	s	s	s	s	p	f	8.2 ± 7.2	11.8 ± 8.4

Mice were infected intracerebrally with 2 x 10^5 PFU of DA virus and were sacrificed on day 45 after infection. Pathologic score (mean ± SD) was determined by examining plastic-embedded spinal cord sections as described (Rodriguez et al., 1986).

genes. Quantitative analysis was performed by sectioning the entire spinal cord from each mouse into 20-25 blocks (1 mm thick). A 1μ section (glycol-methacrylate plastic) was made from each block and graded on a 4 point scale for the presence or absence of inflammation and/or demyelination in each quadrant of every spinal cord coronal section. A maximum pathologic score of 100 represented inflammation and demyelination in every quadrant in each spinal cord section.

There was a marked difference in the extent of inflammation and demyelination between B10.MBR and B10.RBQ1 mice (Table I). Animals with k haplotype alleles in the I region (B10.MBR) had greater extent of pathologic abnormalities compared to matched animals (B10.RBQ1) in which the only difference was the b haplotype alleles in the I region. A possible role for the I region was also noted when comparing B10.RSF3 and B10.RSF5 mice. Again k haplotype alleles in I (B10.RSF3) resulted in more extensive pathology (P<.01, Rank Order Sum Test) compared to B10.RSF5 ($I^{S/P}$). However, there were other strain comparisons [B10.S(8R) vs. B10.ASR2, B10.RKF1 vs. B10.RKF2 and B10.RSF2 vs. B10.RSF4] in which there was no detectable Ir effects even though there was expression of k haplotype I region products. It is of interest that a K region effect on severity of pathology may also be present since B10.RSF3 (K^s) mice showed prominent pathologic changes while less abnormalities were noted in B10.RKF1 (K^k) mice. In this case the I and the D region were kept constant but the K region was varied.

Additional genetic studies will be needed to determine precisely the interaction of various MHC gene products on the severity of demyelination. However, these preliminary experiments suggest that I region genes may influence the severity of disease.

EXPRESSION OF Ia ANTIGENS ON BRAIN CELLS FOLLOWING TMEV INFECTION

In an effort to further clarify the role of Ia antigen on virus-induced demyelination, we performed an immunoelectron microscopic study on spinal cords from mice infected by virus (Rodriguez et al., 1987). We compared the distribution of Ia positive brain cells in B10.S (H-2^s), B10.S(9R) (K^sI^S/K^D^d) and B10.ASR2 ($K^kI^kD^s$) mice. Uninfected mice from these three strains showed very few Ia positive cells in brain as detected by monoclonal antibody 10-2.16 which is specific for s, r, f, and k haplotypes of the I region. These few Ia positive cells had the characteristics of microglial cells which are considered to be brain-derived macrophages. In contrast mice susceptible to TMEV (B10.S and B10.ASR2) showed Ia antigen expression in 20-25% of the glial cells within the infected spinal cord (Fig. 2a,b). The antigens were expressed on astrocytes, endothelial cells and oligodendrocytes. Of particular interest was the novel finding of class II antigen expression by the myelin-producing cell (Fig. 2b). In contrast, B10.S(9R) mice which are resistant to disease had very few Ia positive glial cells. Therefore, susceptible mice with D^s alleles had increased Ia antigen in glial cells whereas resistant mice with D^k allele had low levels similar to uninfected mice. This occurred even though the resistant and susceptible mice had I region haplotype capable of responding to virus and reacting with the monoclonal antibody. Thus increased virus spread in susceptible mice was associated with accompanying demyelination and increased Ia antigen in glial cells. The studies suggested a possible role for antigen presentation by glial cells in TMEV-infection. This correlates with previous studies by us (Rodriguez et al., 1986) and others (Friedman et al., 1987) which have demonstrated a beneficial response of monoclonal antibody therapy to Ia in Theiler's virus-induced demyelination.

TREATMENT OF SUSCEPTIBLE SJL (H-2^s) MICE WITH mAb TO L3T4 AND Lyt2

In order to begin to determine the role of specific T cell subsets in virus-induced demyelination, Rodriguez and Sriram (University of Vermont) treated susceptible mice at various time points of infection with mAb GK1.5 (directed at class II-restricted T cells) or mAb 2.43 (directed at class I-restricted T cells). One milligram of purified antibody given by the intraperitoneal route depleted the corresponding T cell subset in the lymph nodes, spleens and peripheral blood for 6 to 8 weeks. However, no depletion was noted in the thymus. Early treatment with GK1.5 resulted in death, encephalitis and increased demyelination in the majority of mice compared to animals receiving isotype control sera. However, chronic treatment with mAb GK1.5 beginning on day 9 and continued for 35 days resulted in less demyelination and inflammation compared to controls. In contrast, treatment with mAb 2.43 whether begun at time of virus infection or on day 15 (after demyelination was established) resulted in marked diminution of pathologic abnormalities in the spinal cord. The studies indicate an important role for class I-restricted T cells as effectors during the late demyelinating phase of TMEV infection. In addition, class II-restricted T cells may be important in limiting early spread of virus and may provide "help" to class I-restricted T cells during late demyelinating disease.

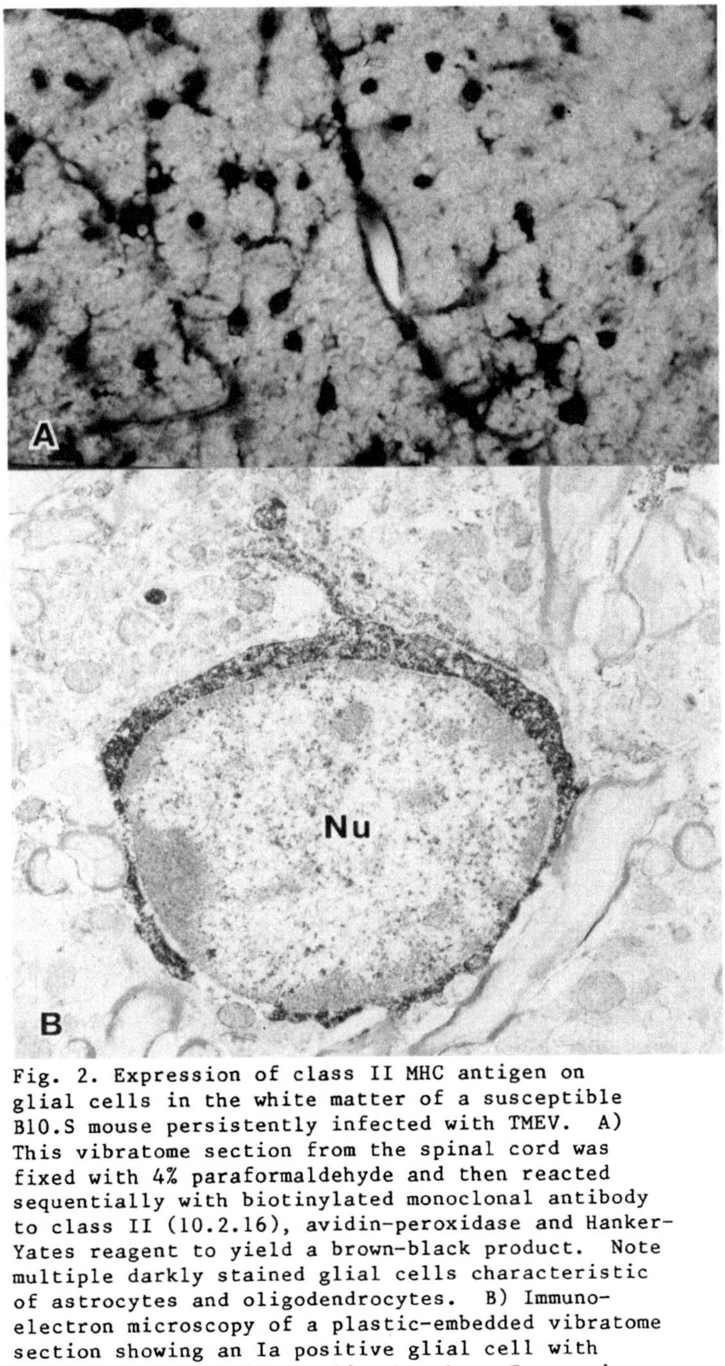

Fig. 2. Expression of class II MHC antigen on glial cells in the white matter of a susceptible B10.S mouse persistently infected with TMEV. A) This vibratome section from the spinal cord was fixed with 4% paraformaldehyde and then reacted sequentially with biotinylated monoclonal antibody to class II (10.2.16), avidin-peroxidase and Hanker-Yates reagent to yield a brown-black product. Note multiple darkly stained glial cells characteristic of astrocytes and oligodendrocytes. B) Immuno-electron microscopy of a plastic-embedded vibratome section showing an Ia positive glial cell with intimate contact with myelin sheaths. Expression of class II antigen on oligodendrocytes after viral infection suggests that this cell may be involved in antigen presentation within the nervous system.

CURRENT HYPOTHETICAL MODEL OF IMMUNE-MEDIATED DESTRUCTION OF MYELIN BY THEILER'S VIRUS

We propose that as a result of intracerebral viral inoculation, viral antigens are presented to T cells in the context of class I and class II MHC glycoproteins (Rodriguez et al., 1986b). The nature of the antigen presenting cells is still to be determined. Our recent experiments suggest that astrocytes, oligodendrocytes, endothelial cells, and macrophages may have the capacity to present viral antigens to T-helper cells in the context of class II MHC products (Rodriguez et al., 1987). Thus far we have been unable to demonstrate by immunocytochemistry class I antigens on brain cells from infected animals with susceptible haplotypes. It is possible that viral antigen fails to be recognized by the immune system in the context of class I antigen during early infection of susceptible mice. This could result in failure to clear virus, thus proceeding to an unaborted persistent infection of myelin-producing cells (oligodendrocyte). L3T4 cells, B cells and immunoglobulins, probably help in protecting against overwhelming encephalitis since treatment with mAb to L3T4 (GK1.5) results in death and/or encephalitis in the majority of animals.

The present role of the immune system during the demyelinating phase of disease is not yet clear. The observation that nude mice from resistant haplotypes (Balb/C) develop demyelination following intracerebral virus inoculation suggests that virus itself without contribution of T cell immunity is able to cause demyelination (Roos and Wollman, 1984; Rosenthal et al., 1986). This probably results from direct lytic injury of the oligodendrocyte. However, the beneficial response of immunosuppression in susceptible mice with cyclophosphamide (Lipton and Dal Canto, 1976; Lipton and Dal Canto, 1977), anti-lymphocyte serum (Roos et al., 1982), cyclosporin A (Rodriguez and Quddus, 1986c) and mAb to Ia (Friedman et al., 1987; Rodriguez et al., 1986) suggests that an immune response to virus antigen or virally-induced "novel" antigens may be important in demyelination.

We favor the hypothesis that persistent infection of oligodendrocytes is critical in pathogenesis (Rodriguez et al., 1983; Rodriguez, 1985; Rodriguez et al., 1986b). The immune system may be contributing to the pathology by at least three possible mechanisms: 1) Immunoglobulin may interact with novel antigen on the surface of oligodendrocytes and injure these cells by activation of complement, antibody-dependent cell-mediated cytotoxicity or activation of macrophages through binding of Fc receptors, 2) Class II-restricted T cells may recognize altered antigen on the surface of oligodendrocytes which have the capacity to express immune response gene products after virus infection; others have suggested that class II-restricted DTH response directed at brain cells other than oligodendrocytes may contribute to demyelination (Clatch et al., 1986; Wisniewski and Bloom, 1975) and 3) Class I-restricted T cells may recognize a novel antigen on glial cells which is seen in the context of class I antigen presenting glycoproteins leading to myelin destruction. The beneficial response of mAb to Lyt2 after demyelination suggests that this is a strong possibility.

SUMMARY

Experimental murine models of human disease have been valuable in helping to understand the molecular genetics of disease pathogenesis. TMEV infection provides one of the best examples of the influence of MHC gene products on the induction of disease. The close similarity of this model to the pathology of multiple sclerosis provides an important impetus to try to unravel the molecular events that lead to myelin breakdown.

REFERENCES

Cash, E., Chammoro, M., and Brahic, M., 1985, Theiler's virus RNA and protein synthesis in the central nervous system of demyelinating mice, Virology, 144:290.

Chamorro, M., Aubert, C., and Brahic, M., 1986, Demyelinating lesions due to Theiler's virus are associated with ongoing central nervous system infection, J. Virol., 57:992.

Clatch, R. J., Melvold, R. W., Miller, S. D., and Lipton, H. L., 1985, Theiler's murine encephalomyelitis virus (TMEV)-induced demyelinating disease in mice is influenced by the H-2D region: Correlation with TMEV-specific delayed-type hypersensitivity, J. Immunol., 135:1408.

Clatch, R. J., Lipton, H. L., and Miller, S. D., 1986, Characterization of Theiler's murine encephalomyelitis virus (TMEV)-specific delayed-type hypersensitivity responses in TMEV-induced demyelinating disease: Correlation with clinical signs, J. Immunol., 136:920.

Daniels, J. B., Pappenheimer, A. M., and Richardson, S., 1952, Observations on encephalomyelitis of mice (DA strain), J. Exp. Med., 96:517.

Dal Canto, M. C., and Lipton, H. L., 1975, Primary demyelination in Theiler's virus infection: An ultrastructual study, Lab. Invest., 33:626.

Dal Canto, M. C., and Lipton, H. L., 1982, Ultrastructural immunohistochemical localization of virus in acute and chronic demyelinating Theiler's virus infection, Am. J. Pathol., 106:20.

Dal Canto, M. C., and Rabinowitz, S. G., 1982a, Experimental models of virus-induced demyelination of the central nervous system, Ann. Neurol., 11:109.

Friedmann, A., Frankel, G., Lorch, Y., and Steinman, L., 1987, Monoclonal anti-I-A antibody reverses chronic paralysis and demyelination in Theiler's virus-infected mice: Critical importance of timing of treatment, J. Virol., 61:898.

Lehrich, J. R., Arnason, B. G. W., and Hochberg, F. H., 1976, Demyelinative myelopathy in mice induced by the DA virus, J. Neurol. Sci., 29:149.

Lipton, H. L., 1975, Theiler's virus infection in mice: An unusual biphasic disease process leading to demyelination, Infect. Immun., 11:1147.

Lipton, H. L., and Dal Canto, M. C., 1976, Theiler's virus-induced demyelination: Prevention by immunosuppression, Science, 192:62.

Lipton, H. L., and Dal Canto, M. C., 1977, Contrasting effects of immunosuppression on Theiler's virus infection in mice, Infect. Immun., 15:903.

Lipton, H. L., and Dal Canto, M. C., 1979, The TO strains of Theiler's viruses cause "slow virus-like" infections in mice, Ann. Neurol., 6:25.

Lipton, H. L., and Dal Canto, M. C., 1979a, Susceptibility of inbred mice to chronic central nervous system infection by Theiler's murine encephalomyelitis virus, Infect. Immun., 26:369.

Lipton, H. L., and Melvold, R., 1984, Genetic analysis of susceptibility to Theiler's virus-induced demyelinating disease in mice, J. Immunol., 132:1821.

Lorch, Y., Friedmann, A., Lipton, H. L., and Kotler, M., 1981, Theiler's murine encephalomyelitis virus group includes two distinct genetic subgroups that differ pathologically and biologically, J. Virol., 40:560.

Rodriguez, M., Leibowitz, J. L., and Lampert, P. W., 1983, Persistent infection of oligodendrocytes in Theiler's virus-induced encephalomyelitis, Ann. Neurol., 13:426.

Rodriguez, M., Leibowitz, J. L., Powell, H. C., and Lampert, P. W., 1983a, Neonatal infection with the Daniels strain of Theiler's murine encephalomyelitis virus, Lab. Invest., 49:672.

Rodriguez, M., 1985, Virus-induced demyelination in mice: "Dying back" of oligodendrocytes, Mayo Clin. Proc., 60:433.

Rodriguez, M., and David, C. S., 1985a, Demyelination Induced by Theiler's Virus: Influence of the H-2 Haplotype, J. Immunol., 135:2145.

Rodriguez, M., Lafuse, W., Leibowitz, J., and David, C. S., 1986, Partial suppression of Theiler's virus-induced demyelination in vivo by administration of monoclonal antibodies to immune response genes products (Ia antigens), Neurol., 36:964.

Rodriguez, M., Leibowitz, J., and David, C. S., 1986a, Susceptibility to Theiler's virus-induced demyelination: Mapping of the gene within the H-2D region, J. Exp. Med., 163:620.

Rodriguez, M., Pease, L. R., and David, C. S., 1986b, Immune-mediated injury of virus-infected oligodendrocytes. A model of multiple sclerosis, Immunol. Today, 7:359.

Rodriguez, M., and Quddus, J., 1986c, Effect of cyclosporin A, silica quartz dust and macrophage protease inhibitors in virus-induced demyelination, J. Neuroimmunol., 13:159.

Rodriguez, M., Pierce, M. L., and Howie, E. A., 1987, Immune response gene products (Ia antigens) on glial and endothelial cells in virus-induced demyelination, J. Immunol., 138:3438.

Roos, R. P., Firestone, S., Wollmann, R., Variakojis, D., and Arnason, B. G. W., 1982, The effect of short-term and chronic immunosuppression on Theiler's virus demyelination, J. Neuroimmunol., 2:223.

Roos, R. P., and Wollmann, R., 1984, DA strain of Theiler's murine encephalomyelitis virus induces demyelination in nude mice, Ann. Neurol. 15:494.

Rosenthal, A., Fujinami, R. S., and Lampert, P. W., 1986, Mechanism of Theiler's virus-induced demyelination in nude mice, Lab. Invest., 54:515.

Theiler, M., 1934. Spontaneous encephalomyelitis of mice - a new virus disease, Science, 80:122.

Wisniewski, H. M., and Bloom, B. R., 1975, Primary demyelination as a non-specific consequence of a cell-mediated reaction, J. Exp. Med. 141:346.

EXPRESSION OF H-2 GENES AND SUSCEPTIBILITY TO PARASITIC INFECTION

Donald L. Wassom, Christopher J. Krco,* and Chella S. David*

School of Veterinary Medicine, University of Wisconsin-Madison, Madison, WI and *The Department of Immunology, Mayo Clinic & Mayo Medical School, Rochester, MN

INTRODUCTION

The term parasitism is difficult to define. Many infectious organisms such as bacteria or fungi, live at the expense of their hosts, yet are not usually regarded as parasites. In contrast, certain protozoans or helminths which live in close association with their hosts, but cause no demonstrable disease, are called parasites nonetheless. For present purposes, the discussion of immunity to parasites will be restricted to immune responses induced in vertebrate hosts following exposure to protozoan, helminth, or arthropod "parasites". While such a distinction is arbitrary, it follows conventional practice. Following a brief discussion of immunity to parasitic infections in very general terms, results from studies of *Trichinella spiralis*-infected mice will be reviewed to provide specific examples of how H-2 genes may influence the outcome of such host-parasite interactions.

Parasites as defined above are antigenically complex, and infection may induce many simultaneous yet independent immune responses. In some cases, cellular or humoral immune products induced by parasite antigens may damage the parasite or may mediate indirect effects by damaging the tissues or cells in which the parasite lives. Consequently, the parasite's ability to live, develop, or reproduce may be impaired. The specific antigens which induce such anti-parasite effects are called functional antigens. Since functional parasite antigens have been difficult to identify and purify in quantities sufficient for detailed immunological analysis, most studies to date have focused on responses to crude antigen preparations or on the in vivo responses induced following active infection. Due to the antigenic complexity of the parasite, and the inability to identify the specific antigens which give rise to functionally significant events, much of the data collected thus far has been phenomenological; the cellular and molecular mechanisms which underlie the observed phenomena remain to be elucidated.

In an attempt to overcome the methodological problems associated with studying complex immune responses in the parasitized host, we adopted a comparative genetic approach. Our approach was based on the belief that significant insights into the mechanisms of anti-parasite immunity might be gained by comparing responses of mice which differed in their ability to resist parasite infection, but were genetically identical, or nearly so, except for the gene(s) responsible for mediating the observed effects. Our studies of *Trichinella spiralis*-infected mice have demonstrated that relevant host genes can be specifically identified. Thus, we are now in a position to utilize this information in studies to elucidate the functional anti-parasite response regulated by these genes.

PARASITE BIOLOGY

Trichinella spiralis is a parasitic worm (Nematode) which can infect most species of mammals. Humans become infected by ingesting improperly cooked meat which harbors infective larval worms. The infective larvae are released when the meat is digested by acid and pepsin in the stomach. Upon entering the small intestine, trypsin further stimulates the worms and they penetrate columnar epithelial cells where they live as adult worms. Due to its size, a single worm may penetrate and occupy a row of 100 or more such cells. Nonetheless, the worm lives in direct contact with host cell cytoplasm and is said to occupy an intramulticellular niche. Development of worms from the larval to the adult stage is extremely rapid with the worms undergoing four molts within the first thirty hours. The adult male and female worms mate, and beginning on day five or six post infection, female worms start giving birth to living young called newborn larvae. A fertilized female worm is capable of producing 100 or more newborn larvae each day that she resides in the small intestine. The newborn larvae enter blood or lymphatic vessels in the gut and are carried by the general circulation to the tissues where they penetrate striated muscles cells and mature to the infective stage. There is an intimate and active association between the worm and the parasitized muscle cell. The infective larvae may live within the muscle cell and retain its infectivity for 30 years or more depending on the longevity of the host. When the infected muscle is ingested by a new host, the cycle can continue.

The *Trichinella*-infected host makes a rapid and vigorous immune response to the developing juvenile and adult worms in the small intestine. This response initiates the expulsion of worms from the gut and thus halts the flow of newborn larvae to the muscle. Additional immune responses directed at reproducing female worms have also been demonstrated, and the production of newborn larvae may be greatly diminished as a result of this response. The number of larvae which successfully enter and develop to the infective stage within muscle cells is a function of at least three factors:

1. How many adult worms establish in the gut and how long they remain prior to being expelled.
2. How many newborn larvae are produced by adult female worms while the worms are resident within the gut.
3. How successful the newborn larvae are in getting from the gut to the muscle.

Once larval worms have entered muscle cells they are generally refractile to the adverse effects of host immune responses despite the fact that the worms are active within these cells and presumably secrete foreign molecules into the immediate environment.

It must be emphasized that all mammals (with rare exceptions) and thus all strains of mice are susceptible to *Trichinella* infection. However, strains or species of hosts may differ markedly in their ability to control such infections once the worms have established.

There are a number of assays which can be used to determine levels of susceptibility to *T. spiralis* infection. In general, resistant hosts have an accelerated expulsion of adult worms from the gut, decreased production of newborn larvae by female worms, and consequently, fewer larvae in their muscles. In addition, cells harvested from the mesenteric lymph nodes of resistant mice proliferate more strongly *in vitro* when cultured with crude *T. spiralis* antigen than do cells from susceptible strains.

Immunologists who study all-or-none genetically controlled responses to well defined antigens may feel uncomfortable evaluating data which reflect relative degrees of susceptibility among individuals which all respond to the infection, but with different kinetics. It is not always appreciated that hosts and parasites have a long evolutionary history during which each has adapted to the other; non-responder phenotypes were not likely favored in the evolutionary process and such hosts were probably killed by the parasites they encountered.

The role of MHC genes in immunity to parasite infection has been most thoroughly explored in studies of mice infected with *T. spiralis*. Prior to these studies, genes within the MHC were not thought to influence levels of susceptibility to infection with helminth or protozoan parasites. However, early attempts to address this question often failed to use hosts expressing a broad range of different MHC haplotypes. Additionally, differences in levels of susceptibility among host strains which shared common MHC genes was often mistaken as evidence that MHC genes played no role in regulating the response observed. In retrospect, it is obvious that MHC genes must be involved in regulating functional anti-parasite responses since virtually all protective responses are T cell dependent.

In addition to MHC genes, genes mapping outside the MHC always play an important role in determining the hosts ability to resist parasite infection. In the mouse, it is likely that H-2 genes regulate the afferent limb of the anti-parasite response and that activated T cells provide the necessary help for other cells which mediate the anti-parasite effects. The ability of effector cells (B cells, macrophages, mast cells, eosinophils, other T cells, etc.) to receive helper T cell signals or to mediate their anti-parasite effects once the signal is received, is probably controlled by the non-MHC-genes. Thus, the host's ability to resist parasite infections is usually determined by multiple genes, and the collective assemblage of these genes determines the host's response phenotype.

H-2 GENES AND IMMUNITY TO *T. SPIRALIS*

Studies of *Trichinella*-infected mice have established that at least two H-2 genes and one or more genes mapping outside the H-2 complex are involved in determining the outcome of experimental infections. One of the H-2-linked genes maps to the I-region and the other maps between S and D. A third gene, probably on chromosome 4, also influences the anti-*Trichinella* response. It is very likely that additional non-H-2-genes are also involved, but the location of these genes is not presently known.

Table 1. The I-A Molecule Appears to Influence the Host Response to *T. spiralis*.

EXPT. NO.	MOUSE STRAIN	H-2 HAPLOTYPE	H-2 LOCI								WORM COUNT ($\pm$ SEM)[a]	PHENOTYPE
			K	A_β	A_α	E_β	E_α	S	D	L		
1[b]	B10.BR	k	k	k	k	k	k	k	k	k	26640 ($\pm$ 3236)	sus
	B10.S	s	s	s	s	s	s	s	s	s	12600 ($\pm$ 646)	res
	B10.S(8R)	as^1	k	k	k	k	s	s	s	s	29120 ($\pm$ 2760)	sus
	B10.HTT	t^3	s	s	s	s	k	k	d	d	14000 ($\pm$ 1050)	res
2[c]	B10.BR	k	k	k	k	k	k	k	k	k	30286 $\pm$ 1291	sus
	B10.A	a	k	k	k	k	k	d	d	d	28680 $\pm$ 2485	sus
	B10.TL	t^1	s	k	k	k	k	k	d	d	29300 $\pm$ 2564	sus
	B10.S	s	s	s	s	s	s	s	s	s	15050 $\pm$ 1024	res

a Total body larval counts 30 days following infection with 150 l_1 larvae of *T. spiralis*.
b Reinterpreted from Wassom et al. (1979); reproduced with permission of the publisher, Springer-Verlag, Berlin.
c Reinterpreted from Wassom et al. (1980); reproduced with permission of the publisher, Academic Press, New York.

The involvement of I-region genes in the anti-Trichinella response was established from studies of H-2 recombinant strains of mice as shown in Table 1. In this series of experiments, mice expressing k alleles at I-region loci were more susceptible to infection than mice expressing s alleles. The relevant gene appears to map to I-A, however it is not clear whether alleles at A_{β} or A_{α} confer different levels of susceptibility upon the host, or if the relevant gene maps to I-A because resistant strains of mice fail to express I-E. It is clear that mice which express cell surface I-E molecules, particularly $I\text{-}E^k$ (E^k_{β} E^k_{α}), are more susceptible to infection than are mice which express only I-A. (see Table 2). As shown in Table 3, susceptibility is inherited as a dominant trait in offspring from susceptible ($I\text{-}E^+$) and resistant ($I\text{-}E^-$) parents.

While mice which express I-A but not I-E are generally resistant to Trichinella infection, this in not invariably so. As shown in Table 4, mice expressing b, s, q, or f alleles at I-region loci (all $I\text{-}E^-$) but expressing d alleles at loci in the D-end of the H-2 complex, are more susceptible to infections than are mice which do not express these D^d alleles. Furthermore, an extensive series of experiments involving b/a (or b/d) and s/a H-2 recombinant strains of mice revealed that the relevant gene maps in the S/D interval rather than to any of the presently assigned H-2 gene loci (see Table 4). This was the first observation that an "immune response gene" maps to this region of the chromosome. The recent mapping of genes encoding tumor necrosis factor and lymphotoxin between S and D, (Muller et al., 1987) and the demonstrated effect of TNF on other parasitic infections (Silberstein and David, 1986; Taverne et al., 1987, Ruddle, 1987) has rekindled interest in our earlier observations. Recently a gene which influences the response to TNP-Ficoll has also been mapped between S and D (Shapiro et al., 1985).

Mice which express cell surface $I\text{-}E^k$ molecules may also be quite resistant to Trichinella infection in some cases. We reported in 1979 that AKR/J mice were resistant to T. spiralis infection despite expressing the $H\text{-}2^k$ haplotype (Wassom et al., 1979). We were therefore interested in Hayes' report that AKR/J mice differed from most other $H\text{-}2^k$ strains in their ability to express $I\text{-}J^k$ molecules on subpopulations of T cells (Hayes, et al. 1984). They reported that AKR/J mice have a defect in a gene (Jt) on chromosome 4, linked to the Fv-1 locus, which influences the expression of $I\text{-}J^k$ molecules. We

Table 2. Association of H-2 Haplotype, Expression of Cell Surface I-E Molecules, and Susceptibility to Infection with T. spiralis.[a]

MOUSE STRAIN	H-2 HAPLOTYPE	I-E EXPRESSION	RESISTANCE INDEX[b]	RESISTANCE PHENOTYPE
B10.BR	k	+	0	sus
B10.P	p	+	-22	sus
B10.RIII	r	+	33	sus
B10	b	-	63	res/int
B10.S	s	-	100	res
B10.M	f	-	104	res
B10.Q	q	-	105	res

a Reproduced from Wassom et al. (1987) with permission of the publisher, Elsevier Science Publishers, Amsterdam, Netherlands.

b RI = $\frac{\text{count for B10.BR - count for B10.? } \times 100}{\text{count for B10.BR - count for B10.S}}$

RI for T. spiralis is calculated on basis of total body larval counts 30 days following per os infection with 150 L_1 larvae as described by Wassom et al. (1983). In a typical experiment, $H-2^k$ mice harbor approximately two-fold more worms than $H-2^s$ mice. The calculated RI, when greater than 100 indicates lower average worm counts than demonstrated for $H-2^s$ mice. A negative index value denotes susceptibility greater than that expressed by $H-2^k$.

tested the strains of mice used by Hayes et al. to identify the Jt gene for their ability to resist T. spiralis infection. AKR-Fv-1^b mice (11th backcross generation) obtained from Dr. E.A. Boyse were compared with AKR/J. As shown in Table 5, AKR-Fv-1^b ($I-J^+$) mice were markedly more susceptible to infection than were AKR/J ($I-J^-$) mice. The two strains are thought to differ only at genes linked to the Fv-1 locus on chromosome 4. Formal genetic analysis must be conducted to confirm whether it is a single gene on chromosome 4 which influences levels of resistance to T. spiralis infection. If levels of susceptibility to infection and the expression of $I-J^k$ molecules on populations of T cells can be assessed concurrently in offspring from crosses between appropriate Fv-1 congenic strains of mice, it should be possible to determine if a common gene mediates both effects.

The influence of $I-E^k$ on $I-J^k$ expression has been assessed in a number of experimental systems (see Moeller 1985; Sumida et al. 1985; Uracz et al. 1985, and Waltenbaugh et al., 1986). Flood et al. (1986), studying transgenic mice, showed that expression of (E_α^k) in

Table 3. Association of Susceptibility to *T. spiralis* Infection in F1 Mice With Expression of *I-E*^{k}.[a]

STRAIN	NO. TESTED	H-2 HAPLOTYPE	I-E^k EXPRESSION	WORM COUNT (± SEM)[b]
B10.BR	17	k	+	51,820 ± 5620[c,d]
B10.Q	22	q	–	25,370 ± 1560
B10.M	20	f	–	28,050 ± 1650
B10.BR x B10.Q	23	k/q	+	41,560 ± 3060[c]
B10.BR x B10.M	22	k/f	+	45,950 ± 2800[d]

a Reproduced from Wassom et al. (1987) with permission of the publisher Elsevier Science Publishers, Amsterdam, Netherlands.
b Total body larval counts 30 days following infection *per os* with 150 L_1 larvae of *T. spiralis* as described by Wassom et al. (1983).
c Significantly more susceptible than B10.Q (p<.05) Students t Test.
d Significantly more susceptible than B10.M (p<.05) Students t Test.

(B6 x SJL)F_1 mice resulted in expression of I-J^k. Neither the B6 or the SJL parent nor the (B6 x SJL)F_1 express I-J^k. These transgenic mice should be extremely valuable in studies to characterize the role of I-E expression on the immune response to parasites.

Several hypothesis to explain how the expression of I-E molecules might confer susceptibility on the host have been put forth in a recent publication (Wassom et al., 1987). The stage is now set to test these hypotheses using a biologically relevant experimental system for which specific genes controlling levels of resistance to infection have been mapped and partially characterized. The data emanating from such studies should provide new insight into how the immune system is regulated following exposure a very complex and potentially lethal antigenic insult.

TABLE 4. A Gene Between S and D Influences Resistance to *T. spiralis* Infection.[a]

EXPT. NO.	MOUSE STRAIN	H-2 HAPLOTYPE	H-2 LOCI								WORM COUNT ($\pm$ SEM)[b]
			K	A_β	A_α	E_β	E_α	S	D	L	
1	B10.Q	q	q	q	q	q	q	q	q	q	23320 ($\pm$ 5467)
	B10.T(6R)	y^2	q	q	q	q	q	q	d	d	42530 ($\pm$ 4034)
2	B10.M	f	f	f	f	f	f	f	f	f	15750 ($\pm$ 1394)
	B10.M(11R)	ap^1	f	f	f	f	f	f	d	d	20301 ($\pm$ 1793)
3	B10.S	s	s	s	s	s	s	s	s	s	15050 ($\pm$ 1024)
	B10.S(7R)	t^2	s	s	s	s	s	s	d	d	24044 ($\pm$ 4936)
	B10.S(23R)	t^{11}	s	s	s	s	s	s	d	d	17260 ($\pm$ 1961)
	B10.S(24R)	t^6	s	s	s	s	s	s	d	d	13833 ($\pm$ 1283)
4	B10.A(18R)	i^{18}	b	b	b	b	b	b	d	d	25033 ($\pm$ 2301)
	B10.S(21R)	i^{21}	b	b	b	b	b	b	d	d	18690 ($\pm$ 2027)
	B10.BAR-5	i^1	b	b	b	b	b	b	d	d	14720 ($\pm$ 1297)
	B10.D2(R107)	i^7	b	b	b	b	b	b	d	d	13000 ($\pm$ 1507)

a Reinterpreted from Wassom et al. (1983) reproduced with permission of the publisher, Blackwell Scientific Publications, Oxford.
b See Table 2.

Table 5. Comparison of AKR/J and AKR-Fv-1b Mice for Susceptibility to *T. spiralis* Infection.[a]

STRAIN	H-2 HAPLOTYPE	I-E[k] EXPRESSION	I-J[k] EXPRESSION[b]	WORM COUNT (± SEM)[c]
AKR/J	k	+	-	13,800 (± 4690)
AKR-Fv-1b	k	+	+	37,610 (± 8740)[d]

a Reproduced from Wassom et al 1987 with permission of the publisher, Elsevier Science Publishers, Amsterdam, Netherlands.
b Hayes et al (1984).
c See Table II.
d Significantly more susceptible than AKR/J (p<.0001) Students t Test.

REFERENCES

Flood, P.M., Benoist, C., Mathis, D., and Murphy, D.B.: Altered I-J phenotype in Eα transgenic mice. Proc Natl Acad Sci, 83:8308-8312, 1986.

Hayes, C.E., Klyczek, K.K., Krum, D.D., Whitcomb, R.M., Hullett, D.A., and Cantor, H.: Chromosome 4 Jt gene controls murine T cell surface I-J expression. Science, 223:559-563.

Moeller, G. ed.: I-J. Immunol Rev vol 83, 1985.

Müller, V., Jongeneel, C.V., Nedospasov, S.A., Fischer-Lindahl, K., and Steinmetz, M.: Tumor necrosis factor and lymphotoxin genes map close to H-2D in the mouse major histocompatibility complex. Nature, 325:265-267, 1987.

Ruddle, N.H.: Tumor necrosis factor and related cytotoxins. Immunol Today, 8:129-130, 1987.

Shapiro, L.H., Dugan, E.S., and Neiderhuber, J.E.: Monoclonal antibody characterization of a unique immune response control locus between H-2 S and D. J Exp Med, 162:1477-1493, 1985.

Silberstein, D.S., and David, J.R.: Tumor necrosis factor enhances eosinophil toxicity to *Schistosoma mansoni* Larvae. Proc Natl Acad Sci, 83:1055-1059, 1986.

Sumida, T., Sado, T., Kojima, M., Ono, K., Kamisaku, H., and Taniguchi, M.: I-J as an idiotype of the recognition component of antigen-specific suppressor T-cell factor. Nature, 316:738-741, 1985.

Taverne, J., Tavernier, J., Fiers, W., and Playfair, J.H.L.: Recombinant tumor necrosis factor inhibits malaria parasites *in vivo* but not *in vitro*. Clin Exp Immunol, 67:1-4, 1987.

Uracz, W., Asano, Y., Abe, R., and Tada, T.: I-J epitopes are adaptively acquired by T cells differentiated in the chimaeric condition. Nature, 316:741-743, 1985.

Waltenbaugh, C., Sun, L., and Lei, H.-Y.: Regulation of immune responses by I-J gene products. VI. Recognition of I-E molecules by I-J-bearing suppressor factors. J. Exp. Med., 163:797-811, 1986.

Wassom, D.L., David, C.S., and Gleich, G.J.: Genes within the major histocompatibility complex influence susceptibility to *Trichinella spiralis* in the mouse. Immunogenetics, 9:491-496, 1979.

Wassom, D.L., David, C.S., and Gleich, G.J.: MHC-linked genetic control of the immune response to parasites: Trichinella spiralis in the mouse. In Skamene E, Kongshavn, P.A.L., and Landy, M. (eds.) "Genetic Control of Natural Resistance to Infection and Malignancy." New York Academic Press pp 75-82, 1980.

Wassom, D.L., Brooks, B.O., Babish, J.G., and David, C.S.: A gene mapping between the S and D regions of the H-2 complex influences resistance to Trichinella spiralis infections of mice. J Immunogenetics, 10:371-378, 1983.

Wassom, D.L., Krco, C.J., and David, C.S.: I-E expression and susceptibility to parasite infection. Immunol Today, 8:39-43, 1987.

THE ROLE OF H-2 GENE COMPLEX IN EXPERIMENTAL AUTOIMMUNE THYROIDITIS

Yi-chi M. Kong and Chella S. David

Department of Immunology and Microbiology
Wayne State University School of Medicine
Detroit, MI and Department of Immunology
Mayo Medical School, Rochester, MN

INTRODUCTION

Susceptibility to experimental autoimmune thyroiditis (EAT) was linked to the H-2 complex in 1971 by the use of inbred strains of independent haplotypes on different backgrounds[1,2]. For example, mice of the k or s haplotype are susceptible (good responder); they develop severe thyroiditis, in addition to autoantibodies to MTg, after immunization with mouse thyroglobulin (MTg) in complete Freund's adjuvant (CFA). In contrast, mice of the b or d haplotype are resistant (poor responder), with little, if any, cellular infiltration in the thyroid, despite the presence of MTg autoantibodies. In the past 10 years, the influence of various H-2 genes on EAT induction and development has been examined in detail. These studies may be grouped into three sections.

DEFINING THE H-2 LINKAGE

The early study on H-2 association with EAT induction was conducted in mice of five different haplotypes on a variety of background genes[1]. Using H-2 recombinant strains available in the early 1970s, the immune response gene to MTg (Ir-Tg) encoding EAT susceptibility was located at the K end[3]. However, it was necessary to ascertain that the K end indeed governed immune responsiveness to MTg and not to mycobacterial antigens in CFA or to MTg epitopes possibly altered by emulsification. Accordingly, we tested several polyclonal activators for their capacity to serve as adjuvant in EAT induction in both susceptible and resistant strains. Bacterial lipopolysaccharide (LPS), given i.v. 3 h after soluble, unaltered MTg, is as effective an adjuvant as CFA in inducing EAT and requires the presence of T cells of susceptible mice for its action[4], as has been shown with CFA[5]. A less potent adjuvant, polyadenylic-polyuridylic acid complex (poly A:U), is efficacious primarily in inducing MTg autoantibody formation in susceptible mice[6]. Table 1 presents data from a direct comparison of the relative efficacy of these polyclonal activators in promoting EAT in susceptible B10.BR mice and their relative ineffectiveness in resistant B10.D2 mice[7]. Extensive thyroid infiltration was observed only in susceptible mice.

To determine if the MHC-based difference in susceptibility to EAT observed in mouse strains on different background genes[1] would remain

Table 1. Effect of Different Adjuvants on EAT Induction in Susceptible and Resistant Mice

Strain	Treatment[a]	Mean $\log_2$ titer $\pm$ SE[b]	Thyroiditis[b] Mean index $\pm$ SE	Thyroiditis[b] No. pos./total
B10.BR(_H-2_[k])	MTg	<1.0	0.0	0/3
	MTg + poly A:U	5.8 $\pm$ 0.4	0.2 $\pm$ 0.1	1/5
	MTg + LPS	9.8 $\pm$ 0.5	1.5 $\pm$ 0.2	6/6
	MTg in CFA	11.0 $\pm$ 0.7	1.0 $\pm$ 0.6	2/3
B10.D2(_H-2_[d])	MTg	<1.0	0.0	0/4
	MTg + poly A:U	<1.0	0.0	0/5
	MTg + LPS	8.2 $\pm$ 0.7	0.0	0/6
	MTg in CFA	11.2 $\pm$ 0.8	0.0	0/5

Adapted from Kong et al.[7]

[a]MTg (20 µg) was given i.v. on d 0, 7; 300 µg poly A:U and 20 µg LPS were injected i.v. 3 h later; and MTg in CFA was injected s.c. on d 0 and 7.

[b]Data from d 28; pathology index on a scale of 0-4 from no infiltration to >80% infiltration and destruction.

unchanged in congenic mice, we tested B10 congenics bearing eleven independent haplotypes[8]. The animals were immunized with MTg plus LPS, a finer discriminator for genetic influences on EAT than CFA[9], and their thyroid pathology was compared in serial sections. Fig. 1 shows that the _k_ and _s_ haplotypes remain susceptible to high incidence of disease, and _b_ and _d_ are resistant with low incidence. As discussed elsewhere[10],

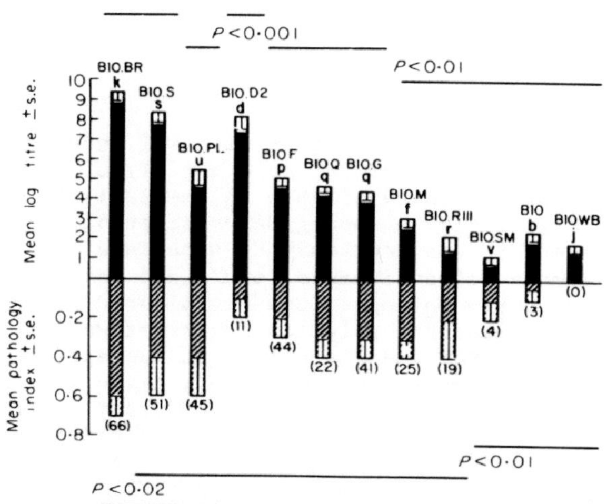

Fig. 1. Autoimmune responses (d 28) to mouse thyroglobulin by B10 cogenic strains with different _H-2_ haplotypes. The number in parentheses is the percentage of animals (17-29 per strain) with thyroid damage. Each horizontal line (continuous or discontinuous) represents strains of the same statistical group and the probability between each group is given. Source: Beisel et al.[8]

the q haplotype on B10 background dropped from susceptible status[1] to intermediate. This lower responsiveness of B10.Q mice, exemplified by lowered MTg antibody titers and reduced severity and incidence of disease when compared with B10.BR and B10.S mice, may, in part, be due to non-H-2 influences[8]. For example, mice of susceptible k haplotype on C3H background had higher pathology and increased incidence of thyroiditis compared with those on B10 background. Whether these differences reflect the input of T cell receptor genes is unknown at present.

Fig. 1 shows further that B10.D2 mice can produce autoantibody levels equivalent to those in susceptible strains, but the incidence of thyroiditis remains low. Although another laboratory has reported their B10.D2 and BALB/c mice, bearing the d haplotype, to be high responders[11], we have consistently found such strains to behave in a resistant fashion, low in thyroid pathology[4,6-8,12] and lacking a T cell proliferative response to MTg stimulation *in vitro*[12-14] (see Table 4), as also observed by others[15,16]. BALB/c mice remain resistant to EAT induction when immnized with purified MTg and LPS, rather than thyroid extract and CFA as employed by others[11].

EAT-susceptible mice can also respond to repeated injections (16x) of MTg over a period of 4 weeks in the absence of any adjuvant[17], although two doses of MTg ranging from 20 µg (Table 1) to 250 µg[4,6] neither induce MTg autoantibodies nor thyroid infiltration. Whereas resistant BALB/c mice showed very low and transient autoantibody production, susceptible C3H mice displayed 100% incidence of high antibody levels and 50% incidence of thyroiditis[17].

Collectively, the above studies show that: 1) The H-2-linked Ir-Tg gene encoding EAT susceptibility holds true for this self antigen regardless of the adjuvant used or if no adjuvant is used. 2) The severity of thyroid damage is unrelated to MTg autoantibody titers, and susceptible mice may have autoantibodies without lesions. 3) As an adjuvant for MTg, LPS (given i.v.) is a finer discriminator for genetic influences than CFA, since lesions are seldom observed in EAT-resistant mice, whereas low[1,4,6] to high[11] incidence of thyroiditis has been reported after CFA treatment.

EXAMINING THE ROLE OF CLASS II GENES

The Ir-Tg gene was located in 1974 at the K end of the H-2 complex[3], which included both the K region (class I genes) and I-A subregion (class II genes). Mapping of Ir-Tg gene to the I-A subregion was not possible until the availability in the early 1980s of B10.MBR strain, an appropriate recombinant between the K region and I-A subregion[10]. As presented in Table 2, the B10.MBR strain retains the capacity of the prototype, B10.BR, to develop EAT, despite carrying the resistant b allele at the K region. Comparisons with the other recombinant strains, such as B10.A(4R), pinpoint the Ir-Tg gene to the I-A subregion.

Two lines of experimental evidence further support locating the Ir-Tg gene at the I-A subregion. One is the testing of congenic K-region mutants of resistant b haplotype to determine if the K region plays any major role in EAT induction. Using LPS as adjuvant, we found all six mutant strains, including B10.C-$H\text{-}2^{bm1}$, to be as resistant to immunization as their B6 prototype[10]. Subsequently, Maron et al.[11] inferred susceptible status to the bm1 mutant after immunization with thyroidextract in CFA. We therefore retested this strain by directly comparing LPS and CFA as an adjunct of MTg in EAT induction. This CFA had been

Table 2. Genetic Mapping of Ir-Tg Gene in H-2 Recombinant Strains

Strain	H-2 Haplotype	K	A	(J)	E	S	D	TL	Mean Log_2 Titer[a] ± SE	Thyroiditis[a] No. pos./total
B10	b	b	b	b	b	b	b	b	1.6 ± 0.3	1/28
B10.BR	k	k	k	k	k	k	k	a	9.5 ± 0.4	21/29
B10.A	a	k	k	k	k	d	d	a	8.5 ± 0.3	12/24
B10.AKM	m	k	k	k	k	k	q	a	7.5 ± 0.7	12/23
B10.MBR	bq1	b	k	k	k	k	q	a	7.0 ± 0.4	21/29
B10.A(4R)	h4	k	k	b	b	b	b	b	9.3 ± 0.4	10/19
B10.A(5R)	i5	b	b	k	k	d	d	a	4.7 ± 0.4	2/10

Modified from Beisel et al.[10]
[a]Data from day 28 postimmunization with MTg + LPS.

especially designed to provide a vigorous autoimmune response[2]. A composite of the findings from four experiments is presented in Table 3. Whereas both antibody titers and disease incidence remain low after immunization with MTg plus LPS, MTg-CFA-immunized mice did show an increased incidence of thyroiditis (47 vs. 17%), in addition to the expected high antibody titers. However, the average pathology index is still quite low. Since class I genes at the K and D regions are involved in thyroid target destruction by cytotoxic T cells (T_C)[18,19] (see next section), the increase in thyroiditis could be related to better recognition/presentation by the bm1 molecule in the presence of the potent adjuvant CFA. The likely presence of a number of H-2 alloantigens in the thyroid extracts incorporated into CFA as used by others[11] probably further enhanced the stimulation. Thus, studies with the K mutants support rather than alter the interpretation that the I-A subregion plays a prime role in initiating the induction of EAT.

Table 3. Comparison of LPS and CFA as Adjuvant on Kinetics of MTg Antibody Response and Thyroid Infiltration in a Low Responder Mutant Strain (B6.C-$H\text{-}2^{bm1}$)[a]

Treatment[b]	Mean Log_2 Titer ± SE on Day				Thyroiditis	
	7	14	21	28	Mean index ± SE	No. Pos./total
20 µg MTg + 20 µg LPS	<1.0	2.1 ± 0.4	2.3 ± 0.3	3.0 ± 0.3	0.2 ± 0.1	6/36
20 µg MTg in CFA	<1.0	7.5 ± 0.9	9.4 ± 0.4	11.1 ± 0.5	0.8 ± 0.2	18/38

[a]Composite table of results from four experiments.
[b]MTg was given i.v. on d 0, 7, followed by LPS i.v. in 3 h; MTg in CFA was given s.c. on the same days.

Table 4. Comparison of T Cell Proliferative Responses of Susceptible (CBA) and Resistant (BALB/c) Mice to Mouse and Human Thyroglobulins

Strain	Immunizing Antigen	[^{3}H]Thymidine Uptake[a] (Mean cpm ± SD) None	MTg 25 μg/ml	HTg 25 μg/ml
CBA	MTg	9,440 ± 1,900	66,500 ± 15,200	50,800 ± 9,520
	HTg	4,060 ± 650	16,900 ± 4,040	56,700 ± 6,040
BALB/c	MTg	260 ± 30	380 ± 80	260 ± 20
	HTg	180 ± 5	310 ± 120	30,900 ± 7,640

Adapted from Simon et al.[14]
[a]Lymph node cells from mice immunized with MTg or HTg in CFA were cultured with MTg or HTg for 6 days.

Another line of evidence corroborating the importance of the *Ir-Tg* gene at the *I-A* subregion is obtained from studies on the *in vitro* activation of T cells and their transfer of autoimmune thyroiditis to normal recipient mice. Only T cells from immunized, EAT-susceptible, but not EAT-resistant, mice proliferate *in vitro* in response to MTg stimulation[12-14]. The proliferative response correlates with lesion development and not with antibody formation ongoing in both susceptible and resistant mice[12]. Thus, it reflects the function, not of helper T cells that aid B cells, but of effector T cells (T_E) in promoting thyroiditis[18-20].

Of further interest is the observation that only T cells from MTg-immunized, susceptible (CBA), but not resistant (BALB/c), mice responded to human(H) Tg stimulation *in vitro*[14] (Table 4). If immunization was with HTg, only CBA, but not BALB/c, mice responded *in vitro* to cross-stimulation with MTg, although both strains showed a response to HTg, apparently to HTg-specific epitopes. Clearly, the *Ir-Tg* gene somehow plays an additional role in the recognition/presentation of shared epitopes on Tg. Table 5 shows further that the *I-E* subregion is not involved in the proliferative response, since monoclonal antibodies to *I-A^k* (Ia.15), but not to *I-E^k* (Ia.7), blocked *in vitro* thymidine uptake.

In vitro activation of either lymph node cells (LNC) or spleen cells (SC) by MTg enables the expansion and differentiation of T_E from immunized mice. These cells are then capable of transferring thyroiditis to syngeneic normal recipients[16,20]. As seen in Table 6, not only MTg, but also HTg, can activate SC to transfer disease to 100% of the recipients. Concanavalin A (Con A)-activated cells are less efficacious in transferring EAT at equivalent cell numbers, probably because many of the activated cells are not MTg-specific and are not retained by the thyroid[9,20]. Similar to the proliferative assay[14] (Table 4 above), T cells from HTg-immunized mice can also be activated *in vitro* by both MTg and HTg to transfer autoimmune thyroiditis[20,21], even though HTg-immunized mice do not develop notable EAT. Moreover, after MTg immunization, bovine and porcine Tg, like MTg and HTg, are good expanders of T_E for adoptive transfer[21]. We conclude therefore that conserved regions are thyroiditogenic. However, T cells recognizing these shared epitopes are subjected to strong suppressive influences *in vivo* and are unable to mount or mediate severe EAT without prior expansion/differentiation *in vitro*.

Table 5. Effect of Ia Antibodies on the Proliferative Response to MTg

Antibodies (10 μg/ml)	[^{3}H]Thymidine Uptake[a] (Mean cpm ± SD) None	MTg (50 μg/ml)	PPD (25 μg/ml)
None	3,610 ± 140	17,860 ± 2,540	105,730 ± 4,780
Anti-I-E^k	4,690 ± 260	23,170 ± 1,280	88,240 ± 9,550
Anti-I-A^k	3,280 ± 280	5,000 ± 60	37,480 ± 10,330
Anti-I-A^d	5,620 ± 250	21,790 ± 2,750	109,200 ± 6,060

[a]Lymph node cells from MTg-CFA immunized CBA/J mice were cultured for 4 days with antigen and monoclonal anti-Ia.

DIFFERENTIATING THE ROLE OF CLASS I GENES

The evidence available thus far indicates the participation of class I genes in EAT, primarily at the effector level. In addition to adoptive transfer of EAT as discussed above, in vitro activated T_E contain T_C precursors, which develop into T_C upon further culture[18,19]. The T_C are Lyt-2$^+$ and require Lyt-1$^+$ cells for expansion/differentiation[18]. As shown in Table 7, T_C derived from LNC of MTg-immunized mice are MTg-specific and destroy CBA, but not BALB/c, thyroid monolayers. This display of strain specificity in target cells is apparently related to class I-antigen restriction seen in cell-mediated lympholysis. Table 8 is an example of such restriction of T_C in EAT, shown by the preincubation of thyroid target cells with antibodies to either K^k or D^k antigen, or with a mixture of both. Each kind of antibody alone reduced cytotoxicity by approximately 50% and both together abrogated cytotoxicity completely[18]. ConA-activated T_C were similarly class I-antigen-restricted as long as the LNC came from MTg-immunized mice[19]. The cells that initiate the adoptive transfer of EAT are L3T4$^+$(Lyt-1$^+$) and are required for the development of Lyt-2$^+$ T_C[18]. Analysis of the kinetics of T cell subsets infiltrating the gland in either thyroid cell suspensions[22] or in situ thyroid sections[23] has verified the presence of both L3T4$^+$ and Lyt-2$^+$ cells in changing ratios. Their relative role in pathogenesis of EAT is under study.

Table 6. Transfer of EAT with MTg-, HTg-, or Con A-Activated Spleen Cells from MTg-Immunized Mice

In Vitro Activation	No. Cells Transferred[a]	Mean Log$_2$ Titer[b] ± SE	Thyroiditis[b] Mean index ± SE	No. pos./total
MTg	10^7	2.8 ± 0.6	2.8 ± 0.1	6/6
HTg	10^7	2.3 ± 0.4	2.0 ± 0.1	6/6
Con A	10^7	2.6 ± 0.5	0.4 ± 0.3	2/5
Con A	3×10^7	3.0 ± 0.5	1.9 ± 0.1	5/5

Adapted from Simon et al.[20]
[a]Donor mice were immunized with MTg + LPS; their spleen cells were cultured for 3 days with MTg (20 μg/ml), HTg (20 μg/ml), or Con A (3 μg/ml), and transferred i.v. into normal recipients.
[b]Determined 14 days following cell transfer.

Table 7. Specificity of T Cell-Mediated Cytotoxicity for Thyroid Monolayers

Immunization	Antigen in Culture	% Specific ^{111}In-Release ± SD from Thyroid Target Cells[a] CBA	BALB/c
MTg in CFA	25 μg MTg/ml	85 ± 12	ND
	50 μg MTg/ml	57 ± 10	3 ± 8
	25 μg BSA/ml	9 ± 5	0 ± 3
	50 μg BSA/ml	14 ± 10	1 ± 1
Saline in CFA	25 μg MTg/ml	8 ± 5	ND

Modified from Creemers et al.[18]
[a]Lymph node cells were collected on day 14 after immunization and incubated *in vitro* for 5 days with MTg or BSA and assayed for cytotoxicity.

Certain *D*-end genes also moderate the severity of thyroiditis by an as-yet unknown mechanism. Since the *a* haplotype, a recombinant of *k* at the *K* end and *d* at the *D* end, is an intermediate responder in EAT[1,3], we immunized recombinant strains, similar at the *I* region but different at the *D* region, with MTg plus LPS[24]. Fig. 2 presents the autoantibody titers and thyroid pathology indices from sample strains bearing the *k* (left graph) or *s* (right graph) allele at the *I* region. It is clear that certain *D*-region genes can moderate both autoantibody titers and extent of thyroid infiltration (A^sD^d), whereas others reduced severity only (A^kD^d, A^kD^q) or had no effect (A^kD^f). The contribution of the *TL* region at the *D* end was ruled out in these[24] and separate experiments[8]. The influence of the *K*-end genes is much less pronounced; some differences in incidence of EAT have been noted when certain *K*-region alleles are superimposed on mice showing a *D*-end effect[10].

Table 8. Class I-Antigen Restriction of Cytotoxic T Cells for Thyroid Target Monolayers

Target Cell Preincubation[a]	% Specific ^{111}In-Release ± SD from Thyroid Target Cells MTg[b]	Con A[c]
Normal mouse serum	66 ± 1	65 ± 11
Mouse anti-*H-2K*^{k}	31 ± 4	36 ± 11
Mouse anti-*H-2D*^{k}	28 ± 2	33 ± 9
Mouse anti-*H-2K*^{k} + anti-*H-2D*^{k}	1 ± 4	0 ± 10

[a]Labeled thyroid cells were washed after incubation with antiserum prior to addition of effector cells.
[b]Lymph node cells from MTg-CFA-immunized CBA mice were activated *in vitro* with MTg (data from Creemers et al.[18]).
[c]Lymph node cells from MTg-CFA-immunized CBA mice were activated *in vitro* with Con A (data from Kong et al.[19]).

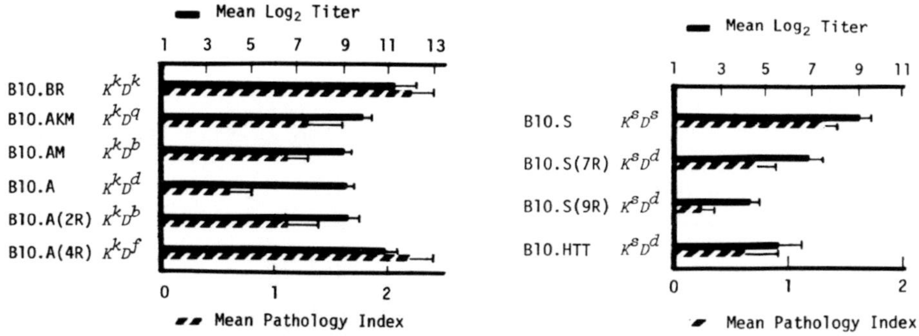

Fig. 2. Influence of D-end genes on autoimmune responses to mouse thyroglobulin in H-2 recombinant strains. The animals were immunized with MTg + LPS on d 0, 7 and sacrificed on d 28. Their thyroids were serially sectioned for pathologic comparisons. Source: Kong et al.[24].

SUMMARY

Experimental autoimmune thyroiditis (EAT) in mice has served as a useful model for hypothyroid Hashimoto's thyroiditis (HT) as well as a prototype for the study of other organ-specific autoimmune diseases. The use of recombinant congenic strains in EAT has enabled the dissection and differentiation of the relative contributions of class I and class II genes within the MHC as well as non-H-2 influences. Such multiple genetic controls more than likely exist in polygenic humans. Some common characteristics shared by murine EAT and HT are: 1) Susceptibility is associated with the MHC; 2) a major thyroid protein, thyroglobulin (Tg), is an autoantigen, and mouse Tg (MTg) induces EAT; 3) autoimmune responses include autoantibody production to Tg, T cell proliferative response to Tg *in vitro* and mononuclear cells in the thyroid infiltrate. The H-2-linked susceptibility to EAT, exemplified by the k or s haplotype and first shown with mouse strains on different backgrounds, has been confirmed with studies in B10 congenics. Susceptibility nd resistance are distinguishable by thyrid infiltration, and not by autoantibody production. Using H-2 recombinant strains, the susceptibility gene, designated Ir-Tg, has been mapped to the I-A subregion. However, the possession of the appropriate I-A allele alone does not necessarily result in disease, since selective D-region genes can moderate both the autoantibody titers and severity of thyroid lesions or reduce severity only. T cells from MTg-immunized mice respond in culture to activation and expansion by MTg and human Tg (shared epitopes). Such *in vitro* activated cells transfer thyroiditis to normal syngeneic recipients and develop cytotoxicity for syngeneic thyroid monolayers. The destruction of thyroid target cells is class I-antigen-restricted. Analysis of the contribution of T cell subsets has implicated both $L3T4^+$ and $Lyt\text{-}2^+$ cells in pathogenesis.

ACKNOWLEDGEMENTS

This work was supported in part by grants from the National Institutes of Health DK 31827. We sincerely thank Drs. Kirk Beisel and Alvaro A. Giraldo for their contribution to Table 3. Secretarial help of Allison Tokman is greatly appreciated.

REFERENCES

1. A.O. Vladutiu and N.R. Rose, Autoimmune murine thyroiditis: relation to histocompatibility (H-2) type. Science, 174:1137(1971).
2. N.R. Rose, F.J. Twarog, and A.J. Crowle. Murine thyroiditis: importance of adjuvants and mouse strain for the induction of thyriod lesions. J. Immunol. 106:698(1971).
3. V. Tomazic, N.R. Rose, and D.C. Shreffler, Autoimmune thyroiditis. IV. Localization of genetic control of the immune response. J. Immunol. 112:965(1974).
4. P.S. Esquivel, N.R. Rose, and Y.M. Kong, Induction of autoimmunity in good and poor responder mice with mouse thyroglobulin and lipopolysaccharide. J. Exp. Med. 145:1250(1977).
5. A.O. Vladutiu, and N.R. Rose, Cellular basis of the genetic control of immune responsiveness to murine thyroglobulin in mice. Cell Immunol. 17:106(1975).
6. P.S. Esquivel, Y.M. Kong, and N.R. Rose, Evidence for thyroglobulin-reactive T-cells in good responder mice. Cell. Immunol. 37:14(1978).
7. Y.M. Kong, F. Audibert, A.A. Giraldo, N.R. Rose, and L. Chedid, Effects of natural or synthetic microbial adjuvants on induction of autoimmune thyroiditis. Infect. Immun. 49:40(1985).
8. K. Beisel, Y.M. Kong, K.S.J. Babu, C.S. David, and N.R. Rose, Regulation of experimental autoimmune thyroiditis: Influence of non-H-2 genes. J. Immunogenetics 9:257(1982).
9. Y.M. Kong, The mouse model fo autoimmune thyroid disease, in: "Immunology of Endocrine Diseases". A.M. McGregor, ed., MTP Press Ltd., Lancaster (1986).
10. K.W. Beisel, C.S. David, A.A. Giraldo, Y.M. Kong, and N.R. Rose, Regulation of experimental autoimmune thyroiditis: mapping of susceptibility to the I-A subregion of the mouse H-2. Immunogenetics 15:427(1982).
11. R. Maron, J. Klein, and I.R. Cohen, Mutations at H-2K or H-2D alter immune response phenotype of autoimmune thyroiditis. Immunogenetics 15:625(1982).
12. I. Okayasu, Y.M. Kong, C.S. David, and N.R. Rose, In vitro T-lymphocyte proliferative response to mouse thyroglobulin in experimental autoimmune thyroiditis. Cell. Immunol. 61:32(1981).
13. P. Christadoss, Y.M. Kong, M. ElRehewy, N.R. Rose, and C.S. David, Genetic control of T-lymphocyte proliferative autoimmune response to thyroglobulin in mice, in:"Genetic Control of Autoimmune Diseases". N.R. Rose, P.E. Bigazzi and N.L. Warner, eds. Elsevier/North-Holland, New York (1978).
14. L.L. Simon, C.J. Krco, C.S. David, and Y.M. Kong, Characterization of the in vitro murine T-cell proliferative responses to murine and human thyroglobulins in thyroiditis-susceptible and -resistant mice. Cell. Immunol. 94:243(1985).

15. J. Salamero and J. Charreire, Syngeneic sensitization of mouse lymphocytes on monolayers of thyroid epithelial cells. IV. Correlation with H-2 haplotypes. Cell Immunol. 78:387(1983).
16. H. Braley-Mullen, M. Johnson, G.C. Sharp, and M. Kyriakos, Induction of experimental autoimmune thyroiditis in mice with in vitro activated splenic T cells. Cell. Immunol. 93,132(1985).
17. M. ElRehewy, Y.M. Kong, A.A. Giraldo, and N.R. Rose, Syngeneic thyroglobulin is immunogenic in good responder mice. Eur. J. Immunol. 11:146(1981).
18. P. Creemers, N.R. Rose, and Y.M. Kong, Experimental autoimmune thyroiditis: in vitro cytotoxic effects of T lymphocytes on thyroid monolayers. J. Exp. Med. 157:559(1983).
19. Y.M. Kong, L.L. Simon, P. Creemers, and N.R. Rose, In vitro T cell proliferation and cytotoxicity in murine autoimmune thyroiditis. Mt. Sinai J. Med. 53:46(1986).
20. L.L. Simon, J.M. Justen, A.A. Giraldo, C.J. Krco, and Y.M. Kong, Activation of cytotoxic T cells and effector cells in experimental autoimmune thyroiditis by shared determinants of mouse and human thyroglobulin. Clin. Immunol. Immunopathol. 39:345(1986).
21. Y.M. Kong, A.A. Giraldo, J.M. Justen, L.L. Simon, and B.E. Fuller, Are conserved regions on thyroglobulin thyroiditogenic? in:"The Thyroid and Autoimmunity". H.A. Drexhage and W.M. Wiersinga, eds., Elsevier Sci. Pub. B.V., Amsterdam (1986).
22. P. Creemers, A.A. Giraldo, N.R. Rose, and Y.M. Kong, T-cell subsets in the thyroids of mice developing autoimmune thyroiditis. Cell. Immunol. 87:692(1984).
23. D. Conaway, A. Giraldo, S. Cobbold, H. Waldmann, V. Potoczak, and Y.M. Kong, In situ analysis of thyroid T cell infiltrates in murine experimental autoimmune thyroiditis. Proc. Fed. Amer. Soc. Exp. Biol. 46:1375(1987).
24. Y.M. Kong, C.S. David, A.A. Giraldo, M. ElRehewy, and N.R. Rose, Regulation of autoimmune response to mouse thyroglobulin: influence of H-2D-end genes. J. Immunol. 123:15(1979).

PRISTANE-INDUCED ARTHRITIS IN MICE: GENETIC REGULATION AND IMMUNITY IN AN EXPERIMENTAL MODEL OF ARTHRITIS

Joan M. Chapdelaine, Janey D. Whalen,
James R. Seibold* and Paul H. Wooley

Immunology Dept., Ayerst Laboratories Research, Inc.
Princeton, NJ 08543 and *Div. of Rheumatology, UMDNJ
Robert Wood Johnson Medical School, New Brunswick, NJ 08903
School, New Brunswick, NJ 08903

ABSTRACT

Intraperitoneal injection of 0.5 ml of pristane (2,6,10,14-tetramethylpentadecane) caused an inflammatory arthritis in certain strains of mice. This arthritis developed in 80% - 100% of BALB/c and DBA/1 mice, but not in DBA/2, B10.RIII, B10.BR, or SWR mice, indicating regulation of susceptibility by both MHC and non-MHC genes. The BALB/c substrains also differed in their susceptibility, with the mice susceptible to ascites formation being less susceptible to arthritis and vice versa. The onset of arthritis was characterized by edema and erythema in one or more peripheral limbs. The arthritic condition persisted for over ten weeks. Several mice developed remissions and recrudescences during the course of the disease. In the majority of animals, joint deformation resulted; however, ankylosis was not detectable. Histological evaluation of the lesions showed synovial hypertrophy and pannus formation, although articular cartilage was not eroded. Periosteitis and erosions of subchondral bone were a frequent finding. Time of onset differed between strains, with DBA/1 mice developing disease 65 - 193 days after injection, and BALB/c mice, 129 - 302 days after injection. Antibodies to type II collagen were detected in sera from 75% of the arthritic mice, whereas no anti-type II antibodies developed in resistant strains. IgM RF was also detected in sera from mice immunized with pristane. Pristane-induced arthritis may represent a new model of RA.

INTRODUCTION

In recent years, several experimental models of rheumatoid arthritis have been developed, including adjuvant arthritis (AA) in rats and collagen-induced arthritis (CIA) in mice (Pearson 1956, Courteney et. al. 1980). These models have been useful in testing potential therapeutic agents and in elucidating the mechanisms involved in the disease process.

Although the injection of Freund's adjuvant into mice does not induce arthritis, it has been observed that pristane (2,6,10,14-tetramethylpentadecane) induces disease (Potter and Wax 1981, Hopkins et.al. 1984). In the course of studying plasmacytoma induction in BALB/c mice by the intraperitoneal administration of this hydrocarbon, Potter and Wax observed that many of the mice developed an arthritis of the ankle and wrist joints. Histological examination of the affected paws showed features characteristic of inflammatory arthritis (Hopkins et.al. 1984, Hopkins et.al. 1985).

We have further investigated the histological, immunological, and genetic features of this model. The data reported here indicate that pristane-induced arthritis (PIA) in mice is quite distinct from adjuvant- and collagen-induced arthritis and exhibits many similarities to rheumatoid arthritis in man.

MATERIALS AND METHODS

Mice. BALB/cByJ, BALB/cJ, DBA/1 LacJ, DBA/2J, B10.RIII, and B10.BR mice were purchased from Jackson Laboratories and maintained in our animal facility. Mice were routinely screened for pathogens and were found to be negative for Sendai virus, mouse Hepatitis virus, and mycoplasma.

Induction and Assessment of PIA. Six- to eight-week-old mice were injected intraperitoneally with 0.5 ml pristane (2,6,10,14-tetramethylpentadecane, Aldrich Chemical Co.). For one year, mice were visually examined weekly for the onset of disease. When arthritis was detected, joints were measured with a constant tension caliper (Schelltaster Syitem, Kroplin, Germany) to follow the progression of joint swelling during the course of the disease. In addition, each arthritic limb was clinically evaluated on a scale of 0 - 3, representing increasing joint swelling and erythema, visible joint distortion, and ankylosis.

Histological Evaluation. Mice were euthanized 10 weeks after the onset of disease, and the limbs were dissected out for histopathologic study. Joints were decalcified and embedded in paraffin blocks. Sections were cut along a longitudinal axis, mounted, and stained with hematoxylin and eosin.

Mitogen Responses. When mice were euthanized, spleens were removed, and single cell suspensions were made. Proliferative responses to Concanavalin A (Con A) or Lipopolysaccharide (LPS) were measured by culturing 2.5 X 10^5 spleen cells with 2.5 μg/ml of Con A or 10 μg/ml LPS in 96-well microtiter plates. After 2 days' incubation at 37°C, wells were pulsed with ^{3}H-thymidine for 18 - 24 hours, then harvested with a PHD cell harvester, and the amount of incorporation was determined.

Serological Analysis. Mice were bled for sera prior to pristane immunization and monthly thereafter. The sera were tested for antibodies to type I and type II collagen, rheumatoid factor, and total immunoglobulin.

ELISA for Anti-type I or II Collagen. Nunc-Immuno II 96-well plates were coated overnight at 4°C with 1.5 μg/well of type I collagen or 3 μg/well of type II collagen. Plates were washed with PBS/0.05% Tween-80, blocked with 0.5% BSA in PBS, and rewashed after 4 hours at 4°C. Sera from pristane-immunized mice were diluted 1:20 in PBS/0.5% BSA. A volume of 100 μl diluted sera was added to the wells and incubated overnight at room temperature. After the plates were washed, 100 μl of a goat anti-mouse Ig labelled with alkaline phosphatase was added to each well and incubated for 1 hour at 37°C. The plates were washed, then developed with 1 M paranitrophenylphosphate, and the absorbance was read at 405 nm on a microplate photometer. The levels of anti-collagen antibody in the test samples were determined by regression analysis from a standard curve.

Rheumatoid Factor Assay. Nunc-Immuno II 96-well plates were coated overnight at 4°C with either 0.4 µg/well IgG (Cappel) or 0.5% BSA in PBS. After washing with PBS/0.05% Tween-80, the plates were blocked with 0.5% BSA in PBS for 4 hours at 4°C. The plates were again washed, and 100 µl of 1:20 dilutions of sera from the pristane-immunized mice were added to to the wells. For each sera sample an IgG- and a BSA-coated well were used. Plates were incubated overnight at 4°C. After the plates were washed, goat anti-mouse IgM labelled with alkaline phosphatase was added to each well, and the plates were again incubated overnight at 4°C. Plates were washed again and developed as described above. Values for RF were obtained by subtracting background BSA binding from IgG binding.

Mancini Radial Immunodiffusion Assay for IgG. Anti IgG, 0.4 mg, (Miles Scientific/ICN) was added to 10 ml of 0.9% agar dissolved in PBS and poured onto plates. Wells were cut, and 20 µl of 1:20 dilutions of reference or sample sera were added to each well. After 24 hours, the diameters of the diffusion rings were measured, and IgG levels were calculated by regression analysis of a standard curve.

RESULTS

Clinical Characteristics of PIA. The disease onset was characterized by edema and erythema, typically of the ankle and distal hindpaw (Fig. 1). Swelling, while consistently present, was less severe than that seen with CIA. Distortion of the involved joints with subluxation and continued swelling, was noted approximately 3 to 4 weeks after onset. Ankylosis was not observed in any of the animals. One unusual finding was the appearance of visible nodules above the ankles in about 10% of the mice.

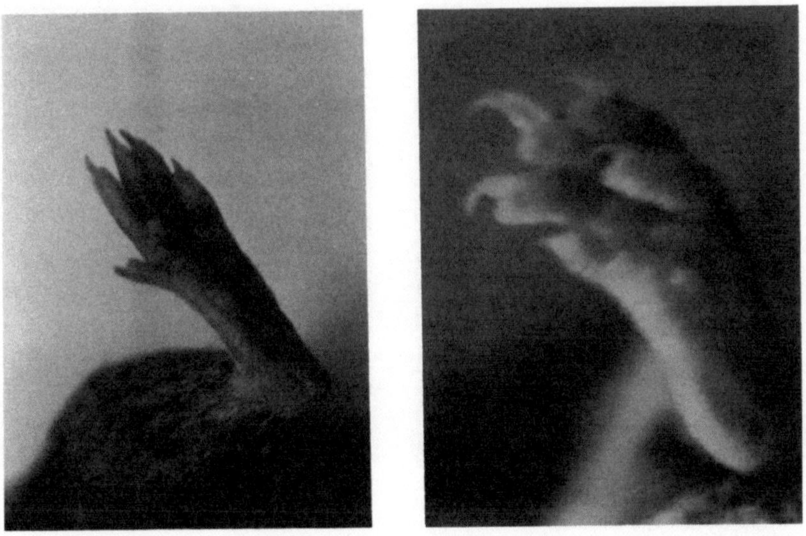

Fig. 1 Comparison of normal and PIA paw. Appearance of a normal mouse hindlimb (A) in contrast to the appearance of a pristane-induced arthritic paw (B).

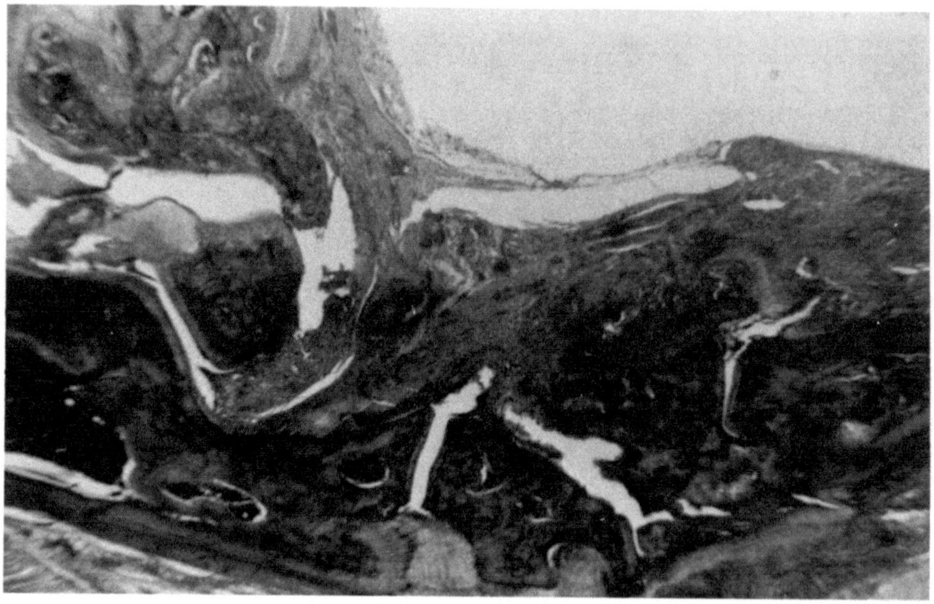

Fig. 2 Histological section of PIA paw. Inflammatory infiltration of the synovium.

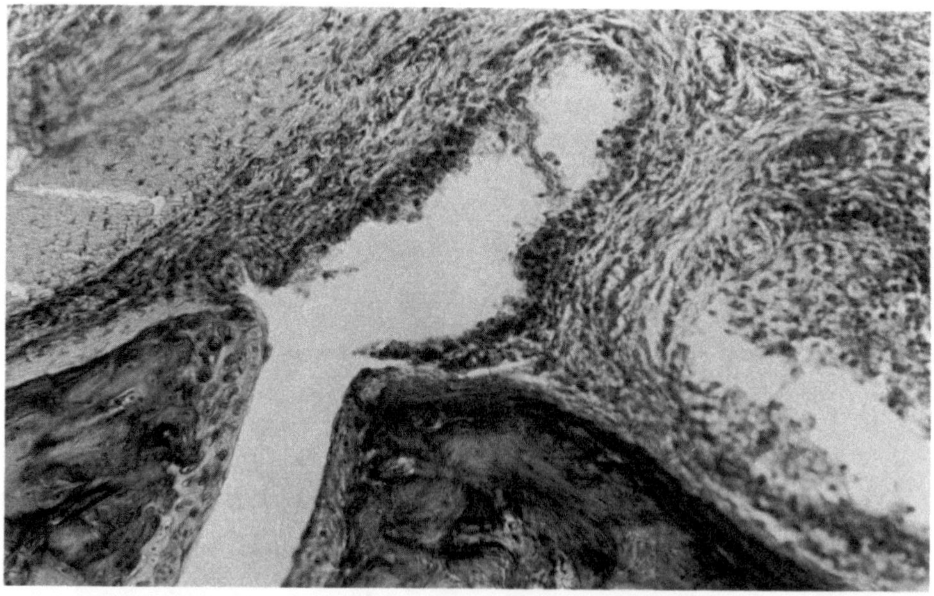

Fig. 3 Histological section of PIA paw. Synovial hypertrophy with monocyte infiltration and pannus formation.

Histopathologic Features of PIA. Figures 2 - 6 illustrate a typical sequence of evolving histopathologic changes in PIA. At early stages, active inflammatory infiltrate of the synovium consisting largely of lymphocytes and monocytes were noted, principally at the margins of the articular capsule (Fig. 2). Subsequently, synovial membrane thickening and monocyte infiltration were noted to increase and, in some cases, pannus-like projections were formed (Fig. 3). Articular cartilage appeared uninvolved but marginal erosions of subchondral bone were frequently noted (Fig. 4). Progressive infiltration of inflammatory pannus into contiguous periosteum and surrounding soft tissues was noted. Subchondral erosions progessively worsened and lead to undermining and destruction of articular cartilage (Fig. 4) and obliteration of the joint.

The nodules of the dorsal hindleg were characterized by necrotic central regions surrounded by palisading arrangements of mononuclear cells, highly reminiscent of human rheumatoid nodules (Fig. 5,6).

Genetic Regulation of Susceptibility. Several strains of mice were studied in this model to determine whether susceptibility to the disease was genetically controlled (Table 1). DBA/1 LacJ and BALB/c mice were the only strains which developed arthritis. Even one year after immunization with pristane, DBA/2, B10.RIII, B10.BR, and SWR mice were clinically free of disease. Since DBA/1 and DBA/2 mice, which are very similar except for H-2, differ in susceptibility, it appears that susceptibility to PIA may be partially controlled by MHC. However, BALB/c mice, which are $H\text{-}2^d$, as are DBA/2 mice, were susceptible, suggesting that there are other non-MHC genes involved in the regulation of the disease.

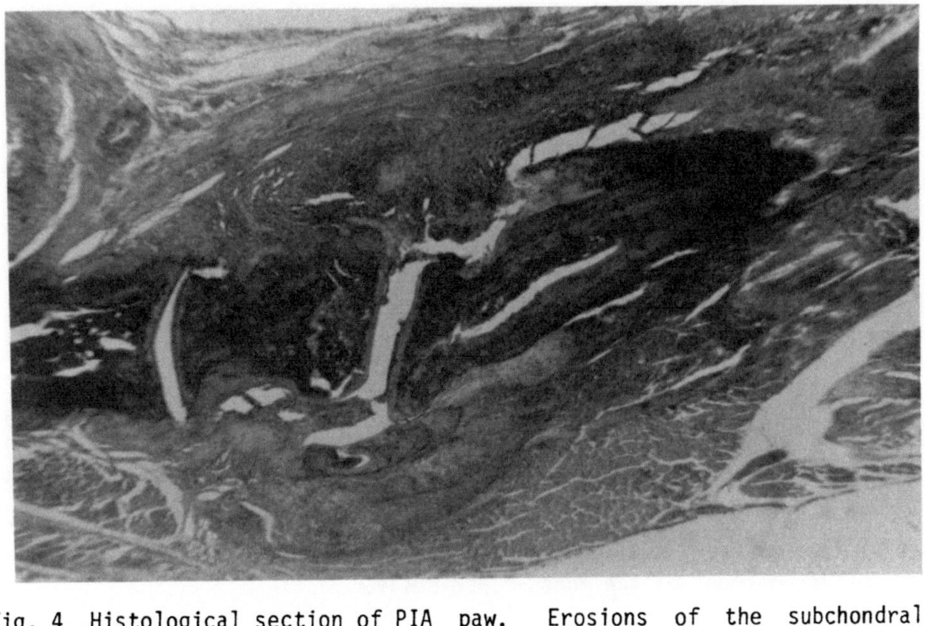

Fig. 4 Histological section of PIA paw. Erosions of the subchondral bone, periosteitis, and destruction of the articular cartilage.

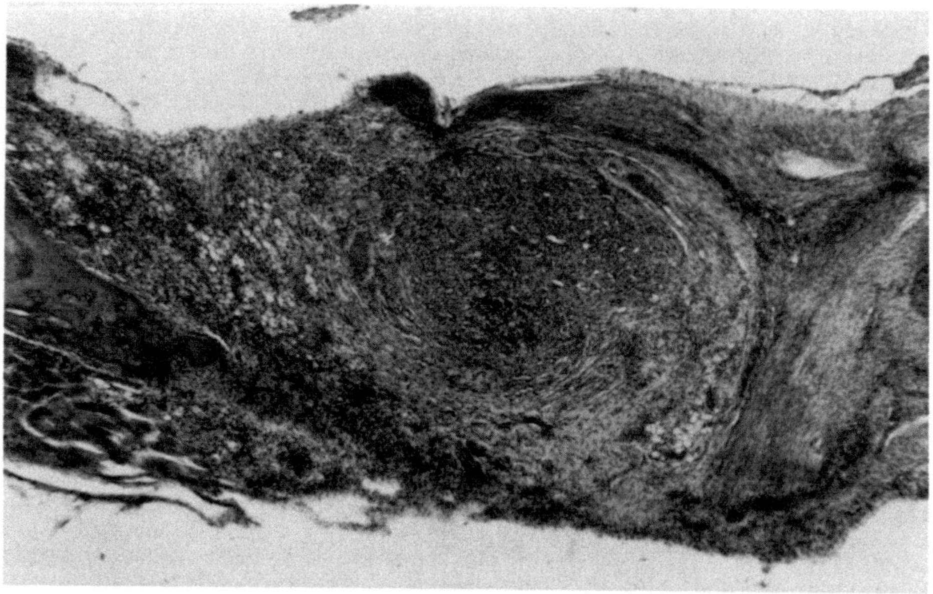

Fig. 5 Histological section of nodule from a PIA paw. The nodules are characterized by a necrotic central region surrounded by a palisading arrangement of mononuclear cells.

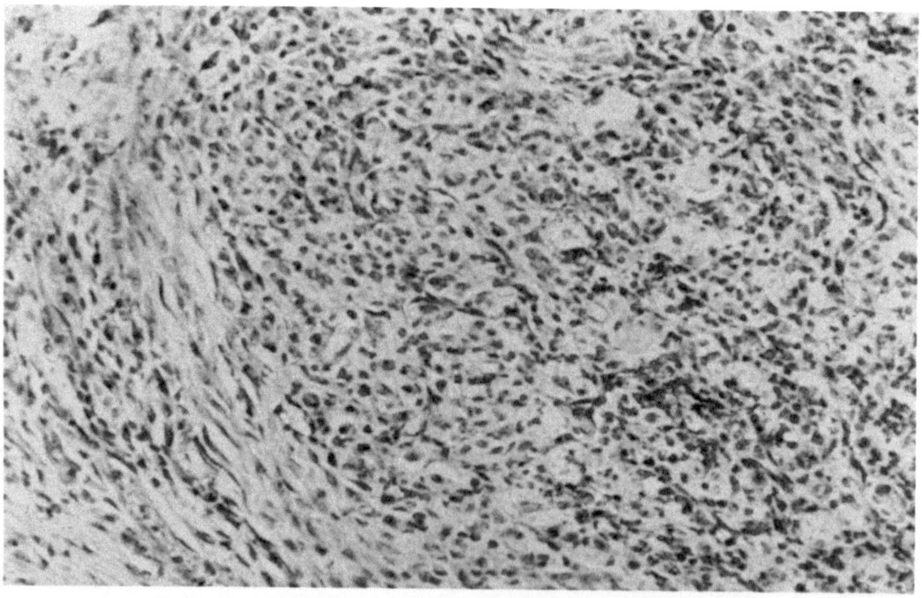

Fig. 6 Histological section of the rheumatoid-like nodule. Palisading arrangement of the mononuclear cells.

Table 1

STRAINS OF MICE TESTED IN PIA

Strain	H-2 Haplotype	Igh-1	Susceptibility PIA	Susceptibility CIA
DBA/1	q	c	+	+
BALB/c	d	a	+	-
B10.RIII	r	b	-	+
DBA/2	d	c	-	-
B10.BR	k	b	-	-
SWR	q	c	-	-

There also appear to be substrain differences, with BALB/c ByJ mice less susceptible than BALB/c J mice (Table 2, Fig. 7). As Potter and Wax (1981) noted, mice that were susceptible to the development of ascites did not develop arthritis and vice versa.

The incidence of disease in susceptible strains was 82% - 100% (Table 2); however, the onset of disease differed between strains (Figure 7). DBA/1 mice developed disease 65 - 193 days after immunization with pristane, while in BALB/c mice onset varied from 129 - 302 days after injection.

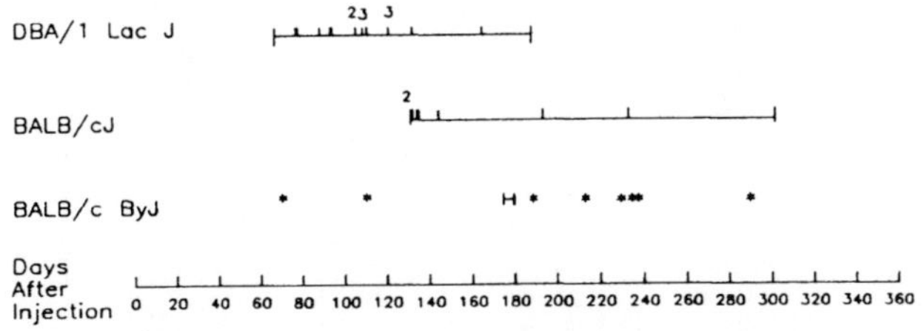

Fig. 7 Onset of PIA. Each hatch mark indicates the onset of arthritis in a mouse. The numbers over the hatch marks indicate the number of onsets on that day. * indicates when an animal died due to ascites.

Table 2

INCIDENCE OF DISEASE

Strain	Arthritis	Ascites	Total
BALB/c J	9	0	9
BALB/c By J	2	8	10
DBA/1 Lac J	18	0	22

Immunological Profile. The sera from the pristane-immunized mice were assayed for a number of auto-antibodies (Table 3). Antibodies to type I collagen were found in the sera from all strains, although not all mice had detectable titers. Type II collagen antibodies were also found in these sera; however, only the susceptible strains and SWR/J mice were positive. Variability in titers between mice within a strain was also observed for these antibodies. In addition, IgM RF was also detected in some mice of some strains. When total IgG levels were measured, the pristane-immunized mice were found to be hypergammaglobulinemic.

Proliferative responses of the spleen cells from these mice to Con A and LPS were also measured. Three to nine weeks after immunization, the response to Con A was greatly reduced (Fig. 8). The response to LPS was also reduced, but to a lesser extent. However, when responses were measured twelve weeks or more after the onset of the disease, the proliferative responses had returned to normal.

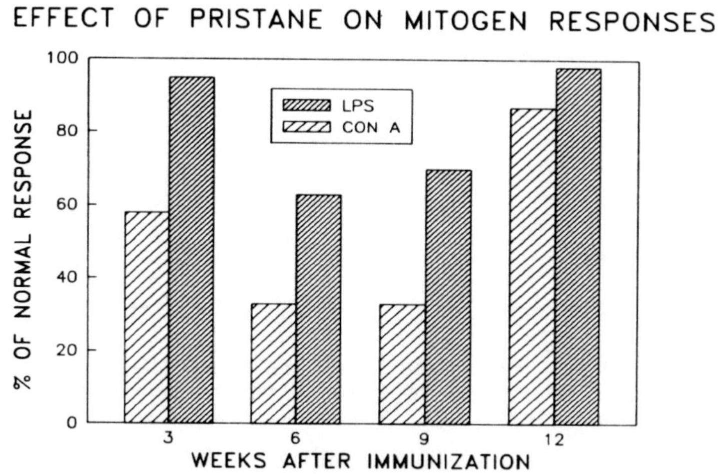

Fig. 8 Effect of pristane immunization on mitogen responses. At each time point, 3 - 4 mice were euthanized, and their spleen cells were individually assayed for response to Con A and LPS. Age-matched control mice were also assayed at each point. Mean responses of the pristane-immunized mice were calculated and compared with the responses seen in the control mice.

Table 3

IMMUNOLOGICAL ABNORMALITIES FOLLOWING PRISTANE INJECTION

Strain	Rheumatoid Factor	Hypergamma-globulinemia	anti-type I collagen	anti-type II collagen
BALB/c	+	+	+	+
DBA/1	-	+	+	+
DBA/2	-	+	+	-
B10.RIII	-	+	+	-
B10.BR	+	+	+	-
SWR	+	+	+	+

DISCUSSION

Pristane-induced arthritis in mice has clinical and histopathologic features similar to those of rheumatoid arthritis and appears to represent a new and useful model of disease. Disease onset is predictable and rheumatoid-like, with synovial inflammation and proliferation progressing to joint instability and distortion. Unlike collagen-induced arthritis, joint ankylosis is not observed. Of great interest is the occurrence, macroscopically and histopathologically, of rheumatoid-like nodules, which have previously not been noted in experimental models of arthritis. Further study is underway to characterize the incidence and natural history of this model better and to define better the sequence of histopathologic changes.

The pattern of strain susceptibility suggests that both MHC and non-MHC genes may influence the development PIA. Several other strains are currently being studied in this model to elucidate further the genetic control of susceptibility. Recently, Bedwell et. al. (1987) reported that the incidence of disease was significantly higher in CBA/Igb mice than in the allotypic congenic strain CBA/H mice, suggesting that a gene linked to the heavy chain immunoglobulin locus controls the development of the disease. However, this finding is not supported by our data. DBA/1 and DBA/2 mice are identical at the Igh-1 locus, yet only DBA/1 mice developed arthritis when immunized with pristane.

Sera from mice immunized with pristane contained autoantibodies to a number of different antigens. Unlike collagen-induced arthritis or adjuvant arthritis, antibodies to both type I and type II collagen could be detected in pristane arthritic animals. In addition, these mice made rheumatoid factor. The presence of RF, anti-type I antibodies, and anti-DNA antibodies makes this model most attractive since these antibodies are also found in sera from patients with rheumatoid arthritis. However, it should be noted that, as in RA, no correlation could be made between the presence of any of the antibodies and the disease, since even the strains that did not develop the disease often had antibody titers. Whether or not any of these antibodies plays a role in the disease is still not clear. However, experiments by Bedwell et. al. (1987) indicate an immunological involvement in the disease process. These experiments showed that irradiated mice injected with pristane failed to develop the disease and that reconstitution of these mice with normal bone marrow cells restored susceptibility.

This new model therefore possesses several unique features also found in RA. Hence, pristane-induced arthritis may prove to be a useful model in which to study the genetic and immunological factors involved in RA.

REFERENCES

Bedwell, A. E., Elson, C. J. and Hinton, C. E.: Immunological involvement in the pathogenesis of pristane-induced arthritis. Scand. J. Immunol. 25: 393-398, 1987.

Courtenay, J. S., Dallman, M. J., Dayan, A. D., Martin, A. and Mosedale, B.: Immunization against heterologous type II collagen induces arthritis in mice. Nature 283: 666-668, 1980.

Hopkins, S. J., Freemont, A. J. and Jayson, M. I. V.: Pristane-induced arthritis in BALB/c mice. I. Clinical and histological features of the arthropathy. Rheumatol. Int. 5: 21-28, 1984.

Hopkins, S. J., Freemont, A. J. and Jayson, M. I. V.: Pristane-induced arthritis in BALB/c mice. Current Topics in Micro. and Immunol. 122: 213-220, 1985.

Pearson, C. M.: Development of arthritis, peri-arthritis and periostitis in rats given adjuvants. Proc. Soc. Exp. Biol. Med. 91: 95-101, 1956.

Potter, M. and Wax, J. S.: Genetics of susceptibility to pristane-induced plasmacytomas in BALB/cAn: Reduced susceptibility in BALB/cJ with a brief description of pristane-induced arthritis. J. Immunol. 127: 1591-1595, 1981.

ROLE OF MHC GENES AND T CELL RECEPTOR GENES IN COLLAGEN INDUCED ARTHRITIS IN MICE

Subhashis Banerjee, Tariq M. Haqqi, Harvinder S. Luthra and Chella S. David

Mayo Clinic and Mayo Medical School, Rochester, MN 55905

Type II collagen induced arthritis (CIA) is an experimental model of autoimmune inflammatory polyarthritis sharing certain similarities with human rheumatoid arthritis (1). It is characterized by redness, swelling and deformity (Fig. 1) in the peripheral joints, following a latent period varying from 3 to 8 weeks after intradermal immunization with native type II collagen (from homologous or heterologous species) in adjuvant. The disease has been described in rats (2), mice (3), and in primates (4). Type II collagen is a "sequestered" antigen present in only a few sites in the body including hyaline cartilage, ears, and vitreous humor of the eye (5). An autoimmune reaction to the type II collagen present in hyaline cartilage of peripheral joints is thought to be the primary etiologic factor in the disease process. Histologically (5), the disease is characterized by the initial deposition of fibrin, followed by infiltration of the synovium with mononuclear and polymorphonuclear cells with synovial hyperplasia and pannus formation (Fig. 2). Cartilage and bone erosions then follow progressing onto the total destruction of the joint with deposition of fibrous tissue and subsequent ankylosis. The acute phase of the disease is thought to be initiated by the deposition of pathogenic anti-type II collagen antibodies on the cartilage followed by activation and deposition of complement in the affected joints, as shown by immunofluorescence (6). Animals depleted of complement fail to develop the disease (7). The acute phase is followed by a chronic destructive phase in which numerous T cells, mostly of helper/inducer phenotype, can be found infiltrating into the synovium (8,9). The central role of T cells in the disease process is shown by the fact that the antibody responses to type II collagen are themselves T-cell dependent (8,10). In addition, nude rats are resistant to the induction of CIA (8). The disease can be passively transferred albeit in a mild and transient form by antibodies (11), as well as by cells (12), T-cell lines and clones (13) derived from arthritic animals. The type II collagen molecule is a triple helix of $\alpha 1(II)$ subunits each having a M.W. approximately 95 kD (14). The presence of specific arthritogenic epitopes on the molecule has been demonstrated earlier (15). At least one of the arthritogenic epitopes has been localized to the cyanogen bromide cleavage fragment 11 (CB11 peptide) of Type II collagen obtained from two different species [chick (16) and bovine (17)]. This peptide has a M.W. of about 25 kD (18). Studies are underway to narrow down the arthritogenic region further on the CB11 peptide.

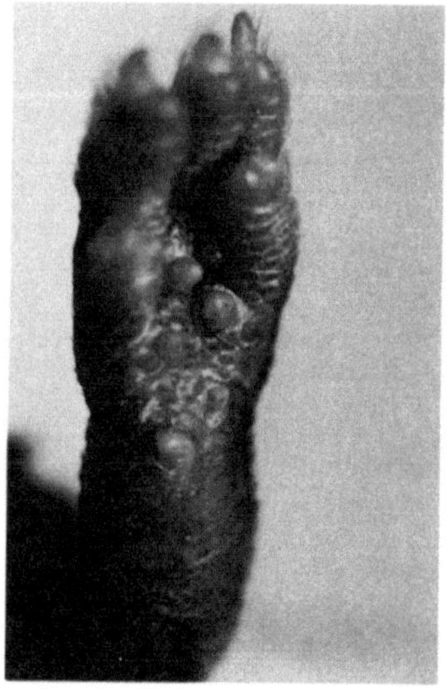

Fig.1 Deformed arthritic rear paw in a mouse immunized with type-II collagen.

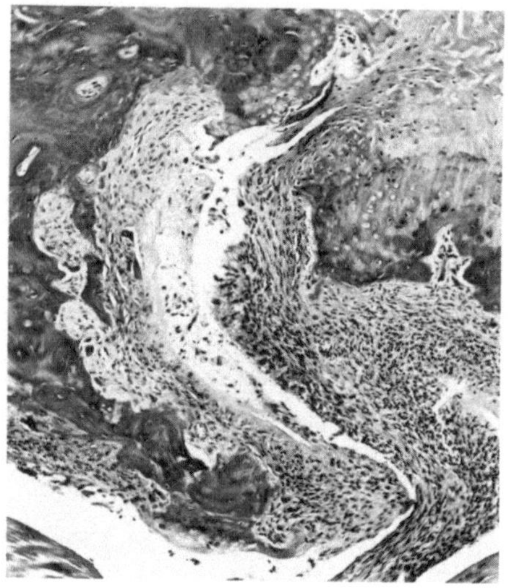

Fig.2 Histopathology of a rear paw with CIA showing mononuclear cell infiltration, and cartilage and bone erosions.

The susceptibility to CIA has earlier been shown to be linked to the MHC regions in mice (3) and rats (19). In mice, only $H\text{-}2^q$ and $H\text{-}2^r$ strains develop this disease, whereas mice of other haplotypes are resistant. This has been demonstrated using various inbred strains and with B10 congenic strains with varying haplotypes. The susceptibility to CIA in $H\text{-}2^q$ and $H\text{-}2^r$ also has been shown to be dependent on the species source of collagen (15). Thus, while B10.Q ($H\text{-}2^q$) and B10.RIII ($H\text{-}2^r$) are both susceptible to arthritis induced with bovine Type II collagen (53% and 73% incidence respectively), B10.Q mice are relatively resistant to porcine type II collagen arthritis (11% incidence) while being susceptible to chick type II collagen arthritis (84% incidence) and conversely B10.RIII mice are resistant to chick type II collagen arthritis (0% incidence) but susceptible to arthritis induced by porcine Type II collagen (95% incidence). This strongly suggests the presence of at least two arthritogenic epitopes located on different sites on chick and porcine type II collagen molecules. The susceptibility to CIA has been further mapped to the I-A subregion in $H\text{-}2^q$ mice using various B10 congenic recombinant strains with crossovers within the H-2 complex (20). Thus, mice with the "q" allele in the I-A subregion, such as B10.T(6R) ($K^qA^qE^qD^d$), B10.DA ($K^qA^qE^qD^s$) and B10.RQB1 ($K^qA^qE^qD^b$) are susceptible to CIA, whereas mice with the "q" allele in the other regions of the H-2 but not in the I-A subregion, such as B10.BYR ($K^qA^kE^kD^b$), B10.AQR ($K^qA^kE^kD^d$), B10.AKM ($K^kA^kE^kD^q$) and B10.MBR ($K^bA^kE^kD^q$) are resistant (Table 1). In addition it has been shown that pretreatment with specific anti-Ia antibodies can suppress or delay the onset of CIA in susceptible strains of mice (21). For instance, pretreatment of B10.Q mice with monoclonal antibody 25-9-17 reactive to $I\text{-}A^q$ causes a decreased incidence (32%) of CIA as compared to a control incidence of 83% ($p<0.01$). Similarly, pretreatment of B10.RIII mice ($H\text{-}2^r$) with M1 112 antibodies reactive to $I\text{-}A^r$ and $I\text{-}E^r$ causes a suppression in incidence of CIA (29%) as compared to controls (87%) ($p<0.001$). This demonstrates the central role of Ia antigens in the induction of pathogenic immune responses in CIA. Studies of susceptibility in F_1 crosses between parents of (susceptible x resistant) haplotypes such as B10.Q x B10.M ($H\text{-}2^f$) showed that in most cases the susceptibility to CIA is inherited as a dominant trait.

Table I

Mapping of CIA susceptibility to the I-A Subregion in Mice

Recombinant Strains	K	I-A	I-E	S	D	Percent Incidence of Arthritis
B10.DA	q	q	q	q	s	65
B10.T(6R)	q	q	q	q	d	55
B10.RQB-1	q	q	q	q	b	75
B10.RQF-1	q	q	q	q	f	70
B10.AKM	k	k	k	k	q	0
B10.RBQ-1	b	b	b	.	q	0
B10.MBR	b	k	k	k	q	0
B10.AQR	q	k	k	d	d	0
B10.BYR	q	k	k	d	b	0

When the studies on H-2^q mice were further extended onto mice with varying backgrounds, it was observed that unlike all other H-2^q strains which were susceptible to CIA, SWR mice (H-2^q) were totally resistant to the induction of disease (Table II). Further, studies on crosses between SWR and other susceptible strains of mice showed that this resistance was a dominant phenomenon with varying degrees of penetrance. Thus, F_1 crosses of (SWR x B10.Q) and (SWR x DBA/1) were relatively resistant to CIA, and (SWR x B10.RIII)F_1 mice had a lower incidence of CIA as compared with the susceptible B10.RIII parent (22). This suggested that either certain important disease permissive genes were absent in the SWR background, or certain disease suppressive genes were present in the SWR background. A role of non-MHC genes in the susceptibility to CIA has similarly been demonstrated in rats (23).

Recently, Behlke and coworkers (24) discovered that SWR mice along with three other inbred strains of mice are T cell receptor (TCR) gene mutants with a large deletion (close to 50% of the known genes) in the V_β gene segments coding for the variable region of the beta chain of the T cell receptor (V_βTCR). The MHC-restricted T cell receptor is a disulfide-linked heterodimer composed of two chains α and β, each having a M.W. of approximately 40-50 kD (25). Each chain consists of variable and constant domains, similar to the immunoglobulin molecule. The specificity of the TCR toward the antigen and MHC is controlled by the variable domains of the α and β chains (26). The variable domains are encoded for by variable (V), diversity (D) and joining (J) region gene segments for β chains and by V and J region gene segments for α chains. The β chain genes are located on chromosome 6 and α chain genes on chromosome 14. Figure 3 illustrates the deletion in the germline V_β TCR genes in SWR mice (27), as compared to the BALB/c germline which has the wild type V_β TCR genes. The deleted V_β genes in SWR are 9, 11, 12, 13 and the 5 and 8 family genes. There are no additional V_β genes to replace those that are deleted in these mice (24). The importance of T cell mediated immune responses in the pathogenesis of CIA has been alluded to earlier. There is increasing evidence in the literature of the restricted usage of V gene segments of the β (and α) chains of the TCR in T cell responses specific to haptens (28) and small antigens (29). The discovery of a large deletion in SWR mice, in an already restricted V_β gene repertoire in mice (24) led us to postulate that these mice were resistant to the induction of arthritis with type II collagen, possibly due to a lack of cellular immune responses to the arthritogenic epitope(s) (15).

Table II
Effect of Non-H-2 Genes on CIA in Mice

Strain	Haplotype	Background	Percent Incidence of Arthritis
B10.Q	$H\text{-}2^q$	C57BL	75
DBA/1	$H\text{-}2^q$	DBA	70
BUB	$H\text{-}2^q$	BUB	77
SWR	$H\text{-}2^q$	Swiss	0

To demonstrate the possible role of T cell receptor (TCR) genes in CIA, crosses were made between two CIA resistant parents, B10 (with the resistant H-2 haplotype - $H\text{-}2^b$, but with the wild type TCR genes) and SWR (with the susceptible H-2 haplotype - $H\text{-}2^q$, but with the mutant form of TCR genes). The mice in the B10 backcrosses, and F_2 hybrids were serotyped for the presence of $H\text{-}2^q$ genes (homozygous or heterozygous) by conventional hemagglutination tests using standard antisera. The $H\text{-}2^q$ mice in these crosses were chosen for the study as it was known earlier that mice homozygous for $H\text{-}2^b$ were resistant to CIA (3). The mice were immunized with 100 µg of native bovine type II collagen in complete Freund's adjuvant intradermally in the base of the tail, boosted with 100 µg of the collagen in incomplete Freund's adjuvant after 3 weeks, and followed up for a period up to 5 months following primary immunization. These were monitored regularly for appearance of arthritis and the course of the disease was ascertained by the measurement of paw thickness with constant tension calipers, and by the appearance of deformity and ankylosis in the affected joint(s). The severity of the disease was graded as per scoring system used earlier (3): grade 1 - redness and swelling in paws, grade 2 - deformity in paws, and grade 3 - ankylosis in the affected joints. Table III summarizes the results showing the appearance of arthritis in all the crosses (30). As expected, mice of both parental strains were totally resistant to CIA.

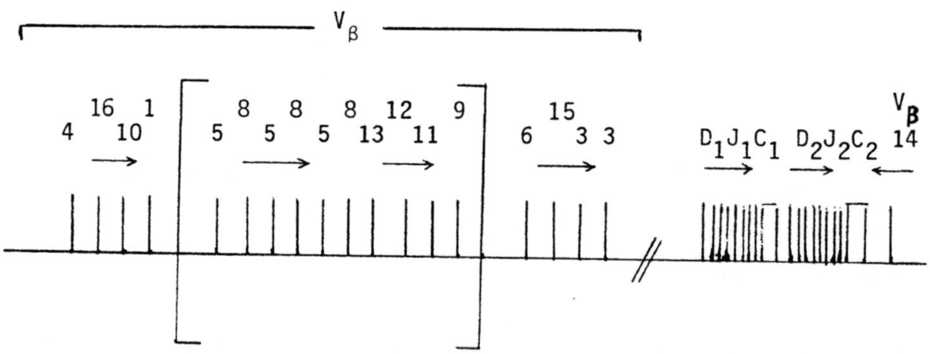

Fig.3 Germline organization of TCR β-chain genes (not drawn to scale) in mouse. The genes are denoted by vertical bars or boxes. The deleted genes in SWR are marked by brackets. Horizontal arrows show transcriptional orientation.

Table III

Incidence of CIA in (SWR x B10) Crosses with $H\text{-}2^q$

	F_1 Hybrid	F_2 Hybrid	B10 Backcross	SWR Backcross
Percent incidence of arthritis	17 (4/24)	52 (13/25)	68 (17/25)	33 (6/18)
Sex ratio of arthritic mice M:F	1:3	10:3	10:7	4:2
$H\text{-}2^{q/q}:H\text{-}2^{q/b}$ ratio of arthritic mice	0:4	6:7	0:17	1:5

To investigate the segregation of V_β TCR genes with disease, the F_2 hybrid mice with arthritis were screened for the presence of $F23.1^+$ T cells in their peripheral blood. F23.1 is an anti-allotypic TCR monoclonal antibody (31) raised in a V_β TCR deletion mutant mouse strain (C57L) after immunization with T cells from a mouse with wild type TCR (Balb.B). This has been shown (32) to stain T cells utilizing the $V_\beta8$ family genes in the β chain of their TCR. Since $V_\beta8$ genes are amongst the 10 genes deleted in SWR, the presence or absence of $F23.1^+$ T cells in the mice was considered to be a useful marker for the absence or presence respectively of the SWR-like deletion in the V_β genes in the respective mice. This was thought to be true provided no recombination had occurred in the germline between the various V_β TCR genes in the F_1 mice at the meiotic stages. Further, since the TCR genes are known to be allelically excluded (33) only half of the number of peripheral blood lymphocytes were expected to stain with this marker in the heterozygous state as compared to the homozygous state. The F23.1 phenotype was ascertained (30) by dual fluorescence flow cytometry (FACS IV) on peripheral blood lymphocytes (from individual mice) purified over a Lymphopaque gradient (Nyegaard Labs, Oslo, Norway) and stained with rat anti-mouse Thy 1.2 with fluoresceinated mouse anti-rat immunoglobulin, and biotinylated F23.1 with streptavidin-phycoerythrin. The percentage of peripheral blood T cells staining with F23.1 was 18% in B10 mice (homozygous for wild type TCR), 0% in SWR mice (TCR mutant) and 10% in the (B10 x SWR)F_1 mice (heterozygous for the wild type TCR). The values in the individual mice in the F_2 hybrids were around 18% suggesting that they were $V_\beta8$ homozygous, 10% suggesting that they were $V_\beta8$ heterozygous, or negative suggesting that they lacked the $V_\beta8$ genes altogether. Table IV summarizes the results of the phenotyping of the F_2 hybrids with arthritis. In the mice which were homozygous for $H\text{-}2^q$ (and were thus similar to SWR), a total of 6 mice were found to have arthritis and all of them had at least one dose of $V_\beta8$ genes as determined by heterozygosity or homozygosity for $V_\beta8$ genes. Thus, there seemed to be a high correlation of the presence of $V_\beta8$ genes and disease in these F_2 hybrid mice with arthritis. Two mice out of 7 $H\text{-}2^{q/b}$ mice with arthritis in the F_2 generation were, however, negative for this phenotype. To rule out the presence of a recombinational "hot spot" within the V_β TCR genes, the tail DNA of these mice are being analyzed by Southern Blot hybridization using specific V_β probes for the presence of V_β genes derived from B10 which are absent in SWR. Preliminary evidence suggests that the above

Table IV

F23.1 ($V_\beta 8$) Phenotype of F_2 Hybrids with Arthritis

MHC	F23.1 Homozygous	F23.1 Heterozygous	F23.1 Negative
$H-2^{q/q}$	2	4	0
$H-2^{q/b}$	1	4	2

"F23.1 negative" mice probably have at least one B10 derived V_β gene in their germline not present in SWR mice. There is also the possibility that the occurrence of $V_\beta 8$ negative mice in the F_2 arthritic mice which were $H-2^{q/b}$, may be due to a presentation of the arthritogenic epitope(s) on type II collagen by hybrid Ia antigens (34), viz. hybrid $I-A^{q/b}$ molecules. These could present antigens to a different set of T cells with TCR which utilize V_β genes present in SWR. Thus, these mice could have the V_β TCR deletion and yet get arthritis. The situation in these mice may therefore not be entirely analogous to that in SWR mice which are homozygous for $H-2^q$. Studies are currently in progress to study the segregation of the V_β TCR genes in the $H-2^{q/q}$ homozygous SWR backcross mice with arthritis to confirm the above findings.

These findings suggest that some of the V_β TCR genes missing in SWR may be important in susceptibility to CIA, as outlined diagrammatically in Figure 4. In the prototypic B10.Q strain which is susceptible to CIA, the arthritogenic epitope on Type II collagen is presented normally by the $I-A^q$ molecules on the antigen presenting cells to the TCR on T cells which can recognize this combination, since B10.Q mice have a complete set of V_β TCR genes. The pathogenic immune response is thus initiated leading to the disease. In B10 mice on the other hand, though T cells of the correct specificity are present, $I-A^b$ molecules cannot present the arthritogenic epitope and therefore the pathogenic immune response is not initiated. Hence, B10 mice are resistant to CIA. In SWR mice by contrast, though $I-A^q$ molecules could present the arthritogenic epitope normally, T cells could fail to recognize it because the TCR necessary for the recognition requires the usage of certain V_β genes in the β chain of TCR which are deleted in SWR. Hence, the SWR mice could be resistant to CIA due to this reason. Further studies are underway with crosses between (C3H x SWR) and (A/Sn x SWR) for studying susceptibility to CIA, to confirm the above findings in the (B10 x SWR) crosses. In addition, crosses between SWR and C57L ($H-2^b$, but with a deletion in the V_β TCR exactly similar (24) to that of SWR) are being made and screened for induction of disease with type II collagen. If the V_β TCR genes missing in SWR (and also missing in C57L) do play a role in CIA susceptibility, then none of the $H-2^{q/q}$ mice in the F_2 hybrids from the latter crosses should develop arthritis. This would further confirm the role of certain V_β TCR genes in the susceptibility to CIA in $H-2^q$ homozygous mice.

In summary, the susceptibility to CIA which is a model of autoimmune disease, has been shown to be linked to the H-2 complex and in particular to the I-A subregion. The role of Ia molecules in the pathogenesis of this disease has been demonstrated. The presence of select epitopes on the Type II collagen molecule necessary for its arthritogenic activity has also been shown. There is now some preliminary evidence that certain T cell receptor genes may also be important in the pathogenesis of CIA, besides MHC antigens.

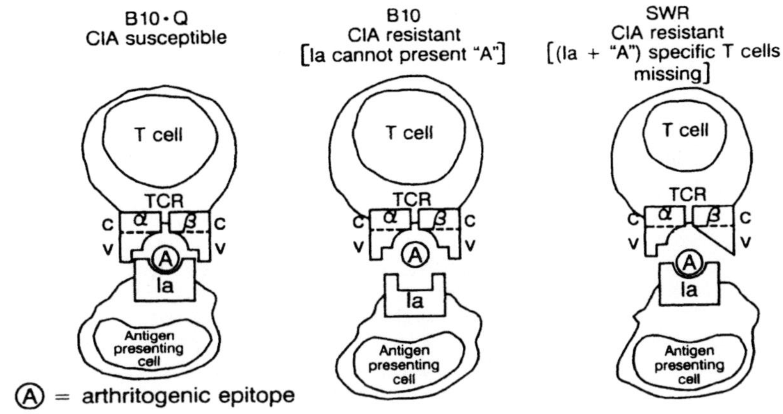

Fig.4 Diagrammatic representation of immune responses to the arthritogenic epitope on type II collagen

REFERENCES

1. Trentham DE. Collagen arthritis as a relevant model for rheumatoid arthtitis. Evidence pro and con. Arthritis Rheum. 25:911-916, 1982.
2. Trentham DE, Townes AS, Kang AH. Autoimmunity to type II collagen: An experimental model of arthritis. J. Exp. Med. 146:857-868, 1977.
3. Wooley PH, Luthra HS, Stuart JM, David CS. Type II collagen induced arthritis in mice. 1. Major histocompatibility complex (I-region) linkage and antibody correlates. J. Exp. Med. 154:688-700, 1981.
4. Cathcart ES, Hayes KC, Gonnerman WA, Lazzari AA, Franzblau C. Experimental arthritis in a non-human primate. I. Induction by bovine type II collagen. Lab Investig. 54:26-31, 1986.
5. Stuart J. Collagen autoimmune arthritis. Ann. Rev. Immunol. 2:199-218, 1984.
6. Kerwar SS, Englert ME, McReynolds RA, Landes MJ, Lloyd JM, Oronsky AL, Wilson FJ. Type II collagen-induced arthritis. Studies with purified anti-collagne immunoglobulin. Arthritis Rheum. 26:1120-1131, 1983.
7. Morgan K, Clague RB, Shaw MJ, Firth SA, Twose TM, Lennox-Holt PJ: Native type II collagen-induced arthritis in the rat. The effect of complement depletion by cobra venom factor. Arthritis Rheum. 24:1356-1362, 1981.
8. Klareskog L, Holmdahl R, Larsson E, Wigzell M. Role of T lymphocytes in collagen II induced arthritis in rats. Clin. Exp. Immunol. 51:117-125, 1983.
9. Holmdahl R, Rubin K, Klareskog L, Dencker L, Gustafsson G and Larsson E. Appearance of different lymphoid cells in synovial tissue and in peripheral blood during the course of collagen-II-induced arthritis in rats. Scand. J. Immunol. 21:197-204, 1985.
10. Nowack H, Hahn E, and Timpl R. Specificity of the antibody response in inbred mice to bovine type I and type II collagen. Immunology 29:621-628, 1975.
11. Wooley PH, Luthra HS, Krco CJ, Stuart JM, David CS. Type II collagen-induced arthritis in mice. II. Passive transfer and suppression by intravenous injection of anti-type II collagen antibody or free native type II collagen. Arthritis Rheum. 27:1010-1017, 1984.

12. Trentham DE, Dynesius RA, David JR. Passive transfer by cells of type II collagen-induced arthritis in rats. J. Clin. Invest. 62:359-365, 1978.
13. Holmdahl R, Klareskog L, Rubin K, Larsson E, Wigzell H. T lymphocytes in collagen II-induced arthritis in mice. Characterizaiton of arthritogenic collagen II-specific T-cell lines and clones. Scand. J. Immunol. 22:295-305, 1985.
14. Kuhn K, Timpl R. Collagens: Molecular and antigenic structure. In: Myelofibrosis and the Biology of Connective Tissue. Alan R. Liss, Inc. New York (1984). pp. 45-59.
15. Wooley PH, Luthra HS, Griffith MM, Stuart JM, Huse A, David CS. Type II collagen induced arthritis in mice. IV. Variations in imunogenetic regulation provide evidence for multiple arthritogenic epitopes on the collagen molecule. J. Immunol. 135:2443-2451, 1985.
16. Terato K, Hasty Ka, Cremer MA, Stuart JM, Townes AS, Kang AH. Collagen-induced arthritis in mice. Localization of an arthritogenic determinant to a fragment of the type II collagen molecule. J. Exp. Med. 162:637-646, 1985.
17. Englert ME, Ferguson KM, Suarez CR, Sapp TM, Oronsky AL, Kerwar SS. Type II collagen arthritis: Identification of arthritogenic epitopes using fractionated anti-collagen IgG. Cell. Immunol. 105:447-453, 1987.
18. Miller EJ. Isolation and characterization of the cyanogen bromide peptides from the α1(II) chain of chick cartilage collagen. Biochemistry 10:3030-3035, 1971.
19. Griffiths MM, Eichwald RJ, Martin JM, Smith CB, Dewitt CW. Immunogenetic control of experimental type II collagen induced arthritis. I. Susceptibility and resistance among inbred strains of rats. Arthritis Rheum. 24:871-879, 1981.
20. Huse A, Wooley PH, Luthra HS, Stuart JM, David CS. New recombinants confirm mapping of susceptibility to type II collagen induced arthritis to the I-A subregion in mice. Fed. Proc. 43:1820, 1984.
21. Wooley PH, Luthra HS, Lafuse WP, Huse A, Stuart JM, David CS. Type II collagen-induced arthritis in mice. III. Suppression of arthritis by using monoclonal and polyclonal anti-Ia antisera. J. Immunol. 134:2366-2374, 1985.
22. Luthra HS, Wooley PH, Dillon AM, Singh SK, Lafuse WP, Krco CJ, Huse A, Stuart JM, Griffiths MM, David CS. Immunogenetics of collagen-induced arthritis (CIA) in mice. A model of autoimmune disease. Ann. N.Y. Acad. Sci. 475:361-363, 1986.
23. Griffiths MM, DeWitt CW. Genetic control of collagen-induced arthritis in rats: The immune response to type II collagen among susceptible and resistant strains and evidence for multiple gene control. J. Immunol. 132:2830-2836, 1984.
24. Behlke MA, Chou HS, Huppl K, Loh DY. Murine T-cell receptor mtuants with deletions of β-chain variable region genes. Proc. Natl. ACad. Sci. USA 83:767-771, 1986.
25. Kronenberg M, Siu G, Hood LE, Shastri N. The molecular genetics of the T-cell antigen receptor and T-cell antigen recognition. Ann. Rev. Immunol. 4:529-591, 1986.
26. Yague J, White J, Coleclough C, Kappler J, Palmer E, Marrack P. The T cell receptor: The α and β chains define idiotype, and antigen and MHC specificity. Cell 42:81-87, 1985.
27. Chou HS, Nelson CA, Godambe SA, Chaplin DD, Loh DY. Germline organization of the murine T-cell receptor β-chain genes. Science 238:545-548, 1987.
28. Hochgeschwender U, Weltzien HU, Eichmann K, Wallace RB, Epplen JT. Preferential expression of a defined T-cell receptor β-chain gene in hapten-specific cytotoxic T-cell clones. Nature 322:376-378, 1986.

29. Fink PJ, Matis LA, McElligott DL, Bookman M, Hedrick SM. Correlations between T-cell specificity and the structure of the antigen receptor. Nature 321:219-226, 1986.
30. Banerjee S, Haqqi TM, Luthra HS, Stuart JM, David CS. Possible role of V_β T cell receptor genes in susceptibility to collagen induced arthritis in mice. J. Exp. Med. (in press).
31. Staerz UD, Rammensee HG, Benedetto JD, Bevan MJ. Characterization of a murine monoclonal antibody specific for an allotypic determinant on T cell antigen receptor. J. Immunol. 134:2994-4000, 1986.
32. Behlke MA, Henkel TJ, Anderson SJ, Lan NC, Hood L, Braciale VL, Braciale TJ, Loh DY. Expression of a murine polyclonal T cell receptor marker correlates with the use of specific members of the $V_\beta 8$ gene segment subfamily. J. Exp. Med. 165:257-262, 1987.
33. Roehm MW, Carbone A, Kushnir E, Taylor BA, Riblet RJ, Marrack P, Kappler JW. The major histocompatibility complex-restricted antigen receptor on T cells: the genetics of expression of an allotype. J. Immunol. 135:2176-2182, 1985.
34. Beck BN, Frelinger JG, Shegeta M, Infante AJ, Cummings D, Hammerling G, Fathman CG. T cell clones specific for hybrid I-A molecules. Discrimination with monoclonal anti-I-A^k antibodies. J. Exp. Med. 156:1186-1194, 1982.

SECTION VII

IMMUNOGLOBULIN GENES AND NATURAL KILLER CELLS

USE OF CONGENIC AND RECOMBINANT INBRED MOUSE STRAINS TO LINK A HIGHLY CONSERVED IDIOTYPE MARKER TO AN Igh-C REGION ALLOTYPE LOCUS AND TO MAP THIS NEW MEMBER OF THE Q52 GENE FAMILY WITHIN THE Igh-V GENE COMPLEX

Sheng-Chang Luo and Richard B. Bankert

Department of Molecular Immunology
Roswell Park Memorial Institute
666 Elm Street, Buffalo, NY 14263 U.S.A.

ABSTRACT

The gene coding for a highly conserved idiotype marker associated with the murine response to the hapten phthalate (Xmp) was linked to the IgCH allotype locus using a pair of congenic resistant mouse strains, CB.20 and BC.8. These two strains of mice produce the same level of anti-phthalate antibody when immunized with phthalate-KLH. However, the idiotype marker identified as CRI-Xmp was found in the anti-phthalate antibody obtained from BC.8 but not CB.20 immune mice. The presence or absence of the CRI-Xmp in the phthalate immune sera of several different wild mouse populations was also monitored. In these studies, we observed some nonconcordance in the expression of the idiotype and the heavy chain allotype marker. This nonconcordance is most likely due to a crossover event occuring between Igh-C and Igh-V gene complexes. Using BXD recombinant inbred strains, the V_H-Xmp was mapped with respect to other known V_H gene markers. Based upon these studies V_H-Xmp was found to map close to the constant region immunoglobulin gene cluster, i.e., between V_H-S14 and V_H-Ox. Preliminary sequence data indicate the V_H-Xmp is a member of the Q52 gene family.

INTRODUCTION

Since this International Symposium was convened in commemoration of the 50th anniversary of the discovery of H-2 antigens, it is appropriate that the majority of contributions to this symposium focus upon the H-2 gene complex and the structure and function of the molecules produced by the genes in this complex. However, it is also important for us to recognize that a portion of the early work of Peter Gorer and George Snell and others on the biology of the H-2 complex had and continues to have a broad and significant positive impact upon numerous other areas of biomedical research. One such example of this is the development of congenic resistant mouse lines. Dr. Snell recognized that in order to initiate a proper genetic analysis of histocompatibility it would be necessary to separate and identify individual histocompatibility loci through mouse lines carrying only one histocompatibility difference. Dr. Snell began to produce the congenic lines in 1946 with the first report appearing in the literature in 1948 (Snell, 1948). These lines which differ at an H-locus and therefore resist each other's skin grafts were called congenic resistant lines. The development of the congenic lines by Snell was perhaps the most significant contribution to transplantation biology since the introduction of inbred strains. Since the original congenic resistant strains, many other partially coisogenic strains have been produced that differ at a variety of selected loci.

Twenty-five years latter, D.W. Bailey also working at The Jackson Laboratory, introduced the concept of recombinant inbred, RI, mice (Baily, 1971). This new concept along with congenic strains are now recognized as two of the major events in the history of the H-2 system. RI strains of mice are those which have been derived from the cross of two unrelated inbred progenitor strains, which have been maintained independently under a regimen of strict inbreeding since the F_2 generation. During the brother-sister mating, some alleles are lost but no other alleles than those present in the original F_2 pair enter into any of those lines. All of the nonlinked genes disperse independently of each other so that each F_2 individual gives rise to a strain expressing a unique distribution pattern, i.e., SDP for strain distribution pattern. In his original publication, Bailey suggested four different experimental applications of the RI strains: 1) to identify H loci, 2) to search for H gene functions, 3) to analyze trails that depend upon replicative observations, and 4) to select marker genes most likely to succeed in locating a new gene by conventional linkage tests.

In the present report, we illustrate how congenic mice and RI mice can be utilized to establish the linkage of an Igh-V gene complex to Igh-C and to genetically map a new V_H gene with respect to previously mapped V_H genes. Idiotypic determinants found on anti-hapten antibodies were used to study this new V_H gene. In conducting such studies, it is essental that the idiotypic marker be polymorphic. We have previously reported that the response to the hapten phthalate in BALB/c mice gives rise to a very heterogeneous group of anti-phthalate antibodies (Bloor et al., 1982), but that a portion (10-30 percent) of these antibodies express a common cross-reactive idiotype we have termed CRI-Xmp (Luo and Bankert, 1985). Subsequently, it was established that the CRI-Xmp was found within phthalate specific antibodies derived from many other inbred strains as well as wild type populations of mice but never observed in the phthalate specific antibodies derived from C57BL/6 mice (Luo and Bankert, 1987). Using two congenic mouse strains and three RI strains, we review the evidence that the V_H gene coding for the CRI-Xmp is linked to a constant region allotype and that this new V_H gene maps close to the constant region of the immunoglobulin gene cluster somewhere between V_H-S14 and V_H-Ox. Preliminary nucleotide sequence data which indicate that V_H-Xmp is in the Q52 gene family are consistent with the genetic map analysis using RI mice.

MATERIALS AND METHODS

Animals. BALB/c, C57BL/6, DBA/2, A/HeHa and C3Hf/HeHa mice were obtained from West Seneca Laboratories, West Seneca, NY. CB6F1 mice (F1 cross between BALB/c and C57BL/6 mice) and BXD recombinant inbred strains of mice were purchased from the Jackson Laboratory, Bar Harbor, ME. Congenic mice BC.8 and CB.20 were a gift from Dr. M. Potter, Bethesda, MD.

Immunogen. The phthalate-keyhole limpet hemocyanin (phthalate-KLH) used as the immunogen was prepared by catalytic reduction of 4-nitrophthalate (Pfaltz and Bauer, Inc.), diazotization of the resulting 4-amino-phthalate and coupling of the diazonium salt to KLH (Mayers et al., 1973).

Immunization. Mice were injected i.p. once with 100 μg of phthalate-KLH in a volume of 0.1 ml emulsified with an equal volume of complete Freund's adjuvant (Difco Laboratories, Detroit, MI). Two weeks later, mice were bled and serum samples were assayed for anti-phthalate antibodies and the expression of 2E9 cross-reactive idiotype.

Purification of monoclonal anti-phthalate antibodies. The gamma globulin was precipitated from serum and ascites fluid, which are derived from mice bearing the phthalate-specific hybridomas, by adding equal volume of 50 percent saturated ammonium sulfate solution. The gamma globulin fraction was passed through a phthalate-coupled Sepharose 4B column (Mayers and Bankert, 1980), and phthalate-specific antibodies were eluted with 0.5 M phthalate, pH 8.0. The eluate fractions containing anti-phthalate monoclonal antibody were dialyzed against many changes of borate-buffered saline for one week to remove the hapten.

Preparation of high-resolution anti-2E9 idiotypic antibodies. Anti-idiotypic antibodies were prepared from rabbit as described by Bloor et al. (1982).

Quantitation of anti-phthalate antibodies in the immune sera. A solid phase radioimmunoassay (RIA) was set up to measure the anti-phthalate antibodies in serum samples from mice immunized with phthalate-KLH. An appropriate anti-phthalate antibody purified from the pooled phthalate immune sera (derived from 14 days after primary immunization) was used to construct a standard curve to quantitate the amount of anti-phthalate antibodies in unknown serum samples.

Competitive radioimmunoassay (RIA). A competitive fluid phase double antibody RIA was performed in the 96-well plastic microtiter plates and radioactive bound immune complexes were harvested rapidly and washed onto a filter by filtration method using a modified cell harvester (Jou et al., 1983). By means of this quick and accurate assay, phthalate specific hybridomas and immune sera derived from various strains of mice were tested for the presence of the 2E9 idiotype. A standard inhibition curve of the binding of ^{125}I-2E9 to anti-idiotype antibody by 2E9 was used to quantitate the amount of 2E9 idiotype in the immune sera.

Sequence of V_H mRNA. mRNA sequence of V_H was obtained from the sequence of cDNA derived from the mRNA of CRI-Xmp$^+$ hybridomas. cDNA was synthesized by primer extension method and sequenced by the chemical degradation method (Maxam and Gilbert, 1977). The detailed procedure for preparing poly A RNA and synthesis of cDNA was previously described (Sood et al., 1986). The oligonucleotide primer: 5' CAGGAGACGAGGGGGAAGAC complementary to a short sequence near the beginning of the constant region of Ig μ mRNA was used for synthesis of cDNA.

RESULTS

Specificity of rabbit anti-idiotype antibody. In an attempt to identify a conserved clonotype within the phthalate specific B cell repertoire, hybridomas were prepared from the spleens of mice that were immunized only once with Xmp-KLH. One monoclonal anti-Xmp antibody (2E9) was purified on a phthalate-coupled affinity column and used to immunize rabbits. High resolution anti-idiotype antibodies were purified by passing the rabbit gamma globulin fraction through a series of affinity columns and finally adsorbing and eluting from a column containing affinity purified 2E9 protein. The specificity of the anti-idiotype reagents was determined using a competitive RIA. The RIA measured (on a weight basis) the ability of other monoclonal anti-phthalate antibodies and myeloma proteins to inhibit the binding of the anti-idiotype antibody to ^{125}I-labeled monoclonal antibody protein. Twenty nanograms of the homologous unlabeled 2E9 (μ,kappa) protein inhibited the binding of anti-2E9 idiotype antibody to ^{125}I-labeled-2E9 by 50 percent, whereas, neither the $gamma_1$,kappa anti-phthalate hybridomas (2C3 or 4C7) or μ,kappa anti-phthalate antibody (4C10) nor the μ,lambda myeloma protein MOPC-104E produced any significant inhibition in the binding at the highest level of unlabeled protein tested (20,000 nanograms).

A cross-reactive idiotype family identified within primary and secondary response hybridomas. Rabbit anti-2E9-idiotype antibodies was used in an attempt to identify a repeat clonotype amongst primary response hybridomas. In the course of this screening, 2E9 positive hybridomas were observed in all subsequent fusion experiments and approximately 25 percent of the primary response μ,kappa phthalate specific hybridomas expressed the 2E9 idiotype.

In view of the apparent conservation of the 2E9 idiotype observed within the primary response hybridomas, the question arose as to whether this idiotype may also be expressed in secondary response hybridomas as well. A total of 70 monoclonal anti-phthalate antibodies (derived from secondary response hybridomas) were assayed. Of this total, six of the antibodies were found to be cross-reactive with the 2E9 idiotype. Two of these purified antibodies (1F4F2 and 1G8F7) and one of the hybridoma culture supernatants (1C2D6) were isotyped as μ,kappa and three other purified monoclonal antibodies (1G1B6, 5E7 and 5A8E3) were isotyped as $gamma_1$,kappa.

Fine specificity analysis of the 2E9 cross-reactive idiotype family. Using an extensive library of phthalate analogs we previously showed that it was possible to assign phthalate specific clones to one of eleven distinct fine specificity sets (Bloor et al., 1982). If, as was suggested from the serological analysis, the combining sites of the IgM and IgG antibodies within 2E9 cross-reactive idiotype family were not subject to somatic variation then one would expect that the three IgM antibodies and the three IgG antibodies would belong to the same fine specificity set as 2E9. This was found to be so. The 2E9 and all of the other six proteins were identified as fine specificity set 2 antibodies. Antibodies in this set are distinguished by the ability of only phthalate and one of the analogs (3-nitrophthalate) to inhibit the

Table 1. Fine Specificity Analysis of 2E9 Cross-reactive Idiotype Family[a]

		Inhibitor				
Clone	Isotype	Phthalate	3-Nitro phthalate	Iso-phthalate	o-sulfo-benzoate	Benzoate
2E9	μ,kappa	+	+	–	–	–
1C2D6	μ,kappa	+	+	–	–	–
1F4F2	μ,kappa	+	+	–	–	–
2D7	μ,kappa	+	+	–	–	–
1G8F7	μ,kappa	+	+	–	–	–
1G1B6	γ_1,kappa	+	+	–	–	–
5A8E3	γ_1,kappa	+	+	–	–	–
5E7	γ_1,kappa	+	+	–	–	–
2C3[b]	γ_1,kappa	+	+	+	–	+

[a] Fine specificity of each clone was measured by the ability of phthalate or each of its analogs to inhibit the binding of the monoclonal antibody to RSA-phthalate coated to 96-well plastic plates. Eighty-five to 100 percent inhibition is indicated by "+", whereas, <10 percent inhibition is indicated by "-". The concentration of phthalate or each of its analogs used as inhibitor was 4×10^{-2}M.

[b] 2C3 is a 2E9 CRI negative monoclonal antibody.

binding of the antibody to phthalate-rabbit serum albumin (Table 1).

Distribution of 2E9 idiotype in other inbred strains of mice and linkage to IgCH allotype locus. In order to determine whether or not the 2E9 idiotype was restricted to BALB/c mice, other inbred strains of mice were immunized with phthalate-keyhole limpet hemocyanin (Xmp-KLH) and their sera were assayed for 2E9 idiotype expression. The presence of 2E9 CRI was determined by measuring the ability of individual phthalate immune serum derived from various mouse strains to inhibit the binding of ^{125}I-2E9 to rabbit anti-2E9 idiotype antibody. The different strains tested and the presence or absence of 2E9 idiotype in the phthalate immune sera of various mouse strains are presented in Fig. 1. The concentration of anti-phthalate antibodies in immune sera (14 days after a single immunization with phthalate-KLH) derived from different strains of mice fell within a range of 212-672 μg/ml of serum. Six inbred strains, in addition to BALB/c, were found to express similar levels of 2E9 idiotype ranging between 24-226 μg/ml of serum and the idiotype expression was shown to be associated exclusively with anti-phthalate

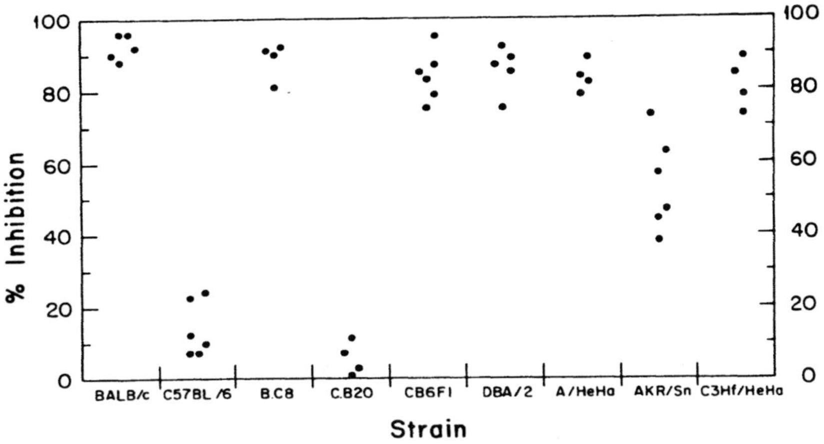

Fig. 1. Strain distribution of 2E9 idiotype in inbred mice. Each spot represents individual phthalate immune serum (bled at day 14 post 1') derived from different inbred strains of mice. The percent inhibition was determined by the ability of individual phthalate immune sera (1:10 dilution) to inhibit the binding of ^{125}I-2E9 to rabbit anti-2E9 idiotype antibody.

antibodies. Only one of the commonly used inbred mouse strains (C57BL/6) was found to be negative for the 2E9 idiotype. The lack of 2E9 idiotype was not due to the inability of the C57BL/6 mice to produce anti-phthalate antibodies in response to phthalate-KLH since these mice produced as much or more anti-phthalate antibody as all other strains tested. One possible explanation for the lack of 2E9 CRI in C57BL/6 mice was that the 2E9 idiotype expression was linked to an IgCH locus since all of the 2E9 positive strains, i.e., BALB/c, DBA/2, C3H and A/HeHa, express identical or cross-reactive Igh-4^a allotypes (Luo and Bankert, 1985) while the one 2E9 idiotype negative strain C57BL/6 expresses an alternative allele at this locus, Igh-4^b. This possibility was confirmed using two congenic mouse strains, BC.8 and CB.20 (Lieberman et al., 1976), which were determined to produce similar amounts of anti-phthalate antibodies following immunization with phthalate-KLH. The first congenic mouse strain BC.8 expresses the same IgCH allotype as BALB/c but possesses the genetic background of C57BL/6. The phthalate immune sera from this strain was found to be positive for 2E9 idiotype (Fig. 1). The other congenic mouse strain CB.20, which expresses the C57BL/6 IgCH allotype and the BALB/c genetic background, did not express the 2E9 idiotype (Fig. 1). It was of interest that the level of 2E9 idiotype in immune CB6F1 hybrid mice were similar to all of the other 2E9 Id^+ strains indicating that gene dosage had no effect upon the idiotype expression.

The one notable exception in the level of idiotype expression amongst the allotype/idiotype positive mice was the AKR mice which were found to express lower levels of the 2E9 idiotype consistently compared to other positive strains (Fig. 1). It is of particular interest to note here that the AKR mice have been shown by Edelman and Gottlieb (1970) to express a polymorphism in their light chains that is not observed in most other strains of mice. The polymorphism in the light chain repertoire could effect the apparent level of 2E9 CRI expression because our rabbit anti-idiotype antibodies were recognizing idiotypic determinants on both light and heavy chains or idiotypic determinants on the heavy chain in association with the light chain.

2E9 idiotype identified in wild mouse populations. In order to determine whether or not there is a concordance between idiotype and allotype expression in the wild mouse population, we surveyed twelve different wild mouse populations for their ability to respond to phthalate-KLH and for their expression of the 2E9 idiotype. These mice were obtained from various areas throughout the world (Luo and Bankert, 1985). All of the twelve different wild type mouse strains produced anti-phthalate antibodies, but only six (MOR, PAC, M. musculus, M. spretus, M. domesticus and M. hortulanus) of these expressed the 2E9 idiotype (Table 2). Two types of nonconcordance between 2E9 idiotype and heavy chain allotype expression were observed. Two of the wild mouse strains (M. musculus Skive, ADH^a and MYL) expressing the $Igh\text{-}4^a$ allotype (reacted with $Igh\text{-}4^a$ specific monoclonal antibodies, 3A9 and 1C10) do not produce the 2E9 idiotype in their pool of anti-phthalate antibodies. Two possible explanations can be made for this nonconcordance between allotype and idiotype expression in the wild type mice. One is that a crossover occurs between the Igh-V gene and the Igh-C gene. The other is that these two wild strains of mice express polymorphism in their light chains and lack the appropriate light chain which is required for the expression of the 2E9 idiotype. Makela et al. (1979) have made a similar observation in which seven wild types of mice which lack the NP^b idiotype were found to have either little or no lambda light chain or have lambda chains different from those lambda chains expressed in inbred mouse strains that secrete the NP^b idiotype. The other example of nonconcordance between 2E9 idiotype and allotype expression was that four out of six ($Igh\text{-}4^a$ allotype negative

Table 2. Expression of 2E9 Idiotype in Wild Mouse Populations

Species Subspecies	Igh-4[a]	Response to Phthalate	Expression of 2E9 Id
MOR	+	+	+
PAC	+	+	+
MYL	+	+	-
M. musculus skive, ADH[D]	+	+	-
M. musculus (Belgrade)	-	+	-
M. musculus (inbred)	-	+	-
M. musculus Castaneus	-	+	-
PWD (inbred)	-	+	-
M. musculus	-	+	+
M. spretus	-	+	+
M. domesticus (Azrou)	-	+	+
M. hortulanus (pancevo)	-	+	+
SM/J (inbred strain)	-	+	+

"+" indicates that mice react with Igh-4[a] allotype specific monoclonal antibody, 3A9 or produce anti-phthalate antibodies or express 2E9 Id in their phthalate-immune sera. "-" indicates that mice do not react with 3A9 or mice are 2E9 Id negative.

strains) were 2E9 idiotype positive. The most probable explanation for this observation is that a crossover has occurred between Igh-V and Igh-C genes. An example of this kind of crossover was found in SM/J mice that expressed the BALB/c-like Igh-V gene repertoire and the b haplotype (C57BL/6-like) of Igh-C gene region (Kipps and Dorf, 1979; Brodear and Riblet, 1984). Consistent with this reported crossover, the SM/J mice were found to express the 2E9 idiotype (Table 2).

Genetic mapping of V_H gene coding for 2E9 idiotype. The series of BXD (C57BL/6 X DBA/2) RI strains of mice repesent a most informative collection of strains with respect to the mapping of Igh-V genes. Based upon the fact that DBA/2 mice express the 2E9 idiotype while C57/BL/6 mice do not, BXD RI strains of mice were used to map the gene encoding the 2E9 idiotype marker within the Igh-V gene locus. As shown in Table 3, a common crossover site has been observed between Sa4 and Sa2 V_H genes in BXD 20 and BXD 27 mice. In BXD 20 another crossover has occurred between (Ox and S14) and (Bg1, Gte, Nb and Np) V_H gene clusters while in BXD 27 there is another crossover site between BCG V_H and Src V_H genes, which has also occurred in BXD 9. Like DBA/2, sera

Table 3. The 2E9 Idiotype Expression in Phthalate Immune Serum From Recombinant Inbred Strains of Mice.

RI Strain	Igh-V Gene Markers											Response to Phthalate	Expression of 2E9 Id
	Src	BCG	Sa2	Sa4	Np	Nb	Gte	Bgl	S14	Ox	Igh-C		
BXD 20	c	c	c X b	b	b	b	b X c	c	c			+	+
BXD 27	b X c		c X b	b	b	b	b	b	b X c			+	-
BXD 9	b X c	c	c	c	c	c	c	c	c	c		+	+

"X" indicates postulated crossover sites; c indicates the DBA/2 allele, and b indicates the C57BL/6 allele (Makela et al., 1979).

derived from these three RI strains of mice also react with mouse $gamma_1$-allotype specific monoclonal antibody 3A9. This confirms that a crossover occurred between Igh-V genes and Igh-C region gene as was previously observed by other investigators. Three BXD RI strains of mice, BXD 20, BXD 27 and BXD 9 were immunized with phthalate-KLH and bled 14 days after a primary immunization. Individual immune sera were tested for anti-phthalate antibody activity and for their ability to inhibit the binding of ^{125}I-2E9 to anti-2E9 idiotypic antibodies. Although all three RI strains of mice were shown to produce anti-phthalate antibodies (52-469 μg/ml), only BXD 20 and BXD 9 strains expressed 2E9 idiotype (Table 3). The data indicate that the V_H-Xmp gene coding for 2E9 idiotype is located near or within the V_H gene cluster of the previously mapped V_H genes (S14 and Ox) and is therefore very close to the Igh-C gene region as shown in Table 3.

Sequence analysis of mRNA coding for V_H of 2E9 (a CRI-Xmp positive monoclonal antibody). cDNA was prepared from the mRNA coding for the immunoglobulin heavy chain produced in the 2E9 hybridoma. The mRNA sequence of V_H was obtained by the chemical degradation method of Maxam and Gilbert. The partial sequence of this molecule is presented in Fig. 2. Here we have compared the 2E9 V_H mRNA sequence with the previously reported mRNA sequence of V_H-Ox_1 from anti-phOx hybridoma NQ2-20.5.3. Based upon this comparison it is apparent that the V_H-Xmp germ-line sequence is identical or very similar to V_H-OX_1. Accordingly we predict that V_H-Xmp is a member of the Q52 gene family. Both the mapping data presented in Table 3 and the partial sequence data in Fig. 2 are consistent with this possibility.

```
              1               5                   10                  15
              Q   V   Q   L   K   E   S   G   P   G   L   V   A   P   S
NQ2-20.5.3    CAG GUG CAG CUG AAG GAG UCA GGA CCU GGC CUG GUG GCG CCC UCA

                              20                  25                  30
              Q   S   L   S   I   T   C   T   V   S   G   F   S   L   T
NQ2-20.5.3    CAG AGC CUG UCC AUC ACU UGC ACU GUC UCU GGG UUU UCA UUA ACC

              _______CDR1_______
                              35                  40                  45
              S   Y   G   V   H   W   V   R   Q   P   P   G   K   G   L
NQ2-20.5.3    AGC UAU GGU GUA CAC UGG GUU CGC CAG CCU CCA GGA AAG GGU CUG
2E9                                       --- --- --- --- --- --- --- ---

                              ________________CDR2__________________
                              50                  55                  60
              E   W   L   G   V   I   W   A   G   G   S   T   N   Y   N
NQ2-20.5.3    GAG UGG CUG GGA GUA AUA UGG GCU GGU GGA AGC ACA AAU UAU AAU
2E9           --- --- --- --- --- --- --- --- --- --- --- --- --- --- --C

              __________________
                              65                  70                  75
              S   A   L   M   S   R   L   S   I   S   K   D   N   S   K
NQ2-20.5.3    UCG GCU CUC AUG UCC AGA CUG AGC AUC AGC AAA GAC AAC UCC AAG
                                                   N
2E9           --- --- --- --- --- --- --- --- --- -A- --- --- --- --- ---

                              80          a   b   c           85
              S   Q   V   F   L   K   M   N   S   L   Q   T   D   D   T
NQ2-20.5.3    AGC CAA GUU UUC UUA AAA AUG AAC AGU CUG CAA ACU GAU GAC ACA
2E9           --- --- --- --- --- --- --- --- --- --- --- --- --- --- ---

                      90              94
              A   M   Y   Y   C   A   R
NQ2-20.5.3    GCC AUG UAC UAC UGU GCC AGA
2E9           --- --- --- --- --- --- ---
```

Fig. 2. Comparison of partial sequence of 2E9 mRNA with that of anti-phOx hybridoma NQ2-20.5.3 (Kaartinen et al., 1983) which is a member of Q52 V_H gene family.

DISCUSSION

In this report, we have demonstrated the presence of the 2E9 idiotype in conventional as well as monoclonal anti-phthalate antibodies derived from BALB/c mice and show here its presence in several other commonly used inbred strains of mice. Analysis of the 2E9 CRI expression in phthalate-immune congenic mice established that the expression of this idiotype is linked to a heavy chain allotype locus. Quantitative analysis of the 2E9 CRI revealed that the level of the idiotype in the immune sera of the positive strains was very similar to BALB/c mice ranging between 24-226 μg/ml amongst individual mice. In contrast to the 2E9 idiotype expression seen in most inbred strains of mice, only six out of twelve wild mouse populations expressed 2E9 idiotype in their phthalate immune sera. And, nonconcordance between 2E9 idiotype and allotype expression was observed in the wild mouse populations. The most likely explanation for this lack of idiotype/allotype concordance is a crossing over between the cluster of constant region genes and the variable region genes.

The mapping of the V_H-Xmp gene with respect to other Igh-V gene markers has placed this new V-gene close to the gene coding for the idiotype identified as Ox and therefore in close proximity to the Igh-C region. Partial sequence of mRNA indicates that V_H-Xmp is a member of Q52 gene family. The proximity of this new V-gene marker to the constant region gene cluster makes it an ideal model with which to test the hypothesis that V genes closest to Igh-C are preferentially expressed in neonates (Yancopoulos et al., 1984 and Perlmutter et al., 1985). If this were true then one would expect that the response to phthalate (and the 2E9 idiotype in particular) would be expressed quite early in ontogeny. Studies which address this possibility are currently in progress.

The highly conserved nature and diverse strain distribution of the 2E9 idiotype expression make the Xmp-KLH a particularly useful model with which to study immune regulation at both the genetic and cellular level. While in many respects this idiotype family resembles the arsonate CRI family, the phthalate idiotype described here is expressed in a much larger number of inbred as well as outbred mouse strains. It also differs from the Ars CRI in that contrary to what has been observed in the Ars system (Hart et al., 1972), the administration of anti-idiotype antibodies prior to immunization consistently results in the enhanced expression of the 2E9 idiotype (Luo and Bankert, 1985). The enhanced expression of 2E9 idiotype occurs independent of the route of administration, with high and low doses of anti-idiotype antibodies, and with site specific as well as conventional anti-idiotypic reagents.

The phthalate model has several additional advantages over other hapten systems due in part to the fact that it exists under physiological conditions as a single molecular species exhibiting two negatively charged immunodominant carboxylate groups (Bankert et al., 1981). In addition to making the molecule highly immunogenic the charged groups eliminate the problem of non-specific hydrophobic interactions that represent potential technical pitfalls that are inherent with several other hapten systems such as 2,4,6-trinitrophenyl (TNP), 2,4-dinitrophenyl (DNP) and 3-nitro-4-hydroxy-5-iodophenylacetic acid (NIP). The problem of hydrophobicity of the ligand is of particular importance when attempting to study membrane events associated with antigen induced activation and regulation of B-lymphocytes. Using a B-cell hybrid that expresses a phthalate specific membrane form of immunoglobulin we have monitored the binding and internalization kinetics of various phthalate-protein conjugates. Our results indicate that phthalate is uniquely suited for these studies due to the absence of non-specific binding to cell membranes.

ACKNOWLEDGMENTS

The authors would like to thank Dr. Verne Chapman for providing wild strains of mice and Dr. B.A. Taylor for helping us to purchase BXD RI strains of mice used in this study. Thanks also go to Mrs. D. Ovak and Mrs. C. Zuber for preparation of the manuscript.

REFERENCES

Baily, D.W., 1971, Recombinant inbred strains. Transplantation 11: 325-327.

Bankert, R.B., Mazzaferro, P.K. and Mayers, G.L.,1981, Hybridomas producing hemolytic plaques used to study the relationship between monoclonal antibody affinity and the efficiency of plaque inhibition with increasing concentrations of antigen. Hybridoma 1 :47-58.

Bloor, A.G., Jou, Y-H., Hoeplinger, C., Gartner, J.E., Mayers, G.L. and Bankert, R.B., 1982, Hapten-specific B cell repertoire probed by hybridoma technology: Selection and characterization of representative clonotypes from the antibody-forming cell pool. J. Immunol. 128: 1443-1449.

Brodeur, P.H. and Riblet, R., 1984, The immunoglobulin heavy chain variable region (Igh-V) locus in the mouse. I. One hundred Igh-V genes comprise seven families of homologous genes. Eur. J. Immunol. 14: 922-930.

Edelman, G.M. and Gottlieb, P.D., 1970, A genetic marker in the variable region of light chains of mouse immunoglobulins. Proc. Natl. Acad. Sci, USA 67: 1192-1199.

Hart, D.A., Wang, A.L., Pawlak, L.L. and Nisonoff, A., 1972, Suppression of idiotypic specificities in adult mice by administration of antiidiotypic antibodies. J. Exp. Med. 135: 1293-1300.

Jou, Y-H., Luo, S-C. and Bankert, R.B., 1983, A filtration double antibody radioimmunoassay that simplifies and semi-automates the isolation of immune precipitates. J. Immunol. Methods 65: 285-292.

Kaartinen, M., Griffiths, G., Markham, A.F., and Milstein, C., 1983, mRNA sequences define an unusually restricted IgG response to 2-phenyloxazolone and its early diversification. Nature 304: 320-324.

Kipps, T.J. and Dorf, M.E., 1979, Genetic mapping of the BGL idiotypic marker within the Igh-V region. Immunogenetics 9: 297-302.

Lieberman, R., Potter, M., Humphrey, W., Jr. and Chien, C.C., 1976, Idiotypes of insulin-binding antibodies and myeloma proteins controlled by genes linked to the allotype locus of the mouse. J. Immunol. 117: 2105-2111.

Luo, S.C. and Bankert, R.B., 1985, Cross-reactive idiotype family observed in the phthalate-specific B cell repertoire of adult BALB/c mice: Diversity of IgM compared with IgG monoclonal anti-phthalate antibodies. J. Immunol. 135: 1252-1258.

Luo, S.C. and Bankert, R.B., 1987, A new cross-reactive idiotype-defined family in the phthalate humoral immune response of mice. I. Linkage of V_H-Xmp to IgCH allotype locus and mapping with respect to other known V_H genes. J. Immunol. 138: 2311-2315.

Luo, S-C. and Bankert, R.B., 1985, Characterization of a new cross-reactive idiotype family and its manipulation in vivo by the administration of anti-idiotype antibodies. Fed. Proc. (Abst.) 44: 1691.

Luo, S-C. and Bankert, R.B., 1985, Monoclonal antibodies specific for the mouse IgG1 allotypic determinants: Reactivity with inbred and outbred mice. Hybridoma 4: 319-329.

Makela, O., Karjalainen, K. and Potter, M., 1979, Evolutionary conservation of a gene which controls the V_H regions of an anti-hapten antibody (Np). Ann. Immunol. (Inst. Pasteur) 130C: 215-223.

Makela, O., Seppala, I.J.T., Pelkonen, J., Kaartinen, M., Cazenave, P.-A. and Gefter, M.L., 1984, Crossing-over frequency in the Igh region of the mouse genome. Ann. Immunol. (Inst. Pasteur) 135C: 169-173.

Mayers, G.L. and Bankert, R.B., 1980, Immunochemistry of monoclonal antibodies. Transpl. Proc. 12: 413-416.

Mayers, G.L., Grossberg, A. and Pressman, D., 1973, Arginine and lysine in binding sites of anti-4-azophthalate antibodies. Immunochemistry 10: 37-41.

Perlmutter, R.M., Kearney, J.F., Chang, S.P. and Hood, L.E., 1985, Developmentally controlled expression of immunoglobulin V_H genes. Science 227: 1597-1600.

Snell, G.D., 1948, Methods for the study of histocompatibility genes. J. Genetics 49: 87-108.

Yancopoulos, G.D., Desiderio, S., Paskind, M., Kearney, J.F., Baltimore, D. and Alt, F., 1984, Preferential utilization of the most D-proximal V_H gene segments in pre-B cell lines. Nature 311: 727-733.

Fc RECEPTOR-LIGAND INTERACTION INDUCES ACTIVATION OF HUMAN NATURAL KILLER CELLS

Ignacio Anegon, Maria Cristina Cuturi,
Giorgio Trinchieri and Bice Perussia

The Wistar Institute of Anatomy and Biology
36th and Spruce Streets
Philadelphia, PA 19104, USA

ABSTRACT

Interaction of NK cells with Sepharose-linked anti-Fc receptor (FcR, CD16 antigen) antibodies inhibits their ability to mediate both spontaneous and antibody-dependent cytotoxicity, whereas bivalent anti-CD16 antibodies enhance spontaneous cytotoxicity. Treatment of cultured NK cells with Sepharose-linked anti-CD16 antibodies induces expression of IL-2 and transferrin (Tf) receptors and of 4F2 antigens and this effect is enhanced in the presence of IL-2 during treatment. Analogously, treatment of NK cells with the anti-CD16 antibodies or immune complexes synergizes with IL-2 in inducing production of IFNγ and TNF. The combined treatment of NK cells with IL-2 and anti-CD16 antibodies induces cytoplasmic accumulation of mRNA transcripts for IL-2R and for the two lymphokines. Nuclear run-on experiments show that gene transcription is induced by the two stimuli. These data indicate that FcR are specialized molecules on NK cell surface that mediate signal transduction upon ligand binding. These effects may be similar to those induced in NK cells upon target cell recognition.

INTRODUCTION

Human Natural Killer (NK) cells are a discrete and homogeneous leukocyte subset bearing a characteristic combination of surface antigens (Trinchieri and Perussia 1984). A germ line configuration of the genes coding for α/β and γ chains of the T cell antigen receptor (TCAR) (Lanier et al. 1986; Tutt et al. 1986), the characteristic presence of a non functional 1.0 Kb transcript of the ß chain gene (Lanier et al. 1986; Tutt et al. 1986; Reynolds et al. 1985) and the lack of expression of the TCAR-associated CD3 surface complex clearly distinguish NK from T cells. A 50-70 Kd low-affinity receptor for the Fc portion of immune complexed IgG (FcR, CD16 molecule) is instead present on NK cells and shares at least one antigenic epitope with a similar, if not identical receptor on polymorphonuclear cells (Perussia et al. 1983a, 1983b; Perussia and Trinchieri 1984). NK cells bind immune complexes [as detected by formation of rosettes with IgG antibody-sensitized erythrocytes (EA7S) or by conjugate formation with antibody-sensitized target cells] and exert antibody-dependent cytotoxicity (Ab-CMC) via the CD16 molecule.

Antibodies to the CD16 molecule inhibit FcR-dependent functions of NK cells but not their spontaneous cytotoxicity (Sp-CMC) (Perussia et al. 1983b; Perussia et al. 1984) indicating that the FcR is not directly involved in binding and recognition of unsensitized target cells. Upon interaction of NK cells with immune complexes, however, their ability to mediate both Ab- and Sp-CMC is diminished (Perussia et al. 1979) and the decrease in Sp-CMC is similar to that following NK cell interaction with sensitive target cells (Perussia and Trinchieri 1981). Antibodies directed to the CD16 molecule induce down-modulation of FcR at the NK cell membrane both when used in bivalent or polyvalent form (Perussia et al. 1983b), mimicking the effect of the natural ligands. These results suggest the possibility that, as in other FcR systems, FcR-ligand interaction on NK cells induces cellular activation.

We now review our data indicating that at least part of the modulatory effects induced by FcR-ligand interaction depends on activation of transcription of specific genes coding for lymphokines and for surface activation antigens involved in NK cell activation and proliferation.

MODULATION OF CYTOTOXIC ACTIVITIES OF NK CELLS UPON INTERACTION WITH ANTI-FcR ANTIBODIES

Enhancement of Sp-CMC was observed when fresh peripheral blood lymphocytes (PBL) were preincubated with anti-CD16 antibodies and washed free of antibody, but not with anti-NKH-1 or with other unrelated antibodies (Fig. 1, left panel). In these experimental conditions anti-CD16 antibodies induce complete down-modulation of the FcR and neither CD16 antigens nor antibodies are detectable at the NK cell surface. $F(ab')_2$ fragments of anti-CD16 antibodies also induced enhancement of Sp-CMC (not shown), indicating that this effect depends on the interaction of the antibody with the specific surface antigen and does not involve binding of the IgG Fc at either the effector or the target cell level. Enhancement of cytotoxicity, as well as FcR down-modulation (Perussia et al. 1983b), is induced only by anti-CD16 antibodies of the IgG1 class (e.g. B73.1, 3G8) but not by those of the IgM class (e.g. Leu 11b, VEP13). Enhancement of cytotoxicity by soluble anti-CD16 and anti-CD3 antibodies has been explained (Van de Griend et al. 1987) by assuming a bridging of target cells bearing FcR to the antibody-coated effector cells with subsequent induction of cytotoxicity. This may, in part, explain the phenomenon observed when intact IgG antibodies are present during cytotoxicity assay, but not when $F(ab')_2$ are used or when the antibodies are removed by washing. In this case, activation of cytotoxicity is induced by triggering of FcR by the antigen-specific portion of the antibody. Morphological changes in NK cell granules upon FcR-ligand interaction are similar to those induced upon NK-target cell interaction (Zarcone et al. 1987), indicating NK cell activation.

When FcR crosslinking is induced at the NK cell membrane using Sepharose-linked anti-CD16 antibodies (Fig. 1, central and right panel) a significant decrease of both Ab-CMC and Sp-CMC is observed. The inhibition of Ab-CMC upon FcR crosslinking can be explained by the disappearance or occupation of FcR induced by anti-FcR antibodies. However, the observations that FcR down-modulation is usually incomplete (Perussia et al. 1983b) and that Sp-CMC is concomitantly inhibited, suggests that crosslinking of FcR at the cell membrane triggers metabolic step(s), common to both Sp- and Ab-CMC, which eventually lead to exhaustion of limiting elements of a common pathway

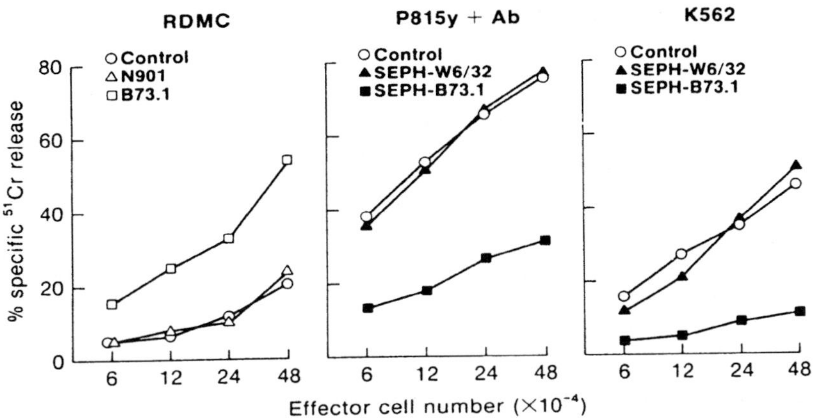

Fig. 1. Modulation of cytotxic activities of NK cells after interaction with anti-FcR (CD16) antibodies. PBL were incubated (18h, 37°C) in medium, o - o, or in medium containing: □ - □ , B73.1, IgG1 0.5 μg/ml; Δ - Δ , N901, ascites 1:2000; ■ - ■ , Sepharose-linked B73.1; ▲ - ▲, Sepharose-linked W6/32. Sepharose beads were detached by vortexing and eliminated from the cell suspension by sedimentation, cells were washed, and Sp- and Ab-CMC were tested (3h-^{51}Cr release assay; Perussia et al. 1983a) against RDMC and K562 or antibody-sensitized P815y target cells, respectively.

involved in cytotoxicity. When NK cells bind to target cells, they undergo modifications, some rapid, including activation of cytotoxic mechanisms and secretion of preformed substances such as pore-forming protein (PFP; Liu et al. 1986) and NK derived cytotoxic factor (NKCF; Wright and Bonavida 1983), and some delayed, including synthesis and release of cytokines (Degliantoni et al. 1985; Wright and Bonavida 1987) and eventual exhaustion of the cytotoxic potential for both Sp- and Ab-CMC (Perussia and Trinchieri 1981). Inhibition of cytotoxicity by anti-CD16 antibodies may depend on a direct secretagogue stimulus mediated through FcR, analogous to the release of mediators of inflammation from basophils upon interaction of IgE-antigen complexes with the Fcε receptor (Metzger and Ishisaka 1982).

Distinct classes of molecules on NK cells might be responsible for target cell recognition in the absence of antibodies and activation of NK cells following binding. The FcR plays an important role in recognition of antibody-sensitized target cells but additional molecules distinct from FcR may also be involved in binding and recognition of these targets. If this were the case, only signals transduced upon simultaneous triggering of the two or more molecular types would be effective in inducing cytotoxicity. FcR-ligand interactions may represent a stimulatory and, possibly subsequent to this, inhibitory signal to NK cells, by the same mechanism as that induced by target cell recognition.

IN VITRO EXPANSION OF NK CELLS

Large numbers of homogeneous NK cell preparations are necessary to directly evaluate whether the CD16 molecule on NK cells serves as a specific signal-transducing molecule and whether its role in NK cell physiology is similar to that of the putative receptor for the target cells. The number of NK cells that can be obtained from peripheral blood is limited; however, stimulation of human peripheral blood mononuclear cells (PBMC) with B lymphoblastoid cell lines (e.g. Daudi cells) results in preferential proliferation of cells with phenotypic characteristics of NK cells (Table I). On average the number of CD16/NKH-1(+) NK cells increases 25-fold after 10-day cultures, whereas the number of CD3/CD5(+) T cells increases only 3-fold. Effective prolifèration of NK cells is not observed in allogeneic mixed leukocyte cultures or in PBMC cultures stimulated by rIL-2, but rIL-2 enhances proliferation of NK cells in Daudi-stimulated PBMC cultures; proliferation of both NK and T cells depends, in part, on endogenous IL-2 production. From these cultures, we can purify by negative selection large numbers of CD16/NKH-1(+) cells that have phenotypic, functional, morphological, and genotypic characteristics of peripheral blood NK cells (Perussia et al. 1987).

FcR CROSSLINKING AT THE NK CELL MEMBRANE INDUCES EXPRESSION OF SURFACE ACTIVATION ANTIGENS

Surface activation antigens are detected on NK cells after 3-4 days of PBMC-Daudi cells culture. At the end of the 10-day culture virtually all NK cells no longer express the activation markers IL-2R (Tac antigen), TfR (Fig. 2) and 4F2 (not shown), although they still express HLA-DR antigens. These NK cells rapidly incorporate ^{3}H-TdR in response to rIL-2, but rIL-2 alone is unable to induce reexpression of Tac antigen or TfR even when used at concentrations (100 U/ml) which induce maximal proliferative response. Upon 18-h incubation with Sepharose-linked anti-CD16 antibodies, expression of FcR is greatly reduced in cultured NK cells, as is the case with those isolated from fresh PBL, and the majority of the cells are induced to express both IL-2R and Tf-R, though at relative low density. The simultaneous presence of IL-2 and Sepharose-linked anti-CD16 antibodies (Figure 2, bottom panels) enhances expression of all activation antigens tested. Similar results are obtained upon culture of NK cells with particulate immune complexes (not shown). No expression of activation antigens was observed on T cells purified by negative selection from the same cultures and similarly treated, or on NK cells treated with antibodies of other specificities (e.g. anti-CD3 or anti-HLA class I, not shown). Induction of surface activation antigens (HLA-DR and IL-2R) was detected by Malavasi et al. (1986) on freshly obtained large granular lymphocytes (LGL) stimulated by Sepharose-linked antibody AB8.28, which detects an antigen distinct from CD16 but possibly associated with it. Our data indicate that specific CD16-ligand interaction is sufficient to induce expression of activation antigens but that maximal expression is achieved only when a second signal (i.e. IL-2) is simultaneously present. It is unlikely that redistribution of an intracellular antigen pool to the membrane occurs under our stimulatory conditions because appearance of the antigen at cell surface requires at least 7 h of incubation. These data indicate that, as is the case for T cells triggered by antibodies to the TCAR-associated molecule CD3 (Isakov et al. 1986), NK cells specifically respond to treatment with anti-CD16 by enhanced expression of the ß chain (Tac antigen) of the IL-2R.

Table I. Expansion of NK cells in vitro upon coculture of PBMC with B lymphoblastoid cell lines.

			Antibody			
Inducer[a]	Cell number ($x10^5$)	Positive cells	3G8 (CD16)	N901 (NKH-1)	OKT3 (CD3)	B36.1 (CD5)
None (day 0)	15.0 ± 0.0[b]	%	21.7 ± 4.4	20.6 ± 5.3	83.4 ± 2.6	83.6 ± 1.3
		number ($x10^5$)	3.2 ± 0.6	3.1 ± 0.8	12.5 ± 0.4	12.5 ± 0.2
Daudi	117.8 ± 39.6	%	67.5 ± 10.8	67.3 ± 12.2	34.1 ± 16.5	31.4 ± 14.1
		number	82.6 ± 32.9	82.2 ± 33.3	34.1 ± 6.8	31.8 ± 6.5
Daudi + rIL-2 (10^2 U/ml)	152.5 ± 54.0	%	70.9 ± 10.4	71.7 ± 11.8	30.9 ± 16.0	27.6 ± 13.5
		number	110.0 ± 43.8	112.9 ± 45.8	41.5 ± 14.6	37.2 ± 12.3
rIL-2 (10^2 U/ml)	18.7 ± 9.6	%	21.3 ± 2.5	23.3 ± 2.0	92.7 ± 1.6	89.4 ± 1.5
		number	3.9 ± 1.9	4.4 ± 2.3	17.5 ± 9.3	16.8 ± 8.8
MLR	10.1 ± 6.1	%	3.6 ± 2.3	4.3 ± 2.7	81.9 ± 2.7	81.3 ± 3.2
		number	0.3 ± 0.2	0.4 ± 0.3	8.2 ± 5.5	8.1 ± 5.3

[a] PBMC (2.5×10^5/ml RPMI 10% FBS) were cultured in the presence of the indicated inducers. The Daudi cells and the allogeneic PBMC used in mixed lymphocyte reaction (MLR), were 50 Gy-irradiated and mixed with PBMC at 1:5 and 2:1 ratios, respectively. After 9 days of culture with an intermediate change of medium, the lymphocytes were collected, counted, and the proportion of NK and T cells determined by indirect immunofluorescence (flow cytometry) using the indicated antibodies.

[b] Figures are mean ± SD of 4 experiments.

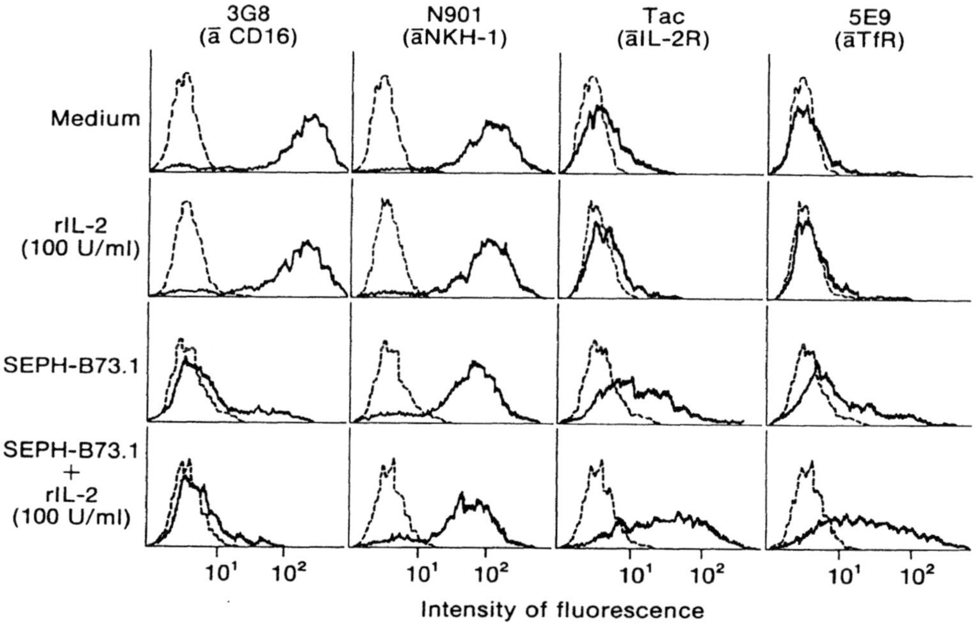

Fig. 2. Interaction of anti-FcR antibodies with FcR on NK cells induces expression of activation antigens. CD3/CD5(-) NK cells were purified by negative selection (Perussia et al. 1983a) from 10-day cultures of PBMC (2.5 x 10^5 cells/ml RPMI-10% FBS) with 50 Gy-irradiated Daudi cells (5:1, PBMC:Daudi) (Perussia et al. 1987). NK cells were incubated (18h, 37°C) in medium in the absence or presence of rIL-2 (10^2 U/ml), Sepharose-linked B73.1 or the two stimuli together. Sepharose beads were detached and eliminated as in Fig. 1, cells were washed, and surface antigens were detected by indirect immunofluorescence (flow cytometry). The histograms in each panel represent the fluorescence of cells treated with an irrelevant (---) or with the indicated antibody (——) and FITC-goat $F(ab')_2$ anti-mouse Ig (Perussia et al. 1983a). x axis, intensity of fluorescence, exponential scale; y axis, number of cells.

NK CELLS PRODUCE LYMPHOKINES UPON FcR (CD16)-LIGAND INTERACTION

Unlike fresh NK cells, the NK cells obtained from 10-day cultures of PBMC with Daudi cells are not or only minimally induced to produce IFNγ upon stimulation with IL-2 (Fig. 3). Low but significant levels of IFNγ and TNF are detected in the supernatants from NK cells stimulated by Sepharose-linked anti-CD16 antibodies but not in those from EA7S-stimulated NK cells. However, both IFNγ and TNF production are synergistically increased by simultaneous exposure of the cells to FcR ligands and IL-2. NK and antigen specificity of this effect was confirmed using T cells and unrelated antibodies (not shown).

Induction of production of IFNγ (Fig. 4) and TNF (not shown) depends, at least in part, on rapid induction and accumulation of cytoplasmic mRNA for the two lymphokines. The 10-day cultured NK cells do not contain detectable IFNγ mRNA; both IL-2 and anti-CD16 antibodies induce minimal accumulation of IFNγ mRNA but the two stimuli combined result in significantly higher accumulation. Because only NK cells are present in our cultures, these data clearly establish that NK cells produce TNF when NK-specific stimuli are used.

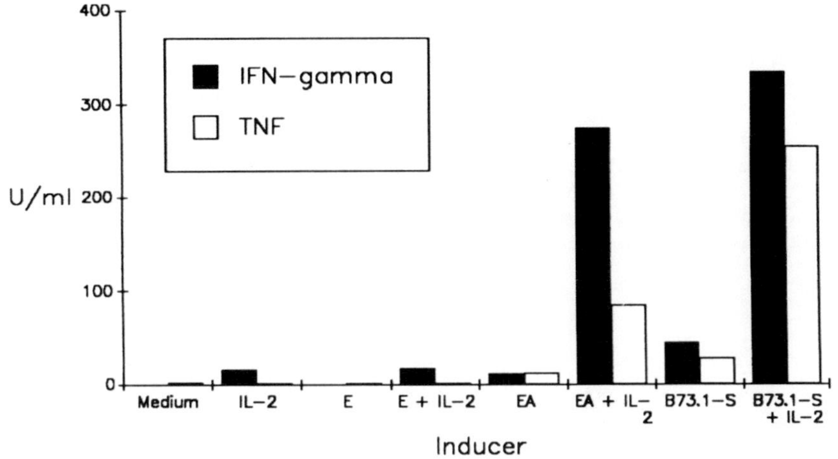

Fig. 3. Interaction of NK cells FcR with FcR ligands induces production of lymphokines. NK cells were purified and incubated with the indicated inducers, as described in Fig. 2. IFNγ and TNF were quantitated by radioimmunoassay (Cuturi et al. 1987; Murphy et al. 1986) in the cell-free supernatants. rIL-2 (100 U/ml); E, bovine erythrocytes; EA, IgG antibody-sensitized E; B73.1-S, Sepharose-linked B73.1.

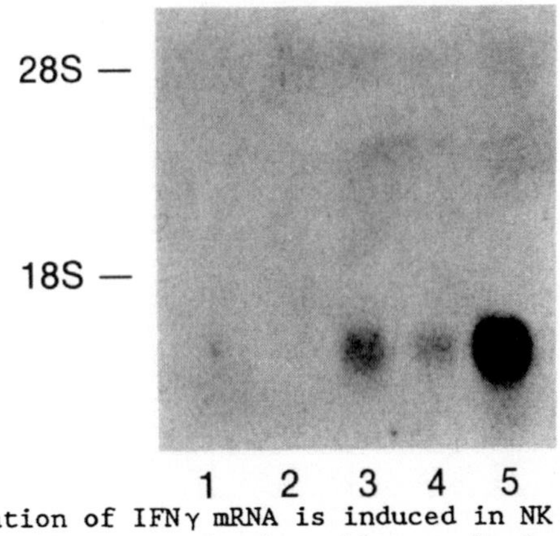

Fig. 4. Accumulation of IFNγ mRNA is induced in NK cells by anti-FcR (CD16) antibodies. Northern blot analysis was performed (Cuturi et al. 1987), using a ^{32}P-labeled nick-translated (Maniatis et al. 1982) IFNγ cDNA probe (pSWIF), on RNA extracted from NK cells purified and stimulated for 1h as described in Fig. 2. Untreated cells, before culture (lane 1); cells cultured in: medium (lane 2), rIL-2 (lane 3), Sepharose-linked B73.1 (lane 4), rIL-2 and Sepharose-linked B73.1 (lane 5).

SIMULTANEOUS STIMULATION OF NK CELLS WITH ANTI-CD16 ANTIBODIES AND IL-2 INDUCES TRANSCRIPTION OF IL-2R AND LYMPHOKINE GENES

Nuclear run-on experiments were performed to define whether the accumulation of RNA transcripts for IL-2R, IFNγ and TNF observed in NK cells stimulated with anti-CD16 antibodies in the presence of the additional IL-2 stimulus is due to induction of gene transcription. As shown in Fig. 5, no evidence for IL-2R gene transcription by 10-day cultured NK cells is detected, whereas the IFNγ and, to a lesser extent, the TNF genes are transcribed in these cells. Transcription of all three genes is induced in NK cells activated for 20 min with anti-CD16 antibodies and IL-2 (with TNF and IFNγ genes at significantly higher rate than IL-2R). Preliminary data from run-on experiments using nuclear RNA from NK cells induced with IL-2 or anti-CD16 antibody alone indicate that transcription of the TNF gene is induced by

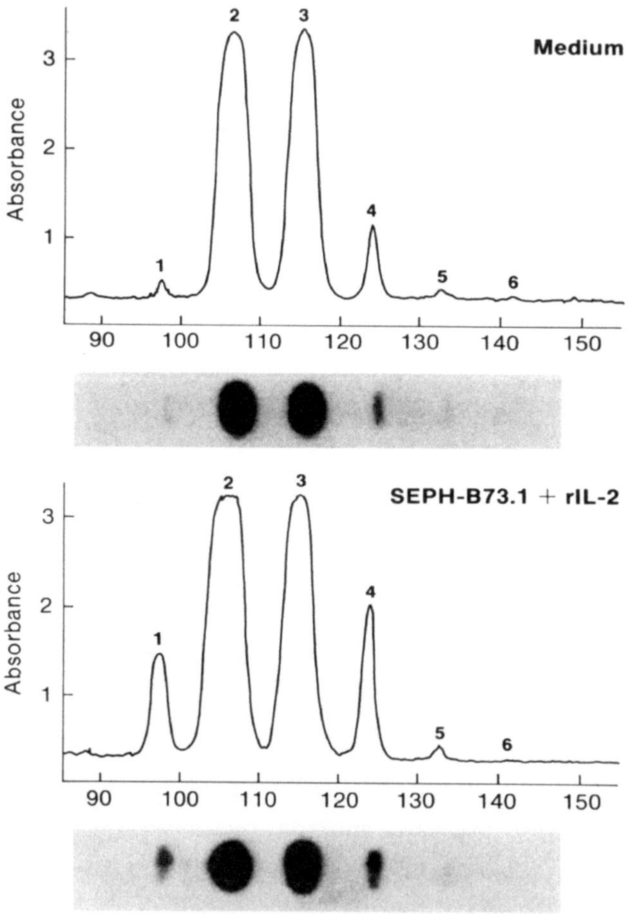

Fig. 5. Treatment of NK cells with anti-CD16 antibodies induces mRNA transcription for IL-2R and lymphokines. NK cells were purified as indicated in Fig. 2 and cultured (20 min) in the absence (top panel) or presence of rIL-2 (10^2 U/ml) and Sepharose-linked B73.1 (bottom panel). Nuclear RNA was extracted (Gariglio et al. 1981) after in vitro elongation (Groudine et al. 1981) from the nuclei (Krönke et al. 1984) and run-on performed. The cDNA probes used to hybridize to ^{32}P-labeled RNA were: 1, TNF; 2, ß actin; 3, pA_{BE} for ribosomal RNA; 4, pSWIF for IFNγ; 5, IL-2R2 for IL-2R; 6, pBR322. The histograms are spectrophotometric readings of the bands in the respective gels.

anti-FcR alone, whereas transcription of IL-2R and IFNγ genes is induced by the two stimuli in combination. A quantitative evaluation of the increased rate of transcription in response to anti-CD16 antibodies, accumulation of cytoplasmic mRNA, and protein expression, however, suggests that induction of transcription is not the only mechanism operating and that postranscriptional effects are also involved, the nature of which remains to be determined. It is also possible that induction of surface activation antigens is mediated by lymphokines (e.g. TNF) which are induced through FcR triggering. Thus an interplay between transcriptional and postranscriptional effect triggered by immune complexes or target cell recognition and secondary effects of the induced lymphokines may contribute to maintain a balance in the state of activation of NK cells.

Acknowledgments: We thank Drs. H.M. Shepard (Genentech), S. Clark (Genetics Institute), W. Greene (NIH), R. Weinmann and P. Curtis (Wistar Institute) for their gifts of the cDNA probes; Drs. J. Griffin (Dana Farber Cancer Institute), T. Waldmann (NIH), and J. Unkeless (Mount Sinai Medical School) for the gift of monoclonal antibodies; J. Faust and J. Urffer for assistance at the cytofluorograph, and M. Kaplan for typing the manuscript. This work was supported, in part, by NIH grants CA10815, CA20833, CA32898, CA37155, and CA40256. Bice Perussia is a Scholar of the Leukemia Society of America.

REFERENCES

Cuturi, M. C., Murphy, M., Costa-Giomi, M. P., Weinmann, R., Perussia, B., and Trinchieri, G.: Independent regulation of tumor necrosis factor and lymphotoxin production by human peripheral blood lymphocytes. J. Exp. Med. 165:1581-1594, 1987

Degliantoni, G., Murphy, M., Kobayashi, M., Francis, M-K., Perussia, B., and Trinchieri, G.: Natural Killer (NK) cell-derived hematopoietic colony-inhibiting activity and NK cytotoxic factor. Relationship with tumor necrosis factor and synergism with immune interferon. J. Exp. Med. 162:1512-1530, 1985

Gariglio, P., Bellard, M., and Chambon, P.: Clustering of RNA polymerase B molecules in the 5' moiety of the adult ß-globin gene of ben erythrocytes. Nucl. Acids Res. 9:2589-2598, 1981

Groudine, M., Peretz, M., and Weintraub, H.: Transcriptional regulation of hemoglobin switching in chicken embryos. Mol. Cell. Biol. 1:281-288, 1981

Isakov, N., Scholz, W., and Altman, A.: Signal transduction and intracellular events in T lymphocyte activation. Immunol. Today 7:271-276, 1986

Krönke, M., Leonard, W. J., Depper, J. M., Arya, S. K., Woong-Staal, F., Gallo, R. C., Waldman, T. A., and Greene, W. C.: Cyclosporin A inhibits T-cell growth factor gene expression at the level of mRNA transcription. Proc. Natl. Acad. Sci. USA 81:5214-5218, 1984

Lanier, L. L., Cwirla, S., Federspiel, N., and Phillips, J. H.: Human natural killer cells isolated from peripheral blood do not rearrange T cell antigen receptor chain genes. J. Exp. Med. 163:209-214, 1986

Liu, C-C., Perussia, B., Cohn, Z. A., and Young, J. D-E.: Identification of a pore-forming protein of human peripheral blood NK cells. J. Exp. Med. 164:2061-2076, 1986

Malavasi, F., Tetta, C., Funaro, A., Bellone, G., Ferrero, E., Collifranzone, A., Della Bona, P., Rusci, R., Matera, L., Camussi, G., and Caligaris Cappio, F.: Fc receptor triggering induces expression of surface-activation antigens and release of platelet-activating factor in large granular lymphocytes. Proc. Natl. Acad. Sci. (USA) 83:2443-2447, 1986

Maniatis, T., Fritsch, E. F., and Sambrook, J.: Molecular cloning: a laboratory manual. Cold Spring Harbor Laboratory, N. Y. 1982

Metzger, J., and Ishizaka, T.: Transmembrane signaling by receptor aggregation: the mast cell receptor for IgE as a case study. Fed. Proc. Am. Soc. Exp. Biol. 41:7-34, 1982

Murphy, M., Loudon, R., Kobayashi, M., and Trinchieri, G.: Gamma interferon and lymphotoxin, released by activated T cells, synergize to inhibit granulocyte-monocyte colony formation. J. Exp. Med. 164:263-279, 1986

Perussia, B., Acuto, O., Terhorst, C., Faust, J., Lazarus, R., Fanning, V., and Trinchieri, G.: Human natural killer cells analyzed by B73.1, a monoclonal antibody blocking FcR functions. II. Studies of B73.1 antibody-antigen interaction on the lymphocyte membrane. J. Immunol. 130:2142-2148, 1983a

Perussia, B., Ramoni, C., Anegon, I., Cuturi, M. C., Faust, J., and Trinchieri, G.: Preferential proliferation of natural killer cells among peripheral blood mononuclear cells cocultured with B lymphoblastoid cell lines. Submitted for publication 1987

Perussia, B., Starr, S., Abraham, S., Fanning, V., and Trinchieri, G.: Human natural killer cells analyzed by B73.1, a monoclonal antibody blocking Fc receptor functions. I. Characterization of the lymphocyte subset reactive with B73.1. J. Immunol. 130:2133-2141, 1983b

Perussia, B., and Trinchieri, G.: Inactivation of natural killer cell cytotoxic activity after interaction with target cells. J. Immunol. 126:754-758, 1981

Perussia, B., and Trinchieri, G.: Antibody 3G8, specific for the human neutrophil Fc receptor, reacts with natural killer cells. J. Immunol. 132:1410-1415, 1984

Perussia, B., Trinchieri, G., and Cerottini, J-C.: Functional studies of Fc receptor-bearing human lymphocytes: effect of treatment with proteolytic enzymes. J. Immunol. 123:681-687, 1979

Perussia, B., Trinchieri, G., Jackson, A., Warner, N. L., Faust, J., Rumpold, H., and Lanier, L. L.: The Fc receptor for IgG on human natural killer cells: phenotypic, functional and comparative studies using monoclonal antibodies. J. Immunol. 133:180-189, 1984

Reynolds, C. W., Bonyhadi, M., Herberman, R. B., Young, H. A., and Hedrick, S. M.: Lack of gene rearrangement and mRNA expression of the beta chain of the T cell receptor in spontaneous rat large granular lymphocyte leukemia lines. J. Exp. Med. 161:1249-1254, 1985

Trinchieri, G., and Perussia, B.: Human natural killer cells: biologic and pathologic aspects. Lab. Invest. 50:489-513, 1984

Tutt, M. M., Kuziel, W. A., Hackett, J. J., Bennett, M., Tucker, P. W., and Kumar, V.: Murine natural killer cells do not express functional transcript of the α, ß, or γ chain genes of the T cell receptor. J. Immunol. 137:2998-3001, 1986

Van De Griend, R. J., Bolhuis, R. L. H., Stoter, G., and Roozemond, R. C.: Regulation of cytolytic activity in $CD3^-$ and $CD3^+$ killer cell clones by monoclonal antibodies (anti-CD16, anti-CD2, anti-CD3) depends on subclass specificity of target cell IgG-FcR. J. Immunol. 138:3137-3144, 1987

Wright, S. C., and Bonavida, B.: Studies on the mechanism of natural killer cytotoxicity. II. Coculture of human PBL with NK-sensitive or resistant cell lines stimulates release of natural killer cytotoxic factors (NKCF) selectively cytotoxic to NK-sensitive target cells. J. Immunol. 130:2479-2483, 1983

Wright, S. C., and Bonavida, B.: Studies on the mechanism of natural killer cell-mediated cytotoxicity. VII. Functional comparison of human natural killer cytotoxic factors with recombinant lymphotoxin and tumor necrosis factor. J.Immunol. 138:1791-1798, 1987

Zarcone, D., Prasthofer, E. F., Malavasi, F., Pistoia, V., LoBuglio, A. F., and Grossi, C.: Ultrastructural analysis of human natural killer cell activation. Blood 69:1725-1736, 1987

V GENE DIVERSITY IN THE MEMORY IMMUNE RESPONSE TO PC-KLH

Mary P. Stenzel-Poore and Marvin B. Rittenberg

Department of Microbiology and Immunology
Oregon Health Sciences University
Portland, OR

ABSTRACT

We report that extensive variable (V) gene diversity is generated in the Balb/c memory response to phosphocholine-keyhole limpet hemocyanin (PC-KLH). Antibodies found in the primary response to PC-KLH (referred to as Group I) express the VH1 gene, are T15 idiotype positive and bind the haptens PC and nitrophenyl PC (NPPC). In contrast, the memory response exhibits new antibodies (Group II) that bind appreciably only NPPC, are T15 idiotype negative and express different VH and VL genes.

VH sequence analysis of a prototype Group II antibody indicates that the M141 VH gene is utilized by this memory-derived hybridoma. This VH gene in association with the Vκ1-3 light chain (L) generates a Group II binding site. The M141 VH gene is also used by four Group II hybridomas that express the lambda-1 (λ1) L chain. Northern and Southern blot analyses indicate that VH gene members of the Q52(M141) and J558 VH families can be used with non-Group I L chains to generate Group II antibodies during immune maturation to PC-KLH. Our findings indicate that the establishment of immune memory in the anti-PC-KLH response is accompanied by the recruitment of B cells using novel VH and VL genes in new associations.

INTRODUCTION

The Balb/c response to PC-KLH begins as a highly focused response that is restricted in V gene usage and idiotype expression.[1-3] The majority of the primary antibodies express the VH1-Vκ22 gene combination which results in the expression of the T15 idiotype, although limited heterogeneity exists due to the utilization of VH1 in association with Vκ24 or Vκ8.[3] The primary antibodies, referred to as Group I, bind the simple haptens PC and NPPC; the latter closely resembles the hapten in the immunizing agent PC-KLH (Fig.1). In contrast to the primary response, antibodies found in the memory response are comprised of two major groups: those resembling the primary antibodies (Group I) and a new population, referred to as Group II, which recognize NPPC and bind poorly to PC.[4-6] Unlike Group I, Group II antibodies are T15$^-$ and dominate the IgG1 and IgG2 isotypes in the PC-KLH memory response whereas Group I antibodies are primarily IgM, IgG3 and IgA.[5] While both Group I and Group II

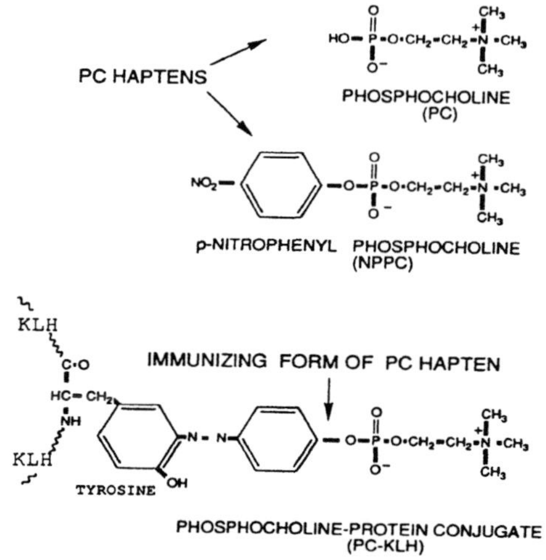

Fig. 1. Immunizing form of hapten in PC-KLH conjugates and its structural relationship to the inhibitory haptens PC and NPPC used to define Group I and Group II anti-hapten antibodies.

antibodies are equally represented in the memory response[6], the primary response is limited to Group I antibodies. Thus, the immune response to PC-KLH begins homogeneously and evolves into a heterogeneous response, one that exhibits a new binding phenotype, idiotype(s) and an isotype preference distinct from those antibodies found in the primary response.

Our laboratory has been investigating the molecular origins of the Group II antibody response to PC-KLH by generating Group II hybridomas. Analysis of their VH and VL utilization revealed that the differences seen in binding specificity were due to differences observed in V gene usage.[7-11] We have determined that VL genes not seen in Group I antibodies are associated with Group II antibodies, particularily Vκ1-3[8] and Vλ1.[10,12] In addition, VL gene products previously found in Group I antibodies of the primary response (Vκ24 and 8) have been observed in Group II antibodies.[13] These findings indicate that the Group II phenotype is due in part to the expression of different light chains.

VH sequence analysis of a prototype Group II hybridoma revealed the use of the Q52 gene family member--M141,[14] a gene that had not previously been observed in the response to PC-KLH.[10] While this hybridoma was shown to utilize the Vκ1-3 L chain in association with VH M141, we have found four additional Group II hybridomas which utilize VH M141 in association with λL chains.

We previously reported use of the VH12 gene, a member of the J558 VH family, in two hybridomas with the Group II binding phenotype.[15] Thus both the Q52 and J558 VH families contribute to diversity generated in the memory response to PC-KLH. These initial studies of VH expression demonstrate that some Group II antibodies observed in the memory response have their origins in novel gene usage and novel gene combinations not seen in the primary stages of the immune response to PC-KLH. These findings indicate that immunological memory to PC-KLH displays a level of genetic complexity not seen in the primary response.

MATERIALS AND METHODS

Immunization and Preparation of Hybridomas

Hybridomas producing anti-PC-KLH antibodies were derived from a fusion of spleen cells from Balb/c mice hyperimmunized with PC-KLH and the nonsecreting myeloma cell line Sp2/0. Specific immunization protocols have been described for the following hybridomas: PCG1-1, aPC-12-3, and PCG1-2 (see ref. 7); PCG1-3;[9] PCG2b-3, PCG2b-4, and PCG3-3 (see ref. 10); aPC-1-56-1 was obtained in the same fusion as that described for aPC-1-111-1;[7] and PCG1-10 was generated in the same fusion as that described for PCG2b-3.[10]

VH Cloning and Sequence Analysis

The VH gene expressed by the hybridoma PCG1-1 was cloned and sequenced as described previously.[10]

Southern Blot Analysis

Genomic DNA was isolated from myelomas and hybridomas as described previously.[10] Southern blot hybridizations were performed as described.[10]

Northern Blot Analysis

Total RNA was obtained from hybridomas using the guanidinium thiocyanate/cesium chloride method[16] modified to obtain both DNA and RNA.[17] 10-15 μg of RNA was electrophoresed through formaldehyde (2.2 M)-agarose gels (1.0%) for 16 hr. The RNA was blotted onto nylon membrane (Biotrans), hybridized and washed as described for Southern blots.[10]

DNA Probes

DNA probes were labeled by random primer extension[18] or nick translation[19] to a specific activity of 0.5-1.0 x 10^9 dpm/μg. The JH specific probe contained JH-1 through JH-4 coding region on a 3.2 kilobase pair (kbp) insert cloned into pBR322.[20] The M141 VH 5' flanking probe was obtained from the cloned VH gene of hybridoma PCG1-1 as described.[10] The M141 VH coding region probe derived from hybridoma PCG1-1 is a 545 bp Hind III/Rsa I fragment containing the leader and VH coding region of the VH gene extending up through amino acid 94 and lacks any JH sequence.

RESULTS AND DISCUSSION

We have cloned and sequenced the productively rearranged JH fragment from a prototype Group II hybridoma, PCG1-1. The 9.5 kbp EcoR1 DNA fragment was obtained from a genomic library constructed from PCG1-1 DNA.[10] The V region sequence was found to be 97% homologous with the VH gene expressed by the myeloma M141; even fewer differences were found when compared with the germline homologue of this gene. The use of the M141 VH gene by a Group II hybridoma is novel in the anti-PC-KLH response and indicates that the Q52 VH gene family from which M141 is derived can participate in this antibody response. The D region was found to be most closely related to the segment-SP2.6[21] which has been seen previously in anti-PC hybridomas of the Group I binding phenotype.[1] The expressed JH region corresponds to JH3 which has rarely been observed in Group I hybridomas since the vast majority of these antibodies are restricted to the expression of JH1. The dominant use of JH1 in Group I antibodies has been thought to indicate that this segment may be important in antigen binding.[1] In support of this notion is the finding that a mutation in the JH region of a PC-binding hybridoma resulted in diminished reactivity with hapten-carrier conjugates while binding to the free hapten PC was unaltered.[22] It was proposed from these observations that the substitution produced a change in the configuration of that portion of the combining site that interacts with a variety of carriers. Thus, the use of a JH segment other than JH1 in a Group II hybridoma may represent an important difference related to the antigen recognition properties that distinguish Group I and Group II antibodies.

In order to determine how extensively the Q52 VH gene family contributes to the Group II response we examined a collection of anti-PC-KLH hybridomas with the Group II binding phenotype for utilization of the M141 VH gene by Southern blot analysis.[10] In addition, Northern blots were probed with the M141 VH coding region to test whether VH members related but not identical to M141 could be expressed by Group II antibodies. Figure 2 shows a Southern blot of four Group II hybridomas compared to the prototype Group II--PCG1-1. A 9.5 kbp JH band representing the productive rearrangement in PCG1-1 is shared by the four Group II hybridomas suggesting that they may all use the VH M141-JH3 gene combination found in PCG1-1. DNA from M141 shows a JH rearrangement slightly smaller (9.0 kbp) consistent with the fact that this myeloma has rearranged the M141 VH gene to the 3'-most JH segment--JH4 yielding the minor difference in this JH band size.

To determine more accurately if the VH rearrangement in PCG1-1 and the four additional Group II hybridomas were derived from the M141 VH germline gene we cloned the 5' flanking region of the PCG1-1 VH gene and used this as a probe to detect rearrangements specific for the M141 VH gene. Re-probing of the Southern blot shown in Figure 2 with the 5' flanking region probe demonstrated that the five hybridomas shared a 9.5

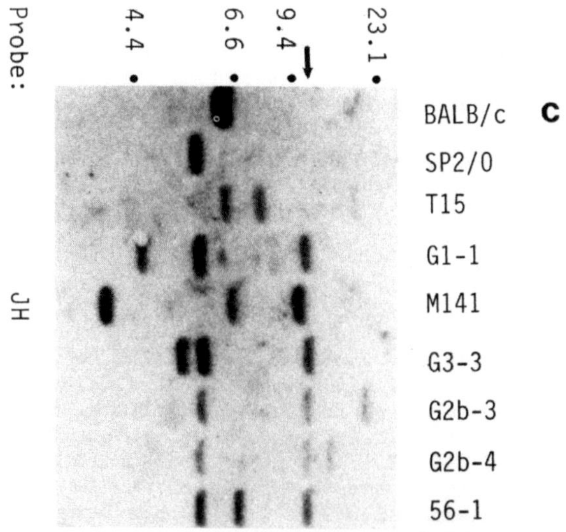

Fig. 2. Southern blot analysis of JH rearrangements in EcoR1 digests of Group II anti-PC-KLH hybridoma DNA. PCG1-1 uses Vκ1-3 and JH3.[10] PCG3-3, PCG2b-2, PCG2b-4 and aPC-56-1 use λ1.[12] M141 is the reference for the Q52 family member, VH M141, rearranged to JH4.[14] (From Stenzel-Poore et al. J. Immunol. in press, 1987)

Table 1. Southern Blot Analysis of VH Gene Rearrangements

Hybridoma/ Myeloma	EcoRl Fragment Sizes in kbp JH[a]	5' VH (M141)[b]
MOPC 141	3.7, 9.0	9.0, 17.0
PCG1-1	4.4, 9.5	9.5, 17.0
PCG2b-3	9.5, 16.5	9.5, 17.0
PCG2b-4	9.5, 12.5	9.5, 17.0
PCG3-3	5.2, 9.5	9.5, 17.0
aPC-1-56-1	6.8, 9.5	9.5, 17.0
PCG1-10	1.6, 3.3	ND
aPC-12-3	2.6, 6.9	ND
PCG1-2	4.6, 5.2, 6.4	ND
PCG1-3	5.2, 5.5	ND

[a] Band size detected using a JH probe; 5.7 kbp band of SP2/0 fusion partner not included.
[b] Band size detected using a 5' flanking probe of VH M141 obtained from hybridoma PCG1-1. 17.0 kbp represents the germline configuration of VH M141.

kbp rearrangement while the myeloma M141 displayed a 9.0 kbp band (not shown); the shared 17.0 kbp band represents the germline configuration of VH M141. Thus all five Group II hybridomas appear to use the M141 VH gene (9.5 kbp band) as was suggested in the JH analysis shown in Figure 2. A summary of the JH and 5'flanking region rearrangements detected in these and other Group II hybridomas is shown in Table I. Interestingly, the four Group II hybridomas other than PCG1-1 which utilize the M141 VH gene express the λ L chain whereas Vκ1-3 is expressed by PCG1-1.[8] It appears that the VH M141 gene can generate a Group II binding site via interaction with either λ or κ L chains. The fact that Vκ1-3 is expressed by 7 of 14 κ-bearing Group II hybridomas (unpublished observations) and its dominance in anti-PC-KLH Group II serum antibodies[23] suggests that it may play an important role in determining the nature of the hapten binding site although it cannot be an essential role since antibodies with a similar fine specificity pattern can be generated with λ L chains. Since we have found both κ and λ L chains in association with the same VH gene structural features common to both light chains may play a critical role in constructing a Group II binding site. Although the use of λ L chains in the anti-PC-KLH memory response is not common in inbred mouse strains, we have now detected them in Balb/c (this report) and (Balb/c x CBA/n)Xid animals.[12,13]

The expression of additional Q52 VH family members by two Group II hybridomas (PCG1-10 and aPC-12-3, Table 1 and 2) was detected by Northern blot analysis using the cloned M141 VH gene from PCG1-1 as a probe. Southern blots of these two hybridomas showed they did not contain the 9.5 kbp JH band characteristic of the M141 VH gene rearrangement thus making it unlikely that they utilize this Q52 member. However, a positive hybridization signal with Northern analysis using the M141 VH gene coding region probe was obtained indicating that a homologous member in the Q52 VH family is expressed by PCG1-10 and aPC-12-3. These two hybridomas use different VL genes; PCG1-10 expresses λ1 and aPC-12-3 has been shown to

Table 2. V Gene Usage in PC-Protein-Binding Hybridomas

Hybridomas	Strain[b]	Group	Inhibition[a] PC	Inhibition[a] NPPC	Heavy Chain	Light Chain[c]	VH Family[d]	Ref.
PCG1-1	B/c	II	-	+	γ1	κ1-3	Q52	7,10
aPC-12-3	B/c	II	-	+	ε	κ1-3	Q52	29
PCG2b-3	B/c	II	-	+	γ2b	λ1	Q52	10,12
PCG2b-4	B/c	II	-	+	γ2b	λ1	Q52	10,12
PCG3-3	B/c	II	-	+	γ3	λ1	Q52	10,12
aPC-56-1	B/c	II	-	+	γ1	λ1	Q52	10,12
PCG1-10	B/c	II	-	+	γ1	λ1	Q52	12
PCG1-2	B/c	II	-	+	γ1	κ24	J558	13
PCG1-3	F1	II	-	+	γ1	κ24	J558	13

a PC or NPPC haptens were used to inhibit antibody binding to PC-histone coated plates in an ELISA as described previously.[5]
b Balb/c (B/c) or CBA/N x Balb/c F1 males (F1) mouse strains.
c Light chain identifications were made by IEF spectrotype analysis and specific anti-κ and λ antisera.[12]
d Q52 VH gene assignments were made by Northern and Southern blot analysis; J558 gene usage was determined by amino acid sequencing.[13]

use Vκ1-3[8] indicating that both light chains can associate with Q52 VH members other than VH M141 to generate a Group II combining site.

It is now clear that VH and VL expression in anti-PC-KLH memory is far more diverse than that observed in the initial phase of the response. We have shown that VH12 of the J558 family[13] and several Q52 VH members[10](and this study) can participate in the establishment of memory to PC-KLH (Table 2); preliminary studies indicate that additional members of the J558 and S107 VH families may also contribute to the Group II response.[11] Thus, immunological memory to PC-KLH is far more complex than was originally viewed. The generation of the Group II binding phenotype is derived in part from a range of VH and VL genes not found in Group I antibodies. In addition, VL genes found in the primary response (Vκ24 and Vκ8) can associate with new VH genes found only in the memory response giving rise to Group II combining sites in their new context. Figure 3 shows the VH and VL associations found thus far in Group I and Group II antibodies. The dominant V gene in Group I antibodies, VH1, can associate with three different VL genes although in the Balb/c PC-KLH response the most common clonotype is VH1/Vκ22. The fact that this VH gene is used by nearly all Group I antibodies observed and that it can associate with more than one VL to generate Group I-like binding sites points to an essential role for the VH chain in hapten binding.

In contrast to Group I antibodies, Group II antibodies express several distinct VH genes and VL genes, although Vκ1-3 may be more frequently observed than other VL genes. We do not know how extensively Vκ24 and Vκ8 are used in the Group II response; their usage in combination with VH genes (J558 family members) not observed in the primary response demonstrates that VL gene elements in the early response can associate with new VH genes to generate related but distinct binding sites that recognize only NPPC and in this context do not bind PC as in

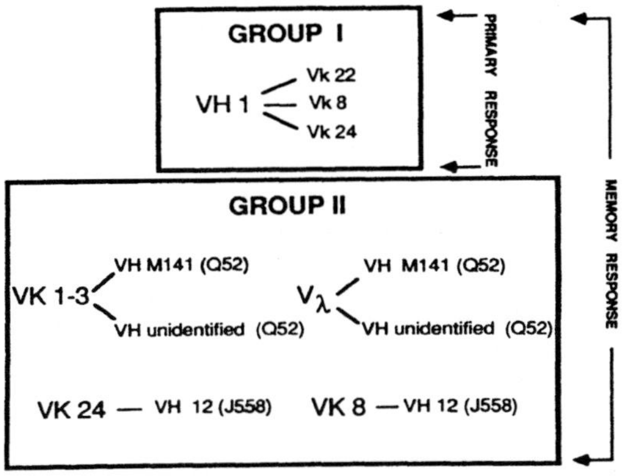

Fig. 3. Summary of VH and VL gene associations in Group I and Group II anti-PC-KLH antibodies in primary and memory responses.

their original context with VH1. Clonotypes which are dominant in these primary responses are thus replaced in memory by other clonotypes some of which express V gene structures related to the primary clonotypes but in new contexts. Moreover, we have found in studies to be reported elsewhere that some Group II antibodies are VH1 gene products. Thus the memory response to PC-KLH represents another example of what has been termed combinational diffusion.[24] In this respect, extensive V gene diversification occuring during the evolution of the memory response to PC-KLH resembles that seen during maturation of the oxazolone response[25,26] and differs sharply from the arsonate response where a single clonotype becomes dominant in the secondary response following a heterogeneous initial response.[27,28]

Group II antibodies appear late and despite the original predominance of Group I antibodies they are expanded to be equally represented among anti-PC-KLH antibodies in the memory response. These findings could easily be explained if the Group II population had a higher affinity for antigen; however, hapten inhibition studies using NPPC indicate that Group I antibodies bind equally well or better to the hapten than do Group II antibodies.[7,29] It is possible that the increase in genetic heterogeneity that characterizes the Group II phenotype may allow a greater degree of tolerance against the deleterious aspects of somatic mutation. Possibly Group I antibodies (T15) are less able to accomodate somatic mutations that would decrease affinity for the PC-protein linkage group which may be involved in binding to PC-protein.

Our findings point to a very strong selection process operating during the development of immunological memory that allows new gene combinations to be recruited in the presence of striking clonotypic dominance by another family of closely related molecules. It is not possible to say whether selection is directed by antigen or anti-idiotypic regulation, or perhaps by more complex mechanisms such as distinct compartmentalization of virgin and memory lymphocytes and/or differential activation requirements. Nevertheless, the memory response to PC-KLH is characterized by a shift toward new gene combinations resulting in increased binding heterogeneity that may serve a fundamental biologic requirement to broaden the antigen recognition potential of B cells entering the memory pool.

REFERENCES

1. R. M. Perlmutter, S. T. Crews, R. Douglas, G. Sorenson, N. Johnson, N. Nivera, P. J. Gearhart, and L. Hood, The generation of diversity in phosphorylcholine-binding antibodies, Adv. Immunol. 35:1 (1984).
2. J. L. Claflin and J. M. Davie, Clonal nature of the immune response to phosphorylcholine. IV. Idiotype uniformity of binding site associated antigenic determinants among mouse antiphosphorylcholine antibodies, J. Exp. Med. 140:673 (1974).
3. R. M. Perlmutter, The molecular genetics of phosphocholine-binding antibodies, in The Biology of Idiotypes, M. I. Greene and A. Nisonoff, ed., Plenum Press, New York (1984)
4. S. P. Chang and M.B. Rittenberg, Immunologic memory to phosphorylcholine in vivo. I. Asymmetric expression of clonal dominance, J. Immunol. 126:975 (1981).
5. S. P. Chang, M. Brown and M. B. Rittenberg, Immunologic memory to phosphorylcholine. II. PC-KLH induces two antibody populations that dominate different isotypes, J. Immunol. 128:702 (1982).
6. S. P. Chang, M. Brown and M. B. Rittenberg, Immunologic memory to phosphorylcholine. III. IgM includes a fine specificity population distinct from TEPC 15, J. Immunol. 129:1559 (1982).
7. S. P. Chang, R. M. Perlmutter, M. Brown, C. H. Heusser, L. Hood and M.B. Rittenberg, Immunologic memory to phosphocholine. I. Hybridomas representative of Group I (T15-like) and Group II (non-T15-like) antibodies utilize distinct VH genes, J. Immunol. 132:1550 (1984).
8. I. Todd, S. P. Chang, R. M. Perlmutter, R. Aebersold, C. Heusser, L. Hood and M.B. Rittenberg, Immunologic memory to phosphocholine. V. Hybridomas representative of Group II antibodies utilize Vκ1-3 gene(s), J. Immunol. 182:1556 (1984).
9. M. Brown, M. Stenzel-Poore and M.B. Rittenberg, Immunologic memory to phosphocholine. VII. Lack of T15 V1 gene utilization in Xid anti-PC hybridomas, J. Immunol. 135:3558 (1985).
10. M. P. Stenzel-Poore, T. J. Hall, C. H. Heusser, C. H. Faust and M. B. Rittenberg, Immunologic memory to PC-KLH: participation of the Q52 VH gene family, J. Immunol. in press September (1987).
11. M. P. Stenzel-Poore and M. B. Rittenberg, V gene heterogeneity accompanies the development of immune memory to phosphocholine (PC). Fed. Proc. 46:1384 (1987).
12. T. J. Hall, M. P. Stenzel-Poore, C. H. Heusser and M. B. Rittenberg, Immunologic memory to phosphocholine-keyhole limpet hemocyanin: use of lambda light chains in antibodies to nitrophenyl-PC, submitted for publication.
13. I. Todd, M. Brown and M. B. Rittenberg, Immunologic memory to phosphorylcholine. VI. Heterogeneity in light chain gene expression, Eur. J. Immunol. 15:177 (1985).
14. H. Sakano, R. Maki, Y. Kurosawa, W. Roeder and S. Tonegawa, Two types of somatic recombination are necessary for the generation of complete immunoglobulin heavy chain genes, Nature 286:676 (1980).
15. M. B. Rittenberg, R. W. Glanville, R. H. Aebersold, S. P. Chang and M. Brown, Immunologic memory to phosphorylcholine (PC). VIII. Expression of the VH-12 gene product in the response to PC-keyhole limpet hemocyanin, Eur. J. Immunol. 16:503 (1986).
16. T. Maniatis, E. F. Fritsch and J. Sambrook, Extraction, purification and analysis of mRNA from eukaryotic cells: guanidinium/cesium chloride method, in Molecular Cloning, Cold Spring Harbor Laboratory, New York (1982).
17. H. Young, Recovery of DNA from guanidinium isothyocyanate-cesium chloride gradients, Focus 6:11 (1984).

18. A. Feinberg and B. Vogelstein, A technique for radiolabeling DNA restriction endonuclease fragments to high specific activity, Analyt. Biochem. 132:6 (1982).
19. P. W. Rigby, J. M. Dieckmann, C. Rhodes and P. Berg, Labeling deoxyribonucleic acid to high specific activity in vitro by nick translation with DNA polymerase, J. Mol. Biol. 113:237 (1977).
20. K. Calame, J. Rogers, P. Early, M. Davis, D. Livant, R. Wall and L. Hood, Mouse Cμ heavy chain immunoglobulin gene segment contains three intervening sequences separating domains, Nature 284:452 (1980).
21. Y. Kurosawa and S. Tonegawa, Organization, structure and assembly of immunoglobulin heavy chain diversity DNA segments, J. Exp. Med. 155:201 (1982).
22. W. D. Cook, S. Rudikoff, A. M. Giusti and M. D. Scharff, Somatic mutation on a cultured mouse myeloma cell affects antigen binding Proc. Natl. Acad. Sci. USA 79:1240 (1982).
23. U. Bruderer, Regulation of antibody isotype expression in mice, Inauguraldissertation Philosophisch-Naturwissenschalftlichen Facultät, der Univesität Basel (1985).
24. T. Manser, L. J. Wysocki, T. Gridley, R. I. Near and M. L. Gefter, The molecular evolution of the immune response, Immunol. Today 6:95 (1985).
25. M. Kaartinen, G. M. Griffiths, A. F. Markham and C. Milstein, mRNA sequences define an unusually restricted IgG response to 2-phenyloxazolone and its early diversification, Nature 304:320 (1983).
26. C. Berek, G. M. Griffiths and C. Milstein, Molecular events during maturation of the immune response to oxazolone, Nature 316:412 (1985).
27. R. I. Near, T. Manser and M. L. Gefter, The generation of major and minor idiotype-bearing families of anti-p-azophenylarsonate antibodies; stochastic utilization of VH gene segments, J. Immunol. 134:2004 (1985).
28. T. Manser, S-H. Huang and M. L. Gefter, Influence of clonal selection on the expression of immunoglobulin variable region genes, Science 226:1283 (1984).
29. C. H. Heusser, J.P.A. Bews, R. Aebersold and K. Blaser, Anti-phosphorylcholine antibodies with a preferred reactivity for either PC or PC-phenyl represent independent expressions. Ann. Immunol. (Inst. Pasteur) 135C:123 (1984).

IMMUNE RECOGNITION OF HUMAN MHC DR2 ANTIGEN

M. Zouhair Atassi*+, Hammad Atassi*
and Robert G. Ulrich+

*Department of Biochemistry and +Department of
Microbiology and Immunology
Baylor College of Medicine
Houston, Texas

INTRODUCTION

The human class II major histocompatibility complex (MHC) antigens are homologues of the murine Ia antigens. Class II HLA glycoproteins have a limited tissue distribution, being found primarily on the macrophage, dendrite cells, B cells and activated T cells, but they may also be induced on other cell types by interferon-γ (Pober et al, 1983). Class II HLA antigens are composed of a dimer of a heavy (33-35 kDa) α chain and a light (27-29 kDa) β chain (Shackelford et al., 1981). Both the α and β subunits are composed of two extracellular domains, each containing a disulfide loop, with the exception of the N-terminal domain of the α chain. Allelic polymorphism is a characteristic of the β chains of DP and DR (Goyert et al., 1982; van Rood et al., 1976; Giles and Capra, 1985) and of both chains of the DQ molecules (Giles and Capra, 1985; Giles et al., 1985).

The specificities of HLA-DR were originally defined by lymphocyte proliferative responses to homozygous typing cells (HTC) (van Rood et al., 1975). At present, alloantisera are the most generally used reagents for typing class II DR and DQ antigens, while DP alleles are still defined by primed lymphocyte typing (PLT) (Shechy et al., 1975). The DR alleles are designated DR1 through DRw10 (Schreuder and van Leeuwen, 1987). The supertypic specificities HLA-DRw52 and HLA-DRw53 are present in several independent DR types as common antigenic determinants (Sorrentino et al., 1985).

There are heterogeneities within any reasonably well-defined DR antigen. HLA-DR2 is divided into several MLR (mixed lymphocyte response) defined or HLA-D specificities, including: Dw2, Dw12, FJO, DB9 and MN2 (Batchelor et al, 1984), along with some serological splits. Based on common DR and DQ two-dimensional electrophoresis patterns Yabe et al. (1987) have classified DR2 into Dw2, Dw12 and DR2.3. The two-dimensional electrophoretic mobility of one DRβ chain is constant within the DR type, while the mobility of the other β chain correlates with the D specificity for those haplotypes examined (Nepom et al., 1983; Nepom et al., 1984). In comparisons of D groups within a DR typing, there are only minor amino acid substitutions in the constant DRβ chain, while the majority of sequence differences are found in the alternative β subunit (Gregerson et al., 1986; Wu et al., 1987). Both DRβ chains of Dw2 and Dw12 types have been shown to function as MHC restriction elements for antigen presentation and as MLR stimulating alloantigens (Sone et al., 1985).

Despite extensive DNA and protein sequence data, classical serological and cellular typing methods cannot unambiguously assign DR antigenic specificities to submolecular regions of the protein. A study of the HLA-DR antigen was therefore undertaken, using methods that have been applied previously in our laboratory to other protein antigens. A series of overlapping synthetic peptides were made, including the entire extracellular sequence of DR2β chain. These peptides were used to screen several anti-DR antisera and human alloantisera for the continuous regions of DR2β that are recognized by these antibodies. Seven antigenic sites were identified within the β subunit, with an eighth site being recognized with some antisera.

MATERIALS AND METHODS

The isolation and purification of the DR2 (αβI) complex and of the individual subunits were carried out as described recently in detail (Ulrich et al., 1987). The synthetic strategy of the 19 overlapping peptides encompassing the entire DR2β chain is shown schematically in Fig. 1.

The structures of the peptides were based on the known amino acid sequence of the β chain (Kratzin et al., 1981). The synthesis, purification and characterization of these peptides were performed as described (Ulrich et al., 1987; Atassi, et al., 1987). The purity of the peptides was checked by high voltage paper electrophoresis and by analytical high performance liquid chromatography (HPLC) on a C18 column, and their structures were confirmed by amino acid analysis.

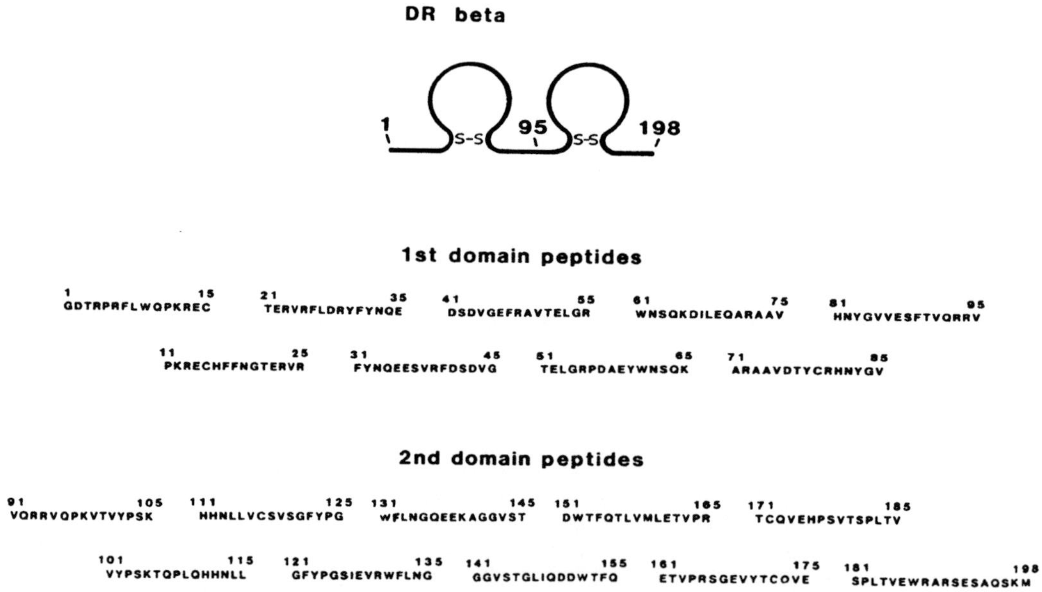

Fig. 1. Covalent structure of the consecutive synthetic overlapping peptides spanning the entire extracellular domains of the DR2β subunit. These peptides were synthesized, purified and characterized as described elsewhere (Ulrich et al., 1987; Atassi et al, 1987).

Antisera against the DR2 complex or the β chain were prepared in chimpanzee and outbred mice and the molecular specificities were studied by quantitative radioimmunoadsorbent titrations as described (Ulrich *et al.*, 1987; Atassi *et al.*, 1987). Double-antibody titrations (Twining and Atassi, 1979) were employed using fixed amounts of prediluted (1:500-1000 v/v, with phosphate-buffered saline (PBS) containing 0.1% bovine serum albumin) unlabeled first antibody (anti-DR) and ^{125}I-labeled second antibody (200 000 cpm) (antiserum against the immunoglobulin species of the first antibody) and increasing amounts of each protein or peptide adsorbent as described (Ulrich et al., 1987). Nonspecific adsorption was determined by titrating, under identical conditions, equivalent volumes of uncoupled Sepharose, and adsorbents of bovine serum albumin, myoglobin, a myoglobin synthetic peptide (residues 87-100) and a nonsense peptide. The binding values of the various adsorbents were corrected for this nonspecific binding. The specificity of binding of antibodies to peptides was confirmed by a number of criteria. Antibodies bound by a peptide carrying a given site were selectively removed by repeated adsorption (about three cycles) with the adsorbent of that peptide, while having no effect on antibody binding by peptides representing other sites. The binding of ^{125}I-labeled anti-DR or anti-β antibodies, by direct antibody titrations (Twining and Atassi, 1979), to the active peptides was not inhibited by a large excess of preimmune or nonimmune IgG. Similarly, ^{125}I-labeled preimmune IgG did not bind to the peptides. Other ^{125}I-labeled non-immunoglobulin proteins did not exhibit any binding with the DR peptides. This was a property found only with Ig from anti-DR antisera.

RESULTS

Binding of anti-DR2 and anti-β chain antibodies to DR2β peptides

Figure 2 summarizes the peptide binding profiles with antisera raised against the isolated DR2 complex in different host species. Figure 3 gives a comparison of the antibody binding profiles to the peptides with antisera against the isolated DR2β chain and against the DR2 complex. Essentially the same regions are recognized by both antisera, with slight differences apparent in the amounts of antibodies directed to the various regions (i.e. the antisera showed some differences in their submolecular immunodominance to the various regions).

Human alloantisera. Four human alloantisera were studied. Two sera had activity directed towards several DR haplotypes (12G2 and 12T8), one was DR2 specific (SK-1) and the fourth (NJ2) was specific for DR1 and DR2. Although the relative amounts of antibodies bound to a given peptide varied with the antisera (Figure 4) antibodies from all four sera bound to peptides 1-15, 81-95, 121-135, 151-165 and 181-198. All sera except NJ2 recognized peptide 51-65. In addition, low levels of antibodies were bound to peptide 101-115 in sera 12G2, 12T8, SK1 and NJ2; to peptide 111-125 in sera 12T8, SK1 and NJ2; to peptide 161-175 in serum NJ2 and to peptide 171-185 in serum 12T8. The remaining peptides showed little or no binding activity. Adsorbents of unrelated proteins and peptides did not bind these antibodies. The specificity of the binding to the peptides was confirmed as described above.

DISCUSSION

The antigenic sites of proteins may comprise residues that are on a continuous segment of the protein chain (Atassi, 1975), or are distant in sequence but, due to the folding of the polypeptide chain, come into close spatial proximity (Atassi, 1978). Therefore, for a protein of an unknown antigenic structure, both alternative site architectures [i.e. continuous or discontinuous (Atassi and Smith, 1978)] should be anticipated. A comprehensive synthetic strategy previously introduced (Kazim and Atassi, 1980) has enabled the relatively rapid localization on a protein of the full profile of the continuous sites of immunological (i.e. T and B cell) activity. The strategy, which is applied here to the extracellular part (residues 1-198) of DR2β chain, consists of the synthesis and investigation of the immunological activity of a series of consecutive overlapping peptides of uniform size and overlaps and which encompass the entire protein chain. It should be stressed that this synthetic peptide strategy has been designed specifically for the localization of continuous antigenic sites.

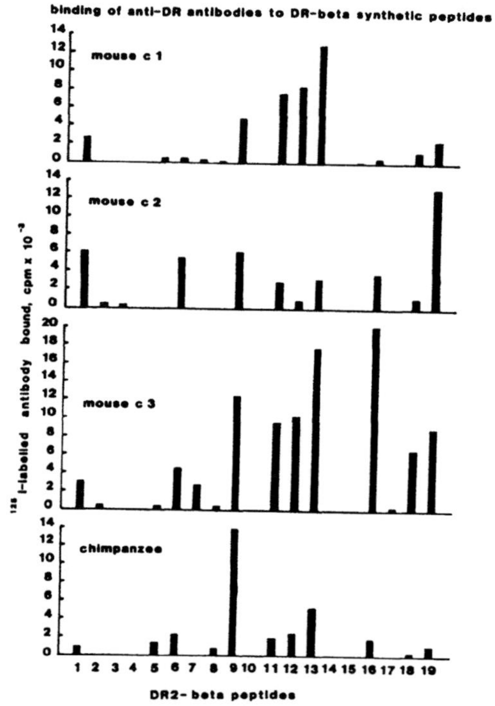

Fig. 2. Summary of the antibody binding results to the DR2β peptides. Values are from triplicate analyses obtained by double antibody radioimmunosorbent titrations, and have been corrected for nonspecific binding to controls (uncoupled sepharose CL4B, myoglobin peptide, bovine serum albumin, nonsense peptide, which were < 4% of added ^{125}I-labelled immune IgG). The DR2β peptides are: (1) 1-15; (2) 11-25; (3) 21-35; (4) 31-45; (5) 41-55; (6) 51-65; (7) 61-75; (8) 71-85; (9) 81-95; (10) 91-105; (11) 101-115; (12) 111-125; (13) 121-135; (14) 131-155; (15) 141-155; (16) 151-165; (17) 161-175; (18) 171-185; (19) 181-198.

The DR2β peptides designed here (Fig. 1) consisted of 15 residues (except for peptide 181-198) with 5-residue overlaps between consecutive peptides. Localization of the antigenic sites from the immunochemical activity of the peptides was done according to the principles previously established (Kazim and Atassi, 1982). The approach does not give the precise boundaries of the sites and further studies with synthetic peptides overlapping within the indicated regions will be required to define the boundaries (Koketsu and Atassi, 1973; Atassi, 1975). Thus, the extracellular part (residues 1-198) of the DR2β chain was found to have seven continuous antigenic sites (three in the first domain and four in the second domain) that are recognized with all the antisera (Ulrich *et al.*, 1987; Atassi *et al.*, 1987). In addition, an eighth antigenic site, occurring in the first domain within residues 63-73, is recognized somewhat weakly with some antisera (Fig. 5). It is necessary to note that residues on the β chain (or other DR chains) outside of the regions assigned to the antigenic sites, but which come in close spatial proximity to site residue(s), or even more distant residues may influence, to various degrees, the reactivities of the sites, through charge-transfer, steric and/or conformational effects (Atassi and Kazim, 1980; Kazim and Atassi, 1980; Twining et al., 1980).

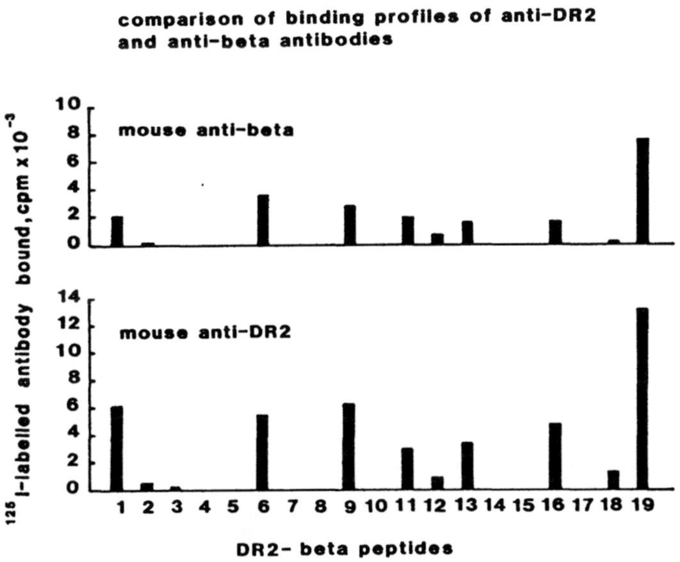

Fig. 3. Comparison of the antibody binding profiles to the DR2β peptides of mouse antisera obtained from immunization with either the isolated DR2β subunit or the DR2 complex. The binding values obtained, and peptides used were as described in the Fig. 2 legend.

The finding that some of the peptides exhibited very low antibody-binding activity indicated the presence of very low antibody responses to regions outside the major antigenic sites of DRβ. Such low level responses interspersed among immunodominant sites have been observed with other proteins (Atassi, 1975; Atassi and Smith, 1978; Yoshioka and Atassi, 1986; Atassi, 1980) and are termed "general background" responses (Atassi, 1980). It was also proposed (Atassi, 1980) that such low level antibodies could be expanded and prepared *in vitro* as monoclonal antibodies (mAb) (Kohler and Milstein, 1975). Indeed, anti-protein mAb have been reported (Atassi, 1984; Metzger et al., 1984) that possess specificities which are not detectable in antisera to the respective protein, and it has been cautioned that mAb should not be used to localize the *in vivo* immunodominant protein regions (Atassi, 1980). It would be necessary to confirm the existence of such specificities in the antisera of the parent animal.

The same regions were recognized by mouse antisera against DR2 or against the isolated β chain. This might suggest that the oligomer is recognized at the subunit level as was found in hemoglobin (Kazim and Atassi, 1982; Yoshioka and Atassi, 1986). However, this question requires more extensive investigations. The mapping of the full continuous antigenic profile of DR2β shows unambiguously that, although their immunodominance varies, the sites are similarly recognized by chimpanzee, and mouse antibodies. Significantly, these are the same sites that are recognized by human alloantibodies. This is in agreement with our previous conclusions that the locations of protein antigenic sites are determined by their conformational locations (Atassi and Kazim, 1978).

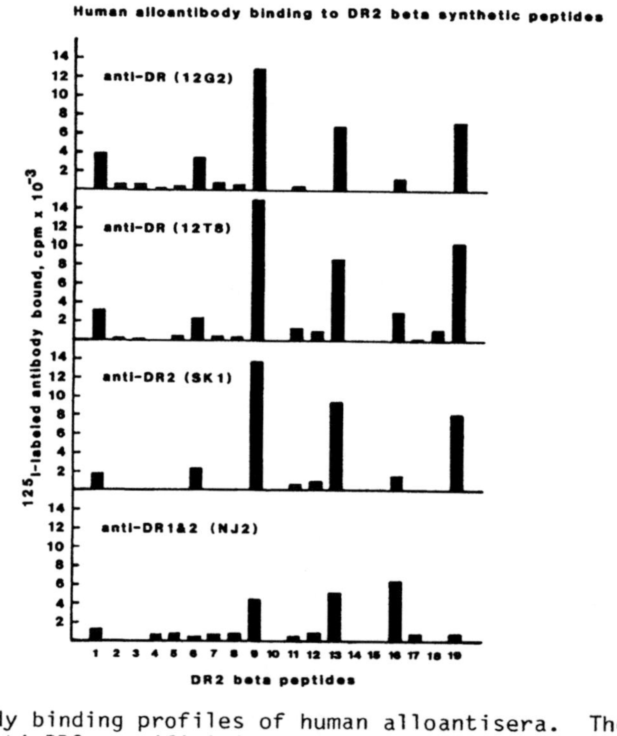

Fig. 4. Antibody binding profiles of human alloantisera. The alloantisera anti-DR2 specificities were determined by standard complement mediated lymphocyte cytolysis assay. The antibody binding values, and DR2β peptides used were as described in the Fig. 2 legend.

Amino acid sequences of the β chains from different DR haplotypes (Tieber et al., 1986; Kratzin et al., 1986) reveal nonconserved regions within residues 9-13, 25-37 and 67-73. The first antigenic site resides within peptide 1-15 and is consistent with a site that might include the polymorphic region 9-13. The antigenic site within region 49-63 is recognized by all the antisera, whereas the site within region 63-73 is recognized by 4 out of 11 antisera. Also, the immunodominant third site within residues 83-93 resides in the most highly conserved region in DR2β. The remaining four sites that occur in the second domain are also in conserved regions. It is therefore concluded that no apparent relationship exists between the locations of the antigenic sites and the polymorphic regions. This was recently discussed in detail (Ulrich et al., 1987). One explanation is that the cytotoxicity assay used to define the specificities of typing sera detects the activities of a minor population of antibodies which are easily lost with dilution whereas the IgM and IgG antibodies that reacted with the peptides were detected at higher dilutions (1:250–1:1000). It is also very likely that the three hypervariable regions may not be entirely present in surface regions of the native protein that are directly accessible to the antibody. This would be similar to the immunoglobulin protein structure present in the V_H and V_L domain interfacial contacts which contain hypervariable residues (Novotny et al., 1983) that are removed from the external medium. Murine class II MHC α–β associations are also strongly influenced by hypervariability within the β1 domain (Germain et al., 1985). The polymorphic regions of the DRβ chain thus may not express unique antigenic sites but may induce conformational effects within the β chain or its association within the αβ complex. Furthermore, as mentioned above, the effect of an amino acid substitution in a protein need not be confined to the immediate region of the substitution, but can also be exerted at distant locations due to charge transfer, steric readjustments and/or regional conformational changes (Twining et al., 1980; Kazim and Atassi, 1980; Atassi and Kazim, 1980). Alternatively, it has been documented that DR sequence variations not detectable serologically may still be detected in some cases by experimental selection and expansion of monoclonal B or T cells (Cairns et al., 1985; Radka et al., 1983).

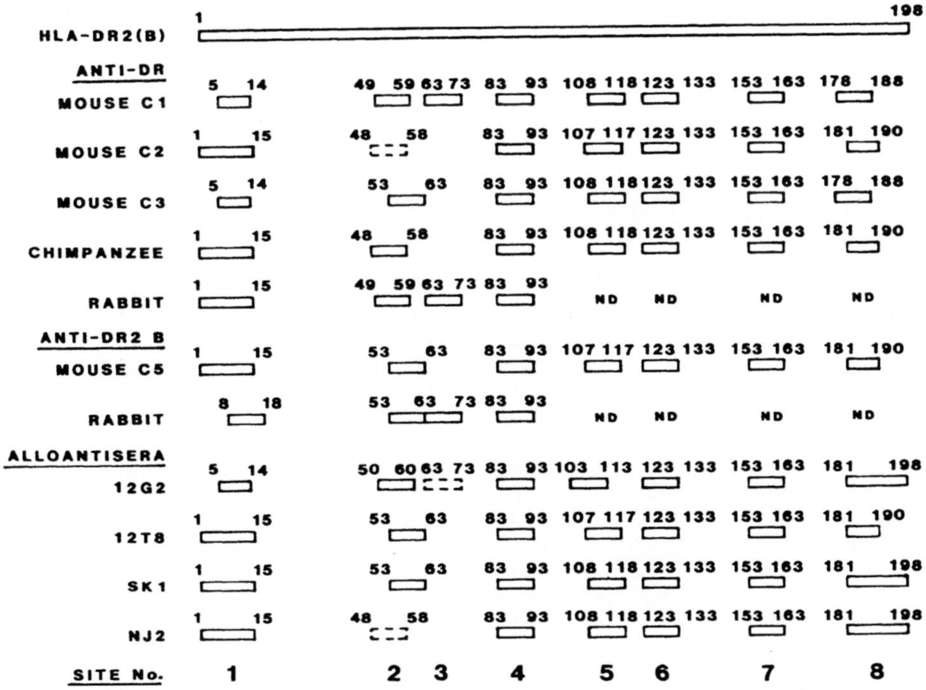

Fig. 5. Schematic diagram showing the antigenic regions on the extracellular part of DR2β subunit that have been localized with human alloantisera and various xenoantisera against the DR2 molecule or the DR2β chain. Regions shown by a broken line are weak antigenic sites with these antisera. (ND) implies that the reactivity of the indicated region with the antiserum was not determined. It is not implied that the antigenic sites comprise the entire size of the regions shown, but rather that they fall within these regions. (Figure is from Atassi et al., 1987).

Monoclonal B and T cell recognition of exon-shuffled class I MHC proteins (Evans et al., 1982; Bluestone et al., 1985; Darsley et al., 1987) has been categorized as either requiring the presence of two protein structural domains or only a single domain. This suggested that the selected alloreactive clones recognized both continuous and discontinuous antigenic sites. However, some of the observed results may be due to the aforementioned effect of amino acid substitutions on protein conformation and/or charge distribution. Our recent studies (Ulrich et al., 1987; Atassi et al., 1987), although not ruling out the existence of discontinuous alloantigenic sites, indicated that continuous sites may play an important role in allorecognition at the polyclonal level.

The study reviewed here is being expanded to examine T cell recognition of the HLA-DR protein as a alloantigenic and as a restriction element for presentation of protein antigens. These synthetic peptides will serve as valuable probes for identifying the molecular regions controlling T cell and class II MHC antigen interactions.

ACKNOWLEDGEMENTS

We thank Drs. Peter Cresswell and Paula Lutz for their generous donations of xenoantisera, and Drs. Marilyn Pollock and Fran Ward for the alloantisera used in this study. This work was supported by the National Institutes of Health (Grant no. AI-21386) and in part by the Welch Foundation (Grant no. Q-994) and due to the award to MZA of the Robert A. Welch Chair of Chemistry.

REFERENCES

Atassi, M.Z. 1975, Immunchem., 12: 423.
Atassi, M.Z. 1978, Immunochem., 15:909.
Atassi, M.Z. 1980, Mol. Cell Biochem., 32:21
Atassi, M.Z. and Kazim, A.L., 1978, in: "Immunobiology of Proteins and Peptides," M.Z. Atassi and A.B. Stavitsky, eds., Plenum, New York.
Atassi, M.Z. and Kazim, A.L., 1980, Biochem. J., 187:163.
Atassi, M.Z. and Smith, J.A. 1978, Immunochem., 15:609.
Atassi, H., Ulrich, R.G., and Atassi, M.Z. 1987, Eur. J. Immunol., 17:497.
Batchelor, J.R., Hors, J., Dodi, I.A., Betuel, H. and Borelli, I. 1984, in: "Histocompatibility Testing," E.D. Albert, ed., Springer-Verlag, Berlin.
Bluestone, J.A., Foo, M., Allen, H., Segal, D., and Flauell, R.A. (1985) J. Exp. Med. 162:268.
Cairns, J.S., Curtsinger, J.M., Dahl, C.A., Freeman, S., Alter, B.J., and Bach, F.H. 1985, Nature, 317:166.
Darsley, M.J., Takahashi, H., Macchi, M.J., Frelinger, J.A., Ozato, K., and Appella, E. (1987) J. Exp. Med. 165:211.
Evans, G.A., Margulies, D.H., Shykind, B., Seidman, J.G., and Ozato, K. (1982) Nature 300:755.
Germain, R.N., Bentley, D.M. and Quill, H. 1985, Cell., 43:233.
Giles, R.C. and Capra, J.D. 1985, Proc. Natl. Acad. Sci. USA, 82:1776.
Giles, R.C., DeMars, R., Chang, C.C. and Capra, J.D., 1985, Proc. Natl. Acad. Sci. USA, 82:1776.
Goyert, S.M., Shiverly, J.F. and Silver, J. 1982, J. Exp. Med., 156:550.
Gregerson, P.K., Shen, M., Song, Q.-L., Merryman, P., Degar, S., Seki, T., Maccari, J., Goldber., D., Murphy, H., Schwenzer, J., Wang, C.Y., Winchester, R.J., Nepom, G.T. and Silver, J. 1986, Proc. Natl. Acad. Sci. USA, 83:2642.
Kazim, A.L. and Atassi, M.Z. 1980, Biochem. J., 191:673.
Kazim, A.L. and Atassi, M.Z. 1982, Biochem. J., 203:201.

Koketsu, J. and Atassi, M.Z. 1973, Biochem. Biophys. Acta, 328:289.
Kratzin, H., Yang, C., Gotz, H., Pauly, E., Kolvel, S., Egert, S., Thinnes, F.P., Wernet, P., Altevogt, P. and Hilschmann, N. 1981, Hoppe-Seyler's Z. Physiol. Chem., 362:1665.
Kratzin, H., Gotz, H., Thinnes, F.P., Kruse, T., Barnikol, H.U., Wernet, P. and Hilschmann, N. 1986, in: "HLA Class II Antigens," B.G. Solheim, E. Moller and S. Ferrone, Springer-Verlag, Berlin.
March, S.E., Parikh, J. and Cuatrecasas, P. 1974, Anal. Biochem., 60:149.
Nepom, B.S., Nepom, G.T., Mickelson, E., Antonelli, P., Hansen, J.A. 1983, Proc. Natl. Acad. Sci. USA., 80:6962.
Nepom, G.T., Nepom, B.S., Wilson, M.E., Mikelson, E., Antonelli, P. and Hansen, J.A., 1984, Hum. Immunol., 10:143.
Novotny, J., Bruccoteri, R., Newell, J., Murphy, D., Haber, E. and Karplus, M. 1983, J. Biol. Chem., 258:14453.
Pober, J.S., Collins, T., Gimbrone, M.A., Jr., Cotron, R.S., Gillin, J.D., Fiers, W., Clayberger, C., Krensky, A.M., Burakoff, S.J. and Reiss, C.S. 1983, Nature, 305:726.
Radka, S.F., Machamer, C., Cresswell, P., Kostyu, D.D., Ward, F.F. and Amos, D.B., 1983, J. Immunol., 130:1863.
Schreuder, G.M.T. and van Leeuwen, A., 1986, in: "HLA Class II Antigens", B.G. Solheim, E. Moller, and S. Ferrone, eds., Springer-Verlag, Berlin.
Shackelford, D.A., Mann, D.L., van Rood, J.J., Ferrara, G.B., and Strominger, J.L., 1981, Proc. Natl. Acad. Sci. USA, 78:4566.
Shechy, M.J., Sondel, P.M., Bach, M.L., Wank, R., and Bach, F.H., 1975, Science, 188:1308.
Sone, T., Tsukamoto, K., Hirayama, K., Nishimura, Y., Takenouchi, T., Aizawa, M. and Sasazuki, T., 1985, J. Immunol., 135:1288.
Sorrentino, R., Lillie, J. and Strominger, J.L., 1985, Proc. Natl. Acad. Sci. USA, 82:3794.
Tieber, V.I., Abruzzini, C.F., Didier, D.K., Schwartz, B.D. and Rotwein, P., 1986, J. Biol. Chem., 261:2738.
Twining, S.S. and Atassi, M.Z., 1979, J. Immunol. Methods, 30:139.
Twining, S.S., Lehmann, H. and Atassi, M.Z., 1980, Biochem. J., 191:681.
Ulrich, R.G., Atassi, H., Lutz, P., Cresswell, P. and Atassi, M.Z., 1987, Eur. J. Immunol., 17:497.
van Rood, J.J., van Leeuwen, A., Keuning, J.J. and Blasse van Oud Alblas, A., 1975, Tissue Antigens, 5:73
van Rood, J.J., van Leeuwen, A., Termijtelen, A. and Keuning, J.J., 1976, Transplant. Rev., 30:122.
Wu, S., Yabe, T., Madden, M., Saunders, T.L. and Bach, F.H., 1987, J. Immunol., 138:2953.
Yabe, T., Reinsmorn, N.L., Wu, S. and Bach, F.M., 1987, Hum. Immunol., 19:127.
Yoshioka, N. and Atassi, M.Z., 1986, Biochem. J., 234:441.

INDEX

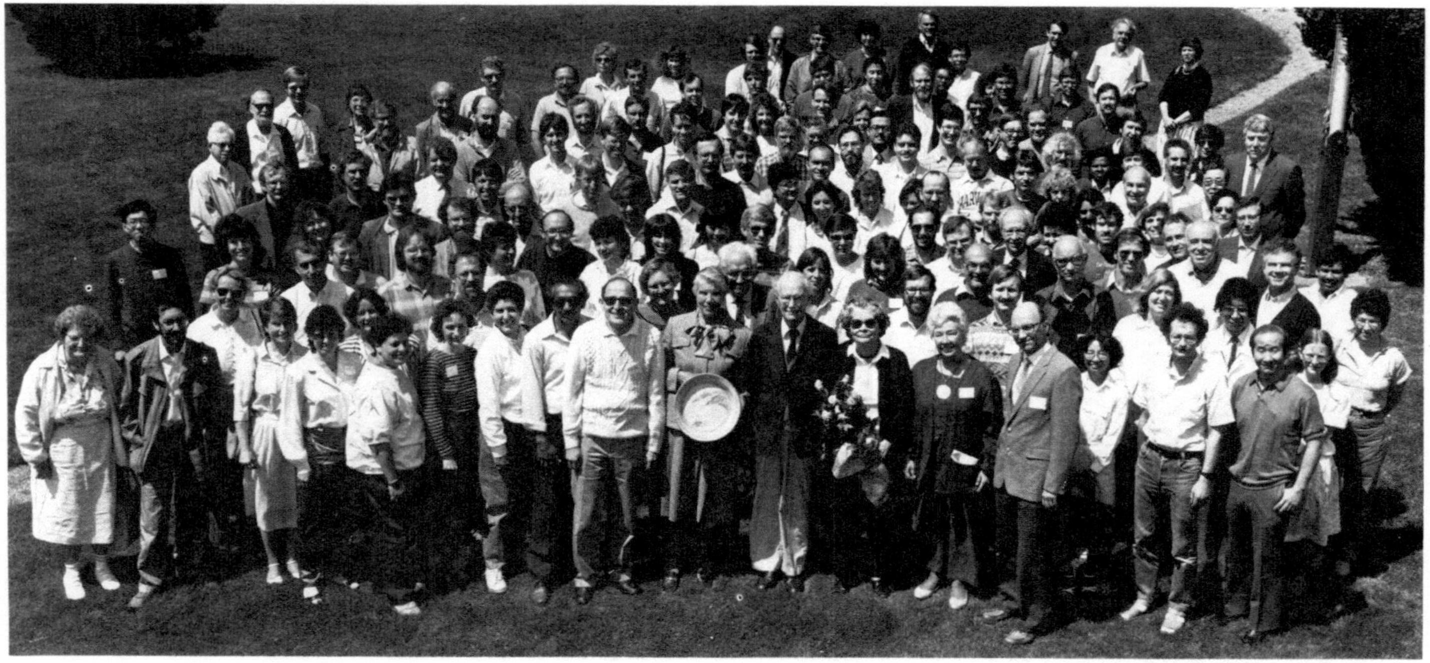

THE WHOLE GROUP

MIX
Papier aus verantwortungsvollen Quellen
Paper from responsible sources
FSC® C105338

If you have any concerns about our products,
you can contact us on
ProductSafety@springernature.com

In case Publisher is established outside the EU,
the EU authorized representative is:
Springer Nature Customer Service Center GmbH
Europaplatz 3, 69115 Heidelberg, Germany

Printed by Libri Plureos GmbH
in Hamburg, Germany